METHODS IN MOLECULAR BIOLOGY

Series Editor
John M. Walker
School of Life and Medical Sciences
University of Hertfordshire
Hatfield, Hertfordshire, UK

For further volumes:
http://www.springer.com/series/7651

For over 35 years, biological scientists have come to rely on the research protocols and methodologies in the critically acclaimed *Methods in Molecular Biology* series. The series was the first to introduce the step-by-step protocols approach that has become the standard in all biomedical protocol publishing. Each protocol is provided in readily-reproducible step-by-step fashion, opening with an introductory overview, a list of the materials and reagents needed to complete the experiment, and followed by a detailed procedure that is supported with a helpful notes section offering tips and tricks of the trade as well as troubleshooting advice. These hallmark features were introduced by series editor Dr. John Walker and constitute the key ingredient in each and every volume of the *Methods in Molecular Biology* series. Tested and trusted, comprehensive and reliable, all protocols from the series are indexed in PubMed.

Methods in Transfusion Medicine

Edited by

Sean R. Stowell and Connie M. Arthur

Division of Transfusion Medicine, Mass General Brigham, Harvard Medical School, Boston, MA, USA

Humana Press

Editors
Sean R. Stowell
Division of Transfusion Medicine
Mass General Brigham
Harvard Medical School
Boston, MA, USA

Connie M. Arthur
Division of Transfusion Medicine
Mass General Brigham
Harvard Medical School
Boston, MA, USA

ISSN 1064-3745 ISSN 1940-6029 (electronic)
Methods in Molecular Biology
ISBN 978-1-0716-5375-3 ISBN 978-1-0716-5376-0 (eBook)
https://doi.org/10.1007/978-1-0716-5376-0

This Humana imprint is published by the registered company Springer Science+Business Media, LLC, part of Springer Nature.
The registered company address is: 1 New York Plaza, New York, NY 10004, U.S.A.

Preface

Blood transfusion is one of the most frequently performed medical interventions in hospitalized patients. Yet, many fundamental questions in the field remain unresolved. Although transfusion can be lifesaving, it also carries inherent risks. A spectrum of complications may occur, ranging from acute hemolytic reactions to metabolic disturbances that can exacerbate a patient's underlying illness. Historically, our mechanistic understanding of these adverse effects has been limited, largely due to the lack of suitable experimental tools and overall methods to examine fundamental aspects of the field. Consequently, many transfusion-related complications have been traditionally managed with supportive care alone. In recent years, however, new experimental approaches have begun to shed light on the biological mechanisms underlying these complications and ways to improve transfusion therapy in general. Some of these discoveries are already shaping clinical practice, while others require further validation. In this volume, an overview is provided of the current models and methodologies used to explore key questions in transfusion medicine. Our goal is to inspire researchers, both within and beyond the field, to help close the remaining knowledge gaps that continue to hinder optimal transfusion practice.

Boston, MA, USA *Sean R. Stowell*
Boston, MA, USA *Connie M. Arthur*

Contents

Contributors

ABRAHAM B. ALTON • *Division of Transfusion Medicine, Mass General Brigham, Harvard Medical School, Boston, MA, USA*
HYUN HYUNG AN • *Department of Cell and Molecular Biology, Perelman School of Medicine at the University of Pennsylvania, Philadelphia, PA, USA*
XIULI AN • *Laboratory of Membrane Biology, New York Blood Center, New York, NY, USA*
AKUA A. APPAH-SAMPONG • *Brigham and Women's Hospital, Harvard Medical School, Boston, MA, USA*
GOWTHAMI M. AREPALLY • *Duke University Medical Center, Durham, NC, USA*
ABHINAV ARNEJA • *Department of Pathology, University of Virginia, Charlottesville, VA, USA*
CONNIE M. ARTHUR • *Division of Transfusion Medicine, Mass General Brigham, Harvard Medical School, Boston, MA, USA*
S. LAWRENCE BAILEY • *Bloodworks Northwest, Research Institute, Seattle, WA, USA*
DIVYA BERI • *Blood-Borne Parasites, Lindsley F. Kimball Research Institute, New York Blood Center, New York, NY, USA*
ANUSHKA BHAT • *Department of Pathology and Immunology, Washington University School of Medicine, St. Louis, MO, USA*
VIJAY G. BHOJ • *Department of Pathology and Laboratory Medicine, Perelman School of Medicine, University of Pennsylvania, Philadelphia, PA, USA; Center for Cellular Immunotherapies, Perelman School of Medicine, University of Pennsylvania, Philadelphia, PA, USA*
BETH BINNINGTON • *Canadian Blood Services, Centre for Innovation, Keenan Research Centre, Toronto, ON, Canada*
MARTIN BOCHENEK • *Bloodworks Northwest, Research Institute, Seattle, WA, USA*
ALEXIS BOSCIA • *Department of Pathology, University of Virginia, Charlottesville, VA, USA*
DONALD R. BRANCH • *Canadian Blood Services, Centre for Innovation, Keenan Research Centre, Toronto, ON, Canada; Department of Laboratory Medicine and Pathobiology, University of Toronto, Toronto, ON, Canada; PolyTech Clermont, Clermont-Ferrand, France; Department of Medicine, University of Toronto, Toronto, ON, Canada*
EMILY BURNETT • *Department of Pathology, University of Virginia, Charlottesville, VA, USA*
JOSE A. CANCELAS • *Hoxworth Blood Center, University of Cincinnati College of Medicine, Cincinnati, OH, USA; Division of Experimental Hematology and Cancer Biology, Cincinnati Children's Hospital Medical Center, University of Cincinnati College of Medicine, Cincinnati, OH, USA; Connell and O'Reilly Families Cell Manipulation Core Facility and Department of Medical Oncology, Dana-Farber Cancer Institute, Harvard Medical School, Boston, MA, USA*
SOFIA CATTANI • *Division of Transfusion Medicine, Mass General Brigham, Harvard Medical School, Boston, MA, USA*
SELENA CEN • *Canadian Blood Services, Centre for Innovation, Keenan Research Centre, Toronto, ON, Canada*
CAITLIN L. CEPEDA • *Division of Transfusion Medicine, Mass General Brigham, Harvard Medical School, Boston, MA, USA*
LI CHAI • *Department of Pathology, Brigham and Women's Hospital, Boston, MA, USA*

ARWEN CHANDLER • *Department of Pathology, University of Virginia, Charlottesville, VA, USA*

CHE-YU CHANG • *Departments of Pathology and Laboratory Medicine, Cedars-Sinai Medical Center, Los Angeles, CA, USA*

DANIEL CHANG • *Department of Pathology, Brigham and Women's Hospital, Boston, MA, USA*

TONI CHANROO • *Aflac Cancer and Blood Disorders Center, Children's Healthcare of Atlanta/Emory University School of Medicine, Atlanta, GA, USA*

RUTH CHOA • *Department of Pathology and Laboratory Medicine, Perelman School of Medicine at the University of Pennsylvania, Philadelphia, PA, USA*

STELLA T. CHOU • *Department of Pathology and Laboratory Medicine, Perelman School of Medicine at the University of Pennsylvania, Philadelphia, PA, USA; Department of Pediatrics, Perelman School of Medicine at the University of Pennsylvania, Philadelphia, PA, USA*

SIMON J. CLEARY • *Institute of Pharmaceutical Science, King's College London, London, UK*

MISCHA L. COVINGTON • *Division of Transfusion Medicine, Mass General Brigham, Harvard Medical School, Boston, MA, USA*

YOELYS CRUZ-LEAL • *Department of Laboratory Medicine, Keenan Research Centre for Biomedical Science, Li Ka Shing Knowledge Institute, St. Michael's Hospital, Toronto, ON, Canada; The Canadian Blood Services Centre for Innovation, Ottawa, ON, Canada*

ANGELO D'ALESSANDRO • *Department of Biochemistry and Molecular Genetics, University of Colorado Denver – Anschutz Medical Campus, Aurora, CO, USA*

YITIAN DAI • *Laboratory of Stem Cell Biology and Engineering Research, New York Blood Center, New York, NY, USA*

PATRICIA E. DAVENPORT • *Department of Newborn Medicine, Boston Children's Hospital, Boston, MA, USA*

SUMAIYA DICKENS • *Center for Transfusion Medicine and Cellular Therapies, Department of Laboratory Medicine and Pathology, Emory University School of Medicine, Atlanta, GA, USA*

BRIAN T. EDELSON • *Department of Pathology and Immunology, Washington University School of Medicine, St. Louis, MO, USA*

STEPHANIE C. EISENBARTH • *The Department of Medicine, Division of Allergy and Immunology, Northwestern University Feinberg School of Medicine, Chicago, IL, USA; Center for Human Immunobiology, Northwestern University Feinberg School of Medicine, Chicago, IL, USA; Department of Laboratory Medicine, Yale University School of Medicine, New Haven, CT, USA; Department of Immunobiology, Yale University School of Medicine, New Haven, CT, USA*

YUPING FAN • *Departments of Pathology, Harvard Medical School and Brigham and Women's Hospital, Boston, MA, USA*

ROSS M. FASANO • *Department of Pathology, Emory University School of Medicine, Atlanta, GA, USA; Department of Pediatrics, Emory University School of Medicine, Atlanta, GA, USA*

EMILY M. FLOWERS • *The Department of Medicine, Division of Allergy and Immunology, Northwestern University Feinberg School of Medicine, Chicago, IL, USA; Center for Human Immunobiology, Northwestern University Feinberg School of Medicine, Chicago, IL, USA*

MEGAN FULLER • *Center for Transfusion Medicine and Cellular Therapies, Department of Laboratory Medicine and Pathology, Emory University School of Medicine, Atlanta, GA, USA*

BETTY GAILLARD • *Vitalant Research Institute, San Francisco, CA, USA*

DAVID R. GIBB • *Cedars-Sinai Medical Center, Los Angeles, CA, USA; Departments of Pathology and Laboratory Medicine, Cedars-Sinai Medical Center, Los Angeles, CA, USA*

LAZARO GIL GONZALEZ • *Department of Laboratory Medicine, Keenan Research Centre for Biomedical Science, Li Ka Shing Knowledge Institute, St. Michael's Hospital, Toronto, ON, Canada*

IDOIA GIMFERRER • *Bloodworks Northwest, Immunogenetics and HLA Laboratory, Seattle, WA, USA*

LAZARO GIL GONZALEZ • *Department of Laboratory Medicine, Keenan Research Centre for Biomedical Science, Li Ka Shing Knowledge Institute, St. Michael's Hospital, Toronto, ON, Canada*

XIAOYU GUAN • *Department of Blood Transfusion, The Third People's Hospital of Chengdu, College of Medicine, Southwest Jiaotong University, Chengdu, China*

HONGJIE GUO • *Antiger Therapeutics Inc, St. Louis, MO, USA*

REBECCA C. HALE • *Division of Transfusion Medicine, Mass General Brigham, Harvard Medical School, Boston, MA, USA*

SHAILAJA HEGDE • *Hoxworth Blood Center, University of Cincinnati College of Medicine, Cincinnati, OH, USA*

ROSARIO HERNÁNDEZ-ARMENGOL • *Cedars-Sinai Medical Center, Los Angeles, CA, USA; Departments of Pathology and Laboratory Medicine, Cedars-Sinai Medical Center, Los Angeles, CA, USA*

BENJAMIN HESTER • *Department of Pathology, University of Virginia, Charlottesville, VA, USA*

LINDSAY K. HILLIS • *Canadian Blood Services, Centre for Innovation, Keenan Research Centre, Toronto, ON, Canada; Department of Laboratory Medicine and Pathobiology, University of Toronto, Toronto, ON, Canada*

MARIE A. HOLLENHORST • *Brigham and Women's Hospital, Harvard Medical School, Boston, MA, USA*

ALAN Y. HSU • *Departments of Pathology, Harvard Medical School and Brigham and Women's Hospital, Boston, MA, USA*

KRYSTALYN E. HUDSON • *Laboratory of Transfusion Biology, Department of Pathology and Cell Biology, Columbia University Irving Medical Center, New York City, NY, USA*

BROCK D. HUGHES • *Division of Transfusion Medicine, Mass General Brigham, Harvard Medical School, Boston, MA, USA*

ZOYA HUSSAIN • *Department of Laboratory Medicine, Keenan Research Centre for Biomedical Science, Li Ka Shing Knowledge Institute, St. Michael's Hospital, Toronto, ON, Canada; Department of Medicine and Laboratory Medicine and Pathobiology, University of Toronto, Toronto, ON, Canada*

SELBY IRELAND • *Department of Pathology, University of Virginia, Charlottesville, VA, USA*

RACHAEL P. JACKMAN • *Vitalant Research Institute, San Francisco, CA, USA; Department of Laboratory Medicine, University of California, San Francisco, CA, USA*

MONTANA JACKSON • *Center for Transfusion Medicine and Cellular Therapies, Department of Laboratory Medicine and Pathology, Emory University School of Medicine, Atlanta, GA, USA*

SHWATINA JAGNARINE • *Laboratory of Transfusion Biology, Department of Pathology and Cell Biology, Columbia University Irving Medical Center, New York, NY, USA*
RYAN P. JAJOSKY • *Division of Transfusion Medicine, Mass General Brigham, Harvard Medical School, Boston, MA, USA*
HAU-MING JAN • *Division of Transfusion Medicine, Mass General Brigham, Harvard Medical School, Boston, MA, USA*
TAKU KAMBAYASHI • *Department of Pathology and Laboratory Medicine, Perelman School of Medicine at the University of Pennsylvania, Philadelphia, PA, USA*
NATALIE E. KANE • *Department of Newborn Medicine, Boston Children's Hospital, Boston, MA, USA*
RICK KAPUR • *Sanquin Research, Department of Experimental Immunohematology, Amsterdam and Landsteiner Laboratory, Amsterdam UMC, University of Amsterdam, Amsterdam, The Netherlands*
SANJAY KHANDELWAL • *Duke University Medical Center, Durham, NC, USA*
SUNGWOONG KIM • *Center for Transfusion Medicine and Cellular Therapies, Department of Laboratory Medicine and Pathology, Emory University School of Medicine, Atlanta, GA, USA*
EMMALENE KYRITSIS • *Laboratory of Transfusion Biology, Department of Pathology and Cell Biology, Columbia University Irving Medical Center, New York, NY, USA*
SADIE LARSON • *Division of Transfusion Medicine, Mass General Brigham, Harvard Medical School, Boston, MA, USA*
ALAN H. LAZARUS • *Department of Laboratory Medicine, Keenan Research Centre for Biomedical Science, Li Ka Shing Knowledge Institute, St. Michael's Hospital, Toronto, ON, Canada; The Canadian Blood Services Centre for Innovation, Ottawa, ON, Canada; Department of Medicine and Laboratory Medicine and Pathobiology, University of Toronto, Toronto, ON, Canada*
JUNE YOUNG LEE • *Departments of Pathology and Laboratory Medicine, Cedars-Sinai Medical Center, Los Angeles, CA, USA*
VIVIEN C. LEE • *Division of Transfusion Medicine, Mass General Brigham, Harvard Medical School, Boston, MA, USA*
LING LI • *Department of Blood Transfusion, The Third People's Hospital of Chengdu, College of Medicine, Southwest Jiaotong University, Chengdu, China*
WENHUI LI • *Division of Transfusion Medicine, Mass General Brigham, Harvard Medical School, Boston, MA, USA*
HSIEN-YA LIN • *Joint Program in Transfusion Medicine, Brigham and Women's Hospital, Harvard Medical School, Boston, MA, USA*
CHANG LIU • *Department of Pathology and Immunology, Washington University School of Medicine, St. Louis, MO, USA; Antiger Therapeutics Inc, St. Louis, MO, USA*
JUN LIU • *Department of Pathology, Brigham and Women's Hospital, Boston, MA, USA*
ZHONG LIU • *Institute of Blood Transfusion, Chinese Academy of Medical Sciences and Peking Union Medical College, Chengdu, China; Key Laboratory of Transfusion Adverse Reactions, Chinese Academy of Medical Sciences, Beijing, China*
CHERYL A. LOBO • *Blood-Borne Parasites, Lindsley F. Kimball Research Institute, New York Blood Center, New York, NY, USA*
MARK R. LOONEY • *Department of Medicine, UCSF, San Francisco, CA, USA*
MELIKA LORIAMINI • *Canadian Blood Services, Centre for Innovation, Keenan Research Centre, Toronto, ON, Canada; Department of Laboratory Medicine and Pathobiology, University of Toronto, Toronto, ON, Canada*

Chance John Luckey • *Department of Pathology, University of Virginia, Charlottesville, VA, USA*

Hongbo R. Luo • *Departments of Pathology, Harvard Medical School and Brigham and Women's Hospital, Boston, MA, USA; Dana-Farber/Harvard Cancer Center, Harvard Medical School and Mass General Brigham, Boston, MA, USA*

Nilam S. Mangalmurti • *Division of Pulmonary, Allergy, and Critical Care, Perelman School of Medicine at the University of Pennsylvania, Philadelphia, PA, USA*

Genevieve Marcoux • *Division of Hematology and Transfusion Medicine, Lund University, Lund, Sweden*

Caroline A. Markmann • *Department of Pathology and Laboratory Medicine, Perelman School of Medicine, University of Pennsylvania, Philadelphia, PA, USA; Center for Cellular Immunotherapies, Perelman School of Medicine, University of Pennsylvania, Philadelphia, PA, USA*

Erika G. Marques de Menezes • *Vitalant Research Institute, San Francisco, CA, USA; Department of Laboratory Medicine, University of California, San Francisco, CA, USA*

James W. McCoy • *Center for Transfusion Medicine and Cellular Therapies, Department of Laboratory Medicine and Pathology, Emory University School of Medicine, Atlanta, GA, USA*

Jelena Medved • *Department of Pathology, University of Virginia, Charlottesville, VA, USA*

Avital Mendelson • *Laboratory of Stem Cell Biology and Engineering Research, New York Blood Center, New York, NY, USA*

Sasikala Muthusamy • *Division of Transfusion Medicine, Mass General Brigham, Harvard Medical School, Boston, MA, USA*

Hirotomo Nakahara • *Division of Transfusion Medicine, Mass General Brigham, Harvard Medical School, Boston, MA, USA; Department of Pathology and Laboratory Medicine, Emory University School of Medicine, Atlanta, GA, USA*

Zahra Naseh • *Center for Transfusion Medicine and Cellular Therapies, Department of Laboratory Medicine and Pathology, Emory University School of Medicine, Atlanta, GA, USA*

Travis Nemkov • *Department of Biochemistry and Molecular Genetics, University of Colorado Denver – Anschutz Medical Campus, Aurora, CO, USA*

Debra K. Newman • *Versiti Blood Research Institute, Milwaukee, WI, USA; Department of Pharmacology, Medical College of Wisconsin, Milwaukee, WI, USA*

Peter J. Newman • *Blood Research Institute, Versiti Blood Center of Wisconsin, Milwaukee, WI, USA; Department of Pharmacology and Toxicology, Medical College of Wisconsin, Milwaukee, WI, USA; Department of Cell Biology, Neurobiology and Anatomy, Medical College of Wisconsin, Milwaukee, WI, USA*

Conrad Niebuhr • *Department of Pathology, University of Virginia, Charlottesville, VA, USA*

Yeniley Ruiz Noa • *Canadian Blood Services, Centre for Innovation, Keenan Research Centre, Toronto, ON, Canada*

Peter A. A. Norris • *Department of Biomedical and Molecular Sciences, Queen's University, Kingston, ON, Canada*

Philip J. Norris • *Vitalant Research Institute, San Francisco, CA, USA; Department of Laboratory Medicine, University of California, San Francisco, CA, USA; Department of Medicine, University of California, San Francisco, CA, USA*

EMILY A. OATMAN • *Division of Traumatology, Surgical Critical Care, and Emergency Surgical Services, Department of Surgery, Perelman School of Medicine at the University of Pennsylvania, Philadelphia, PA, USA*
EMILY OEHRLE • *Division of Transfusion Medicine, Mass General Brigham, Harvard Medical School, Boston, MA, USA*
VICTORIA ORTIZ • *Division of Transfusion Medicine, Mass General Brigham, Harvard Medical School, Boston, MA, USA*
KASHYAP R. PATEL • *Division of Transfusion Medicine, Mass General Brigham, Harvard Medical School, Boston, MA, USA*
ANU PAUL • *Division of Transfusion Medicine, Mass General Brigham, Harvard Medical School, Boston, MA, USA*
KAUSIK PAUL • *Departments of Pathology and Laboratory Medicine, Cedars-Sinai Medical Center, Los Angeles, CA, USA*
GIULIA PAVANI • *Department of Pathology and Laboratory Medicine, Perelman School of Medicine at the University of Pennsylvania, Philadelphia, PA, USA*
ALEQUIS PAVON ORO • *Department of Laboratory Medicine, Keenan Research Centre for Biomedical Science, Li Ka Shing Knowledge Institute, St. Michael's Hospital, Toronto, ON, Canada*
DOMINIQUE PAZ • *Division of Transfusion Medicine, Mass General Brigham, Harvard Medical School, Boston, MA, USA*
FARAHNAZ RAYATDOOST • *Sanquin Blood Supply Foundation, Department Research and Amsterdam UMC location University of Amsterdam, Landsteiner Laboratory, Amsterdam, The Netherlands*
JOHAN REBETZ • *Division of Hematology and Transfusion Medicine, Lund University, Lund, Sweden*
JULIE A. REISZ • *Department of Biochemistry and Molecular Genetics, University of Colorado Denver – Anschutz Medical Campus, Aurora, CO, USA*
JOHN D. ROBACK • *Department of Pathology, Emory University School of Medicine, Atlanta, GA, USA*
MARILIS RODRIGUEZ • *Blood-Borne Parasites, Lindsley F. Kimball Research Institute, New York Blood Center, New York, NY, USA*
JESSELIN J. ROMERO ESCOBAR • *Department of Newborn Medicine, Boston Children's Hospital, Boston, MA, USA*
CLEMENCE SALOU • *Canadian Blood Services, Centre for Innovation, Keenan Research Centre, Toronto, ON, Canada; PolyTech Clermont, Clermont-Ferrand, France*
GURLEEN SANDHU • *Canadian Blood Services, Centre for Innovation, Keenan Research Centre, Toronto, ON, Canada*
LAYAL SAYEGH • *Division of Pulmonary, Allergy, and Critical Care, Perelman School of Medicine at the University of Pennsylvania, Philadelphia, PA, USA*
CATHERINE SCHWARZSCHILD • *Department of Pathology, University of Virginia, Charlottesville, VA, USA*
WILLIAM O. SCOTT • *Division of Transfusion Medicine, Mass General Brigham, Harvard Medical School, Boston, MA, USA*
JOHN W. SEMPLE • *Division of Hematology and Transfusion Medicine, Lund University, Lund, Sweden; Clinical Immunology and Transfusion Medicine, Office of Medical Services, Region Skåne, Lund, Sweden; Departments of Pharmacology, Medicine and Laboratory Medicine and Pathobiology, University of Toronto, Toronto, Canada*
YURIM SEO • *Department of Medicine, UCSF, San Francisco, CA, USA*

YUEXIN SHAN • *Department of Laboratory Medicine, Keenan Research Centre for Biomedical Science, Li Ka Shing Knowledge Institute, St. Michael's Hospital, Toronto, ON, Canada*
ZIYANG SHEN • *Department of Pathology, Brigham and Women's Hospital, Boston, MA, USA*
MARTHA C. SOLA-VISNER • *Department of Newborn Medicine, Boston Children's Hospital, Boston, MA, USA*
ERIN L. SOULE-ALBRIDGE • *Department of Newborn Medicine, Boston Children's Hospital, Boston, MA, USA*
DANIEL STEPHENSON • *Department of Biochemistry and Molecular Genetics, University of Colorado Denver – Anschutz Medical Campus, Aurora, CO, USA*
MORITZ STOLLA • *Bloodworks Northwest, Research Institute, Seattle, WA, USA; Department of Medicine, Division of Hematology and Oncology, University of Washington, Seattle, WA, USA; Department of Laboratory Medicine and Pathology, University of Washington, Seattle, WA, USA; Fred Hutchinson Cancer Center, Clinical Research Division, Seattle, WA, USA*
CARTER J. STOWELL • *Division of Transfusion Medicine, Mass General Brigham, Harvard Medical School, Boston, MA, USA*
SEAN R. STOWELL • *Division of Transfusion Medicine, Mass General Brigham, Harvard Medical School, Boston, MA, USA*
KATELYN STURGIS • *Division of Transfusion Medicine, Mass General Brigham, Harvard Medical School, Boston, MA, USA*
LILLIAN SUN • *Department of Pathology and Laboratory Medicine, Perelman School of Medicine at the University of Pennsylvania, Philadelphia, PA, USA*
ZOYA TAWHIDI • *Department of Laboratory Medicine, Keenan Research Centre for Biomedical Science, Li Ka Shing Knowledge Institute, St. Michael's Hospital, Toronto, ON, Canada; Department of Medicine and Laboratory Medicine and Pathobiology, University of Toronto, Toronto, ON, Canada; The Canadian Blood Services Centre for Innovation, Ottawa, ON, Canada*
MATTHEW R. THAKUR • *The Department of Medicine, Division of Allergy and Immunology, Northwestern University Feinberg School of Medicine, Chicago, IL, USA; Center for Human Immunobiology, Northwestern University Feinberg School of Medicine, Chicago, IL, USA*
TIFFANY A. THOMAS • *Laboratory of Transfusion Biology, Department of Pathology and Cell Biology, Columbia University Irving Medical Center, New York, NY, USA*
GUNNHILDUR THORKELSDOTTIR • *Department of Pathology, University of Virginia, Charlottesville, VA, USA*
KATHERINE H. TIEMEYER • *Yale School of Medicine, New Haven, CT, USA*
TIK NGA TONG • *Canadian Blood Services, Centre for Innovation, Keenan Research Centre, Toronto, ON, Canada; Department of Laboratory Medicine and Pathobiology, University of Toronto, Toronto, ON, Canada*
JOHNSON Q. TRAN • *Vitalant Research Institute, San Francisco, CA, USA; Department of Laboratory Medicine, University of California, San Francisco, CA, USA*
YAIMA TUNDIDOR • *Department of Laboratory Medicine, Keenan Research Centre for Biomedical Science, Li Ka Shing Knowledge Institute, St. Michael's Hospital, Toronto, ON, Canada; The Canadian Blood Services Centre for Innovation, Ottawa, ON, Canada*
MARY VALLECILLO-ZUNIGA • *Division of Transfusion Medicine, Mass General Brigham, Harvard Medical School, Boston, MA, USA*
VICTORIA M. VANCE • *Division of Transfusion Medicine, Mass General Brigham, Harvard Medical School, Boston, MA, USA*

SAMATA P. VARADKAR • *Division of Transfusion Medicine, Mass General Brigham, Harvard Medical School, Boston, MA, USA*
DEMIN WANG • *Versiti Blood Research Institute, Milwaukee, WI, USA; Department of Microbiology and Immunology, Medical College of Wisconsin, Milwaukee, WI, USA*
JUE WANG • *Institute of Blood Transfusion, Chinese Academy of Medical Sciences and Peking Union Medical College, Chengdu, China; Key Laboratory of Transfusion Adverse Reactions, Chinese Academy of Medical Sciences, Beijing, China*
ASHLEE M. WEBBER • *Department of Pathology and Immunology, Washington University School of Medicine, St. Louis, MO, USA*
RENREN WEN • *Versiti Blood Research Institute, Milwaukee, WI, USA; Department of Microbiology and Immunology, Medical College of Wisconsin, Milwaukee, WI, USA*
LUKE L. WESTHOFF • *Division of Transfusion Medicine, Mass General Brigham, Harvard Medical School, Provo, UT, USA*
ADAM WILLIAMS • *The Department of Medicine, Division of Allergy and Immunology, Northwestern University Feinberg School of Medicine, Chicago, IL, USA; Center for Human Immunobiology, Northwestern University Feinberg School of Medicine, Chicago, IL, USA*
COURTNEY A. WINTERS • *Joint Program in Transfusion Medicine, Brigham and Women's Hospital, Harvard Medical School, Boston, MA, USA*
NATHAN D. WITMAN • *Versiti Blood Research Institute, Milwaukee, WI, USA; Department of Microbiology and Immunology, Medical College of Wisconsin, Milwaukee, WI, USA*
ANDRE J. H. WITTIG • *Division of Transfusion Medicine, Mass General Brigham, Harvard Medical School, Boston, MA, USA*
KEVIN DOYOON WON • *Department of Laboratory Medicine, Keenan Research Centre for Biomedical Science, Li Ka Shing Knowledge Institute, St. Michael's Hospital, Toronto, ON, Canada; Department of Medicine and Laboratory Medicine and Pathobiology, University of Toronto, Toronto, ON, Canada*
SHANG-CHUEN WU • *Division of Transfusion Medicine, Mass General Brigham, Harvard Medical School, Boston, MA, USA*
MARIANNE E. M. YEE • *Department of Pediatrics, Emory University School of Medicine, Atlanta, GA, USA*
DANNY YOUNGS • *Bloodworks Northwest, Immunogenetics and HLA Laboratory, Seattle, WA, USA*
MEI YU • *Versiti Blood Research Institute, Milwaukee, WI, USA*
PATRICIA E. ZERRA • *Department of Pathology, Emory University School of Medicine, Atlanta, GA, USA; Department of Pediatrics, Emory University School of Medicine, Atlanta, GA, USA*
HUAN ZHANG • *School of Life Sciences, Zhengzhou University, Zhengzhou, Henan, People's Republic of China*
NANYAN ZHANG • *Blood Research Institute, Versiti Blood Center of Wisconsin, Milwaukee, WI, USA*
LEON ZHENG • *Division of Transfusion Medicine, Mass General Brigham, Harvard Medical School, Boston, MA, USA*
YI ZHENG • *Division of Experimental Hematology and Cancer Biology, Cincinnati Children's Hospital Medical Center, University of Cincinnati College of Medicine, Cincinnati, OH, USA*
HUIYING ZHI • *Versiti Blood Research Institute, Milwaukee, WI, USA*

LU ZHOU • *Versiti Blood Research Institute, Milwaukee, WI, USA; Department of Microbiology and Immunology, Medical College of Wisconsin, Milwaukee, WI, USA*
WEN ZHU • *Versiti Blood Research Institute, Milwaukee, WI, USA; Department of Microbiology and Immunology, Medical College of Wisconsin, Milwaukee, WI, USA; MedSphere Corp, Skokie, IL, USA*

Chapter 1

The Immunology of Transfusion Medicine: Past, Present, and Future

Connie M. Arthur and Sean R. Stowell

Abstract

The identification of alloantigens has been central to understanding how polymorphic variation influences transfusion safety through potential immune incompatibilities between individuals. Patients may possess naturally occurring antibodies that develop within the first few months of life or form alloantibodies after exposure to alloantigens during transfusion or pregnancy. These antibodies complicate the search for compatible blood and increase the risk of hemolytic disease of the fetus and newborn, as well as fetal and neonatal thrombocytopenia. Alloimmune mechanisms can also contribute to transfusion-related acute lung injury and transfusion-associated graft-versus-host disease. Beyond the direct complications of alloimmunity, changes in the metabolic and immunologic characteristics of transfused blood products can affect recipient immune function. In this review, we explore the historical interplay between immunology and transfusion medicine and highlight emerging preclinical and clinical insights into the field, with particular focus on the development and clinical implications of red blood cell alloimmunization.

Key words Transfusion, Blood, Complications, Models, Tools, Experimental approaches

1 Introduction

Early attempts at blood transfusion produced unpredictable results, with some patients benefiting while others suffered life-threatening hemolytic transfusion reactions [1]. This uncertainty was primarily due to a limited understanding of the factors that determined compatibility. Landsteiner's identification of the ABO blood group antigens, the first recognized polymorphisms within the human population, remains the cornerstone of the field of transfusion medicine [1–6]. By demonstrating that human blood could be categorized into distinct groups based on the presence or absence of specific antigens on red blood cells (RBCs), Landsteiner provided the critical framework for understanding blood compatibility and predicting adverse reactions prior to transfusion [1]. As ABO blood group antigens are expressed in a variety of tissues, this understanding also became critical in identifying compatibility for

Sean R. Stowell and Connie M. Arthur (eds.), *Methods in Transfusion Medicine*, Methods in Molecular Biology, vol. 3053, https://doi.org/10.1007/978-1-0716-5376-0_1,

solid organ transplantation [1–8]. Subsequent studies demonstrated the importance of ABO antigens in fetal-maternal health, leading to the routine implementation of ABO testing not only prior to transfusion or transplantation, but also during pregnancy and after birth. While these antigens likely arose as a result of evolutionary selection pressures, they continue to represent the most commonly analyzed polymorphism in the human population [9–12].

2 Alloimmunization in Maternal-Fetal Health

While ABO blood group antigens are the primary immunological barriers in transfusion medicine, they are not the sole target of the immune response to blood products. Alloantibodies can also form against many other RBC polymorphisms [13, 14]. Unlike anti-ABO (H) antibodies, which develop spontaneously within the first few months of life, most other RBC alloantibodies arise only after exposure through transfusion or pregnancy [15–19]. In pregnancy, RBC alloantibodies can cross the placenta and enter fetal circulation, where they may cause hemolysis of fetal RBCs or suppress fetal erythropoiesis. Such immune-mediated injury can result in anemia, which can result in hemolytic disease of the fetus and newborn (HDFN) [20].

Although IgG anti-ABO (H) antibodies can cause HDFN, this condition is typically more severe when antibodies target non-ABO (H) antigens, particularly RhD [21]. This is possibly due to the reduced expression of A and B on fetal RBCs when compared to RhD and other antigens. The development of passive anti-RhD immunoglobulin prophylaxis, which was informed by a series of epidemiologic, translational, and basic science studies [22], has markedly reduced the prevalence of HDFN due to anti-RhD. However, while anti-RhD antibodies can suppress a new alloimmune response, a process known as antibody-mediated immunosuppression (AMIS), there are currently no effective strategies to actively prevent the formation of alloantibodies against other RBC alloantigens. With over 300 different RBC alloantigens [23], the lack of prevention strategies for maternal RBC alloimmunization against other RBC alloantigens is a major gap in maternal-fetal care. These challenges lie in part due to an incomplete understanding of the mechanisms underlying AMIS [24], making it difficult to develop comparable products for targeting other alloantigens [24–26].

The implications of maternal alloimmunization are not confined to RBC alloantigens. Alloantibodies against platelet antigens, which can develop through transfusion or pregnancy, can trigger fetal and neonatal alloimmune thrombocytopenia (FNAIT). Although reduced platelet counts in utero may not impair development, the associated thrombocytopenia increases the risk for severe bleeding at birth, including intracranial hemorrhage [27]. FNAIT remains a challenging clinical problem [28, 29]. Although attempts are being made to generate similar strategies as anti-RhD immunoprophylaxis to prevent FNAIT [30, 31], no analogous AMIS-based strategy currently exists to prevent maternal platelet alloimmunization [32]. While leukoreduction can decrease alloimmunization to human leukocyte antigens (HLAs) [33], it does not prevent immune responses against platelet glycoprotein antigens, which are the primary targets in FNAIT [34–37]. As parental pairing is not typically influenced by blood group compatibility, reducing antigen exposure during pregnancy is not a practical prevention strategy for HDFN or FNAIT. A deeper mechanistic understanding of AMIS is therefore essential to extend this prophylactic strategy to FNAIT and HDFN due to non-RhD alloantigens.

Emerging therapeutic strategies, such as neonatal Fc receptor (FcRn) inhibitors, may offer a complementary approach to reducing HDFN and FNAIT by limiting transfer of maternal antibodies during pregnancy [38–41]. However, as maternal antibodies play an important role in neonatal immune protection, the consequences of broadly reducing antibody transfer remain unclear. Similarly, successive pregnancies could enhance the maternal immune response, which may make it difficult to fully suppress antibody transfer in later gestations. Despite these challenges, recent data support FcRn inhibition as a promising avenue for preventing maternal autoimmunity from impacting fetal development and neonatal outcomes [38, 39].

3 RBC Alloimmunization in the Management of Transfusion-Dependent Patients

In addition to challenges for maternal-fetal health, alloimmunization can complicate the management of patients requiring transfusion [42, 43]. The generation of complex alloantibody profiles or the development of alloantibodies against high-incidence alloantigens can make it difficult to procure compatible blood for transfusion, particularly in time-sensitive situations [44, 45]. These delays may contribute to increased hospital stays, morbidity, and mortality among alloimmunized patients [46, 47]. The urgency of transfusion requirements in these settings may necessitate the use of partially incompatible blood or units that appear compatible but against which patients may have previously developed an alloimmune response that is no longer detectable [48–51]. These later situations can result in a delayed, anamnestic immune response to blood transfusions, leading to accelerated clearance of transfused RBCs that results in a delayed hemolytic transfusion reaction (DHTR) [52–55]. This is partly because healthcare systems can be fragmented, and in the United States in particular there is no national registry for tracking alloantibody formation [56–58], making it difficult for a hospital blood bank to be aware that alloantibodies have previously developed [56, 59]. Despite the ability of anamnestic antibody formation to accelerate the clearance of transfused RBCs, nearly one-third of DHTRs occur in the absence of detectable alloantibodies [53, 60]. This could reflect limitations in methods used clinically or antibody-independent mechanisms [61], demonstrating the need to look beyond alloantibody detection when evaluating potential DHTRs [53, 62]. Implementing hemoglobin electrophoresis could provide a more effective method for determining whether accelerated clearance of transfused RBCs has occurred, particularly after episodic transfusions, where DHTRs are more common [53].

DHTRs in patients with sickle cell disease (SCD) occur more frequently than previously recognized, partly because they often happen at a time distant from the closely monitored transfusion event and can mimic other SCD complications [53]. Recent studies indicate that DHTRs are the most common transfusion reactions in patients with SCD, with a high mortality rate [53]. Severe complications of DHTRs are often due to the tendency of patients with SCD to develop hyperhemolysis, where the patient's own RBCs also experience accelerated clearance [16, 53, 63, 64]. While the mechanisms of hyperhemolysis remain to be fully elucidated, potential changes in macrophage phagocytic activity may contribute to increased RBC clearance in this setting, possibly explaining data suggesting that IL-6 inhibition can reduce RBC removal [65–68]. Release during hemolysis can also exceed the scavenging capacity of hemopexin, which is often saturated due to the chronic hemolysis patients with SCD experience. This can accelerate heme-induced complement activation, which can lead to enhanced C3 fixation on the RBC surface [69–71]. RBCs from patients with SCD are particularly sensitive to complement-induced hemolysis, possibly explaining the increased incidence of hyperhemolysis among these patients [72–84]. Similar to recent findings on IL-6 inhibition [65–68], blocking complement activation has been demonstrated to alleviate excessive hemolysis and mitigate other SCD complications [53, 73, 84, 85]. Hemolysis may also impact erythropoiesis, further complicating management of SCD [86].

4 Increased Recognition of RBC Alloimmunization-Related Complications

The challenges of RBC alloimmunization in transfusion-dependent patients have become increasingly apparent in recent decades. While compatible blood can be found for most patients, repeated transfusions in patients with underlying hemoglobinopathies or other conditions requiring chronic transfusion therapy can lead to the accumulation of alloantibodies and/or the formation of alloantibodies against high-frequency alloantigens not commonly observed in the general population [13, 63]. Patients with SCD appear to be particularly susceptible to RBC alloimmunization [19]. This heightened risk may be attributed to several factors. Genetic differences between donors and recipients increase alloantigen exposure in patients with SCD [87, 88]. However, inflammation at the time of transfusion may be the most pronounced driver in patients with SCD, as evidenced by increased alloimmunization rates following transfusion during complications associated with inflammation but not for other indications, such as stroke [89, 90]. Other patient populations, including patients with systemic lupus erythematosus or myelodysplastic syndrome, are also more likely to develop alloantibodies following transfusion [91–95].

The significance of RBC alloimmunization has become more evident as many patients with SCD and other transfusion-dependent conditions have lived longer [96]. Patients with SCD, in particular in the United States, rarely survived into adolescence prior to the 1970s, reducing the probability that cumulative RBC transfusion exposure would result in alloimmunization and that alloantibodies, once formed, would complicate future transfusions [97, 98]. Similar survival was reported for patients with thalassemia. Chronic transfusion therapy for thalassemia was complicated by iron overload, which improved with the more routine use of chelation therapy in the 1980s [99]. In patients with SCD, transfusions were commonly episodic. It wasn't until the late twentieth century that randomized controlled trials demonstrated the effectiveness of RBC exchange therapy for stroke prevention [100]. As a result, a combination of patients with transfusion-dependent conditions living longer and more transfusion exposure appears to be increasing the frequency of transfusion-related complications due to alloimmunization [44, 45, 47, 58]. However, the complications of RBC alloimmunization extend beyond patients with SCD and thalassemia. Recent data demonstrates that all alloimmunized patients may experience increased susceptibility to complications, longer hospital stays, and higher morbidity and mortality [46].

5 Challenges with Reducing RBC Alloimmunization

Matching alloantigens between donors and recipients beyond ABO and RhD can reduce alloimmunization rates [101, 102]. However, this process is often incomplete and resource intensive, with evidence of breakthrough alloimmunization occurring despite extended matching efforts, in part due to the complexity of many Rh alloantigens [103, 104]. As a result, complementary approaches are needed to actively prevent alloimmunization in at-risk patients.

However, for this to be realized, the factors that dictate the formation of RBC alloantibodies need to be defined [19].

Although nearly all individuals lacking blood group A or B spontaneously generate alloantibodies against these alloantigens in early infancy, the same pattern is not observed in RBC-induced alloantibodies following allogeneic RBC exposure. As there are over 300 different alloantigens, it is highly likely that the vast majority of transfusion recipients are exposed to some allogenic differences between donor and recipient following every single transfusion. Despite this, most RBC transfusions do not result in alloantibody formation. Some chronically transfused patients may receive hundreds of RBC units over their lifetime without generating a detectable alloimmune response, while others develop alloantibodies following early exposure [13, 15, 63]. Patients who develop an alloimmune response are typically called "responders," while those who do not are known as "non-responders." However, this distinction is not always straightforward, as non-responders may eventually become responders after additional allogeneic RBC exposure, and certain indications are much more likely to result in an alloimmune response following allogeneic RBC transfusion (REF Ross and Stella). Studies also suggest that individuals who generate alloantibodies are more likely to develop additional alloantibodies following subsequent transfusions, leading to the concept of "hyperresponders" [105].

While expanding blood matching beyond ABO and RhD to include additional alloantigens can significantly reduce the risk of alloimmunization, as noted above, this approach requires substantial resources beyond conventional transfusion compatibility testing [104, 106]. Recent strategies to prevent alloimmunization are exploring molecular approaches to develop more extensive matching strategies [107–114]. These efforts are expected to be significantly enhanced by advancements in next-generation sequencing and improved bioinformatics tools [115]. To optimize these efforts, while also conserving resources, the identification of factors that predict whether a patient is likely to be a responder or non-responder would allow matching efforts to be directed toward patients who are at the highest risk of alloimmunization [104]. Active prevention strategies would similarly be enhanced by the ability to identify high-risk patients before transfusion occurs.

It is important to note that, beyond being classified as a responder or non-responder, specific patient conditions, such as viral infections or certain complications associated with SCD, can generally increase the risk of alloimmunization [116]. Indeed, while antigen matching is most often achieved during chronic transfusion, acute complications likely warrant the most important consideration. The most effective strategy for reducing alloimmunization after transfusion may therefore involve identifying patients at risk, while specifically targeting transfusion scenarios where the risk of alloimmunization is highest. However, in settings with severe complications like acute chest syndrome, where alloimmunization rates are relatively high, the practicality of matching RBCs becomes particularly challenging due to the urgency of transfusion [89, 90]. This is particularly relevant for centers that rarely see patients with SCD, as they may not typically store alloantigen-negative units or commonly conduct phenotypic or molecular testing for extended antigens [57].

6 Understanding Factors That Influence Alloimmunization

Several studies have aimed to clarify the mechanisms behind the development of alloantibodies, including identifying factors that determine whether an individual is a responder or a non-responder [117, 118]. The responder and non-responder phenomenon is not unique to RBC alloimmunization and has been observed in other contexts, such as platelet alloimmunization and the development of anti-FVIII antibodies (inhibitors), following clotting factor replacement therapy for hemophilia patients [33, 119–123]. These observations suggest that similar principles may govern alloimmune responses in a variety of settings. Several studies have suggested that the distinct behavior of a recipient's immune cells, cytokine responses, recipient inflammation at the time of transfusion, and possible associations with HLA status and other genetic polymorphisms may influence the likelihood of alloimmunization [59, 124–130]. While blood products have been traditionally viewed as lacking adjuvant-like properties, recent studies have suggested that transfusion can trigger immune activation through toll-like receptors [131]. Studies have also shown that retained reticulocytes in transfused RBC units may expose patients to mitochondrial products that mimic microbial stimulation and could therefore trigger immune activation [132]. Refrigerator storage of RBCs may also induce metabolic and other changes that increase their potential to induce immune responses post-transfusion [133–136].

Several studies have identified key differences in the immune cells between responders and non-responders. These differences are evident in whole blood and may stem from variations in cytokine levels, monocyte Fc gamma receptor expression, alterations in T cell chemokine sensitivity, differences in T follicular helper cell (TFH) states, or the proclivity of naïve T cells to become activated following stimulation [64, 137–141], which could in turn influence the likelihood of RBC alloimmunization. Numerous studies have demonstrated that while heme can be a significant modulator of SCD pathogenesis in general [142], heme can also impact immune cell function in a manner that discriminates between responders

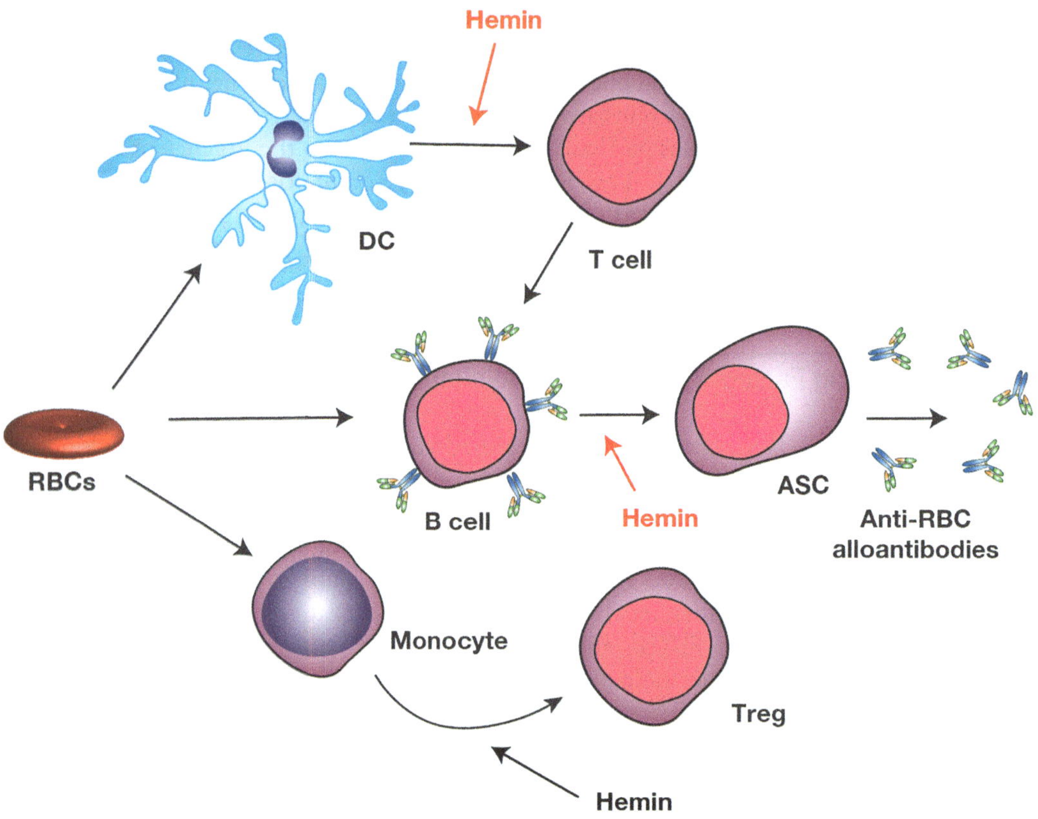

Fig. 1 Hemin impacts the activity of key immune cells involved in RBC alloimmunization. Hemin suppresses T cell activation by dendritic cells (DCs) and inhibits the differentiation of B cells into antibody-secreting cells (ASCs), which are ultimately responsible for producing RBC alloantibodies. In contrast, hemin enhances monocyte-driven regulatory T cell (Treg) function. Through these combined effects, hemin dampens the immune processes that promote alloantibody formation. These pathways are active in individuals who do not develop alloantibodies after transfusion (non-responders) but show reduced sensitivity to hemin in those who generate alloantibodies (responders). This suggests that the responder-non-responder continuum may partly depend on how responsive these immune pathways are to hemin, a mechanism particularly relevant in patients with chronic hemolytic disorders such as sickle cell disease. Red arrows represent inhibition, whereas black arrows represent stimulation of the corresponding process

and non-responders. Heme has the ability to suppress the activity of T cells, B cells, and antigen-presenting cells (APCs) in non-responders while failing to do so in responders [143–146] (Fig. 1). Conversely, heme augments regulatory T cell (Treg) activity in non-responders, while failing to similarly impact Treg function in responders [141], consistent with the ability of Tregs to inhibit RBC alloimmunization [147, 148]. Differences in regulatory B cell activity may also differentiate responders from non-responders [149]. While complications of SCD may be associated with increased hemolysis, in responders, heme's suppressive activity of key immune populations thought to facilitate alloimmunization is less pronounced [143–146], possibly allowing inflammatory signals to occur during these complications unabated by heme's immunosuppressive effects, resulting in a higher rate of alloimmunization [89, 90]. As vaccine responses do not appear to fall along responder-non-responder lines [150], these results highlight the unique nature and distinct pathways engaged during RBC alloimmunization from more commonly studied vaccination. The mechanisms underlying responder and non-responder status to clotting factors, particularly recombinant proteins like Factor VIII that lack known innate immune agonists, remain less clear. However, incorporation of xenoglycan antigens during production of recombinant FVIII products could enhance immune recognition and response [151]. As noted above, recipient inflammation at the time of transfusion, including surgery in the setting of hemophilia, may contribute to innate immune activation that could facilitate alloimmunization [152, 153].

While clinical associations have certainly been helpful in seeking to identify risk factors for alloimmunization, investigating the real-time development of alloantibody formation against RBC alloantigens has proven challenging. Unlike hemophilia A, where antibody development is more commonly examined, patients undergoing RBC transfusions are not typically actively monitored for antibody formation [17, 57]. Instead, RBC alloantibody detection usually occurs only when a transfusion reaction is suspected or when the patient requires an additional transfusion. As patients are only provided ABO and RhD compatible RBCs in the emergent setting, deliberately inducing alloantibodies against non-ABO and RhD alloantigens for experimental purposes is unethical. Similarly, while immune-mediated platelet refractoriness may occur independent of antibodies, alloantibodies that do form against platelet alloantigens are also not actively monitored and therefore often remain undetected until a patient exhibits unresponsiveness to platelet transfusions, prompting an investigation into possible immune-mediated platelet refractoriness [154–156]. However, to target alloimmune responses, identification of early initiating factors that control alloimmunization events is important before downstream pathways amplify the overall response and therefore make prevention strategies more challenging.

In addition to challenges in capturing the immune response to blood products in real time, many of the factors that regulate the development of alloantibodies or alloimmunization in general occur outside the blood compartment in immune tissue [157–160]. As a result, while the consequence of alloimmunization can be observed in blood, the key immune cells that engage and respond to RBC alloantigens primarily exist outside the bloodstream in immune tissue that specializes in developing an immune response [157–160]. The architecture of these tissues plays a crucial role in orchestrating immune responses, as the localization, trafficking, and overall sensitivity of immune cells to various stimuli are heavily influenced by specific characteristics and overall location of these cells in vivo [161, 162]. Given the difficulties in accurately replicating these complex events in patients and the inherent limitations of in vitro models to mimic critical aspects of a developing immune response [163, 164], including the spatial regulation of these responses in general, the utilization of preclinical models has become invaluable. This has been particularly important when examining the intricacies of circulating blood, the interaction between intravenous blood and the immune system, and the resulting consequences of these interactions on alloimmunization and subsequent transfusion [165]. These models offer a complementary approach to many clinical studies and are best used when they identify common and evolutionarily conserved pathways that may hold relevance across mammalian evolution [166–168]. In doing so, these models can aid in the identification of mechanisms that govern alloimmunization and therefore could be targeted to improve prevention and therapeutic strategies.

7 The Use of Preclinical Models in Transfusion Medicine and Related Fields

The use of preclinical models is not new to transfusion medicine. Early studies incubating serum with RBCs were among the first to reveal antigenic differences between species, a finding that likely influenced Landsteiner's exploration of individual variations in RBCs in the human population [169]. Inbred mice were utilized to investigate the genetic factors behind transplant rejection. Through extensive backcrossing and transplant experiments, George Snell and colleagues identified the polymorphic major histocompatibility complex (MHC), which in patients includes HLA and other immune regulators [170]. This discovery helped unravel the complexities of T cell engagement of antigenic peptides presented in a complex with MHC [171], a completely unprecedented mode of immune activation that has transformed medicine as much or more than the discovery of ABO blood group antigens. These findings ultimately provided insight into immune-mediated transplant rejection, platelet refractoriness, and genetic risk factors for RBC alloimmunization [172–174].

Many studies have similarly leveraged animal models to examine the consequences of immune responses to blood transfusion and related areas of medicine. Models of immune thrombocytopenia (ITP) in particular aided in understanding the consequences of antibody engagement of platelets and provided some of the first insight into the unique axis between hemostasis and immunology, concepts that have now extended far beyond the study of ITP and transfusion medicine [175–185]. Models examining the underlying pathology of FNAIT and possible immunoprophylaxis in this setting have also been generated [37, 186–190]. Studies examining the development of autoimmune hemolytic anemia using the New Zealand Black mice, in addition to more recently developed models, have provided important insight into immune dysregulation that can contribute to autoimmunity and the key features of antibodies that drive RBC clearance in vivo [191–198]. Additional studies have outlined the role of immune responses in other conditions, such as heparin-induced thrombocytopenia, that provided important insight into the thrombotic sequelae of more recent conditions, such as COVID-19, providing some insight into the potential role of plasmapheresis in severe COVID-19 clinically [199–208]. The development of preclinical models in these contexts has significantly enhanced our understanding of the immune pathways involved in pathological immune responses to various auto- or allo-antigens.

More recent models have uncovered key features of the overall efficacy and complications following transfusion. Models studying transfusion-associated acute lung injury (TRALI) have uncovered key features of antibodies, cells, lipid mediators, complement, and even the role of the microbiota in dictating this response to transfusion [209–216]. These studies have changed blood donation practice and the overall clinical management of transfusion, which in turn has reduced TRALI incidence [209–218]. Other studies have used the power of mouse genetics to uncover key regulators of RBC metabolism, potentially helping identify donors whose RBCs have superior storage characteristics [219–226]. Additionally, animal models have been employed to develop targeted immunotherapies, such as deleting unwanted B cells or eliminating other immune cells resistant to current treatments [227, 228]. The generation of RBCs and platelets in vitro reflects a blend of emerging technologies with traditional transfusion medicine [229–233]; preclinical models have been employed to determine the efficacy of in vitro-derived or otherwise manipulated blood products for therapeutic purposes [133, 229, 234, 235]. Preclinical models have also investigated developmental differences in response to anemia, thrombocytopenia, and transfusion [236–239], particularly focusing on the sensitivity of preterm infants to transfusion-related complications. Overall, these preclinical models have provided valuable insights into key aspects of transfusion medicine.

8 The Development and Use of Preclinical Models to Study RBC Alloimmunization

Recent studies have also adopted preclinical approaches to study RBC alloimmunization. Current models for RBC alloimmunization range from utilizing antigens like mHEL or human glycophorin A to more complex systems that integrate commonly employed model antigens coupled with a human blood group, such as the HOD system, which incorporates HEL and OVA model antigens with the human blood group Duffy antigen as a chimeric fusion protein [240–245]. Another frequently employed system is the KEL model, comprising various transgenics expressing the human KEL glycoprotein in either Kell or Cellano variants [246], with different transgenic founders producing RBCs that express these antigens at different densities [246–248]. This has allowed for the assessment of antigen levels as a variable influencing RBC alloimmunization and antibody-induced clearance [249–251]. Additional models, including those based on the Duffy antigen alone or the RhD antigen, have been described, although the immune responses in these systems remain to be fully characterized [252, 253]. Collectively, these murine models have provided a useful strategy to study the development and overall consequences of RBC alloimmunization.

Data generated using these preclinical models demonstrates that a variety of downstream pathways may be involved in alloantibody development. Allogeneic RBC transfusion can activate diverse innate immune pathways and engage unique immune components responsible for IgG antibody formation. Key roles have been identified for cytokines such as IL-6 and type I interferons, as well as bridging channel dendritic cells (DCs) and macrophages in the marginal zone, in potentially trapping allogeneic RBCs post-transfusion [131, 251, 254–257]. Notably, bridging channel DCs appear crucial in trafficking antigens to areas optimal for CD4 T cell activation and proliferation [254]. However, not all IgG antibody responses following RBC transfusion require CD4 T cell help. Transfusion of KEL RBCs can induce IgG formation independent of CD4 T cells, a process that appears to rely on complement and complement receptors on B cells [258].

As initial IgM antibody production appears to occur independently of CD4 T cells, early IgM production may allow IgM engagement of transfused RBCs, leading to complement activation and deposition on the RBC surface [258, 259]. In this setting, even if IgG antibodies against a particular antigen are not known to routinely fix complement, the early IgM response, which is not routinely monitored clinically, may fix complement owing to the relative efficiency of IgM antibodies to activate complement when compared to IgG [258]. The ability of IgM to fix complement is likely a product of the overall robustness of the antibody response and the antigen target. The mobility of the antigen and the location of the epitope likely dictate, at least in part, whether IgM engagement can effectively engage C1q and therefore activate complement [69]. Irrespective of the factors that dictate the likelihood of C3 fixation following IgM engagement, C3 deposition on the RBC surface may facilitate binding to complement receptors on antigen-specific B cells during the early phases of the immune response [260, 261]. The magnitude of C3 deposition in this initial stage could potentially be one of several factors influencing the necessity of CD4 T cells in the development of an IgG-mediated immune response. However, as C3 can facilitate antigen removal during the developing immune response [259], this may also introduce a competing process that reduces antigen availability as the immune response unfolds, which, in turn, could affect the overall magnitude of alloantibody formation. As RBC alloimmunization is not monitored in real time, it is very uncommon to detect an evolving IgM immune response following RBC alloantigen exposure, making it difficult to ascertain clinically whether IgM antibody responses and subsequent complement fixation dictate any involvement of CD4 T cells in IgG antibody formation. Prior generation of a CD4 T cell response against surface or intracellular alloantigens can also enhance subsequent immune responses to distinct RBC surface alloantigens [262, 263]. This suggests that immune responses to intracellular determinants, which are not on the RBC surface as discrete antibody targets and therefore not detected by current clinical assays, may provide a common immune target that enhances antibody formation against other alloantigens, thereby providing a possible mechanism that may contribute to the phenomenon of hyperresponders.

Key features of RBCs and recipients that may impact the likelihood of alloimmunization have also been explored using preclinical models. Early studies indicated that refrigerator storage can increase the likelihood of alloantibody formation, with storage of HOD RBCs being the most well studied [264]. However, while storage enhances HOD alloimmunization, storage induces the opposite effect toward KEL, even when both antigens are present on the same RBCs [265]. This dichotomy highlights the distinct immune pathways that can be engaged by different antigens. The ability of storage to enhance alloimmunization against HOD may reflect the impact of accelerated RBC clearance on CD4 T cell activation (Fig. 2). In contrast, as KEL RBCs can induce IgG antibody formation independent of CD4 T cells, enhanced clearance may reduce the likelihood of C3 deposition and B cell engagement, which in turn may reduce the ability of these cells to generate a CD4 T cell-independent IgG response. Although clearance of HOD RBCs would be expected to have a similar effect on B cell engagement, the substantial increase in CD4 T cells may offset any potential decrease in B cell recognition. Inflammation in the recipient at the time of transfusion can also enhance RBC alloimmunization. This may reflect altered RBC uptake and increased immune cell activation following transfusion, leading to enhanced alloimmunization [266, 267]. Although multiple pathways may be involved, type I interferons seem to play a significant role in the ability of recipient inflammation to enhance alloimmunization, especially in settings of viral or lupus-associated inflammation [251, 256, 268].

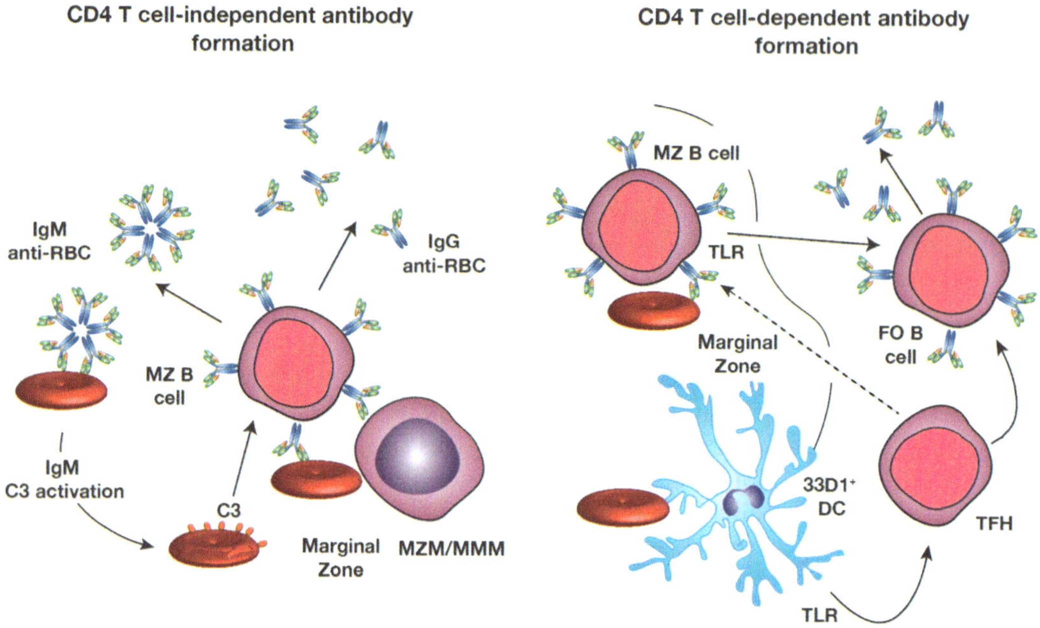

Fig. 2 RBC alloantigens can elicit IgG alloantibody formation through both CD4 T cell-dependent and -independent mechanisms. Marginal zone (MZ) B cells are essential in initiating both types of responses, though the downstream effectors that coordinate each pathway may differ. Complement component 3 (C3), deposited on the RBC surface following initial IgM production, appears to promote MZ B cell class switching in a CD4 T cell-independent manner. Conversely, the uptake of transfused RBCs by 33D1^{+} dendritic cells (DCs) seems critical for activating CD4 T cells, which in turn can facilitate CD4 T cell dependent IgG production. Although these processes occur outside the B cell follicle, several clinical studies suggest that T follicular helper (TFH) and follicular (FO) B cells may also contribute. Additionally, marginal zone macrophages (MZMs) and metallophilic macrophages (MMMs) may play a role in the initial trapping of allogeneic RBCs at the beginning of both pathways

The significance of KEL antigen presentation on the RBC surface to B cells is highlighted by the effect of antigen density on the cell surface, a key factor that can vary among different RBC units [269] (Fig. 3). RBCs with low KEL antigen density (KEL^{lo} RBCs) not only fail to induce anti-KEL alloimmunization, but recipients exposed to these RBCs can become desensitized to the formation of anti-KEL antibodies after subsequent KEL RBC transfusion [249, 270]. However, recipient genetics can modify responsiveness to KEL^{lo} RBC transfusion [271]. In contrast, while transfusion of RBCs with higher levels of the KEL antigen (KEL^{hi} RBCs) may also not trigger a productive IgG response, unlike KEL^{lo} RBC transfusion, inflammation can convert a non-responsive state into responsiveness following KEL^{hi} RBC exposure [251, 256, 268]. Another variable that may influence the immunogenicity of donor RBCs may be the number of reticulocytes present, which can be highly variable among different donors [132]. Studies have shown that retained reticulocytes in

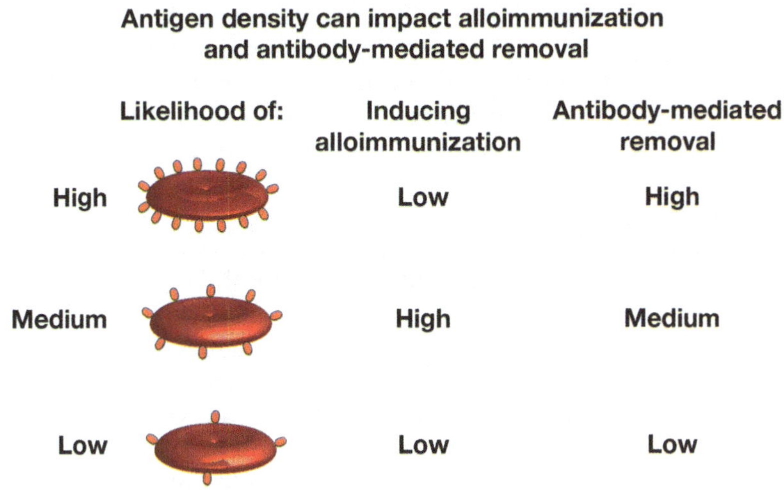

Fig. 3 Antigen density may impact the likelihood of RBC alloimmunization and the consequence of antibody engagement on RBC removal. In a preclinical model that employs RBCs expressing various levels of the KEL antigen, antigen density can influence both the likelihood of IgG alloantibody formation following an initial transfusion and the outcome of incompatible transfusions in recipients previously alloimmunized against KEL. Recipients transfused without inflammation with either high- or low-density KEL RBCs not only fail to generate anti-KEL IgG antibodies but also become resistant to anti-KEL antibody formation when later exposed to medium-density KEL RBCs. In contrast, transfusion with medium-density KEL RBCs readily induces anti-KEL antibody production regardless of prior inflammation. In previously anti-KEL alloimmunized recipients, transfusion of RBCs with different KEL antigen densities results in distinct clearance rates, with high-density KEL RBCs cleared most rapidly and low-density RBCs least. These findings suggest that antigen density not only governs alloantibody induction but also determines the severity of transfusion reactions

donor blood units can trigger RBC alloimmunization, possibly due to retained mitochondria functioning as innate immune activators [132].

While a variety of downstream pathways have been reported to govern alloimmunization, marginal zone (MZ) B cells appear to be central in the initial immune response to blood transfusion [272, 273]. The involvement of MZ B cells is not limited to RBC alloimmunization, as studies have demonstrated that these innate-like B cells appear to play a pivotal role in the development of alloantibodies in a variety of contexts, including alloimmunization following platelet transfusion, FVIII exposure, and even solid organ transplantation [274–276]. MZ B cells are characterized by their lower activation threshold, allowing them to possibly respond to blood-borne antigens even in the absence of potent adjuvants [160, 277–280]. MZ B cells also possess the unique ability to facilitate both CD4 T cell-dependent and independent IgG responses, consistent with the ability of transfused blood products and clotting factor therapeutics to drive distinct responses despite appearing to require a similar initiating node [277, 279, 280]. Given their relatively small contribution to overall B cell numbers [160, 277–280], targeting MZ B cells may offer a promising avenue for preventing alloimmune responses in high-risk patients without completely compromising humoral immunity. However, further research is necessary to fully elucidate the potential of this approach, its associated risks, and, therefore, its clinical applicability.

9 Defining the Consequences of Antibody Engagement

In addition to establishing key nodes for the development of alloantibodies following transfusion, these same models have provided important insight into the consequences of antibody engagement. Early studies demonstrated that antibodies generated following KEL RBC exposure could cause HDFN, providing one of the first mouse models of this disease [247]. Additional studies demonstrated that, following an incompatible transfusion, antibodies could facilitate RBC removal through classical pathways involving Fc receptors or complement [242, 281, 282]. Rapid clearance can lead to elevations in systemic cytokine responses [242], aligning with in vitro findings that show comparable outcomes after antibody-mediated RBC phagocytosis [283]. Antibody isotype and subclass, glycosylation status, affinity for antigen, and the antigen target itself likely influence which antibody effectors are engaged and therefore the overall consequences of incompatible transfusion [284–288]. However, subsequent studies have revealed that antibody binding could paradoxically result in a failure to clear some transfused RBCs due to antibody-mediated antigen removal [241, 289] (Fig. 4). This has been observed to varying degrees in every incompatible transfusion model studied and has also been documented in clinical settings where antibodies are provided therapeutically that engage a patient's RBCs [241, 290–296]. The mechanisms underlying antibody-mediated antigen loss are diverse, with several studies demonstrating that antibodies may enhance proteolytic cleavage of the antigen and/or facilitate trogocytosis of RBC membrane containing the antigen [289, 297]. Fc receptors and complement appear to play a role, but in some settings, neither antibody effector system appears to be required [241, 250, 281, 289–291, 297]. Levels of CD47 on the RBC surface may also influence their sensitivity to antigen loss and RBC clearance following antibody engagement [298]. These findings suggest that antibody-mediated antigen loss could potentially be leveraged to prevent the devastating consequences of incompatible RBC transfusion, particularly in highly alloimmunized individuals who are difficult to transfuse.

While an incompatible RBC transfusion can result in a hemolytic transfusion reaction, passive administration of antibodies in the setting of allogeneic RBC exposure can lead to AMIS

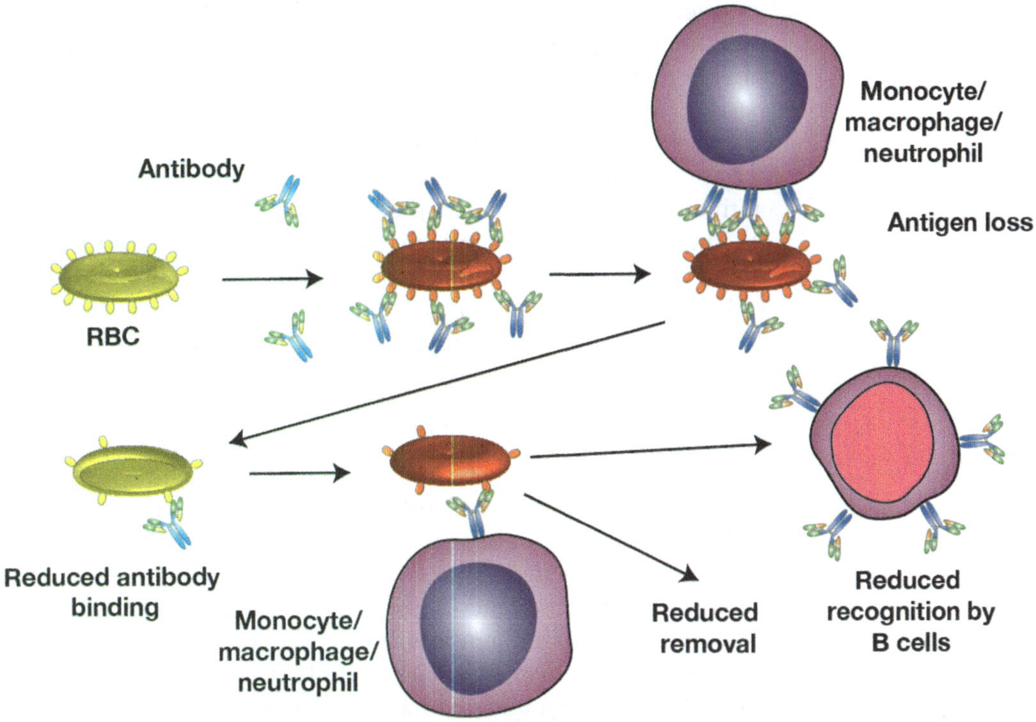

Fig. 4 Antibodies can promote the elimination of a target antigen, thereby modifying the clearance rate of incompatible red blood cells and their ability to initiate an immune response. Antibody-induced antigen removal can occur through various antibody effector mechanisms, such as complement activation and Fc receptor engagement. Once the antigen is removed, the remaining RBCs become less susceptible to further antibody-mediated clearance, even if lower levels of the antigen remain on their surface. Additionally, the loss of antigen may hinder B cells from recognizing and responding to an alloantigen, offering a potential explanation for how antibody-mediated immunosuppression occurs

[24]. Although the mechanisms of AMIS have remained unclear despite its use for the prevention of RhD alloimmunization for decades [24], AMIS is not a uniform outcome of passively administered antibody binding to RBC alloantigens. Instead, some antibody-antigen combinations have been shown to paradoxically enhance antibody formation [249, 287, 288, 299, 300]. While the mechanisms responsible for this remain to be fully uncovered, enhanced RBC uptake by APCs may not only result in their activation, but also an improved CD4+ T cell response [301, 302]. Inclusion of antibodies can even shift an otherwise tolerogenic response toward an augmented antibody response [249], while in other settings, combinations of antibodies can switch an augmented response to AMIS or simply improve AMIS in general [22, 302, 303]. Multiple mechanisms are likely involved in AMIS, including the ability of antibodies to induce antigen loss from the RBC surface [294, 304–307]. However, recipient inflammation at the time of inflammation can also modulate the outcome of antibody

engagement, possibly causing AMIS failure [308]. While antibodies can engage the RBC surface, they can rapidly equilibrate in vivo [309], suggesting that they may not possess the ability to permanently provide steric interference with B cell receptor recognition. Antibody-induced reductions in antigen on the RBC surface may prevent antigen-specific B cells from recognizing RBC-bound antigens or otherwise impact the outcome of antigen engagement. As the density of the antigen on the RBC surface appears to influence B cell responses and eventual antibody production [249, 270], even incomplete elimination of antigen from the RBC surface may modulate the ongoing outcome of alloantigen exposure.

Similar to incompatible RBC transfusion, the antigen target and the antibodies employed may dictate which antibody effector pathways are engaged, which may in turn impact the rate of RBC removal, antigen loss, and other variables that impact whether AMIS, augmentation, or neither occurs following RBC exposure. As antibody-mediated uptake of antigen by APCs may enhance CD4 T cell responses and therefore alloimmunity [301, 302], the rate and extent of antigen loss, along with other recipient factors affecting antigen load and CD4+ T cell activation, may determine whether AMIS or augmented antibody responses occur following RBC exposure. AMIS and augmented responses may therefore in part reflect a dynamic continuum of enhanced components of the immune response (i.e., CD4 T cell activation) and availability of antigen to B cells. This may in part be predicated, at least for some alloantigens, on the number of RBCs to which a recipient is exposed [302]. The relative clearance and degree of antigen loss driven by a particular antibody-antigen pair may also dictate the extent to which antibody engagement influences the immune response to other alloantigens on the same surface not bound by antibody [303, 306, 307, 310–312]. Inflammation at the time of antibody administration may shift this balance by modifying the activation thresholds of immune cells, thereby influencing the range of antigen concentrations required for alloimmunization [308]. While the mechanisms of antibody-induced antigen loss remain to be fully defined, studies have suggested that trogocytosis, a process whereby phagocytes remove just part of the membrane including the antigen without fully phagocytosing a cell, may play a role in antigen removal and AMIS [297]. As a result, while general principles may apply, the mechanisms underlying AMIS or augmented responses following RBC alloantigen exposure may exhibit some degree of antigen specificity due to the diverse consequences of antibody engagement.

Recent clinical studies employing biotinylated RBCs may provide a mechanism to define the consequences of incompatible RBC transfusion following small volume transfusion clinically [313–316], and therefore potentially determine whether similar outcomes occur following small volume exposure of incompatible RBCs in patients. This could be especially important to not only confirm preclinical mechanistic work but also could prove invaluable when seeking to determine whether a given antibody profile in a patient is capable of causing significant RBC clearance following transfusion. This approach may allow the possible transfusion of partially incompatible blood to be assessed, especially in the acute setting where a patient presents with life-threatening anemia but no compatible RBCs can be procured. In this setting, such an approach may provide a complementary strategy to monocyte monolayer tests and may be unique in that it would provide key information regarding the recipient's ability to hemolyze transfused RBCs, which could vary depending on levels of complement, and the overall status and activation of the patient's phagocytes peri-transfusion [317–319].

10 Conclusions

Over the past century, numerous studies have provided insight into key aspects of RBC alloimmunization. These studies initially focused on identifying antigen targets to facilitate compatible unit selection for patients with RBC alloantibodies. As awareness of the complications arising from alloimmunization has grown, research in the field has expanded to include investigation into the process underlying alloantibody formation and the overall consequences of incompatible transfusion. Through a combination of clinical studies, translational research, and preclinical models, emerging themes are shedding light on the factors governing the development and consequences of RBC alloimmunization. The insights gained from these studies hold promise beyond preventing RBC alloimmunization, as similarities exist with alloantibody development against platelets and clotting factor alloantigens. With ongoing advancements in tools and methodologies in various models of RBC alloimmunization and transfusion medicine in general, fundamental understanding of the key regulators in these processes will continue to emerge, potentially leading to improved management and prevention strategies across various settings of alloimmunization and a greater understanding of mammalian biology in general. Similar approaches have been used to gain a deeper understanding of other immune-related transfusion complications, such as platelet refractoriness, TRALI, FNAIT, and transfusion-induced immunomodulatory outcomes more broadly. By integrating both preclinical and clinical studies and employing many of the methods described throughout this volume, significant advances in the scientific understanding of transfusion are likely to emerge.

Conflict of Interest

This work was funded by NIH P01HL171803, R01 HL165975, R01 HL135575, and R01 HL154034. SRS has received speaker and consultant honoraria from Cerus, Grifols, Novartis, Alexion, and Argenx and has received a research grant from Alexion. No other authors have conflicts of interest.

References

1. Storry JR, Olsson ML (2009) The ABO blood group system revisited: a review and update. Immunohematology 25:48–59
2. Landsteiner K (1900) Zentbl Bakt Parasitkde (Abt) 27:357–363
3. Watkins WM (2001) The ABO blood group system: historical background. Transfus Med 11:243–265
4. Stowell SR, Stowell CP (2019) Biologic roles of the ABH and Lewis histo-blood group antigens part II: thrombosis, cardiovascular disease and metabolism. Vox Sang 114:535
5. W. S. Jajosky RP, Zheng L, Jajosky AN, Jajoksy PG, Josephson CD, Hollenhorst MA, Sackstein R, Cummings RD, Arthur CM, Stowell SR (2023) ABO blood group antigens and differential glycan expression: Perspective on the evolution of common human enzyme deficiencies. iScience. in press
6. McRae HL, Millar MW, Slavin SA, Blumberg N, Rahman A, Refaai MA (2021) Essential role of rho-associated kinase in ABO immune complex-mediated endothelial barrier disruption. Biomedicine 9
7. O. M. Arthur CM, Stowell SR, ABO and other carbohydrate blood group systems. C. Cohn, Ed., AABB technical manual (AABB, 21, 2023)
8. Arthur CM SS (2023) The development and consequences of RBC alloimmunization. Ann Rev Pathol. in press
9. Stowell CP, Stowell SR (2019) Biologic roles of the ABH and Lewis histo-blood group antigens part I: infection and immunity. Vox Sang 114:426–442
10. Bansal N, West LJ, Simmonds J, Urschel S (2024) ABO-incompatible heart transplantation-evolution of a revolution. J Heart Lung Transplant 43:1514–1520
11. Urschel S, West LJ (2016) ABO-incompatible heart transplantation. Curr Opin Pediatr 28: 613–619
12. Dean CL, Sullivan HC, Stowell SR, Fasano RM, West LJ, Robitaille N, Josephson CD (2018) Current state of transfusion practices for ABO-incompatible pediatric heart transplant patients in the United States and Canada. Transfusion 58:2243–2249
13. Pirenne F, Floch A, Diop S (2023) Alloimmunisation against red blood cells in sickle cell disease: transfusion challenges in high-income and low-income countries. Lancet Haematol 10:e468–e476
14. Zimring JC, Hudson KE (2016) Cellular immune responses in red blood cell alloimmunization. Hematology Am Soc Hematol Educ Program 2016:452–456
15. Yazdanbakhsh K, Shaz BH, Hillyer CD (2017) Immune regulation of sickle cell Alloimmunization. ISBT Sci Ser 12:248–253
16. Pirenne F, Yazdanbakhsh K (2018) How I safely transfuse patients with sickle-cell disease and manage delayed hemolytic transfusion reactions. Blood 131:2773–2781
17. Tormey CA, Hendrickson JE (2019) Transfusion-related red blood cell alloantibodies: induction and consequences. Blood 133: 1821–1830
18. Zimring JC, Spitalnik SL (2015) Pathobiology of transfusion reactions. Annu Rev Pathol 10:83–110
19. Hudson KE, Fasano RM, Karafin MS, Hendrickson JE, Francis RO (2019) Mechanisms of alloimmunization in sickle cell disease. Curr Opin Hematol 26:434–441
20. de Haas M, Thurik FF, Koelewijn JM, van der Schoot CE (2015) Haemolytic disease of the fetus and newborn. Vox Sang 109:99–113
21. Zwiers C, Slootweg YM, Koelewijn JM, Ligthart PC, van der Bom JG, van Kamp IL, Lopriore E, van der Schoot CE, Oepkes D, de Haas M (2024) Disease severity in subsequent pregnancies with RhD immunization: a nationwide cohort. Vox Sang 119:859–866
22. Stowell SR (2016) Working together to block alloimmunization. Blood 128:1029–1030
23. Arthur CM, Stowell SR (2023) The development and consequences of red blood cell

Alloimmunization. Annu Rev Pathol 18:537–564
24. Brinc D, Lazarus AH (2009) Mechanisms of anti-D action in the prevention of hemolytic disease of the fetus and newborn. Hematology Am Soc Hematol Educ Program 2009: 185–191
25. Vossoughi S, Spitalnik SL (2019) Conquering erythroblastosis fetalis: 50 years of RhIG. Transfusion 59:2195–2196
26. Visser GHA, Di Renzo GC, Spitalnik SL, Motherhood FCS, Newborn H (2019) The continuing burden of Rh disease 50 years after the introduction of anti-Rh (D) immunoglobin prophylaxis: call to action. Am J Obstet Gynecol 221:227 e221–227 e224
27. Salomon O, Rosenberg N (2013) Predicting risk severity and response of fetal neonatal alloimmune thrombocytopenia. Br J Haematol 162:304–312
28. Calandrini C, Verhagen O, Tissoudali A, Homburg CHE, Vessies J, Brussee M, van Beers EH, van der Schoot CE, de Haas M (2025) Real-world performance of a clinical droplet digital polymerase chain reaction assay for non-invasive foetal blood group and platelet antigen genotyping of alloimmunized pregnant women with antibodies directed against RhD, RhE, Rhc, RhC, K1, HPA-1a or HPA-5b: a 1-year experience. Vox Sang 120:170–177
29. de Vos TW, Tersteeg I, Lopriore E, Oepkes D, Porcelijn L, van der Schoot CE, Verweij EJT, Winkelhorst D, de Haas M, van den Akker-van Marle ME (2025) Screening of pregnant women for foetal neonatal alloimmune thrombocytopenia: a cost-utility analysis. Vox Sang 120:178–187
30. Tiller H, Killie MK, Chen P, Eksteen M, Husebekk A, Skogen B, Kjeldsen-Kragh J, Ni H (2012) Toward a prophylaxis against fetal and neonatal alloimmune thrombocytopenia: induction of antibody-mediated immune suppression and prevention of severe clinical complications in a murine model. Transfusion 52:1446–1457
31. Xu X, Chen D, Ye X, Xia W, Xu Y, Chen Y, Shao Y, Deng J, Ding H, Liu J, Wang J, Ni H, Fu Y, Santoso S (2021) Successful prenatal therapy for anti-CD36-mediated severe FNAIT by deglycosylated antibodies in a novel murine model. Blood 138:1757–1767
32. Kumpel BM (2012) Would it be possible to prevent HPA-1a alloimmunization to reduce the incidence of fetal and neonatal alloimmune thrombocytopenia? Transfusion 52: 1393–1397
33. G. Trial to reduce Alloimmunization to platelets study (1997) leukocyte reduction and ultraviolet B irradiation of platelets to prevent alloimmunization and refractoriness to platelet transfusions. N Engl J Med 337:1861–1869
34. de Vos TW, Winkelhorst D, Porcelijn L, Beaufort M, Oldert G, van der Bom JG, Lopriore E, Oepkes D, de Haas M, van der Schoot E (2023) Natural history of human platelet antigen 1a-alloimmunised pregnancies: a prospective observational cohort study. Lancet Haematol 10:e985–e993
35. Oosterhoff JJ, Linty F, Visser R, de Vos T, Hofstede-van Egmond S, van de Weerd M, Porcelijn L, de Haas M, van der Schoot E, Vidarsson G (2024) Generation of human antibodies targeting human platelet antigen (HPA)-1a. Transfusion 64:893–905
36. Zhi H, Ahlen MT, Skogen B, Newman DK, Newman PJ (2021) Preclinical evaluation of immunotherapeutic regimens for fetal/neonatal alloimmune thrombocytopenia. Blood Adv 5:3552–3562
37. Zhi H, Sheridan D, Newman DK, Newman PJ (2022) Prophylactic administration of HPA-1a-specific antibodies prevents fetal/neonatal alloimmune thrombocytopenia in mice. Blood 140:2146–2153
38. Li C, Piran S, Chen P, Lang S, Zarpellon A, Jin JW, Zhu G, Reheman A, van der Wal DE, Simpson EK, Ni R, Gross PL, Ware J, Ruggeri ZM, Freedman J, Ni H (2011) The maternal immune response to fetal platelet GPIbalpha causes frequent miscarriage in mice that can be prevented by intravenous IgG and anti-FcRn therapies. J Clin Invest 121:4537–4547
39. Moise KJ Jr, Ling LE, Oepkes D, Tiblad E, Verweij E, Lopriore E, Smoleniec J, Sachs UJ, Bein G, Kilby MD, Miller RS, Devlieger R, Audibert F, Emery SP, Markham K, Norton ME, Ocon-Hernandez O, Pandya P, Pereira L, Silver RM, Windrim R, Streisand JB, Leu JH, Mirza A, Smith V, Schwartz LB, Tjoa ML, Saeed-Khawaja S, Komatsu Y, Bussel JB, U. S. Group (2024) Nipocalimab in early-onset severe hemolytic disease of the fetus and Newborn. N Engl J Med 391:526–537
40. Chen P, Li C, Lang S, Zhu G, Reheman A, Spring CM, Freedman J, Ni H (2010) Animal model of fetal and neonatal immune thrombocytopenia: role of neonatal fc receptor in the pathogenesis and therapy. Blood 116: 3660–3668
41. Bussel JB, Vander Haar EL, Berkowitz RL (2021) New developments in fetal and

neonatal alloimmune thrombocytopenia. Am J Obstet Gynecol 225:120–127
42. Flegel WA (2016) Red cell alloimmunisation: incidence and prevention. Lancet Haematol 3:e260–e261
43. Yu H, Karafin MS, Tormey CA, Goel R, Spencer BR, Hendrickson JE, Hauser RG (2025) Associations between blood donors, component modifications, and the alloimmunization of transfusion recipients. Transfusion 65:588–603
44. Nickel RS, Hendrickson JE, Fasano RM, Meyer EK, Winkler AM, Yee MM, Lane PA, Jones YA, Pashankar FD, New T, Josephson CD, Stowell SR (2016) Impact of red blood cell alloimmunization on sickle cell disease mortality: a case series. Transfusion 56:107–114
45. Dean CL, Maier CL, Roback JD, Stowell SR (2019) Multiple hemolytic transfusion reactions misinterpreted as severe vaso-occlusive crisis in a patient with sickle cell disease. Transfusion 59:448–453
46. Viayna E, Gehrie EA, Blanchette C, Meny GM, Noumsi G, Huber M, Runken MC (2022) Red cell alloimmunization is associated with increased health care costs, longer hospitalizations, and higher mortality. Blood Adv 6:5655–5658
47. Telen MJ, Afenyi-Annan A, Garrett ME, Combs MR, Orringer EP, Ashley-Koch AE (2015) Alloimmunization in sickle cell disease: changing antibody specificities and association with chronic pain and decreased survival. Transfusion 55:1378–1387
48. Stack G, Tormey CA (2016) Detection rate of blood group alloimmunization based on real-world testing practices and kinetics of antibody induction and evanescence. Transfusion 56:2662–2667
49. Hauser RG, Esserman D, Karafin MS, Tan S, Balbuena-Merle R, Spencer BR, Roubinian NH, Wu Y, Triulzi DJ, Kleinman S, Gottschall JL, Hendrickson JE, Tormey CA (2020) The evanescence and persistence of RBC alloantibodies in blood donors. Transfusion 60:831–839
50. Fasano RM, Miller MJ, Chonat S, Stowell SR (2019) Clinical presentation of delayed hemolytic transfusion reactions and hyperhemolysis in sickle cell disease. Transfus Clin Biol 26:94–98
51. Williams LA 3rd, Lorenz RG, Tahir A, Pham HP, Marques MB (2016) High percentage of evanescent red cell antibodies in patients with sickle cell disease highlights need for a National Antibody Database. South Med J 109:588–591
52. Vidler JB, Gardner K, Amenyah K, Mijovic A, Thein SL (2015) Delayed haemolytic transfusion reaction in adults with sickle cell disease: a 5-year experience. Br J Haematol 169:746–753
53. Narbey D, Habibi A, Chadebech P, Mekontso-Dessap A, Khellaf M, Lelievre JD, Godeau B, Michel M, Galacteros F, Djoudi R, Bartolucci P, Pirenne F (2017) Incidence and predictive score for delayed hemolytic transfusion reaction in adult patients with sickle cell disease. Am J Hematol 92:1340–1348
54. Falguiere C, Allali S, Khazem B, Kamdem A, Arnaud C, Belloy M, Guitton C, Odievre MH, Pertuisel S, Dumesnil C, Guillaumat C, Garrec N, Gauthier A, Mahe P, Soussan-Banini V, Le-Carrer L, Merlin E, David A, Pellegrino B, Paillard C, Brasme JF, Lagarde M, Pirenne F, Pondarre C (2023) Delayed hemolytic transfusion reaction in children with sickle cell disease: first 5-year retrospective study in mainland France. Haematologica 108:889–894
55. Thein SL, Pirenne F, Fasano RM, Habibi A, Bartolucci P, Chonat S, Hendrickson JE, Stowell SR (2020) Hemolytic transfusion reactions in sickle cell disease: underappreciated and potentially fatal. Haematologica 105:539–544
56. Ito S, Pandya A, Hauser RG, Krishnamurti L, Stites E, Tormey C, Krumholz HM, Hendrickson JE, Goshua G (2024) Decreasing alloimmunization-specific mortality in sickle cell disease in the United States: cost-effectiveness of a shared transfusion resource. Am J Hematol 99:570–576
57. Covington ML, Cone-Sullivan JK, Andrzejewski C, Lu W, Thomasson RR, O'Brien K, Brunker PAR, Stowell SR (2022) Unmasking delayed hemolytic transfusion reactions in patients with sickle-cell disease: challenges and opportunities for improvement. Transfusion 62:1662–1670
58. Chang DY, Wankier Z, Arthur CM, Stowell SR (2023) The ongoing challenge of RBC alloimmunization in the management of patients with sickle cell disease. Presse Med 52:104211
59. Karafin MS, Tan S, Tormey CA, Spencer BR, Hauser RG, Norris PJ, Roubinian NH, Wu Y, Triulzi DJ, Kleinman S, Gottschall JL, Hendrickson JE (2019) Prevalence and risk factors for RBC alloantibodies in blood donors in the recipient Epidemiology and Donor Evaluation study-III (REDS-III). Transfusion 59: 217–225

60. Chaplin H Jr, Cassell M (1962) The occasional fallibility of in vitro compatibility tests. Transfusion 2:375–384
61. Gupta GK, Balbuena-Merle R, Hendrickson JE, Tormey CA (2020) Immunohematologic aspects of alloimmunization and alloantibody detection: a focus on pregnancy and hemolytic disease of the fetus and newborn. Transfus Apher Sci 59:102946
62. Parker V, Tormey CA (2017) The direct Antiglobulin test: indications, interpretation, and pitfalls. Arch Pathol Lab Med 141:305–310
63. Pirenne F, Pondarre C (2023) Alloimmunization and hyperhemolysis in sickle cell disease. Hematology Am Soc Hematol Educ Program 2023:653–659
64. Balbuena-Merle R, Curtis SA, Devine L, Gibb DR, Karafin MS, Luckey CJ, Tormey CA, Siddon AJ, Roberts JD, Hendrickson JE (2019) Red blood cell alloimmunization is associated with lower expression of FcgammaR1 on monocyte subsets in patients with sickle cell disease. Transfusion 59:3219–3227
65. Lee LE, Beeler BW, Graham BC, Cap AP, Win N, Chen F (2020) Posttransfusion hyperhemolysis is arrested by targeting macrophage activation with novel use of Tocilizumab. Transfusion 60:30–35
66. Meenan J, Hall R, Badle S, Chatterjee B, Win N, Tsitsikas DA (2022) Tocilizumab in the management of posttransfusion hyperhemolysis syndrome in sickle cell disease: the experience so far. Transfusion 62:546–550
67. Menakuru SR, Priscu A, Dhillon V, Salih A (2022) Acute Hyperhemolysis syndrome in a patient with known sickle cell anemia refractory to steroids and IVIG treated with Tocilizumab and erythropoietin: a case report and review of literature. Hematol Rep 14:235–239
68. Chou ST, Hendrickson JE, Fasano RM (2023) Transfusion therapy for sickle cell disease: what's new? Blood Adv 7:2551–2553
69. Merle NS, Church SE, Fremeaux-Bacchi V, Roumenina LT (2015) Complement system part I - molecular mechanisms of activation and regulation. Front Immunol 6:262
70. Merle NS, Boudhabhay I, Leon J, Fremeaux-Bacchi V, Roumenina LT (2019) Complement activation during intravascular hemolysis: implication for sickle cell disease and hemolytic transfusion reactions. Transfus Clin Biol 26:116–124
71. Merle NS, Paule R, Leon J, Daugan M, Robe-Rybkine T, Poillerat V, Torset C, Fremeaux-Bacchi V, Dimitrov JD, Roumenina LT (2019) P-selectin drives complement attack on endothelium during intravascular hemolysis in TLR-4/heme-dependent manner. Proc Natl Acad Sci USA 116:6280–6285
72. Roumenina LT, Bartolucci P, Pirenne F (2019) The role of complement in post-transfusion hemolysis and Hyperhemolysis reaction. Transfus Med Rev 33:225–230
73. Dumas G, Habibi A, Onimus T, Merle JC, Razazi K, Mekontso Dessap A, Galacteros F, Michel M, Fremeaux Bacchi V, Noizat Pirenne F, Bartolucci P (2016) Eculizumab salvage therapy for delayed hemolysis transfusion reaction in sickle cell disease patients. Blood 127:1062–1064
74. Meuleman MS, Roumenina LT, Grunenwald A (2023) Complement involvement in sickle cell disease. Presse Med 52:104205
75. Roumenina LT, Chadebech P, Bodivit G, Vieira-Martins P, Grunenwald A, Boudhabhay I, Poillerat V, Pakdaman S, Kiger L, Jouard A, Audureau E, Pirenne F, Galacteros F, Fremeaux-Bacchi V, Bartolucci P (2020) Complement activation in sickle cell disease: dependence on cell density, hemolysis and modulation by hydroxyurea therapy. Am J Hematol 95:456–464
76. Wang RH, Phillips G, Medof ME, Mold C (1993) Activation of the alternative complement pathway by exposure of phosphatidylethanolamine and phosphatidylserine on erythrocytes from sickle cell disease patients. J Clin Invest 92:1326–1335
77. Ivy ZK, Belcher JD, Khasabova IA, Chen C, Juliette JP, Abdulla F, Ruan C, Allen K, Nguyen J, Rogness VM, Beckman JD, Khasabov SG, Gupta K, Taylor RP, Simone DA, Vercellotti GM (2023) Cold exposure induces vaso-occlusion and pain in sickle mice that depend on complement activation. Blood 142:1918–1927
78. Wilson WA, Thomas EJ, Sissons JG (1979) Complement activation in asymptomatic patients with sickle cell anaemia. Clin Exp Immunol 36:130–139
79. Chudwin DS, Papierniak C, Lint TF, Korenblit AD (1994) Activation of the alternative complement pathway by red blood cells from patients with sickle cell disease. Clin Immunol Immunopathol 71:199–202
80. Nolasco JG, Nolasco LH, Da Q, Cirlos S, Ruggeri ZM, Moake JL, Cruz MA (2018) Complement component C3 binds to the A3 domain of von Willebrand factor. TH Open 2: e338–e345
81. Vercellotti GM, Dalmasso AP, Schaid TR Jr, Nguyen J, Chen C, Ericson ME, Abdulla F,

Killeen T, Lindorfer MA, Taylor RP, Belcher JD (2018) Critical role of C5a in sickle cell disease. Am J Hematol:1–41

82. Chonat S, Jones JA, Patel SR, Zerra PE, Jeffers LA, Jajosky RP, Arthur CM, Koval M, Joiner CH, Archer DR, Stowell SR (2022) Complement drives acute chest syndrome in a model of sickle cell disease. Blood 140: 8221–8222
83. Chonat S, Jones JA, Patel SR, Briones WM, Schoettler ML, Maarouf M, Jeffers LA, Adisa O, Tan F, Fields E, Sterling MS, Jajosky RP, Verkerke H, Graciaa SH, Foppiani EM, Fasano RM, Zerra PE, Qiu Y, Arthur CM, Lam WA, Ofori-Acquah SF, Koval M, Joiner CH, Archer DR, Stowell SR (2025) Complement is activated in patients with acute chest syndrome caused by sickle cell disease and represents a therapeutic target. Sci Transl Med 17:eadl4922
84. Chonat S, Graciaa S, Shin HS, Newton JG, Quarmyne MO, Boudreaux J, Tang A, Zerra PE, Rollins MR, Josephson CD, Brown C, Joiner CH, Fasano RM, Stowell SR (2020) Eculizumab for complement mediated thrombotic microangiopathy in sickle cell disease. Haematologica 105:2887–2891
85. Chonat S, Quarmyne MO, Bennett CM, Dean CL, Joiner CH, Fasano RM, Stowell SR (2018) Contribution of alternative complement pathway to delayed hemolytic transfusion reaction in sickle cell disease. Haematologica 103:e483–e485
86. Han Y, Gao C, Liu Y, Zhang H, Wang S, Zhao H, Bao W, Guo X, Vinchi F, Lobo C, Shi P, Mendelson A, Luchsinger L, Zhong H, Yazdanbakhsh K, An X (2024) Hemolysis-driven IFNalpha production impairs erythropoiesis by negatively regulating EPO signaling in sickle cell disease. Blood 143:1018–1031
87. Campbell-Lee SA, Kittles RA (2014) Red blood cell alloimmunization in sickle cell disease: listen to your ancestors. Transfus Med Hemother 41:431–435
88. Fasano RM, Meyer EK, Branscomb J, White MS, Gibson RW, Eckman JR (2019) Impact of red blood cell antigen matching on alloimmunization and transfusion complications in patients with sickle cell disease: a systematic review. Transfus Med Rev 33:12–23
89. Fasano RM, Booth GS, Miles M, Du L, Koyama T, Meier ER, Luban NL (2015) Red blood cell alloimmunization is influenced by recipient inflammatory state at time of transfusion in patients with sickle cell disease. Br J Haematol 168:291–300
90. Zheng Y, Gossett JM, Chen PL, Barton M, Ryan M, Yu J, Kang G, Hankins JS, Chou ST (2023) Proinflammatory state promotes red blood cell alloimmunization in pediatric patients with sickle cell disease. Blood Adv 7: 4799–4808
91. Wang L, Xu X, Wang S, Li R, Zhang P (2025) Red blood cell alloimmunization in transfused patients with myelodysplastic syndromes: a retrospective study from northern China. Lab Med 56:22–30
92. Sanz C, Nomdedeu M, Belkaid M, Martinez I, Nomdedeu B, Pereira A (2013) Red blood cell alloimmunization in transfused patients with myelodysplastic syndrome or chronic myelomonocytic leukemia. Transfusion 53:710–715
93. D. Singhal, Kutyna MM, Chhetri R, Wee LYA, Hague S, Nath L, Nath SV, Sinha R, Wickham N, Lewis ID, Ross DM, Bardy PG, L. B. To, Reynolds J, Wood EM, Roxby DJ, Hiwase DK (2017) Red cell alloimmunization is associated with development of autoantibodies and increased red cell transfusion requirements in myelodysplastic syndrome. Haematologica 102:2021–2029
94. Ryder AB, Hendrickson JE, Tormey CA (2016) Chronic inflammatory autoimmune disorders are a risk factor for red blood cell alloimmunization. Br J Haematol 174:483–485
95. Karafin MS, Westlake M, Hauser RG, Tormey CA, Norris PJ, Roubinian NH, Wu Y, Triulzi DJ, Kleinman S, Hendrickson JE, Epidemiology NR, Donor Evaluation S III (2018) Risk factors for red blood cell alloimmunization in the recipient epidemiology and donor evaluation study (REDS-III) database. Br J Haematol 181:672–681
96. Platt OS, Brambilla DJ, Rosse WF, Milner PF, Castro O, Steinberg MH, Klug PP (1994) Mortality in sickle cell disease. Life expectancy and risk factors for early death. N Engl J Med 330:1639–1644
97. Elmariah H, Garrett ME, De Castro LM, Jonassaint JC, Ataga KI, Eckman JR, Ashley-Koch AE, Telen MJ (2014) Factors associated with survival in a contemporary adult sickle cell disease cohort. Am J Hematol 89:530–535
98. Gaston MH, Verter JI, Woods G, Pegelow C, Kelleher J, Presbury G, Zarkowsky H, Vichinsky E, Iyer R, Lobel JS et al (1986) Prophylaxis with oral penicillin in children with sickle cell anemia. A randomized trial. N Engl J Med 314:1593–1599
99. Taher AT, Saliba AN (2017) Iron overload in thalassemia: different organs at different rates. Hematology Am Soc Hematol Educ Program 2017:265–271

100. Adams RJ, McKie VC, Hsu L, Files B, Vichinsky E, Pegelow C, Abboud M, Gallagher D, Kutlar A, Nichols FT, Bonds DR, Brambilla D (1998) Prevention of a first stroke by transfusions in children with sickle cell anemia and abnormal results on transcranial Doppler ultrasonography. N Engl J Med 339:5–11
101. Vichinsky EP, Earles A, Johnson RA, Hoag MS, Williams A, Lubin B (1990) Alloimmunization in sickle cell anemia and transfusion of racially unmatched blood. N Engl J Med 322:1617–1621
102. Chou ST, Jackson T, Vege S, Smith-Whitley-K, Friedman DF, Westhoff CM (2013) High prevalence of red blood cell alloimmunization in sickle cell disease despite transfusion from Rh-matched minority donors. Blood 122: 1062–1071
103. Gerritsma J, Bongaerts V, Eckhardt C, Heijboer H, Nur E, Biemond B, van der Schoot E, Fijnvandraat K, Consortium S (2022) Extended phenotyping does not preclude the occurrence of delayed haemolytic transfusion reactions in sickle cell disease. Br J Haematol 196:769–776
104. Kacker S, Ness PM, Savage WJ, Frick KD, Shirey RS, King KE, Tobian AA (2014) Cost-effectiveness of prospective red blood cell antigen matching to prevent alloimmunization among sickle cell patients. Transfusion 54:86–97
105. Higgins JM, Sloan SR (2008) Stochastic modeling of human RBC alloimmunization: evidence for a distinct population of immunologic responders. Blood 112:2546–2553
106. Zimring JC, Welniak L, Semple JW, Ness PM, Slichter SJ, Spitalnik SL, N. A. W. Group (2011) Current problems and future directions of transfusion-induced alloimmunization: summary of an NHLBI working group. Transfusion 51:435–441
107. van de Weem RHG, Wemelsfelder ML, Luken JS, de Haas M, Niessen R, van der Schoot CE, Hoogeveen H, Janssen MP (2022) Preventing alloimmunization using a new model for matching extensively typed red blood cells. Vox Sang 117:580–586
108. van Sambeeck JHJ, van der Schoot CE, van Dijk NM, Schonewille H, Janssen MP (2022) Extended red blood cell matching for all transfusion recipients is feasible. Transfus Med 32:221–228
109. Joshi SR, Senjaliya SB, Srivastava K, Flegel WA (2020) A resource-conserving serologic and highthroughput molecular approach to screen for blood donors with an IN:-5 phenotype. Immunohematology 36:129–132
110. Carter JH, Flegel WA (2019) Red cell transfusions in the genomics era. Semin Hematol 56:236–240
111. Lane WJ, Westhoff CM, Gleadall NS, Aguad M, Smeland-Wagman R, Vege S, Simmons DP, Mah HH, Lebo MS, Walter K, Soranzo N, Di Angelantonio E, Danesh J, Roberts DJ, Watkins NA, Ouwehand WH, Butterworth AS, Kaufman RM, Rehm HL, Silberstein LE, Green RC, P. MedSeq (2018) Automated typing of red blood cell and platelet antigens: a whole-genome sequencing study. Lancet Haematol 5:e241-e251
112. Lane WJ, Vege S, Mah HH, Lomas-Francis C, Aguad M, Smeland-Wagman R, Koch C, Killian JM, Gardner CL, De Castro M, Lebo MS, Kaufman RM, Green RC, Westhoff CM, MilSeq P (2019) Automated typing of red blood cell and platelet antigens from whole exome sequences. Transfusion 59:3253–3263
113. Montpetit A, Phillips MS, Mongrain I, Lemieux R, St-Louis M (2006) High-throughput molecular profiling of blood donors for minor red blood cell and platelet antigens. Transfusion 46:841–848
114. Veldhuisen B, van der Schoot CE, de Haas M (2009) Blood group genotyping: from patient to high-throughput donor screening. Vox Sang 97:198–206
115. Joseph A, Murray CJ, Novikov ND, Velliquette RW, Vege S, Halls JBL, Mah HH, Dellagatta JL, Comeau E, Aguad M, Kaufman RM, Olsson ML, Guleria I, Stowell SR, Milford EL, Hult AK, Yeung MY, Westhoff CM, Murphey CL, Lane WJ (2023) ABO genotyping finds more a (2) to B kidney transplant opportunities than lectin-based subtyping. Am J Transplant 23:512–519
116. Evers D, van der Bom JG, Tijmensen J, Middelburg RA, de Haas M, Zalpuri S, de Vooght KM, van de Kerkhof D, Visser O, Pequeriaux NC, Hudig F, Zwaginga JJ (2016) Red cell alloimmunisation in patients with different types of infections. Br J Haematol 175:956–966
117. Hendrickson JE, Tormey CA (2016) Understanding red blood cell alloimmunization triggers. Hematology Am Soc Hematol Educ Program 2016:446–451
118. Yazdanbakhsh K (2016) Immunoregulatory networks in sickle cell alloimmunization. Hematology Am Soc Hematol Educ Program 2016:457–461
119. Doshi BS, Rana J, Castaman G, Shaheen MA, Kaczmarek R, Butterfield JS, Meeks SL, Leissinger C, Biswas M, Arruda VR (2021) B cell-activating factor modulates the factor

VIII immune response in hemophilia a. J Clin Invest 131

120. Kaczmarek R, Pineros AR, Patterson PE, Bertolini TB, Perrin GQ, Sherman A, Born J, Arisa S, Arvin MC, Kamocka MM, Martinez MM, Dunn KW, Quinn SM, Morris JJ, Wilhelm AR, Kaisho T, Munoz-Melero M, Biswas M, Kaplan MH, Linnemann AK, George LA, Camire RM, Herzog RW (2023) Factor VIII trafficking to CD4+ T cells shapes its immunogenicity and requires several types of antigen-presenting cells. Blood 142:290–305

121. Zerra PE, Arthur CM, Chonat S, Maier CL, Mener A, Shin S, Allen JWL, Baldwin WH, Cox C, Verkerke H, Jajosky RP, Tormey CA, Meeks SL, Stowell SR (2020) Fc gamma receptors and complement component 3 facilitate anti-fVIII antibody formation. Front Immunol 11:905

122. Khelfa M, Leclerc M, Kerbrat S, Boudjemai YNS, Benchouaia M, Neyrinck-Leglantier D, Cagnet L, Berradhia L, Tamagne M, Croisille L, Pirenne F, Maury S, Vingert B (2023) Divergent CD4 (+) T-cell profiles are associated with anti-HLA alloimmunization status in platelet-transfused AML patients. Front Immunol 14:1165973

123. Meeks SL, Batsuli G (2016) Hemophilia and inhibitors: current treatment options and potential new therapeutic approaches. Hematology Am Soc Hematol Educ Program 2016: 657–662

124. Brantley SG, Ramsey G (1988) Red cell alloimmunization in multitransfused HLA-typed patients. Transfusion 28:463–466

125. Meinderts SM, Sins JWR, Fijnvandraat K, Nagelkerke SQ, Geissler J, Tanck MW, Bruggeman C, Biemond BJ, Rijneveld AW, Kerkhoffs JH, Pakdaman S, Habibi A, van Bruggen R, Kuijpers TW, Pirenne F, van den Berg TK (2017) Nonclassical FCGR2C haplotype is associated with protection from red blood cell alloimmunization in sickle cell disease. Blood 130:2121–2130

126. Sippert EA, Visentainer JE, Alves HV, Rodrigues C, Gilli SC, Addas-Carvalho M, Saad ST, Costa FF, Castilho L (2017) Red blood cell alloimmunization in patients with sickle cell disease: correlation with HLA and cytokine gene polymorphisms. Transfusion 57:379–389

127. Noizat-Pirenne F, Tournamille C, Bierling P, Roudot-Thoraval F, Le Pennec PY, Rouger P, Ansart-Pirenne H (2006) Relative immunogenicity of Fya and K antigens in a Caucasian population, based on HLA class II restriction analysis. Transfusion 46:1328–1333

128. Meinderts SM, Gerritsma JJ, Sins JWR, de Boer M, van Leeuwen K, Biemond BJ, Rijneveld AW, Kerkhoffs JH, Habibi A, van Bruggen R, Kuijpers TW, van der Schoot E, Pirenne F, Fijnvandraat K, Tanck MW, van den Berg TK (2019) Identification of genetic biomarkers for alloimmunization in sickle cell disease. Br J Haematol 186:887–899

129. Gerritsma JJ, Oomen I, Meinderts S, van der Schoot CE, Biemond BJ, van der Bom JG, Fijnvandraat K, S. consortium (2021) Back to base pairs: what is the genetic risk for red bloodcell alloimmunization? Blood Rev 48: 100794

130. Madany E, Lee J, Halprin C, Seo J, Baca N, Majlessipour F, Hendrickson JE, Pepkowitz SH, Hayes C, Klapper E, Gibb DR (2021) Altered type 1 interferon responses in alloimmunized and nonalloimmunized patients with sickle cell disease. EJHaem 2:700–710

131. Soldatenko A, Hoyt LR, Xu L, Calabro S, Lewis SM, Gallman AE, Hudson KE, Stowell SR, Luckey CJ, Zimring JC, Liu D, Santhanakrishnan M, Hendrickson JE, Eisenbarth SC (2022) Innate and adaptive immunity to transfused allogeneic RBCs in mice requires MyD88. J Immunol 208:991–997

132. Thomas TA, Qiu A, Kim CY, Gordy DE, Miller A, Tredicine M, Dzieciatkowska M, Dei Zotti F, Hod EA, D'Alessandro A, Zimring JC, Spitalnik SL, Hudson KE (2023) Reticulocytes in donor blood units enhance red blood cell alloimmunization. Haematologica 108:2639–2651

133. D'Alessandro A, Keele GR, Hay A, Nemkov T, Earley EJ, Stephenson D, Vincent M, Deng X, Stone M, Dzieciatkowska M, Hansen KC, Kleinman S, Spitalnik SL, Roubinian N, Norris PJ, Busch MP, Page GP, Stockwell BR, Churchill GA, Zimring JC (2025) Ferroptosis regulates hemolysis in stored murine and human red blood cells. Blood 145:765–783

134. Zimring JC, Hay AM, Dzieciatkowska M, D'Alessandro A (2024) Molecular communication between red blood cells of different phenotypes during blood storage in mice. Transfusion 64:1762–1771

135. Nemkov T, Key A, Stephenson D, Earley EJ, Keele GR, Hay A, Amireault P, Casimir M, Dussiot M, Dzieciatkowska M, Reisz JA, Deng X, Stone M, Kleinman S, Spitalnik SL, Hansen KC, Norris PJ, Churchill GA, Busch MP, Roubinian N, Page GP, Zimring JC, Arduini A, D'Alessandro A (2024) Genetic

regulation of carnitine metabolism controls lipid damage repair and aging RBC hemolysis in vivo and in vitro. Blood 143:2517–2533

136. Nemkov T, Stephenson D, Erickson C, Dzieciatkowska M, Key A, Moore A, Earley EJ, Page GP, Lacroix IS, Stone M, Deng X, Raife T, Kleinman S, Zimring JC, Roubinian N, Hansen KC, Busch MP, Norris PJ, D'Alessandro A (2024) Regulation of kynurenine metabolism by blood donor genetics and biology impacts red cell hemolysis in vitro and in vivo. Blood 143:456–472
137. Balbuena-Merle R, Santhanakrishnan M, Devine L, Gibb DR, Tormey CA, Siddon AJ, Curtis SA, Gallagher PG, Weinstein JS, Hendrickson JE (2020) Characterization of circulating and cultured Tfh-like cells in sickle cell disease in relation to red blood cell alloimmunization status. Transfus Apher Sci 59: 102778
138. Tamagne M, Pakdaman S, Bartolucci P, Habibi A, Galacteros F, Pirenne F, Vingert B (2021) Whole-blood CCR7 expression and chemoattraction in red blood cell alloimmunization. Br J Haematol 194:477–481
139. Tamagne M, Pakdaman S, Bartolucci P, Habibi A, Galacteros F, Pirenne F, Vingert B (2021) Whole-blood phenotyping to assess alloimmunization status in transfused sickle cell disease patients. Blood Adv 5:1278–1282
140. Vingert B, Tamagne M, Habibi A, Pakdaman S, Ripa J, Elayeb R, Galacteros F, Bierling P, Ansart-Pirenne H, Bartolucci P, Noizat-Pirenne F (2015) Phenotypic differences of CD4 (+) T cells in response to red blood cell immunization in transfused sickle cell disease patients. Eur J Immunol 45: 1868–1879
141. Bao W, Zhong H, Li X, Lee MT, Schwartz J, Sheth S, Yazdanbakhsh K (2011) Immune regulation in chronically transfused Allo-antibody responder and nonresponder patients with sickle cell disease and beta-thalassemia major. Am J Hematol 86:1001–1006
142. Liu Y, Su S, Shayo S, Bao W, Pal M, Dou K, Shi PA, Aygun B, Campbell-Lee S, Lobo CA, Mendelson A, An X, Manwani D, Zhong H, Yazdanbakhsh K (2023) Hemolysis dictates monocyte differentiation via two distinct pathways in sickle cell disease vaso-occlusion. J Clin Invest 133
143. Pal M, Bao W, Wang R, Liu Y, An X, Mitchell WB, Lobo CA, Minniti C, Shi PA, Manwani D, Yazdanbakhsh K, Zhong H (2021) Hemolysis inhibits humoral B-cell responses and modulates alloimmunization risk in patients with sickle cell disease. Blood 137:269–280
144. Godefroy E, Zhong H, Pham P, Friedman D, Yazdanbakhsh K (2015) TIGIT-positive circulating follicular helper T cells display robust B-cell help functions: potential role in sickle cell alloimmunization. Haematologica 100: 1415–1425
145. Godefroy E, Liu Y, Shi P, Mitchell WB, Cohen D, Chou ST, Manwani D, Yazdanbakhsh K (2016) Altered heme-mediated modulation of dendritic cell function in sickle cell alloimmunization. Haematologica 101: 1028–1038
146. Zhong H, Bao W, Friedman D, Yazdanbakhsh K (2014) Hemin controls T cell polarization in sickle cell alloimmunization. J Immunol 193:102–110
147. Bao W, Yu J, Heck S, Yazdanbakhsh K (2009) Regulatory T-cell status in red cell alloimmunized responder and nonresponder mice. Blood 113:5624–5627
148. Yu J, Heck S, Yazdanbakhsh K (2007) Prevention of red cell alloimmunization by CD25 regulatory T cells in mouse models. Am J Hematol 82:691–696
149. Bao W, Zhong H, Manwani D, Vasovic L, Uehlinger J, Lee MT, Sheth S, Shi P, Yazdanbakhsh K (2013) Regulatory B-cell compartment in transfused alloimmunized and non-alloimmunized patients with sickle cell disease. Am J Hematol 88:736–740
150. Nakahara H, Cheedarla N, Verkerke HP, Cheedarla S, Wu SC, Hendrickson JE, Chang A, McLemore ML, El Rassi F, Roback JD, Neish AS, Fasano RM, Stowell SR (2023) Enhanced IgG immune response to COVID-19 vaccination in patients with sickle cell disease. Br J Haematol 202:937–941
151. Arthur CM, Zerra PE, Shin S, Wang J, Song X, Doering CB, Lollar P, Meeks S, Stowell SR (2022) Nonhuman glycans can regulate anti-factor VIII antibody formation in mice. Blood 139:1312–1317
152. Sharathkumar A, Lillicrap D, Blanchette VS, Kern M, Leggo J, Stain AM, Brooker L, Carcao MD (2003) Intensive exposure to factor VIII is a risk factor for inhibitor development in mild hemophilia a. J Thromb Haemost 1: 1228–1236
153. Eckhardt CL, van der Bom JG, van der Naald M, Peters M, Kamphuisen PW, Fijnvandraat K (2011) Surgery and inhibitor development in hemophilia a: a systematic review. J Thromb Haemost 9:1948–1958
154. Forest SK, Hod EA (2016) Management of the Platelet Refractory Patient. Hematol Oncol Clin North Am 30:665–677

155. Hod E, Schwartz J (2008) Platelet transfusion refractoriness. Br J Haematol 142:348–360
156. Arthur CM, Patel SR, Sullivan HC, Winkler AM, Tormey CA, Hendrickson JE, Stowell SR (2016) CD8+ T cells mediate antibody-independent platelet clearance in mice. Blood 127:1823–1827
157. Lewis SM, Williams A, Eisenbarth SC (2019) Structure and function of the immune system in the spleen. Sci Immunol 4
158. Mann ER, Bernardo D, English NR, Landy J, Al-Hassi HO, Peake ST, Man R, Elliott TR, Spranger H, Lee GH, Parian A, Brant SR, Lazarev M, Hart AL, Li X, Knight SC (2016) Compartment-specific immunity in the human gut: properties and functions of dendritic cells in the colon versus the ileum. Gut 65:256–270
159. Klemm A, Tschernig T, Krug N, Pabst R (1998) Lymphocyte subsets in distinct lung compartments show a different ability to produce interferon-gamma (IFN-gamma) during a pulmonary immune response. Clin Exp Immunol 113:252–257
160. Mebius RE, Kraal G (2005) Structure and function of the spleen. Nat Rev Immunol 5: 606–616
161. Attanavanich K, Kearney JF (2004) Marginal zone, but not follicular B cells, are potent activators of naive CD4 T cells. J Immunol 172:803–811
162. Cerutti A, Cols M, Puga I (2013) Marginal zone B cells: virtues of innate-like antibody-producing lymphocytes. Nat Rev Immunol 13:118–132
163. Qiang Y, Sissoko A, Liu ZL, Dong T, Zheng F, Kong F, Higgins JM, Karniadakis GE, Buffet PA, Suresh S, Dao M (2023) Microfluidic study of retention and elimination of abnormal red blood cells by human spleen with implications for sickle cell disease. Proc Natl Acad Sci USA 120:e2217607120
164. Goyal G, Prabhala P, Mahajan G, Bausk B, Gilboa T, Xie L, Zhai Y, Lazarovits R, Mansour A, Kim MS, Patil A, Curran D, Long JM, Sharma S, Junaid A, Cohen L, Ferrante TC, Levy O, Prantil-Baun R, Walt DR, Ingber DE (2022) Ectopic lymphoid follicle formation and human seasonal influenza vaccination responses recapitulated in an organ-on-a-Chip. Adv Sci (Weinh) 9:e2103241
165. Doctor A, Spinella P (2012) Effect of processing and storage on red blood cell function in vivo. Semin Perinatol 36:248–259
166. Hod EA, Arinsburg SA, Francis RO, Hendrickson JE, Zimring JC, Spitalnik SL (2010) Use of mouse models to study the mechanisms and consequences of RBC clearance. Vox Sang 99:99–111
167. Hod EA, Zimring JC, Spitalnik SL (2008) Lessons learned from mouse models of hemolytic transfusion reactions. Curr Opin Hematol 15:601–605
168. Roback JD, Su L, Zimring JC, Hillyer CD (2007) Transfusion-transmitted cytomegalovirus: lessons from a murine model. Transfus Med Rev 21:26–36
169. Hughes-Jones NC, Gardner B (2002) Red cell agglutination: the first description by Creite (1869) and further observations made by Landois (1875) and Landsteiner (1901). Br J Haematol 119:889–893
170. Vandiedonck C, Knight JC (2009) The human major histocompatibility complex as a paradigm in genomics research. Brief Funct Genomic Proteomic 8:379–394
171. Zinkernagel RM, Doherty PC (1974) Restriction of in vitro T cell-mediated cytotoxicity in lymphocytic choriomeningitis within a syngeneic or semiallogeneic system. Nature 248:701–702
172. Aster RH, Jandl JH (1964) Platelet Sequestration in Man. I Methods. J Clin Invest 43: 843–855
173. Aster RH, Jandl JH (1964) Platelet sequestration in Man. Ii. immunological and clinical studies. J Clin Invest 43:856–869
174. Patel R, Terasaki PI (1969) Significance of the positive crossmatch test in kidney transplantation. N Engl J Med 280:735–739
175. Li Q, Marcoux G, Hu Y, Rebetz J, Guo L, Semple E, Provan D, Xu S, Hou M, Peng J, Semple JW (2024) Autoimmune effector mechanisms associated with a defective immunosuppressive axis in immune thrombocytopenia (ITP). Autoimmun Rev 23:103677
176. Johansson K, Maouia A, Rebetz J, Marcoux G, Shannon O, Italiano JE Jr, Narayanan P, Henry S, Shen L, Semple JW (2024) CpG oligonucleotides induce acute murine thrombocytopenia dependent on toll-like receptor 9 and spleen tyrosine kinase pathways. J Thromb Haemost 22:3266–3276
177. Yazdanbakhsh K, Provan D, Semple JW (2023) The role of T cells and myeloid-derived suppressor cells in refractory immune thrombocytopenia. Br J Haematol 203:54–61
178. Kapur R, Semple JW (2023) Binge-reading on immune thrombocytopenia: everything you ever wanted to know. Br J Haematol 201:811–812

179. Semple JW (2010) Animal models of immune thrombocytopenia (ITP). Ann Hematol 89 (Suppl 1):37–44
180. Xu XR, Zhang D, Oswald BE, Carrim N, Wang X, Hou Y, Zhang Q, Lavalle C, McKeown T, Marshall AH, Ni H (2016) Platelets are versatile cells: New discoveries in hemostasis, thrombosis, immune responses, tumor metastasis and beyond. Crit Rev Clin Lab Sci 53:409–430
181. Semple JW, Italiano JE Jr, Freedman J (2011) Platelets and the immune continuum. Nat Rev Immunol 11:264–274
182. Schoenaker JM, Nelson VS, Henderickx JGE, Terveer EM, Jansen AJG, Porcelijn L, Netelenbos T, Schipperus MR, Kapur R (2025) The intestinal flora: the key to unraveling heterogeneity in immune thrombocytopenia? Blood Rev 69:101252
183. Li C, Li J, Li Y, Lang S, Yougbare I, Zhu G, Chen P, Ni H (2012) Crosstalk between platelets and the immune system: old systems with New discoveries. Adv Hematol 2012: 2012, 384685
184. Gil Gonzalez L, Won KD, Tawhidi Z, Cummins E, Cruz-Leal Y, Tundidor Cabado Y, Sachs UJ, Norris PAA, Shan Y, Bhakta V, Li J, Samudio I, Silva-Moreno B, Cerna-Portillo L, Pavon Oro A, Bergqvist P, Chan P, Moorehead A, Sholzberg M, Sheffield WP, Lazarus AH (2024) Human fc gamma receptor IIIA blockade inhibits platelet destruction in a humanized murine model of ITP. Blood Adv 8:1869–1879
185. Khan R, Menard M, Jen CC, Chen X, Norris PAA, Lazarus AH (2020) Inhibition of platelet phagocytosis as an in vitro predictor for therapeutic potential of RBC antibodies in murine ITP. Blood 135:2420–2424
186. Yougbare I, Tai WS, Zdravic D, Oswald BE, Lang S, Zhu G, Leong-Poi H, Qu D, Yu L, Dunk C, Zhang J, Sled JG, Lye SJ, Brkic J, Peng C, Hoglund P, Croy BA, Adamson SL, Wen XY, Stewart DJ, Freedman J, Ni H (2017) Activated NK cells cause placental dysfunction and miscarriages in fetal alloimmune thrombocytopenia. Nat Commun 8:224
187. Vadasz B, Chen P, Yougbare I, Zdravic D, Li J, Li C, Carrim N, Ni H (2015) Platelets and platelet alloantigens: lessons from human patients and animal models of fetal and neonatal alloimmune thrombocytopenia. Genes Dis 2:173–185
188. Li C, Chen P, Vadasz B, Ma L, Zhou H, Lang S, Freedman J, Ni H (2013) Co-stimulation with LPS or Poly I:C markedly enhances the anti-platelet immune response and severity of fetal and neonatal alloimmune thrombocytopenia. Thromb Haemost 110:1250–1258
189. Zhang N, Zhi H, Curtis BR, Rao S, Jobaliya C, Poncz M, French DL, Newman PJ (2016) CRISPR/Cas9-mediated conversion of human platelet alloantigen allotypes. Blood 127:675–680
190. Newman DK, Newman PJ (2024) Antigen-specific immunotherapy for platelet alloimmune disorders. Hum Immunol 85:111172
191. Youssef AR, Shen CR, Lin CL, Barker RN, Elson CJ (2005) IL-4 and IL-10 modulate autoimmune haemolytic anaemia in NZB mice. Clin Exp Immunol 139:84–89
192. Howie HL, Hudson KE (2018) Murine models of autoimmune hemolytic anemia. Curr Opin Hematol 25:473–481
193. Hudson KE, Hendrickson JE, Cadwell CM, Iwakoshi NN, Zimring JC (2012) Partial tolerance of autoreactive B and T cells to erythrocyte-specific self-antigens in mice. Haematologica 97:1836–1844
194. Richards AL, Kapp LM, Wang X, Howie HL, Hudson KE (2016) Regulatory T cells are dispensable for tolerance to RBC antigens. Front Immunol 7:348
195. Wong ASL, Gruber DR, Richards AL, Sheldon K, Qiu A, Hay A, Hudson KE (2020) Tolerization of recent thymic emigrants is required to prevent RBC-specific autoimmunity. J Autoimmun 114:102489
196. Richards AL, Qiu A, Zotti FD, Sheldon K, Usaneerungrueng C, Gruber DR, Hudson KE (2021) Autoantigen presentation by splenic dendritic cells is required for RBC-specific autoimmunity. Transfusion 61: 225–235
197. Dei Zotti F, Qiu A, La Carpia F, Moriconi C, Hudson KE (2021) A New murine model of primary autoimmune hemolytic anemia (AIHA). Front Immunol 12:752330
198. Dei Zotti F, Qiu A, D'Agati VD, Jagnarine S, Kyritsis E, Miller A, Tredicine M, Fliginger D, Stone EF, Panch S, Hudson KE (2024) Mitigation of checkpoint inhibitor-induced autoimmune hemolytic anemia through modulation of purinergic signaling. Blood 144:1581–1594
199. Zhu W, Zheng Y, Yu M, Witman N, Zhou L, Wei J, Zhang Y, Topchyan P, Nguyen C, Wang D, Janecke R, Padmanabhan A, Baumann Kreuziger L, White GC, Hari P, Gu T, Fields AT, Kornblith L, Aster RH, Zhu J, Cui W, Jobe SM, Graham MB, Wang D, Wen R (2024) Prothrombotic antibodies targeting the spike protein's receptor-binding

domain in severe COVID-19. Blood 145: 635–647

200. Zhu W, Zheng Y, Yu M, Wu Y, Wei J, Zhou L, Fu G, Schneider N, Jones C, Irani M, Padmanabhan A, Aster R, Wang D, Wen R (2023) Cloned antibodies from patients with HIT provide new clues to HIT pathogenesis. Blood 141:1060–1069
201. Kanack AJ, Bayas A, George G, Abou-Ismail MY, Singh B, Kohlhagen MC, Splinter NP, Christ M, Naumann M, Moser KA, Smock KJ, Grazioli A, Wen R, Wang D, Murray DL, Padmanabhan A (2022) Monoclonal and oligoclonal anti-platelet factor 4 antibodies mediate VITT. Blood 140:73–77
202. Zheng Y, Zhu W, Haribhai D, Williams CB, Aster RH, Wen R, Wang D (2019) Regulatory T cells control PF4/heparin antibody production in mice. J Immunol 203:1786–1792
203. Padmanabhan A, Jones CG, Curtis BR, Bougie DW, Sullivan MJ, Peswani N, McFarland JG, Eastwood D, Wang D, Aster RH (2016) A novel PF4-dependent platelet activation assay identifies patients likely to have heparin-induced thrombocytopenia/thrombosis. Chest 150:506–515
204. Zheng Y, Yu M, Padmanabhan A, Aster RH, Yuan L, Wen R, Wang D (2015) Critical role of CD4 T cells in PF4/heparin antibody production in mice. Blood 125:1826–1829
205. Zheng Y, Wang AW, Yu M, Padmanabhan A, Tourdot BE, Newman DK, White GC, Aster RH, Wen R, Wang D (2014) B-cell tolerance regulates production of antibodies causing heparin-induced thrombocytopenia. Blood 123:931–934
206. Zheng Y, Yu M, Podd A, Yuan L, Newman DK, Wen R, Arepally G, Wang D (2013) Critical role for mouse marginal zone B cells in PF4/heparin antibody production. Blood 121:3484–3492
207. Padmanabhan A, Jones CG, Bougie DW, Curtis BR, McFarland JG, Wang D, Aster RH (2015) Heparin-independent, PF4-dependent binding of HIT antibodies to platelets: implications for HIT pathogenesis. Blood 125:155–161
208. Maier CL, Nakahara H, Barker NA, Auld SC, Truong AD, Friend S, Caridi-Scheible M, Connor M, Gaddh M, Cobb J, Polly DM, Guarner J, Powell C, Kempton CL, Daniels L, Wynn AT, Sniecinski R, Duncan A, Roback J, Masud T, Conlon S, Wade J, Wong A, Verkerke H, Zerra PE, Butler H, Sullivan HC, Easley KA, Josephson CD, Stowell SR (2025) Therapeutic plasma exchange for fibrinogen-associated hyperviscosity: results of the COVID-19 PLasma EXchange (COPLEX) randomized controlled trial. J Thromb Haemost 23: 1393–1400
209. van der Velden S, van Osch TLJ, Seghier A, Bentlage AEH, Mok JY, Geerdes DM, van Esch WJE, Pouw RB, Brouwer MC, Jongerius I, de Haas M, Porcelijn L, van der Schoot CE, Vidarsson G, Kapur R (2024) Complement activation drives antibody-mediated transfusion-related acute lung injury via macrophage trafficking and formation of NETs. Blood 143:79–91
210. Cleary SJ, Seo Y, Tian JJ, Kwaan N, Bulkley DP, Bentlage AE, Vidarsson G, Boilard E, Spirig R, Zimring JC, Looney MR (2024) IgG hexamers initiate complement-dependent acute lung injury. J Clin Invest 134
211. Cleary SJ, Kwaan N, Tian JJ, Calabrese DR, Mallavia B, Magnen M, Greenland JR, Urisman A, Singer JP, Hays SR, Kukreja J, Hay AM, Howie HL, Toy P, Lowell CA, Morrell CN, Zimring JC, Looney MR (2020) Complement activation on endothelium initiates antibody-mediated acute lung injury. J Clin Invest 130:5909–5923
212. Ortiz-Munoz G, Looney MR (2015) Two-event transfusion-related acute lung injury mouse model. Bio Protoc 5
213. Caudrillier A, Kessenbrock K, Gilliss BM, Nguyen JX, Marques MB, Monestier M, Toy P, Werb Z, Looney MR (2012) Platelets induce neutrophil extracellular traps in transfusion-related acute lung injury. J Clin Invest 122:2661–2671
214. Looney MR, Nguyen JX, Hu Y, Van Ziffle JA, Lowell CA, Matthay MA (2009) Platelet depletion and aspirin treatment protect mice in a two-event model of transfusion-related acute lung injury. J Clin Invest 119:3450–3461
215. Silliman CC, Moore EE, Kelher MR, Khan SY, Gellar L, Elzi DJ (2011) Identification of lipids that accumulate during the routine storage of prestorage leukoreduced red blood cells and cause acute lung injury. Transfusion 51:2549–2554
216. Logdberg LE, Vikulina T, Zimring JC, Hillyer CD (2009) Animal models of transfusion-related acute lung injury. Transfus Med Rev 23:13–24
217. van Wonderen SF, Klanderman RB, Vlaar APJ (2022) Understanding transfusion-related acute lung injury (TRALI) and its complex pathophysiology. Blood Transfus 20:443–445

218. Shaz BH, Stowell SR, Hillyer CD (2011) Transfusion-related acute lung injury: from bedside to bench and back. Blood 117: 1463–1471
219. Hay A, Nemkov T, Gamboni F, Dzieciatkowska M, Key A, Galbraith M, Bartsch K, Sun K, Xia Y, Stone M, Busch MP, Norris PJ, Zimring JC, D'Alessandro A (2023) Sphingosine 1-phosphate has a negative effect on RBC storage quality. Blood Adv 7:1379–1393
220. Howie HL, Hay AM, de Wolski K, Waterman H, Lebedev J, Fu X, Culp-Hill R, D'Alessandro A, Gorham JD, Ranson MS, Roback JD, Thomson PC, Zimring JC (2019) Differences in Steap3 expression are a mechanism of genetic variation of RBC storage and oxidative damage in mice. Blood Adv 3:2272–2285
221. D'Alessandro A, Zimring JC (2025) From metabolomics to transfusion-associated immunomodulation. Curr Opin Immunol 96:102646
222. Dziewulska-Cronk KH, Reisz JA, Hay AM, Nemkov T, Cendali FI, Issaian A, Lamb DR, Palha MS, Legenzov EA, Kao JPY, Walker LA, Tekwani BL, Buehler PW, D'Alessandro A, Zimring JC (2024) Primaquine-5,6-Orthoquinone is directly hemolytic to older G6PD deficient RBCs in a humanized mouse model. J Pharmacol Exp Ther 391:119–129
223. D'Alessandro A, Anastasiadi AT, Tzounakas VL, Nemkov T, Reisz JA, Kriebardis AG, Zimring JC, Spitalnik SL, Busch MP (2023) Red blood cell metabolism in vivo and in vitro. Meta 13
224. Hay A, Dziewulska K, Gamboni F, Nerguizian D, Dzieciatkowska M, Zimring JC, D'Alessandro A (2023) Hypoxic storage of murine red blood cells improves energy metabolism and post-transfusion recoveries. Blood Transfus 21:50–61
225. D'Alessandro A, Howie HL, Hay AM, Dziewulska KH, Brown BC, Wither MJ, Karafin M, Stone EF, Spitalnik SL, Hod EA, Francis RO, Fu X, Thomas T, Zimring JC (2021) Hematologic and systemic metabolic alterations due to Mediterranean class II G6PD deficiency in mice. JCI Insight 6
226. Nemkov T, Sun K, Reisz JA, Song A, Yoshida T, Dunham A, Wither MJ, Francis RO, Roach RC, Dzieciatkowska M, Rogers SC, Doctor A, Kriebardis A, Antonelou M, Papassideri I, Young CT, Thomas TA, Hansen KC, Spitalnik SL, Xia Y, Zimring JC, Hod EA, D'Alessandro A (2018) Hypoxia modulates the purine salvage pathway and decreases red blood cell and supernatant levels of hypoxanthine during refrigerated storage. Haematologica 103:361–372
227. Zhang Z, Markmann C, Yu M, Agarwal D, Rostami S, Wang W, Liu C, Zhao H, Ochoa T, Parvathaneni K, Xu X, Li E, Gonzalez V, Khadka R, Hoffmann J, Knox JJ, Scholler J, Marcellus B, Allman D, Fraietta JA, Samelson-Jones B, Milone MC, Monos D, Garfall AL, Naji A, Bhoj VG (2023) Immunotherapy targeting B cells and long-lived plasma cells effectively eliminates pre-existing donor-specific Allo-antibodies. Cell Rep Med 4:101336
228. Webber AM, Bradstreet TR, Wang X, Guo H, Nelson CA, Fremont DH, Edelson BT, Liu C (2022) Antigen-guided depletion of anti-HLA antibody-producing cells by HLA-fc fusion proteins. Blood 140:1803–1815
229. Tang A, Mendelson A (2021) Recent lessons learned for ex-vivo platelet production. Curr Opin Hematol 28:424–430
230. Shah S, Huang X, Cheng L (2014) Concise review: stem cell-based approaches to red blood cell production for transfusion. Stem Cells Transl Med 3:346–355
231. Olivier E, Zhang S, Yan Z, Bouhassira EE (2024) Stem cell factor and erythropoietin-independent production of cultured reticulocytes. Haematologica 109:3705–3720
232. Gunawardena N, Chou ST (2024) Generation of red blood cells from induced pluripotent stem cells. Curr Opin Hematol 31:115–121
233. An HH, Gagne AL, Maguire JA, Pavani G, Abdulmalik O, Gadue P, French DL, Westhoff CM, Chou ST (2022) The use of pluripotent stem cells to generate diagnostic tools for transfusion medicine. Blood 140:1723–1734
234. Deng J, Lancelot M, Jajosky R, Deng Q, Deeb K, Saakadze N, Gao Y, Jaye D, Liu S, Stowell SR, Cheng L, Roback JD (2022) Erythropoietic properties of human induced pluripotent stem cells-derived red blood cells in immunodeficient mice. Am J Hematol 97: 194–202
235. Hegde S, Akbar H, Wellendorf AM, Nestheide S, Johnson JF, Zhao X, Setchell KD, Zheng Y, Cancelas JA (2024) Inhibition of RHOA activity preserves the survival and hemostasis function of long-term cold-stored platelets. Blood 144:1732–1746
236. Arthur CM, Nalbant D, Feldman HA, Saeedi BJ, Matthews J, Robinson BS, Kamili NA, Bennett A, Cress GA, Sola-Visner M, Jones RM, Zimmerman MB, Neish AS, Patel RM, Nopoulos P, Georgieff MK, Roback JD,

Widness JA, Josephson CD, Stowell SR (2019) Anemia induces gut inflammation and injury in an animal model of preterm infants. Transfusion 59:1233–1245

237. Wallin DJ, Tkac I, Stucker S, Ennis KM, Sola-Visner M, Rao R, Georgieff MK (2015) Phlebotomy-induced anemia alters hippocampal neurochemistry in neonatal mice. Pediatr Res 77:765–771

238. Davenport P, Sola-Visner M (2022) Immunologic effects of red blood cell and platelet transfusions in neonates. Curr Opin Hematol 29:297–305

239. Davenport P, Fan HH, Nolton E, Feldman HA, Lorenz V, Canas J, Acosta-Zaldivar M, Yakah W, Arthur C, Martin C, Stowell S, Koehler J, Mager D, Sola-Visner M (2022) Platelet transfusions in a murine model of neonatal polymicrobial sepsis: divergent effects on inflammation and mortality. Transfusion 62:1177–1187

240. Smith NH, Hod EA, Spitalnik SL, Zimring JC, Hendrickson JE (2012) Transfusion in the absence of inflammation induces antigen-specific tolerance to murine RBCs. Blood 119:1566–1569

241. Zimring JC, Hair GA, Chadwick TE, Deshpande SS, Anderson KM, Hillyer CD, Roback JD (2005) Nonhemolytic antibody-induced loss of erythrocyte surface antigen. Blood 106:1105–1112

242. Hod EA, Cadwell CM, Liepkalns JS, Zimring JC, Sokol SA, Schirmer DA, Jhang J, Spitalnik SL (2008) Cytokine storm in a mouse model of IgG-mediated hemolytic transfusion reactions. Blood 112:891–894

243. Desmarets M, Cadwell CM, Peterson KR, Neades R, Zimring JC (2009) Minor histocompatibility antigens on transfused leukoreduced units of red blood cells induce bone marrow transplant rejection in a mouse model. Blood 114:2315–2322

244. Auffray I, Marfatia S, de Jong K, Lee G, Huang CH, Paszty C, Tanner MJ, Mohandas N, Chasis JA (2001) Glycophorin a dimerization and band 3 interaction during erythroid membrane biogenesis: in vivo studies in human glycophorin a transgenic mice. Blood 97:2872–2878

245. Hartley SB, Crosbie J, Brink R, Kantor AB, Basten A, Goodnow CC (1991) Elimination from peripheral lymphoid tissues of self-reactive B lymphocytes recognizing membrane-bound antigens. Nature 353:765–769

246. Smith NH, Henry KL, Cadwell CM, Bennett A, Hendrickson JE, Frame T, Zimring JC (2012) Generation of transgenic mice with antithetical KEL1 and KEL2 human blood group antigens on red blood cells. Transfusion 52:2620–2630

247. Stowell SR, Henry KL, Smith NH, Hudson KE, Halverson GR, Park JC, Bennett AM, Girard-Pierce KR, Arthur CM, Bunting ST, Zimring JC, Hendrickson JE (2013) Alloantibodies to a paternally derived RBC KEL antigen lead to hemolytic disease of the fetus/newborn in a murine model. Blood 122:1494–1504

248. Stowell SR, Girard-Pierce KR, Smith NH, Henry KL, Arthur CM, Zimring JC, Hendrickson JE (2014) Transfusion of murine red blood cells expressing the human KEL glycoprotein induces clinically significant alloantibodies. Transfusion 54:179–189

249. Jash A, Usaneerungrueng C, Howie HL, Qiu A, Luckey CJ, Zimring JC, Hudson KE (2021) Antibodies to low-copy number RBC alloantigen convert a Tolerogenic stimulus to an immunogenic stimulus in mice. Front Immunol 12:629608

250. Arthur CM, Allen JWL, Verkerke H, Yoo J, Jajosky RP, Girard-Pierce K, Chonat S, Zerra P, Maier C, Rha J, Fasano R, Josephson CD, Roback JD, Stowell SR (2021) Antigen density dictates RBC clearance, but not antigen modulation, following incompatible RBC transfusion in mice. Blood Adv 5:527–538

251. Gibb DR, Liu J, Natarajan P, Santhanakrishnan M, Madrid DJ, Eisenbarth SC, Zimring JC, Iwasaki A, Hendrickson JE (2017) Type I IFN is necessary and sufficient for inflammation-induced red blood cell Alloimmunization in mice. J Immunol 199:1041–1050

252. Campbell-Lee SA, Liu J, Velliquette RW, Halverson GR, Shirey RS, Chaudhuri A, Reid ME, Ness PM, Baldwin WM (2006) The production of red blood cell alloantibodies in mice transfused with blood from transgenic Fyb-expressing mice. Transfusion 46:1682–1688

253. Goossens D, da Silva N, Metral S, Cortes U, Callebaut I, Picot J, Mouro-Chanteloup I, Cartron JP (2013) Mice expressing RHAG and RHD human blood group genes. PLoS One 8:e80460

254. Calabro S, Gallman A, Gowthaman U, Liu D, Chen P, Liu J, Krishnaswamy JK, Nascimento MS, Xu L, Patel SR, Williams A, Tormey CA, Hod EA, Spitalnik SL, Zimring JC, Hendrickson JE, Stowell SR, Eisenbarth SC (2016) Bridging channel dendritic cells

induce immunity to transfused red blood cells. J Exp Med 213:887–896
255. Arneja A, Salazar JE, Jiang W, Hendrickson JE, Zimring JC, Luckey CJ (2016) Interleukin-6 receptor-alpha signaling drives anti-RBC alloantibody production and T-follicular helper cell differentiation in a murine model of red blood cell alloimmunization. Haematologica 101:e440–e444
256. Liu D, Gibb DR, Escamilla-Rivera V, Liu J, Santhanakrishnan M, Shi Z, Xu L, Eisenbarth SC, Hendrickson JE (2019) Type 1 IFN signaling critically regulates influenza-induced alloimmunization to transfused KEL RBCs in a murine model. Transfusion 59:3243–3252
257. Arthur CM, Patel SR, Sharma A, Zerra PE, Chonat S, Jajosky RP, Fasano RM, Patel R, Bennett A, Zhou X, Luckey CJ, Hudson KE, Eisenbarth SC, Josephson CD, Roback JD, Hendrickson JE, Stowell SR (2022) Clodronate inhibits alloimmunization against distinct red blood cell alloantigens in mice. Transfusion 62:948–953
258. Mener A, Patel SR, Arthur CM, Chonat S, Wieland A, Santhanakrishnan M, Liu J, Maier CL, Jajosky RP, Girard-Pierce K, Bennett A, Zerra PE, Smith NH, Hendrickson JE, Stowell SR (2018) Complement serves as a switch between CD4+ T cell-independent and -dependent RBC antibody responses. JCI Insight Nov 15;3(22):e121631
259. Mener A, Arthur CM, Patel SR, Liu J, Hendrickson JE, Stowell SR (2018) Complement component 3 negatively regulates antibody response by modulation of red blood cell antigen. Front Immunol 9:676
260. Sato S, Miller AS, Howard MC, Tedder TF (1997) Regulation of B lymphocyte development and activation by the CD19/CD21/CD81/Leu 13 complex requires the cytoplasmic domain of CD19. J Immunol 159:3278–3287
261. Fearon DT, Carter RH (1995) The CD19/CR2/TAPA-1 complex of B lymphocytes: linking natural to acquired immunity. Annu Rev Immunol 13:127–149
262. Jajosky R, Patel SR, Wu SC, Patel K, Covington M, Vallecillo-Zuniga M, Ayona D, Bennett A, Luckey CJ, Hudson KE, Hendrickson JE, Eisenbarth SC, Josephson CD, Zerra PE, Stowell SR, Arthur CM (2023) Prior immunization against an intracellular antigen enhances subsequent red blood cell alloimmunization in mice. Blood 141:2642–2653
263. Hudson KE, Lin E, Hendrickson JE, Lukacher AE, Zimring JC (2010) Regulation of primary alloantibody response through antecedent exposure to a microbial T-cell epitope. Blood 115:3989–3996
264. Hendrickson JE, Hod EA, Cadwell CM, Eisenbarth SC, Spiegel DA, Tormey CA, Spitalnik SL, Zimring JC (2011) Rapid clearance of transfused murine red blood cells is associated with recipient cytokine storm and enhanced alloimmunogenicity. Transfusion 51:2445–2454
265. Maier CL, Jajosky RP, Patel SR, Verkerke HP, Fuller MD, Allen JW, Zerra PE, Fasano RM, Chonat S, Josephson CD, Gibb DR, Eisenbarth SC, Luckey CJ, Hudson KE, Hendrickson JE, Arthur CM, Stowell SR (2023) Storage differentially impacts alloimmunization to distinct red cell antigens following transfusion in mice. Transfusion 63:457–462
266. Hendrickson JE, Desmarets M, Deshpande SS, Chadwick TE, Hillyer CD, Roback JD, Zimring JC (2006) Recipient inflammation affects the frequency and magnitude of immunization to transfused red blood cells. Transfusion 46:1526–1536
267. Hendrickson JE, Chadwick TE, Roback JD, Hillyer CD, Zimring JC (2007) Inflammation enhances consumption and presentation of transfused RBC antigens by dendritic cells. Blood 110:2736–2743
268. Paul K, Hernandez-Armengol R, Lee JY, Chang CY, Shibata T, Yamashita M, Jefferies C, Gibb DR (2023) Distinct RBC alloantibody responses in type 1 interferon-dependent and -independent lupus mouse models. Front Immunol 14:1304086
269. Patel SR, Maier CL, Zimring JC (2023) Alloantigen copy number as a critical factor in RBC Alloimmunization. Transfus Med Rev 37:21–26
270. Arthur CM, Patel SR, Smith NH, Bennett A, Kamili NA, Mener A, Gerner-Smidt C, Sullivan HC, Hale JS, Wieland A, Youngblood B, Zimring JC, Hendrickson JE, Stowell SR (2017) Antigen density dictates immune responsiveness following red blood cell transfusion. J Immunol 198:2671–2680
271. Jash A, Howie HL, Hay AM, Luckey CJ, Hudson KE, Thomson PC, Ratcliffe SJ, Smolkin M, Zimring JC (2023) Identification of multiple genetic loci associated with red blood cell alloimmunization in mice. Haematologica 108:905–908
272. Patel SR, Gibb DR, Girard-Pierce K, Zhou X, Rodrigues LC, Arthur CM, Bennett AL, Jajosky RP, Fuller M, Maier CL, Zerra PE, Chonat S, Smith NH, Tormey CA, Hendrickson JE, Stowell SR (2018) Marginal zone B

cells induce alloantibody formation following RBC transfusion. Front Immunol 9:2516
273. Zerra PE, Patel SR, Jajosky RP, Arthur CM, McCoy JW, Allen JWL, Chonat S, Fasano RM, Roback JD, Josephson CD, Hendrickson JE, Stowell SR (2021) Marginal zone B cells mediate a CD4 T-cell-dependent extrafollicular antibody response following RBC transfusion in mice. Blood 138:706–721
274. Zerra PE, Cox C, Baldwin WH, Patel SR, Arthur CM, Lollar P, Meeks SL, Stowell SR (2017) Marginal zone B cells are critical to factor VIII inhibitor formation in mice with hemophilia a. Blood 130:2559–2568
275. Couvidou A, Angenieux C, Ruch L, Mangin PH, Gachet C, Maitre B (2023) Marginal zone B cells are responsible for the production of alloantibodies following platelet transfusion in mice. Blood Adv 7:1356–1365
276. Kallarakal MA, Cohen GS, Ibukun FI, Krummey SM (2024) Marginal zone B cells are necessary for the formation of anti-donor IgG after allogeneic sensitization. Transplantation 108:1357–1367
277. Weill JC, Weller S, Reynaud CA (2009) Human marginal zone B cells. Annu Rev Immunol 27:267–285
278. Cinamon G, Zachariah MA, Lam OM, Foss FW Jr, Cyster JG (2008) Follicular shuttling of marginal zone B cells facilitates antigen transport. Nat Immunol 9:54–62
279. Martin F, Kearney JF (2002) Marginal-zone B cells. Nat Rev Immunol 2:323–335
280. Pillai S, Cariappa A, Moran ST (2005) Marginal zone B cells. Annu Rev Immunol 23: 161–196
281. Girard-Pierce KR, Stowell SR, Smith NH, Arthur CM, Sullivan HC, Hendrickson JE, Zimring JC (2013) A novel role for C3 in antibody-induced red blood cell clearance and antigen modulation. Blood 122:1793–1801
282. Schirmer DA, Song SC, Baliff JP, Harbers SO, Clynes RA, Krop-Watorek A, Halverson GR, Czerwinski M, Spitalnik SL (2007) Mouse models of IgG- and IgM-mediated hemolysis. Blood 109:3099–3107
283. Davenport RD, Burdick M, Moore SA, Kunkel SL (1993) Cytokine production in IgG-mediated red cell incompatibility. Transfusion 33:19–24
284. Van Osch TLJ, Oosterhoff JJ, Bentlage AEH, Nouta J, Koeleman CAM, Geerdes DM, Mok JY, Heidt S, Mulder A, Van Esch WJE, Kapur R, Porcelijn L, Van der Schoot CE, De Haas M, Wuhrer M, Voorberg J, Vidarsson G (2022) Fc galactosylation of anti-platelet human IgG1 alloantibodies enhances complement activation on platelets. Haematologica 107:2432–2444
285. Sonneveld ME, Natunen S, Sainio S, Koeleman CA, Holst S, Dekkers G, Koelewijn J, Partanen J, van der Schoot CE, Wuhrer M, Vidarsson G (2016) Glycosylation pattern of anti-platelet IgG is stable during pregnancy and predicts clinical outcome in alloimmune thrombocytopenia. Br J Haematol 174:310–320
286. Kapur R, Della Valle L, Sonneveld M, Hipgrave Ederveen A, Visser R, Ligthart P, de Haas M, Wuhrer M, van der Schoot CE, Vidarsson G (2014) Low anti-RhD IgG-fc-fucosylation in pregnancy: a new variable predicting severity in haemolytic disease of the fetus and newborn. Br J Haematol 166:936–945
287. Shinde P, Howie HL, Stegmann TC, Hay AM, Waterman HR, Szittner Z, Bentlage AEH, Kapp L, Lissenberg-Thunnissen SN, Dekkers G, Schasfoort RBM, Ratcliffe SJ, Smolkin ME, Vidarsson G, van der Schoot CE, Hudson KE, Zimring JC (2020) IgG subclass determines suppression versus enhancement of humoral Alloimmunity to Kell RBC antigens in mice. Front Immunol 11:1516
288. Kumpel BM, Saldova R, Koeleman CAM, Abrahams JL, Ederveen AH, Armour KL, Olovnikova NI, Vidarsson G, Kapur R, Rudd PM, Wuhrer M (2020) Anti-D monoclonal antibodies from 23 human and rodent cell lines display diverse IgG fc-glycosylation profiles that determine their clinical efficacy. Sci Rep 10:1464
289. Mener A, Patel SR, Arthur CM, Stowell SR (2019) Antibody-mediated immunosuppression can result from RBC antigen loss independent of Fcgamma receptors in mice. Transfusion 59:371–384
290. Liepkalns JS, Hod EA, Stowell SR, Cadwell CM, Spitalnik SL, Zimring JC (2012) Biphasic clearance of incompatible red blood cells through a novel mechanism requiring neither complement nor Fcgamma receptors in a murine model. Transfusion 52:2631–2645
291. Liepkalns JS, Cadwell CM, Stowell SR, Hod EA, Spitalnik SL, Zimring JC (2013) Resistance of a subset of red blood cells to clearance by antibodies in a mouse model of incompatible transfusion. Transfusion 53: 1319–1327
292. Zimring JC, Cadwell CM, Chadwick TE, Spitalnik SL, Schirmer DA, Wu T, Parkos CA, Hillyer CD (2007) Nonhemolytic antigen

loss from red blood cells requires cooperative binding of multiple antibodies recognizing different epitopes. Blood 110:2201–2208

293. Stowell SR, Liepkalns JS, Hendrickson JE, Girard-Pierce KR, Smith NH, Arthur CM, Zimring JC (2013) Antigen modulation confers protection to red blood cells from antibody through Fcgamma receptor ligation. J Immunol 191:5013–5025

294. Stowell SR, Arthur CM, Girard-Pierce KR, Sullivan HC, Santhanakrishnan M, Natarajan P, Patel SR, Tormey CA, Zimring JC, Hendrickson JE (2015) Anti-KEL sera prevents alloimmunization to transfused KEL RBCs in a murine model. Haematologica 100:e394–e397

295. Sullivan HC, Gerner-Smidt C, Nooka AK, Arthur CM, Thompson L, Mener A, Patel SR, Yee M, Fasano RM, Josephson CD, Kaufman RM, Roback JD, Lonial S, Stowell SR (2017) Daratumumab (anti-CD38) induces loss of CD38 on red blood cells. Blood 129: 3033–3037

296. Sullivan HC, Arthur CM, Thompson L, Patel SR, Stowell SR, Hendrickson JE, Lazarus AH (2018) Anti-RhD reduces levels of detectable RhD antigen following anti-RhD infusion. Transfusion 58:542–544

297. Cruz-Leal Y, Norris PAA, Gil Gonzalez L, Marjoram D, Wabnitz H, Shan Y, Lazarus AH (2024) Trogocytosis drives red blood cell antigen loss in association with antibody-mediated immune suppression. Blood 143: 807–821

298. C. M. Jajosky RP, Liu J, Chai L, Zerra PE, Chonat S, Stowell SR, Arthur CM, CD47 regulates antigen modulation and red blood cell clearance following an incompatible transfusion Front Immunol. in press, (2025)

299. Jash A, Pridmore T, Collins JB, Hay AM, Hudson KE, Luckey CJ, Zimring JC (2024) Complement C3 and marginal zone B cells promote IgG-mediated enhancement of RBC alloimmunization in mice. J Clin Invest 134

300. Chauhan AR, Nandanwar YS, Ramaiah A, Yelikar KA, Rashmi MD, Sachan R, Mayekar RV, Trivedi YN, Paradkar GV, Patole KP (2019) A Multicenter, Randomized, open-label trial comparing the efficacy and safety of monoclonal anti-Rh (D) immunoglobulin with polyclonal anti-Rh (D) immunoglobulin for the prevention of maternal Rh-Isoimmunization. J Obstet Gynaecol India 69:420–425

301. Gruber DR, Richards AL, Howie HL, Hay AM, Lebedev JN, Wang X, Zimring JC, Hudson KE (2020) Passively transferred IgG enhances humoral immunity to a red blood cell alloantigen in mice. Blood Adv 4:1526–1537

302. Jajosky RP, Patel KR, Allen JWL, Zerra PE, Chonat S, Ayona D, Maier CL, Morais D, Wu SC, Luckey CJ, Eisenbarth SC, Roback JD, Fasano RM, Josephson CD, Manis JP, Chai L, Hendrickson JE, Hudson KE, Arthur CM, Stowell SR (2023) Antibody-mediated antigen loss switches augmented immunity to antibody-mediated immunosuppression. Blood 142:1082–1098

303. Bernardo L, Amash A, Marjoram D, Lazarus AH (2016) Antibody-mediated immune suppression is improved when blends of anti-RBC monoclonal antibodies are used in mice. Blood 128:1076–1080

304. Liu J, Santhanakrishnan M, Natarajan P, Gibb DR, Eisenbarth SC, Tormey CA, Siddon AJ, Stowell SR, Branch DR, Hendrickson JE (2016) Antigen modulation as a potential mechanism of anti-KEL immunoprophylaxis in mice. Blood 128:3159–3168

305. Yu H, Stowell SR, Bernardo L, Hendrickson JE, Zimring JC, Amash A, Uchikawa M, Lazarus AH (2014) Antibody-mediated immune suppression of erythrocyte alloimmunization can occur independently from red cell clearance or epitope masking in a murine model. J Immunol 193:2902–2910

306. Bernardo L, Yu H, Amash A, Zimring JC, Lazarus AH (2015) IgG-mediated immune suppression to erythrocytes by polyclonal antibodies can occur in the absence of activating or inhibitory Fcgamma receptors in a full mouse model. J Immunol 195:2224–2230

307. Cruz-Leal Y, Lazarus AH (2021) Could antigen loss be a potential mechanism to explain antibody-mediated immune suppression? Transfusion 61:1004–1006

308. Escamilla-Rivera V, Santhanakrishnan M, Liu J, Gibb DR, Forsmo JE, Foxman EF, Eisenbarth SC, Luckey CJ, Zimring JC, Hudson KE, Stowell SR, Hendrickson JE (2021) Complement plays a critical role in inflammation-induced Immunoprophylaxis failure in mice. Front Immunol 12:704072

309. Jajosky RP, Ayona D, Mener A, Stowell SR, Arthur CM (2024) Dynamics of antibody engagement of red blood cells in vivo and in vitro. Front Immunol 15:1475470

310. Maier CL, Mener A, Patel SR, Jajosky RP, Bennett AL, Arthur CM, Hendrickson JE, Stowell SR (2018) Antibody-mediated immune suppression by antigen modulation is antigen-specific. Blood Adv 2:2986–3000

311. Wabnitz H, Cruz-Leal Y, Lazarus AH (2023) Antigen copy number and antibody dose can

determine the outcome of erythrocyte alloimmunization inducing either antibody-mediated immune suppression or enhancement in a murine model. Transfusion 63: 696–702

312. Cruz-Leal Y, Marjoram D, Lazarus AH (2018) Erythrocyte saturation with IgG is required for inducing antibody-mediated immune suppression and impacts both erythrocyte clearance and antigen-modulation mechanisms. J Immunol 200:1295–1305

313. Strauss RG, Mock DM, Widness JA, Johnson K, Cress G, Schmidt RL (2004) Posttransfusion 24-hour recovery and subsequent survival of allogeneic red blood cells in the bloodstream of newborn infants. Transfusion 44:871–876

314. Mock DM, Stowell SR, Franco RS, Kyosseva SV, Nalbant D, Schmidt RL, Cress GA, Strauss RG, Cancelas JA, von Goetz M, North AK, Widness JA (2022) Antibodies against biotin-labeled red blood cells can shorten posttransfusion survival. Transfusion 62:770–782

315. Yee MEM, Covington ML, Zerra PE, McCoy JW, Easley KA, Joiner CH, Bryksin J, Francis RO, Lough CM, Patel N, Kutlar A, Josephson CD, Roback JD, Stowell SR, Fasano RM (2024) Survival of transfused red blood cells from a donor with alpha-thalassemia trait in a recipient with sickle cell disease. Transfusion 64:1109–1115

316. Yee MEM, Zerra PE, McCoy JW, Covington ML, Stowell SR, Joiner CH, Lough CM, Delvadia BB, Josephson CD, Roback JD, Fasano RM (2024) Post-transfusion biotin-labeled red blood cell survival studies in pediatric sickle cell disease with antibodies of uncertain significance. Transfusion 64:800–807

317. Tong TN, Cen S, Branch DR (2019) The monocyte monolayer assay: past, present and future. Transfus Med Rev 33:24–28

318. Nance SJT (2023) The monocyte monolayer assay, an in vitro method for prediction of in vivo survival of transfused incompatible red blood cells: a review. Immunohematology 39:61–69

319. Arndt PA, Garratty G (2004) A retrospective analysis of the value of monocyte monolayer assay results for predicting the clinical significance of blood group alloantibodies. Transfusion 44:1273–1281

Chapter 2

Characterization of Platelet and Red Blood Cell Extracellular Vesicles by Spectral Flow Cytometry

Erika G. Marques de Menezes and Philip J. Norris

Abstract

We describe a method to characterize extracellular vesicles (EVs) derived from red blood cells (RBCs) and platelets. This chapter focuses on two widely used techniques: nanoparticle tracking analysis (NTA) and flow cytometry. NTA is particularly well suited to enumerating smaller particles (<200 nm), while flow cytometry techniques generally detect particles >200 nm. The advantage of flow cytometry detection of EVs is that the multiple fluorescent channels allow detection of markers on the surface EVs, which allows determination of their cell of origin. We present methods to isolate EVs for analysis or purify EVs for use in functional analyses based on differential centrifugation. Sensitivity for detection of EVs by flow cytometry varies widely from machine to machine, even within the same class of instruments. We demonstrate how to determine the sensitivity of small particle detection by flow cytometry and present representative data for quantification of RBC and platelet-derived EVs.

Key words Extracellular vesicle, Nanoparticle tracking analysis, Flow cytometry, Red blood cell, Platelet

1 Introduction

Extracellular vesicles (EVs) are membrane-bound particles naturally released from various cell types into the extracellular environment. They play crucial roles in intercellular communication, mediating a range of physiological and pathological processes, including immune responses, inflammation, and cell death [1–3]. The growing interest in EVs stems from their potential as biomarkers for diseases and as therapeutic delivery vehicles. However, their isolation and characterization present significant challenges due to their heterogeneity and the complexity of biological fluids [4]. EVs are generally accepted to range in size from 50 to 1000 nm or roughly 1/200th to 1/10th the size of an average human cell [5]. This small size makes isolation and accurate detection of EVs difficult using conventional techniques such as flow cytometry. We will briefly review common techniques to

Sean R. Stowell and Connie M. Arthur (eds.), *Methods in Transfusion Medicine*, Methods in Molecular Biology, vol. 3053, https://doi.org/10.1007/978-1-0716-5376-0_2,

isolate and characterize EVs, then we will present a protocol based on differential centrifugation for sample preparation and nanoparticle tracking analysis (NTA) and flow cytometry for sample analysis, with a focus on the study of RBC and platelet EVs.

Several methods are commonly employed to isolate EVs, each with its advantages and drawbacks. The choice of method depends on the sample type, the required purity and yield of EVs, and the downstream applications. Differential centrifugation is the most widely used technique for isolating EVs, based on differential centrifugation steps that separate particles by size and density [6]. This method is effective for processing large volumes of samples and is relatively inexpensive. To achieve isolation of small EVs, ultracentrifugation can be employed. However, it has several limitations, including low specificity, potential co-isolation of non-vesicular components, and the requirement for specialized equipment. Density gradient centrifugation can be used to partially separate EVs from other non-vesicular components allowing measurement of EVs and their activity in successive fractions from the density gradient [7]. Compared to differential centrifugation, density gradient centrifugation is time consuming, and the sucrose or iodixanol used in the density gradient could affect the activity of the isolated EVs. Another commonly used technique for EV isolation is size-exclusion chromatography (SEC) [8]. This method isolates EVs based on their size, using a column filled with porous beads. In theory, EVs elute from the column earlier than smaller proteins and other contaminants. However, SEC is limited by the relatively low throughput and potential dilution of the sample, which may require further concentration steps. Precipitation-based methods use polymeric agents, such as polyethylene glycol, to aggregate EVs, which can then be collected by low-speed centrifugation [9]. These methods are simple, scalable, and do not require specialized equipment. However, they can result in co-precipitation of contaminants, such as proteins and lipoproteins. Additionally, the precipitating agents can affect the physical and biochemical properties of EVs. Finally, immunoaffinity capture involves the use of antibodies targeting specific surface markers on EVs to isolate them from complex mixtures [10]. This method can achieve high specificity and purity, making it suitable for isolating specific subpopulations of EVs. However, it is limited by the availability and specificity of antibodies, potential alteration of vesicle function by antibody binding, and relatively high costs.

EVs can be characterized based on their physical characteristics, such as size, abundance, and content (lipid, nucleic acid, and protein) as well as their functional activity, either in biochemical reactions or more commonly by measuring their effects when incubated with target cells. In this chapter, we will focus on the physical characterization of EVs in terms of size, abundance, and surface marker expression. NTA measures the size distribution and concentration of EVs by tracking their Brownian motion under a microscope [11]. NTA requires specialized equipment and is a lower throughput assay compared to flow cytometry. The advantages of NTA include detection of particles in the 50–200 nm range and no need for expensive reagents. NTA is not optimal for detecting larger EVs beyond the 200 nm range, as exemplified by a recent comparison of NTA with transmission electron microscopy for detection of EVs up to 500 nm [12]. Flow cytometry can analyze EVs based on their size, surface markers, and fluorescence properties. It allows for multiparametric analysis and the isolation of specific EV subpopulations [13, 14]. However, conventional flow cytometers have limitations in detecting small EVs (<200 nm) due to their resolution limits. Newer machines, particularly those relying on a violet side-scatter detector, can detect smaller particles, such as polystyrene beads <100 nm, though these beads have a higher refractive index than EVs, making them easier to detect using light scattering methods. Transmission electron microscopy (TEM) provides high-resolution images of EVs, allowing detailed examination of their morphology and size [15]. TEM is considered by some as the gold standard for visualizing EVs and confirming their presence. However, TEM is time-consuming, requires extensive sample preparation, and may introduce artifacts. It also does not provide quantitative data or information about the biochemical composition of EVs. Western blotting and mass spectrometry are also used to analyze the protein composition of EVs. Western blotting allows for the detection of specific proteins, providing qualitative and semi-quantitative data. Mass spectrometry offers comprehensive profiling of the proteome, enabling the identification of a wide range of proteins [16]. However, both techniques require extensive sample preparation, are labor-intensive, and give information about EV populations rather than individual EVs.

2 Materials

2.1 Platelet Processing

1. Whole blood.
2. Anticoagulant (e.g., citrate, EDTA).
3. Centrifuge.
4. 15 mL sterile conical tubes.
5. Adjustable pipettes and tips (p1000, p100, p20).
6. Hemocytometer or automated cell counter.

2.2 Red Blood Cell Processing

1. Whole blood.
2. Phosphate-buffered saline (PBS), without calcium chloride and magnesium chloride, sterile-filtered (Sigma or similar).
3. Anticoagulant (such as EDTA or heparin).

4. Centrifuge.
5. 15 mL sterile conical tubes.
6. Adjustable pipettes and tips (p1000, p100, p20).
7. Hemocytometer or automated cell counter.

2.3 Isolation of EV Subpopulations

1. Platelet and RBC supernatants.
2. Phosphate-buffered saline (PBS), without calcium chloride and magnesium chloride, sterile-filtered (Sigma or similar).
3. Ultrafree MC centrifugal filter with a 0.22 μm pore size (e.g., Millipore or similar).
4. 1.5 mL microcentrifuge tubes.
5. Adjustable pipettes and tips (p1000, p100, p20).
6. 13.2 mL ultra-clear tube suitable for ultracentrifugation (Beckman Coulter or similar).
7. Ultracentrifuge with appropriate rotors (Beckman Coulter or similar).
8. Refrigerated centrifuge.

2.4 Nanoparticle Tracking Analysis

1. Sample containing EVs.
2. Phosphate-buffered saline (PBS), without calcium chloride and magnesium chloride, sterile-filtered (Sigma or similar).
3. Ultrafree MC centrifugal filter with a 0.22 μm pore size (Millipore or similar).
4. 1.5 mL microcentrifuge tubes.
5. Adjustable pipettes and tips (p1000, p100, p20).
6. 5 mL falcon polystyrene tubes.
7. 1 mL syringe for sample handling.
8. Nanosight instrument.

2.5 Size Calibration of Using Apogee and NIST Small Particle Beads

1. ApogeeMix (catalog #1493).
2. Thermo Fisher Scientific NIST traceable PS beads (catalog: #3080A and #3100A).
3. Phosphate-buffered saline (PBS), without calcium chloride and magnesium chloride, sterile-filtered (e.g., Sigma or similar).
4. Ultrafree MC centrifugal filter with a 0.22 μm pore size (Millipore or similar).
5. 5 mL falcon polystyrene tubes.
6. Adjustable pipettes and tips (p1000, p100, p20).
7. Spectral flow cytometer.

2.6 EV Immunophenotyping by Spectral Flow Cytometry

1. Phosphate-buffered saline (PBS), without calcium chloride and magnesium chloride, sterile-filtered (Sigma or similar).
2. Fluorochrome-conjugated monoclonal antibodies from Bio-Legend unless otherwise noted: platelets CD41-BV510, and CD42b-PE/Cy7, tetraspanin protein CD9-APC and CD63-BV421, phosphatidylserine annexin V-BV605 (BD Biosciences), lactadherin-APC, and red blood cells (RBC) CD235a-BV421, and CD108-PE.
3. Ultrafree MC centrifugal filter with a 0.22 μm pore size (Millipore or similar).
4. 5 mL Falcon polystyrene tubes.
5. Adjustable pipettes and tips (p1000, p100, p20).
6. Cytek Aurora or other spectral flow cytometer.

3 Methods

3.1 Platelet Processing

1. Collect 9 mL of whole blood using sterile technique. Use anticoagulant (e.g., EDTA, sodium citrate) and mix blood with the anticoagulant by gently inverting the tube three times.
2. Transfer the whole blood into 15 mL sterile conical tubes and centrifuge the tubes at 350× *g* for 20 min at room temperature. This step separates the blood into two layers: the lower, dark layer of packed red blood cells and the upper yellow of platelet-rich plasma (PRP).
3. Remove the upper PRP layer using a pipette and transfer it to a new sterile tube (*see* **Note 1**).
4. Use a hemocytometer or automated cell counter to determine the concentration of platelets if needed.

3.2 Red Blood Cell Processing

1. Collect 9 mL of whole blood using sterile technique. Use anticoagulant (e.g., EDTA or heparin) to prevent clotting during handling.
2. Transfer the whole blood into 15 mL sterile conical tubes and centrifuge the tubes at 500× *g* for 10 min at 4 °C.
3. Aspirate supernatant, leaving behind a pellet and then resuspend the pellet in PBS. Ensure volume of PBS double the volume of pellet alone.
4. Centrifuge red blood cells (RBCs) at 500× *g* for 10 min at 4 °C.
5. Aspirate supernatant and repeat **steps 3** and **4** two more times for a total of three washes of the RBCs.

6. After the final wash, carefully aspirate supernatant and resuspend the purified RBC pellet of 15 mL sterile conical tubes in an appropriate volume of PBS to achieve the desired concentration (e.g., if the RBD pellet is around 0.5 mL, add 5–10 mL of PBS), and store at 4 °C.
7. Use a hemocytometer or automated cell counter to determine the concentration of RBCs if needed.

3.3 Isolation of EV Subpopulations for Analysis or Functional Studies

1. Transfer 1 mL supernatant from the PRP or RBC incubations to 1.5 mL microcentrifuge tubes.
2. Centrifuge the tubes at 2000× *g* for 10 min at 4 °C. This step will remove cells and large cell fragments, leaving a heterogeneous population of small to medium EVs, including microparticles and ectosomes (*see* **Note 2**).
3. Transfer the supernatant to new 1.5 mL microcentrifuge tubes, being careful not to disturb the pellet.
4. Centrifuge at 13,000× *g* for 30 min at 4 °C. This step will remove most microparticles and ectosomes, leaving small EVs (*see* **Note 3**).
5. Carefully transfer the supernatant, leaving behind some volume to avoid disturbing the pellet, and add the supernatant to ultracentrifuge tubes.
6. Centrifuge at 100,000× *g* for 2 h at 4 °C. This step will generate a pellet containing the small EVs.
7. Aspirate the supernatant and resuspend the pellet in PBS pre-filtered with a 0.22 μm pore-size centrifugal filter.
8. Transfer the purified EVs into 0.22 μm pore-size centrifugal filter tubes and centrifuge using a fixed angle single speed centrifuge (~850× *g*) at 4 °C for 10 min.
9. Collect the purified small EVs from the bottom of the filters, aliquot, and store at −80 °C. Figure 1 shows a schematic of the EV isolation method (*see* **Note 4**).

3.4 Size and Concentration Analyses of EVs by Nanoparticle Tracking Analysis

1. Dilute the EV sample to an appropriate concentration range for analysis. Typically, samples are diluted to achieve a particle concentration within the optimal range of the Nanosight instrument (e.g., 10^7 to 10^9 particles/mL). Samples should be prepared with 1 mL final volume for measurement.
2. Verify that the filtered buffer used to dilute the sample is free from contaminating particles by running it through the instrument with the camera turned to its highest testing setting. No more than five particles/mL should be visualized.
3. Instrument cleaning procedure.
   (a) Prepare a clean solvent solution, such as filtered PBS or deionized (DI) water with a 0.22 μm pore-size filter.

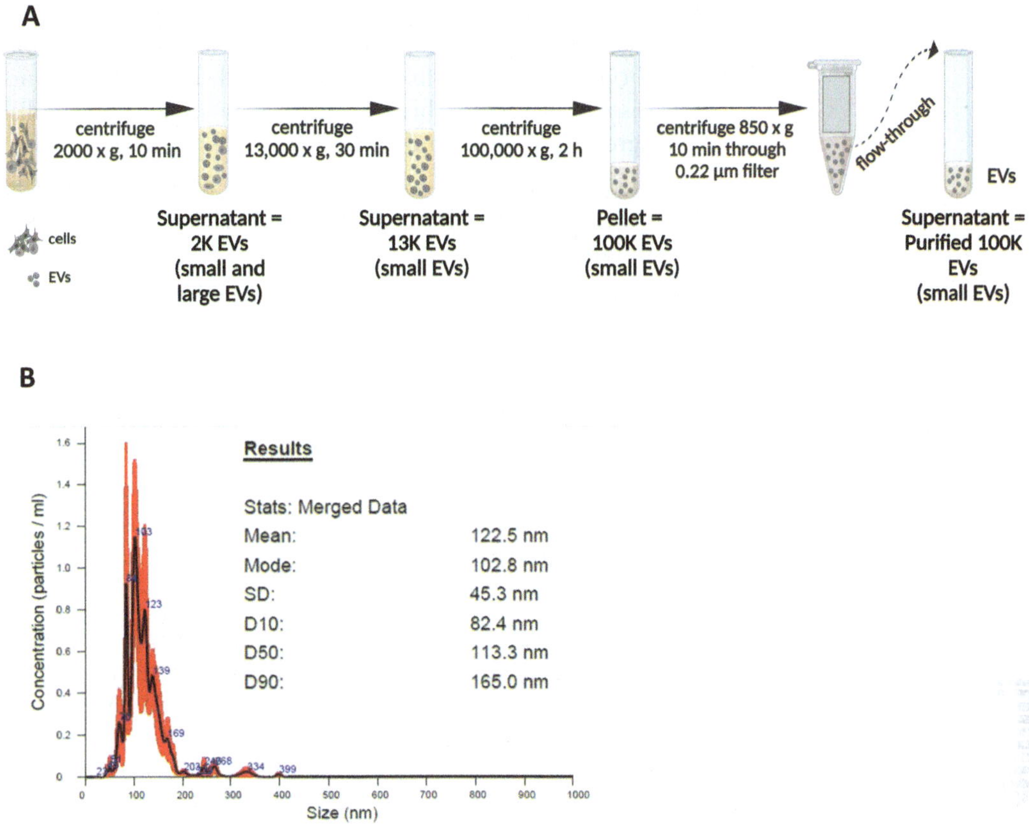

Fig. 1 Isolation and characterization of EVs. (**a**) Schematic of the EV isolation method. (**b**) Representative graph of nanoparticle tracking analysis showing the EV size distribution obtained through ultracentrifugation. This sizing scheme follows convention proposed in an International Society of Extracellular Vesicles position paper [17]. In practice, we find that medium EVs are often found in the 13,000× *g* supernatant. Each laboratory should perform their own sizing analysis to determine EV distribution after differential centrifugation. Figure created with BioRender

(b) Use a syringe or pump to flush the sample line with the clean solvent solution. Ensure that the solvent flows through the entire length of the sample line to thoroughly clean it.

(c) Flush the sample line for an appropriate duration to ensure effective cleaning. Typically, a few minutes of flushing should be sufficient to remove any residual contaminants.

(d) Clean the sample line between each run to prevent cross-contamination.

4. Instrument setup and operation.

   (a) Turn on the Nanosight instrument and allow it to warm up according to the manufacturer's instructions.

(b) Number of image captures: Five is typically adequate for most samples in experiments with low concentration, though more than five can be utilized. For largely monodisperse samples, three captures may suffice to establish agreement between distributions across different runs.

(c) Length of capture: determined by the number of particles on the screen; if fewer than 30 particles are visible, use a duration of 60 s.

(d) Choose the syringe pump flow rate of 30.

(e) Adjust the focus by rotating the knob located on the side of the machine from top to bottom.

(f) Date and time name: leave checked to automatically append the capture date and time to the filename.

(g) Temperature can be activated and set by selecting the respective checkboxes.

(h) Process files after capture and apply the same settings to all videos.

(i) Export the data after the measurement is complete. Figure 2 illustrates a representative graph displaying the nanoparticle tracking analysis of the purified EV particle-size distribution (*see* **Note 5**).

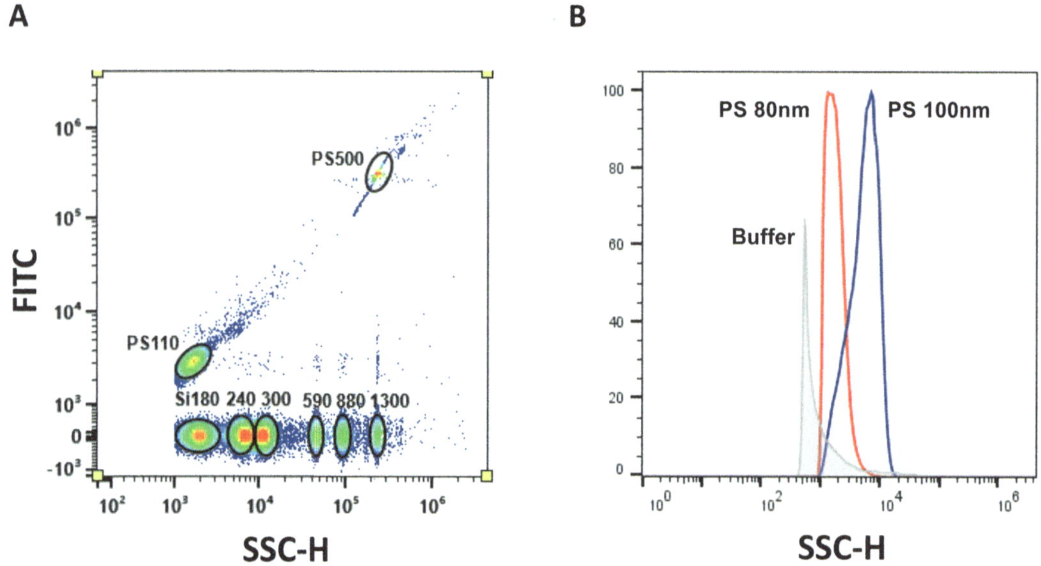

Fig. 2 Sensitive and resolution of small bead populations. (**a**) Apogee beads containing both polystyrene (PS) and silica (Si). (**b**) 80 nm beads are fully resolved above the background and are distinct from the 100 nm beads (NIST traceable polystyrene beads)

3.5 Size Calibration of Using Apogee and NIST Small Particle Beads

1. Prepare the spectral flow cytometer:
   (a) Turn on the flow cytometer.
   (b) Allow the instrument to warm up for 30 min.
   (c) Clean the instrument according to the manufacturer's instructions.
   (d) Prepare Spectro QC beads (one drop of beads in 0.3 mL sheath fluid, DI water, or PBS). Vortex the tube for 5 s to put beads into suspension. Acquire on the instrument shortly after resuspension. Store the diluted beads solution at 4 °C and protect from light.
2. Run reference beads:
   (a) Vortex the vial containing a mixture of non-fluorescent silica beads and fluorescent polystyrene beads, with diameters 180, 240, 590, 880, and 1300 nm diameter with refractive index $\eta = 1.43$ (silica) and two green fluorescent populations (110 and 500 nm) with refractive index $\eta = 1.59$ (polystyrene).
   (b) Prepare the Apogee beads according to the manufacturer's recommendations. Figure 2a demonstrates sensitivity and resolution of small bead detection.
   (c) Additionally, prepare the National Institute of Standards and Technology (NIST) traceable PS bead solution with 80 and 100 nm diameters to calibrate particle sizing according to the manufacturer's instructions. Figure 2b shows 80 nm PS beads can be resolved above the background and from the 100 nm PS beads.
3. Instrument data acquisition:
   (a) Set up the experiment in the SpectroFlo software.
   (b) Use the 405 nm violet laser at a threshold of 1000 arbitrary units.
   (c) Do not use an OR triggering strategy.
   (d) Acquire all samples for 1 min at a low flow rate (~15 μL/min) and set abort rate < 10%. If the flow cytometer boosts the sample during sample loading, ensure that the delay between boosting and data acquisition is sufficiently long to guarantee a stable flow rate.

3.6 EV Immunophenotyping by Spectral Flow Cytometry

1. Sample staining:
   (a) Prior to staining, filter all antibodies to remove aggregates, which can cause false-positive signals.
   (b) Filter the antibodies using a 0.22 μm centrifugal filter at 850× *g* for 5 min at 4 °C, or until the antibody has passed through the filter and no antibody liquid remains on the surface of the filter (*see* **Note 6**).

(c) Optimize the concentration of EVs in the sample (a range of 6–8 serial dilutions is recommended to find the optimum).

(d) Titrate the antibodies to find the optimal concentration of staining reagents. The titration should be performed on a predetermined concentration of EVs (*see* **Note 7**).

(e) Add the appropriate amount of filtered antibody to the EV samples. Mix by pipetting up and down five to eight times. Incubate at 4 °C in the dark for 30 min (*see* **Note 8**).

(f) Dilute the EV samples in 0.22 μm-filtered PBS to appropriate dilutions to avoid swarm detection and high abort rate, and then run immediately (or within the same day) on the flow cytometer (see Subheading 3.5, **step 3**) (*see* **Note 9**). Figure 3 shows representative flow plots of plasma platelet-EV RBC-EV subtypes.

2. Assay controls:

(a) Prepare buffer-only control (0.22 μm-filtered PBS) to quantify the contribution of background noise. Measure the buffer-only sample using the same acquisition settings as for the measurement of the EV samples (*see* **Note 10**).

(b) Prepare buffer with filtered antibodies under the same conditions as the EV samples. Measure the buffer with antibodies using the same settings as for the measurement of the EV samples.

(c) Prepare unstained controls (EVs only) under the same conditions as the stained EV samples to determine at which fluorescence level the fluorescently stained EVs can be differentiated from unstained particles and check for swarm detection induced by unbound reagents. In addition, the unstained samples will be used to ensure accurate unmixing and autofluorescence quantitation by flow cytometry.

4 Notes

1. If desired, activate the platelets by the addition of platelet agonists (e.g., thrombin, collagen) to release growth factors and other bioactive molecules. Add the activation agent to the PRP according to the manufacturer's instructions and incubate for the recommended time at room temperature.
2. For flow cytometry analysis of EVs, we typically use the sample obtained after centrifugation at 2000× *g*, which will contain a mixture of small to large EVs.

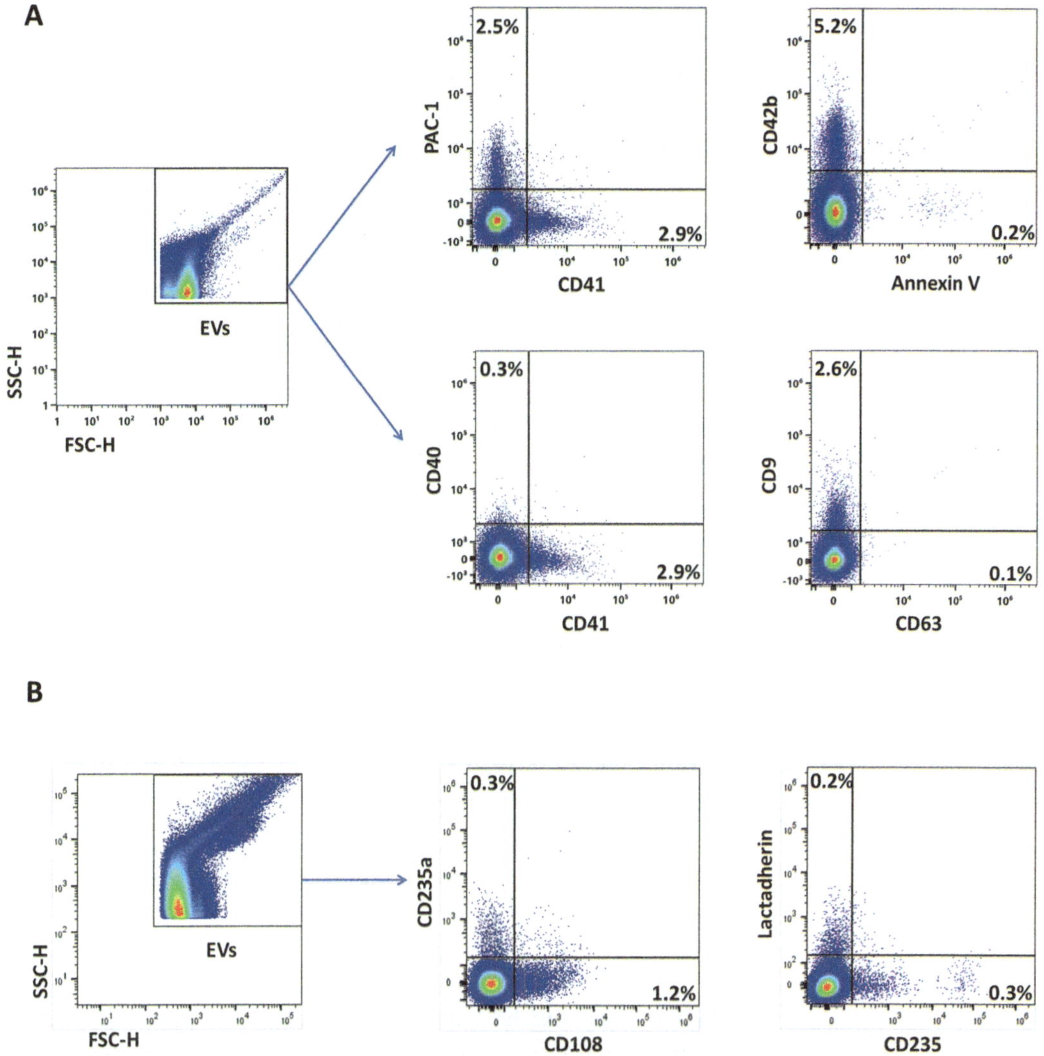

Fig. 3 Characterizing single EVs directly in biofluid by spectral flow cytometry. Representative flow plots showing (**a**) EV markers linked to platelets (CD41a and CD42b), annexin V, which binds to phosphatidyl serine and tetraspanin proteins (CD9 and CD63), and (**b**) red blood cells (CD235a), semaphoring 7a (CD108), and lactadherin, which binds to phosphatidyl serine

3. The use of differential centrifugation speeds does not result in exact size-based separation of EVs. Incorporating orthogonal measurements, such as scanning electron microscopy and dynamic light scattering, can provide insights into the size distribution of EV fractions.
4. For functional studies where EVs are added to target cells to measure effects on cell activation or induction of cell death, we typically purify EVs using the entire protocol through ultracentrifugation and concentration.

5. Nanoparticle analysis typically measures particles under 200 nm in size, and the accuracy of its measurements declines with larger particles, particularly over 500 nm in size [12]. To measure larger EVs, other methods such as dynamic light scattering, laser diffraction, or sensitive flow cytometry.
6. Antibody aggregates, commonly found in commercial preparations, pose a challenge as they can cause false positive events. Employing antibody filtration effectively eliminates these aggregates, enhancing the reliability of the analyses.
7. In the context of flow cytometry analysis of EVs, optimizing antibody concentrations is crucial to strike a balance between achieving sufficient binding sensitivity for accurate detection of target epitopes on EV surfaces and minimizing the risks associated with nonspecific binding and steric hindrance.
8. Detergents are commonly used to confirm if detected events are membrane-enclosed EVs. A detergent lysis step can distinguish non-EV signals or vesicle-mimicking events from other protein complexes. Protein aggregates may appear when analyzing heterogeneous samples such as plasma and serum, or when using reagents that may cause precipitation, such as calcium phosphate. To lyse the EVs post-staining, add 10% NP-40 detergent solution (Thermo Fisher) to the stained EV sample, and then analyze the sample before and after detergent addition using flow cytometry.
9. Serial dilution is crucial for preventing swarm detection in flow cytometry when characterizing EVs. By analyzing data from various dilutions, you can determine the dilution point that maintains single-particle detection without exceeding the optimal abort rate (<10% of the count rate is generally accepted).
10. When analyzing EVs at the limits of a flow cytometer's sensitivity, it is important to provide a reference event rate from a sample containing only the buffer used for diluting EV samples. Additionally, MIFlowCyt-EV can guide researchers in measuring EVs by providing a fundamental reporting structure. This structure includes preanalytical variables, experimental design, sample preparation, assay controls, instrument calibration and data acquisition, and EV characterization. All these aspects should be considered and reported for EV flow cytometry studies.

Conflicts of Interest

The authors have no conflicts of interest to declare that are relevant to the content of this chapter

References

1. Buzas EI, György B, Nagy G et al (2014) Emerging role of extracellular vesicles in inflammatory diseases. Nat Rev Rheumatol 10:356–364. https://doi.org/10.1038/nrrheum.2014.19
2. Robbins PD, Morelli AE (2014) Regulation of immune responses by extracellular vesicles. Nat Rev Immunol 14:195–208. https://doi.org/10.1038/nri3622
3. Rashed MH, Bayraktar E, Helal GK et al (2017) Exosomes: from garbage bins to promising therapeutic targets. Int J Mol Sci 18. https://doi.org/10.3390/ijms18030538
4. Welsh JA, Goberdhan DCI, O'Driscoll L et al (2024) Minimal information for studies of extracellular vesicles (MISEV2023): from basic to advanced approaches. J Extracell Vesicle 13:e12404. https://doi.org/10.1002/jev2.12404
5. Nolte-'t Hoen ENM, van der Vlist EJ, Aalberts M et al (2012) Quantitative and qualitative flow cytometric analysis of nanosized cell-derived membrane vesicles. Nanomedicine 8: 712–720. https://doi.org/10.1016/j.nano.2011.09.006
6. Livshits MA, Khomyakova E, Evtushenko EG et al (2015) Isolation of exosomes by differential centrifugation: theoretical analysis of a commonly used protocol. Sci Rep 5:17319. https://doi.org/10.1038/srep17319
7. Dauros Singorenko P, Chang V, Whitcombe A et al (2017) Isolation of membrane vesicles from prokaryotes: a technical and biological comparison reveals heterogeneity. J Extracell Vesicles 6:1324731. https://doi.org/10.1080/20013078.2017.1324731
8. Böing AN, van der Pol E, Grootemaat AE et al (2014) Single-step isolation of extracellular vesicles by size-exclusion chromatography. J Extracell Vesicles 3. https://doi.org/10.3402/jev.v3.23430
9. Rider MA, Hurwitz SN, Meckes DG (2016) ExtraPEG: a polyethylene glycol-based method for enrichment of extracellular vesicles. Sci Rep 6:23978. https://doi.org/10.1038/srep23978
10. Tauro BJ, Greening DW, Mathias RA et al (2012) Comparison of ultracentrifugation, density gradient separation, and immunoaffinity capture methods for isolating human colon cancer cell line LIM1863-derived exosomes. Methods 56:293–304. https://doi.org/10.1016/j.ymeth.2012.01.002
11. Dragovic RA, Gardiner C, Brooks AS et al (2011) Sizing and phenotyping of cellular vesicles using nanoparticle tracking analysis. Nanomedicine 7:780–788. https://doi.org/10.1016/j.nano.2011.04.003
12. Krishnamachary B, Cook C, Kumar A et al (2021) Extracellular vesicle-mediated endothelial apoptosis and EV-associated proteins correlate with COVID-19 disease severity. J Extracell Vesicle 10:e12117. https://doi.org/10.1002/jev2.12117
13. Nolan JP, Stoner SA (2013) A trigger channel threshold artifact in nanoparticle analysis. Cytometry A 83:301–305. https://doi.org/10.1002/cyto.a.22255
14. Inglis HC, Danesh A, Shah A et al (2015) Techniques to improve detection and analysis of extracellular vesicles using flow cytometry. Cytometry A. https://doi.org/10.1002/cyto.a.22649
15. Kotrbová A, Štěpka K, Maška M et al (2019) TEM ExosomeAnalyzer: a computer-assisted software tool for quantitative evaluation of extracellular vesicles in transmission electron microscopy images. J Extracell Vesicles 8: 1560808. https://doi.org/10.1080/20013078.2018.1560808
16. Greening DW, Xu R, Ji H et al (2015) A protocol for exosome isolation and characterization: evaluation of ultracentrifugation, density-gradient separation, and immunoaffinity capture methods. Methods Mol Biol 1295:179–209. https://doi.org/10.1007/978-1-4939-2550-6_15
17. Mateescu B, Kowal EJK, Van Balkom BWM et al (2017) Obstacles and opportunities in the functional analysis of extracellular vesicle RNA—an ISEV position paper. J Extracell Vesicle 6:1286095. https://doi.org/10.1080/20013078.2017.1286095

Chapter 3

Mouse Models of Platelet Alloimmunization and Refractoriness

Betty Gaillard, Johnson Q. Tran, and Rachael P. Jackman

Abstract

We have established murine models of platelet alloimmunization and refractoriness. Our approaches utilize commonly available strains of mice, along with flow cytometry-based techniques to evaluate the magnitude and quality of the alloimmune response to platelet transfusion and the functional outcomes of these alloresponses. Using these methods, we can evaluate the relative immunogenicity of different blood products, the impact of recipient health on alloimmunization outcomes, and the ability of different interventions to prevent these damaging responses. Here, we discuss the approaches used to prepare platelets for transfusion, measure anti-class I and class II major histocompatibility complex (MHC) alloantibody responses, and assess the ability of these antibodies to mediate platelet refractoriness.

Key words Platelet transfusion, Alloimmunization, Anti-MHC alloantibodies, Platelet refractoriness

1 Introduction

Blood transfusion is one of the most common sources of allogeneic exposure and represents a significant immunological event in the recipient. Transfusion of allogeneic platelets can expose the recipient to a range of donor alloantigens, the most immunogenic of which are the major histocompatibility complex (MHC) antigens also called human leukocyte antigens (HLA) in humans. Class I MHC is expressed at low levels on platelets as well as at high levels on any contaminating leukocytes. Class II MHC is expressed on a subset of contaminating leukoocytes, but not on the platelets themselves. Exposure to these alloantigens via platelet transfusion can result in alloimmunization including the production of alloantibodies. The measured prevalence varies considerably between studies with frequencies of alloimmunization ranging from 7% to 55% following platelet transfusion [1–10]. This risk can be significantly decreased through the use of leukoreduced platelets, as this

Sean R. Stowell and Connie M. Arthur (eds.), *Methods in Transfusion Medicine*, Methods in Molecular Biology, vol. 3053, https://doi.org/10.1007/978-1-0716-5376-0_3,

removes many of the contaminating leukoocytes, but even with leukoreduction alloimmunization remains common.

The presence of alloantibodies can mediate a range of negative outcomes in the recipient including platelet refractoriness and transplant rejection [1, 11–15]. MHC-antibody positive patients who are refractory to subsequent platelet transfusions are generally restricted to MHC-matched platelets which complicates and slows treatment and roughly doubles the per-unit cost of platelets. The presence of anti-MHC antibodies at the time of solid organ transplant can significantly increase the risk of acute rejection of the transplanted tissue, with antibodies against specific HLA loci associated with poor patient outcomes among different types of transplanted tissue [11, 16–19]. Pre-existing anti-MHC antibodies are also associated with a 7.47-fold increase in the failure of hematopoietic stem cell transplants [20]. Furthermore, if these recipients go on to donate blood in the future, the passive transfer of anti-MHC alloantibodies into new recipients is associated with transfusion-related acute lung injury (TRALI) [21, 22].

Evaluating alloimmunization and refractoriness in a clinical setting presents a range of complications. This includes the vast diversity of the MHC genes within populations, the relative inaccessibility of tissue samples, donor and blood product variability, and recipient variability. Recipient variability is broad and includes the number, types, and timing of units given, genetics, underlying health conditions, and additional treatments administered. Animal models help to address these limitations enabling a more controlled reductionist approach, with targeted evaluation of individual variables. Mice in particular offer the advantage of well-defined and controlled genetic backgrounds, well-characterized immune systems, access to different tissues, and wide range of available tools.

Here, we describe our mouse models of platelet alloimmunization and refractoriness. We have used these approaches to assess the relative immunogenicity of different blood products [23–29], the induction of alloimmune tolerance [23, 25, 27, 29, 30], and the impact of recipient health on alloimmunization [31, 32]. These approaches can be used both with commonly available wild-type mouse strains or adapted to a range of congenic or genetically manipulated mice as needed. We outline the basic approaches to preparing platelets for transfusion, measuring alloantibody responses targeting either class I or class II MHC, and evaluating the ability of these alloantibodies to mediate platelet refractoriness.

2 Materials

2.1 Leukoreduced/Non-leukoreduced Platelet Preparation

1. Citrate phosphate dextrose adenine-1 (CPDA-1) collected from WBF Double Blood Bag (Haemonetics).
2. Phosphate-buffered saline (PBS).
3. Lymphocyte separation medium (LSM) density: 1.077–1.080 g/mL (MP Bio).
4. Isoflurane.
5. Anesthesia machine (VetEquip).
6. Induction chamber.
7. Sterile tissue forceps.
8. White blood cell (WBC) syringe filter (Pall Acrodisc).
9. Sterile 5 mL mailing tube.

2.2 Platelet and WBC Counts in Platelet Preparations

1. Veterinary Hematology Analyzer (Heska HT5).

2.3 Transfusion

1. Sterile 27–30-gauge needles with 0.3–1 mL syringes (e.g., Becton Dickinson (BD) insulin syringe).
2. Heat lamp.
3. Mouse restrainer.
4. Clean cage with bedding.
5. Sterile gauze sponges.

2.4 Serum Collection (Non-terminal Samples)

1. 100 μL neutral capillary collection tubes (Sarstedt Minivette).
2. Eppendorf tubes.
3. Heat lamp.
4. Mouse restrainer.
5. Sterile scalpel blade.
6. Clean cage with bedding.
7. Sterile gauze sponges.

2.5 Serum Collection (Terminal Samples)

1. 2 mL microcentrifuge tubes.
2. Eppendorf tubes.
3. Isoflurane.
4. Anesthesia machine (VetEquip).
5. Induction chamber.
6. Sterile tissue forceps.

2.6 Passive Transfer of Alloantibodies

1. 3 mm 0.2 μm cellulose acetate membrane syringe filter (Corning).
2. 1 mL syringe (BD insulin syringe).
3. PBS.

2.7 Platelet Recovery

1. Scale.
2. Flow cytometer (5-laser Cytek Aurora).
3. EDTA capillary collection tubes (Sarstedt Minivette).
4. CD45-BV421 (104) (BD Biosciences).
5. TER-119-APC (TER-119) (BD Biosciences).
6. CD61-PE (2C9.G2) (BD Biosciences).
7. Green fluorescent protein $(GFP)^+$ platelets isolated as described in 2.1 from GFP^+ mice (*see* **Note 1**).
8. PBS.

2.8 Screen for Class I MHC-Specific Alloantibodies

1. Mouse spleen of same class I MHC type as donor.
2. Staining buffer: PBS, 2% fetal calf serum (FCS) or fetal bovine serum (FBS), sterilized through 0.22 μm filter.
3. Frosted slides (Fisher).
4. Petri dishes 60 × 15 mm (Falcon).
5. Cell strainer (100 μm).
6. Red blood cell (RBC) Lysis (BD Pharm Lyse) diluted 1:10 in deionized water.
7. Anti-mouse FcR blocking antibody (2.4G2) (BD Biosciences).
8. Serum samples to screen.
9. IgG3-BV421 (R40-82) (BD Biosciences).
10. IgG2b-PE (RMG2b-1) (BioLegend).
11. IgG2a-APC (RMG2a-62) (BioLegend) (*see* **Note 2**).
12. IgG1-AF488 (RMG1-1) (BioLegend).
13. IgM-PE-Cy7 (RMM-1) (BioLegend).
14. Igκ-APC-Cy7 (RMK-45) (BioLegend).
15. TCRβ-PCP-Cy5.5 (H57-597) (BioLegend).
16. B220-AF700 (RA3-6B2) (BioLegend).
17. Cell counter.
18. 96-well V-bottom plates.
19. Flow cytometer (5-laser Cytek Aurora).

2.9 Differentiation and Activation of Bone Marrow-Derived Dendritic Cells

1. PBS.
2. Beta 2 Microglobulin knock-out (KO) mouse (β2M) such as:

- C.129P2(B6)-$B2m^{tm1Unc}$/J RRID:IMSR_JAX:002420.
- B6.129P2-$B2m^{tm1Unc}$/DcrJ RRID:IMSR_JAX:002087.

3. Sterile petri dishes 100 × 15 mm (VWR).
4. Cell isolation medium dcR10: RPMI-1640, 10% FBS, 1% penicillin-streptomycin, 0.065% α-Monothioglycerol of 1% solution.
5. 10 μg/mL Recombinant Murine granulocyte-macrophage colony-stimulating factor (GM-CSF) (PeproTech).
6. 1 μg/mL Lipopolysaccharides (LPS) from Escherichia coli 0111:B4 (Sigma).

2.10 Screen for Class II MHC-Specific Alloantibodies

1. Class II MHC expressing cells (no class I) of same class II type as donor (refer to 2.9).
2. Staining buffer.
3. Anti-Mouse FcR blocking antibody (2.4G2) (BD Biosciences).
4. Live/Dead Fixable Blue stain (Invitrogen).
5. Serum samples to screen.
6. IgG3-BV421 (R40-82) (BD Biosciences).
7. IgG2b-PE (RMG2b-1) (BioLegend).
8. IgG2a-APC (RMG2a-62) (BioLegend) (*see* **Note 2**).
9. IgG1-AF488 (RMG1-1) (BioLegend).
10. IgM-PE-Cy7 (RMM-1) (BioLegend).
11. Igκ-APC-Cy7 (RMK-45) (BioLegend).
12. F4/80-AF700 (BM8) (BioLegend).
13. CD11c-PerCP-Cy5.5 (N418) (BioLegend).
14. Cell counter.
15. 96-well V-bottom plates.
16. Flow cytometer (5-laser Cytek Aurora).

3 Methods

3.1 Leukoreduced/Non-leukoreduced Platelet Preparation

1. Work using aseptic technique in a biosafety cabinet, and maintain the sample at room temperature during processing (*see* **Note 3**).
2. Add CPDA-1 at 14% of final blood volume to sterile 5 mL mailing tube (*see* **Note 4**).

3. Deeply anesthetize mice by isoflurane inhalation per manufacturer's instructions. Place the mouse inside the induction chamber and secure the lid. Confirm the mouse is under deep anesthesia by checking for a lack of response from a toe pinch.
4. Remove the mouse from the induction chamber.
5. Collect whole blood by exsanguination via orbital enucleation (*see* **Note 5**) into a 5 mL tube with 14% CPDA-1.
6. Euthanize the mouse by cervical dislocation (immediately euthanize mouse by cervical dislocation if mouse wakes from anesthesia during the procedure).
7. Filter blood with a WBC syringe filter per manufacturer's instructions (*see* **Note 6**). (For non-leukoreduced platelets, skip this step)
8. Transfer blood to a 15 mL conical tube.
9. Centrifuge at 200 × g for 15 min (reduced acceleration and deceleration are preferred but not required).
10. Transfer the upper layer (platelets and plasma), the center buffy coat layer (containing platelets and WBCs when present), and top of the bottom layer (RBCs) to a new 15 mL tube.
11. Centrifuge at 200 × g for 15 min.
12. Transfer as much of the clean platelet/plasma layer (top layer) as possible to a new 15 mL tube while avoiding the buffy coat and RBCs and set aside. Measure this platelet/plasma volume.
13. Bring the total volume of the residual tube containing the buffy coat to 10 mL by adding sterile PBS. Then underlayer with 2 mL LSM.
14. Centrifuge this buffy coat tube at 500 × g for 15 min with no brake and low acceleration.
15. Transfer the buffy coat layer into a new 15 mL tube.
16. Wash buffy coat cells with PBS: bring the total volume to 15 mL with PBS, and centrifuge at 500 × g for 5 min with max brake and max acceleration.
17. Discard supernatant and resuspend buffy coat cell pellet in previously isolated platelet/plasma fraction.
18. For non-leukoreduced platelet preparation, if additional WBCs are required, some can be recovered from the RBC fraction left behind at **step 10** by repeating **steps 13–17** on these residual RBCs.

3.2 Platelet and WBC Counts in Platelet Preparations (see Note 7)

1. Aliquot 50 μL non-leukoreduced or leukoreduced platelets into microtube.
2. Count on a hematology analyzer.

   or

3. Count lymphocytes on hemacytometer.
4. Count platelets on flow cytometer with counting beads.

3.3 Transfusion (see Note 8)

1. Warm the recipient mouse under a heat lamp for 3–5 min under observation to dilate the tail vein.
2. Place mouse in a restrainer.
3. Prepare a syringe with 100 μL of prepared platelets (*see* Subheading 3.1).
4. Inject platelets intravenously into mouse through lateral tail vein.
5. Apply gentle pressure to the wound with gauze for 30–45 s to stop bleeding.
6. Return the mouse to a clean cage and observe for 10–15 min.

3.4 Serum Collection (Non-terminal Samples)

1. Warm the mouse under a heat lamp for 3–5 min.
2. Place mouse in restrainer.
3. Cut 1–2 mm from the distal tail at an angle perpendicular to the work surface using a sterile scalpel blade.
4. Collect blood with a capillary tube without anticoagulant and transfer it to an Eppendorf tube. Apply gentle pressure to the wound with gauze for 30–45 s to stop bleeding.
5. Return mouse to a clean cage and observe for 10–15 min.
6. Allow blood to clot at room temperature for 20–30 min.
7. Centrifuge at 10,000 × g for 10 min.
8. Transfer as much serum as possible (it is fine to include some RBCs at this step) to a new Eppendorf tube.
9. Centrifuge at 10,000 × g for 10 min.
10. Transfer the clean serum (avoid the RBC pellet) to a new tube.
11. Aliquot and freeze the serum at −80 °C until ready to use. Avoid excessive freeze/thaw cycles.

3.5 Serum Collection (Terminal Samples)

1. Deeply anesthetize the mouse by isoflurane inhalation (*see* Subheading 3.1, **step 3**).
2. Collect whole blood by exsanguination via orbital enucleation into a 2 mL tube.
3. At the end of the procedure or upon any sign of waking, euthanize the mouse by cervical dislocation.
4. Allow blood to clot for 20–30 min.

5. Centrifuge at 10,000 × g for 10 min.
6. Transfer as much serum as possible (it is fine to include some RBCs at this step) to new Eppendorf tube.
7. Centrifuge at 10,000 × g for 10 min.
8. Transfer clean serum (avoid RBC pellet) to new tube.
9. Aliquot and freeze serum at −80 °C until ready to use. Avoid excessive freeze/thaws.

3.6 Passive Transfer of Alloantibodies

1. Thaw serum, if needed.
2. Sterile filter serum through a 0.2 μm cellulose acetate membrane.
3. Dilute serum with PBS to desired final concentration (*see* **Note 9**).
4. Immediately after transfusion, inject 400 μL diluted serum into the mouse via intraperitoneal injection.

3.7 Platelet Recovery

1. Transfuse mouse as previously described in Subheading 3.3 with GFP^+ platelets (*see* **Note 1**).
2. At 24 h or the desired time point, collect a drop of blood by tail snip using EDTA capillary tubes.
3. Dilute blood by adding 500 μL PBS and mix.
4. Stain 100 μL of diluted blood with 0.5 μL BV421-CD45, 0.5 μL APC-TER-119, and 0.5 μL PE-CD61 antibodies.
5. Analyze by flow cytometry (Fig. 1). Collect a minimum of 10^5 platelet events.
6. Calculate number of platelets expected by multiplying concentration of platelets (*see* **Note 10**) × weight of mouse × 80 μL/g (*see* **Note 11**).
7. Calculate percent recovery by dividing $\%GFP^+$ observed by the percent expected (*see* **Note 12**).

3.8 Screen for Class I MHC-Specific Alloantibodies.

1. Collect the spleen from a donor-type mouse and place it in 5 mL of cold staining buffer in a 15 mL tube. Keep on ice (*see* **Note 13**).
2. Transfer the spleen and staining buffer in a petri dish on ice. Homogenize the spleen between the frosted sides of two frosted slides.
3. Pass cells through a 100 μM cell strainer into a 50 mL tube. Rinse dish and slides with 5 mL cold staining buffer, then pass through the strainer. Transfer cells to a 15 mL tube.
4. Centrifuge at 500 × g for 5 min at 4 °C. Discard the supernatant and resuspend in 1 mL RBC lysis.

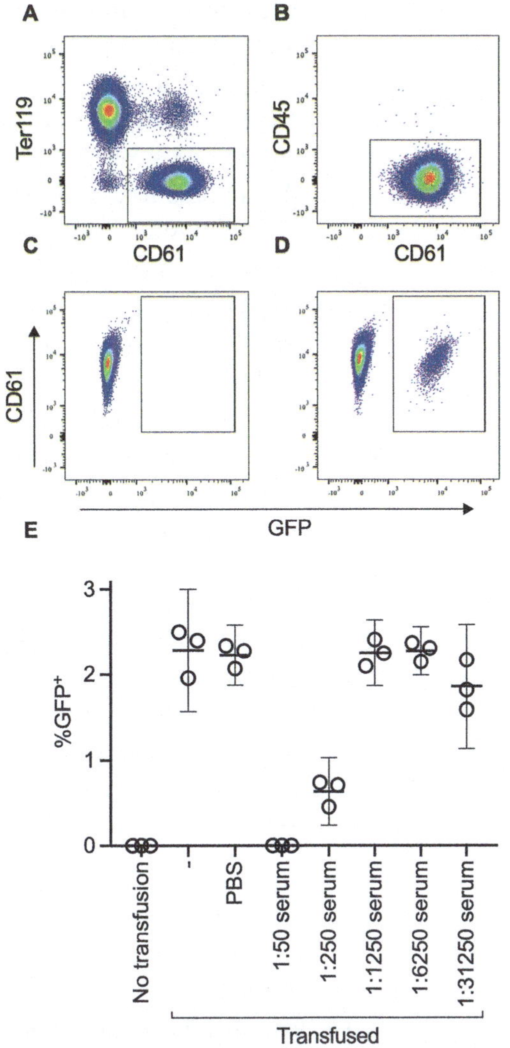

Fig. 1 Detecting platelet refractoriness. Naïve BALB/c mice were given either nothing (-) or a 400 μL intraperitoneal injection of either PBS or diluted serum collected from BALB/c mice that were transfused with B6 platelets, along with a GFP^+ B6 platelet transfusion. A whole blood sample was collected from each mouse 24 h later. Blood was stained with anti-Ter-119 to detect red blood cells, anti-CD61 to detect platelets, and anti-CD45 to detect lymphocytes. A broad FSC/SSC gate was used first (not shown). (**a**) Cells were then gated on $Ter\text{-}119^-CD61^+$ events, then (**b**) on $CD45^-CD61^+$ events to identify platelets, and then the frequency of GFP^+ events within the platelet population was evaluated (%GFP^+). (**c**) An example of a stain from a non-transfused control mouse. (**d**) An example of a stain from a transfusion only control mouse. (**e**) Plots the frequency of GFP^+ donor platelets within the platelet gate by group with means and 95% confidence intervals. For this serum sample, the 1:50 dilution results in complete rejection of platelets, with partial rejection at 1:250, and no rejection with further dilution.

5. Incubate at room temperature for 1 min. Wash cells by bringing the volume up to 14 mL with staining buffer.
6. Centrifuge at 500 × g for 5 min at 4 °C. Discard the supernatant and resuspend with the residual liquid. While resuspending, remove insoluble cell debris. Keep on ice.
7. Measure the total volume and add staining buffer to bring the final volume to 2 mL. Count cells.
8. Adjust to a final concentration of 10^7 cells/mL.
9. Aliquot the total needed volume for experiment and add FcR blocking antibody to cell suspension (1:100). Incubate at 4 °C for 15 min.
10. Aliquot 100 μL of cells per well into a 96-well V-bottom plate for a total of 10^6 cells per well.
11. Prepare serum samples by thawing on ice and vortexing vigorously for 15–30 s. Dilute serum in staining buffer 1:16 (*see* **Note 14**).
12. Centrifuge plate at 500 × g for 5 min at 4 °C. Discard supernatant and resuspend cells in 100 μL diluted serum.
13. Incubate at 4 °C for 45 min. Wash the plate twice and decant the supernatant after each wash.
14. Prepare a cocktail mix of antibodies, including BV421-IgG3 at 2 μL/1 × 10^6 cells, PE-IgG2b at 2 μL/1 × 10^6 cells, APC-IgG2a at 2 μL/1 × 10^6 cells, AF488-IgG1 at 0.25 μL/1 × 10^6 cells, PE-Cy7-IgM at 2 μL/1 × 10^6 cells, APC-Cy7-Igκ at 2 μL/1 × 10^6 cells, PCP-Cy5.5-TCRβ at 0.5 μL/1 × 10^6 cells, AF700-B220 at 0.25 μL/1 × 10^6 cells into 89 μL cold staining buffer. Dilutions should be based on titrations of each antibody.
15. Resuspend cells in 100 μL of the antibody cocktail.
16. Incubate at 4 °C for 30 mins in dark. Wash the plate twice and decant supernatant after each wash.
17. Resuspend cells in 100 μL staining buffer.
18. Analyze by flow cytometry collecting at least 10,000 T cell events (Fig. 2).

3.9 Differentiation and Activation of Bone Marrow-Derived Dendritic Cells

1. Euthanize the β2M KO mouse and collect bone marrow cells using cold PBS into a 15 mL tube as previously described [33]. Keep on ice. Break up clumps and let them settle. Transfer the cell suspension to a new 15 mL tube.
2. Centrifuge at 500 × g for 5 min at 4 °C. Discard supernatant and resuspend cells in 2 mL dcR10. Count the cells.
3. Suspend cells at a concentration of 2 × 10^6 cells/mL.

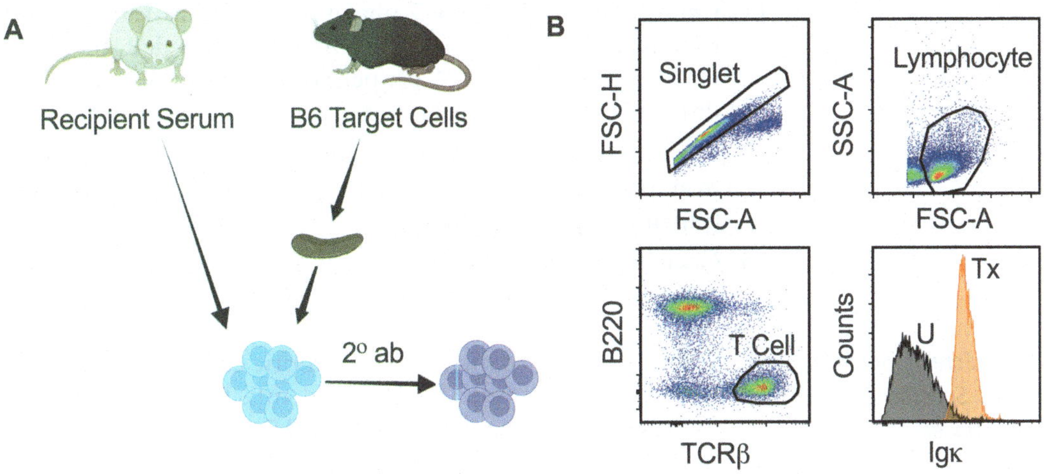

Fig. 2 Detection of anti-class I MHC antibodies. (**a**) Serum from recipient BALB/c mice was used as a primary stain on B6 splenic T cells as target cells, followed by a secondary antibody (2°ab) stain with a cocktail of α-B220, α-TCRβ, α-Igκ, α-IgM, α-IgG1, α-IgG2a, α-IgG2b, and α-IgG3 antibodies to detect total (Igκ) and isotype-specific alloantibodies by flow cytometry. (**b**) Cells were gated on singlet, lymphocyte, and then T cells ($B220^{-}/TCR\beta^{+}$) to identify bound alloantibodies on a BCR^{-}/class II MHC^{-} population that expresses class I MHC. Examples of the signal for the α-Igκ (total) alloantibodies are shown for untreated (U) and transfused (Tx) mice. (This work was originally published in Frontiers in Immunology, Copyright © 2023 Tran, Muench, Gaillard, Darst, Tomayko and Jackman [31])

4. Add 45 mL dcR10, 5 mL cells, and 100 μL GM-CSF to 50 mL tube. Add 10 mL per petri dish. Put in the incubator at 37 °C.
5. After 72 h, replenish cells by adding 10 mL of warm dcR10 with 20 μL GM-CSF to each petri dish. Return to the incubator at 37 °C.
6. After another 72 h, replenish cells by removing 10 mL from each petri dish into a 50 mL tube.
7. Centrifuge this removed volume at 300 × g for 7 min at room temperature to recover the cells. Discard the supernatant and resuspend cells with 10 mL warm dcR10 and 20 μL GM-CSF per petri dish. Add this cell suspension back to the petri dishes and return to the incubator at 37 °C.
8. After another 48 h, replenish cells by removing 10 mL from each petri dish into a 50 mL tube.
9. Centrifuge this removed volume at 300 × g for 7 min at room temperature to recover the cells. Discard the supernatant and resuspend with 10 mL warm dcR10 and 20 μL GM-CSF per petri dish. Add this cell suspension back to the petri dishes and return to the incubator at 37 °C.
10. After another 48 h, collect non-adherent cells from petri dish into 50 mL tubes.

11. Centrifuge at 300 × g for 7 min at room temperature. Discard supernatant and resuspend with 10 mL warm dcR10, 10 μL GM-CSF, and 10 μL LPS per petri dish. Plate cells in new petri dish with 10 mL per plate. Put in the incubator at 37 °C.
12. After 24 h, collect all non-adherent or loosely adherent cells from petri dish surface by rigorous washing into 50 mL tube (pipetting up and down).
13. Centrifuge at 500 × g for 5 min at 4 °C. Discard supernatant and resuspend with 2 mL cold staining buffer. Count cells.

3.10 Screen for Class II MHC-Specific Alloantibodies

1. Suspend bone marrow-derived dendritic cells (*see* Subheading 3.9) at a concentration of 10^7 cells/mL. Centrifuge, decant, and resuspend if necessary (*see* **Note 15**).
2. Aliquot the total needed volume for the experiment and add FcR blocking antibody to the cell suspension (1:100). Add live/dead blue to the cell suspension (1:1000). Incubate in the dark for 15 min at room temperature.
3. Aliquot 100 μL of cells per well into 96-well V-bottom plate to achieve 10^6 cells per well.
4. Prepare serum samples by thawing serum on ice and vortexing vigorously for 15–30 s. Dilute serum in staining buffer 1:16 (*see* **Note 14**).
5. Centrifuge plate at 500 × g for 5 min at 4 °C. Discard supernatant and resuspend cells in 100 μL diluted serum.
6. Incubate at 4 °C for 45 min. Wash plate twice and decant supernatant after each wash.
7. Prepare a cocktail mix of antibodies including BV421-IgG3 at 2 μL/1 × 10^6 cells, PE-IgG2b at 2 μL/1 × 10^6 cells, APC-IgG2a at 2 μL/1 × 10^6 cells, AF488-IgG1 at 0.25 μL/1 × 10^6 cells, PE-Cy7-IgM at 2 uL/1 × 10^6 cells, APC-Cy7-Igκ at 2 μL/1 × 10^6 cells, AF700-F4/80 at 1 μL/1 × 10^6 cells, PCP-Cy5.5-CD11c at 1 μL/1 × 10^6 cells into 87.75 μL/1 × 10^6 cells cold staining buffer. Dilutions should be based on titrations of each antibody. Resuspend cells in 100 μL antibody cocktail.
8. Incubate at 4 °C for 30 mins in dark. Wash plate twice and decant supernatant after each wash.
9. Resuspend cells in 100 μL staining buffer.
10. Analyze by flow cytometry collecting at least 1000 dendritic cells events (Fig. 3).

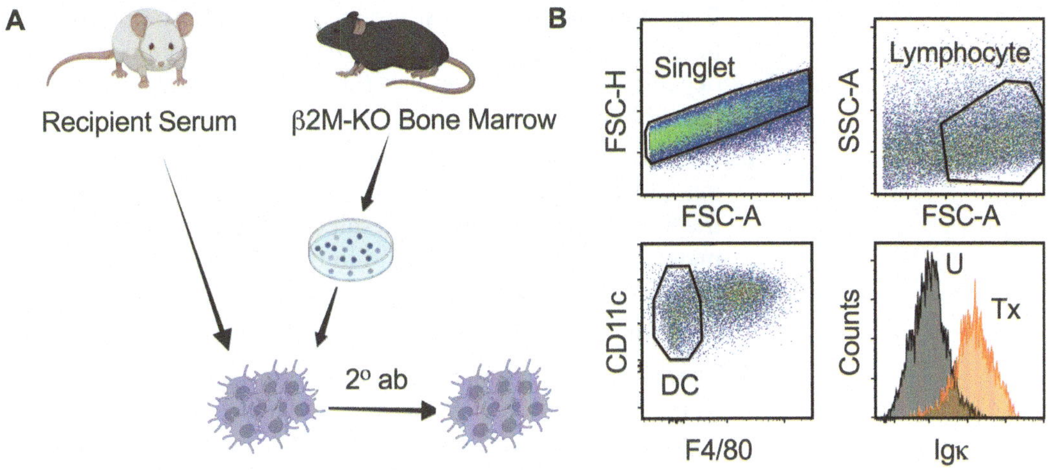

Fig. 3 Detection of anti-class II MHC antibodies. Protocol was similar to anti-class I MHC-antibody screen (Fig. 2) except cultured dendritic cells (DC) from the bone marrow of β2M-KO B6 mice were used as target cells. (B) Cells were gated on singlet, lymphocyte, and then dendritic cells ($CD11c^+/F4/80^-$) to identify bound alloantibodies on a class I MHC^-/class II MHC^+ population. Examples of the signal for the α-Igκ (total) alloantibodies are shown for untreated (U) and transfused (Tx) mice. (This work was originally published in Frontiers in Immunology, Copyright © 2023 Tran, Muench, Gaillard, Darst, Tomayko and Jackman [31])

4 Notes

1. The original GFP mice under the ubiquitin promoter were made on a B6 background (Jackson Labs stock # 004353) and were then crossed back onto a BALB/c background (Jackson Labs stock # 007076). Years later it was discovered that these BALB/c GFP mice were all H-2^b as the GFP had inserted in the MHC locus [34]. This mouse has now been remade on a BALB/c background with the correct H-2^d MHC and is available from Jackson Labs (stock # 034677).
2. Per BioLegend technical data sheet, this anti-IgG2a antibody clone is cross-reactive to both IgG2a (found in BALB/c) and IgG2c (found in B6).
3. Platelets are sensitive to temperature and handling, so care should be taken to keep at room temperature and minimize handling to prevent activation and other functional changes. This is why slower centrifugation speeds are used. Platelet preparations should also be mixed gently by hand avoiding more aggressive techniques such as vortexing.
4. The 14% CPDA-1 is important to prevent clotting. Tubes are prepared prior to blood collection with the volume of CPDA-1 needed to achieve 14% of the total collected volume. For example, for a final blood collection volume of 3 mL, prepare a tube with 420 μL CPDA-1.

5. Collecting blood via cardiac puncture can also be performed; however, this approach generally yields less volume, is more dependent on the skill level of the technician, and may result in more hemolysis.
6. If leukoreduction filters are not available, a leukoreduced product can be made by simply not adding back the buffy coat fraction. However, this will result in a lower platelet count as many of the platelets are found in the buffy coat layer.
7. For C57Bl/6 (B6) and BALB/c mice, typical yields are approximately 3–5 × 10^8 platelets/mL and 5×10^6 WBCs/mL.
8. There can be variability in the immunogenicity of different strain combinations. We have found more potent responses transfusing B6 platelets into BALB/c recipients compared with the inverse. This is despite the higher number of allogeneic alleles going from BALB/c donors into B6 recipients (K^d, D^d, L^d, I-A^d, and I-E^d) versus from B6 donors to BALB/c recipients (K^b, D^b, and I-A^b due to null alleles at L and I-E in B6 mice).
9. Considerations when calculating volume of serum to transfer. We assume a total blood volume of ~1.6 mL and that the serum is approximately half of that total volume, so administration of 400 μL undiluted serum is approximately equivalent to half of the total antibody in the donor mouse. It is suggested that a dose titration be done to determine best dilution and allow one to compare different groups for efficacy as shown in Fig. 1. 400 μL is a reasonable intraperitoneal injection volume for most mice, but this can be adjusted up or down based on dosing needs, animal size, and locally approved animal protocols.
10. The concentration of platelets based on strain can be found at https://phenome.jax.org.
11. Assuming an average total blood volume of a mouse at about 77–80 μL/g [35, 36].
12. Others have used a slightly different approach to assess platelet recovery using tracer RBCs as a reference population. For details see Waterman et al. 2016 [37].
13. For class I MHC expressing target cells, we typically use standard donor-type splenic T cells. These cells do express additional minor antigens beyond the class I MHC, and this can be addressed using congenic mice with donor MHC type on a recipient background. We have done this and compared the minor and major responses and found that the bulk of the response is directed against MHC [27] and therefore feel comfortable using the standard donor-type mice for these evaluations in most scenarios. Peak total antibody responses

are usually around 2 weeks post-exposure for primary responses and around 1-week post-exposure for secondary responses. The kinetics vary slightly for specific isotypes, with IgM peaking earlier and some IgG subsets peaking slightly later with additional variation possible between mouse strains.

14. We use a 1:16 dilution of serum for most of our assays based on initial titrations. Further titrations of samples may be warranted in different settings.
15. Class II MHC molecules are found on dendritic cells, macrophages, and B lymphocytes. As the 10-day dendritic cell cultures are somewhat cumbersome, we have investigated other approaches for generating large numbers of class II MHC expressing cells from our β2m KO mice to use as target cells. B cells are present in the highest numbers but cannot be used, as they all express Ig on their cell surface and would stain positive for many of the secondary reagents regardless of the presence or absence of alloantibody. We have attempted to collect peritoneal macrophages after triggering their recruitment with thioglycolate injection [38, 39], which does increase the yield of harvested peritoneal macrophages, but we found that in our hands, these recruited cells express little to no class II MHC.

Conflict of Interest

This study was funded by NIH NHLBI grant numbers R01 HL144501 and R01 HL133024, and a research grant to Rachael Jackman from Terumo BCT.

References

1. Howard JE, Perkins HA (1978) The natural history of alloimmunization to platelets. Transfusion 18(4):496–503
2. (1997) Leukocyte reduction and ultraviolet B irradiation of platelets to prevent alloimmunization and refractoriness to platelet transfusions. The Trial to Reduce Alloimmunization to Platelets Study Group. N Engl J Med 337(26):1861–1869
3. Andreu G, Fressy P (1995) Transfusion-associated graft-versus-host disease (TA-GVHD): cellular mechanisms and their possible modulation by ultraviolet radiation. Transfus Sci 16(2):109–113
4. Dutcher JP, Schiffer CA, Aisner J, Wiernik PH (1981) Alloimmunization following platelet transfusion: the absence of a dose-response relationship. Blood 57(3):395–398
5. Fauchet R, Genetet B, Gueguen M, Leguerrier A, Rioux C, Logeais Y (1982) Transfusion therapy and HLA antibody response in patients undergoing open heart surgery. Transfusion 22(4):320–322
6. Fisher M, Chapman JR, Ting A, Morris PJ (1985) Alloimmunisation to HLA antigens following transfusion with leucocyte-poor and purified platelet suspensions. Vox Sang 49(5): 331–335
7. Karpinski M, Pochinco D, Dembinski I, Laidlaw W, Zacharias J, Nickerson P (2004) Leukocyte reduction of red blood cell transfusions does not decrease allosensitization rates in potential kidney transplant candidates. J Am Soc Nephrol 15(3):818–824
8. Murphy MF, Metcalfe P, Thomas H, Eve J, Ord J, Lister TA et al (1986) Use of

leucocyte-poor blood components and HLA-matched-platelet donors to prevent HLA alloimmunization. Br J Haematol 62(3): 529–534

9. Schiffer CA, Dutcher JP, Aisner J, Hogge D, Wiernik PH, Reilly JP (1983) A randomized trial of leukocyte-depleted platelet transfusion to modify alloimmunization in patients with leukemia. Blood 62(4):815–820

10. van Marwijk Kooy M, van Prooijen HC, Moes M, Bosma-Stants I, Akkerman JW (1991) Use of leukocyte-depleted platelet concentrates for the prevention of refractoriness and primary HLA alloimmunization: a prospective, randomized trial. Blood 77(1): 201–205

11. Itescu S, Tung TC, Burke EM, Weinberg A, Moazami N, Artrip JH et al (1998) Preformed IgG antibodies against major histocompatibility complex class II antigens are major risk factors for high-grade cellular rejection in recipients of heart transplantation. Circulation 98(8):786–793

12. Massad MG, Cook DJ, Schmitt SK, Smedira NG, McCarthy JF, Vargo RL et al (1997) Factors influencing HLA sensitization in implantable LVAD recipients. Ann Thorac Surg 64(4): 1120–1125

13. Moazami N, Itescu S, Williams MR, Argenziano M, Weinberg A, Oz MC (1998) Platelet transfusions are associated with the development of anti-major histocompatibility complex class I antibodies in patients with left ventricular assist support. J Heart Lung Transplant 17(9):876–880

14. Slichter SJ, Davis K, Enright H, Braine H, Gernsheimer T, Kao KJ et al (2005) Factors affecting posttransfusion platelet increments, platelet refractoriness, and platelet transfusion intervals in thrombocytopenic patients. Blood 105(10):4106–4114

15. Tsau PH, Arabia FA, Toporoff B, Paramesh V, Sethi GK, Copeland JG (1998) Positive panel reactive antibody titers in patients bridged to transplantation with a mechanical assist device: risk factors and treatment. ASAIO J 44(5): M634–M637

16. Schulman LL, Weinberg AD, McGregor C, Galantowicz ME, Suciu-Foca NM, Itescu S (1998) Mismatches at the HLA-DR and HLA-B loci are risk factors for acute rejection after lung transplantation. Am J Respir Crit Care Med 157(6 Pt 1):1833–1837. https://doi.org/10.1164/ajrccm.157.6.9707007

17. Palmer SM, Davis RD, Hadjiliadis D, Hertz MI, Howell DN, Ward FE et al (2002) Development of an antibody specific to major histocompatibility antigens detectable by flow cytometry after lung transplant is associated with bronchiolitis obliterans syndrome. Transplantation 74(6):799–804. https://doi.org/10.1097/01.TP.0000028254.63164.53

18. Reinsmoen NL (2002) Cellular methods used to evaluate the immune response in transplantation. Tissue Antigens 59(4):241–250

19. Sundaresan S, Mohanakumar T, Smith MA, Trulock EP, Lynch J, Phelan D et al (1998) HLA-A locus mismatches and development of antibodies to HLA after lung transplantation correlate with the development of bronchiolitis obliterans syndrome. Transplantation 65(5): 648–653

20. Xie Y, Parekh J, Tang Z, Wu D, Wu X (2021) Donor-specific antibodies and primary graft failure in allogeneic hematopoietic stem cell transplantation: a systematic review and meta-analysis. Transplant Cell Ther 27(8):687 e1–687 e7. https://doi.org/10.1016/j.jtct.2021.04.030

21. Toy P, Lowell C (2007) TRALI--definition, mechanisms, incidence and clinical relevance. Best Pract Res Clin Anaesthesiol 21(2): 183–193

22. Popovsky MA, Moore SB (1985) Diagnostic and pathogenetic considerations in transfusion-related acute lung injury. Transfusion 25(6):573–577

23. Jackman RP, Heitman JW, Muench MO (2020) A small allelic variant in donor class I MHC is sufficient to induce alloantibodies following transfusion of standard or pathogen-reduced platelets in mice. Vox Sang 115(5): 367–376. https://doi.org/10.1111/vox.12897

24. Jackman RP, Muench MO, Heitman JW, Inglis HC, Law JP, Marschner S et al (2013) Immune modulation and lack of alloimmunization following transfusion with pathogen-reduced platelets in mice. Transfusion 53(11):2697–2709. https://doi.org/10.1111/trf.12133

25. Jackman RP, Muench MO, Inglis H, Heitman JW, Marschner S, Goodrich RP et al (2017) Reduced MHC alloimmunization and partial tolerance protection with pathogen reduction of whole blood. Transfusion 57(2):337–348. https://doi.org/10.1111/trf.13895

26. Muench MO, Heitman JW, Inglis H, Fomin ME, Marschner S, Goodrich RP et al (2016) Reduced alloimmunization in mice following repeated transfusion with pathogen-reduced platelets. Transfusion 56(6):1419–1429. https://doi.org/10.1111/trf.13579

27. Tran JQ, Muench MO, Heitman JW, Jackman RP (2019) Allogeneic major histocompatibility complex antigens are necessary and sufficient

for partial tolerance induced by transfusion of pathogen reduced platelets in mice. Vox Sang 114(3):207–215. https://doi.org/10.1111/vox.12756

28. Tran JQ, Muench MO, Heitman JW, Jackman RP (2019) Pathogen reduction with riboflavin and ultraviolet light induces a quasi-apoptotic state in blood leukocytes. Transfusion.. in press

29. Tran JQ, Muench MO, Jackman RP (2020) Pathogen-reduced PRP blocks T-cell activation, induces Treg cells, and promotes TGF-beta expression by cDCs and monocytes in mice. Blood Adv 4(21):5547–5561. https://doi.org/10.1182/bloodadvances.2020002867

30. Tran JQ, Muench MO, Heitman JW, Jackman RP (2019) Pathogen reduction with riboflavin and ultraviolet light induces a quasi-apoptotic state in blood leukocytes. Transfusion 59(11): 3501–3510. https://doi.org/10.1111/trf.15516

31. Tran JQ, Muench MO, Gaillard B, Darst O, Tomayko MM, Jackman RP (2023) Polyinosinic: polycytidylic acid induced inflammation enhances while lipopolysaccharide diminishes alloimmunity to platelet transfusion in mice. Front Immunol 14:1281130. https://doi.org/10.3389/fimmu.2023.1281130

32. Jackman RP, Darst O, Gaillard B, Tran JQ, Tomayko MM, Muench MO (2023) Enhanced alloresponse to platelet transfusion due to immune dysregulation following ablative chemotherapy in mice. Front Immunol 14. https://doi.org/10.3389/fimmu.2023.1281123

33. Mahajan MM, Cheng B, Beyer AI, Mulvaney US, Wilkinson MB, Fomin ME et al (2015) A quantitative assessment of the content of hematopoietic stem cells in mouse and human endosteal-bone marrow: a simple and rapid method for the isolation of mouse central bone marrow. BMC Hematol 15:9. https://doi.org/10.1186/s12878-015-0031-7

34. Liu S, Lockhart JR, Fontenard S, Berlett M, Ryan TM (2020) Mapping the chromosomal insertion site of the GFP transgene of UBC-GFP mice to the MHC locus. J Immunol 204(7):1982–1987. https://doi.org/10.4049/jimmunol.1901338

35. Mitruka BM, Rawnsley HM (1981) Clinical biochemical and hematological reference values in normal experimental animals and normal humans. Masson Pub. USA

36. Harkness JE, Wagner JE (1989) The biology and medicine of rabbits and rodents, 3rd edn. Lea & Febiger

37. Waterman HR, Kapp LM, Munday A, Odem-Davis K, Zimring JC (2016) Transfusion-induced alloimmunization and platelet refractoriness in a mouse model: mechanisms and interventions. Transfusion 56(1):91–100. https://doi.org/10.1111/trf.13270

38. Ray A, Dittel BN (2010) Isolation of mouse peritoneal cavity cells. J Vis Exp (35). https://doi.org/10.3791/1488

39. Ghosn EE, Cassado AA, Govoni GR, Fukuhara T, Yang Y, Monack DM et al (2010) Two physically, functionally, and developmentally distinct peritoneal macrophage subsets. Proc Natl Acad Sci USA 107(6): 2568–2573. https://doi.org/10.1073/pnas.0915000107

Chapter 4

Generation and Use of an Alloantigen-Specific Preclinical Humanized Mouse Model of Fetal and Neonatal Alloimmune Thrombocytopenia

Huiying Zhi, Debra K. Newman, and Peter J. Newman

Abstract

Fetal/neonatal alloimmune thrombocytopenia (FNAIT) is a life-threatening bleeding disorder caused by maternal antibodies targeting a paternally inherited alloantigen present on the surface of fetal platelets. The human platelet alloantigen HPA-1a/HPA-1b, also known as the Pl^{A1}/Pl^{A2} alloantigen, is the most frequently implicated HPA for causing FNAIT in Caucasians. A single Leu33Pro amino acid polymorphism residing within the plexin/semaphorin/integrin (PSI) domain of the integrin β3 subunit (platelet membrane glycoprotein (GP), GPIIIa) is responsible for generating the HPA-1a and HPA-1b epitopes. In mice, the GPIIIa gene encodes a glutamine at position 33, making it challenging to model the alloimmune response, thereby hindering studies on the underlying mechanisms and therapeutic interventions of this alloimmune disorder. This chapter outlines the development and use of a humanized, alloantigen-specific preclinical mouse model of FNAIT, aiming to advance basic and translational research in this field. Basic protocols are provided for (1) generating an HPA-1a transgenic mouse by introducing humanized residues $A_{30}P_{32}L_{33}D_{39}$ within the PSI domain and Q_{470} in the EGF1 domain of mouse integrin β3 using CRISPR/Cas9 gene editing technology, (2) developing a preclinical alloantigen-specific humanized mouse model of FNAIT using the HPA-1a transgenic APLDQ mice, and (3) examining the efficacy of a prophylactic treatment regimen in preventing alloimmunization and FNAIT development using this alloantigen-specific mouse model. This humanized mouse model faithfully recapitulates many clinically important aspects of human FNAIT, serving as a valuable tool for studying the pathophysiological mechanisms underlying the alloimmune response and assessing prophylactic and therapeutic interventions in translational research.

Key words Fetal/neonatal alloimmune thrombocytopenia (FNAIT), Human platelet alloantigen (HPA), Alloimmune response, Integrin β3 subunit, Humanized mouse model, Therapeutic reagents

1 Introduction

Fetal/neonatal alloimmune thrombocytopenia (FNAIT) is a rare but severe alloimmune bleeding disorder, impacting approximately 1 in 350 pregnancies [1, 2]. This condition arises when maternal alloantibodies specifically target fetal platelet alloantigen inherited from the father, resulting in significant destruction of fetal/

Sean R. Stowell and Connie M. Arthur (eds.), *Methods in Transfusion Medicine*, Methods in Molecular Biology, vol. 3053, https://doi.org/10.1007/978-1-0716-5376-0_4,

neonatal platelets [3, 4]. The severity of the disease can vary, with mild cases of thrombocytopenia remaining asymptomatic and resolving without complications, while severe thrombocytopenia can result in life-threatening bleeding during the fetal and neonatal stages. Severe thrombocytopenia occurs in nearly one-third of FNAIT cases, affecting approximately 1 in 1000 to 2500 live births [5, 6]. The severe cases may result in spontaneous or trauma-induced intracranial hemorrhage (ICH), often leading to neurological complications, lifelong disabilities, or even a fatal outcome [7]. Unfortunately, there is currently no preventive treatment for FNAIT. Intravenous immunoglobulin (IVIG), sometimes with concomitant immunosuppressive therapy, is used off-label to prevent thrombocytopenia in subsequent pregnancies for mothers who have previously delivered a baby affected by FNAIT [8, 9].

The fundamental cause of FNAIT lies in the incompatibility between a maternal and fetal human platelet alloantigen (HPA). Naturally occurring amino acid polymorphisms in platelet surface membrane glycoproteins (GPs) are responsible for provoking the alloimmune response in most cases of FNAIT. Over the past six decades, extensive research has identified 37 distinct heritable HPAs distributed across six different glycoproteins (GPs): GPIIb, GPIIIa, GPIbα, GPIbβ, GPIa, and CD109 [1, 10]. Among these, HPA-1a/1b is the most clinically significant cause of FNAIT in the US, accounting for ~80% of FNAIT cases. It is also often linked to ICH and other adverse pregnancy outcomes. The HPA-1a/1b polymorphism is determined by a single amino acid difference at position 33 within the PSI domain of GPIIIa (also known as the integrin β3 subunit) [11]. The HPA-1a allele encodes a leucine at position 33 (L33), whereas HPA-1b encodes a proline (P33). In Caucasians, the allele frequencies for HPA-1a and HPA-1b are 85% and 15%, respectively, with approximately 2% being homozygous for HPA-1b. HPA-1a alloimmunization is strongly associated with the *HLA-DRB3* 01:01 gene* [12–14]. *Approximately* 28% of Caucasians carry the HLA-DRB3*01:01 allele [15]. HPA-1b/b women who are *HLA-DRB3*01:01 positive are at a 25 times higher risk of immunization compared to those who are HLA-DRB3**01:01 negative [16]. The discovery of HPA-1a/1b and associated risk factors has facilitated the development and utilization of molecular genetic technologies for diagnosing FNAIT. A comprehensive understanding of the etiology of FNAIT is essential for developing specific and effective strategies to treat or prevent the condition.

Understanding the etiology of maternal alloimmunization in human patients, especially during pregnancies involving women, fetuses, and neonates, is challenging due to ethical and practical constraints. Mouse models have become invaluable surrogates for studying FNAIT. In mice, the GPIIIa gene encodes glutamine at position 33, making it unsuitable for modeling the alloimmune response. Nevertheless, several animal models have been developed for studying FNAIT. Ni and colleagues were the first to demonstrate that integrin β3-knockout mice develop β3-specific isoantibodies upon injection with wild-type mouse platelets expressing murine integrin β3 [17]. These polyclonal isoantibodies were able to cross the placenta and induce thrombocytopenia in β3-expressing pups [18]. Bakchoul et al. developed a transfusion model by infusing human platelets into immunodeficient NOD/SCID mice to investigate antiplatelet therapeutics [19]. Ghevaert et al. transduced the bone marrow in GPIIIa-deficient mice with a lentiviral vector encoding the human GPIIIa Leu33 allelic isoform, allowing HPA-1a expression, providing a valuable tool to assess therapeutic approaches for FNAIT [20]. These FNAIT mouse models have been invaluable in studying FNAIT, substantially contributing to our understanding of its pathogenesis and aiding in the preclinical evaluation of therapeutic and preventive strategies. However, their inherent limitations in accurately replicating the nature of human alloimmune response hinder the study of underlying mechanisms and the assessment of alloantigen-specific reagents for the prevention or treatment of FNAIT, as well as the translation of these results to the human setting.

To overcome the limitations of previous models, we developed an alloantigen-specific humanized murine model. Using CRISPR-Cas9 gene editing technology, we generated a gene-edited mouse expressing the HPA-1a epitope by introducing humanized residues within the PSI domain and the EGF1 domain of murine integrin β3. Selection of the amino acids necessary to recreate the epitopes recognized by both type I and type II anti-HPA-1a human monoclonal and polyclonal alloantibodies was guided by the previous findings of Barron-Casella et al. [21] and our own study [22] that $T_{30} \rightarrow A$, $S_{32} \rightarrow P$, $Q_{33} \rightarrow L$, $N_{39} \rightarrow D$ within the PSI domain, and $M_{470} \rightarrow Q$ in the EGF1 domain mouse-to-human amino acid substitutions are necessary to support their binding. The resulting so-called APLDQ-allelic form of murine GPIIIa is immunogenic. Wild-type mice immunized with murine APLDQ transgenic platelets either intraperitoneally (IP) with adjuvant or intravenously (IV) without adjuvant elicited a high-titer HPA-1a-specific alloantibody response [23]. We developed a humanized HPA-1a-specific mouse model of FNAIT using APLDQ mice (Fig. 1). Breeding preimmunized wild-type female mice with APLDQ male mice resulted in a maternal APLDQ-specific alloantibody crossing the placenta, leading to severe thrombocytopenia, bleeding, or even death in fetal and neonatal mice [23]. This humanized mouse model faithfully recapitulates clinically important aspects of human FNAIT, providing a valuable tool for studying the pathophysiological mechanisms underlying the alloimmune response and for evaluating potential prophylactic and therapeutic interventions [23–25].

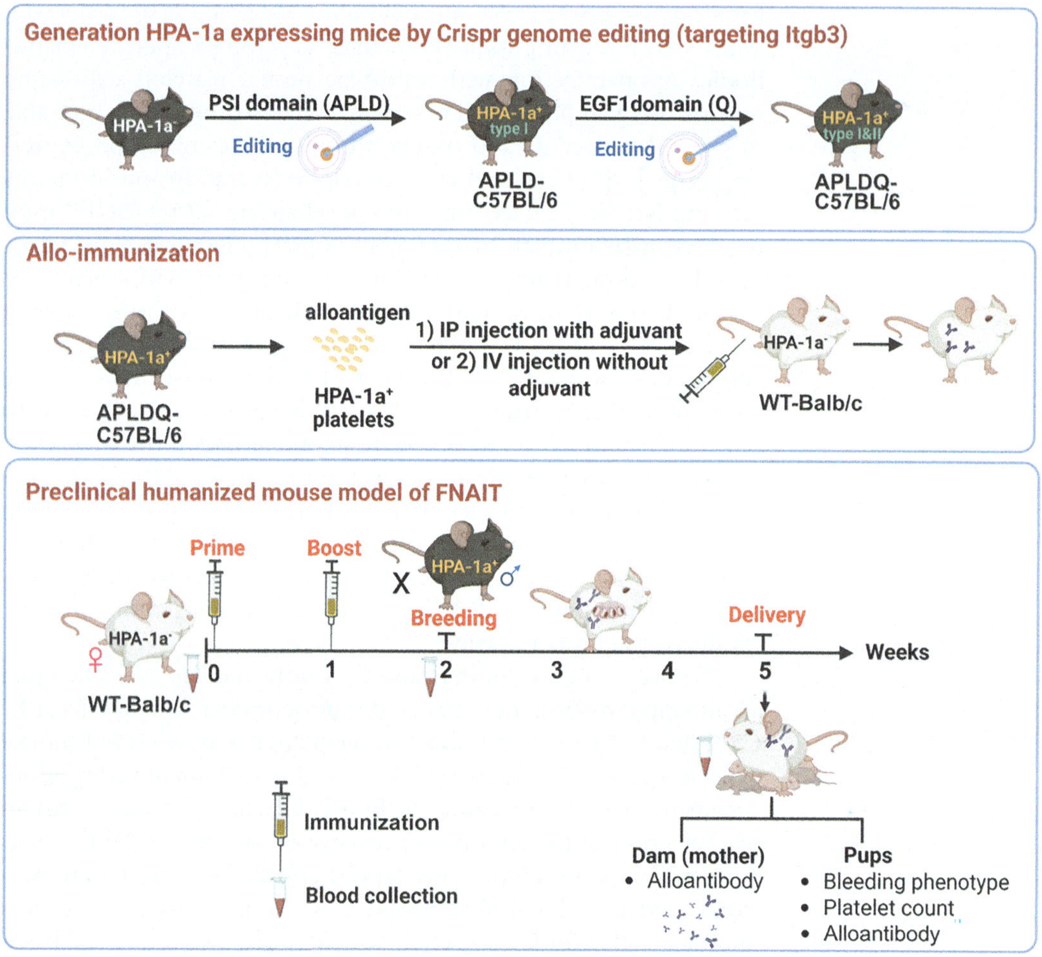

Fig. 1 Schematic overview of the generation of an alloantigen-specific preclinical humanized mouse model of FNAIT. CRISPR-Cas9 gene editing technology was used to generate a transgenic mouse expressing an HPA-1a epitope that could be recognized by both Type I and most Type II HPA-1a antibodies. Humanized "APLD" was first introduced within the PSI domain, followed by the addition of a "Q" in the EGF1 domain of murine integrin β3. Wild-type mice challenged with murine APLDQ transgenic platelets, either intraperitoneally (IP) with adjuvant or intravenously (IV), elicit a high-titer HPA-1a-specific alloantibody response. Breeding preimmunized wild-type female mice with APLDQ male mice results in maternal APLDQ-specific alloantibodies that cross the placenta, leading to severe thrombocytopenia, bleeding, or even death in fetal and neonatal mice. This humanized mouse model faithfully recapitulates clinically important aspects of human FNAIT, providing a valuable tool for studying FNAIT

2 Materials

2.1 Generating a Transgenic Mouse Expressing the HPA-1a Epitope (see Note 1)

1. C57BL/6 N mouse (*see* **Note 2**).
2. MIT online CRISPR tool (http://crispr.mit.edu/).
3. PX459 V2.0 plasmid encoding Cas9 (Addgene).
4. Guide oligoes targeting *ITGB3* gene for generation of APLD GPIIIa mouse:

   Top: 5′- CACCGTTCTCCTTCAGGTTACATCG -3,

   Bottom: 5′- AAACCGATGTAACCTGAAGGAGAAC -3′.
5. BbsI.
6. Quick ligation kit.
7. One Shot™ Stbl3™ competent E. Coli.
8. LB, LB-Agar/Amp plates.
9. Endo-free plasmid maxi kit.
10. Sequencing primer, U6 derived, 5'- GAGGGCCTATTTCC CATGATTCC-3′.
11. ssODN HDR (single-stranded oligodeoxynucleotide homology-directed repair) template encoding GPIIIa T30A, S32P, Q33L, and N39D: 5'- GCCAGGGGGAGGTGACT TACCA

    GCAGGAGGCACAGCCGCCCTAGCTCTGATGTTGACC TTTCCCTCGGGCTCTTCTCTTCATAGGCCTTGCC TCTGGGATCCCCACGCTGTGACCTGAAGGAGAAC CTGCTGAAGGACAATTGTGCTCCAGAGTCTATTG AGTTCCCAGTCAGTGAGGCCCAGATCCTGGAGG CTAGGC-3′.
12. APLD GPIIIa mouse genotyping PCR primer:

    ITGB3 forward primer: 5'-AACCATGGAAGGACCATGAC-3'.

    ITGB3 reverse primer: 5'-CACCCCAGTCCTATCCTGTG-3′.
13. Herculase II Fusion polymerase.
14. 2% TAE agarose gel.
15. Phosphate buffered saline (PBS), pH 7.4.
16. Bovine serum albumin (BSA).
17. Phosphate buffered saline (PBS), pH 7.4, with 1% BSA.
18. Nuclease-free water.
19. Guide oligoes targeting *ITGB3* gene for generation of APLDQ GPIIIa mouse: 5'-CTCCTCAGAGCACTCACACATGG-3′.

20. ssODN HDR template encoding GPIIIa M470Q mutation (ATG > CAA) and TGT > TGC silent mutation:5'-GCCTTCCAGCCCACGCTGCAACAATGGGAACGGACTTTTGAGTGTGGGGTGTGCCGCTGTGACCAGGGCTGGCTGGGGTCCCAATGCGAGTGCTCTGAGGAGGATTACCGACCCTCTCAGCAGGAAGAGTGCAGCCCCAAGGAGGGCCAGCCCATCTGCAGCCA-3′.
21. APLDQ GPIIIa mouse genotyping PCR primer:

    ITGB3 forward primer: 5'- CATTCAGGTGAGCTTTAGTATCGAGGCC-3'.

    ITGB3 reverse primer: 5'-CCCTTTGTAGCGGACGCAGG-3′.

    with PCR product, 424 bp.
22. APLDQ GPIIIa mouse sequencing primer:

    ITGB3 forward primer: 5′- GAGAAGGAGCAGTCTTTCACTATCAAGCC -3'.

    ITGB3 reverse primer: 5′- GCAGGAGAAGTCATCGCACTCAC -3′.
23. Murine monoclonal HPA-1a antibody (mAb) SZ21 (Beckman Coulter Life Sciences).
24. Human monoclonal HPA-1a antibody (mAb) 26.4.
25. FITC-conjugated F(ab')$_2$ Fragment Goat Anti-Mouse IgG.
26. FITC-conjugated F(ab')$_2$ Fragment Goat Anti-Human IgG.
27. 0.2 mL thin-walled PCR tubes.
28. 1.5 mL Eppendorf microcentrifuge tubes.
29. 5 mL polypropylene centrifuge tubes.
30. 15 mL Falcon tubes.
31. Tissue culture dishes.
32. Microcentrifuge.
33. PCR thermal cycler ~~(Bio-Rad Laboratories)~~.
34. Agarose gel electrophoresis systems.
35. Gel imaging system with UV.
36. CO_2 incubator.
37. Centrifuge.
38. Nanodrop (Thermo Fisher Scientific).
39. FACSCelesta™ cell analyzer (BD Biosciences).
40. Accuri C6 flow cytometer (BD Biosciences).
41. FlowJo software.

2.2 Developing a Preclinical Alloantigen-Specific Humanized Mouse model of FNAIT

1. APLDQ-C57BL/6 N mouse.
2. APLDQ-BALB/c mouse (*see* **Note 3**).
3. Female BALB/c mice (7–8 weeks, Charles River Laboratories).
4. Ketamine-xylazine solution.
5. 3.8% sodium citrate solution.
6. 50 μg/mL PGE1.
7. 1 M EDTA.
8. 1× Tyrode–N-2-hydroxyethylpiperazine-N9–2-ethanesulfonic acid (Tyrode-HEPES) buffer.
9. Phosphate buffered saline (PBS), pH 7.4.
10. 70% isopropyl alcohol.
11. Sigma Adjuvant System® S6322.
12. 0.9% saline solution ~~(Sigma)~~.
13. FITC-conjugated $F(ab')_2$ Fragment Goat Anti-Mouse IgG
14. Lancet (3 mm ~ 5 mm).
15. Needles (23–27 gauge; ½ - ⅝ inch).
16. 1.5 mL Eppendorf microcentrifuge tubes.
17. EDTA-coated Microvette blood collection tubes.
18. Heparinized tube microhematocrit capillary.
19. 1 mL syringe, tuberculin, luer slip.
20. Needles (23–27 gauge; ½ - ⅝ inch).
21. 2″ × 2″ gauze.
22. Scil Vet ABC animal counter (Scil Animal Care Company).
23. Vortex mixer.
24. Mouse restrainer.
25. Heat lamp.
26. FACS Celesta™ cell analyzer (BD Biosciences).
27. Accuri C6 flow cytometer (BD Biosciences).
28. FlowJo software.

2.3 Examining the Efficacy of a Prophylactic Treatment Regimen Using the Humanized Preclinical Mouse model of FNAIT

1. General materials for immunization and bleeding are listed above.
2. Female BALB/c mice (7–8 weeks, Charles River Laboratories).
3. APLDQ-C57BL/6 N mouse.
4. Prophylactic treatment regimen.
5. CellTracker™ Green CMFDA.
6. DMSO.
7. Phosphate buffered saline (PBS), pH 7.4.

8. Bovine serum albumin (BSA).
9. Phosphate buffered saline (PBS), pH 7.4, with 1% BSA.
10. Normal human IgG.
11. FITC-conjugated F(ab')$_2$ Fragment Goat Anti-Mouse IgG.
12. Scil Vet ABC Animal Blood Counter (Scil Animal Care Company).
13. FACSCelesta™ cell analyzer (BD Biosciences).
14. FlowJo software.

3 Methods

3.1 Generating a Transgenic Mouse Expressing the HPA-1a Epitope

1. Design guide RNAs (gRNAs) using the CRISPR design tool (http://crispr.mit.edu/) follow the protocol described by Ran et al. [26]. The murine *ITGB3* gene sequence is available as NCBI Gene ID:16416 and GenBank NC 000077.6. Genomic sequencing used for designing the guide is: ctagctctgatgttgacct ttccctcgggctcttctcttcatag ACTTTGTCTCAGGGCTCACCCC GATGTAACCTGAAGGAGAACCTGCTGAAGGACAATTG TGCTCCA (112 bp).
2. Design ssODN HDR as the repair template.
3. **To generate mice expressing the APLD humanized form of muGPIIIa** (Fig. 2a), ssODN HDR template encoding GPIIIa T30A, S32P, Q33L, and N39D mutations also contains 4 silent mutations, 2 of which introduce a diagnostic BamH1 restriction site into the plasmid, while the other 2 mutate the sequence to avoid repetitive digestion of the humanized murine *ITGB3* gene by Cas9 (*see* **Note 4**).
4. Cloning the annealed guide RNA oligos targeting *ITGB3* gene (Fig. 2a) into the BbsI site of the Cas9 expression plasmids PX459 V2.0 using Quick ligation kit. For CRISPR design and detailed cloning protocol, refer to the details provided in the reference protocol [26]. Miniprep each colony and submit for sequencing. Purify PX459 V2.0-*ITGB3* plasmid with correct sequence using Endo-free plasmid maxi kit.
5. C57BL/6 N female mice were superovulated and mated with C57BL/6 N male mice. Fertilized eggs were then collected from the oviducts.
6. The PX459 V2.0-*ITGB3* plasmid (10 ng/mL) and ssODN HDR (5 ng/mL) were injected into the pronuclei of fertilized oocytes. For pronuclear injection, refer to the details provided in the reference protocol [27].
7. Injected zygotes were cultured overnight in potassium simplex optimization medium with amino acids at 37 °C in 5% carbon

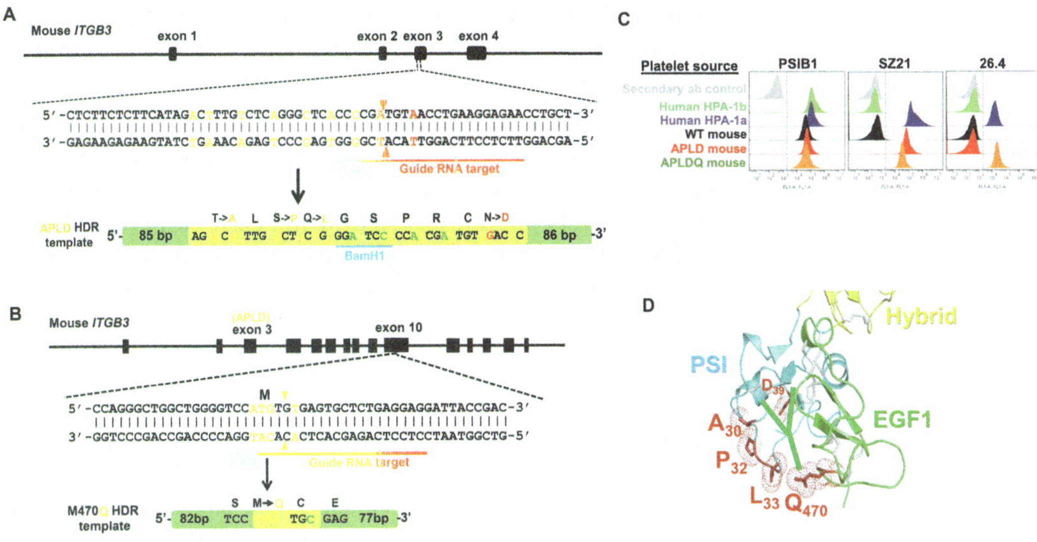

Fig. 2 CRISPR-mediated generation of an HPA-1a-expressing APLDQ mouse. (**a**) Schematic illustration of the *ITGB3* locus, showing the location of the gRNA binding site (red bar), the protospacer adjacent motif (PAM) sequence (magenta bar), and the Cas9 cleavage site (red arrow heads). A 200 bp APLD Homology Directed Repair (HDR) template was designed to introduce the four desired amino acid substitutions (mutated nucleotides labeled in red) and a diagnostic BamH1 restriction site (silent mutation nucleotides labeled in blue) flanked by 80 nucleotide homology arms. The HDR template also introduces nucleotides (green) that encode silent mutations to prevent re-cleavage by Cas9. Pronuclei of C57BL/6 N fertilized eggs was microinjected with the px459 plasmid along with the HDR template to generate the humanized APLD mouse. (**b**) Schematic illustration of the *ITGB3* locus, showing the location of the gRNA binding site (red bar), the protospacer adjacent motif (PAM) sequence (magenta bar), and the Cas9 cleavage site (red arrow heads). A 167 bp Homology Directed Repair (HDR) template was designed to introduce the M to Q amino acid substitutions (mutated nucleotides labeled in red) flanked by 82 and 77 nucleotide homology arms. The HDR template also introduces silent mutations (nucleotides in green) to prevent re-cleavage by Cas9. Cytoplasm of APLD C57BL/6 N fertilized eggs were microinjected with Cas-9 protein and gRNAs along with the HDR template to generate the humanized APLDQ mouse. (**c**) Flow cytometric analysis of the reactivity of HPA-1a-specific antibodies with both human and mouse platelets. Platelets from the indicated species and phenotypes were subjected to reaction with mAbs SZ21 (Type I) and 26.4 (Type II). Note that the humanized APLDQ mouse platelets express an HPA-1a epitope that can be recognized by both mAbs SZ21 and 26.4. (**d**) Structural requirements for binding of the Type II anti-HPA-1a antibody, 26.4, showing the location of the residues that were humanized in the PSI domain and EGF1 domain. (Figure adapted from Zhi et al., Blood Advances 2:3001, 2018)

dioxide and 95% humidified air. Two-cell stage embryos were then transferred into the oviducts of pseudopregnant female mice (*see* **Note 5**).

8. Genomic DNA was isolated from the tails of the pups. Measure DNA concentration with nanodrop.
9. Set up 50 μL PCR reactions using Herculase II Fusion polymerase kit following manufacture's protocol to amplify *ITGB3* gene fragment flanking the targeting locus (717 bp). Each reaction contains 100 ng of genomic DNA collected from **step 7** as template.

10. PCR products were purified using QiaQuick PCR purification kit according to manufacturer's instructions. Elute the DNA in 35 μL distilled water.
11. APLD HDR introduced a BamHI restriction site in the genome, which can be detected by a restriction fragment length polymorphism analysis of the PCR amplicon. Set up a 20 μL BamH1 digestion reaction for each clone as follows: 2 μL of 10× CutSmart buffer, 15 μL of purified PCR products in **step** 7, 0.5 μL of BamH1, and 2.5 μL of distilled water. Keep the reaction at 37 °C for 1 h.
12. Add 4 μL of loading dye to each reaction. Run the digested products on 2% TBE agarose gel.
13. Image the DNA gel under ultraviolet (UV) light to identify the APLD clone which can be cut with BamH1 [22], demonstrating successful incorporation of the HDR oligo. Sequence the remaining PCR amplicon in **step 9** from APLD clone using Sanger sequencing to confirm precise homozygous integration of the HDR sequence.
14. Analyze isolated platelets from the transgenic mice with flow cytometry to confirm the expression of the HPA-1a alloantigen using type I HPA-1a antibody SZ21 [22]. These mice were used to generate mice expressing the APLDQ humanized form of muGPIIIa.
15. **To generate mice expressing the APLDQ humanized form of muGPIIIa,** another round of CRISPR genome editing is conducted using the APLD-GPIIIa mouse (Fig. 2b).
16. Dissect and collect epididymis from APLD-C57BL/6 N mice.
17. Perform IVF using capacitated spermatozoa released from epididymis and oocytes obtained from female mice.
18. Fertilized embryos were injected through cytoplasmic route with a CRISPR targeting cocktail containing active guide RNA molecules (gRNA, 100 ng/μL), one single-stranded oligo deoxynucleotide (ssODN) donor (250 ng/μL), and Cas-9 protein (100 ng/μL).
19. Two-cell stage embryos were then transferred into the oviducts of pseudopregnant female mice.
20. Screen mice born from the microinjection. Genomic DNA was isolated from the tails of the F0 pups. Samples were subjected to PCR amplification and Sanger sequencing using primers listed in the material to screen and confirm ATG > CAA (M470Q) mutation and the TGT > TGC silent mutation in the *ITGB3* locus (*see* **Note 6**).
21. The founders were backcrossed with wild-type B6/N mice to test germline transmission.

22. Analyze isolated platelets from the transgenic mice with flow cytometry to confirm the expression of the HPA-1a alloantigen using both type I HPA-1a antibody SZ21 and type II antibody 26.4 (Fig. 2c and d) (*see* **Note 7**).

3.2 Developing a Preclinical Alloantigen-Specific Humanized Mouse Model of FNAIT

1. **To prepare HPA-1 transgenic (APLDQ) platelets harboring an alloimmune antigen (*see* Note 8),** load a syringe with 100 μL of 3.8% sodium citrate (1/10 volume) and draw mouse whole blood from the inferior vena cava of anesthetized APLDQ-C57BL/6 mice into the syringe using a 23-gauge needle.
2. Dilute the whole blood with an equal volume of 1× Tyrode's buffer.
3. Add PGE-1 to reach a concentration of 50 ng/mL.
4. Centrifuge at 200 × g for 8 min w/o brakes to collect platelet-rich plasma.
5. Add PGE-1 and EDTA to reach final concentrations of 50 ng/mL PGE1 and 1 mM EDTA.
6. Centrifuge at 750 × g for 10 min w/o brakes to pellet platelets.
7. Wash platelets once in Tyrode-HEPES buffer containing 50 ng/mL PGE1 and 1 mM EDTA at pH 7.4.
8. Resuspend platelets in PBS, platelet counts were determined by using a Scil Vet ABC animal counter, ensuring minimal contamination with other blood cells (*see* **Note 9**). Adjust the washed platelet to the desired concentration.
9. **To induce alloimmunization via intraperitoneal injection with adjuvant (*see* Note 10),** add 1 mL of saline to the Sigma Adjuvant System® and vortex several times to mix thoroughly (*see* **Note 11**).
10. Dilute the platelets to a concentration of 1×10^9 cells/mL in PBS. Mix 100 μL of the platelet solution with 100 μL of Sigma adjuvant in an Eppendorf tube.
11. Vortex the Eppendorf tube to resuspend the adjuvant and form an emulsion between the aqueous antigen and oil-based adjuvant. The solution should appear uniformly white with no separation into layers.
12. Draw the solution into a 1.0 mL syringe.
13. Attach a 25-gauge needle to the syringe.
14. Expel any air bubbles present in the syringe barrel or needle by carefully depressing the plunger until the emulsion reaches the needle.
15. Hold the mouse securely with one hand and inject the antigen-adjuvant mix into its peritoneal cavity. Be cautious to avoid accidentally piercing the urinary bladder or large intestines.

16. Wait briefly before withdrawing the needle so that the injected solution does not seep out. Return the animal to its cage and observe for 5 min to ensure its well-being.
17. **To induce alloimmunization via intravenous injection without adjuvant** (*see* **Note 12**)**,** place the BALB/c mice in a separate cage and heat the Balb/c mouse with an infrared lamp to make tail veins easily visible for injection. Ensure the mouse is not overheated.
18. Securely restrain the mouse in the mouse holder.
19. Swab a portion of the tail approximately 1.5 cm below the tail base with alcohol.
20. Attach a 25-gauge needle to a 1.0 mL syringe filled with platelet solution (1×10^8). Expel any air from the syringe to prevent the risk of air embolism. Hold the tail firmly with one hand and carefully insert the needle into a visible vein. Confirm the needle is in the vein and inject slowly.
21. Remove the needle and apply gentle pressure with sterile gauze for 5 s to prevent bleeding. Return the mouse to its cage and observe for 5 min to ensure its well-being.
22. **To test mouse plasma for anti-APLDQ platelet antibodies,** restrain the immunized mouse and use the appropriate size lancet to gently puncture the cheek midway between the ear and the mandible. Collect blood drops from the puncture site (submandibular vein) into EDTA-coated Microvette blood collection tube or a 1.5 mL Eppendorf microcentrifuge tube (containing 3.8% sodium citrate, 1/10 volume).
23. To stop bleeding, apply gentle pressure with sterile gauze for 5 s.
24. Dilute blood with PBS at a 1:3 ratio and centrifuge at 780 × g for 5 min at room temperature.
25. Transfer the plasma to a new microcentrifuge tube.
26. Store plasma samples at −20 °C until analysis of antibody using the following procedure.
27. Draw blood from APLDQ-Balb/c mice and prepare washed platelets, adjust platelet concentration to 1×10^7/mL PBS.
28. Aliquot 25 μL (containing 2.5×10^5 platelet) into each well of 96 well plate.
29. Add 25 μL mouse plasma to the well containing APLDQ-Balb/c platelets.
30. Incubate at room temperature for 30 mins.
31. Wash with 200 μL PBS containing 1% BSA, spin the plate at 320 × g for 5 mins and remove the supernatant.

32. Prepare master mix of FITC-conjugated F(ab')$_2$ fragment goat anti-mouse IgG in PBS containing 1% BSA according to the total number of reactions. Dispense 50 μL of antibody mixture to each reaction. Gently resuspend the platelets by pipetting 2–3 times.
33. Incubate in dark at room temperature for 30 min.
34. Wash with 100 μL of PBS containing 1% BSA, spin the plate at 320 × g for 5 mins and remove the supernatant. Resuspend the platelets in 100 μL of PBS containing 1% BSA.
35. Analyze samples by flow cytometry. Gate on platelets, then analyze the binding of FITC-conjugated F(ab')$_2$ fragment goat anti-mouse IgG in this population with FlowJo software.
36. **To develop a preclinical humanized mouse model of FNAIT,** female BALB/c mice (8–9 weeks old) were immunized with 1×10^8 platelets derived from APLDQ-C57BL/6 N transgenic mice either via intraperitoneal injection with Sigma adjuvant or via intravenous injection without adjuvant (*see* **Note 13** and **14**).
37. One week after the initial immunization (prime), a booster injection was administered. Blood samples were collected from the submandibular region.
38. Collect 100 μL blood from female BALB/c mice via the submandibular vein into EDTA-coated capillary tubes before immunization and 1 week after the boost.
39. Dilute blood with PBS at a 1:3 ratio and centrifuge at 780 × g for 5 min at room temperature. Transfer the plasma to a new microcentrifuge tube. Store plasma samples at −20 °C for future analysis of APLDQ-specific antibody.
40. One week after boost, these preimmunized mice were bred with APLDQ-C57BL/6 N males. Non-immunized BALB/c females and APLDQ-C57BL/6 N males were set up as controls.
41. Within 48 h after birth, pups were monitored for signs of bleeding. Blood samples were collected from the mother (100 μL) and pups (30 μL) via the submandibular vein. Platelet counts of the pups were determined using a Scil Vet ABC Animal Blood Counter. Plasma samples were saved at −20 °C for future analysis of APLDQ-specific antibodies.
42. APLDQ-specific antibody can be detected after immunization (Fig. 3a), the maternal APLDQ-specific alloantibody can cross the placenta and cause severe thrombocytopenia (Fig. 3b), bleeding, or even death in fetal and neonatal mice (Fig. 3c) (*see* **Note 15**). This humanized mouse model faithfully recapitulates many clinically important aspects of human FNAIT (*see* **Note 16**).

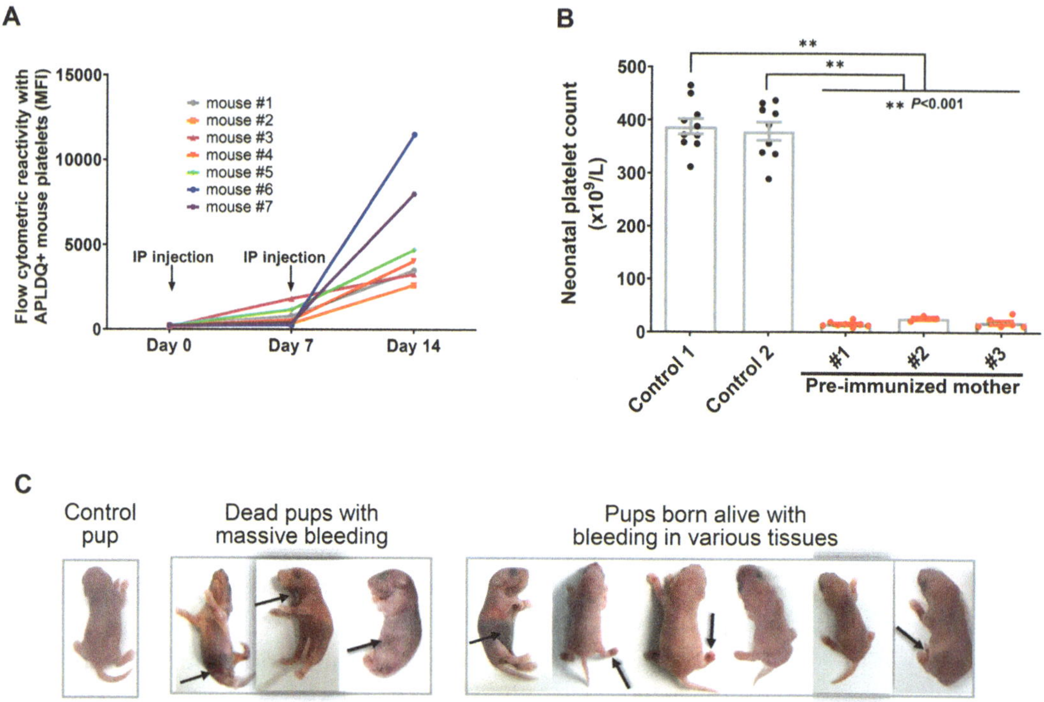

Fig. 3 The APLDQ HPA-1a-positive form of murine GPIIIa is immunogenic and leads to the development of FNAIT. (**a**) Wild-type female BALB/c mice were injected IP with platelets from HPA-1a-transgenic C57BL/6 N mice mixed with Sigma adjuvant at days 0 and 7. Note that all immunized mice developed antibodies that reacted with platelets from HPA-1a-transgenic C57BL/6 N mice. (**b**) Preimmunized wild-type BALB/c mice bred with APLDQ males give birth to severely thrombocytopenic pups. Shown are the platelet counts (mean $\pm$ SEM, $n = 3$–10/group) of neonatal pups within 48 h after birth from three representative BALB/c females that had been pre-immunized with platelets. All the newborn pups were nearly devoid of circulating platelets. Control 1 = platelet counts of pups derived from a female BALB/c mouse that had not been pre-immunized with APLDQ platelets before breeding with an APLDQ C57BL/6 N male. Control 2 = platelet count of pups derived from a wild-type BALB/c female that had been pre-immunized with platelets from an APLDQ-expressing C57BL/6 N mouse before being bred with a wild-type C57BL/6 N male. (**c**) Representative bleeding in pups born to HPA-1a preimmunized WT Balb/c female mice bred with HPA-1a-homozygous males. Arrows identify the abdomen and feet as common sites of bleeding in thrombocytopenic neonatal pups. (Figure adapted from Zhi et al., Blood Advances 5:3552, 2021)

3.3 Examining the Efficacy of a Prophylactic Treatment Regimen Using the Humanized Preclinical Mouse Model of FNAIT

1. **To evaluate the effectiveness of prophylactic agents in eliminating circulating HPA-1a positive APLDQ murine platelets in vivo** (Fig. 4)**,** prepare washed platelets from APLDQ C56BL/6 N mice at a concentration of 1×10^8 cells/mL.
2. Before opening the vial of CellTracker™ Green CMFDA dye (MW 464.9), allow it to warm to room temperature. Dilute CMFDA using high-quality DMSO to create a 5 mM solution.
3. Add 1 μL of 5 mM CMFDA per 1 mL of APLDQ platelet solution (resulting in a final concentration of 5 μM). Incubate the mixture for 45 min at room temperature in the dark.

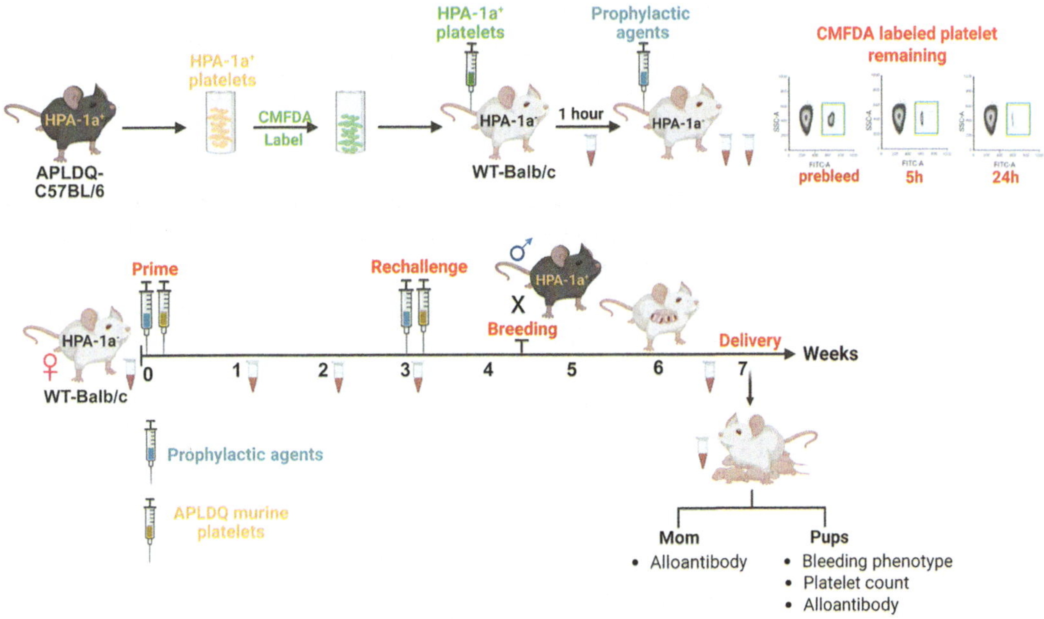

Fig. 4 Protocol for examining the efficacy of prophylactic agents using APLDQ mice. (**a**) Platelets were isolated from APLDQ-C56BL/6 mice, labeled with the cell tracker dye CMFDA, and transfused (1×10^8 CMFDA-labeled platelets per mouse) into WT Balb/c female mice. One hour post-transfusion, antibodies or control reagents were administered via tail vein injection. Blood samples were collected from recipients following platelet transfusion, before antibody injection, and at 5- and 24-h post-antibody injection. The percentage of CMFDA-labeled platelets in whole blood was determined by flow cytometry. Survival of transfused platelets was calculated as the percentage of remaining CMFDA-labeled platelets divided by the initial percentage of CMFDA-labeled platelets. (**b**) WT BALB/c mice received either antibodies or control reagents 1 h prior to transfusion with APLDQ murine platelets. The effectiveness of prophylactic antibodies in preventing alloimmunization to HPA-1a-positive, APLDQ murine platelets was determined by collecting blood samples at specified time points and performing flow cytometry against APLDQ platelets. To determine whether repeat administration of prophylactic agents might provide sustained protection from HPA-1a exposure, BALB/c mice were rechallenged at week three and then bred with APLDQ males at week four. Within 48 h after birth, pups were monitored for signs of bleeding, and platelet counts were measured. Anti-APLDQ antibodies in both the mother and pups were examined

4. Centrifuge the platelet at $320 \times g$ and remove the extra CMFDA dye.
5. Resuspend the CMFDA-labeled platelets in 200 μL PBS transfused to the wild-type (WT) female Balb/c mice.
6. 30 min after the CMFDA-labeled platelet transfusion, blood samples were collected via the submandibular vein.
7. The percentage of CMFDA-labeled platelets in whole blood was determined by flow cytometry. This measurement defines the baseline, with circulating CMFDA-labeled APLDQ platelets set at 100%.
8. One hour after the CMFDA-labeled platelets transfusion, different prophylactic antibodies are administered by IV injection.

9. Blood samples were collected from the submandibular vein 5 and 24 h post-antibody injection.
10. The percentage of CMFDA-labeled platelets remaining in the circulation was determined by flow cytometry.
11. The survival of the transfused labeled platelets was calculated by the percentage of the remaining CMFDA-labeled platelets divided by the beginning percentage of CMFDA-labeled platelets.
12. **To evaluate the effectiveness of prophylactic agents in preventing alloimmunization and FNAIT,** obtain female BALB/c mice (7–8 weeks old) from Charles River and allow them to acclimate for 1 week.
13. Collect 100 μL of blood from female BALB/c mice via the submandibular vein into EDTA-coated capillary tubes before the experiment and prepare plasma as a pre-bleed control.
14. On Day 1, female BALB/c mice receive prophylactic treatment at various concentrations via tail vein injection (diluted in 200 μL PBS). Normal human IgG or PBS is injected as a control.
15. One hour after prophylactic treatment, transfuse these mice with 1×10^8 APLDQ platelets in PBS (*see* **Note 17**).
16. On Days 7, 14, and 21 following platelet transfusion, collect 100 μL of blood and harvest plasma. Examine plasma samples for levels of anti-APLDQ antibodies by flow cytometry analysis using FITC-conjugated $F(ab')_2$ Fragment Goat $(Fab)_2$ Anti-Mouse IgG.
17. On Day 21, administer a second prophylaxis treatment and platelet challenge.
18. On Day 28, breed these female BALB/c mice with APLDQ C57BL/6 N males.
19. Within 48 h after birth, monitor pups for signs of bleeding. Collect blood samples (100 μL from the mother, 30 μL from the pups) via the submandibular vein.
20. Determine platelet counts of the pups using a Scil Vet ABC Animal Blood Counter. Examine plasma samples for levels of anti-APLDQ antibodies.

4 Notes

1. Amino acids on both sides of the polymorphic amino acid 33 in the PSI domain (A30P32L33D39) are required for forming the epitope for the HPA-1a type I antibody. Using CRISPR/Cas9 gene editing technology, we first generated a transgenic

mouse by humanizing residues A30P32L33D39 within the PSI domain. The resulting APLD GPIIIa recreates the HPA-1a epitope for the HPA-1a type I antibody. Amino acids on both sides of the polymorphic amino acid 33 in the PSI domain (A30P32L33D39) and the amino acid glutamine (Q) in the EGF1 domain are required for forming the epitope of the Type II HPA-1a antibody. Starting with our APLD mouse, we introduced one more humanizing residue Q470 within the linearly distant but conformationally close Epidermal Growth Factor (EGF) 1 domain. The resulting APLDQ mouse GPIIIa recreated the HPA-1a epitope for both type I and type II antibodies.

2. All mouse protocols should be approved by your Institutional Animal Care and Use Committee (IACUC) and should be carried out in compliance with the National Institutes of Health Guide for the Care and Use of Laboratory Animals.
3. The APLDQ-BALB/c mouse was obtained by backcrossing APLDQ-C57BL/6 N mice into the BALB/c strain. Using platelets from APLDQ-BALB/c mice enables us to measure anti-APLDQ-specific antibodies in BALB/c mice immunized with APLDQ-C57BL/6 N platelets via flow cytometry analysis.
4. In addition to introducing the target mutation (APLD-GPIIIa), silent mutations need to be incorporated into the guide recognition sequence and/or the PAM sequence of the HDR repair template to prevent repetitive digestion of the repaired genome by Cas9.
5. The APLD humanized mice, expressing the humanized form of APLD-murine GPIIIa, were generated at the transgenic core of the Medical College of Wisconsin, where **steps 5–7** of the procedure were conducted.
6. The APLDQ humanized mice, expressing the humanized form of APLDQ murine GPIIIa, were generated by Applied StemCell, where **steps 17–20** of the procedure were conducted.
7. We also assessed another Type II HPA-1a-specific monoclonal antibody, B2G1, which does not exhibit reactivity with APLDQ platelets. This underscores the complexity of binding specificities that are present in the polyclonal humoral response to the Leu33Pro polymorphism that controls formation of the HPA-1a epitope [22].
8. Naïve female mice do not naturally develop an alloimmune response to the APLDQ platelet alloantigen solely due to pregnancy, even after three consecutive matings with APLDQ homozygous males. Our current FNAIT mouse model requires pre-immunization with HPA-1a platelets. The alloimmune response was induced by administering APLDQ platelets

via different routes: intravenous injection without adjuvant or intraperitoneal injection with adjuvant.

9. Washed APLDQ platelets are utilized as an immune antigen to induce the alloimmune response in our model. However, washed platelets may become contaminated with leukocytes and red blood cells during preparation, potentially influencing the qualitative or quantitative aspects of the immune response. Therefore, it is critical to minimize the presence of leukocytes and red blood cells in the washed platelet preparation.
10. Female BALB/c mice immunized with APLDQ murine platelets via intraperitoneal injection, combined with Sigma adjuvant, elicit a more consistent and robust alloimmune response. This immunization approach results in the pronounced FNAIT phenotype, effectively modeling the human population that has developed alloimmune antibodies before pregnancy. This model is desired for examining the potential efficacy of anti-FNAIT therapeutics.
11. Given that the adjuvant has the potential to induce harmful effects, it is crucial to exercise caution when preparing the adjuvant solution, mixing it with the antigen, and administering the injection.
12. FNAIT is believed to occur when fetal platelets enter the mother's circulation. Female BALB/c mice immunized with APLDQ murine platelets via intravenous injection, without the use of adjuvant, closely mimic the human exposure route. This immunization approach enables us to replicate and investigate alloimmunization and FNAIT induced by fetal-maternal hemorrhage.
13. To establish a humanized preclinical model for FNAIT that closely resembles the human disease, we intentionally crossed Major Histocompatibility Complex (MHC) barriers by using APLDQ platelets from C57BL/6 N mice to immunize the BALB/c mice. While there was a minor degree of reactivity against WT C57BL/6 N platelets, as expected due to differences in class I MHC alleles between the two strains, these antibodies did not induce FNAIT [23].
14. BALB/c and C57BL/6 N mice demonstrate differing responses to antigens, with BALB/c mice showing robust responses to allogeneic platelet antigens, while C57BL/6 N mice exhibit weaker responses [28]. Therefore, BALB/c mice were chosen as recipients for immunization.
15. While severe thrombocytopenia is present in only 25% of neonates born to alloimmunized women (with 3–5% experiencing severe bleeding complications such as intracranial hemorrhage), we observed severe thrombocytopenia in nearly 100% of neonates born to overtly immunized mice. Among them, 10–20% experienced bleeding, possibly due to the

comparatively harsher environmental conditions encountered by neonatal mice.

16. Our first-of-its-kind alloantigen-specific preclinical mouse model of FNAIT, targeting the clinically important HPA-1a alloantigen, faithfully recapitulates many clinically important aspects of human FNAIT. By introducing the APLDQ platelet alloantigen at different times or through different routes, we can model each human subpopulation (Fig. 5) at risk of developing FNAIT. This approach offers a unique and

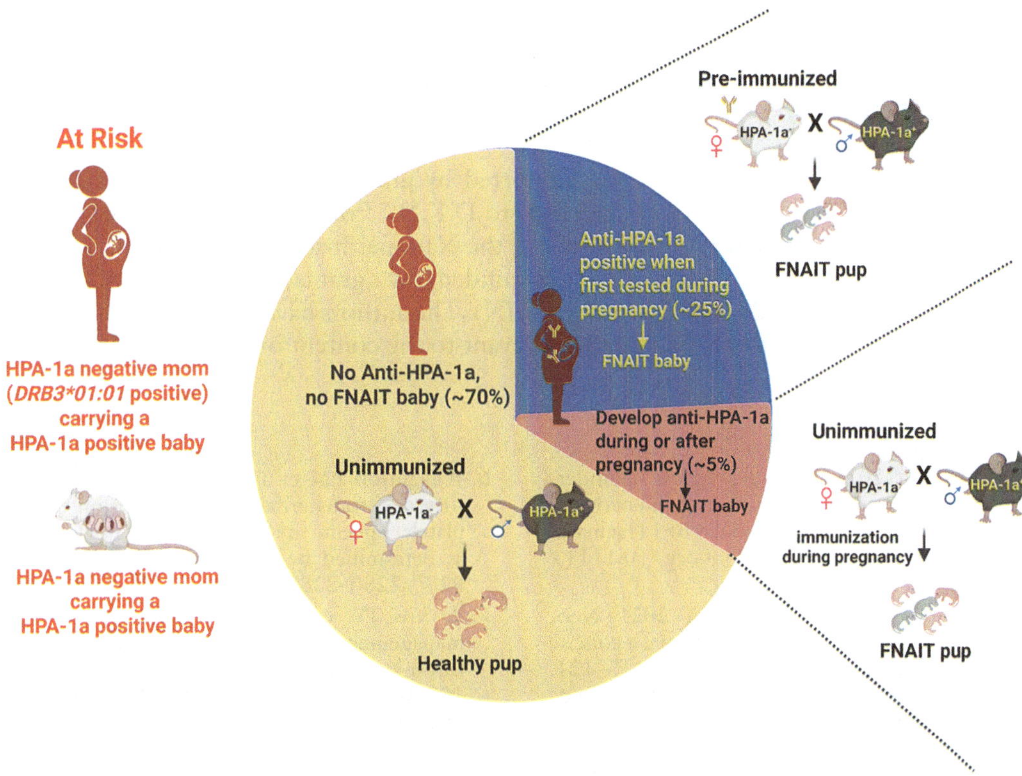

Fig. 5 The HPA-1a-expressing mouse models human subpopulations at risk for developing FNAIT. Naïve, HPA-1a-negative, wild-type (WT) female mice bred with HPA-1a-positive male mice normally do not develop an immune response to HPA-1a during pregnancy, thereby phenocopying the approximately 70% of high-risk HPA-1a-incompatible human pregnancies in which alloantibodies do not develop. WT female mice that have been preimmunized with HPA-1a-positive mouse platelets and then bred with HPA-1a-positive male mice deliver pups with FNAIT, thereby modeling approximately 25% of HPA-1a-incompatible women with pre-existing HPA-1a-specific antibodies whose babies develop FNAIT. Finally, naïve WT female mice that are bred with HPA-positive male mice and then exposed to HPA-1a-positive platelets during pregnancy deliver pups with FNAIT, thereby simulating HPA-1a-incompatible human pregnancies in which alloantibodies develop during or after pregnancy, perhaps because of exposure to HPA-1a as a consequence of small placental hemorrhages or pregnancy loss. The HPA-1a-expressing mouse model may therefore be a valuable tool for studying the pathophysiological mechanisms underlying the maternal alloimmune response to fetal HPA-1a and for assessing the effectiveness of HPA-1a-specific prophylactic and therapeutic interventions for the management of FNAIT

unparalleled opportunity to explore many outstanding issues relevant to the clinical etiology and treatment of FNAIT.

17. The activation status of platelets significantly affects the clearance of the platelets. Transfusing activated platelets into the mice can result in rapid clearance, potentially skewing the platelet clearance results and masking the preventive effects of the prophylactic treatment. Therefore, precautionary measures should be implemented to prevent the activation of washed platelets during preparation. These measures may include using freshly prepared buffers, adding PGE1, handling samples gently, and centrifuging without a break, among others.

Acknowledgments

This study was supported by grants R35-HL139937 (to P.J.N.) and R01-HL169144 (to D.K.N.) from the National Heart, Lung, and Blood Institute of the National Institutes of Health.

This study was funded by grants R35 HL139937 and P01-HL167668 (to PJN). The authors have no conflicts of interest to declare that are relevant to the content of this chapter.

References

1. Curtis BR (2015) Recent progress in understanding the pathogenesis of fetal and neonatal alloimmune thrombocytopenia. Br J Haematol 171(5):671–682. https://doi.org/10.1111/bjh.13639
2. Norton T, Newberry D, Jnah A (2021) Neonatal alloimmune thrombocytopenia: a concise review. Adv Neonatal Care 21(2):115–121. https://doi.org/10.1097/anc.0000000000000775
3. Bussel JB, Vander Haar EL, Berkowitz RL (2021) New developments in fetal and neonatal alloimmune thrombocytopenia. Am J Obstet Gynecol 225(2):120–127. https://doi.org/10.1016/j.ajog.2021.04.211
4. Bussel JB, Primiani A (2008) Fetal and neonatal alloimmune thrombocytopenia: progress and ongoing debates. Blood Rev 22(1):33–52. https://doi.org/10.1016/j.blre.2007.09.002
5. Kjeldsen-Kragh J et al (2007) A screening and intervention program aimed to reduce mortality and serious morbidity associated with severe neonatal alloimmune thrombocytopenia. Blood 110(3):833–839. https://doi.org/10.1182/blood-2006-08-040121
6. Williamson LM et al (1998) The natural history of fetomaternal alloimmunization to the platelet-specific antigen HPA-1a (PlA1, Zwa) as determined by antenatal screening. Blood 92(7):2280–2287
7. de Vos TW et al (2020) Epidemiology and management of fetal and neonatal alloimmune thrombocytopenia. Transfus Apher Sci 59(1):102704. https://doi.org/10.1016/j.transci.2019.102704
8. Wienzek-Lischka S et al (2020) Non-invasive risk-assessment and bleeding prophylaxis with IVIG in pregnant women with a history of fetal and neonatal alloimmune thrombocytopenia: management to minimize adverse events. Arch Gynecol Obstet 302(2):355–363. https://doi.org/10.1007/s00404-020-05618-y
9. Wabnitz H, Khan R, Lazarus AH (2020) The use of IVIg in fetal and neonatal alloimmune thrombocytopenia- principles and mechanisms. Transfus Apher Sci 59(1):102710. https://doi.org/10.1016/j.transci.2019.102710
10. Peterson JA, JG MF, Curtis BR, Aster RH (2013) Neonatal alloimmune

thrombocytopenia: pathogenesis, diagnosis and management. Br J Haematol 161(1): 3–14. https://doi.org/10.1111/bjh.12235

11. Newman PJ, Derbes RS, Aster RH (1989) The human platelet alloantigens, PlA1 and PlA2, are associated with a leucine33/proline33 amino acid polymorphism in membrane glycoprotein IIIa, and are distinguishable by DNA typing. J Clin Invest 83(5):1778–1781. https://doi.org/10.1172/jci114082
12. L'Abbé D et al (1992) Alloimmunization to platelet antigen HPA-1a (PIA1) is strongly associated with both HLA-DRB3*0101 and HLA-DQB1*0201. Hum Immunol 34(2): 107–114. https://doi.org/10.1016/0198-8859(92)90036-m
13. Valentin N et al (1990) HLA-DRw52a is involved in alloimmunization against PL-A1 antigen. Hum Immunol 27(2):73–79. https://doi.org/10.1016/0198-8859(90)90104-W
14. Kjeldsen-Kragh J, Ahlen MT (2020) Foetal and neonatal alloimmune thrombocytopenia—the role of the HLA-DRB3*01:01 allele for HPA-1a-immunisation and foetal/neonatal outcome. Transfus Apher Sci 59(1):102707. https://doi.org/10.1016/j.transci.2019.102707
15. Gragert L, Madbouly A, Freeman J, Maiers M (2013) Six-locus high resolution HLA haplotype frequencies derived from mixed-resolution DNA typing for the entire US donor registry. Hum Immunol 74(10): 1313–1320. https://doi.org/10.1016/j.humimm.2013.06.025
16. Kjeldsen-Kragh J, Olsen KJ (2019) Risk of HPA-1a-immunization in HPA-1a-negative women after giving birth to an HPA-1a-positive child. Transfusion 59(4):1344–1352. https://doi.org/10.1111/trf.15152
17. Ni H et al (2006) A novel murine model of fetal and neonatal alloimmune thrombocytopenia: response to intravenous IgG therapy. Blood 107(7):2976–2983. https://doi.org/10.1182/blood-2005-06-2562
18. Chen P et al (2010) Animal model of fetal and neonatal immune thrombocytopenia: role of neonatal Fc receptor in the pathogenesis and therapy. Blood 116(18):3660–3668. https://doi.org/10.1182/blood-2010-05-284919
19. Bakchoul T et al (2009) Blockade of maternal anti-HPA-1a-mediated platelet clearance by an HPA-1a epitope-specific F(ab') in an in vivo mouse model of alloimmune thrombocytopenia. Transfusion 49(2):265–270. https://doi.org/10.1111/j.1537-2995.2008.01972.x
20. Ghevaert C et al (2013) Recombinant HPA-1a antibody therapy for treatment of fetomaternal alloimmune thrombocytopenia: proof of principle in human volunteers. Blood 122(3): 313–320. https://doi.org/10.1182/blood-2013-02-481887
21. Barron-Casella EA et al (1999) Construction of a human platelet alloantigen-1a epitope (s) within murine glycoprotein IIIa: identification of residues critical to the conformation of the antibody binding site(s). Blood 93(9): 2959–2967
22. Zhi H et al (2018) High-resolution mapping of the polyclonal immune response to the human platelet alloantigen HPA-1a (Pl(A1)). Blood Adv 2(21):3001–3011. https://doi.org/10.1182/bloodadvances.2018023341
23. Zhi H et al (2021) Preclinical evaluation of immunotherapeutic regimens for fetal/neonatal alloimmune thrombocytopenia. Blood Adv 5(18):3552–3562. https://doi.org/10.1182/bloodadvances.2021004371
24. Zhi H, Sheridan D, Newman DK, Newman PJ (2022) Prophylactic administration of HPA-1a-specific antibodies prevents fetal/neonatal alloimmune thrombocytopenia in mice. Blood 140(20):2146–2153. https://doi.org/10.1182/blood.2022015666
25. Mørtberg TV et al (2022) Prevention of fetal/neonatal alloimmune thrombocytopenia in mice: biochemical and cell biological characterization of isoforms of a human monoclonal antibody. Immunohorizons 6(1):90–103. https://doi.org/10.4049/immunohorizons.2100097
26. Ran FA et al (2013) Genome engineering using the CRISPR-Cas9 system. Nat Protoc 8(11):2281–2308. https://doi.org/10.1038/nprot.2013.143
27. Cho A, Haruyama N, Kulkarni AB (2009) Generation of transgenic mice. Curr Protoc Cell Biol. Chapter 19:Unit 19.11. https://doi.org/10.1002/0471143030.cb1911s42
28. Sayeh E et al (2004) Immune responsiveness against allogeneic platelet transfusions is determined by the recipient's major histocompatibility complex class II phenotype. Transfusion 44(11):1572–1578. https://doi.org/10.1111/j.1537-2995.2004.04197.x

Chapter 5

Mouse Model of Hemolytic Disease of the Fetus and Newborn

Hirotomo Nakahara, Sasikala Muthusamy, Rebecca C. Hale, Brock D. Hughes, and Sean R. Stowell

Abstract

Hemolytic Disease of the Fetus and Newborn (HDFN) is caused by the placental transfer of maternal red blood cell (RBC) alloantibodies into the fetal circulation which then targets paternally derived RBC antigens expressed on the fetal RBC. The resulting anemia in the fetus/newborn can lead to grave clinical consequences including hydrops fetalis, kernicterus, and perinatal demise. We have utilized the human KEL transgenic mouse model to study the induction of anti-KEL RBC alloantibodies through pregnancy as well as transfusion and the subsequent placental transfer of anti-KEL RBC alloantibodies into the fetal circulation, causing anemia, hydrops, and fetal/neonatal demise. Here, we describe the methods used to establish the KEL transgenic mouse HDFN model and the assays that evaluate the key pathologic features of HDFN.

Key words Hemolytic Disease of the Fetus and Newborn, HDFN, Pregnancy, Transfusion, RBC alloimmunization, RBC alloantibody, Anemia, KEL, Kell

1 Introduction

Hemolytic disease of the fetus and newborn (HDFN) was originally recognized as erythroblastosis fetalis nearly a century ago and subsequently recognized as an antibody-mediated process driven by fetal-maternal red blood cell (RBC) incompatibility [1–3]. Maternal RBC alloantibody crosses the placenta into the fetal circulation and targets fetal RBCs expressing maternally incompatible, paternally inherited RBC alloantigen resulting in fetal anemia that can progress to hydrops fetalis and perinatal demise. Surviving newborns are at risk of hyperbilirubinemia and kernicterus due to hemolysis from the continued presence of the maternal RBC alloantibody.

The ABO blood group antigens and their corresponding anti-ABO antibodies, first described in 1900, are among the key blood group antigens that can cause incompatibility between individuals

Sean R. Stowell and Connie M. Arthur (eds.), *Methods in Transfusion Medicine*, Methods in Molecular Biology, vol. 3053, https://doi.org/10.1007/978-1-0716-5376-0_5,

[4–6]. Unlike antibodies formed in response to red blood cell (RBC) exposure, anti-ABO antibodies develop within the first few months of life and constitute the primary immunological barrier to transfusion and transplantation. The evolution of ABO blood groups is linked to variations in infectious disease risk and has significant implications for innate immunity against microbes that utilize blood group-like molecular mimicry [7–9]. Since the discovery of ABO antigens, many other antigens have been identified on the surface of RBCs, with the RhD antigen being particularly notable [10]. RhD alloimmunization was quickly identified as the major cause of HDFN. Experiments and clinical trials in the 1960s to prevent RhD alloimmunization by administration of anti-RhD antibody led to the licensing of polyclonal anti-RhD Immune Globulin (RhIG) in North America and Europe in 1968 [11]. Routine antenatal and postnatal RhIG prophylaxis in high-income countries has successfully reduced the rate of RhD alloimmunization in RhD-negative mothers from 16% to <0.2% [12], but the global mortality and morbidity from preventable RhD HDFN remain unacceptably high due to lack of access to quality perinatal care and RhIG prophylaxis in many countries [13–15]. Polyclonal RhIG is derived from a limited supply of RhD hyperimmunized donor plasma and thus is insufficient to fully meet global demands [16]. Additionally, no RhIG equivalent exists to prevent alloimmunization against more than 50 blood group antigens known to cause HDFN [17]. In countries with adequate access to RhIG prophylaxis, HDFN due to ABO, Kell, and other non-RhD blood group incompatibilities now comprise the majority of HDFN cases [18, 19]. Understanding the mechanism by which antibodies against RBC antigens can prevent RBC alloimmunization and HDFN is crucial for the development of novel preventative and therapeutic alternatives beyond polyclonal RhIG [20, 21].

Preclinical animal models have provided crucial insights into factors that govern the formation and consequences of alloantibodies against a variety of alloantigens, including RBC alloantigens [10]. Historically, rabbits were the animal model of choice for the study of HDFN [22–27], but limitations include the requirement to induce RBC alloantibody through immunization rather than pregnancy, as well as the relative lack of immunologic and genetic tools compared to mouse models. While the human RhD transgenic mouse model seems to be an obvious candidate to study RhD HDFN [28], efforts have been hampered by the inability of standard laboratory mice to form RhD-specific antibodies in response to RhD-positive erythrocyte transfusion [29].

The development of new models for studying RBC alloimmunization has significantly enhanced the ability to investigate the underlying principles that govern this process [30–34]. Many studies using these models have provided insight into donor RBCs and recipient characteristics that regulate RBC alloimmunization [35–

44]. Similar models have suggested that common and distinct pathways exist that govern the development and consequences of alloimmune responses to intravascular alloantigens in general [45–47], including similar pregnancy complications due to alloimmunization toward platelet alloantigens [48–54]. Among preclinical models of RBC alloimmunization, the KEL transgenic mouse model was the first animal HDFN model to demonstrate the stimulation of RBC alloantibodies against paternally derived RBC antigens through pregnancy and fully recapitulate the key clinical and pathologic features of HDFN [55, 56]. KEL-negative females develop anti-KEL antibodies when bred with KEL transgenic males, with an increase in anti-KEL antibody titer and a decrease in litter size with successive rounds of pregnancy with delivery of anemic, hydropic, and stillborn pups. Anti-KEL antibody is directly bound to fetal/neonatal RBC and mirrors features specific to KEL HDFN by targeting erythrocyte precursors with suppression of erythropoiesis and relative reticulocytopenia in the pups. Anti-KEL antibody induced through transfusion is also able to undergo placental transfer and cause HDFN. In addition to serving as a useful model for HDFN, the KEL system and other model systems have likewise sought to define mechanisms whereby antibody-mediated immunosuppression (AMIS) occurs [36, 43, 57–59]. These studies suggest that antibody-mediated antigen loss can contribute to AMIS, a process that appears to be mirrored in similar situations clinically.

This chapter provides detailed protocols for studying HDFN using the KEL transgenic mouse model with a focus on characterizing the key immune features and phenotypes of KEL alloimmunization capable of crossing the placenta to cause HDFN. Of note, there are several strains of human KEL transgenic mice with varying levels of KEL antigen expression on the RBC surface that were generated utilizing the same overall genetic approach [40, 56, 60–62]. The human KEL1 (K1) or KEL2 (K2) genes, equivalent to the K or k antigen in the Kell blood group system, respectively, were cloned into an RBC-specific expression vector containing human β-globin regulatory elements, which were then used to generate transgenic mice by pronuclear injection [56]. Originally, three founder lines and their Kell glycoprotein expression levels measured as mean copy numbers were characterized and have now been used in a wide variety of studies examining alloimmunizaton and the consequences of antibody engagement [40, 55, 56, 60–63].

In an effort to streamline the methods shared herein, Part 1 will describe the establishment of the KEL transgenic mouse HDFN model by inducing maternal anti-KEL antibody production through multiple pregnancies (Fig. 1) and an alternative model in which the maternal anti-KEL antibody is induced through multiple transfusions (Fig. 2). The level of anti-KEL IgG in the mother

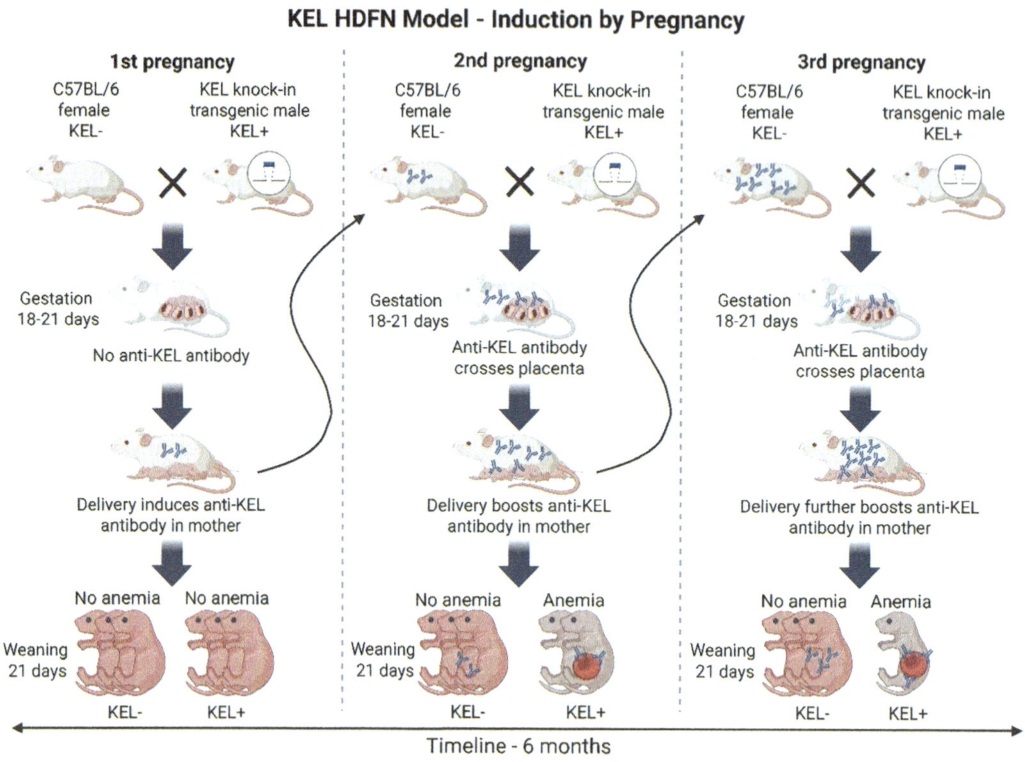

Fig. 1 Schematic representation of the pregnancy-induced KEL HDFN experimental timeline

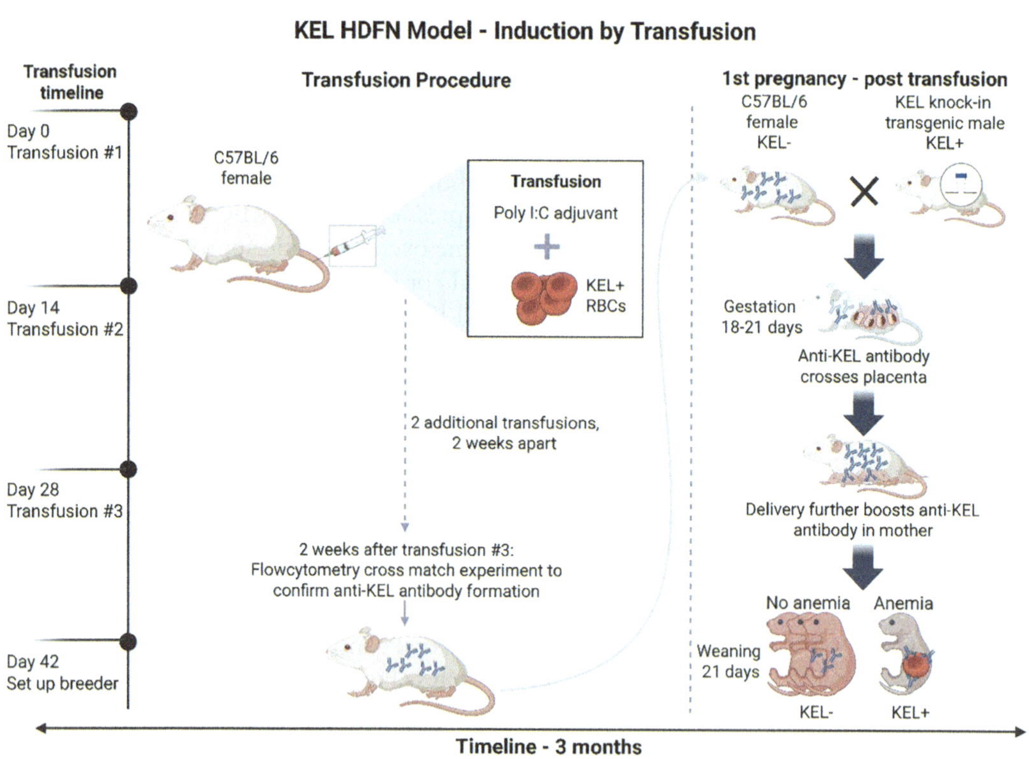

Fig. 2 Schematic representation of the transfusion-induced KEL HDFN experimental timeline

correlates with a decrease in litter size, survival to weaning, and appearance of anemic/hydropic/stillborn pups (Figs. 3, 4 and 5). Part 2 will describe the assays to verify the HDFN phenotype by measurement of anti-KEL IgG by flow cytometry in the KEL immunized mothers, either through pregnancy or

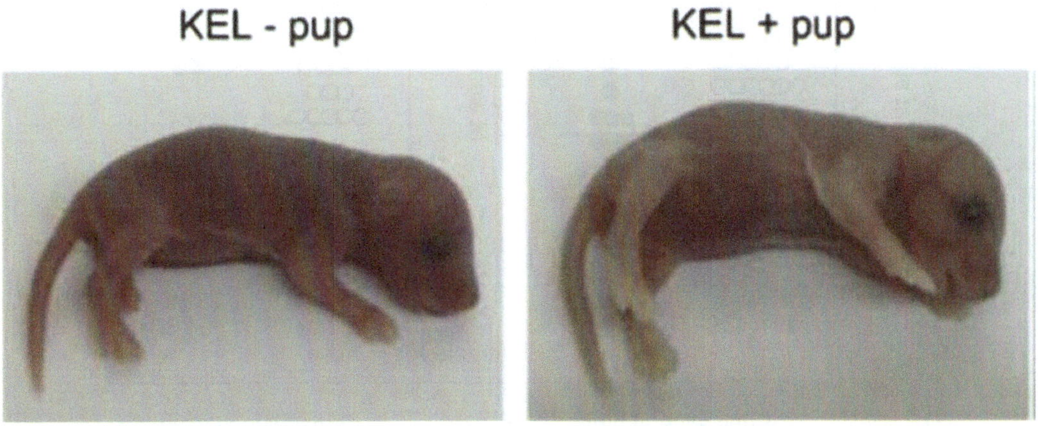

Fig. 3 Photograph of a representative pink KEL-negative and pale KEL-positive pup, hours after birth to a multiparous (third litter) wild-type female mated with a KEL male. (These data were originally published in the journal *Blood.* Stowell et al. [55]. © 2013 by The American Society of Hematology)

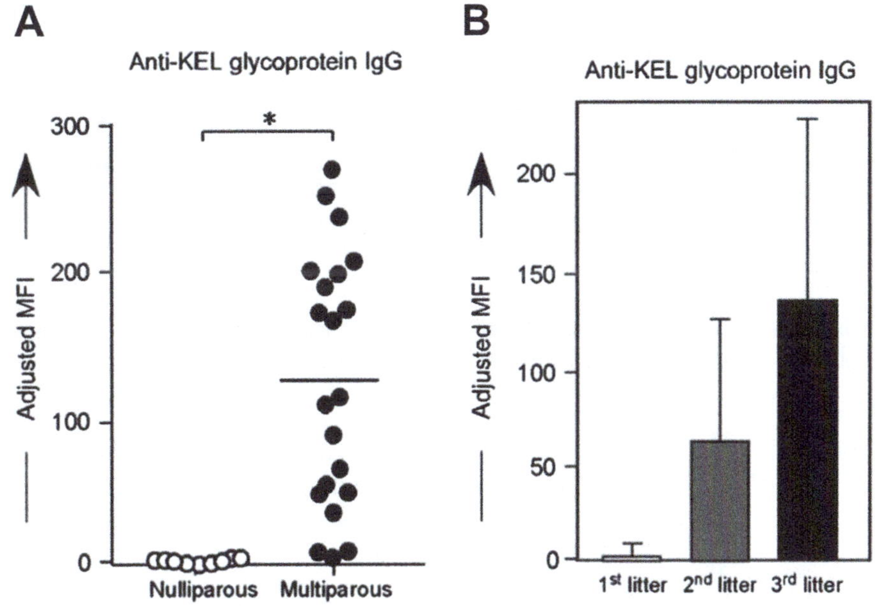

Fig. 4 Anti-KEL red blood cell (RBC) antibodies are detectable in the serum of wild-type females after multiple pregnancies with KEL-positive males. (These data were originally published in the journal *Blood.* Stowell et al. [55]. © 2013 by The American Society of Hematology)

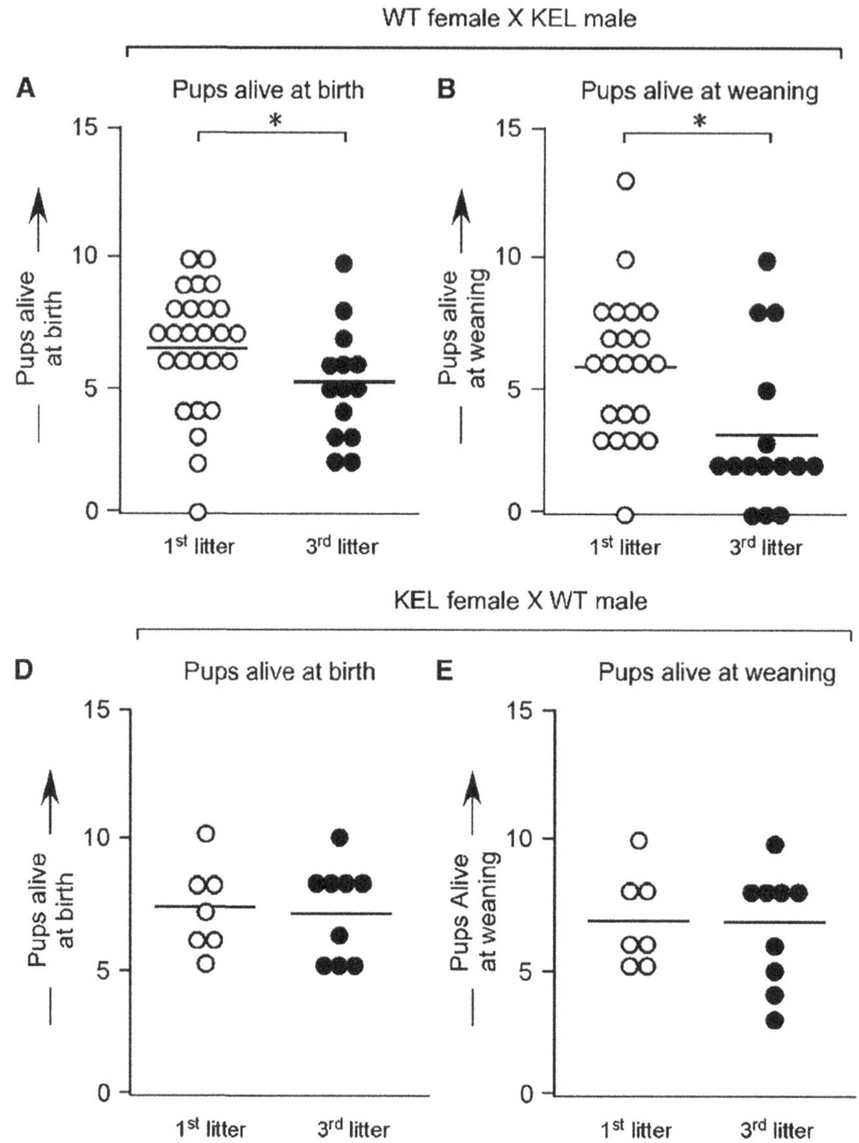

Fig. 5 Smaller successive litters are born to wild-type females mated with KEL males. (These data were originally published in the journal *Blood.* Stowell et al. [55]. © 2013 by The American Society of Hematology)

transfusion (Figs. 4 and 7). Maternal transfer of the anti-KEL IgG across the placenta is measured by flow cytometry of IgG bound to the RBC surface of blood collected from pups (Fig. 6). The principles and methods described in this article should allow for the study of HDFN in other mouse models of RBC alloimmunization.

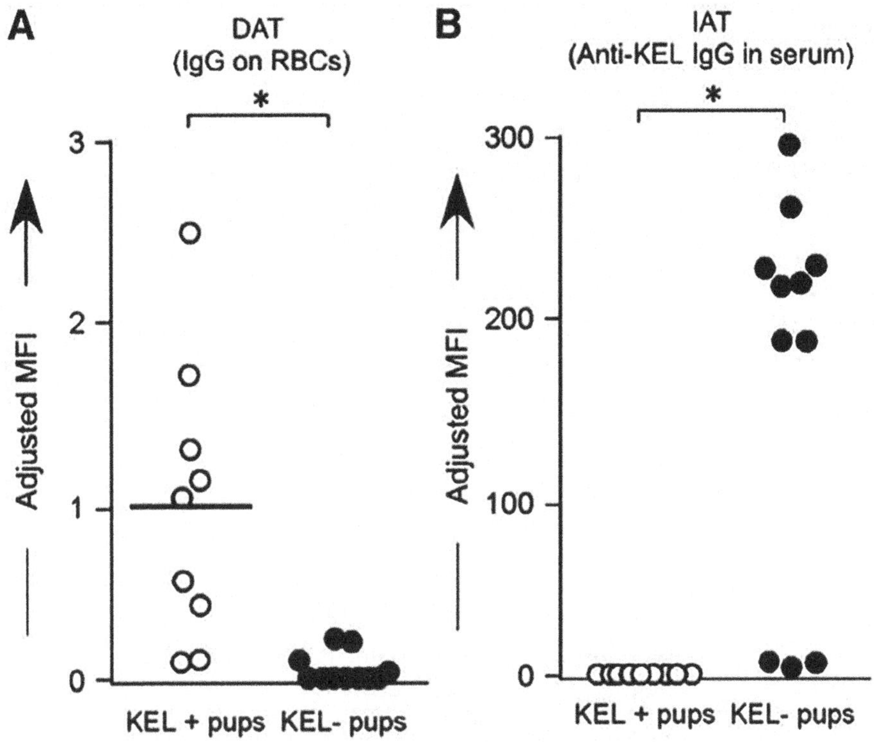

Fig. 6 Maternal anti-KEL IgG crosses the placenta and binds to KEL RBCs of pups. (These data were originally published in the journal *Blood*. Stowell et al. [55]. © 2013 by The American Society of Hematology)

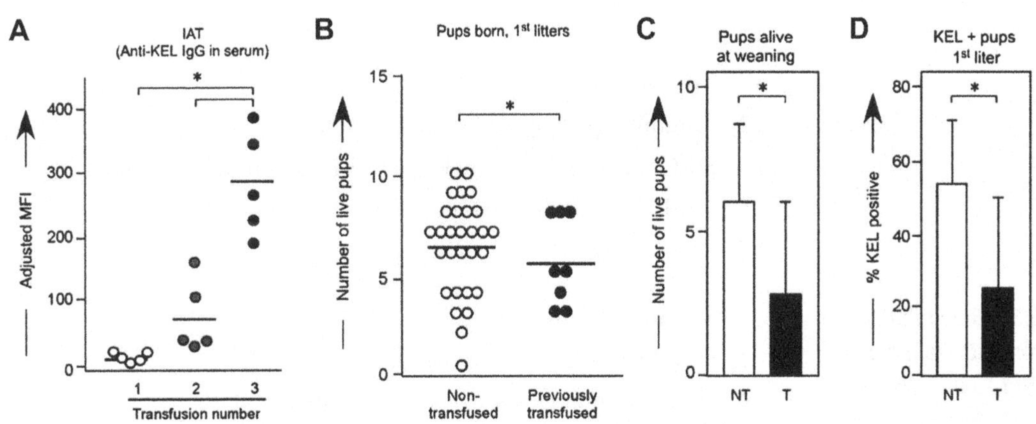

Fig. 7 KEL RBC transfusions induce boostable anti-KEL alloantibodies, which result in adverse pregnancy outcomes. (These data were originally published in the journal *Blood*. Stowell et al. [55]. © 2013 by The American Society of Hematology)

2 Materials

2.1 Induction of Maternal Anti-KEL Antibody by Pregnancy

1. Mice (*see* **Note 1**).
   (a) KEL2 transgenic mice expressing the human KEL glycoprotein (KEL mice).
   (b) C57BL/6 mice (WT mice).

2.2 Induction of Maternal Anti-KEL Antibody by Transfusion

1. Mice (*see* **Note 1**).
   (a) KEL2 transgenic mice expressing the human KEL glycoprotein (KEL mice).
   (b) C57BL/6 mice (WT mice).
2. Donor KEL RBC.
3. Centrifuge tubes and tube holder (tube size depends on amount of donor blood collected).
4. 5 mm lancet.
5. Acid citrate dextrose solution A (ACD-A), sterile.
6. Phosphate buffered saline (PBS), sterile.
7. Poly (I:C) (Amersham).
8. Biosafety cabinet (BSC).
9. Disinfectant and paper towels.
10. Small animal heat lamp, anchored to a support stand using clamps.
11. 70% ethanol.
12. Kimwipes.
13. Mouse restrainer.
14. Magnifying lamp with LED lights.
15. 30 Gauge needles which are 0.5 inches in length, sterile.
16. 1 mL Tuberculin syringe, with Luer slip tip, sterile.
17. Permanent marker.

2.3 Blood Collection for RBC Transfusion and Flow Cytometry DAT (Direct Antiglobulin Test)

1. Biosafety cabinet (BSC).
2. Disinfectant and paper towels.
3. Sterile animal lancets (Fisher Scientific).
   (a) 5 mm for >8-week-old mice.
   (b) 3 mm for younger mice.
4. 4″ × 4″ cotton gauze pad, sterile.
5. Empty mouse cage (recovery cage).
6. Permanent marker.

7. 1.7 mL microcentrifuge tubes and tube holder.
8. Manual pipette and pipette tips.
9. Centrifuge compatible with 1.7 mL microcentrifuge tubes.
10. Acid citrate dextrose solution A (ACD-A).
11. Phosphate buffered saline (PBS).

2.4 Serum Collection for Flow Cytometry IAT (Indirect Antiglobulin Test)

1. Biosafety cabinet (BSC).
2. Disinfectant and paper towels.
3. Sterile animal lancets (Fisher Scientific).
   (a) 5 mm for >8-week-old mice.
   (b) 3 mm for younger mice.
4. 4″ × 4″ cotton gauze pad, sterile.
5. Empty mouse cage (recovery cage).
6. Permanent marker.
7. 1.7 mL microcentrifuge tubes and tube holder.
8. Manual pipette and pipette tips.
9. Centrifuge compatible with 1.7 mL tubes.

2.5 Neonatal Mice Takedown and Blood Collection

1. KIMBLE® Heparinized Micro-Hematocrit Capillary Tubes; Color Red; ID 1.1 mm; Length 75 mm; 90 expansion soda lime glass (VWR).
2. 1.7 mL microcentrifuge tubes.
3. Acid citrate dextrose solution A (ACD-A).
4. Phosphate Buffered Saline (PBS).
5. Pivetal® Isoflurane (Schedule VI controlled substance) (Patterson Veterinary).
6. Breathing Circuits and Accessories, VetEquip®, Complete Dual Procedure Non-Rebreathing Circuit (Fisher Scientific).
7. Razor blades.

2.6 Measurement of Anti-KEL IgG by Flow Cytometry IAT (Indirect Antiglobulin Test)

1. 96-well U-bottom plate.
2. Manual pipette and pipette tips.
3. Multichannel pipette.
4. Phosphate buffered saline (PBS).
5. Buffer Reservoir.
6. Allophycocyanin (APC) AffiniPure Goat Anti-Mouse IgG (subclasses 1 + 2a + 2b + 3), Fcγ Fragment (Jackson ImmunoResearch); any anti-mouse IgG on desired fluorophore.

7. FACS buffer (PBS with 2% BSA and 0.09% EDTA).
8. Centrifuge compatible with 96-well U-bottom plate.
9. Flow cytometer.

2.7 Measurement of Maternal Anti-KEL IgG Placental Transfer by Flow Cytometry DAT (Direct Antiglobulin Test)

1. 96-well U-bottom plate.
2. Manual pipette and pipette tips.
3. Multichannel pipette.
4. Phosphate buffered saline (PBS).
5. Reservoir.
6. Allophycocyanin (APC) AffiniPure Goat Anti-Mouse IgG (subclasses 1 + 2a + 2b + 3), Fcγ Fragment (Jackson ImmunoResearch); any anti-mouse IgG on desired fluorophore.
7. FACS buffer (PBS with 2% BSA and 0.09% EDTA).
8. Centrifuge compatible with 96-well U-bottom plate.
9. Flow cytometer.

2.8 Genotyping for KEL Transgene by PCR (see Note 2)

1. 2–3 mm tail, ear clip, or other tissue biopsy.
2. 50 mM NaOH.
3. 1 M Tris–HCl (pH 8.0).
4. Platinum II Hot-Start Green PCR Master Mix (2×) (Invitrogen).
5. Primers specific for human KEL glycoprotein.
   (a) 5′ forward - GGGGGATCCGCCACCATGGAAGGTGGGGACCAAAGTG.
   (b) 3′ reverse - TTGGAACAGAAGCAGAAAGGAA.
6. Primers specific for mouse G3PDH as control.
   (a) 5′ forward - ACCACAGTCCATGCCATCAC.
   (b) 3′ reverse - TCCACCACCCTGTTGCTGTA.
7. 1 kb Plus DNA ladder (Invitrogen).
8. Ethidium Bromide.
9. 1× TAE buffer.
10. PCR thermocycler.
11. Centrifuges compatible with PCR tubes or 96-well PCR plate.
12. Manual pipette and pipette tips.
13. Multichannel pipette.
14. PCR tube with cap, 8 or 12 PCR strip tubes, or 96-well PCR plate.
15. Agarose gel electrophoresis system.

3 Methods

3.1 Induction of Maternal Anti-KEL Antibody by Pregnancy

1. Set up breeder cages with WT female (2–3 months old) × KEL male per standard animal husbandry conditions. Simultaneously set up breeder cages with age-matched KEL female × WT male as control for change in litter size due to age (*see* **Note 3**).
2. At each birth, count the number of pups alive and carefully observe for stillborn, pale, and/or hydropic appearing pups (Fig. 3). The number of live births should decrease with subsequent pregnancies in the WT female × KEL male breeding pairs, relative to the control breeder pairs (KEL female × WT male).
3. Collect serum from the mother after each birth to evaluate anti-KEL antibody formation by flow cytometry IAT (Subheading 3.4).
4. Track the number of pups alive at weaning. This should also decrease with subsequent pregnancies.
   (a) Neonatal mice takedown and blood collection (Subheading 3.5) can be done to analyze stillborn/anemic pups instead of waiting to wean.
   (b) If KEL male is heterozygous, genotype the pups for KEL transgene by PCR (Subheading 3.8).

3.2 Induction of Maternal Anti-KEL Antibody by Transfusion

3.2.1 Collection of Donor RBCs

1. Calculate adequate volume of blood from KEL mice based on the number of WT females to be transfused. Each transfusion will require 50 μL of KEL RBC (*see* **Note 4**).
2. Collect blood by submandibular bleed into tube pre-filled with ACD (~20% of the total final volume) using a 5 mm lancet (*see* **Note 5**).
3. Following collection, wash blood 3× with sterile PBS, centrifuging at 500 × g for 7–10 min with low/no break. Remove supernatant by careful reverse pipetting between washes (*see* **Note 6**).
4. To obtain packed RBC, pipette repeatedly to resuspend the pellet into residual supernatant.

3.2.2 Antibody Induction and Breeder Setup

1. Pretreat each WT female to be transfused with intraperitoneal injection of 100 μg poly (I:C) approximately 2–4 h prior to transfusion.
2. Transfuse WT female with 50 μL of packed KEL RBC diluted in PBS to 300 μL total volume via lateral tail vein injection.
3. Repeat poly (I:C) and KEL RBC injection every 2–3 weeks.

4. Collect serum 2 weeks after each transfusion to evaluate anti-KEL antibody formation by flow cytometry IAT (Subheading 3.4).
5. Once sufficient anti-KEL antibody formation is observed, set up breeder cages with KEL RBC alloimmunized WT female × KEL male per standard animal husbandry conditions. Simultaneously set up breeder cages with age-matched, un-immunized WT female × KEL male as control (*see* **Note 3**).
6. At birth, count the number of pups alive and carefully observe for stillborn, pale, and/or hydropic appearing pups. The number of live births should be decreased in the KEL RBC alloimmunized WT female × KEL male breeding pairs, relative to the control breeder pairs (un-immunized WT female × KEL male).
7. Track the number of pups alive at weaning. This should also be decreased relative to the control breeder pairs.
   (a) Neonatal mice takedown and blood collection (Subheading 3.5) can be done to analyze placental transfer of maternal IgG into pups instead of waiting to wean.
   (b) If KEL male is heterozygous, genotype the pups for KEL transgene by PCR (Subheading 3.8).

3.3 Serum Collection for Flow Cytometry IAT (Indirect Antiglobulin Test)

1. Collect blood from KEL immunized WT mouse or control WT mouse that is un-immunized into a 1.7 mL tube without ACD-A by performing a submandibular bleed using a 5 mm lancet (*see* **Note 6**).
2. Leave at room temperature for 2 h to clot.
3. Centrifuge the blood at 14,000 × g for 5 min.
4. Transfer the clear supernatant (serum) to a new 1.7 mL tube.
5. Centrifuge the blood at 14,000 × g for 5 min.
6. Transfer the clear supernatant (serum) to a new 1.7 mL tube. Serum can be stored long-term at < −20 °C or used immediately for analysis.

3.4 Neonatal Mice Takedown and Blood Collection for Flow Cytometry DAT (Direct Antiglobulin Test)

1. Place neonatal mouse under isoflurane anesthesia (*see* **Note 4**).
2. Perform a terminal submandibular or retro-orbital bleed using heparin coated capillary tubes and transfer to an empty 1.7 mL microcentrifuge tube containing ACD-A.
3. Centrifuge the blood at 500 × g for 5 min with soft/no brakes to pellet the RBC.
4. Transfer the supernatant (plasma) to a new 1.7 mL microcentrifuge tube. Plasma can be stored long-term at < −20 °C or used immediately for analysis.

5. To obtain packed RBC, wash pelleted RBC 3× with PBS, centrifuging at 500 × g for 5 min with soft/no brakes. Remove supernatant by careful reverse pipetting between washes and resuspend the pellet into residual supernatant after final wash (*see* **Note 7**).
6. Place the pup into an isoflurane chamber. Make sure the pup is under sufficient anesthesia by pinching its toe. If there is no muscle response, decapitate the pup using a razor blade.

3.5 Measurement of Anti-KEL IgG by Flow Cytometry IAT (Indirect Antiglobulin Test)

1. In a 96-well U-bottom plate, for each mouse serum to be tested, add 2 μL of packed RBC from KEL RBC into a well. Add WT RBC into a separate well as a control.
2. Add 10 μL of mouse serum into the corresponding wells (KEL RBC and WT RBC). Mix each well by pipetting up and down using a 10 μL multichannel pipette.
3. Incubate the well plate for 15 min at room temperature.
4. Add 200 μL PBS to each well using a 200 μL multichannel pipette.
5. Centrifuge the plate at 500 × g for 2 min. Visually confirm the pellets are at the bottom of each well and sharply flick out the supernatant.
6. Repeat **Steps 4–5** another 2 times for a total of three washes.
7. Prepare the anti-mouse IgG antibody at a dilution ratio of 1: 100 in FACS buffer (1 μL antibody to 99 μL FACS buffer).
8. Add 25 μL of the prepared anti-mouse IgG antibody solution to each well. Mix each well by pipetting up and down using a 10 μL multichannel pipette.
9. Incubate for 15 min in the dark at room temperature.
10. Add 200 μL PBS to each well using a 200 μL multichannel pipette.
11. Centrifuge the plate at 500 × g for 2 min. Visually confirm the pellets are at the bottom of each well and sharply flick out the supernatant.
12. Repeat **Steps 4–5** another 2 times for a total of three washes.
13. Acquire the sample on the flow cytometer. Determine the anti-KEL IgG level by adjusted mean fluorescence intensity subtracting the background binding signal with control RBCs from that of KEL RBCs.
14. Expected results: IgG will be detectable in serum from KEL immunized mothers through pregnancy or KEL RBC transfusion. IgG will be undetectable in control un-immunized mothers.

3.6 Measurement of Maternal Anti-KEL IgG Placental Transfer by Flow Cytometry DAT (Direct Antiglobulin Test)

1. In a 96-well U-bottom plate, for each pup born to a KEL immunized mother or control un-immunized mother to be tested, add 2 μL of packed RBC or equivalent volume from that pup into a well.
2. Prepare the anti-mouse IgG antibody at a dilution ratio of 1: 100 in FACS buffer (1 μL antibody to 99 μL FACS buffer).
3. Add 25 μL of the prepared anti-mouse IgG antibody solution to each well. Mix each well by pipetting up and down using a 10 μL multichannel pipette.
4. Incubate 15 min in the dark at room temperature.
5. Add 200 μL PBS to each well using a 200 μL multichannel pipette.
6. Centrifuge the plate at 500 × g for 2 min. Visually confirm the pellets are at the bottom of each well and sharply flick out the supernatant.
7. Repeat **Steps 4** and **5** another two times for a total of three washes.
8. Acquire the sample on the flow cytometer.
9. Expected results: IgG will be detectable on RBC of KEL-positive pups born to KEL immunized mothers but will be undetectable in KEL-positive pups born to control un-immunized mothers as well as all KEL-negative pups.

3.7 Genotyping for KEL Transgene by PCR

Protocol adapted from Lopez [64] and Platinum II Taq Hot-Start DNA Polymerase (Invitrogen) manufacturer protocol.

1. Pre-heat PCR thermocycler to 95 °C.
2. Place 2–3 mm tail, ear clip, or other tissue biopsy in each PCR tube as they are obtained.
3. Add 90 μL of 50 mM NaOH to each PCR tube, submerging the entire tissue sample.
4. Incubate in PCR thermocycler at 95 °C for 15 min.
5. Remove from thermocycler and flick tubes (*see* **Note 8**).
6. Neutralize lysate with 10 μL of 1 M Tris–HCl (pH 8.0).
7. Centrifuge the lysate at 14,000 × g for 5 min.
8. The supernatant containing genomic DNA can now be used as the template for PCR. The sample can be kept at < −20 °C for long-term storage.
9. Prepare sufficient PCR master mix for 20 μL PCR reaction per mouse sample.

10. Aliquot 18 μL of master mix into new PCR tubes at RT.
11. Transfer 2 μL of genomic DNA from tissue lysate to PCR tubes.
12. Mix well by flicking the tubes and briefly centrifuge to remove liquid from lid.
13. Place PCR tubes into PCR thermocycler.
14. Cycling protocol for human KEL-specific PCR (*see* **Note 9**).

Component	Volume
Platinum II Hot-Start PCR Master Mix (2×)	10 μL
10 μM forward primer	0.4 μL
10 μM reverse primer	0.4 μL
Nuclease-free water	7.2 μL

PCR cycle	Step	Temperature	Time
1	Denaturation	94 °C	2 min
35	Denaturation	94 °C	15 s
	Annealing	60 °C	15 s
	Extension	68 °C	45 s
Hold		4 °C	Indefinitely

15. The PCR product can be kept at 4 °C for up to a week, or < −20 °C for long-term storage before agarose gel electrophoresis.
16. The Platinum II Hot-Start PCR Master Mix (2×) already contains loading dye, allowing the PCR product to be directly loaded into agarose gel wells for electrophoresis.
17. For each row of wells containing PCR product, reserve an extra well for addition of 1 kb DNA ladder with loading buffer, per manufacturer protocol.
18. Run gel electrophoresis, adjusting voltage and time based on equipment and band resolution.
19. Use the appropriate gel viewer or imaging apparatus to identify bands.
20. For KEL-negative samples, set up PCR with the mouse G3PDH-specific primer pairs as a control.

4 Notes

1. For the KEL transgenic mouse, the KEL2B strain [56] aka KEL^{med} [63] aka KEL-$K2_{med}$ [60] is the only KEL strain with published data demonstrating the HDFN phenotype. Another consideration is the use of KEL homozygote vs. heterozygote males in the breeder setup. The WT female × KEL homozygote male breeding pair will produce an all KEL-positive litter which may show a more apparent HDFN phenotype (more pups affected) but setup of an age-matched control will be necessary. The WT female × KEL heterozygote male breeding pair will produce KEL-negative littermate controls, but the KEL phenotype of the pups will need to be verified by PCR.
2. We list the previously published primers for KEL genotyping [56], but our lab outsources routine mouse genotyping to a commercial vendor that designed proprietary primers based on provided genomic information. For design of optimized primers, refer to precise transgene integration site of KEL-$K2_{med}$ strain [60].
3. In the pregnancy-induced model, the expected length of time from setup of breeder pairs to weaning of third litter is approximately 6 months to account for multiple rounds of pregnancy/weaning (Fig. 1). In the transfusion-induced model, the expected length of time from immunization to weaning of first litter is approximately 3 months (Fig. 2). In both setups, females of 2–3 months of age should be used to account for decrease in fertility due to advanced maternal age.
4. Be sure to abide by IACUC guidelines at your institution.
5. Donor mice can be bled multiple times using this non-terminal technique. Be sure to clearly identify mice that are bled and keep track of the volume and frequency of blood collected from each donor. Do not exceed IACUC guidelines for blood collection.
6. Anticoagulated whole blood can be temporarily stored at 4 °C prior to transfusion but should be used on the same day to avoid confounding effects from RBC storage lesions.
7. It is best to stain RBCs within a few hours after collection; however, successful staining has been performed in our hands on RBCs stored at 4 °C in PBS for up to 3 days prior to staining.
8. Flick the PCR tube to verify sufficient incubation. The tissue sample should partially break apart, and the liquid should be cloudy. Incubate for longer if necessary.

9. The Platinum II PCR buffer contains isostabilizing molecules that allow for universal primer annealing temperature at 60 °C. If using other PCR systems, thermocycler conditions may need to be adjusted.

Conflict of Interest

This work was funded by NIH P01HL171803, R01 HL165975, and R01 HL135575. SRS has received speaker and consultant honoraria from Cerus, Grifols, Novartis, Alexion, and Argenx, and has received a research grant from Alexion. No other authors have conflicts of interest.

References

1. Diamond LK, Blackfan KD, Baty JM (1932) Erythroblastosis fetalis and its association with universal edema of the fetus, icterus gravis neonatorum and anemia of the newborn. J Pediatr 1(3):269–309
2. Levine P et al (1941) The role of iso-immunization in the pathogenesis of erythroblastosis fetalis. Am J Obstet Gynecol 42(6): 925–937
3. Naiman JL (2001) On Dr. Louis K. Diamond's 1932 article and subsequent contributions to erythroblastosis fetalis. J Pediatr Hematol Oncol 23(8):550–553
4. Storry JR, Olsson ML (2009) The ABO blood group system revisited: a review and update. Immunohematology 25(2):48–59
5. Joseph A et al (2023) ABO Genotyping finds more A(2) to B kidney transplant opportunities than lectin-based subtyping. Am J Transplant 23(4):512–519
6. Jajosky RP et al (2023) ABO blood group antigens and differential glycan expression: perspective on the evolution of common human enzyme deficiencies. iScience 26(1):105798
7. Wu SC et al (2022) Innate immune Galectin-7 specifically targets microbes that decorate themselves in blood group-like antigens. iScience 25(7):104482
8. Blenda AV et al (2022) Galectin-9 recognizes and exhibits antimicrobial activity toward microbes expressing blood group-like antigens. J Biol Chem 298(4):101704
9. Jan HM et al (2024) Galectin-4 antimicrobial activity primarily occurs through its C-terminal domain. Mol Cell Proteomics 23(5):100747
10. Arthur CM, Stowell SR (2023) The development and consequences of red blood cell alloimmunization. Annu Rev Pathol 18:537–564
11. Bowman J (2003) Thirty-five years of Rh prophylaxis. Transfusion 43(12):1661–1666
12. Practice Bulletin No (2017) 181: prevention of Rh D alloimmunization. Obstet Gynecol 130(2):e57–e70
13. Visser GHA et al (2019) The continuing burden of Rh disease 50 years after the introduction of anti-Rh(D) immunoglobin prophylaxis: call to action. Am J Obstet Gynecol 221(3): 227 e1–227 e4
14. Bhutani VK et al (2013) Neonatal hyperbilirubinemia and Rhesus disease of the newborn: incidence and impairment estimates for 2010 at regional and global levels. Pediatr Res 74 Suppl 1(Suppl 1):86–100
15. Zipursky A, Paul VK (2011) The global burden of Rh disease. Arch Dis Child Fetal Neonatal Ed 96(2):F84–F85
16. Verweij E et al (2024) Monoclonal RhD prophylaxis: high time to evaluate efficacy. Lancet 403(10429):806–807
17. (2018) ACOG Practice Bulletin No. 192: Management of alloimmunization during pregnancy. Obstet Gynecol 131(3):e82–e90
18. Yu D et al (2023) Live birth prevalence of hemolytic disease of the fetus and newborn in the United States from 1996 to 2010. AJOG Glob Rep 3(2):100203
19. Sugrue RP et al (2024) Maternal red blood cell alloimmunization prevalence in the United States. Blood Adv
20. Cruz-Leal Y, Marjoram D, Lazarus AH (2017) Prevention of hemolytic disease of the fetus and newborn: what have we learned from animal models? Curr Opin Hematol 24(6):536–543

21. Hendrickson JE, Delaney M (2016) Hemolytic disease of the fetus and newborn: modern practice and future investigations. Transfus Med Rev 30(4):159–164
22. Heard DH, Hinde IT, Mynors LS (1949) An experimental study of haemolytic disease of the newborn due to isoimmunization of pregnancy. J Hyg (Lond) 47(2):119–131
23. Moise KJ Jr et al (1998) An animal model for hemolytic disease of the fetus or newborn in New Zealand white and New Zealand red rabbits: newborn effects. Am J Obstet Gynecol 179(5):1353–1358
24. Moise KJ Jr et al (1995) An animal model for hemolytic disease of the fetus and newborn. I. Alloimmunization techniques. Am J Obstet Gynecol 173(1):51–55
25. Moise KJ Jr et al (1995) An animal model for hemolytic disease of the fetus and newborn. II. Fetal effects in New Zealand rabbits. Am J Obstet Gynecol 173(3 Pt 1):747–753
26. Kellner A, Hedal EF (1953) Experimental erythroblastosis fetalis in rabbits. I. Characterization of a pair of allelic blood group factors and their specific immune isoantibodies. J Exp Med 97(1):33–49
27. Kellner A, Hedal EF (1953) Experimental erythroblastosis fetalis in rabbits. II. The passage of blood group antigens and their specific isoantibodies across the placenta. J Exp Med 97(1):51–60
28. Goossens D et al (2013) Mice expressing RHAG and RHD human blood group genes. PLoS One 8(11):e80460
29. Bernardo L et al (2014) RhD specific antibodies are not detectable in HLA-DRB1(*)1501 mice challenged with human RhD positive erythrocytes. Adv Hematol 2014:470242
30. Hod EA, Zimring JC, Spitalnik SL (2008) Lessons learned from mouse models of hemolytic transfusion reactions. Curr Opin Hematol 15(6):601–605
31. Zimring JC et al (2005) Nonhemolytic antibody-induced loss of erythrocyte surface antigen. Blood 106(3):1105–1112
32. Zimring JC et al (2007) Nonhemolytic antigen loss from red blood cells requires cooperative binding of multiple antibodies recognizing different epitopes. Blood 110(6):2201–2208
33. Hod EA et al (2008) Cytokine storm in a mouse model of IgG-mediated hemolytic transfusion reactions. Blood 112(3):891–894
34. Mener A et al (2018) Complement serves as a switch between CD4+ T cell-independent and -dependent RBC antibody responses. JCI Insight 3(22)
35. Arneja A et al (2016) Interleukin-6 receptor-alpha signaling drives anti-RBC alloantibody production and T-follicular helper cell differentiation in a murine model of red blood cell alloimmunization. Haematologica 101(11): e440–e444
36. Qiu A et al (2022) FcgammaRIV is required for IgG2c mediated enhancement of RBC alloimmunization. Front Immunol 13:972723
37. Soldatenko A et al (2022) Innate and adaptive immunity to transfused allogeneic RBCs in mice requires MyD88. J Immunol 208(4): 991–997
38. Thomas TA et al (2023) Reticulocytes in donor blood units enhance red blood cell alloimmunization. Haematologica 108(10):2639–2651
39. Jash A et al (2024) Complement C3 and marginal zone B cells promote IgG-mediated enhancement of RBC alloimmunization in mice. J Clin Invest 134(8)
40. Arthur CM et al (2017) Antigen density dictates immune responsiveness following red blood cell transfusion. J Immunol 198(7): 2671–2680
41. Jajosky R et al (2023) Prior immunization against an intracellular antigen enhances subsequent red blood cell alloimmunization in mice. Blood 141(21):2642–2653
42. Zerra PE et al (2021) Marginal zone B cells mediate a CD4 T-cell-dependent extrafollicular antibody response following RBC transfusion in mice. Blood 138(8):706–721
43. Jajosky RP et al (2023) Antibody-mediated antigen loss switches augmented immunity to antibody-mediated immunosuppression. Blood 142(12):1082–1098
44. Jajosky RP et al (2024) Dynamics of antibody engagement of red blood cells in vivo and in vitro. Front Immunol 15:1475470
45. Arthur CM et al (2016) CD8+ T cells mediate antibody-independent platelet clearance in mice. Blood 127(14):1823–1827
46. Zerra PE et al (2017) Marginal zone B cells are critical to factor VIII inhibitor formation in mice with hemophilia A. Blood 130(23): 2559–2568
47. Arthur CM et al (2022) Nonhuman glycans can regulate anti-factor VIII antibody formation in mice. Blood 139(9):1312–1317
48. Newman DK, Newman PJ (2024) Antigen-specific immunotherapy for platelet alloimmune disorders. Hum Immunol 85(6):111172
49. Zhi H et al (2022) Prophylactic administration of HPA-1a-specific antibodies prevents fetal/ neonatal alloimmune thrombocytopenia in mice. Blood 140(20):2146–2153

50. Tiller H et al (2012) Toward a prophylaxis against fetal and neonatal alloimmune thrombocytopenia: induction of antibody-mediated immune suppression and prevention of severe clinical complications in a murine model. Transfusion 52(7):1446–1457
51. Xu X et al (2021) Successful prenatal therapy for anti-CD36-mediated severe FNAIT by deglycosylated antibodies in a novel murine model. Blood 138(18):1757–1767
52. Zhi H et al (2021) Preclinical evaluation of immunotherapeutic regimens for fetal/neonatal alloimmune thrombocytopenia. Blood Adv 5(18):3552–3562
53. Li C et al (2011) The maternal immune response to fetal platelet GPIbalpha causes frequent miscarriage in mice that can be prevented by intravenous IgG and anti-FcRn therapies. J Clin Invest 121(11):4537–4547
54. Chen P et al (2010) Animal model of fetal and neonatal immune thrombocytopenia: role of neonatal fc receptor in the pathogenesis and therapy. Blood 116(18):3660–3668
55. Stowell SR et al (2013) Alloantibodies to a paternally derived RBC KEL antigen lead to hemolytic disease of the fetus/newborn in a murine model. Blood 122(8):1494–1504. https://doi.org/10.1182/blood-2013-03-488874
56. Smith NH et al (2012) Generation of transgenic mice with antithetical KEL1 and KEL2 human blood group antigens on red blood cells. Transfusion 52(12):2620–2630
57. Jash A et al (2021) Antibodies to low-copy number RBC alloantigen convert a tolerogenic stimulus to an immunogenic stimulus in mice. Front Immunol 12:629608
58. Maier CL et al (2018) Antibody-mediated immune suppression by antigen modulation is antigen-specific. Blood Adv 2(21):2986–3000
59. Mener A et al (2019) Antibody-mediated immunosuppression can result from RBC antigen loss independent of Fcgamma receptors in mice. Transfusion 59(1):371–384
60. Jash A et al (2023) The role of RBC antigen transgene integration sites on RBC biology in mice. Transfusion 63(1):239–248
61. Gibb DR et al (2017) Type I IFN is necessary and sufficient for inflammation-induced red blood cell alloimmunization in mice. J Immunol 199(3):1041–1050
62. Patel SR, Maier CL, Zimring JC (2023) Alloantigen copy number as a critical factor in RBC alloimmunization. Transfus Med Rev 37(1): 21–26
63. Arthur CM et al (2021) Antigen density dictates RBC clearance, but not antigen modulation, following incompatible RBC transfusion in mice. Blood Adv 5(2):527–538
64. Lopez ME (2012) A auick, no frills approach to mouse genotyping. Bio Protoc 2(15)

Chapter 6

Anti-platelet Factor 4/Heparin Antibody Production in a Mouse Immunization Model

Mei Yu, Renren Wen, and Demin Wang

Abstract

Heparin-induced thrombocytopenia (HIT) is the most prevalent form of drug-induced, immune-mediated thrombocytopenia. It involves the production of antibodies that target platelet factor 4 (PF4) in complex with heparin, leading to platelet activation. The pathogenesis of HIT is not fully understood, primarily due to the limitations of studying human patients. To bridge this gap and gain a deeper understanding of the mechanisms behind HIT antibody generation, researchers developed a murine model using immunization with mouse PF4 (mPF4)/heparin complexes. Here, we provide a detailed methodology for inducing mPF4/heparin antibodies in C57BL/6 mice and validating the immunization process. Through these techniques, we identified the critical subset of B cells responsible for producing mPF4/heparin-specific antibodies, as well as other immune cells essential for regulating this production. This immunization-based mouse model of HIT is a valuable tool for studying the immunopathogenesis of the condition.

Key words Heparin-induced thrombocytopenia, Platelet factor 4/heparin-specific antibody, Mouse model

1 Introduction

Heparin-induced thrombocytopenia (HIT) is the most common immune-mediated drug-induced thrombocytopenia resulting from heparin treatment [1]. HIT occurs in approximately 0.5–1% of patients treated with unfractionated heparin within 3 to 6 days of treatment [2]. Despite the development of low-molecular-weight heparin and several new anticoagulants, heparin continues to be widely used, affecting over 20,000 patients annually in the USA [3]. It is estimated that 20–64% of HIT patients experience thrombosis, with mortality rates ranging from 6% to 53% across various clinical retrospective studies [4]. Thus, HIT remains a significant adverse drug reaction today.

Despite significant progress in the study of HIT, its pathogenesis remains not fully understood. Heparin binds to platelet factor 4 (PF4), causing a conformational change that exposes epitopes

Sean R. Stowell and Connie M. Arthur (eds.), *Methods in Transfusion Medicine*, Methods in Molecular Biology, vol. 3053,
https://doi.org/10.1007/978-1-0716-5376-0_6,

recognized by anti-PF4/heparin antibodies [5]. These antigen–antibody complexes bind to the cellular Fcγ receptor (FcγRIIA) on platelets, monocytes, and neutrophils [6, 7], leading to the activation of platelets and other immune cells, and ultimately resulting in thrombocytopenia and a high risk of thrombosis [8]. However, only a subset of patients receiving heparin treatment develop anti-PF4/heparin antibodies, and an even smaller fraction produce pathogenic antibodies capable of activating platelets [9]. Studies have shown that the antibody response in HIT patients differs from the classic humoral immune response. Typically, IgM antibodies, indicative of a primary immune response, are produced within 5–10 days of antigen exposure, followed by IgG antibodies. In HIT, however, high titers of IgG antibodies are generated soon after initial heparin treatment [2]. Most anti-PF4/heparin antibodies in HIT patients are of the IgG1 isotype, with a smaller proportion being IgG2 [10]. Additionally, HIT patients appear to lack immunologic memory against the PF4/heparin complex, differing from the classic immune response [11, 12]. These unique features of HIT indicate that its immunogenesis is complex but crucial for understanding its pathogenesis.

Several animal models have been developed to elucidate the intriguing pathogenesis of HIT. Immunizing mice with patient-derived HIT IgGs induces mouse antibodies against PF4/heparin, resulting in thrombocytopenia following unfractionated heparin injection [13, 14]. The immunized mice develop anti-idiotypic antibodies against the human HIT antibodies, functionally resembling the human HIT antibody. Additionally, human FcγRIIA and PF4 double transgenic mice injected with KKO, a mouse monoclonal IgG2b antibody against human PF4 (hPF4)/heparin, develop thrombocytopenia and thrombosis, recapitulating the symptoms in HIT patients [15]. However, these models depend on the administration of human or mouse antibodies rather than antigens, which differs from the real cause of HIT. To better replicate the immunogenesis of HIT, a model using wild-type C57BL/6 mice as recipients, with mouse PF4 and heparin complex (mPF4/heparin) serving as the antigens for immunization, has been developed. Antibodies against the mPF4/heparin complex are rapidly generated and share the serologic and functional features of human HIT antibodies [16–18] (Fig. 1). Using this mouse model, our group demonstrated that MZ B cells are critical for PF4/heparin-specific antibody production, and T cells are required for the production of anti-PF4/heparin antibodies [19, 20]. Furthermore, our studies elucidated the important roles of B-cell tolerance and Treg in controlling PF4/heparin-specific antibody production [21, 22]. In summary, this murine immunization model provides a valuable approach to elucidate the immunogenesis and pathogenesis of HIT.

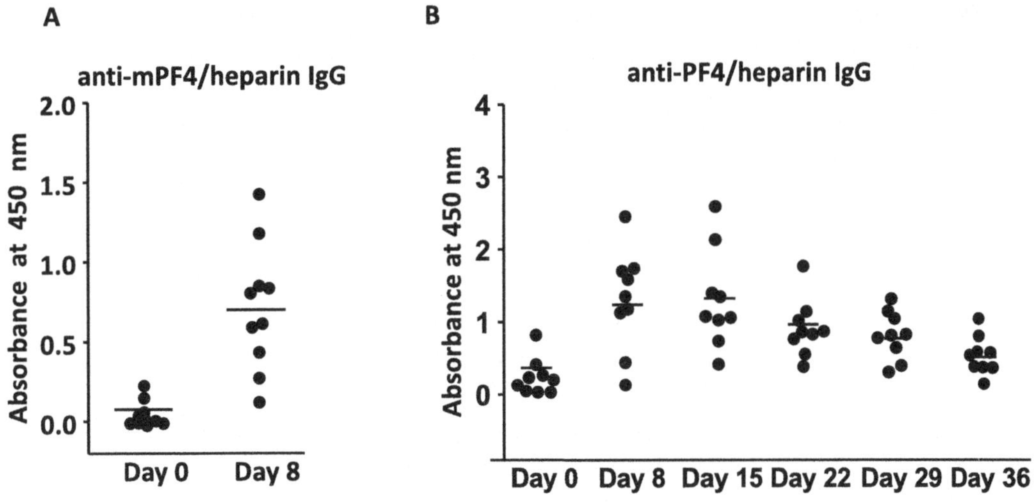

Fig. 1 Anti-mouse platelet factor 4 (mPF4)/heparin antibody production in C57BL/6 mice following mPF4/heparin immunization. (**a**) C57BL/6 mice immunized with mPF4/heparin (molar ratio 2.6:1) via the retro-orbital route daily for 5 days elicited optimal immune responses that mimic human heparin sensitization. (**b**) Six- to 8-week-old C57BL/6 mice were immunized intravenously via the retro-orbital route with 100 μL of PF4/heparin. Sera were collected on Days 8, 15, 22, 29, and 36 post-immunization. PF4/heparin-specific IgG levels in the sera were measured by ELISA. Consistent Anti-mPF4/heparin antibody production can be detected in C57BL/6 mice in our studies that are reported previously [19–22]

2 Materials

2.1 Baseline Blood Collection from Mice Prior to Immunization

1. C57BL/6 Mice: 8–10 mice from The Jackson Laboratory.
2. Animal Lancets: 4.0 mm lancets from Goldenrod.
3. Isoflurane: provided by Piramal Healthcare (NDC 66794-013-10).
4. Sterile Eppendorf Tubes: 1.5 mL tubes.

2.2 Preparation of Reagents for Immunization

1. Hanks' balanced salt solution (HBSS; 10X): GIBCO (Cat. No. 14185, Invitrogen).
2. Purified mouse PF4: Protein Foundry LLC (Product No. PFP068).
3. Heparin: Millipore-Sigma (Cat. No. H3393-100KU).
4. A 0.22 μm Syringe Filter: Corning (Part No. 431219).
5. Sterile Eppendorf Tubes: 1.5 mL tubes.

2.3 Performing Immunization Via Retro-Orbital Injection

1. Isoflurane.
2. Isoflurane evaporator.
3. Syringe with 27.5-gauge needle (Becton-Dickinson Part No. 305109).

2.4 Bleeding Mice After Immunization

1. Animal lancets: 4.0 mm lancets from Goldenrod.
2. Sterile Eppendorf tubes: 1.5 mL tubes.

2.5 ELISA Assay for Anti-PF4/H Antibodies Detection

1. A 96-well flat-bottom immuno plate (NUNC, Product No. 96).
2. Purified mouse PF4 (Protein Foundry LLC, Product No. PFP068).
3. Heparin (Millipore-Sigma, Product No. H3393-100KU).
4. 1X Phosphate Buffered Saline (PBS).
5. Tris-buffered saline with 0.05% Tween-20 (TBS-T) (Fisher, Product No. BP337-500).
6. PBS with 10% Fetal Calf Serum (FCS) (GIBCO HI-FBS, Cat. No. 10082-147 Invitrogen).
7. Horseradish peroxidase (HRP)-conjugated secondary anti-mouse antibodies for targeted isotypes (e.g., goat anti-mouse IgG gamma chain, HRP-labeled, Sigma, Cat. No. 3673).
8. 3,3',5,5'-Tetramethylbenzidine (TMBZ) substrate solution (A +B) (KPL, Cat. No. 50-76-01, 50-65-00).
9. 1N Sulfuric acid (H_2SO_4).
10. Microplate Shaker.
11. Absorbance Microplate Reader.

3 Methods

3.1 Baseline Blood Collection from Mice Prior to Immunization

1. Place the mouse in an anesthesia induction chamber and anesthetize using isoflurane.
2. Once anesthetized, remove the mouse from the chamber. Restrain it by holding the skin over the shoulders and behind the ears.
3. Using a lancet, make a shallow puncture (1–2 mm depth) in the submandibular (facial) vein. Blood will begin to flow immediately.
4. Collect 0.1–0.2 mL of blood into an Eppendorf tube.
5. Apply gentle pressure to the puncture site with a gauze sponge to stop the bleeding.
6. Return the mouse to its cage and monitor it until it fully recovers from anesthesia.
7. Perform the blood collection procedure on 8-10 C57BL/6 mice (*see* **Note 1**).

3.2 Preparation of Reagents for Immunization

1. Dilute the 10X HBSS solution to 1X by using deionized distilled water (ddH_2O).
2. Filter the diluted 1X HBSS using a 0.22 μm syringe filter.
3. Dilute mPF4 with the filtered 1X HBSS to a final concentration of 1 mg/mL.
4. Filter the diluted mPF4 solution using a 0.22 μm syringe filter and aliquot the filtered mPF4 solution. Store the aliquots at − 20 °C (*see* **Note 2**).

3.3 Fresh Preparation of mPF4 and Heparin Complex for Daily Injection

1. Prepare the mPF4/heparin solution in 1X HBSS with a final concentration of mPF4 at 200 μg/mL and heparin at 4 U/mL for injection. Each mouse will receive 100 μL of this solution (*see* **Note 3**). Sequentially add HBSS, mPF4, and then heparin (*see* **Note 4**).
2. Do not vortex the solution. Instead, gently rotate the tube several times, then incubate at room temperature for 1 h (*see* **Note 5**).
3. Transfer the mPF4/heparin mixture into a syringe fitted with a 27.5G needle.

3.4 Retro-Orbital Injection

1. Anesthetize the mouse using an isoflurane evaporator supplied with oxygen (*see* **Note 6**).
2. Once the mouse has lost its limb reflexes, remove it from the induction chamber and place the nose cone over the mouse's face.
3. Inject 100 μL of the mPF4/heparin mixture in HBSS via the retro-orbital vein (*see* **Note 7**).
4. Return the mouse to its cage with fresh air and monitor it until it fully recovers from anesthesia.
5. Repeat the anesthesia and injection procedure for each subsequent mouse.
6. Perform the injection for five consecutive days, from Day 1 to Day 5 (*see* **Note 8**).

3.5 Bleed the Mice After Immunization

1. Bleed the mice on Days 8, 15, 22, 29, and 36, collecting 0.1–0.2 mL of blood from each mouse each time.
2. Allow the collected blood to coagulate for 30 min at room temperature.
3. Transfer the tubes to the refrigerator for overnight storage.
4. Centrifuge the blood samples at 5000 rpm for 5 min. Carefully transfer the top layer of serum without disturbing or aspirating the clotted blood cells.
5. Aliquot the serum and store it at −80 °C. Avoid repeated freezing and thawing.

3.6 ELISA Assay for Detecting Anti-PF4/H Antibodies

1. Coat a 96-well plate with 10 μg/mL PF4 and 0.4 U/mL heparin in PBS. Add 100 μL of this solution to each well and incubate on a shaker at room temperature overnight (*see* **Note 9**).
2. Wash the plate three times with TBS/0.05% Tween-20 and slap the plate several times between each wash.
3. Block the plate by adding 200 μL of 10% FCS/PBS to each well and incubate at room temperature for 2 h.
4. Repeat the washing step three times with TBS/0.05% Tween-20 and slap the plate several times between each wash.
5. Dilute mouse sera 1:100 in 10% FCS/PBS. Prepare negative controls using serum from unimmunized mice and prepare positive controls using standardized anti-mPF4/heparin antibodies or previously tested anti-mPF4/heparin positive mouse serum. Use 10% FCS/PBS as a blank control.
6. Add 100 μL of mouse sera, negative control, positive control, and blank control to each well in duplicate. Incubate on a shaker at room temperature for 1 h.
7. Wash the plate three times with TBS/0.05% Tween-20 and slap the plate several times between each wash.
8. Dilute HRP-conjugated secondary antibodies (specific for the isotype of interest) 1:500 in 10% FCS/PBS.
9. Add 100 μL of diluted secondary antibody to each well. Incubate on a shaker at room temperature for 1 h.
10. Wash the plate three times with TBS/0.05% Tween-20 and slap the plate several times between each wash.
11. Develop the signal by adding 100 μL of TMBZ (A+B), prepared by mixing Solution A substrate and Solution B peroxidase at a 1:1 ratio, to each well. Incubate at room temperature for 1 h without shaking.
12. Stop the reaction by adding 50 μL of 1N H_2SO_4 to each well.
13. Read the absorbance of the plate at 450 nm using a microplate reader.

4 Notes

1. The immune response varies from 20% to 60% due to different lots of PF4. Therefore, use 8–10 mice to ensure statistically significant results after immunization.
2. After thawing a new vial of mPF4, vortex thoroughly to fully recover the protein.
3. Prepare enough reagent for two additional mice to account for any loss during injection.

4. The order of adding reagents is critical for forming the mPF4/ heparin complex.
5. Gently rotate the reagents by hand to mix; do not vortex. The formation of a white, cloudy precipitate indicates successful complex generation.
6. An isoflurane evaporator with oxygen flow is highly recommended for retro-orbital injections, as it provides better control over anesthesia depth and duration. To prevent hypothermia, place the mouse on a warming pad or blanket during the injection.
7. Insert the needle at a 30° angle into the corner of the eye to a depth of 1/10 inch. Tilt the needle to a horizontal level, then insert it 1/10 inch deeper until it goes under the eyeball. Inject the reagent, ensuring it enters the vessels under the eyeball. A small amount of blood may appear after a correct injection, but this is not always the case.
8. It has been shown that a 5-day injection schedule significantly increases the production of anti-mPF4/heparin antibodies compared to 4-day or 1-day schedules [18].
9. Prepare the reagent as for immunization, but use PBS. Do not filter, and leave at room temperature for 10 min to allow complex formation. Rotate the tube to mix the reagents; do not vortex.

Conflict of Interest

This work is supported in part by NIH grants AI079087 (D.W.), HL130724 (D.W.), HL148120 (R.W.), HL161127 (R.W.), and HL167668 (R.W., D.W.). The authors have no financial conflicts of interest.

References

1. Warkentin TE, Kelton JG (2001) Temporal aspects of heparin-induced thrombocytopenia. N Engl J Med 344:1286–1292
2. Warkentin TE, Sheppard JA, Moore JC, Cook RJ, Kelton JG (2009) Studies of the immune response in heparin-induced thrombocytopenia. Blood 113:4963–4969
3. Dhakal B, Kreuziger LB, Rein L, Kleman A, Fraser R, Aster RH, Hari P, Padmanabhan A (2018) Disease burden, complication rates, and health-care costs of heparin-induced thrombocytopenia in the USA: a population-based study. Lancet Haematol 5:e220–e231
4. Arepally GM, Padmanabhan A (2021) Heparin-induced thrombocytopenia: a focus on thrombosis. Arterioscler Thromb Vasc Biol 41:141–152
5. Brandt S, Krauel K, Gottschalk KE, Renné T, Helm CA, Greinacher A, Block S (2014) Characterisation of the conformational changes in platelet factor 4 induced by polyanions: towards in vitro prediction of antigenicity. Thromb Haemost 112:53–64
6. Kelton JG, Sheridan D, Santos A, Smith J, Steeves K, Smith C, Brown C, Murphy WG (1988) Heparin-induced thrombocytopenia: laboratory studies. Blood 72:925–930

7. Chong BH, Fawaz I, Chesterman CN, Berndt MC (1989) Heparin-induced thrombocytopenia: mechanism of interaction of the heparin-dependent antibody with platelets. Br J Haematol 73:235–240
8. Warkentin TE, Sheppard JA, Moore JC, Moore KM, Sigouin CS, Kelton JG (2005) Laboratory testing for the antibodies that cause heparin-induced thrombocytopenia: how much class do we need? J Lab Clin Med 146:341–346
9. Nazi I, Arnold DM, Warkentin TE, Smith JW, Staibano P, Kelton JG (2015) Distinguishing between anti-platelet factor 4/heparin antibodies that can and cannot cause heparin-induced thrombocytopenia. J Thromb Haemost: JTH 13:1900–1907
10. Denomme GA, Warkentin TE, Horsewood P, Sheppard JA, Warner MN, Kelton JG (1997) Activation of platelets by sera containing IgG1 heparin-dependent antibodies: an explanation for the predominance of the Fc gammaRIIa "low responder" (his131) gene in patients with heparin-induced thrombocytopenia. J Lab Clin Med 130:278–284
11. Potzsch B, Klovekorn WP, Madlener K (2000) Use of heparin during cardiopulmonary bypass in patients with a history of heparin-induced thrombocytopenia. N Engl J Med 343:515
12. Selleng K, Schutt A, Selleng S, Warkentin TE, Greinacher A (2010) Studies of the anti-platelet factor 4/heparin immune response: adapting the enzyme-linked immunosorbent spot assay for detection of memory B cells against complex antigens. Transfusion 50:32–39
13. Blank M, Cines DB, Arepally G, Eldor A, Afek A, Shoenfeld Y (1997) Pathogenicity of human anti-platelet factor 4 (PF4)/heparin in vivo: generation of mouse anti-PF4/heparin and induction of thrombocytopenia by heparin. Clin Exp Immunol 108:333–339
14. Blank M, Eldor A, Tavor S, Ziporen L, Cines DB, Arepally G, Afek A, Shoenfeld Y (1999) A mouse model for heparin-induced thrombocytopenia. Semin Hematol 36:12–16
15. Reilly MP, Taylor SM, Hartman NK, Arepally GM, Sachais BS, Cines DB, Poncz M, McKenzie SE (2001) Heparin-induced thrombocytopenia/thrombosis in a transgenic mouse model requires human platelet factor 4 and platelet activation through FcgammaRIIA. Blood 98: 2442–2447
16. Suvarna S, Rauova L, McCracken EK, Goss CM, Sachais BS, McKenzie SE, Reilly MP, Gunn MD, Cines DB, Poncz M, Arepally G (2005) PF4/heparin complexes are T cell-dependent antigens. Blood 106:929–931
17. Suvarna S, Espinasse B, Qi R, Lubica R, Poncz M, Cines DB, Wiesner MR, Arepally GM (2007) Determinants of PF4/heparin immunogenicity. Blood 110:4253–4260
18. Suvarna S, Qi R, Arepally GM (2009) Optimization of a murine immunization model for study of PF4/heparin antibodies. J Thromb Haemost: JTH 7:857–864
19. Zheng Y, Yu M, Podd A, Yuan L, Newman DK, Wen R, Arepally G, Wang D (2013) Critical role for mouse marginal zone B cells in PF4/heparin antibody production. Blood 121:3484–3492
20. Zheng Y, Yu M, Padmanabhan A, Aster RH, Yuan L, Wen R, Wang D (2015) Critical role of CD4 T cells in PF4/heparin antibody production in mice. Blood 125:1826–1829
21. Zheng Y, Wang AW, Yu M, Padmanabhan A, Tourdot BE, Newman DK, White GC, Aster RH, Wen R, Wang D (2014) B-cell tolerance regulates production of antibodies causing heparin-induced thrombocytopenia. Blood 123:931–934
22. Zheng Y, Zhu W, Haribhai D, Williams CB, Aster RH, Wen R, Wang D (2019) Regulatory T cells control PF4/Heparin antibody production in mice. J Immunol 203:1786–1792

Chapter 7

Microscopy-Based Methods for Measuring Platelet and Red Blood Cell Phagocytosis

Alequis Pavon Oro, Zoya Tawhidi, Zoya Hussain, Yoelys Cruz-Leal, Yaima Tundidor, Lazaro Gil Gonzalez, Yuexin Shan, Peter A. A. Norris, and Alan H. Lazarus

Abstract

Phagocytosis plays a pivotal role in diseases involving the accelerated removal of platelets and erythrocytes from the circulation and can be mediated by antibodies through the mononuclear phagocyte system. In autoimmune conditions such as immune thrombocytopenia and autoimmune hemolytic anemia, autoantibodies target self-antigens on platelets or red blood cells. Similarly, in alloimmune diseases like fetal and neonatal alloimmune thrombocytopenia and hemolytic disease of the fetus and newborn, maternal alloantibodies can target platelet or erythrocyte antigens, leading to cytopenias. Phagocytosis can be facilitated by Fc gamma receptors on macrophages, which bind to the Fc region of IgG that sensitizes these platelets or erythrocytes. Understanding the mechanisms of phagocytosis is crucial, as it can significantly drive the pathophysiology of autoimmune and alloimmune diseases. In this chapter, we detail confocal and phase contrast microscopy-based methods for quantifying antibody-mediated phagocytosis of platelets and erythrocytes, respectively.

Key words Platelets, Red blood cells, Phagocytosis, Phagocytic index, Confocal microscopy, Phase Contrast microscopy

1 Introduction

Phagocytosis can play a pivotal role in diseases involving platelet or erythrocyte clearance by the mononuclear phagocyte system (MPS). This system, particularly in the spleen and liver, includes macrophages with a high capacity to engulf these cells, contributing to various hematologic conditions. In autoimmune disorders such as immune thrombocytopenia (ITP) and autoimmune hemolytic anemia (AIHA), autoantibodies trigger the phagocytosis of platelets and erythrocytes, respectively [1, 2]. Platelet glycoproteins (GP), such as GPIIb/IIIa [3] and GPIb/IX [4], are commonly targeted antigens in ITP. Similarly, in alloimmune diseases, such as

Sean R. Stowell and Connie M. Arthur (eds.), *Methods in Transfusion Medicine*, Methods in Molecular Biology, vol. 3053, https://doi.org/10.1007/978-1-0716-5376-0_7,

fetal and neonatal alloimmune thrombocytopenia (FNAIT) and hemolytic disease of the fetus and newborn (HDFN), maternal alloantibodies can target fetal platelets or erythrocytes, leading to their elimination [5, 6].

Phagocytosis triggered by IgG is often facilitated by Fc gamma receptors (FcγRs), which interact with the Fc region of IgG bound to antigens on the surfaces of platelets and erythrocytes. Human FcγRs vary in their affinity for IgG, with FcγRI regarded as a "high affinity" receptor, and FcγRIIA, FcγRIIC, FcγRIIIA, and FcγRIIIB regarded as "low affinity" receptors. Using in vitro phagocytosis assays, such as confocal and phase contrast microscopy-based methods described in this article, FcγRI and FcγRIII have been demonstrated to be the predominant drivers of platelet and erythrocyte phagocytosis [7–9].

The Monocyte Monolayer Assay (MMA) is another in vitro phagocytosis method that has been used for many years in clinical testing laboratories to predict the survival of transfused incompatible erythrocytes [10]. However, unlike the assay provided here, which focuses primarily on direct measurement of phagocytosis by macrophages, the MMA specifically uses human monocytes to form a monolayer, allowing assessment of erythrocyte-monocyte interactions in the context of antibody-mediated phagocytosis. The MMA has been particularly useful in transfusion medicine for evaluating the clinical relevance of alloantibodies against erythrocyte antigens. It can quantify the degree of phagocytosis and has shown good correlation with clinically significant antibodies, making it a reliable tool for predicting the potential for hemolytic transfusion reactions. However, the use of monocytes rather than true macrophages in the MMA presents certain limitations. Blood monocytes are not typically implicated in the physiological destruction of erythrocytes, as this function is predominantly carried out by tissue macrophages in organs like the spleen and liver. Additionally, monocytes only express FcγRIII on a very small proportion of cells, and FcγRIIIA appears to play a role in erythrocyte clearance [11]. Thus, while the MMA provides valuable insights and correlates well with clinical outcomes, it may not entirely reflect the complex dynamics of erythrocyte phagocytosis. Readers interested in utilizing the MMA for their studies are directed to publications Boligan et al. [12] and Dean et al. [13] for detailed protocols and guidelines. These resources provide comprehensive instructions and considerations for implementing the MMA in clinical and research settings.

Current therapeutic strategies for ITP patients include intravenous immunoglobulin (IVIg) and, less commonly, anti-D immunoglobulin (anti-D) for RhD-positive patients. Although the mechanism of action of IVIg has not been fully elucidated, one of the downstream effects of IVIg is FcγR blockade and/or inhibition of phagocytosis. Similarly, the therapeutic effect of anti-D is also thought to involve or result in FcγR blockade [14] where erythrocytes sensitized with anti-D could potentially competitively occupy FcγRs, diverting the MPS from destroying platelets [15]. Prior work from our laboratory has demonstrated that inhibition of platelet phagocytosis was a valuable in vitro tool to determine the therapeutic potential of a number of anti-erythrocyte antibodies in murine ITP [16].

In conclusion, phagocytosis is a central pathogenic process in multiple IgG-dependent autoimmune and alloimmune diseases. Studying phagocytosis is critical to understanding these diseases. By targeting the pathways involved in the clearance of platelets and erythrocytes, potential treatments can aim to preserve these cells in circulation and mitigate associated symptoms, thereby advancing drug development for diseases such as ITP, AIHA, FNAIT, and HDFN. High-quality phagocytosis assays are valuable tools for screening the properties of autoantibodies and alloantibodies in platelet and erythrocyte diseases. An advantage of the methods detailed here is that virtually any primary or cultured macrophage can be used in this assay, offering the flexibility to genetically manipulate the macrophages. In this chapter, we describe two in vitro microscopy-based methods for quantifying phagocytosis of platelets (confocal microscopy) and erythrocytes (phase contrast microscopy).

2 Platelet Phagocytosis by Confocal Microscopy

2.1 Materials

2.1.1 Cell Culture of THP-1-CD16A Cells (or THP-1 Cells)

1. THP-1 cells stably expressing FcγRIIIA (THP-1-CD16A) or THP-1 cells (*see* **Note 1**).
2. Roswell Park Memorial Institute (RPMI) 1640 medium (Gibco, USA, Catalog# 11875093): 23.8 mM sodium bicarbonate and 2 mM L-glutamine; store at 4 °C.
3. Complete RPMI medium: RPMI 1640 medium supplemented with 10% heat-inactivated fetal bovine serum (Wisent Bioproducts, Canada, Catalog# 090-150), 100 IU/mL penicillin, 10 mg/mL streptomycin (Wisent Bioproducts, Canada, Catalog# 450-201 EL), 2 mM gluta-plus (Wisent Bioproducts, Canada, Catalog# 609-066 EL); store at 4 °C.
4. Puromycin (Gibco, USA, Catalog# A1113803) if using THP-1-CD16A: prepare stock solution 10 mg/mL in double-distilled water (ddH_2O) and store at −20 °C for up to 6 months (*see* **Note 2**).
5. Phorbol 12-Myristate 13-Acetate (PMA) (BioShop, Canada, Catalog# 16561-29-8): prepare stock solution 1.0 mg/mL in DMSO (Invitrogen, USA, Catalog# D12345) and store at −20 °C for up to 6 months (*see* **Note 3**).

6. Olympus CK40 inverted phase-contrast microscope (Olympus America Incorporation, USA) or another microscope with similar properties.
7. CO_2 cell culture incubator set to 5% CO_2 and 37 °C.
8. 24-well polystyrene clear flat-bottom-treated cell culture plate (Corning, USA) or other cell culture plates with the same properties (*see* **Note 4**).
9. Polystyrene tissue culture-treated T-75 flasks filter cap (Corning, USA), or other flasks with the same properties.
10. Conical sterile tubes (50 mL).
11. Hemocytometer (e.g., Neubauer chamber) (Fisher Scientific, CA, Catalog# 02-671-51A).
12. For assessing platelet phagocytosis by confocal microscopy: Glass coverslips (0.16–0.19 mm thickness and 12 mm diameter) (Fisher Scientific, CA, Catalog# 50949008).

2.1.2 Platelet Purification

1. BD Vacutainer™ Glass Venous Blood Collection Tubes with Acid Citrate Dextrose, Solution A, Yellow-Cap (8.5 mL) (VWR, CA, Catalog# 364606) (*see* **Note 5**).
2. Phosphate Buffered Saline Solution (PBS) without calcium and magnesium, pH: 7.4 (Gibco, USA, Catalog# 10010023).
3. Prostaglandin E1 (PGE1) (Sigma-Aldrich, USA, Catalog# 745-65-3): prepare a stock solution at 1.0 mg/mL in PBS and store at −30 °C up to 12 months.
4. Platelet counter, such as the Z2 or M3/M4/M4e Coulter counter (Beckman Coulter™, USA), automated hematology analyzer (e.g., poch-100i), or other method to enumerate platelets.
5. PBS with 0.1% EDTA (PBS-0.1% EDTA).
6. ISOTON™ II Diluent (Beckman Coulter™, USA, Catalog# 15-655-119).
7. Microcentrifuge tubes (1.5 mL).
8. Polypropylene round bottom tubes (5.0 mL).
9. Conical sterile tubes (15 mL).
10. Accuvette tubes, if using a Coulter counter (Beckman Coulter, USA).

2.1.3 Fluorescent Labeling of Platelets

1. 5-Chloromethylfluorescein diacetate (CMFDA) (Thermo Fisher Scientific, USA, Catalog# C7025): prepare a stock solution of 10 mM CMFDA in DMSO and store at −20 °C for up to 6 months (*see* **Note 6**).
2. PGE1 (1.0 mg/mL).

3. Microcentrifuge, such as an Eppendorf Centrifuge 5415 C (Eppendorf, CA).
4. Tube roller CRR-08X CAPP Rondo (CAPP, Germany) or another product with similar properties.

2.1.4 Sensitization of Platelets

1. Antibody with specificity for human platelets capable of triggering phagocytosis. For example, anti-human CD41/CD61 antibody (clone A2A9/6) (BioLegend, USA, Catalog# 359804) works well to trigger phagocytosis of platelets in this model (*see* **Notes 7** and **8**). Platelets sensitized with anti-HPA-1a standard (NIBSC, UK, Catalog# 03/152) can also be used to trigger phagocytosis. In addition, serum samples from patients with ITP can also be considered, but not all ITP patients have antibodies capable of triggering in vitro phagocytosis [7].
2. Normal human sera (NHS) (e.g., VWR, CA, Catalog# 10152-222); store at 4 °C.
3. PBS.
4. Microcentrifuge such as an Eppendorf Centrifuge 5415 C (Eppendorf, CA).
5. Tube roller CRR-08X CAPP Rondo (CAPP, Germany) or another product with similar properties.
6. Microcentrifuge tubes (1.5 mL).

2.1.5 Platelet Phagocytosis

1. Fluorescent anti-platelet antibody such as Alexa Fluor 647-conjugated anti-CD42a (GPIX) antibody (clone GRP-P) (Bio-Rad, CA, Catalog# MCA1227A647) to help distinguish internalized platelets from surface-bound platelets: prepare a stock solution of 0.5 mg/mL in PBS and store at 4 °C (*see* **Notes 8** and **9**).
2. Dako Fluorescence Mounting Medium (Agilent Technologies, USA, Catalog# S302380).
3. 4,6-diamidino-2-phenylindole (DAPI) nucleic acid stain (Cell Signaling Technology, USA, Catalog# 4083S) to identify the nucleus of the macrophages, which helps with the identification of macrophages; store at 4 °C for up to 12 months.
4. Freshly prepared mounting media (Dako-DAPI). Once the platelet phagocytosis experiment has been started and you get to about **Step 10** (*see* Subheading 2.2.5), start to prepare the mounting media. In a microcentrifuge tube, add 0.6 mL of Dako fluorescence mounting medium followed by 2.0 μL of DAPI (final concentration of 1.0 μg/mL of DAPI).
5. PBS.
6. 4% paraformaldehyde (PFA) in PBS.
7. Glass microscopy slides (Fisher Scientific, CA).

8. Kimwipes (Fisher Scientific, CA).
9. CO_2 cell culture incubator set to 5% CO_2 and 37 °C.

2.1.6 Quantification of Platelet Phagocytosis by Confocal Microscopy

1. Confocal microscope equipped with a high-powered lens. We use a spinning-disc confocal microscope with a 63× (oil immersion) objective (numerical aperture 1.47) with differential interference contrast (DIC) and laser fluorescence (488 nm, 647 nm excitation) on a Quorum multi-modal imaging system (Quorum Technologies, Canada) equipped with 50 micrometer pinhole spinning disc and an ORCA-Flash 4.0 V2 PLUS sCMOS camera.
2. Imaris image software V10.0.0 (Bitplane, UK) or an equivalent software system.

2.2 Methods

2.2.1 Cell Culture of THP-1-CD16A Cells (or THP-1 Cells)

1. Grow THP-1 or THP-1-CD16A monocytes in T-75 flasks with 15 mL of complete RPMI medium in the presence of 5% CO_2 at 37 °C. Specifically for THP-1-CD16A, we recommended growing the cells in complete RPMI medium with 5.0 μg/mL puromycin. Allow cells to grow at a concentration of ~1.5×10^6 cells/mL (*see* **Note 10**).
2. Determine the concentration of THP-1-CD16A cells. We count the cells using a hemocytometer and an inverted microscope under a 10× objective (*see* **Note 11**). Mix 10 μL of the cell suspension with 90 μL of pre-warmed complete RPMI medium (dilution 1:10) and add 10 μL of the suspension to the hemocytometer.
3. **Platelet phagocytosis:** Place coverslips into the wells of a 24-well plate and sterilize them by exposing them to UV light in a biosafety cabinet for 30 min.
4. For both the platelet and erythrocyte (or red blood cells, RBCs) phagocytosis assays, seed monocytes at 2.5×10^5 cells/well in 1.0 mL complete RPMI medium containing 100 ng/mL PMA for macrophage differentiation (*see* **Note 3**). For a full 24-well plate, in a 50 mL conical tube, we add 24 mL of cells at 2.5×10^5 cells/mL (6.0×10^6 cells) in pre-warmed complete RPMI medium and then add 2.4 μL of PMA at 1.0 mg/mL to the conical tube to achieve a final concentration of 100 ng/mL. The cells and PMA are then mixed, and 1.0 mL of the mixture is pipetted into each well of the plate. Incubate the plate for 24 h in 5% CO_2 at 37 °C.
5. After the above incubation, remove all the media containing the PMA (*see* **Note 3**) and then wash the cells twice to remove residual PMA by sequentially adding and removing 1.0 mL of pre-warmed complete RPMI without PMA to each well. Incubate the plate for 24 h in complete RPMI in the presence of 5% CO_2 at 37 °C.

2.2.2 Platelet Purification

1. Collect approximately 9.0 mL of blood into a Yellow-Cap BD Vacutainer™ tube (*see* **Note 5**).
2. Aliquot the blood into three 5.0 mL tubes with ~3.0 mL each and centrifuge at 400 × *g* for 8 min (8 acceleration, 1 brake). By dividing the total volume into three tubes, the supernatant platelet-rich plasma (PRP) recovery is easier.
3. Take as much of the PRP as possible (~1.0–1.5 mL from each 5.0 mL tube) using a pipette without disturbing the RBC pellet and combine these PRPs into a clean 15 mL tube (~3.0–4.5 mL final volume of supernatant PRP).
4. Enumerate the platelets using a Coulter counter or other equipment such as a complete blood count analyzer. In our facility, we prepare a 1:5000 dilution of PRP in ISOTON with a final volume of 50 mL and transfer 10 mL of the dilution to an accuvette tube for counting in a Coulter counter.
5. Increase the volume of the combined PRP (you should have 3.0–4.5 mL; from **Step 3**) by adding PBS-0.1% EDTA to bring the volume to 5.0 mL, and then add 1.0 μL of PGE1 at 1.0 mg/mL to achieve a final concentration of 200 ng/mL. Both EDTA and PGE1 help prevent platelet activation.
6. Centrifuge the PRP at 800 × *g* for 10 min (8 acceleration, 1 brake) and discard the supernatant using a pipette; avoid disturbing the platelet pellet.
7. Resuspend the platelet pellet to a final concentration of 4.0×10^8 platelets/mL in PBS-0.1% EDTA, considering the platelet count performed in **Step 4**. Add additional PGE1 again to achieve a final concentration of 200 ng/mL.

2.2.3 Fluorescent Labeling of Platelets

1. Add 2.0 μL of 10 mM CMFDA per mL of platelet solution at 4.0×10^8 platelets/mL (20 μM final CMFDA concentration). Mix gently by pipetting and cover the tube with aluminum foil (*see* **Note 12**). Place the tube on a roller for 45 min at room temperature.
2. Wash the labeled platelets by adding 5.0 mL of PBS WITHOUT EDTA and 0.5 μL of PGE1 at 1.0 mg/mL.
3. Centrifuge at 800 × *g* for 10 min (8 acceleration, 8 brake) and discard the supernatant using a pipette; avoid disturbing the platelet pellet.
4. Wash the labeled platelet pellet by adding 5.0 mL of PBS WITHOUT EDTA/PGE1 to remove any residual EDTA/CMFDA/PGE1 (*see* **Note 13**).
5. Centrifuge at 800 × *g* for 10 min (8 acceleration, 8 brake). Discard the supernatant using a pipette; avoid disturbing the platelet pellet.
6. Prepare the labeled platelet solution at a concentration of 4.0×10^8 platelets/mL in PBS.

2.2.4 Sensitization of Platelets

1. Mix 50 μL of the labeled platelet solution (4.0×10^8 platelets/mL) and 50 μL of the anti-platelet antibody solution [CD41/CD61 antibody (clone A2A9/6) at 10 μg/mL in PBS] in a microcentrifuge tube and cover the tube with aluminum foil. As a control, platelets sensitized with an IgG isotype-matched control should be included. Platelets sensitized with 50 μL of anti-HPA-1a standard (NIBSC, UK, Catalog# 03/152) can also be used to trigger phagocytosis. In this latter case, the same volume of NHS should be used as a negative control.
2. Place the tubes in a roller and rotate for 30 min at room temperature.
3. Wash the platelets by adding 1.0 mL of PBS to each microcentrifuge tube and centrifuge at $800 \times g$ for 5 min (8 acceleration, 8 brake).
4. Discard the supernatant carefully using a pipette; avoid disturbing the pellet. Add 0.1 mL of PBS to the tubes; this should result in a 2.0×10^8 platelets/mL solution (*see* **Note 14**).

2.2.5 Platelet Phagocytosis

Once the monocytes have differentiated into macrophages from Subheading 2.2.1, the platelet phagocytosis assay can begin. Note that the macrophages on the coverslips can sometimes be easy to dislodge. So, be careful in the washing steps not to directly pipette the washing solution with force onto the coverslips. Try to gently add liquid at the edge of the coverslips. For the aspiration steps, likewise, avoid the rapid aspiration of the liquid from the coverslip area where the macrophages are seeded.

1. Remove the 24-well plate from the incubator and wash off the complete RPMI medium (*see* **Note 15**).
2. Add 0.1 mL/well of the sensitized-platelet solution at 2.0×10^8 platelets/mL directly to each coverslip and then add 0.4 mL/well of fresh pre-warmed complete RPMI medium (maintaining an 80:1 ratio of platelets:macrophages) (*see* **Notes 16** and **17**). Allow phagocytosis to proceed for 1 h in the presence of 5% CO_2 at 37 °C.
3. Remove the plate from the incubator and place it on ice to stop the phagocytosis. Aspirate the medium completely (*see* **Note 15**).
4. Add 0.5 mL/well of ice-cold PBS to wash the macrophages and remove free platelets.
5. Aspirate the PBS (*see* **Note 15**).
6. Repeat **Steps 4** and **5** washing steps.
7. Add 0.5 mL/well of 4% PFA. Incubate at 4 °C for 25 min in the dark (cover the plate with aluminum foil).
8. Aspirate the PFA (*see* **Note 15**) and add 0.5 mL/well of ice-cold PBS to wash off excess PFA.

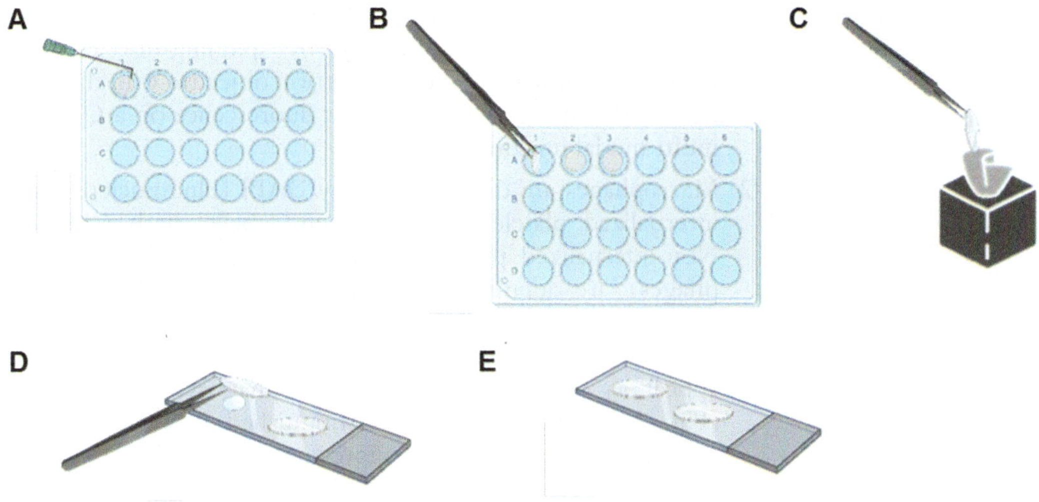

Fig. 1 Illustration showing a step-by-step laboratory procedure for removing the coverslip with cells from the 24-well plate in the platelet phagocytosis assay by confocal microscopy. (**a**) Separate the coverslip from the bottom of the well using a 22G needle with a slightly bent tip, as shown. (**b**) Remove the coverslip with the attached cells from the well using a tweezer. (**c**) Dab the edge of the coverslip on a Kimwipe to remove the excess PBS. (**d**) Drop Dako-DAPI fluorescent mounting media onto a glass microscopy slide. (**e**) Lay the coverslip onto the Dako-DAPI drop with the cells face down and in contact with the mounting media

9. Aspirate the PBS and add 0.35 mL of Alexa Fluor 647-conjugated anti-CD42a (GPIX) antibody (clone GRP-P) (anti-platelet antibody at a 1:50 dilution in PBS) to stain the non-phagocytized platelets attached to the macrophage surface but not internalized. Incubate the plate for 30 min at room temperature in the dark (cover the plate with aluminum foil).
10. Aspirate the anti-platelet antibody and add 1.0 mL/well of PBS to wash the cells (*see* **Note 15**). Repeat this step twice and remove PBS. *(At this point in the assay, prepare the fresh Dako-DAPI mounting media.)*
11. Carefully remove the coverslip with the attached cells from a well with a tweezer and dab the coverslip edge on a Kimwipe to remove excess PBS (Fig. 1).
12. Add a small drop of Dako-DAPI fluorescent mounting media onto a glass microscopy slide. Lay the coverslip onto the Dako-DAPI droplet (the side of the coverslip where the cells are attached must be in contact with mounting media) and NOT wipe up excess medium.
13. Leave coverslips mounted for 24 h or overnight at room temperature in a dry and dark environment to allow Dako polymerization (Dako will NOT polymerize properly at 4 °C). Slides can be stored for up to 1 month at 4 °C once the polymerization is complete (*see* **Notes 18** and **19**).

2.2.6 Quantification of Platelet Phagocytosis by Confocal Microscopy

1. Phagocytosis is quantified by confocal microscopy. In our laboratory, the slides are assessed by spinning-disc confocal microscopy under a 63× oil immersion objective with differential interference contrast and laser fluorescence on a Quorum multi-modal imaging system.
2. Macrophages are distinguished by DAPI (blue nucleus), and internalized platelets appear green, labeled with CMFDA. Non-internalized platelets (bound to the surface of macrophages) are identified as red stained with Alexa Fluor 647-conjugated anti-CD42a (GPIX) antibody (clone GRP-P). Areas of red and green co-localization in the merge appear as orange-yellow (e.g., non-phagocytosed platelets) (Fig. 2). Platelets are also distinguished from internalized microparticles or platelet aggregates by their size, which range from 1.5 μm to 3.5 μm.
3. At least four different images should be taken near the center of each well to image 500 macrophages. We perform Z-stacking every 0.33 μm with >30 stacking pictures taken for each image. This not only allows us to help determine whether platelets are inside the macrophage but also allows us to count all of the platelets in any plane of the macrophage.
4. Z-stacked images are 3D reconstructed for analysis using Imaris v10.0.0 (Bitplane, UK). Surface-bound platelets are distinguished from phagocytosed platelets by 3D reconstruction and Alexa Fluor 647-conjugated anti-CD42a (GPIX) antibody (clone GRP-P) staining. The platelet phagocytic index (PPI) is calculated as follows:

   [(total number of internalized platelets) / (total number of macrophages counted)] × 100 (*see* **Note 20**).

3 RBC Phagocytosis by Phase Contrast Microscopy

3.1 Materials

3.1.1 Cell Culture of THP-1-CD16A Cells (or THP-1 Cells)

Cell culture materials are common for both platelet phagocytosis by confocal microscopy and RBC phagocytosis by phase contrast microscopy. *See* Subheading 2.1.1.

3.1.2 RBC Purification

1. BD Vacutainer™ Plastic Blood Collection Tubes with K_2EDTA, Lavender-Cap (10 mL), (VWR, CA, Catalog# 367863) or Blood Transfer and Storage Bags, example Charter MedicalBags, (150 mL, 600 mL, or 1000 mL) (VWR, CA, Catalog# MSPP-T3101, MSPP-T3106, or MSPP-T3107). These bags are used for the collection, storage, processing, transport, separation, and administration of blood and its components.

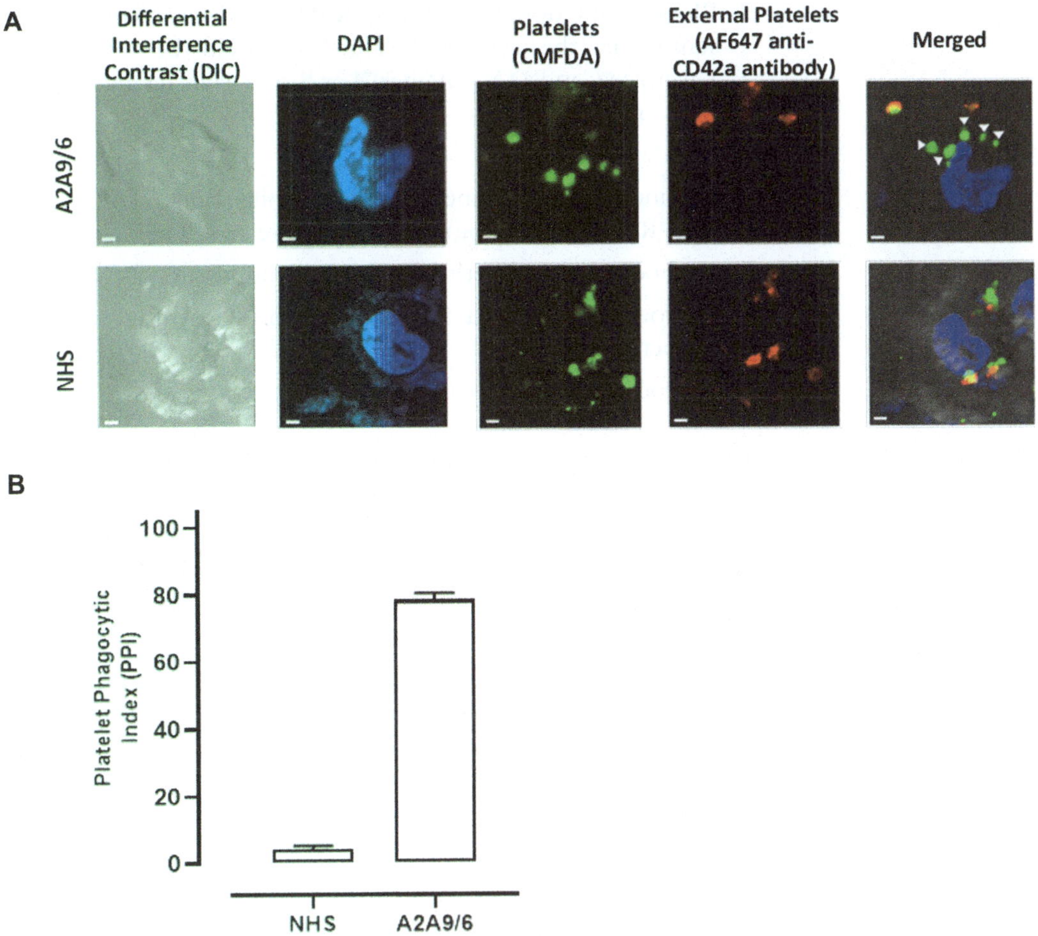

Fig. 2 Antibody-mediated platelet phagocytosis quantified by confocal microscopy. THP-1-CD16A macrophages were incubated with platelets sensitized with anti-human CD41/CD61 antibody (clone A2A9/6) at 10 μg/mL for 1 h at 37 °C with 5% CO_2. Normal human sera (NHS) was included as a control, although an isotype control would be more appropriate. (**a**) Representative images of macrophages and platelets in each condition. Phagocytosis was visualized by spinning-disc confocal microscopy under a 63× objective with differential interference contrast (DIC) and laser fluorescence. Macrophage nuclei were distinguished with DAPI (blue), and platelets were labeled with the cytoplasmic dye CMFDA (green). Platelets that were not internalized were identified post-phagocytosis using Alexa Fluor 647 (AF647)-conjugated anti-CD42a (GPIX) antibody (clone GRP-P) (red). Merged channels with DIC images are shown in the last panel. Areas of red and green co-localization in the merge appear as orange-yellow (e.g., non-phagocytosed platelets). Examples of engulfed platelets (white arrow heads) are observed in green within macrophages. Four images were taken and Z-stacked to be 3D reconstructed using Imaris V10.0.0. Platelets were defined by size (1.5–3.5 μm) to differentiate them from internalized microparticles or platelet aggregates. The scale bar represents 3.0 μm. (**b**) Platelet Phagocytic Index (PPI) calculated for each condition, as indicated on the x-axis. The bars represent the PPI ± SEM of three independent experiments

2. Blood from donors who are RhD positive (if you will be sensitizing the cells with anti-D) should be taken in a Lavender-Cap BD Vacutainer™ or Blood Transfer and Storage Bags (*see* **Note 5**).
3. PBS.
4. Glycine buffered saline for RBC stabilization (ID-CellStab) (Bio-Rad, CA, Catalog# 005650); store at 4 °C.
5. Hemocytometer or other method to enumerate RBCs.
6. Microcentrifuge such as an Eppendorf Centrifuge 5415 C (Eppendorf, CA).
7. Microcentrifuge tubes (1.5 mL).

3.1.3 RBC Sensitization

1. Antibodies specific for antigens on the RBC surface, which are capable of triggering phagocytosis:
   - Anti-E complete blood typing serum, human WHO International Standard (NIBSC, UK, Catalog# W1005): prepare stock solution as directed by the NIBSC instructions (*see* **Note 8**).
   - Polyclonal anti-human Rho (D) antibody (anti-D, also called RhIg) (WinRho® SDF, Rhophylac, or another commercially available anti-D preparation; store at 4 °C (*see* **Note 8**).
2. Complete RPMI medium; store at 4 °C.
3. PBS.
4. Microcentrifuge such as an Eppendorf Centrifuge 5415 C (Eppendorf, CA).
5. Tube roller CRR-08X CAPP Rondo (CAPP, Germany) or another product with similar properties.
6. Microcentrifuge tubes (1.5 mL).

3.1.4 RBC Phagocytosis

1. PBS.
2. Distilled water (dH_2O).
3. 10× PBS (Gibco, USA, Catalog# 70011044), for the RBC lysis step.
4. 4% paraformaldehyde (PFA) (Sigma-Aldrich, USA, Catalog# 28906) in PBS: prepare 4% PFA by diluting 16% PFA solution in PBS and store at 4 °C for up to 3 months.
5. CO_2 cell culture incubator set to 5% CO_2 and 37 °C.

3.1.5 Quantification of RBC Phagocytosis by Phase Contrast Microscopy

1. EVOS FLoid Imaging System (Thermo Fisher Scientific, USA) or an equivalent system.
2. Commercial image analysis software such as ImageJ (NIH, USA) [17, 18] (*see* **Note 21**).

3.2 Methods

3.2.1 Cell Culture of THP-1-CD16A Cells (or THP-1 Cells)

Differentiation of THP-1-CD16A monocytes into macrophages is common for both platelet phagocytosis by confocal microscopy and RBC phagocytosis by phase contrast microscopy. *See* Subheading 2.2.1.

3.2.2 RBC Purification

1. Collect blood in a Lavender-Cap BD Vacutainer™ tube from donors who express the target antigen of interest (e.g., RhD antigen-positive blood when anti-D will be used). Immediately invert the tube 8–10 times post-collection to ensure thorough mixing with the anticoagulant and keep at room temperature.
2. Centrifuge the tube at 1200 × *g* for 10 min without brake. Blood should optimally be centrifuged within 2 h of collection.
3. Discard the plasma using a pipette. If you wish to keep the RBCs beyond one day, we suggest aliquoting the RBCs into microcentrifuge tubes and diluting them 1:1 (v/v) with RBC: ID-CellStab. RBCs diluted in ID-CellStab can be stored at 4 °C for up to 1 month. However, it is not necessary to dilute the RBCs in ID-CellStab if the phagocytosis assay will be performed on the same day.
4. Transfer 0.1 mL of RBCs or 0.2 mL of RBCs diluted in ID-CellStab (for a 24-well plate) to a microcentrifuge tube, add 1.0 mL of PBS, centrifuge at 300 × *g* for 3 min and discard the supernatant using a pipette without disturbing the RBC pellet. Repeat this step twice (it may be necessary to wash the cells more than twice if hemolysis is observed).
5. Resuspend the RBC pellet with 0.1 mL of PBS.
6. Enumerate the RBCs using a hemocytometer or other equipment. In our facility, we prepare a 1:20,000 dilution of RBC in PBS with a final volume of 1.0 mL for counting in a Guava EasyCyte flow cytometer.
7. Prepare the RBC-solution at a concentration of 5.0×10^8 RBC/mL in PBS.

3.2.3 RBC Sensitization

1. Mix 50 μL of the RBC-solution (5.0×10^8 RBC/mL) and 50 μL of a sensitizing anti-RBC antibody at the desirable concentration(s) [e.g., polyclonal anti-D is highly effective at 9.0 international units (IU)/mL (generally corresponding to 1.8 μg/mL)]. As controls, RBCs mixed with NHS, IVIg, isotype control antibodies, or PBS (non-sensitized RBC) should also be included. Further controls can use antigen-negative blood. Place the tubes containing the mixture in a roller for 45 min at room temperature (*see* **Note 22**).
2. Add 1.0 mL of PBS to each microcentrifuge tube and centrifuge at 300 × *g* for 3 min.

3. Remove the supernatant carefully using a pipette without disturbing the pellet and add 50 μL of pre-warmed complete RPMI medium to the pellet (the cell concentration should be roughly 5.0×10^8 RBC/mL).

3.2.4 RBC Phagocytosis

Once the monocytes have differentiated into macrophages according to Subheading 2.2.1, the RBC phagocytosis assay can begin.

1. Remove the 24-well plate containing the macrophages from the incubator and replace the complete RPMI medium with 0.5 mL/well of fresh pre-warmed complete RPMI medium (*see* **Note 15**).
2. Add 10 μL/well of sensitized RBCs at 5.0×10^8 RBC/mL (maintaining a 20:1 ratio of RBCs:macrophages) (*see* **Notes 16** and **23**). Incubate the plate for 30 min (some laboratories use longer incubation times) in the CO_2 incubator.
3. Remove the 24-well plate from the incubator and place it on ice to stop phagocytosis. Aspirate the medium completely (*see* **Note 15**).
4. Add 0.5 mL/well of ice-cold PBS followed by aspiration of the PBS to wash the macrophages and remove some of the non-phagocytized and free RBCs (*see* **Note 15**).
5. Add 0.45 mL/well of dH_2O to hypotonically lyse the remaining free/non-phagocytosed RBC in the well (*see* **Note 24**).
6. After 1 min of exposure to dH_2O, add 0.05 mL/well of 10×PBS to restore tonicity.
7. Aspirate the PBS (*see* **Note 15**) and add 0.5 mL/well of ice-cold PBS to wash the macrophages.
8. Aspirate the PBS and add 0.5 mL/well of 4% PFA (*see* **Note 15**). Incubate at 4 °C for 25 min in the dark (cover the plate with aluminum foil).
9. Remove the 4% PFA (*see* **Note 15**) and add 0.5 mL/well of ice-cold PBS to wash the macrophages.
10. Aspirate the PBS and add 0.25 mL/well of fresh PBS (*see* **Note 15**).
11. At least four different and non-overlapping images should be taken near the center of each well at a magnification sufficient to allow the macrophages with the engulfed RBCs to be visualized. We recommend you count at least 500 macrophages/well. The plate can be stored for up to 15 days at 4 °C.

3.2.5 Quantification of RBC Phagocytosis by Phase Contrast Microscopy

1. Phagocytosed RBCs are easily distinguishable inside macrophages with a relatively spherical shape and dark color (Fig. 3, white arrow heads).

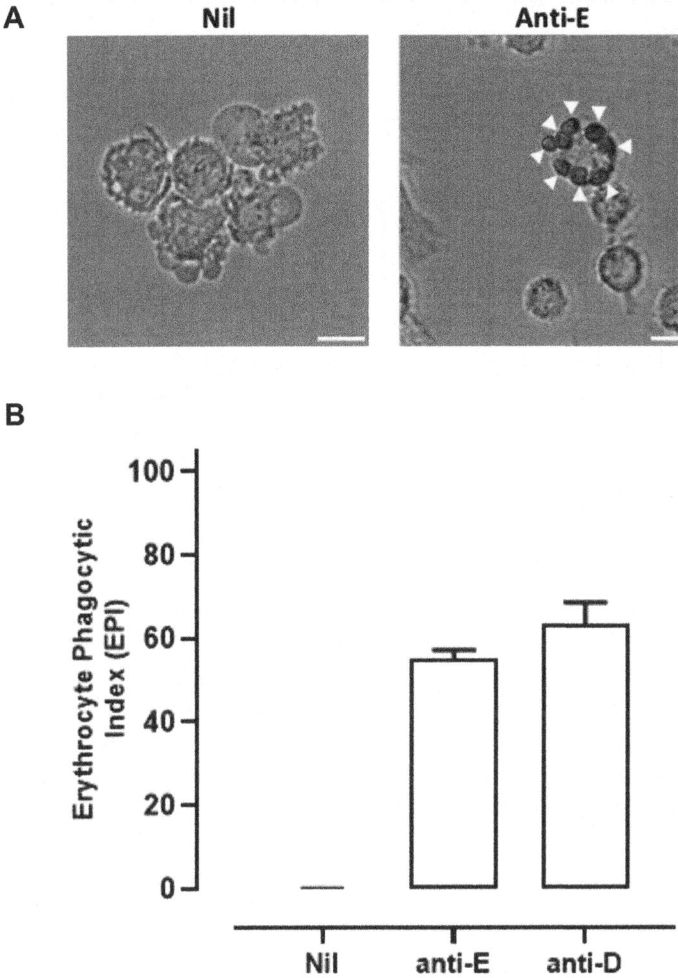

Fig. 3 Antibody-mediated red blood cell (RBC) phagocytosis quantified by phase contrast microscopy. THP-1-CD16A macrophages were incubated with RBCs sensitized with a 1:10 dilution of anti-E complete blood typing serum or anti-D IgG at 9.0 international units (IU)/mL (~1.8 μg/mL of anti-D) for 30 min at 37 °C with 5% CO_2. Non-sensitized RBC (Nil) were included as a control. (**a**) Representative images of macrophages in each condition. Examples of engulfed erythrocytes (white arrow heads) are observed as dark spheres within macrophages. The scale bar represents 20 μm. (**b**) Erythrocyte Phagocytic Index (EPI) calculated for each condition, as indicated on the x-axis. The bars represent the EPI ± SEM of three independent experiments

2. To quantify the level of phagocytosis induced in each condition, the erythrocyte phagocytic index (EPI) is calculated as follows:

   [(total number of internalized erythrocytes) / (total number of macrophages counted)] × 100 (*see* **Note 20**).

4 Notes

1. Phagocytosis can be performed with a number of different phagocytosis-competent cell lines, as well as with primary macrophages [7, 8]. This protocol is focused on measuring phagocytosis using either THP-1 cells (ATCC TIB-202) or THP-1-CD16A cells (ATCC CRL-3575), which are both human cells. The major difference between these two cell lines is that THP-1 cells meaningfully express FcγRI and FcγRIIA, while THP-1-CD16A cells also express FcγRIIIA, which is a major FcγR involved in both erythrocyte and platelet clearance. In addition, other types of macrophages, as well as other macrophage cell lines, such as murine RAW 264.7 along with murine reagents, can also be used with minor modifications to this assay.
2. Puromycin is an antibiotic used to select and maintain FcγRIIIA expression in THP-1-CD16A cells.
3. **Warning:** The phorbol ester PMA used in this study is a potent tumor promoter and should be handled with extreme caution. Be sure to follow your institution's safety guidelines and protocols when using PMA. Appropriate safety measures should include but are not limited to the use of personal protective equipment (PPE) such as gloves, lab coats, and eye protection. If available, work with PMA should be conducted in a biological safety cabinet which exhausts air outside. All waste materials contaminated with PMA should be disposed of in accordance with institutional hazardous waste disposal guidelines.
4. Polystyrene flat-bottom plates of other sizes can also be easily used. If a different plate format is desired (e.g., 48-well plate), use 1.3×10^5 cells per cm^2 of culture area of the plate.
5. **Warning:** Human blood is a potentially dangerous biological agent owing to its potentially infectious agent content. Be sure to follow your institution's safety guidelines when using any component from human blood.
6. Before opening the CMFDA vial to prepare the stock solution, allow the product to warm to room temperature. Dissolve the lyophilized dye in DMSO using a vortex and ensure that all contents of the dye tube are spun down to the bottom before freezing.
7. The anti-human CD41/CD61 (clone A2A9/6) is an IgG2a kappa mouse monoclonal antibody that recognizes CD41/CD61, also known as GPIIb/IIIa, a member of the integrin receptor family expressed by platelets and megakaryocytes.

These phagocytosis experiments should be performed with azide-free antibodies, as azides interfere with cellular respiration and dramatically affect the results. In addition, antibodies that have low endotoxin levels are highly recommended. For sensitization, we generally use 5.0 μg/mL of most monoclonal antibodies to sensitize platelets.

8. Avoid repeated freeze-thaw cycles of antibodies.
9. The anti-human CD42a (GPIX) antibody (clone GRP-P) is an IgG1 mouse monoclonal antibody that recognizes CD42a, also known as GPIX, a surface marker expressed by platelets and megakaryocytes. This antigen is different from that recognized by the previous antibody used in the sensitization step. Fluorescently labeled antibodies should be protected from light exposure to reduce the risk of photobleaching.
10. We suggest growing THP-1 or THP-1-CD16A cells at the indicated concentrations because macrophage marker expression in response to PMA is optimal at this cell density [19].
11. If using an inverted microscope and a hemocytometer to count the THP-1-CD16A cells, use phase contrast to more easily distinguish the cells and count the number of cells per mL [20, 21].
12. After staining with CMFDA, platelets must be protected from light to avoid photobleaching. We use aluminum foil for this purpose.
13. EDTA must be completely removed to prevent calcium chelation when platelets are incubated with human serum.
14. It is important to resuspend the solution without generating bubbles. To do this, add 100 μL, reduce the pipette volume to 50 μL, and pipette the platelets up and down until the platelets are completely resuspended without any noticeable clumps.
15. The aspiration steps in the phagocytosis process can be performed using a pipette or vacuum system. We recommend using a pipette to ensure that aspiration occurs more slowly, helping ensure that macrophages are not detached from the plate.
16. Rock plates several times to completely distribute and mix.
17. The ratio of 80:1 per well is as follows: 2.0×10^7 platelets:2.5×10^5 macrophages in 24-well plate.
18. Store slides in a low-humidity fridge. High-humidity fridges will cause accumulation of water around the edges of the coverslips and can weaken the mounting. If imaging after storage at 4 °C, leave out at room temperature for a few hours prior to imaging to allow the re-solidification of Dako.

19. We suggest imaging within 1 week after the completion of the experiment because the photostability under Dako is ~1 month, according to the manufacturer.
20. The selection of statistical tests must be compatible with the data distribution: parametric (t-test or ANOVA) or non-parametric (*Mann-Whitney* U-test or *Kruskal-Wallis* test) and with the number of experimental groups. For example, two groups (t-test or *Mann-Whitney* U-test) and multiple groups (ANOVA or *Kruskal-Wallis* test).
21. Image analysis can be performed using the freely available Java-based Fiji platform, which includes additional preloaded plugins. To count the number of phagocytized particles, plugins such as the Cell Counter plugin or the Analyze Particle plugin may be used [17, 18].
22. Avoid longer incubation, because it may lead to clumping.
23. The ratio of 20:1 per well is as follows: 5.0×10^6 RBC:2.5×10^5 macrophages in 24-well plate.
24. RBCs burst in the presence of water. Macrophages could be damaged if the incubation time with dH_2O is prolonged for more than 1 min.

Conflict of Interest

Funding: This research was supported by The Canadian Blood Services (Intramural Research Grant Program, to AHL), funded by the federal government (Health Canada) and provincial and territorial ministries of health. YT is supported by a Canadian Blood Services Postdoctoral Fellowship Program award. The views herein do not necessarily reflect the views of the federal, provincial, or territorial governments of Canada. The authors declare no conflicts of interest relevant to the content of this manuscript. AHL has research funding from argenx (paid to the institution), outside the submitted work.

References

1. González-López TJ, Provan D, Bárez A et al (2023) Primary and secondary immune thrombocytopenia (ITP): time for a rethink. Blood Rev 61(101112):101112. https://doi.org/10.1016/j.blre.2023.101112
2. Mulder FVM, Evers D, de Haas M et al (2023) Severe autoimmune hemolytic anemia; epidemiology, clinical management, outcomes and knowledge gaps. Front Immunol 14. https://doi.org/10.3389/fimmu.2023.1228142
3. van Leeuwen EF, van der Ven JT, Engelfriet CP, von dem Borne AE (1982) Specificity of autoantibodies in autoimmune thrombocytopenia. Blood 59(1):23–26. https://doi.org/10.1182/blood.v59.1.23.23
4. Kiefel V, Santoso S, Kaufmann E, Mueller-Eckhardt C (1991) Autoantibodies against platelet glycoprotein Ib/IX: a frequent finding in autoimmune thrombocytopenic purpura. Br J Haematol 79(2):256–262. https://doi.org/10.1111/j.1365-2141.1991.tb04530.x

5. Christensen RD, Bahr TM, Ilstrup SJ, Dizon-Townson DS (2023) Alloimmune hemolytic disease of the fetus and newborn: genetics, structure, and function of the commonly involved erythrocyte antigens. J Perinatol 43(12):1459–1467. https://doi.org/10.1038/s41372-023-01785-3
6. Stam W, Wachholz GE, de Pereda JM, Kapur R, van der Schoot E, Margadant C (2023) Fetal and neonatal alloimmune thrombocytopenia: current pathophysiological insights and perspectives for future diagnostics and treatment. Blood Rev 59(101038): 101038. https://doi.org/10.1016/j.blre.2022.101038
7. Norris PAA, Segel GB, Burack WR et al (2021) FcγRI and FcγRIII on splenic macrophages mediate phagocytosis of anti-glycoprotein IIb/IIIa autoantibody-opsonized platelets in immune thrombocytopenia. Haematologica 106(1):250–254. https://doi.org/10.3324/haematol.2020.248385
8. Gil Gonzalez L, Fernandez-Marrero Y, Norris PAA et al (2022) THP-1 cells transduced with CD16A utilize Fcγ receptor I and III in the phagocytosis of IgG-sensitized human erythrocytes and platelets. PLoS One 17(12): e0278365. https://doi.org/10.1371/journal.pone.0278365
9. Armour KL, Smith CS, Ip NCY et al (2014) Clearance of human IgG1-sensitised red blood cells in vivo in humans relates to the in vitro properties of antibodies from alternative cell lines. PLoS One 9(10):e109463. https://doi.org/10.1371/journal.pone.0109463
10. Nance SJT (2023) The monocyte monolayer assay, an in vitro method for prediction of in vivo survival of transfused incompatible red blood cells: a review. Immunohematology 39(2):61–69. https://doi.org/10.21307/immunohematology-2023-010
11. Miescher S, Spycher MO, Amstutz H et al (2004) A single recombinant anti-RhD IgG prevents RhD immunization: association of RhD-positive red blood cell clearance rate with polymorphisms in the FcgammaRIIA and FcgammaIIIA genes. Blood 103(11): 4028–4035. https://doi.org/10.1182/blood-2003-11-3929
12. Boligan KF, Sandhu G, Branch DR (2022) Methods to evaluate the potential clinical significance of antibodies to red blood cells. Curr Protoc 2(8). https://doi.org/10.1002/cpz1.504
13. Dean MM, Tran TV, Ji Y et al (2020) Development of a semi-automated monocyte monolayer assay (MMA) to determine the clinical significance of red cell alloantibodies. J Immunol 204(1_Suppl):86.55–86.55. https://doi.org/10.4049/jimmunol.204.supp.86.55
14. Debré M, Griscelli C, Bonnet MC et al (1993) Infusion of Fcγ fragments for treatment of children with acute immune thrombocytopenic purpura. Lancet 342(8877):945–949. https://doi.org/10.1016/0140-6736(93)92000-j
15. Crow AR, Lazarus AH (2008) The mechanisms of action of intravenous immunoglobulin and polyclonal anti-d immunoglobulin in the amelioration of immune thrombocytopenic purpura: what do we really know? Transfus Med Rev 22(2):103–116. https://doi.org/10.1016/j.tmrv.2007.12.001
16. Khan R, Menard M, Jen CC, Chen X, Norris PAA, Lazarus AH (2020) Inhibition of platelet phagocytosis as an in vitro predictor for therapeutic potential of RBC antibodies in murine ITP. Blood 135(26):2420–2424. https://doi.org/10.1182/blood.2019003646
17. Schneider CA, Rasband WS, Eliceiri KW (2012) NIH Image to ImageJ: 25 years of image analysis. Nat Methods 9(7):671–675. https://doi.org/10.1038/nmeth.2089
18. Schindelin J, Arganda-Carreras I, Frise E et al (2012) Fiji: an open-source platform for biological-image analysis. Nat Methods 9(7): 676–682. https://doi.org/10.1038/nmeth.2019
19. Phuangbubpha P, Thara S, Sriboonaied P, Saetan P, Tumnoi W, Charoenpanich A (2023) Optimizing THP-1 macrophage culture for an immune-responsive human intestinal model. Cells 12(10). https://doi.org/10.3390/cells12101427
20. Zhang M, Gu L, Zheng P et al (2020) Improvement of cell counting method for Neubauer counting chamber. J Clin Lab Anal 34(1):e23024. https://doi.org/10.1002/jcla.23024
21. EMS. Technical data sheets neubauer haemocytometry. Electron Microscopy Sciences. Web cite. https://www.emsdiasum.com/docs/technical/datasheet/68052-14. Accessed July 7, 2024

Chapter 8

Miniaturized In Vitro Transfusion Model

Erin L. Soule-Albridge, Jesselin J. Romero Escobar, Natalie E. Kane, Martha C. Sola-Visner, and Patricia E. Davenport

Abstract

We have created a miniaturized in vitro model of transfusion using neonatal (cord blood) and adult blood to investigate the immune and hemostatic changes that occur when a neonate receives a transfusion of functionally different adult platelets. These techniques allow us to model neonatal thrombocytopenia using neonatal cells (from cord blood) and create platelet concentrates of either neonatal or adult origin to mechanistically interrogate how the developmental state of the transfused platelets influences the hemostatic and/or immune responses of neonates to transfusion. These methods utilize common in vitro techniques that have been tailored for the unique characteristics of cord blood. Using this model, investigators can simulate platelet transfusions into a thrombocytopenic patient and investigate the effects of platelet transfusions in a human system.

Key words Platelet transfusion, Neonatal, Cord blood, Miniaturized transfusion, Thrombocytopenia

1 Introduction

Thrombocytopenia occurs in 18–35% of neonates admitted to the neonatal intensive care unit (NICU), and the incidence increases to 70% in the most premature neonates born with a weight <1000× g [1–3]. These same infants also have the highest incidence of intracranial bleeding of any patient population, and as a result it has historically been accepted that preterm neonates should be transfused at higher platelet counts than older children and adults, in hopes of preventing bleeding. Over the past 20 years, multiple retrospective and observational studies have suggested that liberal neonatal platelet transfusion practices do not prevent bleeding and, instead, may be associated with harm [4–10]. In 2019, the results from the largest randomized controlled trial of neonatal platelet transfusion thresholds (the PlaNet-2 trial) were published. This study randomized 660 neonates <34 weeks' gestational age to receive platelet transfusions for platelet counts $<50 \times 10^9$/L

Sean R. Stowell and Connie M. Arthur (eds.), *Methods in Transfusion Medicine*, Methods in Molecular Biology, vol. 3053,
https://doi.org/10.1007/978-1-0716-5376-0_8,

(high threshold group) or <25 × 10^9/L (low threshold group) and found an increased incidence of the primary combined outcome of death or major bleeding in the 28 days following randomization in the high threshold arm [11]. Among secondary outcomes, infants randomized to the high threshold group also had a higher incidence of bronchopulmonary dysplasia (chronic lung disease of prematurity), and upon 2-year follow-up, these same infants had worse neurodevelopmental outcomes and an increased need for supplemental oxygen or respiratory support compared to infants randomized to the low threshold arm [12].

The mechanisms underlying the potential harm associated with neonatal platelet transfusion are an active area of research. Neonatal and adult platelets are functionally distinct from each other, due to differences in surface receptor expression and downstream signaling that result in a comparatively hypo-reactive neonatal platelet [13]. Thus, it has been hypothesized that the transfusion of adult platelets into the unique physiologic environment of the preterm neonate might result in a "developmental mismatch" between the transfused platelets and the recipient, with potential negative consequences [14]. Furthermore, it is now well established that, in addition to their hemostatic functions, platelets are active immune cells [15]. How the immune functions of platelets change over development and whether a developmental mismatch in platelet immune function contributes to the harm associated with neonatal platelet transfusion is just beginning to be investigated [16–18].

Rigorous clinical investigation into these mechanistic questions is difficult, if not impossible, due to the small size, small blood volumes, and intensive care required by infants born preterm. Thus, in vitro models using human *neonatal* cells are essential to better understand the cellular interactions and mechanisms underlying neonatal diseases and responses to therapies. It is not always appropriate to use adult cells as surrogates for neonatal cells, given the major developmental differences between neonatal and adult cellular biology and physiology, including in the hemostatic and immune systems. The accessibility of large volumes of placental cord blood makes it an ideal source from which we can isolate and study neonatal cells. While cord blood is not a perfect surrogate for blood drawn directly from a neonate after birth (which cannot be collected in large volumes), it is superior to using adult cells. Using cord blood from healthy full-term deliveries and adult blood drawn from healthy adult donors, we developed a miniaturized in vitro model of neonatal thrombocytopenia and platelet transfusion (*see* Fig. 1 for an overview). Importantly, this method can be used to not only model the developmental mismatch that occurs when neonates receive a transfusion of functionally different adult platelets but also to model what would happen if a neonate received a transfusion of neonatal platelets. This is currently not possible in clinical practice but could become a reality in the future. Using this model, investigators can examine the immune and hemostatic

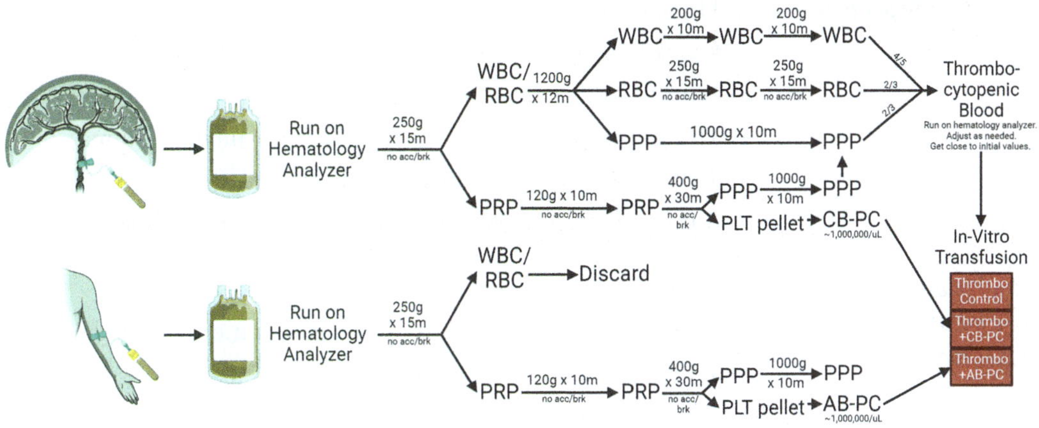

Fig. 1 Schematic overview of component isolation and thrombocytopenic blood creation. acc/brk acceleration or brake, WBC white blood cell, RBC red blood cell, PRP platelet-rich plasma, PPP platelet poor plasma, PLT platelet, CB cord blood, AB adult blood, PC platelet concentrate, Thrombo thrombocytopenic blood

effects of platelet transfusions and the role of developmental differences in platelet function in the context of the unique neonatal physiology.

2 Materials

2.1 Prefilled Sodium Citrate Syringe Preparation

1. Trisodium citrate.
2. 4-(2-hydroxyethyl)-1-piperazineethanesulfonic acid (HEPES).
3. Double-deionized water (ddH_2O).
4. Stir plate and stir bar.
5. Hydrogen chloride (HCl) (recommended 0.5M).
6. Sodium hydroxide (NaOH) (recommended 0.05M).
7. 0.22 μm polyvinylidene fluoride (PVDF) filter (or another suitable filter).
8. 30 mL sterile syringes.

2.2 Blood Collection

1. Cord Blood
   (a) Access to fresh cord blood (usually through scheduled C-sections).
   (b) Prefilled sodium citrate syringes.
   (c) 21G needle.
   (d) Premoistened alcohol wipes.
2. Adult Blood
   (a) Prefilled sodium citrate syringes.
   (b) 21G needle.
   (c) Blood drawing supplies (tourniquet, gauze, alcohol swabs, bandages, etc.).

2.3 Blood Separation

1. Hematology analyzer.
2. Centrifuge with an option for no acceleration and brake.
3. Normal saline (0.9% sodium chloride).
4. 10 μg/mL prostaglandin E1 (PGE-1) (Millipore Sigma).
5. 15 and 50 mL polypropylene conical vials.
6. 8 mL Falcon polystyrene round bottom tubes (Corning).

2.4 Platelet Concentrate Preparation

1. Hematology analyzer.
2. Centrifuge with an option for no acceleration and brake.
3. 10 μg/mL PGE-1 (Millipore Sigma).
4. 15 and 50 mL polypropylene conical vials.

2.5 Thrombocytopenic Blood Creation

1. Hematology analyzer.
2. Red blood cell (RBC), white blood cell (WBC), and platelet-poor plasma (PPP) components from previous separation steps.

2.6 In Vitro Transfusion

1. Thrombocytopenic blood from previous step.
2. Platelet concentrate (PC) from previous step (or an alternate platelet product).
3. Flasks, dishes, or well plates.
4. 37 °C incubator with 5% CO_2 and an electric outlet.
5. Mixer that can be placed in the incubator.

2.7 Measurements of Potential Outcomes

1. Tests of hemostasis
   (a) Thromboelastography (TEG)
      1. Calcium chloride
      2. TEG machine (Haemscope)
   (b) Platelet Function Analyzer (PFA-100®)
      1. PFA-100® (Siemens)
2. Measurement of cellular markers by flow cytometry
   (a) 1X BD FACS lysing solution (BD Biosciences)
   (b) Flow antibodies (e.g., BD Biosciences, BioLegend)
   (c) Flow cytometry machine (such as an LSRFortessa) (BD Biosciences)
3. Plasma measurements (cytokines, etc.)
   (a) Benchtop centrifuge

3 Methods

3.1 Prefilled Sodium Citrate Syringe Preparation

1. Prepare buffered trisodium citrate (0.109M ~ 3.2% trisodium citrate, 0.05M HEPES).
2. Mix on stir plate until dissolved.
3. Adjust pH to 7 with HCl or NaOH as needed.
4. Store at 4 °C.
5. Sterile filter before use with a 0.22 μm PVDF filter.
6. Add 3.33 mL of buffered sodium citrate into a 30 mL syringe for a 1:9 ratio.
7. Cap and store at 4 °C until use.

3.2 Blood Collection

1. Cord Blood
   (a) Bring prefilled sodium citrate syringes to room temperature before blood collection.
   (b) Obtain placenta from OBGYN team with cord clamp in place after delivery.
   (c) Wipe down the cord and the surface of the placenta with premoistened wipes.
   (d) Using the 21G needle (*see* **Note 1**) attached to the syringe, insert the needle into a large vessel on the cord of the placenta and slowly draw blood into the syringe.
   (e) Mix blood through gentle inversion of the syringe
2. Adult Blood
   (a) Bring prefilled sodium citrate syringe to room temperature before blood collection.
   (b) Obtain consent from healthy adult volunteer.
   (c) Draw blood from a healthy adult volunteer by routine procedure. Briefly, place a tourniquet over the upper arm, cleanse the antecubital area with a fresh alcohol swab twice, insert a 21G needle (*see* **Note 1**) attached to a prefilled syringe into the identified vein, remove the tourniquet, and slowly draw back on the syringe until full. Once blood is collected, remove and retract the needle, apply pressure to the site with sterile gauze, and apply a bandage. Mix blood in syringe through gentle inversion.

3.3 Separation of Blood into Individual Components

1. Run the cord blood (CB) and adult blood (AB) sample on a hematology analyzer to obtain starting red blood cell (RBC), white blood cell (WBC), hematocrit (HCT), hemoglobin (HGB), and platelet (PLT) levels (*see* **Note 2**).

2. Place both the CB and AB in separate 50 mL conical vials and centrifuge at 250× *g* for 15 min without acceleration or brake (*see* **Note 3**).
3. Remove the top layer of platelet-rich plasma (PRP) from each, avoiding any RBC or WBC contamination, and place in new 15 mL conical vials keeping CB and AB separate.
4. Add 3.57 μL of 10 μg/mL PGE-1 for every 1 mL of PRP to each.
5. Centrifuge the CB and AB PRP + PGE-1 at 120× *g* for 10 min without acceleration or brake to pellet any remaining WBC or RBC.
6. Transfer the top layer of pure CB and AB PRP to new 15 mL conical vials for the platelet concentrate preparation (*see* Subheading 3.4, **step 1** Platelet Preparation below).
7. Discard the remaining adult blood from Subheading 3.3, **step 3** above, keeping the cord blood for Subheading 3.3, **step 8**.
8. Place remaining cord blood (from Subheading 3.3, **step 3**) in an 8 mL Falcon tube and centrifuge at 1200× *g* for 12 min, resulting in three layers—a platelet poor plasma (PPP) top layer, a middle layer of WBCs, and a bottom layer of RBCs (*see* **Note 3**).
9. Remove the top layer of PPP and place in a new 15 mL conical vial.
10. Spin the PPP at 1000× *g* for 10 min to pellet any residual cells.
11. Remove the PPP and place in a new tube, discarding the cellular pellet.
12. Next, remove the middle layer of WBCs (taking some RBCs to maximize the WBC extraction), place in an 8 mL Falcon tube and add ~7 mL of normal saline.
13. Centrifuge WBC and saline at 200× *g* for 10 min to wash the WBC component.
14. Discard the supernatant and re-suspend the WBCs in ~7 mL of normal saline. Repeat the centrifugation at 200× *g* for 10 min and discard the supernatant, saving the washed WBC component for Subheading 3.5, **step 1**.
15. Next, centrifuge the remaining blood from Subheading 3.3, **step 12** (containing RBCs) at 250× *g* for 15 min without acceleration or brake.
16. Remove and discard the supernatant containing any residual WBC or plasma.
17. Wash the RBCs in ~2–5 mL normal saline and repeat centrifugation at 250× *g* for 15 min without acceleration or brake. Discard the supernatant, keeping the washed RBC component for Subheading 3.5, **step 1**.

3.4 Platelet Concentrate Preparation

1. Take the CB and AB PRP isolated in Subheading 3.3, **step 6** above.
2. Using the hematology analyzer, obtain platelet counts from both the CB and AB PRP to calculate the final volume of resuspension fluid needed to create the desired final platelet concentration (we use a target concentration of 1,000,000 platelets/μL).
3. To both CB and AB PRP, add 3.57 μL of 10 μg/mL PGE-1 for every 1 mL of PRP.
4. Centrifuge CB and AB PRP at 400× *g* for 30 min without acceleration or brake to pellet the platelets (*see* **Note 4**).
5. Remove the PPP supernatant from both and place in new 15 mL conical vials, saving the platelet pellets for resuspension.
6. Centrifuge CB and AB PPP at 1000× *g* for 10 min to pellet any remaining cells.
7. Remove the CB and AB PPP and place in new 15 mL conical vials, discarding the cellular pellet.
8. Add the CB PPP to that isolated in Subheading 3.3, **step 11** (above).
9. Gently resuspend the CB and AB platelet pellets in the calculated amount of their respective PPP (from **step 2** above), forming the CB and AB platelet concentrates (in plasma).
10. Confirm final platelet concentration on hematology analyzer.

3.5 Thrombocytopenic Cord Blood Creation

1. Combine the cord blood components by adding ~4/5 of the washed WBC (from Subheading 3.3, **step 13** above), ~2/3 of the PPP (from Subheading 3.3, **step 11** and Subheading 3.4, **step 8** above), and ~2/3 of the washed RBC (from Subheading 3.3, **step 16** above) together in a 50 mL conical vial to make thrombocytopenic CB.
2. Run a sample of the newly created thrombocytopenic CB on hematology analyzer to measure the RBC, HCT, HGB, WBC, and PLT components.
3. Adjust, adding more of the CB PPP, RBC, and WBC components as needed until the RBC, WBC, HCT, and HGB are within 10% of initial values measured in the whole blood sample (from Subheading 3.3, **step 1**) and the platelet count is reduced to around 50,000/μL (*see* **Note 5**).
4. Run the final thrombocytopenic CB sample on the hematology analyzer and record values (*see* **Note 6**).

3.6 In Vitro Transfusion

1. In a flask, dish, or well plate, add the desired volume of thrombocytopenic blood (in a T25 flask, we add 8 mL of thrombocytopenic CB).

2. Add the desired volume of platelet concentrate to thrombocytopenic blood (we typically add 1.5 mL of platelet concentrate to the 8 mL of blood) (*see* **Note 7**).
3. Mix gently by rocking.
4. Save ~2 mL of blood to analyze hemostatic functions.
5. Incubate at 37 °C, under constant rocking motion for the desired amount of time (time will vary depending on outcomes measured).

3.7 Measurements of Potential Outcomes (see Note 8)

1. Tests of hemostasis [19].
   - (a) Thromboelastography (TEG)
     - (a) Measured immediately after mixing.
     - (b) Recalcify 340 μL of blood with 20 L of 0.2M calcium chloride inside the preheated TEG plastic cup.
     - (c) Record variables measured from TEG.
   - (b) Platelet Function Analyzer-100 (PFA-100®)
     - (a) Measured immediately after mixing.
     - (b) Add 800 μL of blood to appropriate test cartridge and follow manufacturer's instructions.
     - (c) Record closure times in response to collagen and epinephrine (CT-Epi) and/or collagen and ADP (CT-ADP).
2. Measurement of cellular markers by flow cytometry
   - (a) Can be measured 3–4 h after initial mixing.
   - (b) Lyse 120 μL of blood in 1 mL of cold BD FACS Lyse.
   - (c) Allow samples to stand for 10 min at RT to allow RBCs to lyse.
   - (d) Centrifuge lysed samples at 500× *g* for 5 min, removing and discarding supernatant.
   - (e) Stain for desired cell markers (*see* **Note 9**).
   - (f) Run samples on flow machine.
3. Plasma measurements (cytokines, etc.)
   - (a) Can be measured 12–24 h after initial mixing.
   - (b) Centrifuge ~1 mL of blood in an Eppendorf at 2800× *g* for 10 min.
   - (c) Remove the PPP supernatant and place in a new Eppendorf, leaving the cellular component behind to discard.
   - (d) Aliquot and freeze PPP at −80 °C until analysis.

4 Notes

1. To minimize platelet activation during the blood draw, a 21G needle and gentle mixing is used to reduce shear forces.
2. Thrombocytopenic blood generation, while developed for cord blood, also works in adult blood.
3. PPP, WBC, and RBC centrifugation steps happen simultaneously or within quick succession of each other if only one centrifuge is available. Do not wait to finish one component before starting on the next.
4. Using multiple centrifuges simultaneously is recommended so that blood component separation and platelet concentrate preparation can occur simultaneously.
5. To adjust, add more washed WBCs to increase the WBC components, more washed RBCs to increase all values (since it still contains some WBC and platelets), and more PPP to decrease all values through dilution.
6. From a starting volume of 30 mL, the final thrombocytopenic blood volume will be about 15–25 mL.
7. This ratio models the transfusion of 10–15 mL/kg of platelets into a neonate with a blood volume of 80 mL/kg.
8. The outcomes provided here are only examples and will change depending on the questions being asked.
9. For example, it can measure platelet–monocyte or platelet–neutrophil aggregates.

Conflict of Interest

P.D. receives support from NIH/NHLBI K99 HL156051. M.S.V. receives support from NIH/NHLBI P01-HL046925. No other conflicts of interest related to this work to report.

References

1. Christensen RD et al (2006) Thrombocytopenia among extremely low birth weight neonates: data from a multihospital healthcare system. J Perinatol 26(6):348–353
2. Castle V et al (1986) Frequency and mechanism of neonatal thrombocytopenia. J Pediatr 108(5 Pt 1):749–755
3. Andrew M et al (1987) Clinical impact of neonatal thrombocytopenia. J Pediatr 110(3): 457–464
4. Del Vecchio A et al (2001) Platelet transfusions in the neonatal intensive care unit:factors predicting which patients will require multiple transfusions. Transfusion 41(6):803–808
5. Garcia MG et al (2001) Epidemiologic and outcome studies of patients who received platelet transfusions in the neonatal intensive care unit. J Perinatol 21(7):415–420
6. Bonifacio L et al (2007) Thrombocytopenia related neonatal outcome in preterms. Indian J Pediatr 74(3):269–274

7. Kenton AB et al (2005) Platelet transfusions in infants with necrotizing enterocolitis do not lower mortality but may increase morbidity. J Perinatol 25(3):173–177
8. Baer VL et al (2007) Do platelet transfusions in the NICU adversely affect survival? Analysis of 1600 thrombocytopenic neonates in a multi-hospital healthcare system. J Perinatol 27(12): 790–796
9. Patel RM et al (2019) Platelet transfusions and mortality in necrotizing enterocolitis. Transfusion 59(3):981–988
10. Elgendy MM et al (2021) Platelet transfusion and outcomes of preterm infants: a cross-sectional study. Neonatology 118(4):425–433
11. Curley A et al (2019) Randomized trial of platelet-transfusion thresholds in neonates. N Engl J Med 380(3):242–251
12. Moore CM et al (2023) Two-year outcomes following a randomised platelet transfusion trial in preterm infants. Arch Dis Child Fetal Neonatal Ed:F1–F6
13. Ferrer-Marin F, Sola-Visner M (2021) Neonatal platelet physiology and implications for transfusion. Platelets:1–9
14. Davenport P (2023) Neonatal platelet transfusions: more than meets the eye. Pediatr Res 94: 1864
15. Koupenova M, Livada AC, Morrell CN (2022) Platelet and megakaryocyte roles in innate and adaptive immunity. Circ Res 130(2):288–308
16. Maurya P et al (2023) Transfusion of adult, but not neonatal, platelets promotes monocyte trafficking in neonatal mice. Arterioscler Thromb Vasc Biol 43:873–885
17. Davenport P et al (2022) Platelet transfusions in a murine model of neonatal polymicrobial sepsis: divergent effects on inflammation and mortality. Transfusion 62(6):1177–1187
18. Thom CS et al (2023) Quantitative label-free mass spectrometry reveals content and signaling differences between neonatal and adult platelets. J Thromb Haemost 22(5):P1447–P1462
19. Ferrer-Marin F et al (2011) Effects of in vitro adult platelet transfusions on neonatal hemostasis. J Thromb Haemost 9(5):1020–1028

Chapter 9

Mouse Models of Immune Thrombocytopenia

Genevieve Marcoux, John W. Semple, Rick Kapur, and Johan Rebetz

Abstract

There is an extensive body of literature related to animal models of various immune thrombocytopenic conditions. These include those related to the autoimmune bleeding disorder immune thrombocytopenia (ITP), the alloimmune disorder of pregnancy, and the fetal and neonatal alloimmune thrombocytopenia (FNAIT). It appears that many of these models either confirm what has been found in the human disorders or, in some instances, are the first to describe a phenomenon related to immune thrombocytopenia that is of relevance in human medicine. These clinically relevant models will undoubtedly play a significant role in understanding the pathogenesis of the human disorders and the development of novel therapeutics. This chapter will describe the various animal models of ITP and FNAIT and the basic methodology on how to create them.

Key words Immune thrombocytopenia (ITP), Animal models, Passive ITP, Active ITP, Fetal and neonatal thrombocytopenia, Methodology

1 Introduction

There are several conditions where the immune system targets platelets and causes clinical sequelae. For example, immune thrombocytopenia (ITP) is the most common hematological autoimmune disorder caused by immune-mediated destruction of platelets and megakaryocytes (MKs) that can lead to bleeding, fatigue, and a probability of thrombosis [1–5]. On the other hand, fetal and neonatal alloimmune thrombocytopenia (FNAIT) arises during pregnancy when a platelet-antigen positive fetus is carried by an antigen-negative mother who generates alloantibodies against the antigen [6, 7]. These alloantibodies can cross the placenta and induce thrombocytopenia in the fetus, possibly leading to intracranial hemorrhage [6–8]. Furthermore, patients transfused with platelets can generate alloantibodies against the mismatched human leukocyte antigen (HLA) antigens on the donor platelet which can lead to rapid transfused platelet destruction and refractoriness to further transfusions [9, 10]. In other

Sean R. Stowell and Connie M. Arthur (eds.), *Methods in Transfusion Medicine*, Methods in Molecular Biology, vol. 3053, https://doi.org/10.1007/978-1-0716-5376-0_9,

cases, thrombocytopenia can be induced by various drugs or infections [11–13]. All of these immune responses can cause potentially life-threatening scenarios primarily related to excessive bleeding. While many different animals have been used in platelet immunity studies, this chapter will highlight the various murine models of ITP and FNAIT and discuss the methodologies used to establish these models.

1.1 Mouse Models of Primary ITP

ITP is a heterogeneous disorder characterized by immune-mediated destruction and impaired production of platelets, resulting in thrombocytopenia and an increased risk of bleeding [1, 2, 14]. Despite advances in treatment, the underlying mechanisms of ITP remain incompletely understood, necessitating the development of animal models to study disease pathogenesis and explore novel therapeutic strategies. ITP is not a unique disorder to humans as the veterinary literature has many reports of primary chronic ITP affecting various domesticated animals including, dogs, cats, and domestic livestock [15–17]. On the contrary, however, there are no laboratory research animal models of spontaneous autoimmune ITP, and this may be due to the differences in breeding schemes for domesticated verses laboratory animals, e.g., line breeding versus inbreeding. Thus, mouse models of ITP are not true autoimmune platelet models but are contrived by inducing allogeneic or xenogeneic immune responses against platelets. For example, probably the first use of mice to study ITP was performed by Ebbe et al. [18] in 1970, where injection of rabbit anti-mouse platelet serum caused a profound thrombocytopenia after 2 days, which subsequently recovered; this likely represents the first demonstration of the passive model of murine ITP. Since then, hundreds of papers have been published on various methods to induce passive murine ITP [19–21].

1.2 Murine Passive ITP

Passive ITP is the oldest and classic model that simply involves the administration of anti-platelet antibodies leading to thrombocytopenia that resembles human ITP. The advantage of this model is its simplicity and acuteness (thrombocytopenia is usually induced within 1 day), and thus it is amenable to testing therapeutics (e.g., IVIg) for antibody-mediated thrombocytopenia. Disadvantages include, for example, a thrombocytopenia that is transient and begins to quickly subside after its nadir is observed after a single dose of anti-platelet antibody. This can be alleviated by using a dose-escalation protocol where multiple increasing doses of the antiplatelet antibody are administered on a routine basis. In addition, there is not an anti-platelet T-cell component of passive thrombocytopenia (like in human ITP). This can be alleviated by using an active model of ITP (*see* below). Furthermore, most monoclonals that induce passive ITP do not necessarily spontaneously bleed as one would expect [22]. However, multiple injections of small doses of certain anti-GPIIbIIIa monoclonal antibodies (e.g., clones JON1, JON2, Jon3) induce Fc-dependent intestinal bleeding [22]. Of interest, using extremely high doses of MWReg30 (anti-mouse CD41, 550–5000 ug/kg) induce hypothermia and acute lung injury in passively administered mice [23]. In addition to thrombocytopenia, some monoclonal antibodies (e.g., MWReg30) can also induce megakaryocyte (MK) damage, while others cannot [24]. Each new monoclonal antibody used will have to be tested for this MK-destructive capability.

1.3 Fetal and Neonatal Alloimmune Thrombocytopenia

Fetal and neonatal alloimmune thrombocytopenia (FNAIT) is characterized by the maternal immune system producing antibodies against fetal platelets, leading to their destruction. This immune-mediated thrombocytopenia can result in severe complications, including intracranial hemorrhage and even fetal death. FNAIT occurs due to the incompatibility between maternal and fetal platelet antigens. Platelets express various antigens, known as human platelet antigens (HPAs), which can differ between the mother and the fetus. When the fetus inherits a paternal antigen that the mother lacks, her immune system may recognize these fetal platelets as foreign. This leads to the production of maternal alloantibodies that cross the placenta and target fetal platelets for destruction. Understanding the pathophysiology, diagnosis, and management of FNAIT is crucial for improving outcomes in affected pregnancies.

2 Materials

2.1 Passive Immunization ITP Model

1. Mice: Any inbred mouse strain can be used for the induction of passive ITP, but BALB/c, C57BL/6, and CD1 strains are the most commonly used strains (*see* **Note 1**).
2. Monoclonal anti-platelet antibody: Clone MWReg30 [a rat IgG1κ anti-mouse platelet GPIIb (CD41) monoclonal antibody], sourced from various commercial sources (e.g., BioLegend, BD, Merck, Bio X Cell] (*see* **Note 2**).
3. Polyclonal anti-platelet antibodies. Anti-mouse platelet antisera can be commercially obtained or generated by immunizing various species (e.g., rat, rabbit, or guinea pig) with murine platelet transfusions beforehand (*see* **Note 3**).
4. Minivettes (Starstedt) with added preservatives (EDTA or citrate).
5. Ketamine or isoflurane.
6. Hemacytometer.
7. Bone fixative (B+ fixative; BBC Biochemicals).
8. 10% nitric acid.

9. Paraffin.
10. Hematoxylin and eosin (H&E).
11. Light microscope.
12. Phosphate buffered saline (PBS) (*see* **Note 4**).

2.2 Active (Platelet-Induced) ITP Model

1. Mice: Platelet antigen KO animal (*see* **Note 5**).
2. Minivettes (Starstedt) with added preservatives (EDTA).
3. Ketamine or isoflurane.
4. Hemacytometer.
5. Bone fixative (B+ fixative; BBC Biochemicals).
6. 10% nitric acid.
7. Paraffin.
8. Hematoxylin and eosin (H&E).
9. Light microscope.
10. PBS.
11. Citrate-phosphate-dextrose solution with adenine (CPDA) (*see* **Note 6**).

2.3 Fetal and Neonatal Thrombocytopenia (FNAIT Model)

1. Female CD61 KO mice (B6.129S2-*Itgb3*^{tm1Hyn}/JSemJ, JAX stock #008819) on the C57BL/6 background are available from Jackson Laboratories (Bar Harbor, ME) (*see* **Note 7**).
2. Male C57BL/6 mice (JAX Strain #:000664) are available from the Jackson Labs (Bar Harbor, ME).
3. Minivettes (Starstedt) with added preservatives (e.g., EDTA, citrate).
4. Ketamine or isoflurane.
5. Hemacytometer.
6. Bone fixative (B+ fixative; BBC Biochemicals).
7. 10% nitric acid.
8. Paraffin.
9. Hematoxylin and eosin (H&E).
10. Light microscope.
11. PBS.
12. CPDA.

3 Methods

3.1 Passive Immunization ITP Model (see Note 8)

1. Weigh each mouse for baseline measure (*see* **Note 9**).
2. Bleed mice for baseline platelet count (*see* below).
3. Inject anti-platelet antibody into recipient (*see* **Note 10**).

4. If prevention or treatment strategies are being examined, inject treatment modality (e.g., IVIG) either before or after anti-platelet antibody depending on experimental setup (*see* **Note 11**).
5. If vasodilation assistance is required for bleeding for baseline and each subsequent time point, place a heat lamp over the occupied mouse cage for ~5 min to warm the mouse, making sure the animal does not overheat.
6. Place the mouse in a restraining device (a cut 50 cc polystyrene centrifuge tube with the conical end cut to allow the nose to protrude is ideal) with hind legs free.
7. Remove hair from caudal surface of thigh with clippers (if necessary) and swab the site with alcohol.
8. Apply petroleum jelly to the collection site (*see* **Note 12**).
9. Grasp the fold of skin between the tail and thigh; the saphenous vein is found on the caudal surface of the thigh.
10. Apply pressure to the leg above the knee on the thigh, and puncture the vein at a ~ 45° angle with a 23–25 gauge needle or lancet and collect drops of blood with a Minivette as they appear.
11. Apply pressure with gauze until hemostasis occurs. Monitor mouse for 5–10 min to ensure bleeding has stopped.
12. Obtain peripheral blood for platelet enumeration at the desired time points post anti-platelet antibody injection by saphenous vein blood draw using Minivettes (Starstedt) that have added preservatives (EDTA or citrate) (*see* **Note 13**).
13. Using a hemacytometer, enumerate the platelet count of the isolated peripheral blood (*see* **Note 14**).
14. Sacrifice mice 24 h post antibody injection to enumerate megakaryocyte numbers (*see* **Note 15**).
15. Remove muscle tissue and isolate each femur.
16. Remove each epiphysis to extract bone marrow and place in bone fixative (B+ fixative).
17. Decalcify bone in 10% nitric acid for 2 h.
18. Stain with hematoxylin and eosin (H&E).
19. Enumerate megakaryocytes by microscopic evaluation using 40× objective lens with the numerical aperture of objective lens set at 0.75 (*see* **Note 16**).

3.2 Active (Platelet-Induced) ITP Model

1. To harvest platelets, WT mice are anesthetized (e.g., intraperitoneal ketamine injection or inhalation of isoflurane) [25, 26] and whole blood (WB) drawn by cardiac puncture into Ca++/Mg++-free phosphate-buffered saline containing citrate-phosphate-dextrose solution with adenine (CPDA).

2. Blood volume obtained by cardiac puncture (usually 600–1000 uL) is added to PBS with CPDA into to the syringe at an approximately 1:7 dilution (e.g., for 1 mL of blood, add 143 uL of CPDA solution to the syringe).
3. The WB is pooled and diluted with sterile PBS (Ca++/Mg++-free) at a ratio of 1:2 of WB:PBS and centrifuged at 150× *g* for 15 min at 20 °C, and the platelet-rich plasma (PRP) is collected.
4. The PRP is washed two times by centrifuging at 4500× *g* for 5 min at 20 °C, and the washed platelets are resuspended in PBS (Ca++/Mg++-free), counted and their concentration adjusted to 10^9 cells/mL (stock platelet solution).
5. Transfuse 10^8 WT platelets into KO mouse weekly (100 uL of stock platelet solution iv into lateral tail vein) for 4 weeks.
6. On day −1, SCID mice screened to ensure the absence of IgG (*see* **Note 17**) are depleted of natural killer (NK) cells by an ip infusion of 50 uL of a rabbit anti-asialo GM1 antibody (Wako Pure Chemical Industries, Ltd).
7. On day 0, the SCID mice are subjected to 200 cGy total body γ irradiation to inhibit recipient innate immune responses.
8. Within 3 h of irradiation, mice are bled from the saphenous vein for prebleed platelet counts and then injected intraperitoneally with 100 uL of the immune KO splenocyte preparations (*see* **Note 18**).
9. If prevention or treatment strategies are being examined, inject treatment modality (e.g., IVIG) before or after splenocyte injection.
10. At the time points indicated, if vasodilation assistance is required for bleeding, place a heat lamp over the occupied mouse cage for ~5 min to warm the mouse, making sure the animal does not overheat.
11. Place the mouse in a restraining device (a cut 50 cc polystyrene centrifuge tube with the conical end cut to allow the nose to protrude is ideal) with hind legs free.
12. Remove hair from caudal surface of thigh with clippers (if necessary) and swab the site with alcohol.
13. Apply petroleum jelly to the collection site (*see* **Note 12**).
14. Grasp the fold of skin between the tail and thigh; the saphenous vein is found on the caudal surface of the thigh.
15. Apply pressure to the leg above the knee on the thigh and puncture the vein at a ~ 45° angle with a 23–25 gauge needle or lancet and collect drops of blood with a Minivette as they appear.
16. Apply pressure with gauze until hemostasis occurs. Monitor mouse for 5–10 min to ensure bleeding has stopped.

17. Obtain peripheral blood for platelet enumeration at regular time points post splenocyte injection by saphenous vein blood draw using Minivettes (Starstedt) that have added preservatives, e.g., EDTA, citrate (*see* **Note 5**).
18. Using a hemacytometer, enumerate the platelet count in isolated peripheral blood (*see* **Note 6**).
19. Sacrifice mice 24 h post antibody injection.
20. Remove muscle tissue and isolate each femur.
21. Remove each epiphyses to extract bone marrow and place in bone fixative.
22. Decalcify bone in 10% nitric acid for 2 h.
23. Stain with hematoxylin and eosin (H&E).
24. Enumerate megakaryocytes by microscopic evaluation using 40× objective lens with the numerical aperture of objective lens set at 0.75 (*see* **Note 16**).

3.3 Fetal and Neonatal Thrombocytopenia (FNAIT Model) (see Note 19)

1. WT mice are anesthetized (e.g., intraperitoneal ketamine injection or inhalation of isoflurane) [25, 26] and whole blood (WB) is drawn by cardiac puncture into Ca++-/Mg++-free phosphate-buffered saline (PBS, *see* **Note 4**) containing citrate-phosphate-dextrose solution with adenine (CPDA) (*see* **Note 4**).
2. The WB is pooled and diluted with sterile PBS (Ca++-/Mg++-free) at a ratio of 1:2 of WB:PBS and centrifuged at 150× *g* for 15 min at 20 °C, and the platelet-rich plasma (PRP) is collected.
3. The PRP is washed two times by centrifuging at 4500× *g* for 5 min at 20 °C, and the washed platelets are resuspended in PBS (Ca++-/Mg++-free), counted, and their concentration adjusted to 10^9 cells/mL (stock platelet solution).
4. Transfuse female CD61 KO mice weekly with 10^8 C57BL/6 J platelets (100 uL of stock platelet solution iv into lateral tail vein) for 4 weeks (*see* **Note 20**).
5. Upon completion of alloimmuniation schedule, bled via the saphenous vein and the drawn blood allowed to clot for 4 h at room temperature.
6. Centrifuge the clotted whole blood at 13,400× *g* for 5 min and collect the serum.
7. Examine serum for anti-mouse CD61 IgG (*see* **Note 21**).
8. Mate immunized and control (non-immunized) CD61 KO dams with CD61+ C57BL/6 J sires in a standard two male to three female ratio, and pregnancies are monitored. After delivery, platelet counts, bleeding diatheses, and anti-CD61 antibodies can be measured as outlined above (*see* **Note 22**).

4 Notes

1. Additionally, outbred mouse strains can also be used. Both male and female mice can be used, and their age usually ranges between 8 and 12 weeks. For statistical analysis, usually groups of at least five mice are used. Obtain mice and acclimatize for at least 1 week before beginning the protocol.
2. In theory, any anti-mouse platelet monoclonal antibody can be used in the passive model, but each new antibody will have to be titrated and tested for its ability to induce thrombocytopenia [24]. For monoclonal antibodies, the most commonly used clone used in passive ITP studies is clone MWReg30 [a rat IgG1κ anti-mouse platelet GPIIb (CD41) monoclonal antibody], sourced from various commercial sources (e.g., BioLegend, BD, Merck, Bio X Cell].
3. Anti-mouse platelet antisera can be commercially obtained or generated by immunizing various species (e.g., rat, rabbit, or guinea pig) with murine platelet transfusions beforehand. Empirically, the dose of platelets and number of transfusions will have to be determined to generate a high-titer anti-platelet antiserum. Usually, a 100 uL of a stock platelet solution (10^9 platelets/mL) is transfused, and 3 to 4 weekly transfusions are a good starting point to generate the antisera.
4. PBS can be purchased or made. If PBS is to be made, begin with 800 mL of distilled water in a 1 L graduated cylinder (with stirrer). Measure out and add 8 g of NaCl. Add 1.44 g of Na_2HPO_4, 0.2 g of KCl, and 0.24 g of KH_2PO_4. Bring the pH to 7.4 or 7.2 (depending on the application) using HCl. Add distilled water until the total volume reaches 1 liter. Sterilize in an autoclave on a liquid cycle. Store at room temperature.
5. The active ITP model involves immunizing a platelet antigen knockout (KO) mouse with wild-type (WT) platelets, and once immunized, the KO mouse spleen cells are transferred to an immunodeficient mouse strain that becomes thrombocytopenic. This was first performed by Chow et al. [27], who utilized platelet GPIIIa (CD61) KO mice as the recipients of WT platelet transfusions. When the immune spleen cells from these mice were transferred to mice with severe combined immunodeficiency (SCID), a profound thrombocytopenia occurred that lasted for the entire 4-week protocol [27]. By first depleting various lymphocyte populations in the spleen cells, it was determined that the thrombocytopenia induction was dependent on CD4+ T cells and was mediated by both antibodies and cytotoxic T cells (CTL) [27]. Of interest, this model showed that antibody-mediated thrombocytopenia was sensitive to IVIg therapy, whereas the T cell–mediated

thrombocytopenia was not [27]. This same model has also been performed using CD41 KO mice as the source of spleen cells and these mice induce an identical phenotype as the CD61 model [28]. The advantage of this model is that the thrombocytopenia is dependent on both antibody- and T cell-dependent mechanisms and closely mimics characteristics similar to human ITP. Thus, one can determine whether novel therapies may be efficacious in ITP and whether the therapy affects either antibody- or T cell-mediated ITP (or both). This model has been shown to respond to various therapies similarly to patients with ITP, and these therapies include IVIg, Staph Protein A, anti-CD20 (Rituximab), thrombopoietin receptor agonists (TPO-RA), and platelet transfusions to name a few [27, 29–32]. The main disadvantage of this model is that there can be excessive bleeding depending on the spleen cell dose, which needs to be carefully titrated, and this does not mimic typical human ITP [27].

6. CPDA can be purchased or made. If CPDA is to be made, we typically generate 100 mL by adding 0.299 g citric acid (anhydrous), 2.630 g sodium citrate (dihydrate), 0.222 g sodium phosphate monohydrate, 3.190 g dextrose monohydrate, 0.0275 g adenine to 95 mL of sterile water and then mix and add additional sterile water to achieve 100 mL.

7. CD61 KO mice (B6.129S2-*Itgb3*^{tm1Hyn}/JSemJ, JAX stock #008819) on the C57BL/6 background are available from Jackson Laboratories (Bar Harbor, ME). C57BL/6 SCID mice (B6.Cg-*Prkdc*^{scid}/SzJ, JAX stock #001913) are available from the Jackson Labs (Bar Harbor, ME). It is important that the SCID recipient mice exactly match the H-2 haplotype of the KO mice to avoid any unwanted anti-MHC responses after transfer. The BALB/c CD61 KO mouse was generated by Richard Hynes and was extensively used as an active model of ITP but it is no longer available This active model has also been performed with CD41 KO mice with very similar results to the CD61 KO model [28].

8. In some instances, a longer period of thrombocytopenia is desired, and to achieve this, Katsman et al. [33] developed a dose escalation model of passive ITP that increases the thrombocytopenic period to at least 6 days. The dose of MWReg30 was gradually increased over time as follows (based on our group's dosages; each lab will have to optimize the dosages): first does of 100 μg/kg on days 0 and 1, 150 μg/kg on day 2, 200 μg/kg on day 3, 250 μg/kg on day 4, and 300 μg/kg on day 5. These escalations in dosage maintain a more robust thrombocytopenia for up to 6 days. A typical platelet count curve is shown in Fig. 1.

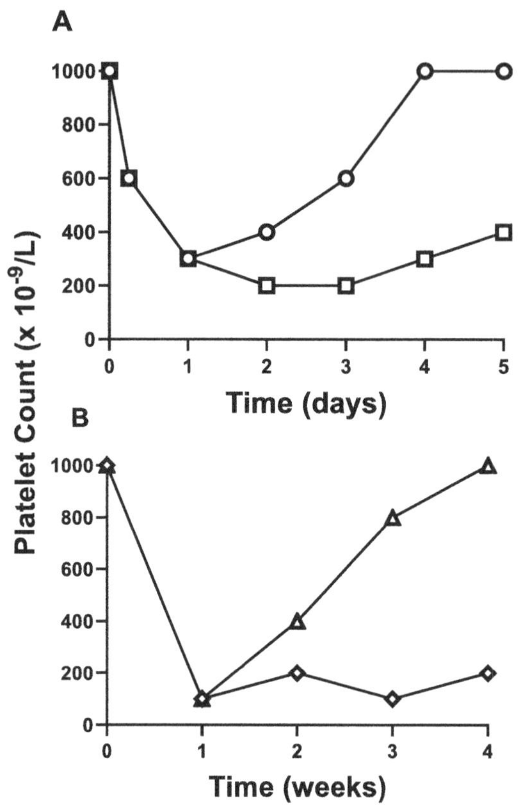

Fig. 1 Typical platelet counts in (**a**) passive models of ITP (○, MWReg30 passive model, single injection; □, MWReg30 dose escalation model, multiple injections) and (**b**) active model of ITP (Δ, control transfer with naïve splenocytes; ◇, transfer with anti-CD61 immune splenocytes). The thrombocytopenia at week 1 in control and test curves is due to the pre-conditioning irradiation

9. The method of saphenous vein blood sampling included in this protocol has been developed in the Semple Lab. The volume of blood removed and the frequency of sampling should be based on the total blood volume of the animal (72 mL/kg), usually no more than 7.5% of the total volume per week. Sample volumes and the total number of samples should be kept to the minimum necessary, and proper consideration should be given to microsampling [34]. It is often helpful to weigh mice and bleed them for baseline platelet counts by using the saphenous vein bleed as it is the least stressful bleeding technique and allows small draws of blood (approximately 100 uL) for accurately determining the platelet counts (this also ensures that the mice do not become anemic with larger draws of blood).
10. While various antibodies can be used, an example strategy is to inject mice with 100–200 ug/kg MReg30 at time zero either intraperitoneally (ip) or intravenously (iv) (both routes will induce thrombocytopenia with the iv route causing a more

acute platelet drop (usually within minutes). After injection, mice can then be bled at various time points, e.g., 6-, 12-, 24-, and 48-h post-injection and platelet counts monitored. A typical platelet count curve is shown in Fig. 1.

11. Passively induced ITP can be treated with various drugs (e.g., IVIg, steroids, and anti-CD20 therapy). The drugs can be administered either prophylactically (before the administration of MWreg30) or therapeutically (after the MWReg30 administration). Dosages and routes will need to be optimized, but for most drugs like IVIg, the ip route is preferred. All reagents and doses must be first optimized so that the desired amount of thrombocytopenia is achieved.
12. We find that this aids in the formation of a large bead of blood.
13. Mice can be bled for estimating platelets counts by various ways, e.g., retrobulbar venous plexus, heart, inferior vena cava, jugular vein, carotid artery, tail, or lateral saphenous veins [25, 26]. We find that the saphenous bleed is best in that it is the least stressful on the mouse and reduces platelet activation. Blood collection is usually performed under general anesthesia (e.g., intraperitoneal ketamine injection or inhalation of isoflurane) [25, 26].
14. Normal murine platelet counts usually range from 600 to 1200 × 10^9 platelets/L, and there are various methods to count murine platelets [25, 26]. In addition to hemocytometers, flow cytometry (with counting beads), Coulter counters, and hematology analyzers can be used [26]. One will have to optimize their method of platelet collection and counting techniques to obtain precise results.
15. ITP is also characterized by abnormalities in bone marrow megakaryocytes. Some anti-platelet monoclonal antibodies (e.g., MReg30) not only induce thrombocytopenia but also cause abnormalities in bone marrow MK [24].
16. We find it helpful to take images of 10 random non-overlapping fields (450 μm × 320 μm/field) throughout each slide from each mouse [30]. The images can then be randomized and blindly assigned to individuals who are trained in megakaryocyte enumeration. The megakaryocyte count of each mouse can then be calculated as the mean value of the 10 fields.
17. The SCID mouse sera have to be screened for the presence of murine IgG by an enzyme-linked immunoabsorbent assay (ELISA) (commercially available or an in-house assay will suffice). Any mouse with a serum IgG concentration greater than 20 ug/mL is deemed "leaky" and should be removed from the experiment.

18. It is important to also isolate control spleen cells from naïve mice for a negative transfer control. The dose of the spleen cells transferred depends on the KO immunization titers and needs to be appropriately adjusted. For example, for fresh spleen cells from a highly immunized KO mouse (IgG anti-platelet titers >1:6400), it is advisable to begin a dose of 5×10^4 spleen cells/SCID mouse ip. This dose may have to be adjusted if the SCID mice bleed severely. A typical platelet count curve is shown in Fig. 1. Immune KO spleen cells can be frozen in liquid nitrogen and used at a later date. Keep in mind that the efficacy of ITP induction will decrease but we have used spleen cells frozen for up to 5 years with good success. Dosages will have to be tested for each frozen batch.
19. The original murine FNAIT model was originally generated using female CD61 KO mice immunized with WT platelets and then mated with CD61+ males [35]. The resulting CD61+ pups were severely affected with thrombocytopenia and bleeding [35].
20. Zhi et al. [36] recently described the development of a APLDQ GPIIIa mouse FNAIT model, wherein transgenic mice expressing the human HPA-1a alloantigenic epitope on the murine GPIIIa backbone are used. C57BL/6 mice expressing murine GPIIIa harboring T30 → A, S32 → P, Q33 → L, N39 → D, and M470 → Q (referred to as APLDQ GPIIIa) express the HPA1 alloantigen. They reported that immunization of wild-type (WT) female mice with platelets from the APLDQ GPIIIa transgenic mice induced high-titer anti–HPA-1a alloantibodies that can cross the placenta and induce the clinical features of FNAIT [37]. Additionally, they went on to demonstrate that treating the female APLDQ GPIIIa dams with HPA-1a–specific antibodies could prevent FNAIT [38]. These transgenic mice are superior to the CD61 KO FNAIT model because the APLDQ mouse model is a true biallelic preclinical model to replicate the intended patient population of an HPA-1a– patient bearing an HPA-1a+ fetus [38]. At this time, however, it is not clear if these mice are available for distribution. Nonetheless, this model is also set up in the same way as the CD61 KO FNAIT model. In order to induce FNAIT in the above models, the female CD61 KO or APLDQ mice must be pre-immunized before mating because natural pregnancies between a CD61 KO dams and a CD61+ sires do not lead to FNAIT; the dam needs to be primed against CD61 prior to pregnancy.
21. IgG1 and IgG2a anti-CD61 antibodies were detected by incubating a 1:100 dilution of sera with C57BL/6 platelets at room temperature for 1 h, centrifuged at 600× *g* for 15 min, and washed with phosphate-buffered saline (PBS). The bound

antibodies were detected with a FITC-conjugated goat anti–mouse IgG, rat anti–mouse IgG1, and IgG2a, respectively, and analyzed on a flow cytometer. A value for anti-platelet IgG levels can be calculated as a fold increase ratio. Fold mean fluorescent intensity (MFI) of test serum/MFI of preimmune serum.

22. Whole blood (10 uL) is isolated from either adult mice (saphenous bleeding) or pups (carotid bleeding) and diluted into 990 uL of PBS-CPDA. Dilute the blood in PBS to a final dilution of 1:12000. A total of 20 to 30 uL of whole blood from the pups can be collected after carotid bleeding for platelet counts and antibody detection.

Acknowledgments

This work was supported by grants from the Swedish Research Council (VR, 2021-01310, 2021-2025) and Avtal om Läkarutbildning och Forskning (ALF) to JWS. G.M. was supported by a Fellowship from the Fonds de recherche en santé du Québec (FRQS).

Author Contributions G.M wrote the first draft, J.W.S. provided financial resources, and J.W.S., R.K, and J.R edited the manuscript.

Conflict of Interest Statement The authors declare no competing interests.

References

1. Neunert C, Terrell DR, Arnold DM, Buchanan G, Cines DB, Cooper N, Cuker A, Despotovic JM, George JN, Grace RF, Kühne T, Kuter DJ, Lim W, McCrae KR, Pruitt B, Shimanek H, Vesely SK (2019) American Society of Hematology 2019 guidelines for immune thrombocytopenia. Blood Adv 3(23):3829–3866. https://doi.org/10.1182/bloodadvances.2019000966. PubMed PMID: 31794604
2. Provan D, Arnold DM, Bussel JB, Chong BH, Cooper N, Gernsheimer T, Ghanima W, Godeau B, González-López TJ, Grainger J, Hou M, Kruse C, McDonald V, Michel M, Newland AC, Pavord S, Rodeghiero F, Scully M, Tomiyama Y, Wong RS, Zaja F, Kuter DJ (2019) Updated international consensus report on the investigation and management of primary immune thrombocytopenia. Blood Adv 3(22):3780–3817. https://doi.org/10.1182/bloodadvances.2019000812. PubMed PMID: 31770441; PMCID: PMC6880896
3. Zufferey A, Kapur R, Semple JW (2017) Pathogenesis and therapeutic mechanisms in immune thrombocytopenia (ITP). J Clin Med 6(2). https://doi.org/10.3390/jcm6020016
4. Delshad M, Davoodi-Moghaddam Z, Pourbagheri-Sigaroodi A, Faranoush M, Abolghasemi H, Bashash D (2024) Translating mechanisms into therapeutic strategies for immune thrombocytopenia (ITP): lessons from clinical trials. Thromb Res 235:125–147. Epub 20240206. https://doi.org/10.1016/j.thromres.2024.02.005. PubMed PMID: 38335568
5. Moulinet T, Moussu A, Pierson L, Pagliuca S (2024) The many facets of immune-mediated thrombocytopenia: principles of

immunobiology and immunotherapy. Blood Rev 63:101141. Epub 20231111. https://doi.org/10.1016/j.blre.2023.101141. PubMed PMID: 37980261

6. Barg A, Bonstein L (2023) New horizons in fetal and neonatal alloimmune thrombocytopenia. Semin Thromb Hemost 49(4): 402–408. Epub 20221111. https://doi.org/10.1055/s-0042-1757900. PubMed PMID: 36368687
7. Stam W, Wachholz GE, de Pereda JM, Kapur R, van der Schoot E, Margadant C (2023) Fetal and neonatal alloimmune thrombocytopenia: current pathophysiological insights and perspectives for future diagnostics and treatment. Blood Rev 59:101038. Epub 20221222. https://doi.org/10.1016/j.blre.2022.101038. PubMed PMID: 36581513
8. Kjeldsen-Kragh J, Bengtsson J (2020) Fetal and neonatal alloimmune thrombocytopenia-new prospects for fetal risk assessment of HPA-1a-negative pregnant women. Transfus Med Rev 34(4):270–276. Epub 20200916. https://doi.org/10.1016/j.tmrv.2020.09.004. PubMed PMID: 33039264
9. Pavenski K, Freedman J, Semple JW (2012) HLA alloimmunization against platelet transfusions: pathophysiology, significance, prevention and management. Tissue Antigens 79(4): 237–245. Epub 2012/03/06. https://doi.org/10.1111/j.1399-0039.2012.01852.x. PubMed PMID: 22385314
10. Saris A, Pavenski K (2020) Human leukocyte antigen alloimmunization and alloimmune platelet refractoriness. Transfus Med Rev 34(4):250–257. Epub 20201007. https://doi.org/10.1016/j.tmrv.2020.09.010. PubMed PMID: 33127210
11. Khandelwal S, Arepally GM (2016) Immune pathogenesis of heparin-induced thrombocytopenia. Thromb Haemost 116(5):792–798. Epub 20160728. https://doi.org/10.1160/th16-01-0074. PubMed PMID: 27465274; PMCID: PMC6260829
12. Warkentin TE (2023) Autoimmune heparin-induced thrombocytopenia. J Clin Med 12(21). Epub 20231103. https://doi.org/10.3390/jcm12216921. PubMed PMID: 37959386; PMCID: PMC10649402
13. Fogagnolo A, Campo GC, Mari M, Pompei G, Pavasini R, Volta CA, Spadaro S (2022) The underestimated role of platelets in severe infection a narrative review. Cells 11(3). Epub 20220126. https://doi.org/10.3390/cells11030424. PubMed PMID: 35159235; PMCID: PMC8834344
14. Provan D, Semple JW (2022) Recent advances in the mechanisms and treatment of immune thrombocytopenia. EBioMedicine 76:103820. Epub 20220121. https://doi.org/10.1016/j.ebiom.2022.103820. PubMed PMID: 35074629; PMCID: PMC8792416
15. LeVine DN, Brooks MB (2019) Immune thrombocytopenia (ITP): pathophysiology update and diagnostic dilemmas. Vet Clin Pathol 48(Suppl 1):17–28. Epub 20190919. https://doi.org/10.1111/vcp.12774. PubMed PMID: 31538353
16. Gershwin LJ (2018) Current and newly emerging autoimmune diseases. Vet Clin North Am Small Anim Pract 48(2):323–338. Epub 20171214. https://doi.org/10.1016/j.cvsm.2017.10.010. PubMed PMID: 29248206
17. Spurlock NK, Prittie JE (2011) A review of current indications, adverse effects, and administration recommendations for intravenous immunoglobulin. J Vet Emerg Crit Care (San Antonio) 21(5):471–483. https://doi.org/10.1111/j.1476-4431.2011.00676.x. PubMed PMID: 22316195
18. Ebbe S, Stohlman F Jr (1970) Stimulation of thrombocytopoiesis in irradiated mice. Blood 35(6):783–792. PubMed PMID: 5427248
19. Neschadim A, Branch D (2015) Mouse models of autoimmune diseases: immune thrombocytopenia. Curr Pharm Des 21. https://doi.org/10.2174/1381612821666150316123436
20. Neschadim A, Branch DR (2016) Mouse models for immune-mediated platelet destruction or immune thrombocytopenia (ITP). Curr Protoc Immunol 113:15.30.1–15.30.13. Epub 20160401. https://doi.org/10.1002/0471142735.im1530s113. PubMed PMID: 27038460
21. Semple JW (2010) Animal models of immune thrombocytopenia (ITP). Ann Hematol 89 Suppl 1:37–44. Epub 20100325. https://doi.org/10.1007/s00277-009-0882-8. PubMed PMID: 20336297
22. Nieswandt B, Bergmeier W, Rackebrandt K, Gessner JE, Zirngibl H (2000) Identification of critical antigen-specific mechanisms in the development of immune thrombocytopenic purpura in mice. Blood 96(7):2520–2527. PubMed PMID: 11001906
23. Nieswandt B, Echtenacher B, Wachs FP, Schröder J, Gessner JE, Schmidt RE, Grau GE, Männel DN (1999) Acute systemic reaction and lung alterations induced by an antiplatelet integrin gpIIb/IIIa antibody in mice. Blood 94(2):684–693. PubMed PMID: 10397735
24. Guo L, Kapur R, Aslam R, Hunt K, Hou Y, Zufferey A, Speck ER, Rondina MT, Lazarus

AH, Ni H, Semple JW (2018) Antiplatelet antibody-induced thrombocytopenia does not correlate with megakaryocyte abnormalities in murine immune thrombocytopenia. Scand J Immunol 88(1):e12678. Epub 2018/06/02. https://doi.org/10.1111/sji.12678. PubMed PMID: 29855061

25. Im JH, Muschel RJ (2017) Protocol for murine/mouse platelets isolation and their reintroduction in vivo. Bio Protoc 7(4): e2132. Epub 20170220. https://doi.org/10.21769/BioProtoc.2132. PubMed PMID: 34458453; PMCID: PMC8376615
26. Jirouskova M, Shet AS, Johnson GJ (2007) A guide to murine platelet structure, function, assays, and genetic alterations. J Thromb Haemost 5(4):661–669. https://doi.org/10.1111/j.1538-7836.2007.02407.x. PubMed PMID: 17403200
27. Chow L, Aslam R, Speck ER, Kim M, Cridland N, Webster ML, Chen P, Sahib K, Ni H, Lazarus AH, Garvey MB, Freedman J, Semple JW (2010) A murine model of severe immune thrombocytopenia is induced by antibody- and CD8+ T cell-mediated responses that are differentially sensitive to therapy. Blood 115(6):1247–1253. Epub 2009/12/17. https://doi.org/10.1182/blood-2009-09-244772. PubMed PMID: 20007808
28. Li X, Wang SW, Feng Q, Hou Y, Lu N, Ma CH, Gao CJ, Hou M, Peng J (2019) Novel murine model of immune thrombocytopaenia through immunized CD41 knockout mice. Thromb Haemost 119(3):377–383. Epub 20190110. https://doi.org/10.1055/s-0038-1677032. PubMed PMID: 30630213
29. Guo L, Kapur R, Aslam R, Speck ER, Zufferey A, Zhao Y, Kim M, Lazarus AH, Ni H, Semple JW (2016) CD20+ B-cell depletion therapy suppresses murine CD8+ T-cell-mediated immune thrombocytopenia. Blood 127(6):735–738. Epub 2015/11/12. https://doi.org/10.1182/blood-2015-06-655126. PubMed PMID: 26556550
30. Guo L, Yang L, Speck ER, Aslam R, Kim M, McKenzie CG, Lazarus AH, Ni H, Hou M, Freedman J, Semple JW (2014) Allogeneic platelet transfusions prevent murine T-cell-mediated immune thrombocytopenia. Blood 123(3):422–427. Epub 2013/11/22. https://doi.org/10.1182/blood-2013-08-523308. PubMed PMID: 24258817
31. Kapur R, Catalina MD, Aslam R, Speck ER, Francovitch RF, Semple JW (2018) A highly purified form of staphylococcal protein a alleviates murine immune thrombocytopenia (ITP). Br J Haematol 183(3):501–503. Epub 2017/10/20. https://doi.org/10.1111/bjh.14985. PubMed PMID: 29048127
32. Kapur R, Aslam R, Speck ER, Rebetz JM, Semple JW (2020) Thrombopoietin receptor agonist (TPO-RA) treatment raises platelet counts and reduces anti-platelet antibody levels in mice with immune thrombocytopenia (ITP). Platelets 31(3):399–402. Epub 20190530. https://doi.org/10.1080/09537104.2019.1624709. PubMed PMID: 31146647
33. Katsman Y, Foo AH, Leontyev D, Branch DR (2010) Improved mouse models for the study of treatment modalities for immune-mediated platelet destruction. Transfusion 50(6): 1285–1294. Epub 20100115. https://doi.org/10.1111/j.1537-2995.2009.02558.x. PubMed PMID: 20088841
34. Diehl KH, Hull R, Morton D, Pfister R, Rabemampianina Y, Smith D, Vidal JM, van de Vorstenbosch C (2001) A good practice guide to the administration of substances and removal of blood, including routes and volumes. J Appl Toxicol 21(1):15–23. https://doi.org/10.1002/jat.727. PubMed PMID: 11180276
35. Ni H, Chen P, Spring CM, Sayeh E, Semple JW, Lazarus AH, Hynes RO, Freedman J (2006) A novel murine model of fetal and neonatal alloimmune thrombocytopenia: response to intravenous IgG therapy. Blood 107(7): 2976–2983. Epub 2005/12/01. https://doi.org/10.1182/blood-2005-06-2562. PubMed PMID: 16317099; PMCID: PMC1895387
36. Zhi H, Ahlen MT, Thinn AMMMM, Weiler H, Curtis BR, Skogen B, Zhu J, Newman PJ (2018) High-resolution mapping of the polyclonal immune response to the human platelet alloantigen HPA-1a (PlA1). Blood Adv 2(21):3001–3011. https://doi.org/10.1182/bloodadvances.2018023341
37. Zhi H, Ahlen MT, Skogen B, Newman DK, Newman PJ (2021) Preclinical evaluation of immunotherapeutic regimens for fetal/neonatal alloimmune thrombocytopenia. Blood Adv 5(18):3552–3562. https://doi.org/10.1182/bloodadvances.2021004371. PubMed PMID: 34470046; PMCID: PMC8945581
38. Zhi H, Sheridan D, Newman DK, Newman PJ (2022) Prophylactic administration of HPA-1a-specific antibodies prevents fetal/neonatal alloimmune thrombocytopenia in mice. Blood 140(20):2146–2153. https://doi.org/10.1182/blood.2022015666. PubMed PMID: 35881848; PMCID: PMC9837438

Chapter 10

Methods to Examine Complement Activation by HIT Immune Complexes

Sanjay Khandelwal and Gowthami M. Arepally

Abstract

Current assays for measuring complement activation by immune complexes (ICs) are largely indirect, non-specific, and employ non-physiologic conditions. To address these drawbacks, we developed methods for measuring the complement activating effects of ICs that cause heparin induced thrombocytopenia (HIT), a blood clotting disorder. These assays rely on the formation of in situ ICs in undiluted healthy donor plasma and/or whole blood as a physiologic source of complement. Once formed, complement-bound ICs in plasma or whole blood are detected using immunocapture and/or flow-based assays. While these methods are designed to study the complement activating properties of HIT ICs, the immunocapture and flow-based assays can be readily extended to other ICs of known composition.

Key words PF4, Heparin, Complement, Immunocapture, Flow cytometry, ELISA, Plasma, Whole blood, Immune complexes, Antigen, Antibody

1 Introduction

It is recognized that immune complexes (ICs) are potent activators of the classical pathway of complement, generating both soluble and IC-bound complement activation fragments [1, 2]. To date, methods for interrogating complement activation by ICs are largely indirect: hemolytic assays of total complement activity as measured by the CH50 [3], release of soluble complement activation products by ELISA [4], detection of C1q bound to ICs using radioactivity [5] or immunoassays [6], and/or flow cytometric assays of C3-bound ICs to cell-lines [7]. While these methods assess complement activating capacity of ICs, they lack specificity, are often conducted under non-physiologic conditions with limited amounts of complement, and/or are performed in disease states marked by complement consumption.

Sean R. Stowell and Connie M. Arthur (eds.), *Methods in Transfusion Medicine*, Methods in Molecular Biology, vol. 3053,
https://doi.org/10.1007/978-1-0716-5376-0_10,

To circumvent these limitations, we developed assays to directly examine ICs of known composition, using immunocapture and/or flow-based methods. These assays are optimized for detection of ICs formed in heparin induced thrombocytopenia (HIT), a life-threatening clotting disorder caused by IgG antibodies to multivalent complexes of platelet factor 4 (PF4) and heparin (H) [8–12].

The principle of these assays rests on the generation of in situ ICs in undiluted healthy donor plasma and/or whole blood. Undiluted, anticoagulated plasma or whole blood is used as a physiologic source of complement and complement regulatory proteins. The ICs are formed by addition of patient plasma or patient-derived antibodies (antibody source) and target antigens to undiluted healthy donor plasma/whole blood (complement source; *see* Fig. 1). Once ICs are formed in situ, complement-opsonized ICs are either detected using a sandwich immunoassay or detected on the cell-surface by flow cytometry.

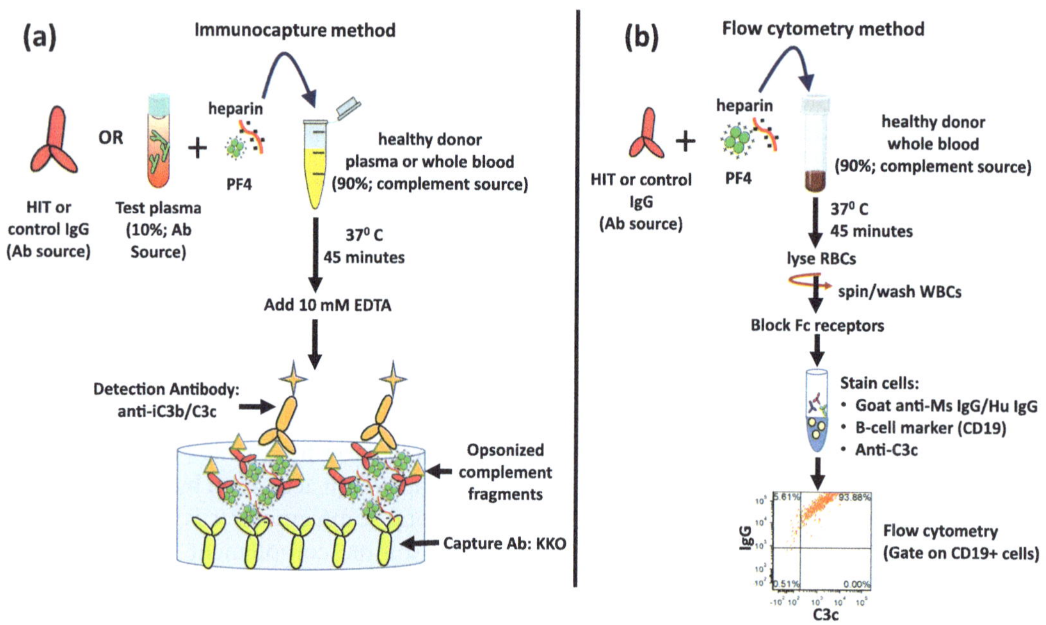

Fig. 1 Schema of complement activation assays by HIT immune complexes. (**a**) Immunocapture method. Healthy donor whole blood or plasma is incubated with antigen (PF4 and heparin) and antibodies (Abs) or patient plasma (as a source of Abs) for 45 min at 37 °C, followed by the addition of EDTA to inhibit further complement activation. ICs are captured by using the KKO antibody, and IC-bound C3c is detected with an anti-human C3c antibody. If healthy donor whole blood is used instead as a source of complement, plasma supernatant is separated from whole blood by centrifugation before adding EDTA. (b) Flow cytometry method. Whole blood from a healthy donor is incubated with antigens and Abs as described for the immunocapture assay. After red cell lysis, washing, and blocking of Fc receptors, white cells are stained with Abs against mouse or human IgG, CD19 (B-cells), and C3c. Deposition of IgG and C3c is determined on B-cells (CD19 + cells) by flow cytometry

For the immunocapture assay, complement-fixed ICs are captured from plasma using an antigen-specific monoclonal or polyclonal antibody, followed by detection of bound complement activation fragments (iC3b/C3c or C4b, etc.) using labeled antibodies directed to complement proteins. The flow-based assay detects complement-opsonized ICs that bind to cell-surface complement receptors (CRs, such as CR2 or CD21 on B-cells or CR3 on neutrophils/monocytes). Whereas the immunocapture assays can be performed in healthy donor plasma or whole blood and require antigen-specific antibodies for capturing ICs, the flow-based assays can only be performed in healthy donor whole blood due to a requirement for white cells. The flow-based assay does not need antigen-specific antibodies, as this technique relies only on detecting components of the ICs on the cell-surface, either human or mouse IgG and associated complement fragments.

The methods outlined in this protocol permit investigation of a variety of IC and complement interactions, including, but not limited to, the complement activating properties of ICs derived from patient samples, molecular and structural determinants of complement activation, biochemical regulation of complement activation, and effects of complement inhibitors. The utility of these assays is shown in the accompanying figures demonstrating the complement activating properties of IgG from HIT patients (Fig. 2) or other ICs (Fig. 3), investigating the effects of complement inhibitors (Fig. 4a), generating inhibitory concentration curves (Fig. 4b), and measuring the binding of ICs to the cell-surface (Fig. 6).

Protocols for the following methods are described below:

- Immunocapture method.
- Flow cytometry method.

2 Materials

2.1 Immunocapture Method

2.1.1 Complement Activation in Plasma or Whole Blood

Measurement of Complement Activation by Immunocapture Assay

1. Fresh or frozen healthy donor plasma prepared from healthy donor whole blood collected in acid-citrate-dextrose solution A (ACD-A) or whole blood collected in ACD-A {Baxter Healthcare Corporation, Deerfield, IL, Trisodium citrate, 22.0 g/L (85.3 mM), citric acid, 8.0 g/L (41.6 mM), and dextrose, 24.5 g/L (136 mM)} using the ratio of ACD-A to blood as 1:7 (v/v) (*see* **Notes 1–4**).
2. 1.5 mL micro-centrifuge tubes.
3. Capture antibody: Anti-PF4/H antibody (KKO, a monoclonal anti-PF4/heparin antibody [13]; catalog # CL2767AP, Cedarlane).

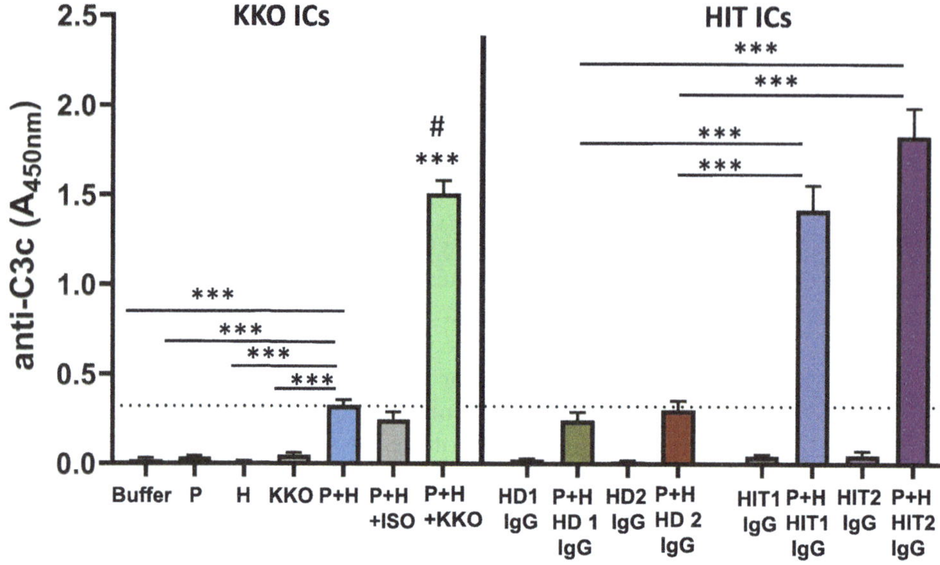

Fig. 2 Immunocapture assay for detecting complement activation by HIT immune complexes: Plasma from a healthy donor was incubated with various reagents, including PF4 (P,25 μg/mL), heparin (H,1 U/mL), KKO (50 μg/mL), isotype antibody (ISO, 50 μg/mL), HIT or HD IgG (500 μg/mL) as shown in the graph. After a 45-min incubation at 37 °C, further complement activation was quenched by the addition of 10 mM EDTA, and immunocapture was performed using KKO (2 μg/mL) as the capture antibody and anti-C3c as the detection antibody, as described in Subheading 3.1.2. Plasma incubated with antigens (P or H alone) or antibodies alone (KKO, HD, or HIT IgG) did not show C3c binding. When plasma is incubated with P + H complexes or with ICs consisting of KKO + P + H or HIT IgG + P + H, C3c can be detected on captured ICs. Whereas P + H complexes elicit some complement activation due to binding IgM in donor plasma as previously described [14], ICs consisting of KKO (KKO + P + H) or HIT IgG (HIT IgG + P + H) show markedly higher complement activation. ***$p < 0.0001$ using the one-way ANOVA with Tukey's multiple comparisons test. #p values relative to all conditions to the left

4. Patient and control antibodies (purified IgG or frozen plasma/ serum samples).
5. Platelet factor 4 (PF4, Abcam).
6. Heparin (H; 100 U/mL; Elkins-Sinn Inc.,).
7. 37° C thermal convection or dry-bath incubator (e.g., Quincy Lab Thermal incubator, Quincy Lab).
8. EDTA (Invitrogen).
9. 96-well ELISA plate (Thermo Scientific).
10. Phosphate buffered saline (PBS; 137 mM NaCl, 2.7 mM KCl, 10 mM Na2HPO4,1.8 mM KH2PO4, without calcium and magnesium; pH 7.4).
11. Bovine serum albumin fraction V (BSA; Millipore Sigma).

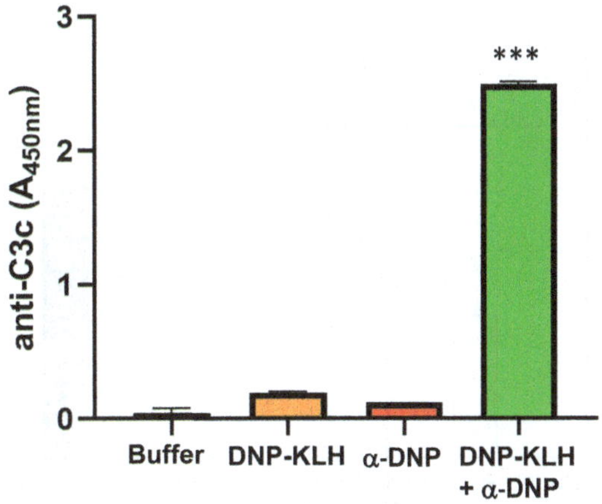

Fig. 3 Complement activation by DNP-KLH and α-DNP antibody ICs as determined by an immunocapture assay: Plasma from a healthy donor was incubated with buffer, anti (α)-DNP antibody alone (100 μg/mL), DNP-KLH antigen (25 μg/mL) alone, or with a combination of α-DNP antibody (100 μg/mL) and DNP-KLH (25 μg/mL) for 45 min at 37 °C followed by the addition of 10 mM EDTA to quench further complement activation. Immunocapture was performed using α-DNP antibody (2 μg/mL) as the capture antibody and anti-C3c as the detection antibody, as described in Subheading 3.1.2. Plasma incubated with antigen (DNP-KLH) or antibody alone (α-DNP) did not have bound C3c, but α-DNP ICs formed by α-DNP and DNP-KLH had a significant amount of bound C3c. ***$p < 0.0001$ relative to all conditions on the graph, using the one-way ANOVA with Tukey's multiple comparisons test

12. ELISA washing buffer: Tris-buffered saline/Tween 20, TBST, 20 mM Tris, 150 mM NaCl, 0.05% (v/v) Tween® 20 detergent.
13. Blocking buffer: 1% BSA/PBS.
14. Sample dilution buffer: 1% BSA/PBS/10 mM EDTA.
15. Biotin-conjugated anti-human C3c antibody (e.g., catalog # A701, Quidel Ortho, San Diego, CA) (*see* **Notes 4** and **6**).
16. Horseradish peroxidase conjugated streptavidin (SAv HRPO, e.g., catalog #554066, BD Biosciences).
17. Developing reagents: TMB peroxidase substrate and peroxidase substrate solution B (Sera Care).
18. Stop solution: 1N H2SO4.
19. ELISA plate reader (capable of reading absorbance at 450 nm, e.g., Spectra Max M2, Molecular Devices).
20. Benchtop centrifuge (capable of 300 × g spins) with adapters to hold micro-centrifuge tubes.

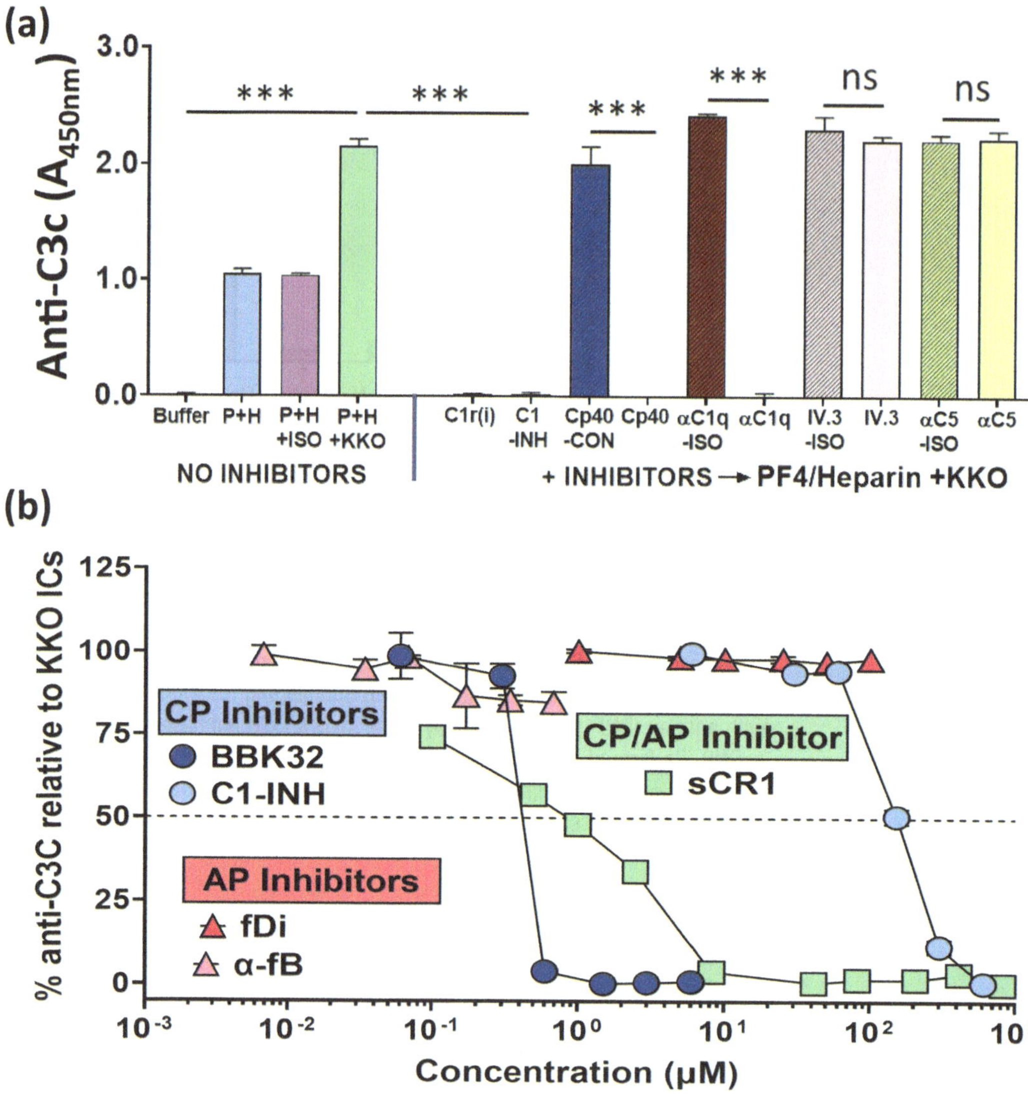

Fig. 4 Effects of complement inhibitors using the immunocapture assay. (**a**) Effects of complement inhibitors on complement activation by KKO ICs. Healthy donor plasma was pre-incubated with complement inhibitors (BBK32, a small molecule C1 inhibitor, 25 μg/mL), C1-esterase inhibitor (C1-INH, 100 μg/mL), Cp40 (a C3 inhibitor, 20 μM), anti-C1q blocking antibody (300 μg/mL), IV.3 (10 μg/mL), an FcγRIIA blocking antibody, anti-C5 monoclonal antibody (50 μg/mL) or isotype controls before adding PF4(P)/heparin(H) antigen and KKO. As shown, C3 activation was inhibited by C1/C3 blocking agents but not by anti-C5 or anti-FcγRIIA. ***$p < 0.0001$, ns = not significant, using the one-way ANOVA with Tukey's multiple comparisons test. (**b**) Inhibitory concentration curve of complement inhibitors. The inhibitory concentration leading to half-maximal C3c generation (IC50) was determined in the immunocapture assay by incubating healthy donor whole blood with increasing concentrations (x-axis) of complement inhibitors as indicated in the graph. Pre-incubation of whole blood with inhibitors was followed by addition of PF4, H, and KKO to form in situ ICs, and complement activation measured as described in Subheading 3.1.2. Classical pathway (CP) and CP/alternative pathway (AP) inhibitors inhibited complement activation, but AP pathway-specific inhibitor had no effect. The graph shows the C3c generated relative to KKO ICs (PF4/H/KKO). (Figure 4a adapted from Blood [9] with permission from the American Society of Hematology. Figure 4b adapted from Journal of Thrombosis and Haemostasis [11] with permission from the International Society on Thrombosis and Haemostasis)

2.2 Flow Cytometry Method

2.2.1 Complement Activation in Whole Blood

Staining of the Ccells for ICs (IgG), CD19, and C3c

1. Fresh healthy donor whole blood collected in ACD-A (*see* details in Subheading 2.1.1.1) (*see* **Notes 1–2**).
2. Sterile 12 × 75 mm, 5 mL polystyrene round bottom test tubes with cap (Falcon, Corning).
3. Non-sterile 12 × 75mm, 5 mL polystyrene round bottom test tubes (fluorescence-activated cell sorting tubes, FACS tubes, Falcon, Corning).
4. 37 °C thermal convection or dry-bath incubator.
5. Heat inactivated fetal bovine serum (HI FBS, Hyclone).
6. Fluorescence-activated cell sorting buffer (FACS buffer, 2% HI FBS/ PBS).
7. ACK (ammonium-chloride-potassium) lysing buffer (e.g., catalog # A1049201, ThermoFisher Scientific).
8. Human Fc block reagent (e.g., catalog # 564220 BD Biosciences) or Intravenous immunoglobulin (IVIG, catalog # NDC44206–436-05, Grifols).
9. Fluorescently conjugated antibodies to:
   - CD19: eFluor™ 450 conjugated mouse anti-human CD19 antibody (Clone HIB19, e.g., catalog # 48–0199-42).
   - C3c: Fluorescein isothiocyanate (FITC) conjugated rabbit polyclonal anti-human C3c antibody (e.g., catalog # Ab4212 from Abcam) (*see* **Note 5**).
   - Mouse or human IgG: Fluorescently conjugated (Alexa Fluor 647) secondary antibodies: Goat anti-mouse IgG (H + L), (e.g., catalog No. 21335) or goat anti-human IgG (H + L; e.g., catalog #21445 from Invitrogen).
10. PBS, pH 7.4.
11. 1% Paraformaldehyde, prepared fresh in FACS buffer from the stocks of 4% Paraformaldehyde in PBS, pH 7.4.
    - 4% Paraformaldehyde (w/v) prepared from paraformaldehyde powder (catalog # P6148 Millipore Sigma) in 1× PBS, pH 7.4; aliquoted and stored in −20 °C (*see* **Note 7**).
12. Patient and control antibodies (purified IgG).
13. PF4 (Abcam).
14. Heparin (Elkins-Sinn Inc.).
15. Flow cytometer (BD Canto or any other brand/model flow cytometer with three lasers (405, 488, and 633 nm) and having capability to acquire FSC, SSC, and three fluorescent markers (*See* **Note 8**).
16. Benchtop centrifuge with adapters to hold 5 mL tubes (capable of up to 350 × g spins).

3 Methods

3.1 Immunocapture Method (Schema Shown in Fig. 1a)

3.1.1 Complement Activation in Plasma or Whole Blood

1. The following methods describe assays with a final volume of 100 μL.
2. Prepare micro-centrifuge tubes for control and test conditions:
   (a) Prepare single or duplicate tubes for relevant controls. For our assays, this includes buffer only, antigen only (e.g., PF4 alone or heparin alone), and antibody only (KKO and isotype).
   (b) Prepare tubes for test conditions of ICs and isotype controls. For our assays, this includes tubes for ICs formed by antibody (KKO or isotype) and antigen (PF4 and heparin).
3. Add 90 μL of healthy donor plasma or whole blood to each micro-centrifuge tube containing control or test conditions (*see* **Note 9**).
4. To limit complement activation until ICs are formed, add the following components to plasma/whole blood in the following sequence:
   (a) If using complement inhibitors or blocking antibodies, add these first to plasma/whole blood and incubate for 20–30 min at room temperature to ensure adequate blocking of proteins. If complement inhibitors or blocking antibodies are not being used, skip to the next Step (4b).
   (b) Add buffer and antigens to designated micro-centrifuge tubes. We typically use PF4 (25 μg/mL) ± heparin (1 U/mL).

   The antigen for KKO and HIT antibodies is a complex of PF4/heparin.

   (c) Add antibodies (KKO 50 μg/mL) or isotype controls to designated tubes. If using patient or control plasma, add 10% v/v to designated tubes. Final total volume of inhibitors/antigen/antibody added in this section (4a-4c) should be about 10 μL added to 90 μL volume of healthy donor plasma or whole blood (total final volume = 100 μL). Larger volumes of reagents (inhibitors/antigen/antibody) will dilute complement and complement regulatory proteins present in healthy donor plasma or whole blood.
   (d) Add required buffer (PBS) to make up the final reaction volume to 100 μL for all conditions.
5. Tap all tubes to mix the content and incubate the tubes at 37 °C for 45 min (*see* **Notes 10** and **11**).

(a) If using the whole blood in Step 3, spin the whole blood after incubations at 300 × g for 5 min and collect the plasma supernatant as sample.

6. Add EDTA to a final concentration of 10 mM to inhibit any further complement activation and incubate at room temperature for 10 min.
7. Plasma could be stored at -80 °C for future analysis or can be used directly to measure complement activation as described in Subheading 3.1.2.

3.1.2 Measurement of Complement Activation by Immunocapture Assay

1. Coat a 96-well microtiter plate with capture antibody overnight.
   (a) For our assay, we typically use KKO at 2 μg/mL in PBS.
   (b) Add 100 μL of diluted antibody to each well of the 96-well plate.
   (c) Incubate the plate at room temperature overnight on a rotating or shaker platform.
2. Wash the plate 3–5 times with ELISA washing buffer (TBST). Tap to remove excessive fluid in between washes.
3. Block the wells by adding 200 μL of blocking buffer (1% BSA/PBS) to each well.
4. Incubate 2 hours at room temperature.
5. Wash the plate 5 times with ELISA washing buffer (TBST). Tap to remove excessive fluid in between washes.
6. Load 100 μL of samples to each well in triplicate.
   (a) Dilute plasma samples containing controls or test ICs from 3.1.1 at a 1:50 dilution in 1% BSA/PBS/10 mM EDTA.
   (b) If frozen plasma samples are being used, thaw the samples at room temperature before making dilutions.
   (c) Prepare blank wells using 100 μL of sample dilution buffer (1% BSA/PBS/10 mM EDTA) in triplicate.
7. Incubate the plate for 1 hour at room temperature.
8. Wash plate 5 times with ELISA washing buffer (TBST). Tap to remove excessive fluid in between washes.
9. Add biotin-conjugated anti-C3c antibody diluted (1:1500) in blocking buffer (1% BSA/PBS).
10. Incubate for 1 hour at room temperature.
11. Wash plate 5 times with ELISA washing buffer (TBST). Tap to remove excessive fluid in between washes.
12. Add SAv HRPO diluted (1:2000) in blocking buffer (1% BSA/PBS).

13. Incubate for 30 min at room temperature.
14. Wash five times with ELISA washing buffer (TBST). Tap to remove excessive fluid in between washes.
15. Calculate volume needed for peroxide developing reagent solution which is added at 100 μL/well.
16. Just before using, prepare peroxide developing reagent by mixing equal volume of TMB peroxidase substrate and peroxidase substrate solution B.
17. Add 100 μL peroxide developing reagent to each well.
18. Allow to develop at room temperature for 10–30 min, depending on the speed of color development for wells containing KKO immune complexes.
19. Stop reaction by adding 50 μL of 1 N 1 N H2SO4 to each well.
20. Read the absorbance at 450nm(A450nm) using the ELISA plate reader.
21. Subtract the blank values from all other conditions.
22. Use the A450nm as values of relative complement activation.
23. *Expected results shown in* Figs. 2 and 4 (*see* **Notes 12–14**).

3.2 Methods: Flow Cytometry Method (Schema Shown in Fig. 1b)

3.2.1 Complement Activation in Whole Blood

1. The following methods describe assays with a final volume of 200 μL and detect binding of KKO or HIT ICs to B-cells by measuring the binding of anti-mouse or human IgG and anti-C3c antibodies to B-cells.
2. Obtain the healthy donor fresh whole blood in ACD-A as described above in Subheading 2.1.1.1.
3. Prepare 5 mL polystyrene round bottom test tubes (with cap) for control and test conditions as follows:
   (a) Prepare single or duplicate tubes for relevant controls. For our assays, this includes buffer only, antigen only (e.g., PF4 alone or heparin alone), and antibody only (KKO or isotype).
   (b) Prepare tubes for test conditions of ICs and isotype controls. For our assays, this includes tubes for ICs formed by antibody (KKO, or isotype) and antigen (PF4 and heparin).
4. Add 180 μL of healthy donor whole blood, to 5 mL polystyrene round bottom test tubes (with cap).
5. To limit complement activation until ICs are formed, add the following components to fresh whole blood in the following sequence:

(a) If using complement inhibitors or blocking antibodies, add these first to whole blood to ensure adequate blocking of proteins. If complement inhibitors or blocking antibodies are not being used, skip to next Step (5b).

(i) Incubate for 20–30 min at room temperature.

(b) Add buffer and antigens to the designated tubes. We typically use PF4 (25 μg/mL) and heparin (1 U/mL).

(c) Add antibodies (KKO 50 μg/mL or HIT IgG 500 μg/mL) or isotype controls to designated tubes. Final volume of reagents added in these substeps (5a-5c) should be about 20 μL for a 200 μL final volume, as larger volumes of reagents will dilute whole blood as well as complement and complement regulatory proteins.

(d) Add required buffer (PBS) to make up the final reaction volume same (200 μL) for all conditions.

6. Tap the tube to mix the content.
7. Incubate the tubes at 37 °C for 45 min.
8. Immediately proceed to staining of the cells (Subheading 3.2.2).

3.2.2 Staining of the Cells for ICs (IgG), CD19, and C3c.

1. After completion of whole blood incubations, lyse the red blood cells in samples as follows:

(a) Add ACK lysis buffer to each tube (about 3 mL/200 μL of blood).

(b) Mix the tubes gently and keep at room temperature for 5 min.

(c) Spin the tubes at 300 × g without break for 5 min.

(d) Decant the liquid or remove the liquid by suction.

2. Wash the cells two times with FACS buffer (2% FBS/PBS).

(a) Resuspend cells in 3 mL of FACS buffer in the tubes and tap the tube 3–4 times to mix.

(b) Spin the tubes at 340 × g for 5 min.

(c) Decant the liquid or remove the liquid by suction.

(d) Repeat steps a-c again.

Resuspend pellet in 280 μL of FACS buffer with IVIG (final IVIG 4 mg/mL) or human Fc block (1:20 dilution) to block the Fc receptors on the cells (*see* **Note 15**).

3. Add 70 μL of cell suspension (from Step 3) to individual FACS tubes as follows for staining.
   (a) One tube without fluorescent antibodies to identify unstained cells.
   (b) One tube each for individual antibodies as single color controls (e.g., only eFluor 450 anti-human CD19 or FITC anti-human C3c, etc.) for adjusting compensation (*see* **Notes 8** and **16**).
   (c) Experimental tubes containing all three labeled antibodies (e.g., eFluor 450 anti-human CD19, FITC anti-human C3c, and AF647 goat anti-human IgG) to examine deposition of complement and IgG to B-cells (*see* **Notes 17** and **18**).
4. Incubate the FACS tubes with cells at 4 °C for 10 min.
5. Add fluorescently conjugated secondary anti-mouse or anti-human IgG antibody (final dilution 1:500), based on the species composition of ICs in Subheading 3.2.1, **step 5**, to the designated tubes. *See* ***Note 19*** *for the rationale for sequential antibody staining. From here on, minimize ambient light exposure.*
6. Incubate the cells at 4 °C for 30 min in dark.
7. Wash the cells two times with FACS buffer as described in Subheading 3.2.2, **step 2**.
8. Add 70 μL of FACS buffer to each tube.
9. Add fluorescently conjugated anti-human CD19 (final dilution 1:45) and/or anti-human C3c antibody (final dilution 1:100); (*see* **Notes 19** and **20**).
10. Incubate the cells at 4 °C for 30 min.
11. Wash the cells two times with FACS buffer as described in Subheading 3.2.2, **step 2**.
12. After last washing, tap the tubes to dislodge the cell pellet and resuspend in 200 μL of FACS buffer, if directly analyzing by flow, or in 200 μL 1% paraformaldehyde, if analyzing later by flow. After resuspending, tap the tube again to reduce the aggregate formation.

Samples resuspended in 1% paraformaldehyde can be stored at 4 °C in dark until acquisition of the samples by flow cytometer for up to 48 hours.

13. Use the standard settings for white blood cells acquisition (linear scale for FSC and SSC and log scale for fluorescent marker) and store 10,000 events in the lymphocyte gate. The gating strategy for B-cell analysis is shown in Fig. 5.
14. Expected results shown in Fig. 6 (*see* **Note 21**).

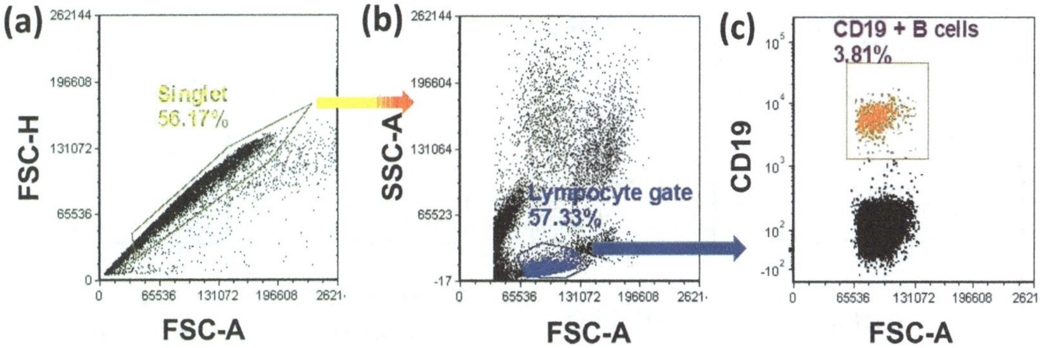

Fig. 5 Gating strategy for identifying B-cells in whole blood samples. (**a**) Identify single cell populations: Single cell population is gated based on the FCS-H and FSC-A. Cells with proportional FSC-H and FSC-A values are considered single cells. (**b**) Identify total lymphocyte population. Lymphocyte population is identified on the SSC-A and FSC-A plot from the single cell gate. Lymphocytes have lower FSC and SSC. (**c**) Identify B-cells in total lymphocyte population. CD19-positive B-cells are gated from the lymphocyte population by plotting FSC-A vs CD19. B-cells are subsequently analyzed for deposition of C3c and mouse or human IgG using respectively labeled antibodies

4 Notes

1. In our hands, the citrate concentrations in ACD or sodium citrate do not significantly limit the complement activating properties of HIT ICs. It is possible that citrate concentrations of commonly used anticoagulants may limit complement activation by less potent ICs; additional testing using alternative anticoagulants may be needed for ICs that do not activate complement in immunocapture or flow assays as described in this protocol.
2. When using fresh plasma or whole blood as a source of complement, samples should be used within 2 hours of collection. If using frozen plasma as a source of complement, avoid repeated freeze and thaw cycles of plasma by freezing small aliquots of plasma after collection.
3. We preferentially use plasma prepared from whole blood collected in ACD-A anticoagulant, as we get lower background, but plasma prepared from blood collected in sodium citrate anticoagulant (3.2% Sodium Citrate BD Vacutainer blood collection tubes (BD)) or serum can also be used, but may be associated with higher background complement activation in buffer and/or control conditions. Plasma should be separated at high speed (2000 × g for 15 min) to avoid platelet activation.

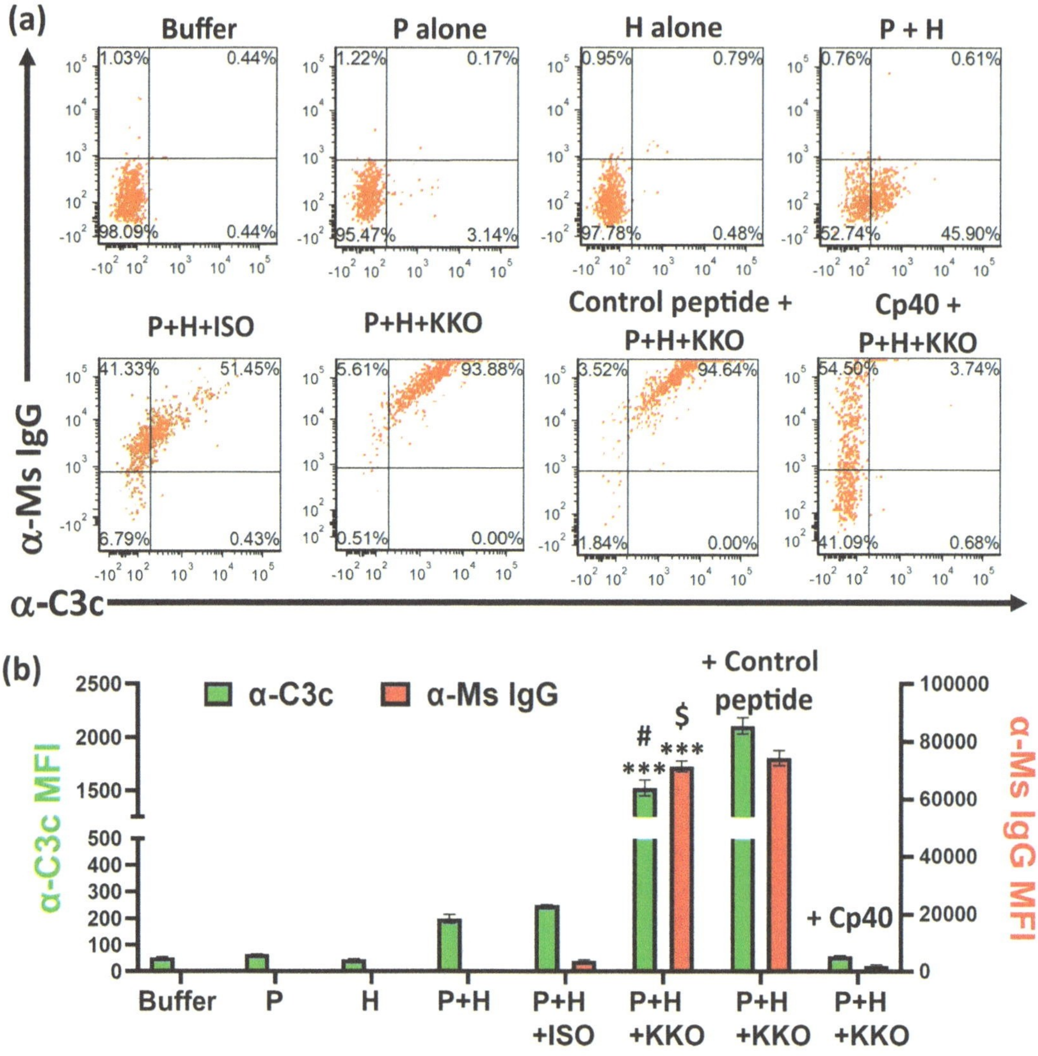

Fig. 6 Complement-dependent deposition of KKO ICs on B-cells: (**a**) Dot plots showing complement-dependent binding of KKO ICs to B-cells. Upper panel shows dot plots of gated B-cells from whole blood incubated with buffer, PF4 (P) alone, heparin (H) alone or PF4/heparin (P + H), while lower panel shows gated B-cells from whole blood conditions incubated with antigen (P+ H) and antibodies (Isotype, ISO or KKO) in the absence or presence of a C3 inhibitor (Cp40) or control peptide. Anti-C3c staining is shown on the x-axis, and anti-mouse IgG is shown on the y-axis. Incubation of whole blood with antigens alone shows minimal C3c deposition on B-cells, while incubation with antigen and antibody shows significant C3c and IgG deposition on B-cells in a rocket shape, indicating a tight correlation of C3c with IgG deposition. Inhibition of complement by Cp40 completely inhibits the deposition of complement and IgG on the B-cells. (**b**) Analysis of mean fluorescent intensity (MFI) from data shown in Panel (**a**). MFI for C3c and IgG was markedly increased on B-cells in whole blood incubated with P + H + KKO. A small amount of C3c deposition is seen with P and H, as natural IgM binds to P/H and activates complement. Pre-incubation of whole blood with Cp40 (20 μM), but not the control peptide, completely inhibits the deposition of complement and IgG on the B-cells. *** $p < 0.0001$, using the one-way ANOVA with Tukey's multiple comparisons test. # C3c relative to all other conditions and $, Ms. IgG relative to all other conditions except control peptide + P + H + KKO. (Part of Fig. **a** adopted from Blood [9] (after permission from the American Society of Hematology))

4. This ex-vivo assay can also be performed in plasma from other species (e.g., mouse, rat, monkey) by using species-specific anti-complement antibodies.
5. Detection antibodies can be varied to detect other complement fragments bound to the IC or cells, including C3d, C4d, C4b, etc.
6. Soluble degradation products such as C3a, C5a, C5b-9, and C1s-C1 inhibitor complexes are also generated in the ex-vivo assays and can be measured using commercial immunoassays.
7. After thawing, 4% paraformaldehyde can be stored at 4 °C for up to 1 month.
8. For fluorescently conjugated antibodies which are used for staining cells in Subheading 3.2.2, we use fluorophores (eFluor™ 450, FITC, and Alexa Fluor 647) which show very minimal or no spectral overlap with each other. However, if there are limitations due to flow cytometer capabilities (such as two laser flow cytometers) different combinations of fluorophores could be used (e.g., phycoerythrin (PE), FITC, and Alexa Fluor 647) with appropriate measures to adjust compensation.
9. Healthy donor plasma volume may be scaled up or down depending on the needs of the experiment. If using whole blood, the final plasma volume for immunocapture assay will be ~30–40% of the blood volume, depending on the donor's hematocrit.
10. These assays are adaptable for measuring complement activation by ICs other than HIT ICs. As proof of principle, we can detect complement activation by ICs formed by rabbit anti-dinitrophenyl (DNP) antibody and DNP-keyhole limpet hemocyanin (KLH) antigen. Results of the immunocapture assay using rabbit anti-DNP antibody as a capture antibody are shown in Fig. 3. If developing complement activation assays of other ICs, we recommend titrating antigen and antibody concentrations in the immunocapture assay to identify the optimal concentration of antigen and antibody that elicits complement activation.
11. For assays employing 45-min incubation times, sterile conditions are not needed, but if incubating longer for other analyses (e.g., cytokine analysis), sterile conditions should be maintained.
12. Plasma supernatant from whole blood incubations can be used for various cytokine analyses by using ELISA or multiplex cytokine assays. For cytokine measurements, whole blood incubations with ICs should be longer, depending on the cytokine of interest (typically, we use 6–24 hours).

13. As shown in Fig. 2, when using healthy donor plasma as a complement source, anti-C3c generated by KKO ICs should be 7–ten-fold higher than buffer alone, heparin alone, PF4 alone, or KKO alone, and 3–six-fold higher than PF4/heparin antigen alone. When using healthy donor whole blood as a complement source, A450nm values are generally half of values seen with healthy donor plasma as a complement source.
14. Background complement activation can be expected with PF4/H antigenic complexes due to non-specific binding by circulating natural IgM in healthy donor plasma/blood [14]. However, C3c generation should be markedly higher with ICs formed by monoclonal anti-PF4/heparin or HIT IgG.
15. For assays of ICs containing human IgG, use human Fc block instead of IVIG, as IVIG contains human IgG that will bind secondary antibodies.
16. For the single color control tubes, the fluorescent antibody should bind to the cell-surface; e.g., B-cells with bound KKO ICs will be positive for CD19, mouse IgG, and C3c, and therefore can serve as single color controls for either anti-CD19, anti-mouse IgG, or anti-C3c).
17. The methods for examining C3c/IC deposition on B-cells can be readily adapted to measuring C3c/IC deposition on other white cells by using cell-specific markers (e.g., CD14 for monocytes, CD3 for T-cells, and CD66b for neutrophils).
18. This assay can also detect cellular activation, as indicated by upregulation of activation markers such as MHC II, CD11b, CD69, and CD86 on B-cells, monocytes, and neutrophils, or tissue factor on monocytes [14]. The incubation time should be adjusted based on the specific activation marker being studied.
19. A two-step sequential staining protocol is necessary to examine the deposition of ICs (IgG) and complement on the cell-surface, as described in Subheading 3.2.2. Secondary antibodies to mouse or human IgG may bind or have cross-reactivity to other primary antibodies (e.g., to anti-C3c or anti-CD19) used for the staining. If interested in only examining complement deposition without the need for staining IgG, or alternatively, if the antibody contributing to IC formation is directly labeled (e.g., KKO-FITC), then cells can be directly stained in one step with a cell-specific marker antibody and appropriate anti-complement antibodies.
20. Use of fluorescently conjugated antigens like PF4 or heparin allows visualization and co-localization of antigen, antibody, and complement on the cells.

21. Healthy donor whole blood incubated with PF4/H/KKO ICs induces significant deposition of complement (C3c) and IgG on B-cells as seen in the dot plots (Fig. 6a) and column graph (Fig. 6b), which may be 30–35-fold higher than buffer alone, heparin alone, or PF4 alone. PF4/heparin induces deposition of complement on B-cells due to non-specific binding of natural IgM in the healthy donor blood [14], but complement deposition is about ten-fold higher in the PF4/H/KKO conditions. The dot plot analysis (Fig. 5a) for PF4/H/KKO conditions shows a rocket shape for C3c and IgG deposition, indicating co-deposition of ICs and complement to the cells.

Acknowledgments

These studies were supported by the National Institutes of Health, National Heart, Lung, and Blood Institute grants R01HL136512 (G.M.A.) and R01HL151730 (G.M.A.), and Department of Defense grant GRANT13955374 (SK).

Conflict of Interest This study was funded by the National Institutes of Health, National Heart, Lung, and Blood Institute [R01HL136512 (G.M.A.) and R01HL151730 (G.M.A.)], National Institute of Allergy and Infectious Diseases [R21-AI175743 (G.M.A)], and Department of Defense [13,955,374 (SK)]. Gowthami Arepally has received a research grant from Sanofi, Novartis, Momenta, and Hikari.

Gowthami Arepally has received consultant fees from Alexion Pharmaceuticals, Inc., a subsidiary of AstraZeneca, and Otsuka Pharmaceutical Factory, Inc., and receives royalties from Biokit.

References

1. Merle NS, Church SE, Fremeaux-Bacchi V, Roumenina LT (2015) Complement system part I - molecular mechanisms of activation and regulation. Front Immunol 6:262. https://doi.org/10.3389/fimmu.2015.00262
2. Theofilopoulos AN, Dixon FJ (1980) Immune complexes in human diseases: a review. Am J Pathol 100:529–594
3. Fust G, Csecsi-Nagy M, Medgyesi GA, Kulics J, Gergely J (1976) Study of the interaction between monoclonal IgM proteins and the complement system. Immunochemistry 13:793–800. https://doi.org/10.1016/0019-2791(76)90178-6
4. Mollnes TE, Jokiranta TS, Truedsson L, Nilsson B, Rodriguez de Cordoba S, Kirschfink M (2007) Complement analysis in the 21st century. Mol Immunol 44:3838–3849. https://doi.org/10.1016/j.molimm.2007.06.150
5. Nydegger UE, Lambert PH, Gerber H, Miescher PA (1974) Circulating immune complexes in the serum in systemic lupus erythematosus and in carriers of hepatitis B antigen. Quantitation by binding to radiolabeled C1q. J Clin Invest 54:297–309. https://doi.org/10.1172/JCI107765
6. Wener MH (2014) Tests for circulating immune complexes. In: Eggleton P, Ward FJ

(eds) Systemic lupus erythematosus: methods and protocols. Springer New York, New York, NY, pp 47–57

7. Theofilopoulos AN, Dixon FJ (1979) The biology and detection of immune complexes. Adv Immunol 28:89–220. https://doi.org/10.1016/s0065-2776(08)60800-7
8. Khandelwal S, Johnson AM, Liu J, Keire D, Sommers C, Ravi J, Lee GM, Lambris JD, Reis ES, Arepally GM (2018) Novel immunoassay for complement activation by PF4/heparin complexes. Thromb Haemost 118: 1484–1487. https://doi.org/10.1055/s-0038-1660858
9. Khandelwal S, Barnes A, Rauova L, Sarkar A, Rux AH, Yarovoi SV, Zaitsev SS, Lambris JD, Myoung SS, Johnson A, Lee GM, Duarte M, Poncz M, Arepally GM, Cines DB (2021) Complement mediates binding and procoagulant effects of ultralarge HIT immune complexes. Blood 138:2106–2116. https://doi.org/10.1182/blood.2020009487
10. Khandelwal S, Lee GM, Hester CG, Poncz M, McKenzie SE, Sachais BS, Rauova L, Kelsoe G, Cines DB, Frank M, Arepally GM (2016) The antigenic complex in HIT binds to B cells via complement and complement receptor 2 (CD21). Blood 128:1789–1799. https://doi.org/10.1182/blood-2016-04-709634
11. Barnes AP, Khandelwal S, Sartoretto S, Myoung S, Francis SJ, Lee GM, Rauova L, Cines DB, Skare JT, Booth CE Jr, Garcia BL, Arepally GM (2022) Minimal role for the alternative pathway in complement activation by HIT immune complexes. J Thromb Haemost 20:2656–2665. https://doi.org/10.1111/jth.15856
12. Khandelwal S, Arepally GM (2016) Immune pathogenesis of heparin-induced thrombocytopenia. Thromb Haemost 116:792–798. https://doi.org/10.1160/TH16-01-0074
13. Arepally GM, Kamei S, Park KS, Kamei K, Li ZQ, Liu W, Siegel DL, Kisiel W, Cines DB, Poncz M (2000) Characterization of a murine monoclonal antibody that mimics heparin-induced thrombocytopenia antibodies. Blood 95:1533–1540
14. Khandelwal S, Ravi J, Rauova L, Johnson A, Lee GM, Gilner JB, Gunti S, Notkins AL, Kuchibhatla M, Frank M, Poncz M, Cines DB, Arepally GM (2018) Polyreactive IgM initiates complement activation by PF4/heparin complexes through the classical pathway. Blood 132:2431–2440. https://doi.org/10.1182/blood-2018-03-834598

Chapter 11

Cloning of Antibodies from Patients with Heparin-Induced Thrombocytopenia

Lu Zhou, Nathan D. Witman, Wen Zhu, Demin Wang, and Renren Wen

Abstract

We discuss two antibody cloning protocols—single B-cell culture (Nojima culture) and single B-cell expression cloning—to isolate antibodies associated with heparin-induced thrombocytopenia (HIT) from patients displaying clinical manifestations of the condition. The objective of the antibody cloning study is to provide valuable insights into the molecular mechanisms underlying the B-cell response and antibody-mediated pathogenesis in HIT, aiming to improve the diagnosis and management of this condition.

Key words Antibody, Cloning, Recombinant, B-cells, Heparin-induced thrombocytopenia, Nojima culture, Single B-cell expression cloning

1 Introduction

Recent technological advancements in producing antigen-specific monoclonal antibodies from human B-cells have significantly enhanced the isolation and characterization of human antibodies that respond to self-antigens or pathogens. This progress has contributed substantially to developing antibody-based therapies and facilitated a deeper mechanistic understanding of immune responses in human diseases [1]. Common methods for isolating human monoclonal antibodies include (1) combinatorial display libraries, (2) single B-cell expression cloning, (3) memory B-cell immortalization, (4) single B-cell culture, and (5) immunization of human immunoglobulin transgenic mice [2]. This chapter describes our methods using a single B-cell culture approach (specifically, the Nojima culture) and single B-cell expression cloning (Fig. 1) to clone heparin-induced thrombocytopenia (HIT)-associated antibodies from patients experiencing clinical manifestations of HIT.

Sean R. Stowell and Connie M. Arthur (eds.), *Methods in Transfusion Medicine*, Methods in Molecular Biology, vol. 3053, https://doi.org/10.1007/978-1-0716-5376-0_11,

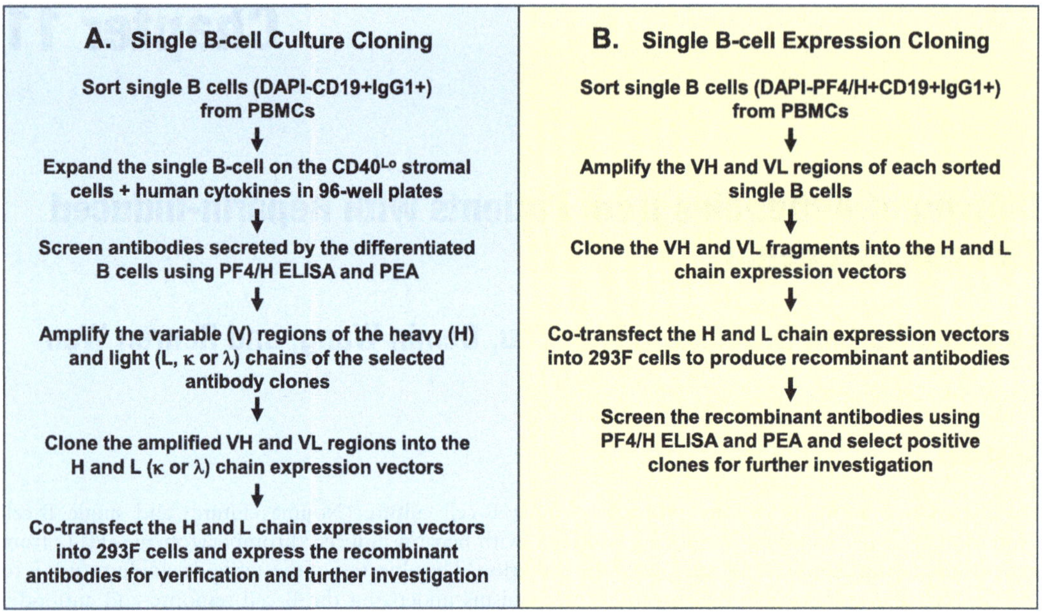

Fig. 1 Flowcharts of (**a**) single B-cell culture cloning and (**b**) single B-cell expression cloning methods

HIT is the most common drug-induced thrombocytopenia, frequently linked with severe arterial or venous thrombosis and thromboembolism [3, 4]. HIT affects approximately 1 in 1500 hospitalized patients who receive heparin in the US, with an increased incidence following major surgery and administration of unfractionated heparin [5–7].

HIT is characterized by the development of IgG antibodies (primarily IgG1) specific to the platelet chemokine platelet factor 4 (PF4) when it binds to heparin (PF4/H) or other anionic substances [8, 9]. However, not all patients with antibodies reactive to PF4/H complexes in solid-phase binding assays experience HIT [10–12]. Functional assays that detect antibodies capable of inducing platelet activation, such as the serotonin release assay [7, 13–16] or P-selectin expression assay (PEA) [17–19], are more specific for HIT diagnosis. However, these platelet functional tests, requiring intact and functional platelets, are time-consuming and limit their usefulness for timely treatment decisions. Consequently, initiating treatment for HIT is often based primarily on clinical 4Ts scores or antibody binding results without the benefit of platelet functional assays [20]. Failure to diagnose HIT in an affected patient poses a significant risk of catastrophic thrombosis [21]. Conversely, an erroneous diagnosis of HIT can prolong hospital stays, increase costs, and needlessly expose a patient to treatments with serious side effects.

Characterizing the molecular properties that distinguish "pathogenic" antibodies from seemingly non-pathogenic ones that recognize PF4/H complexes but fail to activate platelets would enhance our understanding of HIT pathogenesis and potentially lead to improved diagnostic tests and management of this condition. Therefore, we cloned PF4/H-reactive IgG1 antibodies from HIT patients, generated recombinant antibodies from these clones, and characterized their functional and molecular properties. We identified specific sequence motifs in the heavy chain complementarity-determining region 3 that distinguish "pathogenic" (platelet-activating) antibodies from non-activating, presumably non-pathogenic ones and suggest possible new approaches to the diagnosis and treatment of HIT [22].

We modified protocols for single B-cell expression cloning [23, 24] and Nojima culture cloning methods [25, 26] reported previously to clone antibodies associated with HIT [22]. The single B-cell expression cloning protocol enables the cloning of antibodies from both antigen-specific memory B-cells and plasmablasts actively producing antibodies. In contrast, the Nojima culture cloning protocol only permits cloning from memory B-cells. However, the single B-cell expression cloning protocol is more technically challenging and laborious, and it requires more B-cells than the Nojima culture protocol. Therefore, our study used the Nojima culture cloning protocol to clone most antibodies identified in HIT patients [22].

2 Materials

2.1 Nojima Culture Cloning Protocol

2.1.1 MS-40L^{lo} Cell Preparation

1. MS-40L^{lo} cells.
2. Iscove's Modification of DMEM (IMDM) (Corning, 10016CV).
3. Fetal Bovine Serum (FBS) (HyClone, SH30070.03).
4. 100X Penicillin Streptomycin Solution (Corning, 30002CI), Tissue culture dish (TPP Techno Plastic Products, 93100).
5. 2-Mercaptoethanol (2-ME) (Sigma Aldrich, M3148).
6. Phosphate buffered saline (PBS) (Corning, 21040CV).
7. 0.05% Trypsin-EDTA (Corning, 25052CI).

2.1.2 Single B-Cell Sorting

1. RPMI-1640, [+] L-Glutamine (Corning, 10040CV).
2. Fetal Bovine Serum (FBS) (Hyclone, SH30070.03).
3. HEPES Buffer (Corning, 2506CI).
4. Sodium Pyruvate (Corning, 25000CI).
5. MEM nonessential amino acid (Corning, 25025CI).
6. 2-Mercaptoethanol (2-ME) (Sigma Aldrich, M3148).
7. 100X Penicillin Streptomycin Solution (Corning, 30002CI).

8. APC-anti-human CD19 Antibody (Biolegend, 302212).
9. PE-anti-human IgG1 antibody (SouthernBiotech, 9054-09).
10. 4′,6-Diamidino-2-Phenylindole, Dihydrochloride (DAPI) (Invitrogen, D1306).
11. Fluorescence activated cell sorter- BD FACSAria™ III Cell Sorter.

2.1.3 Nojima Culture

1. Phosphate buffered saline (PBS) (Corning, 21040CV).
2. 0.05% Trypsin-EDTA (Corning, 25052CI).
3. Iscove's Modification of DMEM (IMDM) (Corning, 10016CV).
4. Fetal Bovine Serum (FBS) (HyClone, SH30070.03).
5. 100X Penicillin Streptomycin Solution (Corning, 30002CI).
6. 2-Mercaptoethanol (2-ME) (Sigma Aldrich, M3148).
7. Tissue culture dish (TPP Techno Plastic Products, 93100).
8. RPMl-1640, [+] L-Glutamine (Corning, 10040CV).
9. HEPES Buffer (Corning, 25060CI).
10. Sodium Pyruvate (Corning, 25000CI).
11. MEM nonessential amino acid (Corning, 25025CI).
12. Recombinant human IL-2 (PeproTech, 20002).
13. Recombinant Human IL-4 (PeproTech, 20004).
14. Recombinant Human IL-21 (PeproTech, 20021).
15. Recombinant Human BAFF (PeproTech, 31013).
16. Sodium azide (Sigma Aldrich, S2002).
17. TRIzol Reagent (Invitrogen, 15596018).

2.1.4 Screening for the Antibody Function

IgG Enzyme-Linked Immunosorbent Assay (ELISA)

1. Goat anti-human IgG (Southern Biotech, 204001).
2. Phosphate buffered saline (PBS) (Corning, 21040CV)96.
3. 96-well ELISA plate (Thermo Scientific, 442404).
4. Polysorbate 20 (Tween 20) (Fisher Bioreagents, BP337500).
5. Bovine serum albumin (BSA) (Sigma Aldrich, A9647).
6. Goat-anti-human IgG-HRP (Southern Biotech, 204005).
7. KPL Peroxidase Substrate Solution B (Sera Care, 51200038).
8. KPL TMB Peroxidase Substrate (Sera Care, 51200049).
9. Sulfuric acid (Sigma Aldrich, 339741).

PF4/H ELISA

1. Recombinant Human CXCL4/PF-4 (Protein Foundry, LN00366).
2. Heparin sodium salt from porcine intestinal mucosa (Sigma Aldrich, H3393).

3. Phosphate buffered saline (PBS) (Corning, 21040CV).
4. Polysorbate 20 (Tween 20) (Fisher Bioreagents, BP337500).
5. Bovine serum albumin (BSA) (Sigma Aldrich, A9647).
6. Goat-anti-human IgG-HRP (Southern Biotech, 204005).
7. KPL Peroxidase Substrate Solution B (Sera Care, 51200038).
8. KPL TMB Peroxidase Substrate (Sera Care, 51200049).
9. 96-well ELISA plate (Thermo Scientific, 442404).
10. Sulfuric acid (Sigma Aldrich, 339741).

P-Selectin Expression Assay (PEA)

1. Platelet-rich plasma (PRP, ordered from Versiti Biomaterials).
2. Prostaglandin E1(PGE1) (Sigma Aldrich, A5515).
3. Phosphate buffered saline (PBS) (Corning, 21040CV).
4. Bovine serum albumin (BSA) (Sigma Aldrich, A9647).
5. Recombinant Human CXCL4/PF-4 (Protein Foundry, LN00366).
6. Heparin sodium salt from porcine intestinal mucosa (Sigma Aldrich, H3393).
7. Anti-CD32B (Clone IV.3, FcgRIIa-blocking monoclonal antibody, manufactured at the Versiti Blood Research Institute).
8. PE-conjugated Anti-Hu/Mo CD62P (Invitrogen, 12062682).
9. Alexafluor647-conjugated anti-CD41b (Clone MBC290.5, manufactured at the Versiti Blood Research Institute).

2.1.5 Production of Recombinant Antibodies from the Nojima Culture

PCR Amplification of the Variable Regions of the Heavy (VH) and Light (VL) Chains of the Antibodies [25]

1. TRIzol Reagent (Invitrogen, 15596018).
2. RNase-free water (ThermoFisher, AM9906).
3. Maxima Enzyme Mix (Thermo Scientific, K1641).
4. 5x Reaction Mix (Thermo Scientific, K1641).
5. 2x DreamTaq Green MasterMix (Thermo Scientific™, K1081).

Cloning of VH and VL Regions into the Expression Vectors

1. The NCBI GenBank accession numbers for the heavy (H) chain, k light chain, and l light chain expression vectors are FJ475055, FJ475056, and FJ517647, respectively. They are available upon request.
2. 10x FastDigest buffer (Thermo Scientific™, B64).
3. FastDigest SalI (Thermo Scientific™, FD0644).
4. FastDigest Pfl23II (Thermo Scientific™, FD0854).
5. FastDigest XhoI (Thermo Scientific™, FD0694).

6. FastDigest BshTI (Thermo Scientific™, FD1464).
7. Ambion™ Nuclease-Free Water (Life Technologies, AM9937).
8. FastAP Thermosensitive Alkaline Phosphatase (Thermo Scientific™, EF0654).
9. QIAquick Gel Extraction Kit (50) (QIAGEN, 28704).
10. NEBuilder 2x Mastermix (New England Biolabs, E2621L).

Transformation and Plasmid Purification

1. NEB 5-alpha Competent E. coli cells (New England Biolabs, C2987H).
2. SOC medium (New England Biolabs, B9020S).
3. Miniprep kit (QIAGEN, 27104).
4. Ampicillin (Sigma Aldrich).

Antibody Production and Purification

1. Expi293 ExpressionTM Medium (Gibco, A1435101).
2. 100X Penicillin Streptomycin Solution (Corning, 30002CI).
3. ExpiFectamineTM 293 Transfection Kit (Gibco, A14525).
4. Opti-MEM™ I Reduced Serum Medium (Gibco, 31985070).
5. Sodium azide (Sigma Aldrich, S2002).
6. Protein A beads (Cytiva MabSelect SureTM, 17543801).
7. Chromatography spin column (Bio-Rad Micro Bio-Spin Chromatography column, 732-6204).

2.2 Single B-Cell Expression Cloning

Materials in addition to those already listed for cell sorting in Subheading 2.1:

2.2.1 Single B-Cell Sorting

1. BV510 anti-human CD3 antibody (BD Bioscience, 563109).
2. FITC labeled heparin (H-FITC) (ThermoFisher, H7482).
3. 96-well PCR plate (USA Scientific, 1402-9500).
4. Recombinant Human CXCL4/PF-4 (Protein Foundry, LN00366).
5. RNase-free water (ThermoFisher, AM9906).
6. 1 M Tris pH 8.0 (ThermoFisher, AM9855G).
7. RNasin (Promega, N2615).
8. RNase-free sealing tape (Sigma, TMO232698).

2.2.2 Single B-Cell RT-PCR and Antibody Cloning

1. IGEPAL (Sigma, I8896).
2. RNasin (Promega, N2615).
3. One-step RT-PCR kit (Qiagen, 210212).
4. RNase-free water (ThermoFisher, AM9906).

5. DNA-OFF cleaning solution (Fisher Scientific, MP11QD0500).
6. DreamTaq Green Master Mix 2X (ThermoFisher, K1081).
7. Exo-CIP™ Rapid PCR Cleanup Kit (NEB Lab, E1050L).

3 Methods

3.1 Nojima Culture Cloning Protocol

3.1.1 MS-40L^{lo} Cell Preparation [27]

1. Prepare MS-40^{lo} cells from cryopreserved stock.
2. Pre-warm MS-40L^{lo} culture medium (IMDM supplemented with 10% FBS, 1% Pen Strep, and 55 mM 2-ME) to 37 °C.
3. Thaw frozen MS-40L^{lo} cells at 37 °C in a water bath. Once thawed, transfer the cell suspension dropwise into a 15 mL tube containing 9 mL of pre-warmed culture medium. Mix gently.
4. Count the cells and centrifuge at 150× *g* for 5 min.
5. Discard the supernatants and resuspend the cells in pre-warmed culture medium to a final concentration of 1×10^6/mL. Mix thoroughly.
6. Plate 0.5–1 × 10^6 cells in 10 mL culture medium in a 10 cm tissue culture dish. Incubate at 37 °C in a CO_2 incubator for 2–3 days.
7. After 3 days of incubation, carefully aspirate the culture supernatants and gently wash the cells by adding 10 mL of pre-warmed PBS.
8. Remove the PBS, then add 3 mL of 0.05% Trypsin-EDTA. Incubate for 3 min at 37 °C in a CO_2 incubator to detach cells.
9. Add 7 of mL pre-warmed culture medium to neutralize the trypsin-EDTA and transfer the cell suspension into a 15 mL centrifuge tube.
10. Count the cells and centrifuge at 150× *g* for 5 min.
11. Discard the supernatant and resuspend the pellet in pre-warmed culture media to a final concentration of 1×10^6/mL. Mix thoroughly.
12. Plate 1×10^6 cells in 10 mL culture medium into a 10 cm dish. Incubate at 37 °C in a CO_2 incubator for 2–3 days.
13. Repeat Steps 1–3 to maintain the MS-40^{lo} cell line.

3.1.2 Single B-Cell Sorting

1. Warm the B-cell culture medium (BCM: RPMI-1640 supplemented with 10% FBS, 55 μM 2-ME, 1% Pen Strep, 10 mM HEPES, 1 mM Sodium Pyruvate, and 1% MEM nonessential amino acid) to 37 °C.

2. Thaw a vial of cryopreserved peripheral blood mononuclear cells (PBMCs) from a HIT patient at 37 °C using a water bath and transfer the cells to a 15 mL tube containing 9 mL of pre-warmed culture medium, adding slowly dropwise while mixing thoroughly.
3. Count the cells and centrifuge at 1200 rpm for 5 min.
4. Remove the supernatant and stain the cells ($<2x10^7$ cells/mL) in a mixture of fluorescently labeled antibodies, including APC-anti-CD19 (50 μg/mL) and PE-anti-IgG1 (0.5 mg/mL), both diluted at 1:200. Incubate the cells for 30 min at 4 °C in the dark.
5. Wash the cells by adding 2–3 volumes of BCM and centrifuging at 1200 rpm for 5 min. Carefully remove the supernatant without disturbing the cell pellet.
6. Resuspend the cells in BCM to achieve 5–10 × 10^6 cells/mL. Add DAPI at a 1:5000 dilution.
7. Sort $DAPI^-CD19^+IgG1^+$ cells for a Nojima culture using the BD FACSAria™ III Cell Sorter (see the next Subheading 3.1.3).

3.1.3 Nojima Culture [25, 26]

Day—1

1. The MS-$40L^{lo}$ cells that have been passaged 1–2 times after thawing are used as feeder cells for Nojima culture.
2. Prepare the MS-$40L^{lo}$ cells as described in the "MS-$40L^{lo}$ cell preparation" method. Resuspend the cells at 3 × 10^4/mL in BCM and add 100 μL/well into 96-well plate.
3. Incubate the plates at 37 °C overnight in a CO_2 incubator.

Day 0

1. Warm BCM to 37 °C and use it to prepare a 2x recombinant human cytokine mixture with 80 U/mL IL-2 and 20 ng/mL each of IL-4, IL-21, and BAFF.
2. Add 100 μL/well of the cytokine mixture to each well of the 96-well plate seeded with MS-$40L^{lo}$ cells on Day—1.
3. Sort a single $DAPI^-CD19^+IgG1^+$ B-cell into each well of the 96-well plate containing the prepared MS-$40L^{lo}$ cells.
4. Culture the single B-cell at 37 °C in a CO_2 incubator.

Days 4 and 8

1. Warm BCM to 37 °C and prepare a 1x recombinant human cytokine mixture containing 40 U/mL IL-2 and 10 ng/mL each of IL-4, IL-21, and BAFF.
2. Replace 100 μL of culture media with 100 μL of the fresh 1x recombinant human cytokine mixture (*see* **Note 1**).
3. Place the culture plates back in the CO_2 incubator.

Day 12

1. Warm BCM to 37 °C and prepare a 1x recombinant human cytokine mixture.
2. Replace 100 μL of culture media with 200 μL of the 1x recombinant human cytokine mixture.
3. Place the culture plates back in the CO_2 incubator.

Days 15, 18, and 21

1. Warm BCM to 37 °C and prepare a 1x recombinant human cytokine mixture.
2. Replace 200 μL of culture media with 200 μL of the fresh 1x recombinant human cytokine mixture.
3. Place the culture plates back in the CO_2 incubator.

Day 25

1. Harvest all culture supernatants into new 96-well plate using a fresh pipette tip for each well to avoid cross-contamination.
2. Add 2.5 mL of 10% sodium azide (final concentration ~ 0.1%) into each well and store the plates at 4 °C for immediate use within 1 week or at −20 °C for longer storage.
3. After harvesting the culture supernatant, add 200 mL of TRIzol Reagent to each well of the B-cells left at the bottom of the culture plates.
4. Store the plates at −80 °C for subsequent amplification of the VH and VL regions of the antibodies.

3.1.4 *Antibody Screening*

IgG ELISA

1. Plate 50 mL goat anti-human IgG (1 mg/mL), diluted at 1: 5000 in PBS, overnight in each well of a 96-well ELISA plate with gentle shaking at room temperature.
2. Bring all reagents and samples to room temperature (18–25 °C) before use (*see* **Note 2**).
3. Discard the solution and wash each well three times with 200 mL PBS containing 0.1% Tween. Ensure thorough removal of liquid at each step. After the last wash, remove any remaining wash buffer by inverting the plate and blotting it against clean paper towels.
4. Incubate the plate for 2 h with 200 mL PBS containing 0.1% Tween and 3% BSA with gentle shaking.
5. Discard the solution and add 50 mL of supernatant collected on Day 25 of the B-cell culture. Cover wells and incubate for 1 h at room temperature with gentle shaking.
6. Discard the solution. Repeat the washing procedures as in **step 3**.

7. Add 50 μL of HRP-goat-anti-human IgG (0.5 mg/mL), diluted at 1:5000 in PBS with 0.1% Tween and 3% BSA, to each well. Cover wells and incubate for 45 min at room temperature with gentle shaking.
8. Discard the solution. Repeat the washing procedures as in **step 3**.
9. Add 100 μL per well of TMBZ (A + B) (KPL) by mixing solution A (TMB Peroxidase Substrate) and solution B (Peroxidase Substrate Solution B) at a 1:1 ratio. Cover wells and incubate for 30 min at room temperature in the dark.
10. Add 50 μL of Stop Solution (1 N H_2SO_4) to each well. Read absorbance at 450 nm immediately.

PF4/H ELISA

1. Plate 50 mL of PBS containing 10 mg/mL PF4 and 0.4 U/mL heparin into each well of a 96-well ELISA plate and incubate overnight at room temperature with gentle shaking.
2. Follow the Steps 2–10 described in the IgG ELISA method.

PEA [28]

1. Bring all reagents and samples to room temperature (18–25 ° C) before use.
2. Add 10 μL PGE1 (50 ng/mL) into 10 mL platelet-rich plasma (PRP) and incubate at room temperature for 15 min.
3. Centrifuge 10 mL PRP at 150× *g* for 15 min without braking.
4. Collect the top 3 mL of PRP into a new tube and centrifuge at 1000× *g* for 15 min with a break.
5. Remove supernatant and resuspend platelets in 600 μL PBS containing 1% BSA.
6. Count platelets using a cell counter.
7. Dilute platelets to a final concentration of 200,000/μL with PBS containing 1% BSA.
8. Incubate platelets (100,000/μL) with 150 μg/mL PF4 at room temperature for 20 min.
9. Add 10 μL of the platelet and PF4 mixture into 40 μL of the culture supernatant collected on Day 25 of the B-cell culture and incubate at room temperature for 1 h.
10. Add 10 μL of a staining mix containing pre-diluted (1:200) PE-conjugated anti-CD62P (0.2 mg/mL) and Alexafluor647-conjugated anti-CD41b (0.2 mg/mL) antibody in PBS containing 1% BSA.
11. Incubate for 20 min at room temperature in the dark.
12. After 20 min of incubation, add 200 μL of PBS containing 1% BSA, followed by flow cytometry analysis.

3.1.5 Production of Recombinant Antibodies

PCR Amplification of the VH and VL of the Antibodies

1. Extract total RNA from the selected cryopreserved B-cells stored in TRIzol Reagent according to the manufacturer's recommendation.
2. Synthesize cDNA using Maxima Enzyme Mix according to the manufacturer's recommendation.
3. Prepare separately VH, Vk, and Vl primer mixes containing 10 μM of each primer to amplify VH, Vk, and Vl regions:

   VH primer mix: 10 μM of each VH and JH primers.
   Vk primer mix: 10 μM of each Vk and Jk primers.
   Vl primer mix: 10 μM of each of Vl and Cl primers (*see* **Note 3**).
4. For each PCR reaction, add the following into a sterile, RNase-free PCR tube on ice:

   Nuclease-free H_2O, 7.5 μL.
   2x DreamTaq Green MasterMix, 12.5 μL.
   Chain-specific primer mix, 2.5 μL.
   0.02–2 mg/mL cDNA, 2.5 μL.
5. PCR program:
   - Initial denaturation, 94 °C for 4 min.
   - Cycling reactions (40 cycles):

     Denaturation, 94 °C for 30 s.
     Annealing, 58 °C for 30 s.
     Extension, 72 °C for 45 s.
     Final extension, 72 °C for 8 min.
   - Hold at 4 °C.
6. Run 2 μL of PCR product on a 1% agarose gel to confirm a successful reaction and to check for contamination in the negative control wells. PCR bands should be around 350–450 bps, depending on the chain length.

Cloning of the VH and VL Regions into the Expression Vectors Using Gibson Assembly

1. Linearization of the H, k, and l chain expression vectors for cloning:
   - Make the reaction mix to linearize the expression vectors:

     10x FastDigest buffer, 5 μL.
     Chain-specific restriction enzyme, 2.5 μL (SalI for H chain, Pfl23II/BsiWI for k chain, and XhoI for l chain).
     Common restriction enzyme, 2.5 μL of BshTI/AgeI.
     H, k, or l chain expression plasmid, 5 μg.
     Add nuclease-free water to reach a final volume of 50 μL.
   - Incubate the reaction at 37 °C for 15 min.
   - Add 2.5 μL FastAP and incubate at 37 °C for 10 min.
   - Heat-inactivate at 80 °C for 10 min.

- Run the linearized vectors on a 1.2% agarose gel (100 V for 5 min, then 75 V for 75 min) and cut them from the gel.
- Extract the linearized vectors using a gel extraction kit following the manufacturer's recommendation, and elute the DNA with 40 μL elution buffer.
- Quantify the linearized plasmids by Nanodrop.

2. Gibson assembly reaction mix.

   NEBuilder 2x Mastermix, 5 μL.
   Linearized expression vector (H, k, or l chain), 25 ng.
   PCR product (VH, Vk, or Vl), 1 μL.
   Add nuclease-free water to adjust the total volume to 10 μL.

3. Incubate the reaction in the PCR machine at 50 °C for 1 h. The assembled product can be stored at −20 °C.

Transformation and Plasmid Purification

1. NEB 5-alpha competent E. coli were used for bacterial transformation with the expression plasmid using the High Efficiency Transformation Protocol with ampicillin.
2. Pick three colonies for each transfection for further culture.
3. Purify the plasmid using the QIAGEN miniprep kit following the manufacturer's recommendation.
4. Sequence the plasmid DNA using the SP6 primer to verify the VH, Vk, or Vl sequences (SP6: ATTTAGGTGACACTATAG).

Antibody Production and Purification

1. The Expi293F™ cells used for recombinant antibody production were cultured in Expi293™ Expression Medium supplemented with 1% Pen Strep at 37 °C according to the manufacturer's recommendation.
2. The ExpiFectamine™ 293 Transfection kit was used for cell transfection and antibody production according to the manufacturer's protocol.
3. Protein A beads were used for antibody purification from the culture supernatant, following the manufacturer's instructions (Table 1).

3.2 Single B-Cell Expression Cloning Protocol

3.2.1 Single B-Cell Sorting

Preparation of PBMCs

1. The procedures for thawing PBMCs are the same as described in Method 1.
2. Stain the cells ($<2 \times 10^7$ cells/mL) in a mixture of fluorescently labeled antibodies, including APC-anti-CD19, BV510-anti-human CD3, and PE-anti-IgG1, diluted at 1:200 and PF4/H-FITC complexes. Incubate the cells for 30 min at 4 °C in the dark (*see* **Note 4**).
3. The procedures for preparation of cells for sorting after staining are the same as described in Method 1.

Table 1
PCR primers for the cloning steps in both the Nojima culture cloning and single B-cell expression cloning methods

VH cloning primers	
VH1/5/7	ATCCTTTTTCTAGTA GCAACTGCAACCGGTGTACAT TCCGAGGTGCAGCTGGTGCAG
VH3	ATCCTTTTTCTAGTAGCAACTGCAACCGGTGTACATTCTGAGGTGCAGC TGGTGGAG
VH3-23	ATCCTTTTTCTAGTAGCAACTGCAACCGGTGTACATTCTGAGGTGCAGC TGTTGGAG
VH4	ATCCTTTTTCTAGTAGCAACTGCAACCGGTGTACATTCCCAGGTGCAGC TGCAGGAG
VH4-34	ATCCTTTTTCTAGTAGCAACTGCAACCGGTGTACATTCCCAGGTGCAGC TACAGCAGTG
VH3-9/30/33	ATCCTTTTTCTAGTAGCAACTGCAACCGGTGTACATTCTGAAGTGCAGC TGGTGGAG
VH6-1	ATCCTTTTTCTAGTAGCAACTGCAACCGGTGTACATTCCCAGGTACAGC TGCAGCAG
JH1/2	GGAAGACCGATGGGCCCTTGGTCGACGCCTGAGGAGACGGTGACCAG
JH4/5	GGAAGACCGATGGGCCCTTGGTCGACGCTGAGGAGACGGTGACCAG
JH3	GGAAGACCGATGGGCCCTTGGTCGACGCTGAAGAGACGGTGACCATTG
JH6	GGAAGACCGATGGGCCCTTGGTCGACGCTGAGGAGACGGTGACCGTG

Vk cloning primers	
Vk1	ATCCTTTTTCTAGTAGCAACTGCAACCGGTGTACATTCTGACATCCAGA TGACCCAGTC
Vk1-9/1-13	ATCCTTTTTCTAGTAGCAACTGCAACCGGTGTACATTCAGACATCCAG TTGACCCAGTCT
Vk1D-43/1-8	ATCCTTTTTCTAGTAGCAACTGCAACCGGTGTACATTGTGCCATCCGGA TGACCCAGTC
Vk2	ATCCTTTTTCTAGTAGCAACTGCAACCGGTGTACATGGGGATATTGTGA TGACCCAGAC
Vk2-28/2-30	ATCCTTTTTCTAGTAGCAACTGCAACCGGTGTACATGGGGATATTGTGA TGACTCAGTC
Vk3-11/3D-11	ATCCTTTTTCTAGTAGCAACTGCAACCGGTGTACATTCAGAAATTGTG TTGACACAGTC
Vk3-15/3D-15	ATCCTTTTTCTAGTAGCAACTGCAACCGGTGTACATTCAGAAATAGTGA TGACGCAGTC
Vk3-20/3D-20	ATCCTTTTTCTAGTAGCAACTGCAACCGGTGTACATTCAGAAATTGTG TTGACGCAGTCT

(continued)

Table 1 (continued)

Vk cloning primers	
Vk4–1	ATCCTTTTTCTAGTAGCAACTGCAACCGGTGTACATTCGGACATCGTGA TGACCCAGTC
Jk1/2/4	AAGACAGATGGTGCAGCCACCGTACGTTTGATYTCCACCTTGGTC
Jk3	AAGACAGATGGTGCAGCCACCGTACGTTTGATATCCACTTTGGTC
Jk5	AAGACAGATGGTGCAGCCACCGTACGTTTAATCTCCAGTCGTGTC

Vl cloning primers	
Vl1	ATCCTTTTTCTAGTAGCAACTGCAACCGGTTCCTGGGCCCAGTCTGTGC TGACKCAG
Vl2	ATCCTTTTTCTAGTAGCAACTGCAACCGGTTCCTGGGCCCAGTCTGCCCTGAC TCAG
Vl3	ATCCTTTTTCTAGTAGCAACTGCAACCGGTTCTGTGACCTCCTATGAGCTGAC WCAG
Vl4/5	ATCCTTTTTCTAGTAGCAACTGCAACCGGTTCTCTCTCSCAGCYTGTGCTGACTCA
Vl6	ATCCTTTTTCTAGTAGCAACTGCAACCGGTTCTTGGGCCAATTTTATGCTGACTCAG
Vl7/8	ATCCTTTTTCTAGTAGCAACTGCAACCGGTTCCAATTCYCAGRCTGTGGTGACYCAG
Cl	TGTTGGCTTGAAGCTCCTCACTCGAGGGYGGGAACAGAGTG

Sorting Single B-Cells

1. During cell staining, make a fresh catch buffer. Each 10 μL catch buffer contains 9.65 μL RNase-free water, 0.1 μL 1 M pH 8.0 Tris–HCl, and 0.25 μL RNasin.
2. Use a multi-channel pipette to add 10 mL catch buffer to each well of the 96-well PCR plate. Perform the procedures in an RNase-free hood and seal the plates with RNase-free sealing tape.
3. Single live PF4/H-binding IgG1$^+$ B-cells (-DAPI$^-$CD3$^-$CD19$^+$IgG1$^+$PF4/H$^+$) were sorted by BD FACSAria™ III Cell Sorter into 96-well plate containing catch buffer. Seal the plates with RNase-free sealing tape.
4. Store the plates at −80 °C immediately after sorting.

3.2.2 Single B-Cell RT-PCR and Antibody Cloning

First PCR (One-Step RT-PCR)

1. Make a 5′ and 3′ primer mix with 200 nM of each primer for the first PCR to separately amplify VH, Vk, and Vl regions. The final concentration of each primer in each reaction is 20 nM. Refer to Table 2 for the sequences of the first PCR primers.

Table 2
Primers for the first and second PCRs were used in the single B-cell expression cloning

VH primers for the first PCR	
5′ L-VH 1	ACAGGTGCCCACTCCCAGGTGCAG
5′ L-VH 2	ACAGGGGTCTTGTCCCAGRTCACC
5′ L-VH 3	AAGGTGTCCAGTGTGARGTGCAG
5′ L-VH 4/6	CCCAGATGGGTCCTGTCCCAGGTGCAG
5′ L-VH 5	CAAGGAGTCTGTTCCGAGGTGCAG
3′ HuIgG-const	TCTTGTCCACCTTGGTGTTGCT

Vk primers for the first PCR	
5′ L Vk 1/2	ATGAGGSTCCCYGCTCAGCTGCTGG
5′ L Vk 3	CTCTTCCTCCTGCTACTCTGGCTCCCAG
5′ L Vk 4	ATTTCTCTGTTGCTCTGGATCTCTG
3′ Ck 543–566	GTTTCTCGTAGTCTGCTTTGCTCA

Vl primers for the first PCR	
5′ L Vl 1	GGTCCTGGGCCCAGTCTGTGCTG
5′ L Vl 2	GGTCCTGGGCCCAGTCTGCCCTG
5′ L Vl 3	GCTCTGTGACCTCCTATGAGCTG
5′ L Vl 4/5/9	GGTCTCTCTCSCAGCYTGTGCTG
5′ L Vl 6	GTTCTTGGGCCAATTTTATGCTG
5′ L Vl 7	GGTCCAATTCYCAGGCTGTGGTG
5′ L Vl 8	GAGTGGATTCTCAGACTGTGGTG
3′ Cl	CACCAGTGTGGCCTTGTTGGCTTG

VH primers for the second PCR	
5′ VH3a-sense	SARGTGCAGCTGGTGGAG
5′ VH3b-sense	GAGGTGCAGCTGTTGGAG
5′ VH1/5/7-sense	CTGCAACCGGTGTACATTCCGAGGTGCAGCTGGTGCAG
5′ VH4-sense	CTGCAACCGGTGTACATTCCCAGGTGCAGCTGCAGGAG
3′ Cgamma (IgG)	AGTAGTCCTTGACCAGGCAGCCCAG

(continued)

Table 2
(continued)

Vk primers for the second PCR	
5′ Pan Vk	ATGACCCAGWCTCCABYCWCCCTG
3′ Ck 494–516	GTGCTGTCCTTGCTGTCCTGCT

Vl primers for the second PCR	
5′ AgeI Vl1	CTGCTACCGGTTCCTGGGCCCAGTCTGTGCTGACKCAG
5′ AgeI Vl2	CTGCTACCGGTTCCTGGGCCCAGTCTGCCCTGACTCAG
5′ AgeI Vl3	CTGCTACCGGTTCTGTGACCTCCTATGAGCTGACWCAG
5′ AgeI Vl4/5	CTGCTACCGGTTCTCTCTCSCAGCYTGTGCTGACTCA
5′ AgeI Vl6	CTGCTACCGGTTCTTGGGCCAATTTTATGCTGACTCAG
5′ AgeI Vl7/8	CTGCTACCGGTTCCAATTCYCAGRCTGTGGTGACYCAG
3′ XhoI Cl	CTCCTCACTCGAGGGYGGGAACAGAGTG

2. Make a master mix for the one-step RT-PCR to separately amplify VH, Vk, and Vl regions. Each 14 μL master mix contains:

   Nuclease-free water, 3 μL.
   5x Qiagen One-Step RT-PCR buffer, 5 μL.
   10 mM dNTPs, 1 μL.
   0.5% IGEPAL, 1.5 μL.
   RNasin, 0.1 μL.
   Qiagen one-step RT Enzyme Mix, 1 μL.
   First PCR primer mix, 2.5 μL.

3. Thaw the plates containing the sorted single B-cells from −80 °C on ice and add 14 μL of the master mix to each well for one-step RT-PCR, so the total volume in each well is around 25 μL.

4. The One-step RT-PCR program:
   - RT reaction, 50 °C for 30 min.
   - Initial denaturation, 94 °C for 15 min.
   - Cycling reactions (50 cycles):

     Denaturation, 94 °C for 20 s.
     Annealing, 55 °C for 30 s.
     Extension, 72 °C for 60 s.
   - Keep at 4 °C.

   The plates can be stored at −20 °C after the reaction (*see* **Note 5**).

Second PCR

1. Make a 5′ and 3′ primer mix with 3.8 μM of each primer for the second PCR to separately amplify VH, Vk, and Vl regions. The final concentration of each primer in the reaction is 380 nM. Refer to the primer tables below for the sequences of the second PCR primers.
2. Make a master mix for the second PCR to amplify VH, Vk, and Vl regions individually.

   2X DreamTaq Green MasterMix, 12.5 μL.
   5′ and 3′ primer mix, 2.5 μL.
   Nuclease-free water to 7.5 μL.
   The first PCR product for VH, Vk, or Vl is 2.5 μL.
3. Run the second PCR program. Plates can be stored at 4 °C.
   - Initial denaturation, 94 °C for 4 min.
   - Cycling reactions (50 cycles):

     Denaturation, 94 °C for 30 s.
     Annealing, 57 °C for 30 s.
     Extension, 72 °C for 45 s.
     Final extension, 72 °C for 10 min.
   - Keep at 4 °C.
4. Run 2 μL of product on a 1.2% agarose gel (130 V, 25 min). Successful reactions are identified by a band at approximately 400 bp. Generate a list of wells that have a heavy chain amplicon and at least one light chain amplicon. Only antibodies with both VH and VL regions amplified will be cloned (*see* **Note 6**).
5. Clean 5 μL of the PCR products for sequencing.
   - PCR cleanup reaction contains:

     dH2O 0.7 μL.
     NEB buffer 0.7 μL.
     CIP (10 units/ul) 0.1 μL.
     ExoI 0.5 μL.
     Second PCR product: 5 μL.
   - Incubate at 37 °C for 30 min.
   - Incubate at 80 °C for 20 min.
6. Sequence with the 5′ primers used in the second PCR (VH3a/b-sense, VH1/5/7-sense, VH4-sense, Pan Vk, and XhoI Cl primers).

Cloning PCR

1. Before setting up the cloning PCR, use NCBI's IgBLAST database to determine the exact V and J genes used by each antibody's VH and VL regions. V gene identity determines the forward primer for the cloning PCR, and J gene identity determines the reverse primer. Many primers target conserved sequences for more than one gene segment. For example, the human VH1/5/7 primer is used to amplify all V genes from

the VH1, VH5, or VH7 families. The human VH3 primer is used to amplify all V genes from the VH3 family except VH3–23, which uses the VH3-23 primer. Refer to Table 1 in method 1 for the primers used in this reaction.

2. Cloning PCR mix:

   2X DreamTaq Green MasterMix, 12.5 μL.
   5′ primer, 10 μM 1 μL.
   3′ primer, 10 μM 1 μL.
   Add nuclease-free water to 9 μL.
   First PCR product: 1.5 uL (*see* **Note** 7)

3. Run the following cloning PCR program. Plates can be stored at 4 °C.
   - Initial denaturation, 94 °C for 4 min.
   - Cycling reactions (40 cycles):

     Denaturation, 94 °C for 30 s.
     Annealing, 58 °C for 30 s.
     Extension, 72 °C for 45 s.
     Final extension, 72 °C for 8 min.
   - Keep at 4 °C.

4. Run 2 μL of PCR product on a 1% agarose gel to confirm a successful reaction and to check for contamination in the negative control wells.

Refer to the systems and protocols used for bacteria transformation, cell transfection, and antibody production, screening, and purification in Method 1.

4 Notes

1. Add the medium carefully and gently to avoid disturbing the MS-40L^{lo} feeder cell layer.
2. We recommend running all standards and samples at least in duplicate.
3. Incorporate a template-free negative control into each primer master mix. Refer to Table 1 for the sequences of the primers.
4. PF4/H-FITC complexes are made by mixing 20 mg/mL PF4 + 4 mg/mL H-FITC and left at room temperature for 2 h before staining.
5. To prevent contamination, it's crucial to take precautions such as refraining from touching the interior of Eppendorf tubes, minimizing airflow around open racks, and wiping pipettes and surfaces with the DNA-OFF cleaning solution before use. The first PCR product serves as the template DNA for both the second PCR and the cloning PCR. Subsequently, the product

of the second PCR undergoes sequencing, while the product of the cloning PCR is utilized for further cloning steps.

6. There should be no bands at 400 bp in the negative control wells. Infrequently, the kappa and lambda PCRs will both produce a positive result.
7. Include a template-less negative control for each master mix of primers to ensure no contamination.

Acknowledgments

We thank Dr. Garnett Kelsoe (Duke University) for giving us the CD40L^{lo} stromal cell line and a detailed protocol for Nojima culture. We also thank Dr. Patrick Wilson (Cornell University) for helping us establish the single B-cell expression cloning system.

Conflicts of Interest This study was funded by [NIH] [R01HL148120 and R01HL161127]. Other than the NIH grant, the authors have no conflicts of interest to declare that are relevant to the content of this work.

References

1. Julien JP, Wardemann H (2019) Antibodies against plasmodium falciparum malaria at the molecular level. Nat Rev Immunol 19(12): 761–775
2. Walker LM, Burton DR (2018) Passive immunotherapy of viral infections: 'super-antibodies' enter the fray. Nat Rev Immunol 18(5): 297–308
3. Arepally GM (2017) Heparin-induced thrombocytopenia. Blood 129(21):2864–2872
4. Warkentin TE (1999) Heparin-induced thrombocytopenia: a ten-year retrospective. Annu Rev Med 50:129–147
5. Dhakal B et al (2018) Disease burden, complication rates, and health-care costs of heparin-induced thrombocytopenia in the USA: a population-based study. Lancet Haematol 5(5):e220–e231
6. Pishko AM, Cuker A (2017) Heparin-induced thrombocytopenia in cardiac surgery patients. Semin Thromb Hemost 43(7):691–698
7. Warkentin TE et al (1995) Heparin-induced thrombocytopenia in patients treated with low-molecular-weight heparin or unfractionated heparin. N Engl J Med 332(20): 1330–1335
8. Staibano P et al (2017) The unique immunological features of heparin-induced thrombocytopenia. Br J Haematol 177(2):198–207
9. Arepally GM, Cines DB (2020) Pathogenesis of heparin-induced thrombocytopenia. Transl Res 225:131–140
10. Litvinov RI et al (2013) Distinct specificity and single-molecule kinetics characterize the interaction of pathogenic and non-pathogenic antibodies against platelet factor 4-heparin complexes with platelet factor 4. J Biol Chem 288(46):33060–33070
11. Vayne C et al (2017) Beneficial effect of exogenous platelet factor 4 for detecting pathogenic heparin-induced thrombocytopenia antibodies. Br J Haematol 179(5):811–819
12. Warkentin TE et al (2011) Laboratory testing for heparin-induced thrombocytopenia: a conceptual framework and implications for diagnosis. J Thromb Haemost 9(12):2498–2500
13. Lo GK, Sigouin CS, Warkentin TE (2007) What is the potential for overdiagnosis of heparin-induced thrombocytopenia? Am J Hematol 82(12):1037–1043
14. Warkentin TE (2011) How I diagnose and manage HIT. Hematology Am Soc Hematol Educ Program 2011:143–149

15. Morel-Kopp MC et al (2012) Validation of whole blood impedance aggregometry as a new diagnostic tool for HIT: results of a large Australian study. Thromb Haemost 107(3): 575–583
16. Sheridan D, Carter C, Kelton JG (1986) A diagnostic test for heparin-induced thrombocytopenia. Blood 67(1):27–30
17. Padmanabhan A et al (2016) A novel PF4-dependent platelet activation assay identifies patients likely to have heparin-induced thrombocytopenia/thrombosis. Chest 150(3):506–515
18. Samuelson Bannow BT et al (2020) A prospective, blinded study of a PF4-dependent assay for HIT diagnosis. Blood. https://doi.org/10.1182/blood.2020008195
19. Eichler P et al (1999) First workshop for detection of heparin-induced antibodies: validation of the heparin-induced platelet-activation test (HIPA) in comparison with a PF4/heparin ELISA. Thromb Haemost 81(4):625–629
20. Cuker A, Cines DB (2012) How I treat heparin-induced thrombocytopenia. Blood 119(10):2209–2218
21. Kelton JG, Warkentin TE (2008) Heparin-induced thrombocytopenia: a historical perspective. Blood 112(7):2607–2616
22. Zhu W et al (2023) Cloned antibodies from patients with HIT provide new clues to HIT pathogenesis. Blood 141(9):1060–1069
23. Wardemann H et al (2003) Predominant autoantibody production by early human B cell precursors. Science 301(5638):1374–1377
24. Smith K et al (2014) Corrigendum: rapid generation of fully human monoclonal antibodies specific to a vaccinating antigen. Nat Protoc 9(12):2903
25. Kuraoka M et al (2016) Complex antigens drive permissive clonal selection in germinal centers. Immunity 44(3):542–552
26. McCarthy KR et al (2018) Memory B cells that cross-react with group 1 and group 2 influenza a viruses are abundant in adult human repertoires. Immunity 48(1):174–184.e9
27. Luo XM et al (2009) Engineering human hematopoietic stem/progenitor cells to produce a broadly neutralizing anti-HIV antibody after in vitro maturation to human B lymphocytes. Blood 113(7):1422–1431
28. Padmanabhan A et al (2015) A modified PF4-dependent, CD62p expression assay selectively detects serotonin-releasing antibodies in patients suspected of HIT. Thromb Haemost 114(6):1322–1323

Chapter 12

A Detailed Protocol to Induce and Treat Passive Immune Thrombocytopenia in Mice

Yaima Tundidor, Lazaro Gil Gonzalez, Kevin Doyoon Won, Alequis Pavon Oro, Yuexin Shan, and Alan H. Lazarus

Abstract

Immune thrombocytopenia (ITP) is an autoimmune disorder characterized by the destruction of platelets through autoantibody-mediated mechanisms in most patients. Mouse models of ITP can serve as valuable tools for emulating key facets of human ITP pathology and facilitating the exploration of both conventional and innovative therapeutic strategies. This chapter outlines a passive model for inducing ITP using anti-platelet antibodies, with thrombocytopenia assessed by peripheral blood platelet enumeration. Furthermore, we detail a method of how to mitigate the thrombocytopenia in this model through the administration of intravenous immunoglobulin (IVIg).

Key words Murine model, Glycoprotein IIbIIIa, CD41, Cytopenia, Platelet destruction, Rabbit anti-platelet serum

1 Introduction

The autoimmune disease immune thrombocytopenia (ITP) is a hematologic disorder mainly characterized by autoantibody-mediated destruction of platelets, leading to a decreased platelet count and an increased risk of bleeding [1, 2]. Although there are a number of mechanisms that can contribute to the thrombocytopenia in ITP, it is widely accepted, for the most part, that antibody-sensitized platelets are recognized and phagocytosed through Fc gamma receptors (FcγR) expressed on macrophages [3]. In addition, other FcγR-independent mechanisms can also contribute to thrombocytopenia [4].

Conventional therapies, such as corticosteroids, intravenous immunoglobulin (IVIg), and Rho(D) immune globulin (otherwise referred to as anti-D), have long served as cornerstones in the management of ITP, exerting their effects through modulation of the immune response and suppression of platelet destruction

Sean R. Stowell and Connie M. Arthur (eds.), *Methods in Transfusion Medicine*, Methods in Molecular Biology, vol. 3053, https://doi.org/10.1007/978-1-0716-5376-0_12,

[5, 6]. Other therapies, such as Fostamatinib (a Syk inhibitor), were first demonstrated to be successful in a passive ITP model prior to successful use in patients with ITP [7].

Mouse models of ITP constitute a valuable tool for studying the immunopathogenesis of the disease as well as addressing mechanisms of potential treatments to control it. Conventional treatments such as IVIg have demonstrated their efficacy in mouse models of ITP, mirroring the results obtained in ITP patients and highlighting the utility of these models. Most mouse models of ITP are based on the administration of anti-platelet antibodies, which are injected into the animals to induce thrombocytopenia, representing a passive model of the disease [8].

Among the various antibodies used in passive ITP models, the most commonly used is the rat anti-mouse CD41 antibody (clone MWReg30, rat IgG1:κ), which targets GPIIb/IIIa, often an antigen target in patients with ITP. Repeated administration of the anti-CD41 antibody provokes prolonged thrombocytopenia that can, to some extent, mimic chronic human ITP [9]. However, a sustained condition of thrombocytopenia can potentially drive increases in the megakaryocyte compartment, generating compensatory increases in platelet production, increasing the baseline platelet count beyond day three in some mice [9]. That is why potential treatments are often first evaluated prophylactically versus models requiring a stable nadir platelet count before therapy. For those who wish to cause prolonged thrombocytopenia, the reader is referred to Neschadim et al. [10], which provides a method to help sustain thrombocytopenia over several days.

Here, we present a comprehensive protocol for inducing ITP through a single-dose administration of MWReg30. Additionally, we provide information on two alternative anti-platelet antibodies: a rabbit anti-mouse platelet serum and the monoclonal antibody (6A6) targeting murine platelets. The rabbit anti-mouse platelet serum is a commercially available polyclonal serum, which recognizes multiple unknown antigens on mouse platelets [11]. In contrast, 6A6 is thought to target two related and uncharacterized murine platelet surface proteins of approximately 100 kDa and 43 kDa [12] and is known to induce rapid in vivo platelet clearance [13]. Furthermore, we provide insights into ameliorating thrombocytopenia in passive ITP through prophylactic administration of IVIg.

The model outlined in this manuscript equips researchers with essential knowledge to utilize a passive model of murine ITP, thereby facilitating the exploration of novel treatment strategies in this area.

2 Materials

2.1 ITP Induction

1. Anti-murine platelet antibodies or serum (*see* **Note 1**).
   1.1 Purified rat anti-mouse CD41 antibody, clone MWReg30 (IgG1) (BD Pharmingen, 553847).
   1.2 Anti-mouse platelet polyclonal rabbit serum (Cedarlane, CLA31440).
   1.3 Mouse anti-mouse platelet antibody, clone 6A6 (*see* **Note 2**).
2. Sterile phosphate buffered saline without calcium and magnesium (PBS) (WISENT INC, 311-010-CL).
3. 1.5 mL microcentrifuge tubes.
4. 5 mL Polypropylene round-bottom Falcon tubes (Falcon, 352063).
5. Female C57BL/6 mice (The Jackson Laboratory) or female CD1 mice (Charles River) (age: 5–12 weeks) (*see* **Note 3**).
6. Heating Pad.
7. Mouse restraint tube.
8. 1 mL syringe.
9. Syringe needles 30G.
10. Gauze.
11. Ethanol 70%.

2.2 Bleeding of Mice to Evaluate Thrombocytopenia

1. Citrate phosphate dextrose solution with adenine (CPDA) (Sigma, C4431-10 × 50 mL).
2. PBS.
3. 1.5 mL microcentrifuge tubes.
4. In-house made conical mouse restrainer (*see* **Note 4**) (Fig. 1).
5. Electric clippers (e.g., Wahl cordless pet clipper or Andis Proclip AGC2).
6. Syringe needles, 27G.
7. P20 pipette with tips.
8. Gauze.
9. Centrifuge.
10. P1000 pipette with tips.

2.3 Platelet Counting

2.3.1 M3/M4 Coulter Counter or Z2 Coulter Counter

1. Vials with Caps, 25 mL (Beckman Coulter Accuvette™ ST Sampling, A35473).
2. Isoton II diluent (Beckman Coulter, C96980); we recommend 0.2 μM filtering the solution.

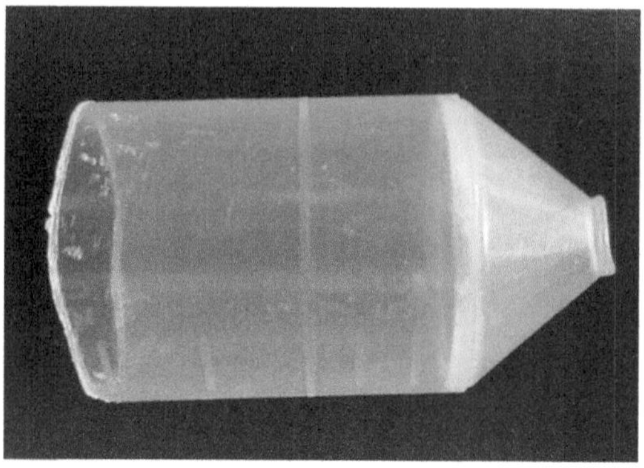

Fig. 1 An in-house mouse restrainer was made with a 50 mL centrifuge tube by cutting the tube around the 20 mL label. The conical tip of the tube must also be cut off to allow the mouse to breathe while restrained. After cutting the restrainer, a flame was used to dull all of the sharp edges

3. 10 mL Serological pipette and pipette controller.
4. P200 pipettes and tips.
5. Platelet counter, M3, M4, or Z2 Coulter Counter (Beckman Coulter).

2.3.2 Flow Cytometry

1. PBS.
2. 5 mL Polystyrene round-bottom Falcon tubes (Falcon, 352008).
3. Pipettes and tips.
4. Flow cytometer.

2.4 ITP Amelioration Using IVIg

1. Intravenous human immunoglobulin, IVIg. We have tested a number of different clinical grade IVIg preparations and have not noticed major differences in their ability to increase platelet counts in this model.
2. PBS.
3. 1.5 mL microcentrifuge tubes.
4. 5 mL Polypropylene round-bottom Falcon tubes (Falcon, 352,063).
5. 1 mL syringes.
6. Syringe needles 30G and 27G.
7. Heating pad.
8. Gauze.
9. Ethanol 70%.
10. Female C57BL/6 mice (The Jackson Laboratory) or female CD1 mice (Charles River) (age: 5–12 weeks).
11. Mouse restraint tube.

3 Methods

3.1 ITP Induction

1. Prepare the anti-mouse platelet antibody in an appropriate container (*see* **Note 5**).
   1.1 MWReg30: Make a solution of the antibody sufficient to treat the number of mice you wish to use, 2–4 μg in 100 μL of sterile PBS per mouse (*see* **Note 6**).
   1.2 Anti-mouse platelet polyclonal rabbit serum: 15 μL in 100 μL of sterile PBS per mouse (*see* **Note 7**).
   1.3 Antibody 6A6: 3 μg in 100 μL of sterile PBS per mouse.
2. Separate the mice into the different treatment groups.
   2.1 Group 1: Untreated mice. These mice will be manipulated in the same way as compared to mice in Group 2 but will not receive any ITP-inducing antibody (control; normal platelet count).
   2.2 Group 2: Mice that will receive the anti-mouse platelet antibody (ITP group).
3. Intravenous administration of anti-mouse platelet antibody (*see* **Note 8**).
   3.1. Inside a laminar flow hood, place the mice (groups 1 and 2) in a fresh cage partially positioned on top of a heating pad for 10 min (*see* **Note 9**).
   3.2. During this time, clean the mouse restrainer, fill the syringe with the antibodies (make sure to eliminate all bubbles), and position the needle (30G) with the hole facing up.
   3.3. Place the mice (group 2) in the restrainer and wipe the tail with gauze soaked in 70% ethanol to sanitize the tail and facilitate the visualization of the lateral vein.
   3.4. Administer the anti-platelet antibodies intravenously (group 2).
   3.5. Apply gauze and gentle pressure to the vein for as long as needed to stop the bleeding (group 2).
   3.6. Return the mice to the cage for 2–24 h to allow thrombocytopenia to develop (*see* **Note 10**).

3.2 Bleeding the Mice to Evaluate Thrombocytopenia

1. Prepare a solution of 10% CPDA in PBS (5 mL of CPDA and 45 mL of PBS) (*see* **Note 11**).
2. Fill 1.5 mL microcentrifuge tubes with 990 μL of 10% CPDA (one tube per mouse).
3. After 2–24 h of ITP induction, bleed the mice (groups 1 and 2) via the saphenous vein [14] (Fig. 2) (*see* **Note 12**).

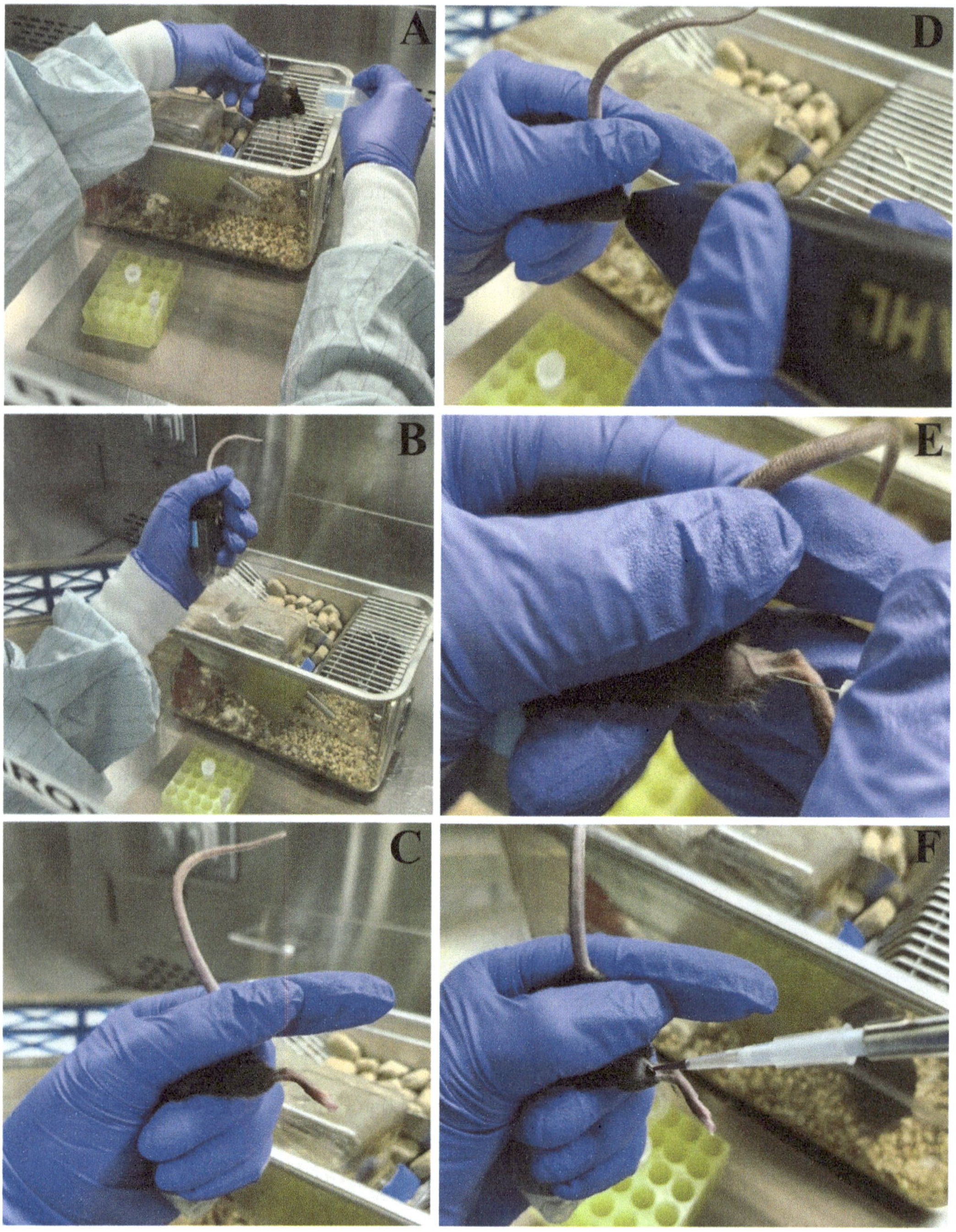

Fig. 2 Step by step procedure of saphenous vein sampling. Coax the mouse into a conical restrainer (**a**, **b**). Once the mouse is in the restrainer, isolate one of its rear legs (**c**). Shave its leg, being careful not to make any nicks or cuts (**d**), find the vein as shown, and induce a small surface puncture wound (do not go deep into the leg) with a 27G needle (**e**) and take precisely 10 μL of blood from the surface of the leg with a P20 pipette tip (**f**)

3.1 At the time point desired to evaluate thrombocytopenia in the mice, coax the mouse headfirst into a conical restrainer and isolate one of its rear legs.

3.2 Shave the mouse's leg and find the vein (Fig. 2; panel E).

3.3 Puncture the vein only to the extent needed with a 27G needle (do not go deep into the leg).

3.4 Once the vein starts to bleed and a bead of blood starts to form on the skin, take exactly 10 μL of blood with a P20 pipette tip and suspend it in the tubes pre-filled with 990 μL of 10% CPDA (blood dilution 1/100) (*see* **Notes 13** and **14**).

3.5 Apply gauze and gentle pressure on the saphenous vein for as long as needed to allow the wound to clot. Make sure the bleeding has completely stopped before returning the animal to its cage.

4. To separate the platelets from the other cellular components of blood (mostly erythrocytes), centrifuge the tubes at 170 g for 2 min, acceleration 8 and brake 0 (*see* **Note 15**).

5. Take the supernatant (containing the platelets, or platelet rich plasma) with a P1000 pipette tip and place it in a new 1.5 mL microcentrifuge tube, ensuring that the platelets are well mixed. To avoid erythrocyte contamination, do not disrupt the pellet (Fig. 3).

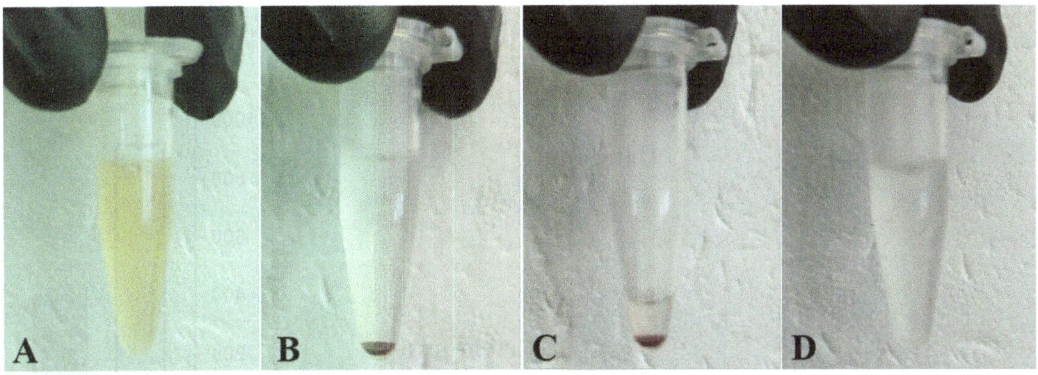

Fig. 3 Separation of platelets from the other cellular components of blood. The vials containing 10 μL of blood suspended in 990 μL of 10% CPDA (**a**) were centrifuged at 170 g for 2 min to separate the platelet supernatant fluid from the erythrocyte pellet (**b**). The supernatant was collected carefully without disrupting the pellet (**c**). It is critically important to ensure that the amount of remaining supernatant fluid is very consistent between all of the samples, as platelets will be in this supernatant. There is somewhat of an art form in consistently removing as much supernatant as possible without disturbing the pellet. In the picture shown, this would be the absolute maximum volume of supernatant that can be left in the sample. The supernatant fluid containing the platelets was transferred to a new clean tube for counting (**d**)

3.3 Platelet Counting (See Note 16)

3.3.1 M3/M4 Coulter Counter or Z2 Coulter Counter

1. Turn on the M3 Coulter Counter and the computer after the machine has loaded a platelet template (*see* **Note 17**); wash the electrodes twice by running a vial with 10 mL of Isoton II diluent.
2. To prepare the platelet sample for counting, dilute the platelets at a 1:50 ratio in Isoton II diluent. This is achieved by transferring 200 μL of platelet rich plasma into 9.8 mL of Isoton II diluent in capped vials.
3. Mix gently by inversion, run all of the samples, and save the results (*see* **Note 18**).
4. After running all the samples and saving the data, analyze the results with the software provided with the Coulter counter (Fig. 4) (*see* **Note 19**).

3.3.2 Flow Cytometry

1. Prepare and save a platelet template according to the attributes of your machine/software.
   1.1 Run a sample and gate the platelet population according to the parameters of cell size (FSC) and granularity (SSC) (Fig. 5) (*see* **Note 20**).
   1.2 To ensure you are counting platelets, it is recommended to include several (separate) control and ITP samples labeled with a fluorescent anti-platelet antibody to verify the platelet population (*see* **Note 21**).
2. Dilute the samples at a 1:10 ratio with PBS in 5 mL polystyrene round-bottom Falcon tubes by adding 50 μL of platelet rich

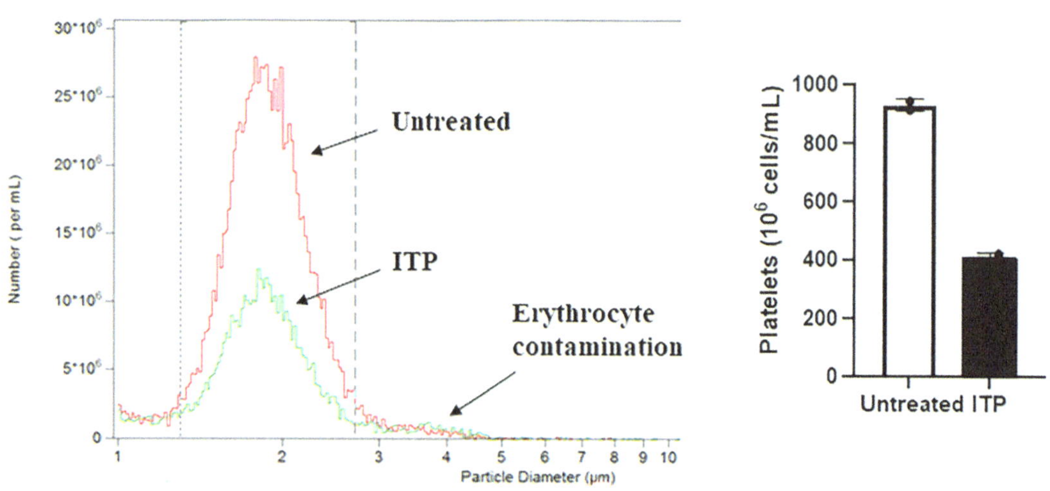

Fig. 4 Platelet count in normal and ITP mice. C57BL/6 mice were either untreated or injected with 15 μL of polyclonal rabbit anti-mouse platelet serum to induce thrombocytopenia. Two hours post-injection, the mice were bled, and platelets were counted using an M3 Coulter counter. Some Coulter counters (eg., Z2) provide a platelet number on a digital display that can be used for the platelet count; however, it is important not just to rely on this number but also to look at the distribution of platelets in the sample to ensure quality data

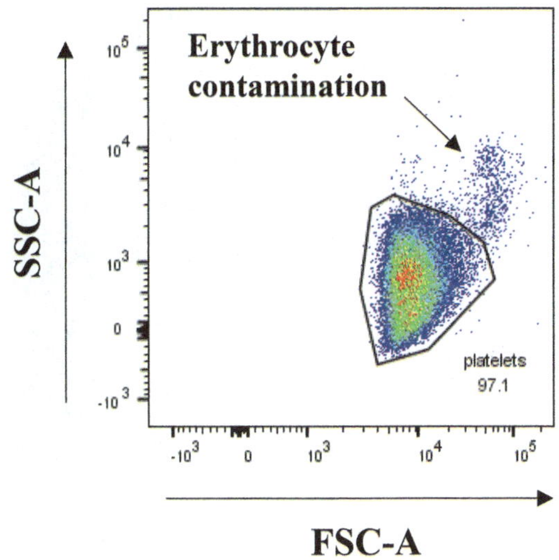

Fig. 5 Flow cytometry platelet gate. C57BL/6 mice were bled, and platelet rich plasma was obtained by centrifugation. Platelets were detected by flow cytometry according to the parameters of cell size (FSC) and granularity (SSC)

plasma to 450 μL of PBS. Considering the previous 1:100 dilution of blood in CPDA, the final platelet dilution is 1:1000.

3. Set up the flow cytometer by loading the platelet template.
4. Acquire the diluted sample and measure the number of platelets passing through the pre-set forward scatter/side scatter gate. Wait around 6 s (until the flow rate becomes stable) before commencing the two-minute based platelet count.
5. Record the platelet count over a two-minute period and use this data in conjunction with the sample flow rate to derive the platelet count, as previously described [15] (*see* **Notes 22** and **23**).
6. Analyze the data using appropriate software (e.g., FlowJo) and visualize the results using an analysis software (e.g., Prism GraphPad or Excel) (*see* **Note 24**).

3.4 ITP Amelioration Using IVIg

1. Prepare the IVIg as follows:

   Remove the amount of IVIg from the bottle corresponding to a dose of 2 g IVIg/kg body weight (*see* **Note 25**).
2. Divide the mice into four different groups.

   Group 1: Untreated (Control; normal platelet count).

   Group 2: Anti-mouse platelet antibody (ITP).

   Group 3: IVIg + anti-mouse platelet antibody (treatment group).

   Group 4: IVIg only (IVIg control).

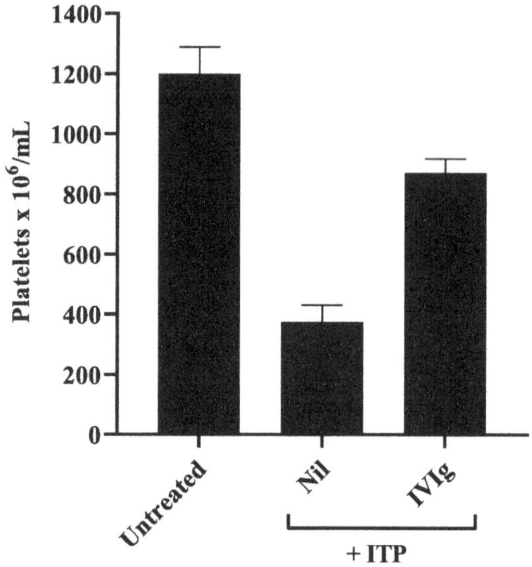

Fig. 6 IVIg ameliorates an antibody-induced passive model of ITP. CD1 mice were either left untreated or intravenously injected with MWReg30 (2 μg/mouse; + ITP) to induce passive ITP. Two hours before the MWReg30 administration, animals either were left untreated (Nil) or, in the IVIg group, received an intraperitoneal injection of IVIg (50 mg). Platelet counts were measured 24 h post-MWReg30 treatment using an M3 Coulter counter. In this MWReg30-induced thrombocytopenic model, significant thrombocytopenia can be observed 10 min after antibody injection, with consistent thrombocytopenia occurring between 1 and 2 h. Only a minimal recovery in platelet counts occurs in the absence of IVIg by 24 h [20]

3. Administer the IVIg by the intraperitoneal route (groups 3 & 4) (*see* **Note 26**).
4. Two hours after IVIg treatment, proceed to induce ITP in groups 2 and 3 with the selected anti-mouse platelet antibody, following the steps described in Subheading 3.1 (*see* **Note 27**).
5. Bleed the mice for platelet counting 2 and/or 24 h after the ITP induction and/or the interval desired (Subheading 3.2).
6. Determine the number of platelets/mL as described (Subheading 3.3) (Fig. 6).

4 Notes

1. While the focus of this manuscript is on antibodies that result in thrombocytopenia due to Fcγ receptor-mediated thrombocytopenia, essentially any antibody that would be expected to cause thrombocytopenia in a mouse could be potentially studied. While it is always best practice to use antibodies that are

low endotoxin and azide free, people over the years in our lab have made mistakes and used normal antibodies and even some therapeutic antibodies that had azide present in them. Oddly, we have not noticed that this has made a difference in the model.

2. The plasmids encoding the heavy and light chains of 6A6 IgG2a/c were gifts from Prof. Falk Nimmerjahn at the University of Erlangen-Nuremberg, Germany. The antibody was produced and purified in our laboratory.
3. A large number of different mouse strains have been successfully used in this model [16]. Essentially, any mouse strain that is amenable to thrombocytopenia in response to the antibody or mechanism of thrombocytopenia being examined can potentially be utilized. We have chosen to mostly use female mice when possible, as they demonstrate less aggression toward each other in the cage. This decreases the probability of thrombocytopenia occurring due to inflammatory responses or wound healing associated with recovery from aggressive behavior.
4. The conical animal restrainer can be made by cutting a 50-mL conical polypropylene tube near the 20 mL marking. Then, cut off some of the conical tip to allow the mouse to breathe. Flame the cut edges to smooth them and avoid hurting the animals (Fig. 1).
5. Example: 1.5 mL microcentrifuge or 5 mL Polypropylene round-bottom Falcon tubes; these containers will allow you to load a 1 mL syringe more easily during **step 3**.
6. For each mouse strain and antibody utilized, the amount of antibody required for inducing thrombocytopenia should be experimentally determined. We have found that injecting 2–4 μg/mouse is generally sufficient to obtain a level of thrombocytopenia that provides useful results. The antibody can be administered either through the intravenous route or the intraperitoneal route in this model.
7. There have been a number of different polyclonal rabbit serums available for inducing thrombocytopenia over the years. Each lot of serum must be individually evaluated in a dose-response study, as the results can be quite variable between different lots.
8. The advantage of administering the antibody by the intravenous route is that it is very easy to see that the antibody is being successfully injected. Many people, however, have difficulty in being able to find and inject the vein. It is also possible to inject the antibody by the intraperitoneal route for those familiar with that injection. In this case, however, a larger injection volume (200–250 μL) is recommended.

9. This step facilitates vein dilatation while allowing the mice to move back-and-forth between the warmer and cooler parts of the cage.
10. Depending on the mouse strain and other conditions, the thrombocytopenia generally becomes noticeable by 15–30 min, with the two-hour time point resulting in the maximal amount of thrombocytopenia and only a very modest recovery by 24 h. If you wish to look at prolonged thrombocytopenia, the mice should be injected with the anti-platelet antibody every 24 h.
11. This solution, if filter sterilized, can be stored at 4 °C and used for further experiments.
12. The mice can be sampled to look at the development of thrombocytopenia several times; however, one must be careful not to overbleed the mice.
13. After puncturing the vein, allow at least one drop of blood to flow. Quickly and accurately collect 10 μL of blood from the surface of the leg using a pipette, ensuring that the sample is taken promptly to prevent coagulation.
14. If the blood does not form a nice bead on the skin, allowing you to easily pipette it off, you can rub a small amount of Vaseline on the skin prior to puncture to help facilitate the blood forming a bead.
15. It is important to set the centrifuge to slow down without brakes to prevent disruption of the pellet.
16. Obtaining an accurate platelet count can be the most challenging part of this model. For many years, we used a FACScan flow cytometer and relied on the calibrated flow rate of our machine (~12.8 μL/min) to count platelets over a two-minute time base. Quality control samples from representative normal and ITP mice should be stained with fluorescent anti-platelet antibodies to verify the accuracy of the FSC/SSC-based platelet population. Only 1 of 3 FACScan cytometers that we had access to gave reliable and reproducible results, likely due to very careful cleaning procedures and maintenance of the machine. We later purchased a Guava flow cytometer specifically for the purpose of counting platelets. Although this flow cytometer was excellent at counting other cell populations, for some reason, the machine was not able to reproducibly count platelets. In addition, we have used various clinical hematology analyzers meant for human subjects, a Hemavet, and most recently, Z2 and M3 Coulter counters. Each of these techniques has its pluses and minuses. The hematology analyzers meant for human platelets were very reproducible, but mouse platelets are smaller than human platelets, and these machines

cut off the mouse platelet population, losing roughly 20–30% of the platelets in the sample. Most recently, we have used Z2 and M3 Coulter counters and found them to be reliable and inexpensive per sample to run.

17. The platelet template is created by the Counter Coulter technician during equipment and software installation and includes a number of parameters, including specifying the aperture size, the electrolyte (e.g., Isoton II), measurement settings, threshold current, gain, etc. This template should be tailored by the technician to count mouse platelets.
18. Between samples, wash the electrodes thoroughly with double distilled water and run a vial with 10 mL of Isoton II diluent until the reported background value (i.e., Sigma) on the display screen is less than 250.
19. The software provides the platelet count in cells/mL. It is important to visualize the distribution of the platelets in the samples to ensure that you are counting platelets rather than contaminating erythrocytes or debris. Typical mouse platelet size for the buffers and mice we use is between 1.3 μm and 2.7 or 2.8 μm (Fig. 4). If the experiment has worked well, you will see a diminution in the platelet peak of the ITP mice, as shown. Depending on the nature of the experiment, sometimes platelet microparticles can be seen to the left of the main peak (not shown).
20. If one is counting the platelet rich plasma using the method described, the main population observed should be platelets. Minor contamination with erythrocytes can be observed, and it can sometimes be challenging to distinguish debris and platelet microparticles from the actual platelets (Fig. 5).
21. Platelet enumeration by flow cytometry can be performed with the inclusion of a fluorescent anti-platelet antibody in each sample [9, 15]; however, this can also sometimes affect the actual platelet count in the sample.
22. Flow rate can either be calculated by you or provided by the technician during the flow cytometer's preventative maintenance; you generally need to request this information from the technician before they perform the maintenance.
23. Considerations for flow cytometry: It is important to highlight that flow cytometers using pressure-based fluidics can undergo variations in pressure, including a burst of pressure during the first few seconds of acquisition. For these reasons, one must be very careful in interpreting the data to assess platelet counts. We have routinely run control samples at the beginning of the experiment and again rerun the same samples at the end of the experiment to ensure the reliability and consistency of the flow

cytometer. Some groups have found it helpful to add calibrator beads of known concentration into the sample. By calculating a ratio of the number of beads observed on the cytometer to the expected number of beads added into the sample, it is possible to calculate the concentration of the particles of interest. For more details on using beads to calibrate and standardize platelet counting, the reader is referred to Robert et al. [17]. Another approach used by some groups is employing a conversion factor, which is obtained by comparing the platelet count obtained by cytometry to that obtained on an electronic machine platelet counter (e.g., hematology analyzer) [9].

Flow cytometers using a volumetric-based fluidics system (syringe or peristaltic pump) can provide absolute cell counts (cells/mL). Since the exact sample volume can be measured in these machines, they should be a reliable choice.

24. Any method that accurately gives a reliable platelet count can be potentially considered. We have provided instructions for an M3 Coulter counter as well as some general guidance on the use of a flow cytometer. In addition, it is technically possible to use a hemocytometer [18]. In addition, there are a number of hematology analyzers capable of measuring platelets in a mouse (e.g., Hemavet). Challenges with counting mouse platelets using any technique include problems with platelet clumping, resulting in false thrombocytopenia, inaccuracy of the machine employed, or using a machine that is poorly maintained.
25. For example, if you are using 10% IVIg and injecting mice that weigh 25 grams on average, inject a volume of 500 μL of pure IVIg. Do not dilute the IVIg in a buffer, as this could cause aggregate formation, affecting the results. If you wish to do a dose-response study, use a lower volume of IVIg. An IVIg buffer control and/or protein control should be used as appropriate.
26. IVIg can also be administered by the intravenous route if desired. In this case, because 500 μL of IVIg would overwhelm the mouse circulatory system, the total amount should be split into three injections given 30 min apart.
27. Selecting the appropriate ITP model is crucial based on the thrombocytopenic pathway you intend to evaluate. For studying inhibitors targeting macrophages, any of the three antibodies mentioned here can be used to induce passive ITP. To specifically evaluate FcγRIII-mediated thrombocytopenia, the model utilizing MWReg30 is ideal. MWReg30 is a rat IgG1 whose Fc portion binds to mouse FcγRIII, but not to other activating FcγRs. If the goal is to initiate thrombocytopenia via FcγRIV, the 6A6-mouse IgG2a/c subtypes are preferable due to their selective interaction with FcγRIV [19].

Funding

This research was supported by The Canadian Blood Services (Intramural Research Grant Program, to AHL), funded by the federal government (Health Canada) and provincial and territorial ministries of health. YT is supported by a Canadian Blood Services Postdoctoral Fellowship Program award. KDW was supported by a Canada Graduate Scholarship from the Canadian Institutes of Health Research (CIHR). The views herein do not necessarily reflect the views of the federal, provincial, or territorial governments of Canada. The authors declare no conflicts of interest relevant to the content of this manuscript. AHL has research funding from argenx (paid to the institution), outside the submitted work.

References

1. Li J, Sullivan JA, Ni H (2018) Pathophysiology of immune thrombocytopenia. Curr Opin Hematol 25:373–381
2. Semple JW, Rebetz J, Maouia A, Kapur R (2020) An update on the pathophysiology of immune thrombocytopenia. Curr Opin Hematol 27:423–429
3. Li G, Gao L, Ma R, Tian W, Mingzhi L (2019) Associations between FCGR polymorphisms and immune thrombocytopenia: a meta-analysis. Scand J Immunol 89:e12758
4. Swinkels M et al (2018) Emerging concepts in immune thrombocytopenia. Front Immunol 9: 880
5. Schwab I, Nimmerjahn F (2013) Intravenous immunoglobulin therapy: how does IgG modulate the immune system? Nat Rev Immunol 13:176–189
6. Shock A, Humphreys D, Nimmerjahn F (2020) Dissecting the mechanism of action of intravenous immunoglobulin in human autoimmune disease: lessons from therapeutic modalities targeting Fcγ receptors. J Allergy Clin Immunol 146:492–500
7. Podolanczuk A, Lazarus AH, Crow AR, Grossbard E, Bussel JB (2009) Of mice and men: an open-label pilot study for treatment of immune thrombocytopenic purpura by an inhibitor of Syk. Blood 113:3154–3160
8. Zufferey A, Kapur R, Semple JW (2017) Pathogenesis and therapeutic mechanisms in immune thrombocytopenia (ITP). J Clin Med 6:16
9. Katsman Y, Foo AH, Leontyev D, Branch DR (2010) Improved mouse models for the study of treatment modalities for immune-mediated platelet destruction. Transfusion (Paris) 50: 1285–1294
10. Neschadim A, Branch DR (2015) Mouse models of autoimmune diseases: immune thrombocytopenia. Curr Pharm Des 21:2487–2497
11. Liew PX, Lee W-Y, Kubes P (2017) iNKT cells orchestrate a switch from inflammation to resolution of sterile liver injury. Immunity 47: 752–765.e5
12. Mizutani H, Engelman RW, Kurata Y, Ikehara S, Good RA (1993) Development and characterization of monoclonal antiplatelet autoantibodies from autoimmune thrombocytopenic purpura-prone (NZW x BXSB)F1 mice. Blood 82:837–844
13. Nimmerjahn F, Ravetch JV (2005) Divergent immunoglobulin g subclass activity through selective Fc receptor binding. Science 310: 1510–1512
14. Hem A, Smith AJ, Solberg P (1998) Saphenous vein puncture for blood sampling of the mouse, rat, hamster, gerbil, Guinea pig, ferret and mink. Lab Anim 32:364–368
15. Crow AR, Song S, Semple JW, Freedman J, Lazarus AH (2001) IVIg inhibits reticuloendothelial system function and ameliorates murine passive-immune thrombocytopenia independent of anti-idiotype reactivity. Br J Haematol 115:679–686
16. Crow AR, Amash A, Lazarus AH (2015 Jun) CD44 antibody-mediated amelioration of murine immune thrombocytopenia (ITP): mouse background determines the effect of FcγRIIb genetic disruption. Transfusion 55(6 Pt 2):1492–1500

17. Robert S et al (2009) Standardization of platelet-derived microparticle counting using calibrated beads and a Cytomics FC500 routine flow cytometer: a first step towards multicenter studies? J Thromb Haemost 7:190–197
18. Thibodeaux J, Roussel J, Adkinson R, Goodeaux L (1989) An efficient procedure for manual platelet counting. Vet Rec 125:417–419
19. Nimmerjahn F, Bruhns P, Horiuchi K, Ravetch JV (2005) FcgammaRIV: a novel FcR with distinct IgG subclass specificity. Immunity 23: 41–51
20. Jen Chao Ching (Mark) (2015) Thesis: anemia mediated by an anti-erythrocyte antibody is not closely linked to the amelioration of murine passive immune thrombocytopenia (ITP) [see figure 21 on page 80 of the thesis]. https://tspace.library.utoronto.ca/handle/1807/94510. University of Toronto, Toronto

Chapter 13

Platelet Transfusions in Murine Models of Neonatal Thrombocytopenia

Jesselin J. Romero Escobar, Natalie E. Kane, Erin L. Soule-Albridge, Martha C. Sola-Visner, and Patricia E. Davenport

Abstract

We have created a neonatal murine model of platelet transfusion to study the biological effects of platelet transfusions given to neonates. This model replicates the "developmental mismatch" that occurs when human preterm neonates receive a transfusion of functionally different adult platelets. These methods utilize common in vivo techniques that have been tailored for the small size of P1-P10 pups. Using this model and blood draw/analysis methods, investigators can prepare a washed, resting platelet transfusion product and transfuse it into a clinically relevant neonatal mouse model to interrogate both the hemostatic and immune functions of platelets and platelet transfusions in this important clinical context.

Key words Platelet transfusion, Neonatal mouse, Retro-orbital transfusion, Retro-orbital bleed, Facial-vein puncture

1 Introduction

Thrombocytopenia occurs in 18–35% of neonates admitted to the neonatal intensive care unit (NICU), and the incidence increases to 70% in the most premature neonates born with a weight <1000 g [1–3]. These same infants also have the highest incidence of intracranial bleeding of any patient population, and as a result it has historically been accepted that preterm neonates should be transfused at higher platelet counts than older children and adults, in hopes of preventing bleeding. Over the past 20 years, multiple retrospective and observational studies have suggested that liberal neonatal platelet transfusion practices do not prevent bleeding and instead, may be associated with harm [4–10]. In 2019, the results from the largest randomized controlled trial of neonatal platelet transfusion thresholds (the PlaNet-2 trial) were published. This study randomized 660 neonates <34 weeks' gestational age to receive platelet transfusions for platelet counts $<50 \times 10^9/L$

Sean R. Stowell and Connie M. Arthur (eds.), *Methods in Transfusion Medicine*, Methods in Molecular Biology, vol. 3053,
https://doi.org/10.1007/978-1-0716-5376-0_13,

(high threshold group) or < 25 × 10^9/L (low threshold group) and found an increased incidence of the primary combined outcome of death or major bleeding in the 28 days following randomization in the high threshold arm [11]. Among secondary outcomes, infants randomized to the high threshold group also had a higher incidence of bronchopulmonary dysplasia (chronic lung disease of prematurity), and upon 2-year follow up, these same infants had worse neurodevelopmental outcomes and an increased need for supplemental oxygen or respiratory support compared to infants randomized to the low threshold arm [12].

The mechanisms underlying the potential harm associated with neonatal platelet transfusion are an active area of research. Neonatal and adult platelets are functionally distinct from each other, due to differences in surface receptor expression and downstream signaling that result in a comparatively hypo-reactive neonatal platelet [13]. Thus, it has been hypothesized that the transfusion of adult platelets into the unique physiologic environment of the preterm neonate might result in a "developmental mismatch" between the transfused platelets and the recipient, with potential negative consequences [14]. Furthermore, it is now well established that, in addition to their hemostatic functions, platelets are active immune cells [15]. How the immune functions of platelets change over development and whether a developmental mismatch in platelet immune function contributes to the harm associated with neonatal platelet transfusion is just beginning to be investigated [16–18].

Rigorous clinical investigation into these mechanistic questions is difficult, if not impossible, due to the small size, very small blood volumes, and intensive care required by infants born preterm. Thus, pre-clinical models are essential to understand the mechanisms behind neonatal diseases and to discover therapies or alternative approaches that minimize harm. It is no longer acceptable for adult mice to be used as models of neonatal disease, as the unique physiologic state of a neonate is crucial to our understanding of their pathology and to our ability to translate pre-clinical findings to the care of preterm infants in the NICU. To investigate the hemostatic and immunological effects of platelet transfusions in a developmentally appropriate animal model, we developed a neonatal murine model of platelet transfusion and methods for serial and terminal blood collection, including the potential for blood reconstitution to maximize the testing that can be carried out in these extremely small blood samples. These methods can be used in pups as young as P1-P10 and recapitulate the developmental mismatch that occurs when adult platelets are transfused into preterm neonates.

2 Materials

2.1 Solutions Preparation

1. Tyrode's buffer without calcium (store at 4 °C): 137 mM sodium chloride (NaCl), 0.43 mM sodium dihydrogen phosphate (NaH_2PO_4), 2.7 mM potassium chloride (KCl), 12 mM sodium bicarbonate ($NaHCO_3$), 5 mM 4-(2-hydroxyethyl)-1-piperazineethanesulfonic acid (HEPES), and 1 mM magnesium dichloride hexahydrate ($MgCl_2 \times 6H_2O$).
2. 20 U/mL sodium heparin in 1X tris-buffered saline (TBS) (store at 4 °C) (Boston BioProducts).
3. 10 U/mL apyrase (Sigma-Aldrich*)* in Tyrode's buffer (store at −20 °C).
4. Citrate theophylline adenosine dipyridamole (CTAD): 0.109 M sodium citrate, 15 mM theophylline, 3.7 mM adenosine, and 0.198 mM dipyridamole. Diluted 1:10 in 0.9% sodium chloride (normal saline) (store at 4 °C in dark).

2.2 Murine Adult (Donor) Terminal Retro-Orbital Blood Collection

1. Tyrode's buffer without calcium (store at 4 °C).
2. Heparin-coatedHeparin glass capillary tubes (Fisherbrand).
3. 20 U/mL sodium heparin in 1X TBS (stored at 4 °C) (Boston BioProducts).
4. Isoflurane.
5. Euthanasia materials required by your animal facility.

2.3 Murine Fresh Washed Platelet Preparation

1. 20 U/mL sodium heparin in 1X TBS (store at 4 °C).
2. Tyrode's buffer without calcium (store at 4 °C).
3. Heat block.
4. 10 U/mL apyrase in Tyrode's buffer (store at −20 °C).
5. 0.9% sodium chloride (normal saline).
6. Hematology analyzer (*see* **Note 1**).
7. Bench top centrifuge.
8. Parafilm.

2.4 Murine Retro-Orbital Transfusion

1. 6 mm × 31G, 3/10 mL, insulin syringe with ultrafine needle.
2. Calibrated 20 μL pipette and tips (dedicated for use in animal facility only).
3. Washed murine adult donor platelets (collected and prepared fresh).
4. Phosphate buffered saline (PBS), pH 7.4.
5. Isoflurane.

2.5 Murine Neonatal Serial Facial Vein Blood Collection

1. CTAD diluted 1:10 in normal saline (store at 4 °C in dark).
2. 1.5 mL Eppendorf tubes.
3. Calibrated 20 μL pipette and tips (dedicated for use in animal facility only).
4. Hematology analyzer.
5. ½ inch × 27G, 1 mL TB Syringe (Slip Tip with BD Precision Glide Needle).

2.6 Murine Neonatal Terminal Retro-Orbital Blood Collection

1. Tubes with K_2E (EDTA coated tubes) (BD Microtainer).
2. Disposable glass micropipettes (capillary blood collection tubes) (VWR International).
3. Hematology analyzer.

2.7 Murine Neonatal Plasma Separation and Storage

1. Calibrated 20 and 200 μL pipette and tips.
2. Eppendorf tubes.
3. 0.5 mL microcentrifuge tubes
4. Murine whole blood collected in EDTA-coated tubes.
5. Bench top centrifuge.
6. Ice.

2.8 Murine Neonatal Whole Blood Cell Resuspension and Freezing Protocol

1. Murine whole blood collected in EDTA-coated tubes.
2. Calibrated 200 μL pipette and tips.
3. 1.5 mL Eppendorf tubes.
4. Bench top centrifuge.
5. 5% bovine serum albumin (BSA) in PBS.
6. 20% dimethyl sulfoxide (DMSO) in RPMI 1640 medium (Gibco).
7. 95% isopropanol.
8. 0.5 mL cryovials.
9. Cryogenic freezing container (Thermo Fisher Scientific Nalgene).

3 Methods

3.1 Solution Preparation

1. Tyrode's buffer without calcium (store at 4 °C): 137 mM NaCl, 0.43 mM NaH_2PO_4, 2.7 mM KCl, 12 mM $NaHCO_3$, 5 mM HEPES, 1 mM $MgCl_2 \times 6H_2O$ combined at 35 °C.
2. 20 U/mL sodium heparin in 1X TBS (stored at 4 °C):
3. 10 U/mL apyrase in Tyrode's buffer without calcium (stored at −20 °C). To limit freeze thaw cycles, store stock at 100 and 10 U/mL working solution in 10 μL aliquots.

4. CTAD stock is diluted 1:10 in normal saline and stored at 4 °C in the dark. For the CTAD stock solution, combine 0.109 M sodium citrate, 15 mM Theophylline, 3.7 mM Adenosine, 0.198 mM Dipyridamole, and mix rigorously. Store this photosensitive stock solution at room temperature, covered in foil (*see* **Note 2**).

3.2 Terminal Adult Murine Retro-Orbital Blood Collection

1. For each donor, place 300 μL of heparin (20 U/mL) into 1.5 mL Eppendorf tubes, and keep the heparin on lab bench to warm to room temperature.
2. In the animal facility, deeply anesthetize mice with isoflurane.
3. Break the tip off both ends of the heparin-coated capillary tubes to create segments that are about 12 mm in length from each end.
4. Insert the blunt (unbroken) end of the heparin-coated capillary tube into the retro-orbital space and allow drops of blood to flow freely into the Eppendorf containing heparin until 700 μL of blood has been collected (you will have a total of 1 mL of blood and heparin in the Eppendorf) (Fig. 1).
5. Invert the tube to mix gently.
6. Sacrifice mouse either by CO_2 or cervical dislocation.

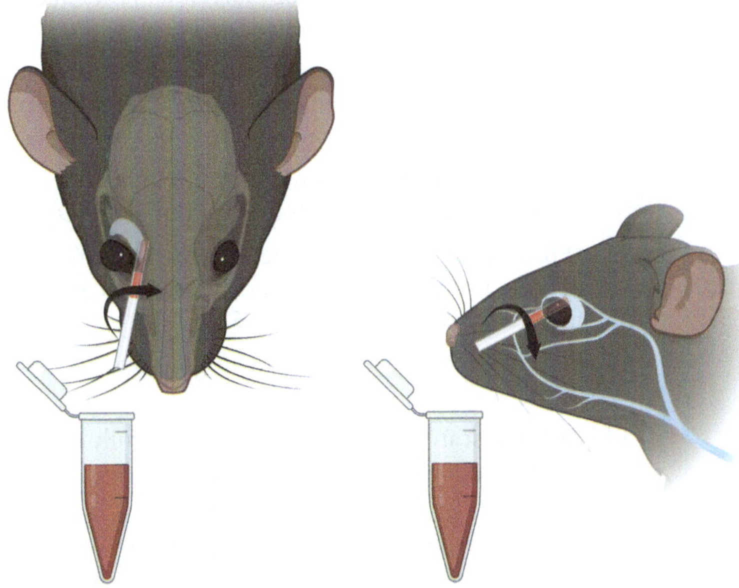

Fig. 1 Retro-orbital bleed in adult mice. Heparin-coated capillary tube can be twisted counterclockwise or clockwise, depending on investigator preference

3.3 Murine Platelet Wash

1. Set heat block to 37 °C and place three 1 mL aliquots of Tyrode's buffer without calcium into warmer (*see* **Note 3**).
2. Add 300 μL of heparin (20 U/mL) to Eppendorf tubes containing just collected adult donors' blood (see above).
3. Centrifuge heparinized blood for 6 min at 200× *g* at 27 °C.
4. To maximize platelet recovery, use a 1000 μL pipette to remove 900 μL of platelet-rich plasma (PRP) and red blood cells (RBC) and transfer to a new Eppendorf tube containing 300 μL of heparin.
5. Centrifuge again for 6 min at 100× *g* at 27 °C.
6. With a 1000 μL pipette, carefully remove PRP 250 μL at a time and place into a new, empty 1.5 mL Eppendorf tube; avoid any RBC contamination.
7. Pellet platelets by centrifuging sample for 5 min at 800× *g* at 27 °C.
8. Add 5 μL of 10 U/mL apyrase to two of the tubes containing 1 mL of Tyrode's warming in the heat block (final concentration of apyrase in Tyrode's is 0.2 U/mL).
9. Carefully discard the supernatant while not disturbing the platelet pellet. Gently (to not activate the platelets) re-suspend the pellet in Tyrode's buffer with apyrase, combining all re-suspended donor platelet aliquots in a total of 1 mL Tyrode's buffer with apyrase (*see* **Note 4**).
10. Dilute 10 μL of platelet suspension in 90 μL of normal saline and run on hematology analyzer to obtain the platelet concentration.
11. Place the Eppendorf containing the remainder of the platelet suspension in the heat block for 10 min to rest.
12. While resting, calculate the volume of Tyrode's buffer with apyrase needed to re-suspend platelets to achieve the desired final concentration (*see* **Note 5**).
13. Pellet platelets again by centrifuging for 5 min at 800× *g* at 27 °C.
14. Again, discard the supernatant and carefully re-suspend platelet pellet in calculated volume of Tyrode's with apyrase.
15. Dilute 10 μL of final platelet suspension in 90 μL of normal saline and run on hematology analyzer to verify the final platelet concentration.
16. Wrap tubes containing Tyrode's buffer (without apyrase) and washed platelets in parafilm and transport to animal facility held tightly in closed fist (to keep warm) for transfusion (*see* **Note 6**).

3.4 Neonatal Mouse Transfusion

1. Record the weight of the mouse to administer the desired volume of transfusion (*see* **Note 7**).
2. Place the mouse under isoflurane anesthesia (*see* **Note 8**).
3. Carefully resuspend platelet suspension (or desired transfusion produce) with a 20 μL pipette and then draw up the desired transfusion volume using a 6 mm × 31G, 3/10 mL, insulin syringe with ultrafine needle (*see* **Note 9**).
4. Gently invert the syringe (needle up) and tap to remove any air bubbles.
5. In the youngest mice (P1-P10), the eye will be fused shut and can either be opened (by gently scraping a needle tip across the aperture) or kept closed for transfusion (*see* **Note 10**).
6. In the youngest mice, the procedure is best performed with one person holding the pup on their side (eye up) so that the individual transfusing can use both hands to hold and advance the syringe in a controlled manner.
7. Slowly, inject the platelets into the retro-orbital space behind the medial corner of the eye, using a new needle for each mouse to avoid contamination of the platelet suspension.
8. For sham transfusions, transfuse Tyrode's buffer with no apyrase into the control group mice following the identical technique.
9. Monitor transfused mice closely until they fully recover from anesthesia.

3.5 Murine Neonatal Serial Facial Vein Blood Collection (for Small Volumes)

1. Prepare 1.5 mL Eppendorf tubes with either 90 or 95 μL of CTAD (or liquid anticoagulant of choice) for a ten-fold or 20-fold dilution of the blood sample, respectively.
2. Prepare one Eppendorf tube with 1 mL CTAD to prime needles and pipette tips.
3. Prime the 1/2 × 27G, 1 mL TB syringe needle by drawing up ~500 μL of CTAD and push a small volume through the needle tip.
4. Set a 20 μL pipette to the desired blood collection volume and prime with CTAD (*see* **Note 11**).
5. Place the mouse on its side, stabilizing its head, and identify the facial vein (Fig. 2).
6. Using the CTAD primed TB needle, prick the mouse's facial vein creating a small bubble of blood on the surface of the skin.
7. Expel the CTAD from the pipette and collect the desired volume of blood (either 10 or 5 μL) and immediately add to the prepared CTAD tubes and carefully mix sample.

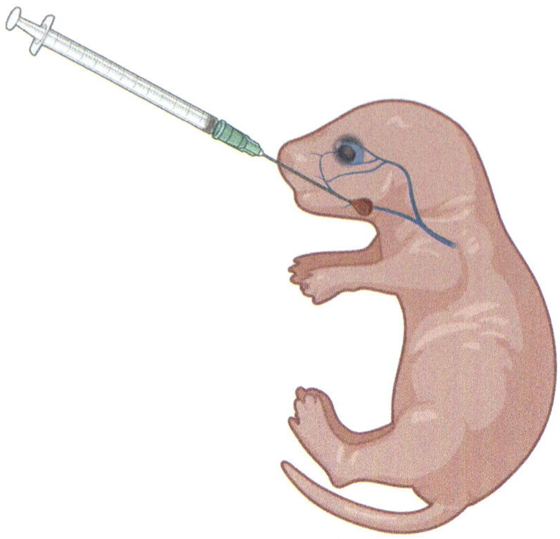

Fig. 2 Facial-vein puncture in newborn mice

8. Hold pressure to area of facial vein puncture until bleeding has stopped.
9. For each mouse, re-prime the TB needle by expelling a small volume and use a new pipette tip, priming with CTAD.
10. Run diluted samples on hematology analyzer or perform desired experiment immediately after collection.

3.6 Murine Neonatal Terminal Retro-Orbital Blood Collection (for Large Volumes)

1. Place pup under deep isoflurane anesthesia.
2. Break the tip off both ends of the heparin-coated capillary tubes to create segments that are about 6 mm in length from each end.
3. For the youngest pups (P1-P10), the eye will be fused shut. Carefully open it using a needle tip to break away the skin cells along the aperture.
4. Insert the blunt (unbroken) end of the heparin-coated capillary tube into the retro-orbital space and allow drops of blood to flow freely into the EDTA-coated tube until the desired amount of blood is collected (*see* **Note 12**).
5. Lightly tap the tube to ensure all blood has contacted EDTA coating.
6. Sacrifice mouse either by CO_2 or decapitation (depending on the age).

3.7 Murine Neonatal Sample Processing: Plasma Separation

1. Retro-orbitally bleed pups into EDTA-coated tubes (as above).
2. Transfer the anticoagulated blood into new Eppendorf tubes.
3. Centrifuge blood for 10 min at 3000× *g* to separate platelet-poor plasma (PPP).

4. Put all samples on ice and carefully pipette the plasma supernatant to new Eppendorf tubes, careful to not contaminate sample with cellular fraction.
5. Aliquot desired volume of plasma into microcentrifuge tubes and freeze at −80 °C for future use.

3.8 Murine Neonatal Whole Blood Cell Resuspension and Freezing Protocol

1. Retro-orbitally bleed pups into EDTA-coated tubes (as above).
2. Transfer the anticoagulated blood into new Eppendorf tubes.
3. Centrifuge blood for 10 min at 3000× *g* to separate PPP from the cellular component.
4. Remove the plasma and store (if desired), as above.
5. Re-suspend the cellular fraction with a volume equal to that of the removed plasma using 5% BSA or FBS.
6. Use cells immediately for flow cytometry studies. If flow cytometry studies will be performed in batches at a later date, resuspend cells again 1:1 with 20% DMSO in RPMI.
7. For each sample, quickly aliquot 100 μL of the cellular suspension into 0.5 mL cryovials (*see* **Note 13**).
8. Place cryovials into the cryogenic freezing container filled with isopropanol and immediately transfer to −80 °C freezer.
9. After 24 h, remove cryovials and place into −80 °C freezer or a liquid nitrogen tank for a maximum of 4 weeks.

4 Notes

1. The hematology analyzer used in this protocol is the Sysmex XN-1000; however, another analyzer could be used as well.
2. CTAD is photosensitive, so it should be stored in the dark. This solution should have a pale-yellow color, and if the liquid becomes clear, it is no longer viable. Dissolution of all materials into a homogenous solution is difficult, so stir vigorously.
3. When planning the experiment, the number of mice that will be transfused should be considered when preparing the platelet product. In the present experiments, the number of adult mice bled is one additional to the number of neonatal mice to be transfused. Prepare three tubes of Tyrode's buffer for bleeding less than five mice. If bleeding more than five mice, you will need five tubes of Tyrode's buffer.
4. If four donors are bled, re-suspend each in 250 μL and add together. Do not combine more than five platelet aliquots in 1 mL (200 μL is the minimum volume needed to re-suspend the pellet without activating the platelets). If more than five

donors are needed, create multiple 1 mL platelet suspensions to avoid exceeding five samples per suspension.

5. We create a suspension of 5×10^6 platelets/μL, but this can be adjusted depending on experimental goals.
6. Washed platelets become activated over time, so it is important to begin transfusions immediately after platelets have been prepared and to transfuse platelets quickly to minimize time lapse.
7. We transfuse 10 μL/g of a 5×10^6/μL platelet solution to mimic a 15 mL/kg transfusion administered to a neonate, accounting for the three- to fivefold higher platelet counts of mice compared to humans.
8. Hypothermia cannot be used as a method of anesthesia since it can induce platelet dysfunction and thrombocytopenia.
9. When conducting the platelet transfusion, use a new needle for every mouse to avoid dipping a dirty needle into the platelet suspension. Make sure to keep platelets warm to prevent activation and transfuse platelet groups first to minimize the time platelets spend sitting after the wash.
10. In the youngest mice (P1-P3) platelets can also be transfused into the facial vein, which is clearly visible at this age (Fig. 2).
11. We collect between 1 and 10 μL in P1-P10 pups and aim for a 1:10 dilution. If unable to obtain 10 μL of blood, then use a 1:20 dilution of blood into CTAD (5 μL blood into 95 μL of CTAD). The reading from the hematology analyzer will be less accurate if the 1:20 dilution is used. Normal saline can be used in substitution of CTAD, but this does not function to prevent coagulation and might cause platelet activation and clumping.
12. Use glass capillary tubes as opposed to plastic so it is possible to break tubes into smaller segments with clean edges. We typically can collect at least 150 μL of blood from P5-P10 pups. For adults, 700 μL blood is typically collected, for P10 mice 250 μL blood is typically collected.
13. Once DMSO has been added, the samples should be frozen as soon as possible because DMSO has some toxicity to cells.

Conflict of Interest

P.D. receives support from NIH/NHLBI K99 HL156051. M.S.V. receives support from NIH/NHLBI P01-HL046925. No other conflicts of interest related to this work to report.

References

1. Christensen RD et al (2006) Thrombocytopenia among extremely low birth weight neonates: data from a multihospital healthcare system. J Perinatol 26(6):348–353
2. Castle V et al (1986) Frequency and mechanism of neonatal thrombocytopenia. J Pediatr 108(5 Pt 1):749–755
3. Andrew M et al (1987) Clinical impact of neonatal thrombocytopenia. J Pediatr 110(3): 457–464
4. Del Vecchio A et al (2001) Platelet transfusions in the neonatal intensive care unit:factors predicting which patients will require multiple transfusions. Transfusion 41(6):803–808
5. Garcia MG et al (2001) Epidemiologic and outcome studies of patients who received platelet transfusions in the neonatal intensive care unit. J Perinatol 21(7):415–420
6. Bonifacio L et al (2007) Thrombocytopenia related neonatal outcome in preterms. Indian J Pediatr 74(3):269–274
7. Kenton AB et al (2005) Platelet transfusions in infants with necrotizing enterocolitis do not lower mortality but may increase morbidity. J Perinatol 25(3):173–177
8. Baer VL et al (2007) Do platelet transfusions in the NICU adversely affect survival? Analysis of 1600 thrombocytopenic neonates in a multihospital healthcare system. J Perinatol 27(12): 790–796
9. Patel RM et al (2019) Platelet transfusions and mortality in necrotizing enterocolitis. Transfusion 59(3):981–988
10. Elgendy MM et al (2021) Platelet transfusion and outcomes of preterm infants: a cross-sectional study. Neonatology 118(4):425–433
11. Curley A et al (2019) Randomized trial of platelet-transfusion thresholds in neonates. N Engl J Med 380(3):242–251
12. Moore CM et al (2023) Two-year outcomes following a randomised platelet transfusion trial in preterm infants. Arch Dis Child Fetal Neonatal Ed:F1–F6
13. Ferrer-Marin F, Sola-Visner M (2021) Neonatal platelet physiology and implications for transfusion. Platelets:1–9
14. Davenport P (2023) Neonatal platelet transfusions: more than meets the eye. Pediatr Res 94: 1864
15. Koupenova M, Livada AC, Morrell CN (2022) Platelet and megakaryocyte roles in innate and adaptive immunity. Circ Res 130(2):288–308
16. Maurya P et al (2023) Transfusion of adult, but not neonatal, platelets promotes monocyte trafficking in neonatal mice. Arterioscler Thromb Vasc Biol 43:873–885
17. Davenport P et al (2022) Platelet transfusions in a murine model of neonatal polymicrobial sepsis: divergent effects on inflammation and mortality. Transfusion 62(6):1177–1187
18. Thom CS et al (2023) Quantitative label-free mass spectrometry reveals content and signaling differences between neonatal and adult platelets. J Thromb Haemost 22(5):P1447–P1462

Chapter 14

Quantification of Human Platelet Clearance In Vitro and in Xenotransfused Animals

Shailaja Hegde, Yi Zheng, and Jose A. Cancelas

Abstract

We have utilized macrophage-dependent and hepatocyte-dependent phagocytosis assays as well as in vivo xenotransfusion experiments to determine the survival and rate of clearance of stored platelets in several conditions that include cold storage and the use of a novel preservative solution. Our novel preservative solution targets RHOA, a key signaling GTPase that controls refrigeration-induced storage damage. Using these approaches, the outcome of fluorescently labeled human platelets can be analyzed for their potential to be cleared by integrin-dependent phagocytes, lectin-binding domain-dependent hepatocytes or in circulation of thrombocytopenic, innate- and adaptive immunity–deficient animals.

Key words Platelet storage, Additive solution, RHOA, inhibitor, R-(S-)G-04, Survival, Clearance, Phagocytosis

1 Introduction

Platelets collected for transfusion are typically stored at room temperature (RT) for 5–7 days. Storage at room temperature facilitates the growth of small inocula of bacteria that may contaminate the blood product during the process of phlebotomy. This poses challenges in ensuring an adequate just-in-time supply for patient care, especially cancer patients in whom multiple doses of platelets are required for bleeding prophylaxis and/or therapy. Despite efforts to minimize bacterial contamination through storage duration limitations and pathogen reduction techniques [1], the risk of sepsis (severe infection) from contaminated platelets remains a concern. The short shelf-life of RT stored platelets limits their availability for transfusion and results in a logistical nightmare for blood centers that face the paradox of having alternate situations of excess of inventory, resulting in wastage, and situations of significant shortage, impairing appropriate health care [2].

Sean R. Stowell and Connie M. Arthur (eds.), *Methods in Transfusion Medicine*, Methods in Molecular Biology, vol. 3053, https://doi.org/10.1007/978-1-0716-5376-0_14,

Alternatively, platelets can be stored refrigerated for civilian use for up to 14 days [3]. Unfortunately, refrigerated platelets are rapidly cleared from circulation after transfusion and are only approved for transfusion of bleeding patients in whom standard room-temperature stored platelets are not available or not practical. Cold-stored circulating platelets are cleared by host macrophages and hepatocytes through integrin-mediated and lectin-binding receptor–mediated phagocytosis [4, 5].

A modified protocol to store refrigerated platelets, which is gentle to platelets and able to prevent their cold-induced storage lesion, could significantly prevent the growth of microorganisms, potentially allowing storage for longer periods, increasing safety of the existing inventory, reducing wastage, and facilitating the development of a healthy inventory of platelets ready-to-use at any time, even in underserved and poor-resource communities.

The small GTPase RHOA is critical for various signaling pathways within platelets, including receptor signaling and modulation of platelet receptors. This small GTPase plays essential roles in regulating platelet function both in terms of activation and adhesion [6]. Through rational and structure–activity relationship approaches, novel reversible inhibitors of RHOA activity have been identified [7, 8]. These inhibitors have relatively low affinity for the small GTPase substrates but effectively mitigate platelet storage lesions and rapid clearance post-transfusion when platelets are cold-stored ex vivo [9]. Pharmacologic inhibition of RHOA, mimicking the effects of genetic targeting, allows for cold storage of human platelets while preserving their survival and clotting activity to levels comparable to room-temperature stored platelets upon transfusion [9]. In this chapter, we will describe two main experimental approaches that helped us identify the potential benefit of RHOA inhibition in the prevention of cold-storage-induced human platelet clearance in preclinical, in vitro and in vivo models. First, a macrophage-mediated and hepatocyte-mediated phagocytosis assay is employed to quantify platelet clearance in vitro, and second, a preclinical animal model to analyze platelet survival in thrombocytopenic, innate- and adaptive-immune system–deficient mice is described.

2 Materials

2.1 Platelet Preparation

2.1.1 Preparation and Storage of Human Platelet Products

1. Whole blood (WB; units obtained through cooperating Blood Center) (*see* **Note 1**).
2. Transfer bags (*see* **Note 2**).
3. Platelet Additive Solution (PAS-E); we recommend PAS-3M (Grifols) (*see* **Note 3**).
4. Acrodose PL Leukocyte Reduction Filter.

Special Equipment

1. Blood banking centrifuge (Thermo Scientific RC 3BP Plus).
2. Plasma expressor.
3. Helmer horizontal agitator (PF900h or PF48h).

2.1.2 Platelet Labeling with Carboxyfluorescein Succinimidyl Ester

1. HEPES buffered solution (HBS), containing 119 mM NaCl, 5 mM KCl, 25 mM HEPES buffer, 2 mM $CaCl_2$, 2 mM $MgCl_2$, and 6 g/L glucose; pH 7.4.
2. Carboxyfluorescein succinimidyl ester (CFSE, Thermo-Fisher Scientific).
3. Anti-hCD61 PE antibody (BD Biosciences).
4. Fetal Bovine Serum (FBS, Atlanta Biologicals, Flowery Branch, GA).
5. Phosphate buffered saline (PBS); pH 7.5.

2.2 Platelet Phagocytosis

1. THP1 cells (ATCC, Manassas).
2. HepG2 cells (ATCC, Manassas).
3. RPMI-1 (Thermo-Fisher Scientific).
4. DMEM (Thermo-Fisher Scientific).
5. Fetal Bovine Serum (Atlanta Biologicals, Flowery Branch, GA).
6. Phosphate buffered saline (PBS); pH 7.5.
7. Penicillin (10,000 IU/mL)/Streptomycin (10 mg/mL) (Thermo-Fisher Scientific).
8. Transforming growth factor-beta (TGF-β) (R&D systems).
9. 25-(OH) 2-vitamin D3 (Sigma-Aldrich).
10. Phorbol-myristate acetate (PMA, Sigma-Aldrich).
11. Cell culture 0.05% trypsin/0.53% EDTA solution (Thermo-Fisher Scientific).
12. Anti-human CD68 antibody (Cat# 565595, BD Biosciences).
13. Anti-human CD11b antibody (CD11b; Cat# 557321, BD Biosciences).
14. Tissue culture plates (6-well and 24-well) (Costar).
15. Cell culture incubator (37 °C, 10% CO_2, 100% humidity).

Special Equipment

1. Flow Cytometer

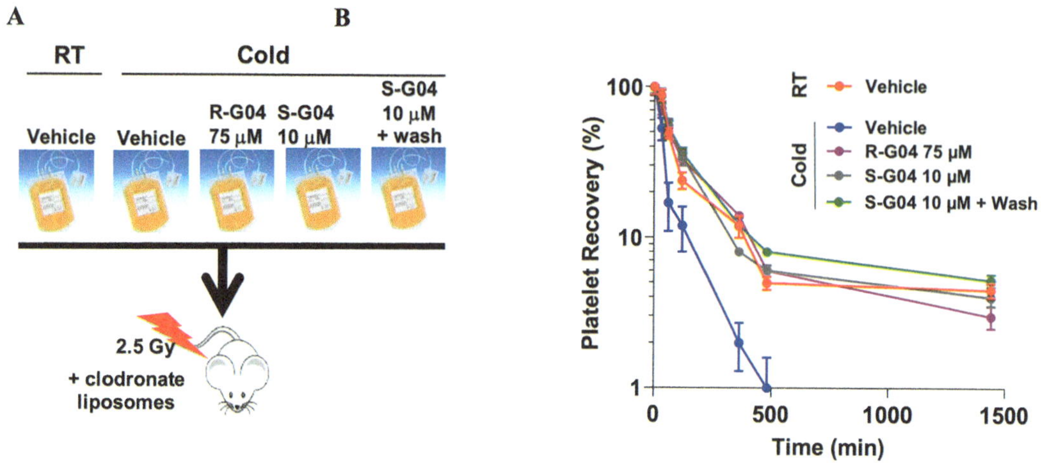

Fig. 1 Cold Storage Impairs Platelet Recovery In Vivo, Rescued by S-G04 Treatment with Post-Storage Wash Under Irradiation and Macrophage Depletion Conditions

2.3 In Vivo Platelet Survival

2.3.1 Mouse Conditioning and Transfusion (See Fig. 1)

1. ^{137}Cs γ Irradiator (J.L. Shepherd).
2. NOD/SCID/γc−/−(NSG) mice (males and females, 6–10 week old).
3. Chlodronate liposomes (Cat # CP-005-005, Liposoma).
4. 0.5 mL syringes.
5. 27 1/2-gauge needles.
6. Ca/Mg-free phosphate buffered saline (PBS, Thermo-Fisher).
7. Anti-murine Gr1 antibody (Cat#551460, BD Biosciences).
8. Anti-F4/80 antibody (Cat#566787, BD Biosciences).
9. Heparinized microhematocrit capillaries.
10. Isoflurane for inhalation anesthesia.
11. PharmLyse (Cat # 555899, BD Biosciences).

2.3.2 Platelet Survival Analysis

1. Heparinized microhematocrit capillaries.
2. Isoflurane for inhalation anesthesia.
3. 0.5 mL EDTA tubes.
4. Anti-hCD61 PE antibody (Cat # 555754, BD Biosciences).
5. PharmLyse (Cat # 555899, BD Biosciences).
6. Ca/Mg-free phosphate buffered saline (PBS, Thermo-Fisher).
7. GraphPad Prism version 10.0.0. for Windows, GraphPad Software, Boston, Massachusetts USA, www.graphpad.com.

3 Methods

3.1 Platelet Preparation

3.1.1 Preparation and Storage of Human Platelet Pooled Products

1. To generate platelet-rich plasma (PRP), pack WB units with all accessory bags (including filter) into centrifuge buckets of a blood banking centrifuge and centrifuge according to steps outlined below (see Table 1).
   (i) Centrifuge each of the collected units through a first centrifugation at 1000× *g* followed by separation of the platelet layer into separate bags (*see* **Notes 1** and **3**).
   (ii) After this first centrifugation, use plasma expressors to isolate PRP from red blood cells (RBCs) and let this rest for 30 min before proceeding to the second spin.
   (iii) After rest, centrifuge collected PRP a second time at 2500× *g* to deplete plasma (*see* **Note 4**). In detail, WB units were packed with all accessory bags into centrifuge buckets (including the filter) and spun in a blood banking centrifuge (Thermo Scientific RC 3BP Plus) using the following settings:
2. A reduced volume of 20 mL (assessed by weight; transformation: 1.03 g/mL) of plasma should be left for platelet resuspension in each unit.
3. Add a total of 40 mL of the additive solution PAS-E (PAS-3 M, Grifols Inc., Barcelona, Spain) to each unit for a final ratio of 67% PAS-E/33% plasma [10].
4. Pool five ABO identical platelet concentrates in a 600 mL transfer bag and leukocyte deplete through an Acrodose PL Leukocyte Reduction Filter within 2 h after starting the centrifugation process.
5. Split pooled platelets are split on Day 1 into sterile docked into 300 mL transfer bags, made of PVC with Tris (2-ethylhexyl) trimellitate (TOTM) plasticizer (Transfer Grifols 300 bags, Ref # 721293, Barcelona, Spain).

Table 1
Platelet-rich plasma (PRP) preparation in Thermo Scientific RC3 BP Plus blood banking centrifuge

Centrifugation order	Speed (× g)	Time (mins)	Brake setting	Temp (°C)
1	1000	4	OFF	23.0 ± 2
REST	Resting PRP for 30 min before proceeding to spin #2			
2	2500	6	5	23.0

6. After collection and reconstitution with additive solution, leave single platelet units to rest for 2 h (unagitated) and then move each to a shaker for 24–30 h under agitation conditions (60 cycles per minute) at room temperature (20–24 °C) or cold (1–4 °C) under the same agitation conditions in Helmer PF900h or Helmer PF48h horizontal agitators.
7. Each aliquot should contain a minimum of 5×10^{10} platelets with a range between 5.1 and 6.4×10^{10} platelets.
8. Alqiuots of 5-mL from the split platelet components were obtained by sterile docking (Terumo welder TSCD-II, Lakewood, CO) of 25 mL pouches (Fresenius-Kabi, Lake Zurich, IL or Grifols, Barcelona, Spain) at different time points for analysis. No more than three different days of storage were analyzed from the same products, after Day 1 (*see* **Note 5**).
9. After sampling, the platelet pools were immediately returned to their storage conditions.

3.1.2 Platelet Labeling with CFSE

1. Collect 2 mL of platelet-rich plasma (PRP) (containing ~5×10^8 platelets/mL) from each sample bag that has been stored with vehicle control (containing 0.05% DMSO) of specific inhibitors and centrifuged for 15 min at 180× *g*.
2. Collect the supernatant and centrifuge the samples for 8 min at 450× *g*.
3. Decant the supernatant and resuspend the platelets in 5 mL HBS and centrifuge the platelets.
4. For the washing step, wash the platelets one more time with HBS.
5. Platelet counts are obtained in a Sysmex XN-100 Hematology Analyzer (Lincolnshire, IL) with Blood Banking module and platelets are resuspended in 1 mL PBS.
6. Stain the platelets with CFSE (10 μM final concentration) diluted in PBS by incubating at 37 °C for 10 min.
7. Wash the platelets with PBS one time by centrifuging the platelets for 5 min at 450× *g*. Resuspend the platelets in 1 mL PBS.

3.2 Platelet Phagocytosis

3.2.1 Phagocytosis Assay Using THP1 Cells

1. Culture THP-1 cells in suspended DMEM supplemented with 10% fetal bovine serum (R&D, Minneapolis, MN), 2 mM glutamine (Life Technologies, Waltham, MA), 100 IU/mL penicillin, 0.1 mg/mL streptomycin (see **Note 6**).
2. Transfer 10,000 THP-1 cells to 24-well plates and allow them to adhere 24 h. Starve the cells for 30 min prior to start the experiments.

3. Upon fresh confluency, differentiate using 1 ng/mL TGF-β1 (R&D) and 50 nM 1, 25-$(OH)_2$-vitamin D3 (Sigma-Aldrich) for 24 h.
4. Activate the adherent macrophages by the addition of 15 ng/mL phorbol-myristate acetate (PMA, Sigma-Aldrich) for 15 min.
5. Stain each of the sample groups of platelets with CFSE as described earlier (see Subheading 3.1.2), wash the CFSE stained platelets and proceed to step 5 to overlay on top of the THP1 cells.
6. Overlay 1×10^7 CFSE labeled platelets stored in different conditions per THP-1 cell coated well and incubate for 30 min at 37 °C in a 5% CO_2 incubator.
7. Detach the monocyte layer by treatment with 0.05% trypsin/0.53% EDTA. Centrifuge the cell pellets and quantify the percentage of THP-1 cells containing CFSE-labeled platelets by flow cytometry (Fig. 2).

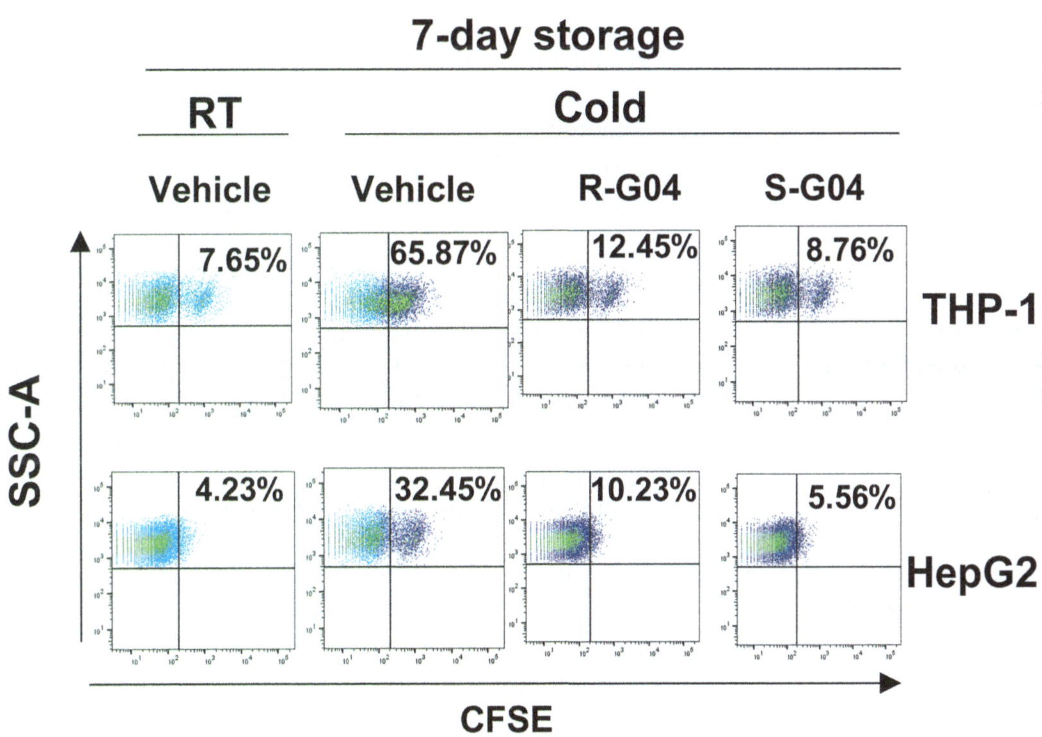

Fig. 2 Cold Storage–Induced Alterations in CFSE/SSC-A Cell Populations Are Mitigated by R-G04 and S-G04 Treatments in THP-1 and HepG2 Cells

3.2.2 Phagocytosis Assay Using HepG2 Cells

1. Culture HepG2 cells in αMEM, 10% fetal bovine serum, 100 IU/mL penicillin, and 0.1 mg/mL streptomycin (*see* **Note 6**).
2. Upon subconfluency (80%), trypsinize with 0.05% trypsin/ 0.53% EDTA solution.
3. Transfer 10,000 HepG2 cells per well to 24-well plates and allow them to adhere for 24 h.
4. Starve the cells in medium with no serum for 30 min prior to starting the experiments.
5. Overlay 1×10^7 CFSE-labeled platelets (see Subheading 3.1.2) with different conditions per well and incubate for 30 min at 37 °C.
6. Remove the nonadherent and extracellular adhered platelets by three washes with calcium-free PBS.
7. After the incubation period, wash the monolayers of HepG2 cells three times. Dissociate the HepG2 cells from the well using 0.05% trypsin/0.53% EDTA solution and quantify the percentage of HepG2 cells containing CFSE-labeled platelets by flow cytometry (Fig. 2).

3.3 In Vivo Platelet Survival

3.3.1 Mouse Conditioning and Transfusion

Irradiation of NSG Mice

1. Irradiate (sublethal 2.5 Gy) NSG mice 7 days before the infusion to induce moderate thrombocytopenia. We used a 137-Cesium source irradiator.
2. Analyze the CBC of each mouse using an automatic blood counter, and platelet counts should be around 350,000/mm^3.

Injection of Chlodronate and PBS Liposomes to NSG Mice

1. Inject 200 μL of Chlodronate liposomes (Cat# C-005, Liposoma) per mouse through intraperitoneal administration 72 h. Prior to infusion of platelets.
2. Follow steps listed in Subheading 3.3.1.3 below to analyze the macrophage depletion in the peripheral blood by flow cytometry using mouse Gr1 and F4/80 antibodies.

Flow Cytometry Analysis of Macrophage Depletion

1. Bleed each mouse (50 μL) in EDTA tubes by retro-orbital bleeding.
2. Add 2 mL of Red Blood Cell (RBC) lysis buffer (Thermo-Fisher, Cat #00-4333-57) to the flow cytometry tubes.
3. Add 20 μL of blood from each mouse to these tubes and vortex hard for 30 s. Incubate at room temperature for 10 min.
4. Collect the cells by centrifuging the tubes at 1700 rpm for 5 min.

5. Wash the cells in FACS buffer (PBS + 1% FBS + 0.05 mM sodium EDTA).
6. Stain the cells with mouse Gr1 and F4/80 antibodies by adding 2 μL of antibodies/sample in 200 μL of sample buffer and incubate for 15 min at room temperature.
7. Wash the cells with 2 mL of FACS buffer, decant the tubes, resuspend the cells in 500 μL of FACS buffer, and perform flow cytometry analysis.

Preparation of Human PRP Pooled Platelets for Platelet Infusion into NSG Mice

1. Two milliliter of human platelets (containing ~$2 \times 10^6/mm^3$) from each sample bag are stored with Vehicle (containing 0.05% DMSO) or inhibitor in each storage condition.
2. Stain each of the sample groups of platelets with CFSE as described above (see Subheading 3.1.2) and resuspend in PBS.
3. Infuse 1×10^9 platelets/mouse through tail vein of conditioned mice (see above).

3.3.2 Platelet Survival Analysis

Analysis of the Platelet Recovery In Vivo

1. Bleed (heparin-coated capillaries through retro-orbital bleeding; 25 μL; in EDTA tubes) mice under isoflurane anesthesia at different time points post-infusion.
2. Add 5 μL of blood to FACS tube and add 200 μL of PBS.
3. Stain the blood samples with anti-hCD61 antibody for 15 min.
4. Lyse red blood cells with PharmLyse solution as recommended by the manufacturer.
5. Dilute the samples by adding 700 μL of PBS and analyze the samples by using flow cytometry gating for CFSE$^+$ hCD61$^+$ samples and calculate the percentages of the donor platelet recovery.

Statistical Analysis of Platelet Recovery In Vivo

1. Data are presented as normalized ratio to time 0 (which is obtained within 1 min after the infusion of platelets).
2. Area under the curve analysis was estimated using Graphpad Statistical package.

4 Notes

1. Whole blood is collected using automated HemoFlow devices (500 ± 50 mL) and processed at room temperature within 8 h after collection following the manufacturers' instructions and Blood Center standardized operating procedures. Donors had not had any aspirin intake for at least 48 h before the donation.
2. Transfer bags of 300 mL, made of PVC with Tris (2-ethylhexyl) trimellitate (TOTM) plasticizer (Transfer Grifols 300 bags, Barcelona, Spain), can be used. Alternatively, 150 mL Charter

Medical CXP-500 bags (non-DEHP, polyolefin, gas permeable; Winston-Salem, NC) can also be used for storage at RT and in refrigerated conditions. Other transfer bags commercially available are expected to perform similarly. Experience with single-donor platelets collected with the Trima Accel v7.0 (Terumo BCT, Lakewood, CO) provides similar results.

3. PAS-3 (Fresenius-Kabi) could also be used in place of PAS-3M.
4. As an alternative to isolating PRP from whole blood units, platelet-rich plasma pooled (ABO group identical), whole-blood–derived platelets (Acrodose, Hemonetics Inc., Quincy, MA) can be used. Similarly, buffy-coat–derived platelet pools or Revios (TerumoBCT, Lakewood, CO)-generated platelet pool products can also be used. Alternatively, single-donor apheresis products collected in Trima Accel (Terumo BCT) or Amicus systems (Fresenius-Kabi, Lake Zurich, IL) can also be used.
5. All experiments were performed with platelets allowed to rewarm at room temperature for 15 min.
6. THP-1 and HepG2 cells should be used within 10 passages after receiving them from ATCC and always passed at 80% confluency.

Conflict of Interest Statement

This study was funded by NHLBI P01 HL158688, NCI R01 CA237016, and NIDDK R01 DK124115. Jose A Cancelas and Yi Zheng have equity and received consultant honoraria from Preservation Bio/OG4.

References

1. FDA (2022) Important information for blood establishments and tranfsusion services regarding bacterial contamination of platelets for transfusion. https://www.fda.gov/media/123448/download#:~:text=FDA%20has%20established%20regulations%20to%20address%20the%20control
2. Dunbar NM (2015) Modern solutions and future challenges for platelet inventory management. Transfusion 55:2053–2056. https://doi.org/10.1111/trf.13192
3. FDA (2023) Alternative procedures for the manufacture of cold-stored platelets intended for the treatment of active bleeding when conventional platelets are not available or their use is not practical: guidance for industry. https://www.fda.gov/media/169714/download#:~:text=FDA%20(we)%20is%20issuing%20this%20guidance%20to%20provide
4. Hoffmeister KM et al (2003) The clearance mechanism of chilled blood platelets. Cell 112:87–97. https://doi.org/10.1016/s0092-8674(02)01253-9
5. Rumjantseva V et al (2009) Dual roles for hepatic lectin receptors in the clearance of chilled platelets. Nat Med 15:1273–1280. https://doi.org/10.1038/nm.2030
6. Schoenwaelder SM et al (2002) RhoA sustains integrin alpha IIbbeta 3 adhesion contacts under high shear. J Biol Chem 277:14738–14746. https://doi.org/10.1074/jbc.M200661200
7. Dandamudi A et al (2023) Structure-activity relationship analysis of Rhosin, a RhoA GTPase

inhibitor, reveals a new class of antiplatelet agents. Int J Mol Sci 24. https://doi.org/10.3390/ijms24044167

8. Shang X et al (2012) Rational design of small molecule inhibitors targeting RhoA subfamily Rho GTPases. Chem Biol 19:699–710. https://doi.org/10.1016/j.chembiol.2012.05.009
9. Hegde S et al (2024) Inhibition of RHOA activity preserves the survival and hemostasis function of long-term cold stored platelets. Blood. https://doi.org/10.1182/blood.2023021453
10. Hegde S, Wellendorf AM, Zheng Y, Cancelas JA (2021) Antioxidant prevents clearance of hemostatically competent platelets after long-term cold storage. Transfusion 61:557–567. https://doi.org/10.1111/trf.16200

Chapter 15

Tracking and Testing Transfused Versus Endogenous Platelets with Biotin or Human Leukocyte Antigen

S. Lawrence Bailey, Martin Bochenek, Danny Youngs, Idoia Gimferrer, and Moritz Stolla

Abstract

Platelet transfusions are a critical and life-saving intervention utilized in bleeding patients and those at risk of bleeding. The laboratory assessment of fresh or stored platelets, both before and after transfusion, is of interest in licensing and basic science research. Platelets can be given either allogeneic (i.e., from a genetically different donor) or autologous (i.e., donor and recipient are the same, or genetically identical). In this protocol, we demonstrate how to distinguish circulating endogenous platelets from transfused platelets using biotinylation (useful for autologous and allogeneic transfusions) and HLA antibodies (practical in allogeneic transfusion scenarios) to differentiate between circulating endogenous and transfused platelets. Our described methodology not only enables the tracking of platelets but also facilitates post-transfusion functional assessment and the evaluation of platelet function post-transfusion using flow cytometry.

Key words Platelet transfusion, Platelet function, Platelet HLA, Biotin, Platelet storage, Human platelets, Platelet labeling

Abbreviations

PRP	Platelet Rich Plasma
PPP	Platelet Poor Plasma
PLT	Platelet or Platelet Count
WB	Whole Blood
MTB	Modified Tyrode's Buffer
RBC	Red Blood Cells
CBC	Complete Blood Count
LTA	Light Transmission Aggregometry

Sean R. Stowell and Connie M. Arthur (eds.), *Methods in Transfusion Medicine*, Methods in Molecular Biology, vol. 3053,
https://doi.org/10.1007/978-1-0716-5376-0_15,

1 Introduction

Platelets are transfused to bleeding patients and those at risk of bleeding (Fig. 1). They can be stored for up to 7 days for transfusion. Platelet transfusions are among the most frequently performed hospital procedures, and ~2.5 million platelet doses were distributed in the U.S. in 2021 [1]. Approximately 50% of all platelets are given to actively bleeding patients, and 50% are given for prophylaxis, i.e., to prevent bleeding [2]. Notably, a national survey reveals a shift in the utilization of blood components. While the use of red blood cells has been declining over the last few years, the demand for platelets has shown a slight but significant increase of 7.3% [1].

The function of platelets after storage and transfusion is poorly understood. The FDA prioritizes platelet circulation time over the function of stored platelets for licensing purposes. Radiolabeling with isotopes such as chromium-51 and indium-111 is the gold standard for measuring platelet recovery and survival [3]. However, other methods to trace platelets have been described, including biotinylation [4], mitochondrial DNA [5], and HLA [6]. Each procedure has specific advantages and disadvantages in certain testing scenarios. For example, biotinylation and HLA typing

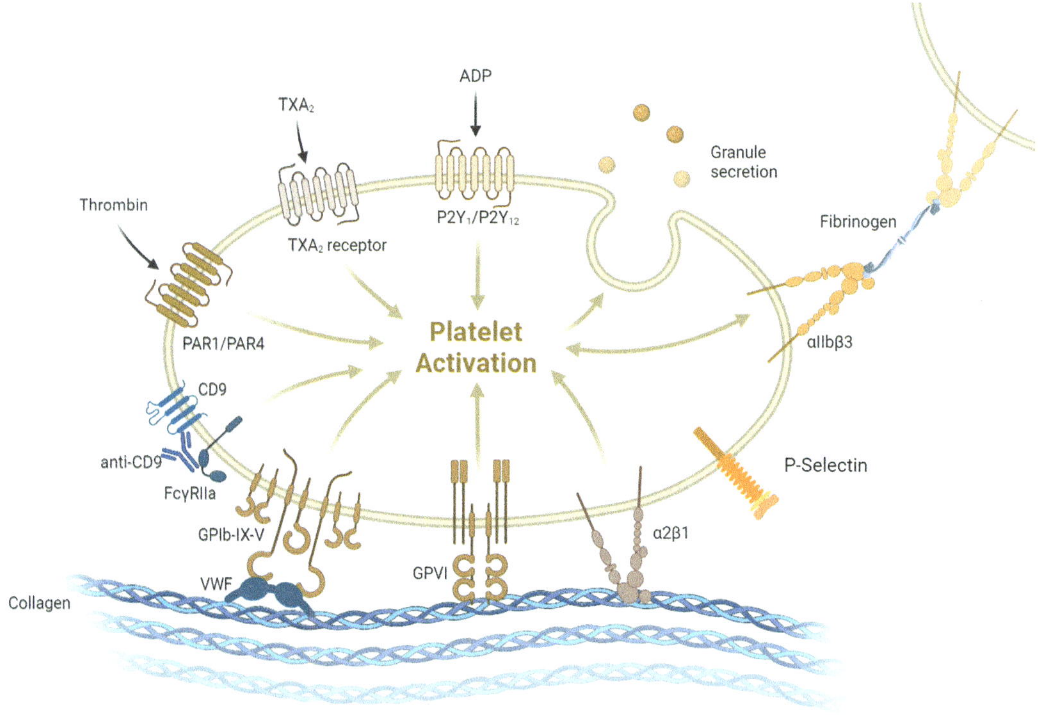

Fig. 1 Overview and examples of platelet activation pathways evaluated

enable the identification of endogenous and transfused platelets by flow cytometry, whereas tracing radiolabeled platelets requires a gamma counter and does not permit platelet function testing after transfusion [7]. However, separation based on differences in HLA expression and mitochondrial DNA can only be used after allogeneic transfusion (if both recipient and donor differ enough to allow for separation), in contrast to radiolabeling and biotinylation.

The protocol at hand describes a method for distinguishing between endogenous and transfused platelets and performing functional testing on both populations after transfusions. We opted to include the separation of transfused and endogenous platelets based on HLA differences (more likely to be beneficial in the allogeneic transfusion scenario) and biotinylation (applicable to the autologous and allogeneic transfusion scenarios). This protocol can be applied to in vitro transfusion models [8], xenotransfusions [9], and clinical trials with allogeneic transfusions, e.g., to bleeding surgery patients, trauma patients, and thrombocytopenic patients, and to studies with healthy human volunteers, where allogeneic transfusions are unethical.

We validated an array of anti-HLA antibodies, all conjugated to the same fluorophore. With this panel of antibodies, we ran the assays on both the donor-stored platelets and recipient blood to identify a single platelet HLA mismatch. This mismatch between donor and recipient platelet HLA subclass can be used to discriminate between patient endogenous versus transfused platelets by flow cytometry.

Then, the appropriate HLA antibody was used in a multicolor flow cytometry assay to assess functional and phenotypic differences between transfused and endogenous platelets with and without agonist stimulation. Possible non-HLA platelet membrane surface antibody targets were included: GPIbα, GPVI, phosphatidylserine, activated conformation of αIIbβ3, and P-selectin.

2 Materials

2.1 Special Reagent Preparation

2.1.1 Labeling Lactadherin Using Rapid DyLight 405 Lightning Link Kit

1. Lactadherin: Made in house with Bovine Lactadherin (Cellsystems, #BLANC-1200).
2. DyLight 405 Rapid Lightning Link (abcam, #ab201798).
3. Flow Cytometry Staining Buffer (ThermoFisher, #00-4222-26).
4. PBS (Ca++ free).
5. 2 mL screw cap tube.

2.1.2 Modified Tyrode's Buffer

1. 50mLFalcon tube
2. NaCl.
3. HEPES.
4. Glucose.
5. BSA.
6. MgCl2.
7. KCl.
8. NaH2PO4.

2.2 Platelet Preparation

2.3 Agonist Preparation

2.4 Flow Cytometry Assay

1. Cytometer with violet, blue, yellow-green, and red lasers (we use CytoFlex LX in a VSSC configuration—Beckman Coulter).
2. Uncoated 96-well plate for use in cytometer.
3. Calibrated pipettes and tips (P2 through P1000, recommend including a P10).
4. 1.7 mL Eppendorf tubes, racks
5. Flow Cytometry Staining Buffer (ThermoFisher, #00-4222-26).
6. IC Fixation Buffer (ThermoFisher, #00-0222-49).
7. PBS (Ca++ free).
8. Acetic Acid (0.1 M).
9. Modified Tyrode's Buffer (*see* Subheading 3.1.2).

List of Antibodies

10. PE—GPVI (BD, 565241).
11. BV421—CD42b (BD, 740075).
12. PerCP-Cy5.5—CD61 (BD, 564173).
13. PE—CD62P (BD, 555524).
14. DyLight 405—Lactadherin: Made in house with: Bovine Lactadherin (Cellsystems, #BLANC-1200) and DyLight 405 Rapid Lightning Link (abcam, #ab201798) and diluted with flow cytometry staining buffer.
15. FITC—PAC-1 (BD, 340507).

Table 1
Outline of agonists and doses

Agonist:	Target:	Proxy for:	Units	Stock	High dose[a]	High dose (10X)
ADP	P2Y1, P2Y12	ADP	uM	1000	1.0	10
Trap-6	Par-1	Thrombin	uM	3200	5.0	50
CRP	GPIV	Collagen	ug/mL	3000	0.3	3
U46619	Thromboxane A_2 Receptor (TP)	Thromboxane A_2 (TXA_2)	uM	10000	1.0	10
Ristocetin	GPIb (alpha & beta)	vWF modifier	mg/mL	125	1.5	15
anti-CD9	CD9	Fc receptor activation	ug/mL	1000	10.0	100
Par4 Peptide	Par-4	Thrombin	uM	50,000	100.0	1000
CLEC2 (AYP1)	CLEC2	Podoplanin	ug/mL	500	1.0	10
PAF-C16	PAF 5	PAF	uM	1000	0.2	2

[a]This is the highest tested dose concentration in the final label/activation reaction and generally has a strong activation profile in a normal subject. The 10X is also provided, as it is the "working" concentration that is mixed into the label/activation reaction. Note, these are sometimes very steep dilutions and may require a few intermediate dilutions to ensure pipetting accuracy

16. APC—CD63 (Invitrogen, A15712).
17. APC—HLA-A2 (BioLegend, 343307).
18. APC—HLA-A3 (Invitrogen, 17-5754-42).
19. APC—HLA-B7 (BioLegend, 372405).
20. APC—HLA-B8 (Miltenyi Biotec, 130-126-633).
21. APC—Streptavidin (BioLegend, 405204).
22. BV421 Isotype (BD, 56436).
23. FITC Isotype (BD, 340755).
24. PE Isotype (BD, 340760).
25. APC Isotype (BD, 340442).

List of Agonist (See Table 1)

26. TRAP-6 (Bio-Techne, 3497).
27. CRP-XL (CambCol Laboratories, Cambridge, UK).
28. U46619 (TOCRIS, 1932).

29. ADP (Chronolog, #384).
30. Ristocetin (Chronolog, #396).
31. Anti-CD9 (abcam, AB2215).
32. Par4 Peptide (GenScript, RP11529).
33. CLEC2—clone: AYP1 (BioLegend, 372002).
34. PAF-C16—(Cayman Chemical, 60900).

3 Methods

3.1 Special Reagent Preparation

3.1.1 Labeling Lactadherin Using Rapid DyLight 405 Lightning Link Kit

1. Reconstitute the Lactadherin in 100 uL PBS.
2. Follow the manufacturer's instructions for the labeling kit and add 10 uL of the modifier reagent supplied to the resuspended Lactadherin.
3. Add this mixture to the DyLight 405 Conjugation Mix labeling tube supplied and wait at least 15 min.
4. Add 10 uL of the Quencher reagent supplied and wait 5 min.
5. Take this mixture to a light sealed 2 mL screw cap tube and add 565 uL of the flow cytometry staining buffer (final concentration is 73 pg/uL).
6. This can be kept for 18 months in the fridge.

3.1.2 Modified Tyrode's Buffer

1. Modified Tyrode's Buffer (MTB) has a lot of small variations among labs; this is the one we use:

			g/1 L	**g/500 mL**
NaCl	**137**	**mM**	**8.00**	**4.00**
HEPES	20	mM	4.76	2.38
Glucose	5.6	mM	1.01	0.51
BSA	1	g/L	1.00	0.50
$MgCl_2$	1	mM	0.20	0.10
KCl	2.7	mM	0.20	0.10
NaH_2PO_4	3.3	mM	0.47	0.24

2. Adjust pH to 7.4.
3. Filter and aliquot 40 mL into 50 mL Falcon tubes and freeze at −80 °C until needed.
4. Ensure the MTB is at room temperature prior to use.

3.2 Platelet Preparation

3.2.1 From Citrated Whole Blood: Make a "Dirty" PRP

1. Make PRP within 4 h of collection, leaving citrate collected whole blood undisturbed while preparing labeling mixes and agonists.
2. Centrifuge ~1 mL citrated whole blood in a microcentrifuge for 5 min at 100× *g*.
3. Take supernatant (the PRP) while avoiding the pelleted blood cell layer (RBCs and buffy coat). If some RBC is taken up that is okay, the goal is to gently separate the majority of the RBCs.
4. Obtain a platelet count (PLT), either by use of an automated analyzer to get a CBC, or in the absence of dedicated equipment, a hemacytometer can be used. Ensure PLT concentration is <300 K/uL; if higher, dilute with MTB or plasma (PPP) derived from additional WB spun at 2000× *g* (*see* **Note 1**).

3.2.2 From Apheresis Bag

1. Take small aliquot (ensure sterility from a closed system bag that is intended for later use). The amount needed is rather small, 5 mL should work for platelets and plasma for diluting the sample, or as little as 1 mL if diluting with MTB.
2. Count for CBC and dilute PLT concentration to <300 K/uL, with MTB or PPP derived from additional apheresis platelets spun at 2000× *g* (*see* **Note 1**).

3.3 Agonist Preparation: (See Note 2)

3.3.1 ADP

1. Follow manufactures' instructions for reconstitution. Typically, this leads to a concentration that is useful for LTA or WBA (this assay often runs in tandem with those tests), which will be the stock concentration for long-term storage. Keep in aliquots suitable for that task if required at −80 °C for up to a year.
2. From the freezer, warm a stock concentration tube until unfrozen.
3. Dilute the stock concentration to 10X desired testing concentration with PBS.
4. Store 10X desired testing concentration in refrigerator for up to 8 h prior to testing.

3.3.2 TRAP-6

1. Adding 179.9 uL ddH_2O to 1 mg lyophilized TRAP will make a 3.2 mM stock. Store at −80 °C in 10 uL aliquots for up to a year.
2. From the freezer, warm a stock concentration tube until unfrozen. *DO NOT REFREEZE* stock tube.
3. Dilute the stock concentration to 10X desired testing concentration with PBS.
4. Store 10X desired testing concentration in refrigerator for up to 5 h prior to testing.

3.3.3 CRP-XL

1. Stored at −20 °C at 3 mg/mL in 10 uL aliquots.
2. Dilute 10 uL of CRP in 990uL 0.1 M acetic acid. This can be refrozen once in 50 uL aliquots at −20 °C.
3. From this new dilution, dilute 5 uL in 45 uL PBS—this makes 10X. Use within 5 h and refrigerate when not using.

3.3.4 U46619

1. Adding 285 uL ddH_2O to 1 mg U46619 will make a 10 mM stock. Store at −80 °C in 10 uL aliquots for up to a year.
2. From the freezer, warm a stock concentration tube until unfrozen.
3. Dilute the stock concentration to 10X the desired testing concentration with PBS.
4. Store 10X desired testing concentration in the refrigerator for up to 5 h prior to testing.

3.3.5 Ristocetin

1. Follow manufactures instructions for reconstitution. Typically, this leads to a concentration that is useful for LTA or WBA (this assay often runs in tandem with those tests), which will be the stock concentration for long-term storage. Keep in aliquots suitable for that task if required at −80 °C for up to a year.
2. From the freezer, warm a stock concentration tube until unfrozen.
3. Dilute the stock concentration to 10X desired testing concentration with PBS.
4. Store 10X desired testing concentration in refrigerator for up to 5 h prior to testing.

3.3.6 Anti-CD9

1. Arrives from manufacturer ready to be used. Store in refrigerator.
2. Dilute the stock concentration to 10X desired testing concentration with PBS.
3. Store 10X desired testing concentration in refrigerator for up to 5 h prior to testing.

3.3.7 Par4 Peptide

1. Adding 147 uL ddH_2O to 5 mg lyophilized Par4 peptide will make a 50 mM stock. Store at −80 °C in 6 uL aliquots for up to a year.
2. From the freezer, warm a stock concentration tube until unfrozen. *DO NOT REFREEZE* stock tube.
3. Dilute the stock concentration to 10X desired testing concentration with PBS.
4. Store 10X desired testing concentration in refrigerator for up to 5 h prior to testing.

3.3.8 CLEC2 (AYP1)

1. Arrives from manufacturer ready to be used. Store in refrigerator.
2. Dilute the stock concentration to 10X desired testing concentration with PBS.
3. Store 10X desired testing concentration in refrigerator for up to 5 h prior to testing.

3.3.9 PAF-C16

1. Add 1.91 mL PBS to 1 mg PAF-C16 to make a 1 mM stock. Store at −80 °C in 10 uL aliquots for up to a year.
2. From the freezer, warm a stock concentration tube until unfrozen. *DO NOT REFREEZE* stock tube.
3. Dilute the stock concentration to 10X desired testing concentration with PBS.
4. Store 10X desired testing concentration in refrigerator for up to 5 h prior to testing.

3.4 Flow Cytometry Assay

The flow assay is a two-pronged approach using (1) a tube looking at GPVI and CD42b to detect the levels of expression and (2) at least 2 tubes looking at a) a tube with no agonist to detect phosphatidyl serine (PS) positivity (Lactadherin), integrin activation (CD61, Pac1), alpha granule secretion (CD62p), and as a wild card (when the use of the APC channel is not needed for population differentiation), dense granule secretion (CD63) as well as b) up to 8 (tested) separate agonist tubes, often under a couple of concentrations. Additionally, there will be two isotype tubes, one for the surface markers tube and one for the agonist induced activation markers tubes. We also include a no color control tube (*see* **Note 3**).

3.4.1 Assay Setup

Make a master mix for the surface marker tubes and the agonist induced activation marker tubes according to Table 2. (*see* further detail in Subheading 3.4.1.1, 3.4.1.2 and 3.4.1.3 below) (*see* **Notes 4** and **5**).

Surface Expression Assay (No Agonist) Setup

1. Make master mix (U1), enough for every sample and timepoint in your experiment as well as a small additional amount for adsorption loss, with a 1X (90 uL) of: (*see* **Note 6**).
   (a) 87.0 uL Stain Buffer
   (b) 0.3 uL PerCP-cy5—CD61
   (c) 0.2 uL PE—GPVI
   (d) 2.5 uL BV421—CD42b
2. In a labeled 1.7 mL Eppendorf tube, for each sample, pipette 90 uL of U1 master mix.
3. This has been validated for storage for 24 h when kept in the dark and refrigerated.

Table 2
Pipetting schematic

For 1X (per tube, volumes in uL)								
	Unstim 1 (U1)	**Unstim 2 (U2)**	**Stim 1 (S1)**	**Stim 2 (S2)**	**Stim etc....**	**Iso U1**	**Iso U2**	**No color**
Stain buffer	87.0	70.2	70.2	70.2	70.2	86.6	81.8	90.0
PerCP-cy5—CD61	0.3	0.3	0.3	0.3	0.3	0.3	0.3	
PE—GP6	0.2							
BV421—CD42b	2.5							
PE—CD62p		2.5	2.5	2.5	2.5			
DyLight 405—Lactadherin		2.0	2.0	2.0	2.0			
Fitc—Pac1		5.0	5.0	5.0	5.0			
APC—CD63								
PBS		10.0						
Stim 1 (diluted to 10X final)			10.0					
Stim 2 (diluted to 10X final)				10.0				
Stim etc.[a] (diluted to 10X final)					10.0			
APC—ISO								
PE—ISO						0.6	2.5	
FITC- ISO							5.0	
BV421—ISO						2.5	0.4	
Dirty PRP	10.0	10.0	10.0	10.0	10.0	10.0	10.0	10.0
Final reaction volume	100.0	100.0	100.0	100.0	100.0	100.0	100.0	100.0

[a]Repeat as needed to include all stimulation conditions

Activation Surface Marker Expression Assay (Agonist) Setup

1. Make master mix (U2), enough for all the no agonist and each agonist being tested for all timepoints in your experiment as well as a small additional amount for adsorption loss, with a 1X (80uL) of:
   (a) 70.2 uL Stain Buffer
   (b) 0.3 uL PerCP-cy5—CD61
   (c) 2.5 uL PE—CD62P
   (d) 2.0 uL DyLight 405—Lactadherin

   (e) 5.0 uL FITC—PAC-1
   (f) *If using the wild card slot for CD63.
      (i) Reduce the stain buffer amount from 70.2 uL to 65.2 uL.
      (ii) Add 5.0 uL APC-CD63.
2. In a labeled Eppendorf tube, for each sample, agonist, agonist concentration, and no agonist control, pipette 80 uL of U2 master mix.
3. This has been validated for storage for 24 h when kept in the dark and refrigerated.

Isotype and Unlabeled Tube Setup

1. Isotype U1 (Iso U1)—90 uL:
   (a) 86.6 uL Stain Buffer
   (b) 0.3 uL PerCP-cy5—CD61
   (c) 0.6 uL PE—Isotype
   (d) 2.5 uL BV421—Isotype
2. Isotype U2 (Iso U2)—90 uL:
   (a) 80.2 uL Stain Buffer
   (b) 0.3 uL PerCP-cy5—CD61
   (c) 2.5 uL PE—Isotype
   (d) 5.0 uL FITC—Isotype
   (e) 2.0 uL BV421—Isotype (*see* **Note 12**)
   (f) *If using the wild card slot for CD63
      (i) Reduce the stain buffer amount from 80.2 uL to 75.2 uL
      (ii) Add 5.0 uL APC Isotype
3. Unlabeled Tube—90uL:
   (a) 90.0 uL Stain Buffer.

3.4.2 Running the Assay

1. For the U1, nothing is added while the agonist tubes are finished being set up.
2. For each agonist tube add:
   (a) Tube (U2)—10 uL PBS (this is the no agonist tube), mixing gently with pipette.
   (b) Tube (S1)—10 uL of 10X agonist 1, at highest concentration, mixing gently with pipette.
      (i) If doing more than 1 concentration, the next tube would be S1b, S1c, etc.
   (c) Tube (S2)—10 uL of 10X agonist 2, at highest concentration, mixing gently with pipette.

(i) If doing more than 1 concentration, the next tube would be S2b, S2c, etc.

(d) Do this for all agonists and concentrations in assay in like fashion (i.e., S3, S4, S4b, etc., *see* **Note 7**).

3. For the Iso U1, Iso U2, and No color tubes, nothing is added while the agonist tubes are finished being set up.
4. With all tubes now ready for PRP, pipette 10 uL of PRP to each tube, mixing gently with pipette.
   (a) Start a 15-min timer after first tube and continue to aliquot the PRP to each subsequent tube working at a quick but steady pace.
   (b) After last tube is mixed, note the time left on the timer.
      (i) Take the time elapsed and divide by the total number of tubes to make a mental note of the time per tube.
5. Close each lid and place in the dark at room temperature with no agitation.
6. As the time is about to elapse, retrieve the samples from the dark and open the lids of the tubes.
7. After timer elapses, flood each tube with 900 uL of cold IC Fix /PBS mix (5 parts IC Fix to 4 parts PBS).
   (a) Add this to each tube at the same time per tube as you added the PRP (*see* **Note 8**).
8. Place in fridge for 30 min to 3 h.
9. Centrifuge each tube for 5 min at 2000× *g*; decant the supernatant (*see* **Note 9**).
10. If analysis will be happening imminently, resuspend in 0.4 mL PBS and plate samples (200 uL per well) for your run, storing for up to 48 h to analyze. Else, resuspend in 1 mL flow cytometry staining buffer if there will be a second label by HLA or biotinylation for population differentiation (see next section). If analyzing now, retain the tubes with leftover cells in the fridge; this should be enough to replate again if there is a need to rerun the samples.

3.4.3 Second Label HLA Analysis—When Using HLA as a Discriminator for Donor Versus Recipient Platelets

1. Follow **steps 2–14** below to screen for HLA mismatch between the donor and the recipient (*see* **Note 10**).
2. From a pre-transfusion recipient blood sample, you may already have made a "dirty" PRP, if not make one:
   (i) Make PRP within 4 h of collection, leaving citrate collected whole blood undisturbed while preparing labeling mixes and agonist.
   (ii) Centrifuging ~1 mL citrated whole blood in a microcentrifuge for 5 min at 100× *g*.

(iii) Take PRP (some RBC is okay)—the goal is to gently separate the majority of the RBCs.

(iv) Count on CBC and ensure PLT concentration is <300 K/uL; if higher, dilute with MTB or plasma derived from additional WB spun at 2000× *g*.

3. From a segment of the donor apheresis unit, cut the tubing (taking all necessary splash precautions) and drain into an Eppendorf tube.
4. Set up two Eppendorf tubes, each with 900 uL of cold IC Fix/PBS mix (5 parts IC Fix to 4 parts PBS).

   (i) Label one recipient PRP and add 50 uL recipient PRP to tube.

   (ii) Label one donor PRP and add 10 uL donor PRP to tube.

5. Place in fridge for 30 min to 3 h.
6. Centrifuge each tube for 5 min at 2000× *g*; decant the supernatant (*see* **Note 9**).
7. Resuspend in 1 mL flow cytometry staining buffer, place in fridge, and use for further steps within 48 h.
8. Set up 4 master mix tubes (each is enough for three labeling tubes).

   (a) Tube A2

   (i) 1.5 uL APC-HLA-A2

   (ii) 268.5 uL flow cytometry staining buffer

   (iii) Mix by pipetting and aliquot 90 uL to two wells on a 96-well plate; one well will be used for the donor and one well for the recipient.

   (b) Tube A3

   (i) 5.6 uL APC-HLA-A3

   (ii) 264.4 uL flow cytometry staining buffer

   (iii) Mix by pipetting and aliquot 90 uL to two wells on same 96-well plate; one well will be used for the donor and one well for the recipient.

   (c) Tube B7

   (i) 2.8 uL APC-HLA-B7

   (ii) 267.2 uL flow cytometry staining buffer

   (iii) Mix by pipetting and aliquot 90 uL to two wells on same 96-well plate; one well will be used for the donor and one well for the recipient.

   (d) Tube B8

   (i) 2.3 uL APC-HLA-B8

   (ii) 267.7 uL flow cytometry staining buffer

(iii) Mix by pipetting and aliquot 90 uL to two wells on same 96-well plate; one well will be used for the donor and one well for the recipient.

9. Set up an isotype antibody gradient using the APC isotype with three concentrations to match the concentrations of the HLA antibody in **step 8**.
   (a) Make the following three wells using the same 96-well plate
      (i) Well iso 1
         1. 15.0 uL APC Isotype
         2. 165.0 uL flow cytometry staining buffer
      (ii) Well iso 1/2
         1. 90.0 uL flow cytometry staining buffer
      (iii) Well iso 1/4
         1. 90.0 uL flow cytometry staining buffer
   (b) Take 90 uL from well iso 1 and mix into well iso 1/2 with gentle pipetting.
   (c) Take 90 uL from well iso 1/2 and mix into well iso 1/4 with gentle pipetting.
   (d) Take 90 uL from well iso 1/4 and throw away.
10. Make another isotype gradient by repeating **step 3** in new wells; one set will be used for the donor and one set for the recipient.
11. With seven tubes (A2, A3, B7, B8, and three isotype antibody gradients) for both donor and recipient:
   (a) Aliquot 10 uL of donor PRP into the donor set.
   (b) Aliquot 10 uL of recipient PRP into the recipient set.
12. Set a timer for 15 min and place in the dark at room temperature with no agitation.
13. After timer elapses, flood each well with 150 uL PBS.
14. Analyze samples on flow cytometer to determine if a suitable HLA difference exists between donor and recipient platelets. Use the strongest difference if more than one exists, and ideally it is also preferable to have a positive donor/negative recipient difference.
15. After HLA screen is complete, centrifuge each tube from **step 10** of Subheading 3.4.2 for 5 min at 2000× *g*; decant the supernatant (*see* **Note 9**).
16. Add 80 uL flow cytometry staining buffer to each tube and resuspend by gentle pipette mixing.

17. Set up the HLA master mix using the selected HLA marker, enough for every sample and timepoint in your experiment as well as a small additional amount for adsorption loss, with a 1X (50 uL) of:
    (a) If HLA-A2 is selected
        (i) 0.5 uL APC-HLA-A2
        (ii) 49.5 uL flow cytometry staining buffer
        (iii) Mix by quick vortexing.
    (b) If HLA-A3 is selected
        (i) 1.9 uL APC-HLA-A3
        (ii) 48.1 uL flow cytometry staining buffer
        (iii) Mix by quick vortexing.
    (c) If HLA-B7 is selected
        (i) 0.9 uL APC-HLA-B7
        (ii) 49.1 uL flow cytometry staining buffer
        (iii) Mix by quick vortexing.
    (d) If HLA-B8 is selected
        (i) 0.8 uL APC-HLA-B8
        (ii) 49.2 uL flow cytometry staining buffer
        (iii) Mix by quick vortexing.
18. Plate 50 uL of each sample tube in 96-well plate that will be used for flow cytometry; also plate the isotypes and no label controls as well as a donor only well (*see* **Note 11**).
19. Using a multichannel pipette, add 50 uL of the prepared master mix of selected APC-HLA antibody to each well with gentle mixing, except for the unlabeled well, which gets 50 uL PBS.
20. Let the label reaction go for at least 20 min (up to an hour has been tested) in the dark and unagitated.
21. Flood each well with 150 uL PBS and analyze on flow cytometer.

3.4.4 Second Label Biotin Labeled Platelet Analysis—When Using Biotin as a Discriminator Between Platelet Populations

1. Make a dilution of APC-Streptavidin, enough for 50 uL per sample for all samples being analyzed, plus a bit extra for adsorption loss. For 1X:
    (a) 49.4 ul flow cytometry staining buffer.
    (b) 0.6 uL of APC-Streptavidin.
    (c) Vortex briefly and centrifuge briefly to mix and collect at the bottom of the tube.
    (d) Spin each sample tube for 5 min at 2000 g; decant the supernatant (*see* **Note 9**).

2. Add 80 uL flow cytometry staining buffer to each tube and resuspend by gentle pipette mixing.
3. Pipette 50 uL of each tube in a 96-well plate that will be used for flow cytometry; also pipette isotypes and no label controls as well as a donor only well.
   (a) Retain the tubes with leftover cells in the fridge; this should be enough to replate again if there is need to rerun the samples.
4. Using a multichannel pipette, add 50 uL of the prediluted APC- Streptavidin to each well with gentle mixing, except for the unlabeled well, which gets 50 uL PBS.
5. Let the label proceed for at least 15 min, in the dark and unagitated.
6. Flood each well with 150 uL PBS and analyze on a flow cytometer.

4 Notes

1. The assay was originally created to be used for subject samples in a study where the subjects received platelets after cardiac surgery. As such, the PRPs from these subjects were always <300 K. When the concentration is higher, the amounts of antibodies and agonists may need to be adjusted to reflect this. However, it is easy to adjust samples down to an appropriate sub 300 K concentration, which also ensures that larger clumping is avoided, and, depending on the goals of the experiments, it is often appropriate to have matched concentrations across samples.
2. Make agonist dilutions at 10X the final reaction concentration to be used.
3. Each label/reaction tube is final label reaction volume of 100 uL.
4. Due to our flow cytometer's detection capabilities, using the fluorochromes chosen (PE, FITC, PerCP-Cy5, BV421/ Dylight 405, and APC) does not require compensation; these colors also have wide commercial availability for our selected antibodies. We predict using fluorochrome selectors that other combinations may be possible, allowing up to seven colors with minimal crossover; however, off-the-shelf options for many of the targets in these colors are not available (indeed, there are not even available labeling kits for some of the colors). Concentrations of the platelets detected per volume are also evaluable without beads, allowing for the detection of clumping.

5. Depending on the amounts of samples being run, this assay can be antibody and agonist intensive. However, with the antibodies listed, we have found that after running antibody titrations, we can use less than the manufacturer-recommended amounts. While using less almost always results in a lower staining index (SI), in many cases even with a lower SI, it can be high enough that positives remain well over negatives. Accordingly, we usually went with a dilution that retained 2/3rds of the manufacture's recommended amounts of SI. Similarly, agonists are often made at a much higher concentration for aggregometry, but in this flow assay much less is used.
6. There is an open FITC slot here if you have another surface marker of interest to add; just reduce the amount of stain buffer by the amount of new antibody added. Also include FITC Isotype in the equivalent concentration to your Iso U1 setup later.
7. When setting up experiments and selecting agonists, it is helpful to run agonist dose curves so that an adequate dose able to differentiate between populations can be selected. Here we might go with dose 1 as a high dose, dose 2 as a middle dose, and dose 3 as a dose where we expect little activation. *See* Fig. 2.
8. This ensures that each tube is reacted for the same time. This is done easily with a count-up timer.
9. We typically decant by the flick method over the sink, but it can also be done with a transfer pipette.

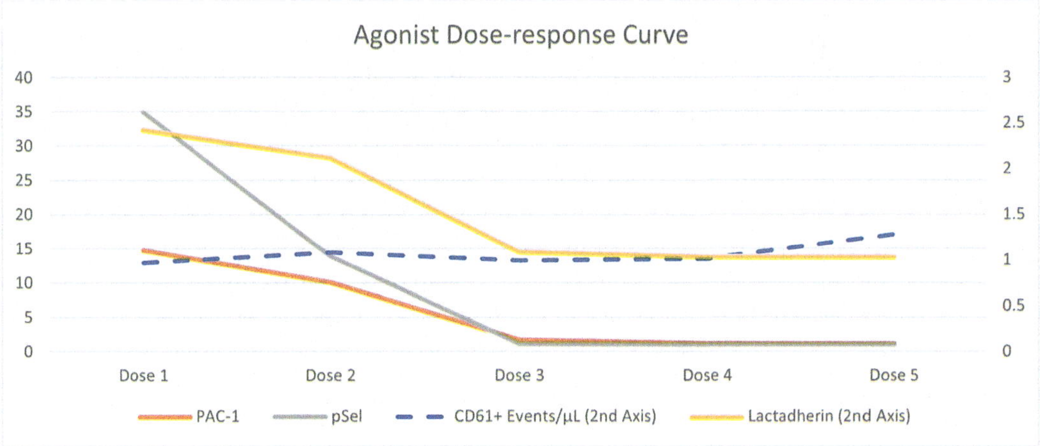

Fig. 2 Example agonist dose-response curve

10. In order to establish an HLA mismatch, either the HLA MHC class I of both the donor and recipient must be known or a mismatch can also be detected after the transfusion, as long as a segment from the donor unit can be retained from the recipient and you have access to pre-transfusion recipient PRP (often from a pre-transfusion time point).
11. Retain the tubes with leftover cells in the fridge; this should be enough to replate again if there is a need to rerun the samples.
12. BV421 and DyLight 405 have very similar emission spectrums, and we feel comfortable using the BV421 iso for both with our 405 laser in the 450/45 window—one could use a DyLight 405 iso instead if they wanted.

Conflicts of Interest

Moritz Stolla has received research grants from Cerus Corp. and Terumo BCT. All other authors have no conflicts of interest to declare that are relevant to the content of this chapter.

References

1. Free RJ, Sapiano MRP, Ortiz JLC, Stewart P, Berger J, Basavaraju SV (2023) Continued stabilization of blood collections and transfusions in the United States: findings from the 2021 National Blood Collection and utilization survey. Transfusion 63(S4):S8–S18. PMCID: PMC10543447
2. Gottschall J, Wu Y, Triulzi D, Kleinman S, Strauss R, Zimrin AB, McClure C, Tan S, Bialkowski W, Murphy E, Ness P, Study for the NRE and DE (REDS-III) (2020) The epidemiology of platelet transfusions: an analysis of platelet use at 12 US hospitals. Transfusion 60(1):46–53. PMID: 31850522
3. Collaborative TBE for ST (BEST) (2006) Platelet radiolabeling procedure. Transfusion 46(s3): 59S–66S
4. Stohlawetz P, Horvath M, Pernerstorfer T, Nguyen H, Vondrovec B, Robisch A, Eichler HG, Spitzauer S, Jilma B (1999) Effects of nitric oxide on platelet activation during plateletpheresis and in vivo tracking of biotinylated platelets in humans. Transfusion 39(5):506–514. PMID: 10336001
5. Doescher A, Petershofen EK, Hertenstein B, Kraemer D, Casper J, Schmidt J, Müller TH (2015) Quantification of transfused PLTs. Transfusion 55(1):55–63. PMID: 25056505
6. Hughes DL, Evans G, Metcalfe P, Goodall AH, Williamson LM (2005) Tracking and characterisation of transfused platelets by two colour, whole blood flow cytometry. Br J Haematol 130(5):791–794. PMID: 16115139
7. van der Meer PF, Tomson B, Brand A (2010) In vivo tracking of transfused platelets for recovery and survival studies: an appraisal of labeling methods. Transfus Apher Sci 42(1): 53–61. PMID: 19931490
8. Ferrer Marin F, Chavda C, Lampa M, Michelson AD, Frelinger AL, Sola-Visner M (2011) Effects of in vitro adult platelet transfusions on neonatal hemostasis. J Thromb Haemost 9(5): 1020–1028. PMCID: PMC3130591
9. Bailey SL, Bochenek M, Chauhan A, Miller B, Stolla M (2024) Biotin labeling allows for post-transfusion functional assessment of stored human platelets in mice. Transfusion 64: 1306. PMID: 38757806

Chapter 16

Analysis of Biotinylated Red Blood Cells Following Transfusion

Mischa L. Covington, Patricia E. Zerra, Samata P. Varadkar, Dominique Paz, Rebecca C. Hale, Connie M. Arthur, John D. Roback, Ross M. Fasano, Marianne E. M. Yee, and Sean R. Stowell

Abstract

Patients with sickle cell disease (SCD) can present with numerous complications, primarily associated with red blood cell (RBC) turnover, hemolysis, and associated immune pathway activation. While RBC transfusions can alleviate some of the most severe complications, the survival of transfused RBCs in chronically transfused patients varies significantly. To address this, novel protocols combining RBC biotinylation with flow cytometric detection have been developed, enabling more precise measurements of post-transfusion RBC survival. In an effort to elucidate the half-life of transfused RBCs in chronically transfused patients, cell-surface biotinylation has been integrated with Annexin V staining as a proof of concept. This approach allows for the examination of both RBC survival and changes in RBC lipid distribution, which often accompany cellular removal, providing valuable insights into the complex dynamics of RBC transfusions in patients with SCD.

Key words Red blood cells (RBCs), Sickle cell anemia, Transfusion and blood storage, Biotinylated RBCs (BRBCs), RBC lifespan, Flow cytometry, Immune pathways

1 Introduction

Sickle cell disease (SCD) is an umbrella term that includes several hemoglobinopathies that lead to a change in morphology and normal function of red blood cells (RBCs). One such condition is hemoglobin SCD, commonly seen in patients of African descent, in which a missense point mutation occurs in the hemoglobin beta gene on chromosome 11p15.5, which results in the replacement of glutamic acid by valine, leading to the formation of HbS instead of HbA [1]. The reduced solubility of HbS leads to polymerization and formation of rod-like structures when the RBCs experience hypoxia. The conformational change in hemoglobin makes the RBCs rigid and sickle shaped, which leads to occlusion in small

Sean R. Stowell and Connie M. Arthur (eds.), *Methods in Transfusion Medicine*, Methods in Molecular Biology, vol. 3053, https://doi.org/10.1007/978-1-0716-5376-0_16,

blood vessels and causes severe vascular and cardiopulmonary complications [2]. This condition is also associated with autoimmune hemolytic anemia, which can lead to immune-mediated removal of sickled RBCs by autoantibodies [3].

In patients with SCD, acute triggers such as illness, trauma, or cold temperatures precipitate sickling and cause ischemia and acute inflammation in tissues [4]. Moreover, the release of free heme from sickled RBCs leads to activation of multiple immune pathways, including complement, further exacerbating pain and thrombosis in SCD patients [5–11]. Patients with SCD frequently require blood transfusions during acute episodes to restore oxygen-carrying capacity and alleviate vaso-occlusion [12]. In addition to the formation of autoantibodies, transfusion of donor RBCs can cause the formation of alloantibodies against donor RBC antigens, particularly during the acute episodes when the immune system is primed to generate an antibody response. Alloimmunization can significantly complicate transfusion outcomes, leading to increased morbidity and mortality [13–18].

While a variety of preclinical models have begun to provide insight into key factors that may govern and influence the overall likelihood of alloimmunization, including numerous studies that have begun to highlight the distinct facets of this process and the overall complexity of the pathways involved [19–33], SCD patient immune activation and alloantibody formation are hypothesized to cause increased clearance of transfused donor RBCs. This can be particularly pronounced in patients who have become previously allosensitized as a result of transfusion or pregnancy [34, 35]. RBC alloimmunization may be distinct from key features of immune pathways that govern alloantibody formation following exposure to other intravascular alloantigens, which have been highlighted in numerous studies that have examined various aspects of this process [36–45], although common pathways may certainly exist. Antibodies that develop in response to prior alloantigen exposure can evanesce to undetectable levels, making it difficult for transfusion medicine services to detect prior alloimmunization [46–48]. When this occurs, patients may inadvertently be re-exposed to the same alloantigen, leading to delayed hemolytic transfusion reactions (DHTRs) [49, 50]. DHTRs are particularly life-threatening and occur much more frequently than previously appreciated, likely due to the temporal separation of the reaction from the transfusion event when adverse transfusion reactions are no longer being actively monitored and presentations can often mimic common complications of SCD [17, 51, 52].

To assess the rate of donor RBC clearance and the markers associated with increased removal, we developed flow cytometric antibody panels to analyze phosphatidylserine expression, a common removal signal on the surface of RBCs and the survival of transfused donor RBCs over time. While HbA measurements can provide a general understanding of the survival of transfused RBCs

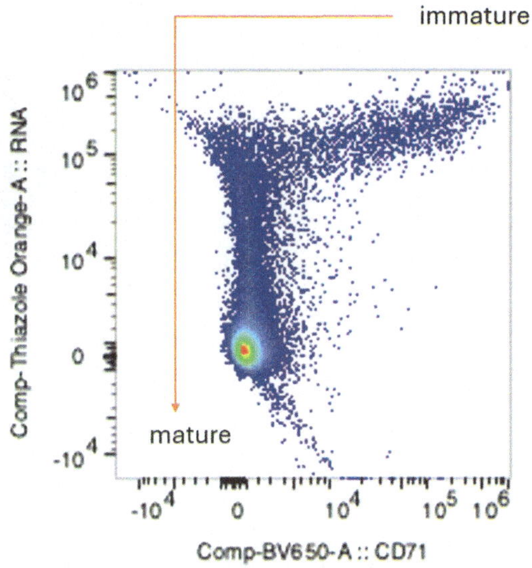

Fig. 1 Detecting immature red blood cells (RBCs)/reticulocytes. Pseudocolor dot plot of flow cytometric data for whole blood samples from sickle cell disease (SCD) patients. CD71 marks the most immature RBCs, whereas thiazole orange (TO, which labels RNA) additionally captures reticulocytes. The most immature RBC progenitors express both CD71 and stain positive for thiazole orange. As RBCs mature, they first lose CD71 expression, then gradually lose TO staining over time as their RNA content decreases. Mature RBCs are negative for both CD71 and TO staining

[53], a way to track transfused RBCs (as opposed to the patient's endogenous RBCs) is by biotinylating a small percentage of donor RBCs (BRBCs) prior to transfusion and following the transfused donor BRBCs over time using fluorescent antibodies against biotin and RBC markers. Small aliquots of different donor RBC units are labeled with varying densities of biotin for identification on Day 0. These labeled aliquots are then transfused into the patient along with the majority of unlabeled donor RBCs (*see* Figs. 1 and 2) [54]. Glycophorin A is a glycoprotein present on erythrocytes and erythroid precursors and binds the CD235a receptor on RBCs. Streptavidin noncovalently binds biotin. These two markers are used together in this protocol to differentiate transfused BRBCs from endogenous patient RBCs. In addition to tracking the percentage of BRBCs relative to total RBCs over time, our panels are designed to assess temporal changes and associations between various RBC markers that have been implicated in modulating RBC survival. Given the role of phosphatidylserine exposure in cellular turnover in other settings where several studies have demonstrated that changes in the surface of a cell can alter sensitivity to factors capable of including cellular turnover [55, 56], we can investigate changes in Annexin V, which can detect cell-surface phosphatidylserine, in the post-transfusion period (*see* Fig. 3) [54, 57].

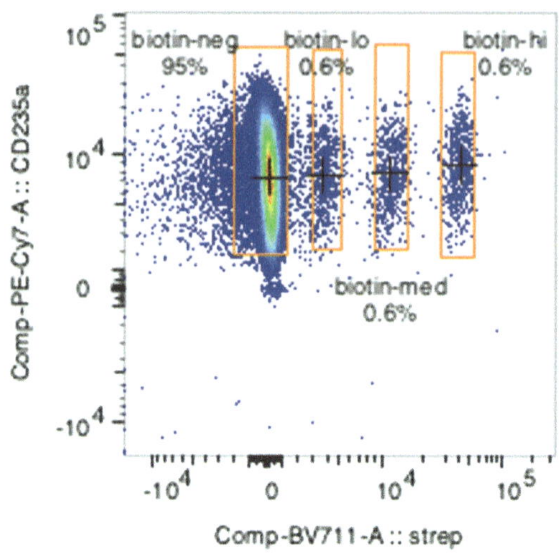

Fig. 2 Identifying biotin-labeled donor red blood cells (RBCs). Antibodies against streptavidin and CD235a, a marker for human RBCs, are used to identify and designate gates for biotin-negative, low-density biotin, medium-density biotin, and high-density biotin–labeled RBCs. Each biotin-labeled population came from a different donor pRBC unit (and represents a small percentage of the transfused RBCs). The data shown are from a patient transfused with three different units of packed RBCs on day 0. Biotin-negative population includes a mix of the various transfused donor units (the majority of donor RBCs are unlabeled) and the patient's endogenous RBCs [4]

2 Materials

2.1 Wash RBCs

1. Blood sample.
2. Microcentrifuge tubes.
3. 1 mL PBS.

2.2 Thiazole Orange (TO) Staining (Will Only Be Used with Panel A)

1. 0.4 mM TO (*see* **Note 1**).
2. Rotisserie.

2.3 Prepare Master Mixes for Each Panel and Staining (Each Sample Will Have Three Wells, One per Panel for Panels A and B)

1. 96-well plate V-Bottom plate.
2. BD Brilliant Stain Buffer.
3. Primary antibodies: *see* Tables 1 and 2 for all primary antibodies used for staining for each panel.
4. 2% BSA/PBS wash buffer.

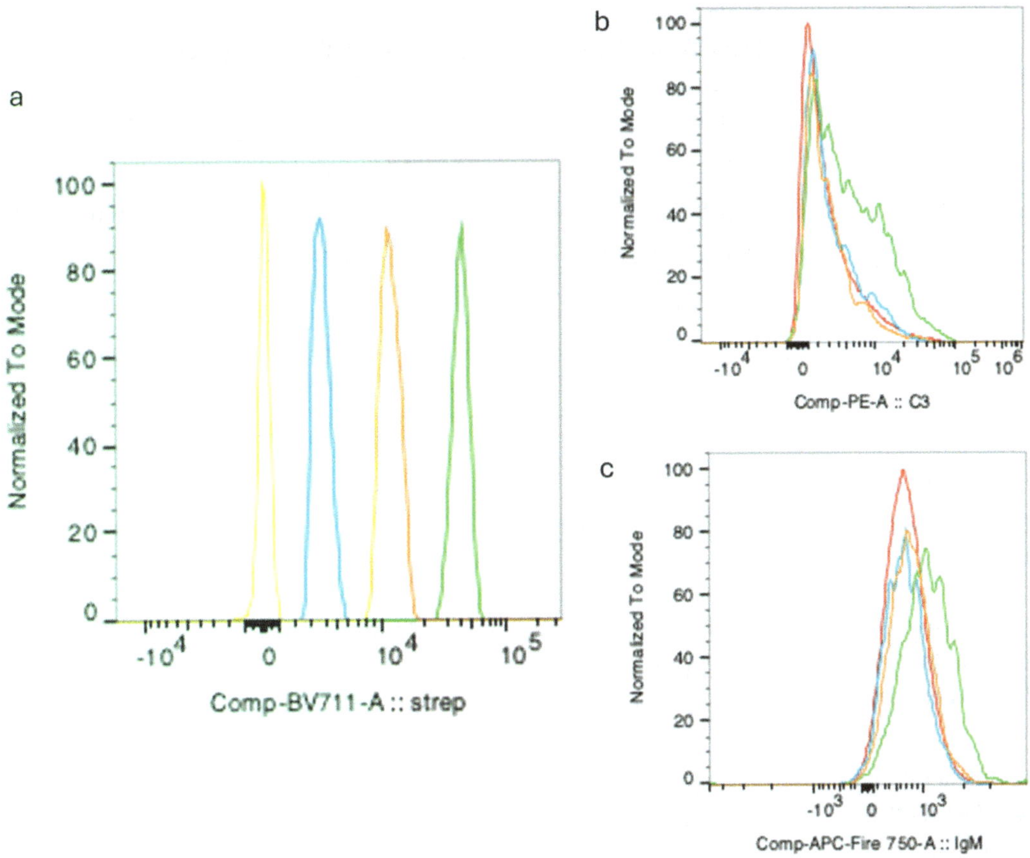

Fig. 3 Red blood cell (RBC) clearance markers in different transfused donor units. The different transfused donor RBC populations along with endogenous RBCs (three donor RBC populations) are represented as histograms according to (**a**) biotin density on the cell surface. Red: no biotin, Blue: low-density biotin, Orange: medium-density biotin, Green: high-density biotin. Example figures show fluorescence intensity of (**b**) C3 and (**c**) IgM on the various RBC populations at 3 weeks post-transfusion. For this particular sample, both IgM and C3 are enriched on the high-biotin donor RBCs compared to RBCs from the other two donor units and the patient's endogenous RBCs

Table 1
Panel A staining—use 1.5 μL of packed thiazole orange-labeled cells

Marker	Color	Dilution
RNA	Thiazole orange	Preincubation
CD235a	PE-Cy7 (tandem)—*see* **Note 3** for tandem dyes	1:100
Streptavidin	BV711 (tandem)	1:100
C3 total	PE	1:100
CD71	BV650 (tandem)	1:200
IgG	AF647	1:100
IgM	APC-Fire750 (tandem)	1:25

Table 2
Panel B staining—use 1.5 μL of packed thiazole orange-labeled cells

Marker	Color	Dilution
RNA	Thiazole orange	Preincubation
CD235a	PE-Cy7 (tandem)	1:100
Streptavidin	BV711 (tandem)	1:100
C3 total	PE	1:100
CD71	BV650 (tandem)	1:200
Annexin V[a]	AF647	1:25

[a]Do not add in the first round of staining; add separately later in the second round

2.4 Data Collection Part 1

1. Flow cytometer.

2.5 Subsequent Stain for AnnV for Panel B Samples

1. 1× Annexin V buffer (*see* **Note 2**).
2. Annexin V BV605.
3. 2% BSA/PBS wash buffer.

2.6 Data Collection Part 2 for AnnV for Panel B Samples

1. Flow cytometer.

3 Methods

3.1 Wash RBCs

1. Aliquot 50 μL of whole blood sample into a microcentrifuge tube containing 1 mL of PBS.
2. Centrifuge the tubes at 300 RCF (g) at room temperature for 4 min.
3. Aspirate off the supernatant carefully.
4. Wash two more times with 1 mL PBS. Centrifuge the tubes at 300 RCF (g) at room temperature for 4 min so that the RBCs are packed at the bottom.
5. Carefully suction off most of the supernatant until ~200 μL of supernatant and packed RBCs are left.

3.2 Thiazole Orange Staining (TO—Will Only Be Used with Panel A)

1. Make 1 mL TO staining solution per sample: To 1 mL of PBS in an Eppendorf add 10 μL of 0.4 mM TO (1:100 dilution) (*see* **Note 1**).
2. Aliquot 1 mL of TO staining solution per Eppendorf for each reaction/sample.

3. Using a 10 μL pipette tip, carefully pipette 7.5 μL of washed RBCs (taken from the bottom) into the 1 mL TO staining solution-containing tube per reaction/sample.
4. Rotate the microfuge tubes containing 7.5 μL washed RBC + 1 mL TO staining solution on rotisserie at room temperature for 60 min in the dark (cover the tubes with foil).
5. Centrifuge the tubes at 300 RCF (g) at room temperature for 4 min. Aspirate off the supernatant until packed TO-stained RBCs are left.

3.3 Prepare Master Mixes for Each Panel and Staining (Each Sample Will Have Three Wells, One per Panel for Panels A, B, and C)

1. Prepare master mixes for each panel in Brilliant Stain Buffer per Tables 1 and 2.
2. Aliquot 25 μL of master mix to required number of wells (depending on the number of samples) in a 96-well V-Bottom plate.
3. Pipette in indicated volumes (*see* Table 2) of washed packed RBCs for Panel B and Panel C and TO-labeled RBCs for Panel A (*see* Table 1). Mix well with a multichannel pipette.
4. Stain in the dark, stationary at room temperature for 30 min.
5. Add 200 μL of 2% BSA/PBS wash buffer (wash 1).
6. Centrifuge at 400 RCF (g) at room temperature for 3 min in a plate spinner. Quickly flip the plate over a sink with forceful wrist flick to dump off the supernatant and leave RBCs in the well (*see* **Note 4**).
7. Wash once more with 2% BSA/PBS (wash 2). Centrifuge at 400 RCF (g) at room temperature for 3 min in plate spinner. Give a quick flip to the plate over a sink to dump off supernatant.
8. Resuspend in 200 μL of 2% BSA/PBS (three washes total).

Panels for Staining and Flow Cytometry

3.4 Subsequent Stain for AnnV for Panel B Samples

1. Centrifuge at 400 RCF (g) at room temperature for 3 min in a plate spinner. Give a quick flip to the plate over a sink to dump off the supernatant.
2. Wash panel B samples twice with 200 μL Annexin V buffer. Centrifuge at 400 RCF (g) at room temperature for 3 min in plate spinner. Give a quick flip to the plate over a sink to dump off supernatant just prior to adding AnnV master mix so that residual packed RBCs at the bottom of the well are not left dry for too long.
3. Prepare master mix for staining.
   (a) Annexin V BV605 diluted 1:25 in 1× of special AnnV staining buffer (no calcium chelators nor EDTA, contains optimal Ca^{2+} concentration which is critical for AnnV:PS binding.) (*see* **Note 2**).

4. Aliquot AnnV staining master mix 25 μL/well on top of previously stained panel B reaction wells (supernatant dumped out, only packed RBCs remaining at bottom of well). Mix well.
5. Stain in the dark, stationary at room temperature for 30 min.
6. Add 200 μL of 2% BSA/PBS (wash 1).
7. Centrifuge at 400 RCF (g) at room temperature for 3 min in plate spinner. Give a quick flip to the plate over a sink to dump off supernatant.
8. Wash once more with 2% BSA/PBS (wash 2). Centrifuge at 400 RCF (g) at room temperature for 3 min in plate spinner. Give a quick flip to the plate over a sink to dump off supernatant.
9. Resuspend in 200 μL of 2% BSA/PBS (3 washes total).

3.5 Data Collection Part 1

1. Run samples on flow cytometer according to manufacturer guidelines.

4 Notes

1. 0.4 mM TO should be stored at 4 °C. Reconstitute lyophilized TO in DMSO to make a 4 mM stock, which should be stored at −80 °C, from which you can dilute 1:10 to make 0.4 mM stock. Prewarm 0.4 mM TO stock to 37 °C in a water bath ahead of time (minimum 5 min) to help with dissolving precipitates. Vortex then quick spin down at max speed in tabletop microcentrifuge afterward. One can use 1:1000 dilution of 0.4 mM TO if fresh, but if it is not fresh and has precipitation, use 1:100.
2. Make sure the buffer is 1× (10× diluted in dH_2O).
3. For tandem conjugated fluorescent antibodies, there may be a lot-to-lot variation in fluorescence emission spectra. The investigator should aim to perform all flow cytometric analyses using the same antibody lot or readjust compensation parameters/ controls when changing lots.
4. It is recommended to practice this step beforehand with unstained control RBCs to prevent losing cells from slow/ inefficient plate flip. Alternatively, carefully aspirate off supernatant between washes.

Conflict of Interest

This work was funded by NIH P01HL171803, R01 HL165975, R01 HL135575, and R01 HL154034. SRS has received speaker and consultant honoraria from Cerus, Grifols, Novartis, Alexion, and Argenx and has received a research grant from Alexion. No other authors have conflicts of interest.

References

1. Brandow AM, Liem RI (2022) Advances in the diagnosis and treatment of sickle cell disease. J Hematol Oncol 15(1):20. https://doi.org/10.1186/s13045-022-01237-z. Epub 20220303. PubMed PMID: 35241123; PubMed Central PMCID: PMCPMC8895633
2. Kavanagh PL, Fasipe TA, Wun T (2022) Sickle cell disease: a review. JAMA 328(1):57–68. https://doi.org/10.1001/jama.2022.10233
3. Chaturvedi S, DeBaun MR (2016) Evolution of sickle cell disease from a life-threatening disease of children to a chronic disease of adults: the last 40 years. Am J Hematol 91(1): 5–14. https://doi.org/10.1002/ajh.24235
4. Ansari J, Gavins FNE (2019) Ischemia-reperfusion injury in sickle cell disease: from basics to therapeutics. Am J Pathol 189(4): 706–718. https://doi.org/10.1016/j.ajpath.2018.12.012. PubMed PMID: 30904156; PubMed Central PMCID: PMCPMC6446225
5. Dumas G, Habibi A, Onimus T, Merle JC, Razazi K, Mekontso Dessap A et al (2016) Eculizumab salvage therapy for delayed hemolysis transfusion reaction in sickle cell disease patients. Blood 127(8):1062–1064. https://doi.org/10.1182/blood-2015-09-669770. Epub 20160112. PubMed PMID: 26758914
6. Meuleman MS, Roumenina LT, Grunenwald A (2023) Complement involvement in sickle cell disease. Presse Med 52(4):104205. https://doi.org/10.1016/j.lpm.2023.104205. Epub 20231114. PubMed PMID: 37972851
7. Merle NS, Boudhabhay I, Leon J, Fremeaux-Bacchi V, Roumenina LT (2019) Complement activation during intravascular hemolysis: implication for sickle cell disease and hemolytic transfusion reactions. Transfus Clin Biol. 26(2):116–124. https://doi.org/10.1016/j.tracli.2019.02.008. Epub 20190222. PubMed PMID: 30879901
8. Merle NS, Paule R, Leon J, Daugan M, Robe-Rybkine T, Poillerat V et al (2019) P-selectin drives complement attack on endothelium during intravascular hemolysis in TLR-4/heme-dependent manner. Proc Natl Acad Sci U S A. 116(13):6280–6285. https://doi.org/10.1073/pnas.1814797116. Epub 20190308. PubMed PMID: 30850533; PubMed Central PMCID: PMCPMC6442544
9. Chonat S, Graciaa S, Shin HS, Newton JG, Quarmyne MO, Boudreaux J et al (2020) Eculizumab for complement mediated thrombotic microangiopathy in sickle cell disease. Haematologica. 105(12):2887–2891. https://doi.org/10.3324/haematol.2020.262006. Epub 20201201. PubMed PMID: 33256394; PubMed Central PMCID: PMCPMC7716365
10. Chonat S, Quarmyne MO, Bennett CM, Dean CL, Joiner CH, Fasano RM et al (2018) Contribution of alternative complement pathway to delayed hemolytic transfusion reaction in sickle cell disease. Haematologica. 103(10):e483–e4e5. https://doi.org/10.3324/haematol.2018.194670. Epub 20180524. PubMed PMID: 29794144; PubMed Central PMCID: PMCPMC6165824
11. Ghosh S, Adisa OA, Chappa P, Tan F, Jackson KA, Archer DR et al (2013) Extracellular hemin crisis triggers acute chest syndrome in sickle mice. J Clin Invest 123(11):4809–4820. https://doi.org/10.1172/JCI64578. PubMed PMID: 24084741; PubMed Central PMCID: PMCPMC3809772
12. Howard J (2016) Sickle cell disease: when and how to transfuse. Hematol Am Soc Hematol Educ Program 2016(1):625–631. https://doi.org/10.1182/asheducation-2016.1.625. PubMed PMID: 27913538; PubMed Central PMCID: PMCPMC6142434
13. Viayna E, Gehrie EA, Blanchette C (2024) Alloimmunization in myelodysplastic syndrome is associated with higher healthcare costs, longer hospitalizations, and increased mortality. Transfusion 64(9):1640–1647. https://doi.org/10.1111/trf.17966. Epub 20240807. PubMed PMID: 39109551
14. Viayna E, Gehrie EA, Blanchette C, Meny GM, Noumsi G, Huber M et al (2022) Red cell alloimmunization is associated with increased health care costs, longer hospitalizations, and higher mortality. Blood Adv 6(20): 5655–5658. https://doi.org/10.1182/bloodadvances.2022006982. PubMed PMID: 35939787; PubMed Central PMCID: PMCPMC9582716
15. Telen MJ, Afenyi-Annan A, Garrett ME, Combs MR, Orringer EP, Ashley-Koch AE (2015) Alloimmunization in sickle cell disease: changing antibody specificities and association with chronic pain and decreased survival. Transfusion. 55(6 Pt 2):1378–1387. https://doi.org/10.1111/trf.12940. Epub 20141201. PubMed PMID: 25444611; PubMed Central PMCID: PMCPMC4451450
16. Nickel RS, Hendrickson JE, Fasano RM, Meyer EK, Winkler AM, Yee MM et al (2016) Impact of red blood cell alloimmunization on sickle cell disease mortality: a case series. Transfusion. 56(1):107–114. https://doi.org/10.1111/trf.13379. Epub 20151028. PubMed PMID: 26509333
17. Thein SL, Pirenne F, Fasano RM, Habibi A, Bartolucci P, Chonat S et al (2020) Hemolytic transfusion reactions in sickle cell disease:

underappreciated and potentially fatal. Haematologica. 105(3):539–544. https://doi.org/10.3324/haematol.2019.224709. Epub 20200206. PubMed PMID: 32029505; PubMed Central PMCID: PMCPMC7049330

18. Narbey D, Habibi A, Chadebech P, Mekontso-Dessap A, Khellaf M, Lelievre JD et al (2017) Incidence and predictive score for delayed hemolytic transfusion reaction in adult patients with sickle cell disease. Am J Hematol 92(12): 1340–1348. Epub 20171031. https://doi.org/10.1002/ajh.24908
19. Soldatenko A, Hoyt LR, Xu L, Calabro S, Lewis SM, Gallman AE et al (2022) Innate and adaptive immunity to transfused allogeneic RBCs in mice requires myD88. J Immunol. 208(4):991–997. https://doi.org/10.4049/jimmunol.2100784. Epub 20220117. PubMed PMID: 35039331; PubMed Central PMCID: PMCPMC10107373
20. Arneja A, Salazar JE, Jiang W, Hendrickson JE, Zimring JC, Luckey CJ (2016) Interleukin-6 receptor-alpha signaling drives anti-RBC alloantibody production and T-follicular helper cell differentiation in a murine model of red blood cell alloimmunization. Haematologica. 101(11): e440–e4e4. https://doi.org/10.3324/haematol.2016.149278. Epub 20160804. PubMed PMID: 27662015; PubMed Central PMCID: PMCPMC5394864
21. Jash A, Usaneerungrueng C, Howie HL, Qiu A, Luckey CJ, Zimring JC et al (2021) Antibodies to low-copy number RBC alloantigen convert a tolerogenic stimulus to an immunogenic stimulus in mice. Front Immunol. 12: 629608. https://doi.org/10.3389/fimmu.2021.629608. Epub 20210312. PubMed PMID: 33777014; PubMed Central PMCID: PMCPMC7994621
22. Jash A, Pridmore T, Collins JB, Hay AM, Hudson KE, Luckey CJ et al (2024) Complement C3 and marginal zone B cells promote IgG-mediated enhancement of RBC alloimmunization in mice. J Clin Invest. 134(8). https://doi.org/10.1172/JCI167665. Epub 20240415. PubMed PMID: 38618959; PubMed Central PMCID: PMCPMC11014669
23. Shinde P, Howie HL, Stegmann TC, Hay AM, Waterman HR, Szittner Z et al (2020) IgG subclass determines suppression versus enhancement of humoral alloimmunity to kell RBC antigens in mice. Front Immunol. 11:1516. https://doi.org/10.3389/fimmu.2020.01516. Epub 20200716. PubMed PMID: 32765523; PubMed Central PMCID: PMCPMC7378678
24. Escamilla-Rivera V, Santhanakrishnan M, Liu J, Gibb DR, Forsmo JE, Foxman EF et al (2021) Complement plays a critical role in inflammation-induced immunoprophylaxis failure in mice. Front Immunol. 12:704072. https://doi.org/10.3389/fimmu.2021.704072. Epub 20210625. PubMed PMID: 34249009; PubMed Central PMCID: PMCPMC8270673
25. Jajosky RP, Ayona D, Mener A, Stowell SR, Arthur CM (2024) Dynamics of antibody engagement of red blood cells in vivo and in vitro. Front Immunol. 15:1475470. https://doi.org/10.3389/fimmu.2024.1475470. Epub 20241128. PubMed PMID: 39669570; PubMed Central PMCID: PMCPMC11634868
26. Zerra PE, Patel SR, Jajosky RP, Arthur CM, McCoy JW, Allen JWL et al (2021) Marginal zone B cells mediate a CD4 T-cell-dependent extrafollicular antibody response following RBC transfusion in mice. Blood 138(8):706–721. https://doi.org/10.1182/blood.2020009376. PubMed PMID: 33876205; PubMed Central PMCID: PMCPMC8394907
27. Mener A, Patel SR, Arthur CM, Chonat S, Wieland A, Santhanakrishnan M et al (2018) Complement serves as a switch between CD4+ T cell-independent and -dependent RBC antibody responses. JCI Insight 3(22). https://doi.org/10.1172/jci.insight.121631. Epub 20181115. PubMed PMID: 30429364; PubMed Central PMCID: PMCPMC6302935
28. Arthur CM, Patel SR, Smith NH, Bennett A, Kamili NA, Mener A et al (2017) Antigen density dictates immune responsiveness following red blood cell transfusion. J Immunol. 198(7): 2671–2680. https://doi.org/10.4049/jimmunol.1601736. Epub 20170301. PubMed PMID: 28250159; PubMed Central PMCID: PMCPMC5777137
29. Patel SR, Gibb DR, Girard-Pierce K, Zhou X, Rodrigues LC, Arthur CM et al (2018) Marginal zone B cells induce alloantibody formation following RBC transfusion. Front Immunol. 9:2516. https://doi.org/10.3389/fimmu.2018.02516. Epub 20181116. PubMed PMID: 30505302; PubMed Central PMCID: PMCPMC6250814
30. Jajosky RP, Patel KR, Allen JWL, Zerra PE, Chonat S, Ayona D et al (2023) Antibody-mediated antigen loss switches augmented immunity to antibody-mediated immunosuppression. Blood 142(12):1082–1098. https://doi.org/10.1182/blood.2022018591. PubMed PMID: 37363865; PubMed Central PMCID: PMCPMC10541552
31. Jajosky RP, Covington ML, Liu J, Chai L, Zerra PE, Chonat S et al (2025) CD47 regulates antigen modulation and red blood cell clearance following an incompatible

transfusion. Front Immunol. 16:1548548. https://doi.org/10.3389/fimmu.2025.1548548. Epub 20250404. PubMed PMID: 40255405; PubMed Central PMCID: PMCPMC12006802

32. Chonat S, Jones JA, Patel SR, Briones WM, Schoettler ML, Maarouf M et al (2025) Complement is activated in patients with acute chest syndrome caused by sickle cell disease and represents a therapeutic target. Sci Transl Med 17(807):eadl4922. https://doi.org/10.1126/scitranslmed.adl4922. Epub 20250716. PubMed PMID: 40668893
33. Maier CL, Jajosky RP, Patel SR, Verkerke HP, Fuller MD, Allen JW et al (2023) Storage differentially impacts alloimmunization to distinct red cell antigens following transfusion in mice. Transfusion. 63(3):457–462. https://doi.org/10.1111/trf.17251. Epub 20230127. PubMed PMID: 36708051; PubMed Central PMCID: PMCPMC10414794
34. Higgins JM, Sloan SR (2008) Stochastic modeling of human RBC alloimmunization: evidence for a distinct population of immunologic responders. Blood. 112(6):2546–2553. https://doi.org/10.1182/blood-2008-03-146415. Epub 20080605. PubMed PMID: 18535200
35. Jajosky R, Patel SR, Wu SC, Patel K, Covington M, Vallecillo-Zuniga M et al (2023) Prior immunization against an intracellular antigen enhances subsequent red blood cell alloimmunization in mice. Blood 141(21):2642–2653. https://doi.org/10.1182/blood.2022016588. PubMed PMID: 36638335; PubMed Central PMCID: PMCPMC10356576
36. Zerra PE, Cox C, Baldwin WH, Patel SR, Arthur CM, Lollar P et al (2017) Marginal zone B cells are critical to factor VIII inhibitor formation in mice with hemophilia A. Blood. 130(23):2559–2568. https://doi.org/10.1182/blood-2017-05-782912. Epub 20171004. PubMed PMID: 28978569; PubMed Central PMCID: PMCPMC5721282
37. Arthur CM, Zerra PE, Shin S, Wang J, Song X, Doering CB et al (2022) Nonhuman glycans can regulate anti-factor VIII antibody formation in mice. Blood 139(9):1312–1317. https://doi.org/10.1182/blood.2020009210. PubMed PMID: 34019619; PubMed Central PMCID: PMCPMC8900271
38. Arthur CM, Patel SR, Sullivan HC, Winkler AM, Tormey CA, Hendrickson JE et al (2016) CD8+ T cells mediate antibody-independent platelet clearance in mice. Blood. 127(14):1823–1827. https://doi.org/10.1182/blood-2015-10-673426. Epub 20160119. PubMed PMID: 26787734; PubMed Central PMCID: PMCPMC4825415
39. Li C, Piran S, Chen P, Lang S, Zarpellon A, Jin JW, et al. The maternal immune response to fetal platelet GPIbalpha causes frequent miscarriage in mice that can be prevented by intravenous IgG and anti-FcRn therapies. J Clin Invest. 2011;121(11):4537–4547. doi: https://doi.org/10.1172/JCI57850. Epub 20111024. PubMed PMID: 22019589; PubMed Central PMCID: PMCPMC3204841
40. Chen P, Li C, Lang S, Zhu G, Reheman A, Spring CM et al (2010) Animal model of fetal and neonatal immune thrombocytopenia: role of neonatal Fc receptor in the pathogenesis and therapy. Blood. 116(18):3660–3668. https://doi.org/10.1182/blood-2010-05-284919. Epub 20100720. PubMed PMID: 20647570
41. Xu X, Chen D, Ye X, Xia W, Xu Y, Chen Y et al (2021) Successful prenatal therapy for anti-CD36-mediated severe FNAIT by deglycosylated antibodies in a novel murine model. Blood 138(18):1757–1767. https://doi.org/10.1182/blood.2021011131. PubMed PMID: 34041523; PubMed Central PMCID: PMCPMC8701625
42. Vadasz B, Chen P, Yougbare I, Zdravic D, Li J, Li C et al (2015) Platelets and platelet alloantigens: lessons from human patients and animal models of fetal and neonatal alloimmune thrombocytopenia. Genes Dis 2(2):173–185. https://doi.org/10.1016/j.gendis.2015.02.003. PubMed PMID: 28345015; PubMed Central PMCID: PMCPMC5362271
43. Newman DK, Newman PJ (2024) Antigen-specific immunotherapy for platelet alloimmune disorders. Hum Immunol 85(6):111172. https://doi.org/10.1016/j.humimm.2024.111172. Epub 20241108. PubMed PMID: 39520801; PubMed Central PMCID: PMCPMC11637901
44. Zhi H, Sheridan D, Newman DK, Newman PJ (2022) Prophylactic administration of HPA-1a-specific antibodies prevents fetal/neonatal alloimmune thrombocytopenia in mice. Blood 140(20):2146–2153. https://doi.org/10.1182/blood.2022015666. PubMed PMID: 35881848; PubMed Central PMCID: PMCPMC9837438
45. Zhi H, Ahlen MT, Skogen B, Newman DK, Newman PJ (2021) Preclinical evaluation of immunotherapeutic regimens for fetal/neonatal alloimmune thrombocytopenia. Blood Adv

5(18):3552–3562. https://doi.org/10.1182/bloodadvances.2021004371. PubMed PMID: 34470046; PubMed Central PMCID: PMCPMC8945581

46. Tormey CA, Hendrickson JE (2019) Transfusion-related red blood cell alloantibodies: induction and consequences. Blood. 133(17):1821–1830. https://doi.org/10.1182/blood-2018-08-833962. Epub 20190226. PubMed PMID: 30808636; PubMed Central PMCID: PMCPMC6484385

47. Siddon AJ, Kenney BC, Hendrickson JE, Tormey CA (2018) Delayed haemolytic and serologic transfusion reactions: pathophysiology, treatment and prevention. Curr Opin Hematol 25(6):459–467. https://doi.org/10.1097/MOH.0000000000000462. PubMed PMID: 30124474

48. Stack G, Tormey CA (2016) Detection rate of blood group alloimmunization based on real-world testing practices and kinetics of antibody induction and evanescence. Transfusion 56(11):2662–2667. https://doi.org/10.1111/trf.13704. Epub 20160709. PubMed PMID: 27394029

49. Covington ML, Cone-Sullivan JK, Andrzejewski C, Lu W, Thomasson RR, O'Brien K et al (2022) Unmasking delayed hemolytic transfusion reactions in patients with sickle-cell disease: challenges and opportunities for improvement. Transfusion 62(8): 1662–1670. https://doi.org/10.1111/trf.16967. PubMed PMID: 35778994. Epub 20220702

50. Dean CL, Maier CL, Chonat S, Chang A, Carden MA, El Rassi F et al (2019) Challenges in the treatment and prevention of delayed hemolytic transfusion reactions with hyperhemolysis in sickle cell disease patients. Transfusion 59(5):1698–1705. https://doi.org/10.1111/trf.15227. Epub 20190308. PubMed PMID: 30848512

51. Vidler JB, Gardner K, Amenyah K, Mijovic A, Thein SL (2015) Delayed haemolytic transfusion reaction in adults with sickle cell disease: a 5-year experience. Br J Haematol. 169(5): 746–753. Epub 20150305. PubMed PMID: 25753472. https://doi.org/10.1111/bjh.13339

52. Dean CL, Maier CL, Roback JD, Stowell SR (2019) Multiple hemolytic transfusion reactions misinterpreted as severe vaso-occlusive crisis in a patient with sickle cell disease. Transfusion 59(2):448–453. https://doi.org/10.1111/trf.15010. Epub 20181109. PubMed PMID: 30412270

53. Yee MEM, Josephson CD, Winkler AM, Webb J, Luban NLC, Leong T et al (2018) Hemoglobin A clearance in children with sickle cell anemia on chronic transfusion therapy. Transfusion. 58(6):1363–1371. https://doi.org/10.1111/trf.14610. Epub 20180417. PubMed PMID: 29664198; PubMed Central PMCID: PMCPMC6021219

54. Yee MEM, Zerra PE, McCoy JW, Covington ML, Stowell SR, Joiner CH et al (2024) Post-transfusion biotin-labeled red blood cell survival studies in pediatric sickle cell disease with antibodies of uncertain significance. Transfusion 64(5):800–807. https://doi.org/10.1111/trf.17800. Epub 20240320. PubMed PMID: 38506450; PubMed Central PMCID: PMCPMC11088511

55. Stowell SR, Karmakar S, Stowell CJ, Dias-Baruffi M, McEver RP, Cummings RD (2007) Human galectin-1, -2, and -4 induce surface exposure of phosphatidylserine in activated human neutrophils but not in activated T cells. Blood. 109(1):219–227. https://doi.org/10.1182/blood-2006-03-007153. Epub 20060829. PubMed PMID: 16940423; PubMed Central PMCID: PMCPMC1785076

56. Stowell SR, Arthur CM, Mehta P, Slanina KA, Blixt O, Leffler H et al (2008) Galectin-1, -2, and -3 exhibit differential recognition of sialylated glycans and blood group antigens. J Biol Chem. 283(15):10109–10123. https://doi.org/10.1074/jbc.M709545200. Epub 20080123. PubMed PMID: 18216021; PubMed Central PMCID: PMCPMC2442294

57. Yee MEM, Covington ML, Zerra PE, McCoy JW, Easley KA, Joiner CH et al (2024) Survival of transfused red blood cells from a donor with alpha-thalassemia trait in a recipient with sickle cell disease. Transfusion. 64(6):1109–1115. https://doi.org/10.1111/trf.17857. Epub 20240501. PubMed PMID: 38693059; PubMed Central PMCID: PMCPMC11144116

Chapter 17

Examination of Antigen-Specific B Cell Responses to Red Blood Cell Transfusion

Leon Zheng, Hirotomo Nakahara, Sofia Cattani, Victoria M. Vance, Emily Oehrle, Connie M. Arthur, Ryan P. Jajosky, and Sean R. Stowell

Abstract

Various models have been developed to study red blood cell (RBC) alloimmunization. While studies using these models have primarily examined general features of this response, identifying key characteristics of antigen-specific B cells is critical when seeking to define regulators of alloimmune responses. Unlike analysis of antigen-specific T cells, which requires peptide loaded in the appropriate major histocompatibility class structure, B cells recognize native antigens, which requires the generation of tools that incorporate individual antigens into multimeric constructs to enhance B cell receptor recognition. While a wide variety of models have now been generated to study the developing immune response to blood group antigens, the use of tetramers has most commonly been applied to the hen egg lysozyme (HEL), ovalbumin (OVA), and Duffy (HOD) model system. We will examine the development and use of B cell tetramers for the purpose of studying antigen-specific B cell responses following RBC transfusion.

Key words Antigen-specific B cells, RBC transfusion, B cell subsets, Tetramers

1 Introduction

Transfusion of blood products can provide a lifesaving intervention. Despite this, differences in alloantigen expression between individuals can form the basis of immune incompatibility between individuals [1–3]. Indeed, immune reactions resulting in hemolytic transfusion reactions were the first barrier to successful blood transfusions. It was not until the discovery of ABO blood group antigens and corresponding anti-ABO antibodies that the underlying basis for immune incompatibility between blood donors became apparent. As a result of this discovery, ABO antigens and anti-ABO antibodies became the foundation of compatibility testing for transfusion, and eventually, transplantation.

Following the initial discovery of ABO blood group antigens, studies identified additional alloantigens that can trigger

Sean R. Stowell and Connie M. Arthur (eds.), *Methods in Transfusion Medicine*, Methods in Molecular Biology, vol. 3053, https://doi.org/10.1007/978-1-0716-5376-0_17,

alloimmune responses. Unlike anti-ABO antibodies, which naturally develop within the first few months of life, alloantibodies against other alloantigens typically form only after exposure through pregnancy or blood transfusion [2, 4, 5]. Indeed, while ABO antigens are the most common source of incompatibility between donors and recipients, more than 300 RBC alloantigens have been identified that can form the basis of alloimmune responses, resulting in hemolytic transfusion reactions or the development of hemolytic disease of the fetus and newborn (HDFN) [6]. As a result, while blood group antigens likely evolved due to selection pressures from infectious diseases and possibly other factors that have consequences on host immunity against microbes that decorate themselves in mimics of these blood group antigens [7–9], the impact of these polymorphisms is particularly evident in patients who require transfusion or who experience pregnancy complications in the form of HDFN [2, 4, 5].

The effects of RBC alloimmunization can be especially difficult to manage in patients who require long-term transfusion therapy [10]. Unlike alloimmunization against platelets or clotting factors, where alloimmune response renders products ineffective without causing additional negative effects following infusion [11–14], transfusing incompatible RBCs can lead to acute or delayed hemolytic transfusion reactions, which may result in significant complications that can result in death [15–18]. Although the exact pathophysiology of hemolytic transfusion reactions is not yet fully understood, elevated levels of free heme that accompany these reactions likely contribute to the downstream events that result in complications that accompany hemolytic transfusion reactions. Initial studies demonstrated that heme can activate toll-like receptors [19], leading to immune cell activation and inflammation. More recent research indicates that heme can also activate the alternative complement pathway [20–25], causing additional inflammation and injury. Supporting the potential role of complement in some hemolytic transfusion reactions, complement inhibition appears to improve clinical outcomes in patients with sickle cell disease (SCD) who experience complications, including delayed hemolytic transfusion reactions [26–28].

Matching common alloantigen targets (e.g., C, c, E, e, K, k) for patients with sickle cell disease (SCD) has reduced the formation of alloantibodies [29–32]. However, as these approaches are not able to fully prevent alloimmunization, complementary strategies are necessary. Because RBC alloantigens vary with respect to structure and propensity to induce alloantibody formation, the identification of the pathways responsible for the initiation of alloimmunization would be predicted to enhance the development of strategies to prevent antibody formation against a wide variety of alloantigens [1–3].

To develop a more comprehensive understanding of the key immune regulators that govern RBC alloimmunization, numerous clinical studies have identified risk factors that may increase the likelihood of alloantibody formation following exposure to allogenic blood products [33–39]. These studies have highlighted donor and recipient characteristics that can affect RBC alloimmunization [40]. To enhance these findings and offer a way to study key immune populations not easily accessible through peripheral blood alone, a wide variety of preclinical models and overall approaches have also been developed to investigate various aspects of RBC alloimmunization [41–45]. Through these models, studies have uncovered key features of recipients, such as B and T cell populations, innate signaling pathways, and antigen-presenting cells, and many other factors that can drive RBC alloimmunization [46–52]. Additional studies, many of which have utilized similar model systems, have also identified key characteristics of RBCs, including the potential impact of product modifications, antigen density, and other RBC features, that may influence alloimmunization [52–56]. Comparable mechanisms have been examined in a variety of other studies and suggest that similar pathways may contribute to the development of an alloimmune response against other antigens, suggesting that general themes may emerge, although the precise processes and the extent to which antibodies are required in the outcomes of alloimmunization may vary [12–14, 57, 58]. These models have also been used to a wide variety of studies to examine the outcome of antibody engagement following transfusion and in doing so also provided valuable insights into the actual consequences of RBC alloimmunization [59–67], with key features of incompatible transfusion having been likewise observed in the clinical setting where antibodies that target RBCs are employed. Similar studies, using a variety of approaches and model systems, have explored the mechanisms by which antibodies may prevent the formation of new antibodies [68–78], often referred to as antibody-mediated immunosuppression. Each of these studies illustrate the utility of model systems and the ability of use distinct preclinical approaches to define the mechanisms whereby antibodies can suppress alloimmunization.

To prevent RBC alloimmunization, the key B cell populations responsible for alloantibody development need to be identified [79]. Many studies employ various techniques to examine B cell populations broadly, including potential activation changes that may occur after exposure to allogeneic RBCs. However, to understand the effects of alloantigen exposure on the specific B cell populations that generate the alloantigen-specific responses to blood transfusions, reagents are needed to analyze antigen-specific B cell populations (Fig. 1). While T cell tetramers are created by loading peptides onto the relevant MHC, most B cells recognize antigens in their intact form [80]. Consequently, the

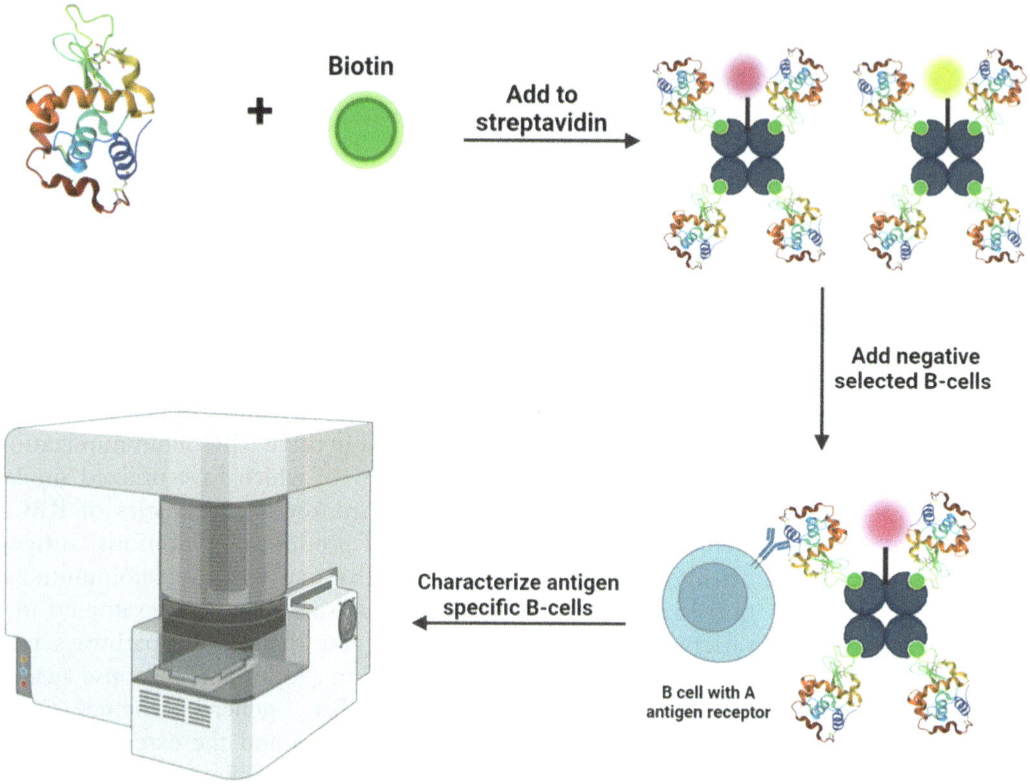

Fig. 1 Identifying HEL-specific B cells by binding of two HEL B cell tetramers, each with a different fluorophore. These cells should not bind to the nonspecific BSA B cell tetramer, which is also labeled with a distinct fluorescent dye (not shown in the figure)

tetramerization of B cell antigens typically requires the use of the target antigen as a native structure. Herein, we outline the development and application of B cell tetramers to investigate antigen-specific responses to blood transfusion in preclinical models using the HEL, OVA, and Duffy (HOD) model system.

2 Materials

2.1 Synthesis of B Cell Tetramers

1. HEL.
2. BSA.
3. Phosphate-buffered saline (PBS) or other amine-free buffer with pH 7–8.
4. Desalting columns or dialysis units.
5. Sulfo-NHS-LC biotin (*see* **Note 1**).
6. Metal spatula.
7. 1.7 mL Eppendorf tubes.

8. Electronic scale.
9. Ultrapure water.
10. Zeba™ Dye and Biotin Removal Spin Columns.
11. Nanodrop (to determine protein concentration).
12. APC-conjugated Streptavidin (APC-SAv).
13. PE-SAv.
14. FITC-SAv.
15. Variable-speed benchtop microcentrifuge.
16. 15 mL conical tubes (for use with 2 mL and 5 mL spin columns).
17. 50 mL conical tubes (for use with 10 mL spin columns).

2.2 Validating and Using the B Cell Tetramers

1. Both HEL tetramers and the BSA tetramer.
2. B6 mice.
3. MD4 mouse.
4. HOD mice.
5. 5.5 mm animal lancet.
6. ACD-A.
7. 5 mL Eppendorf tubes.
8. 50 mL conicals.
9. 4″ × 4″ gauze.
10. 1 mL Tuberculin syringes.
11. 30-gauge 0.5″ needle.
12. Manual pipettes and pipette tips.
13. 70 μm cell-strainer attachment for a 50 mL conical.
14. RBC lysis buffer.
15. PBS.
16. Zombie Yellow live/dead viability dye.
17. BV750 conjugated anti-mouse B220 antibody.
18. PE-Dazzle 594 conjugated anti-mouse CD3 antibody.
19. Flow cytometer.
20. Optional: high-performance liquid chromatography column (HPLC).

3 Methods

3.1 Synthesis of B Cell Tetramers

1. Decide how many mmol of protein (e.g., HEL and BSA) to biotinylate (*see* **Note 2**).
   (a) HEL and BSA have molecular weights of ~14.3 kDa and 66.4 kDa, respectively.

2. Read the manufacturer's instructions for biotinylation but consider making adjustments (*see* **Notes 3** and **4**).
3. Separately incubate HEL and BSA with sulfo-NHS-LC biotin.
   (a) This can be done at room temperature for 30 min or at 4 °C for 2 h.
4. Use a biotin removal column, according to the manufacturer's instructions, to remove free (unbound) biotin.
5. Use a nanodrop to determine the protein concentrations.
6. Determine the mmol concentration of the biotinylated proteins.
7. Mix the biotinylated proteins with fluorescent SAv molecules.
   (a) In the first 1.7 mL Eppendorf, add the desired mmols of biotinylated HEL to be reacted with SAv-PE.
   (b) In the second tube, add biotinylated HEL to be reacted with SAv-APC.
   (c) In the third tube, add biotinylated BSA to be reacted with SAv-FITC.
   (d) Divide the mmols of biotinylated protein in each tube by four to get the number of mmol of SAv that needs to be added (*see* **Note 5**).
   (e) Add one tenth of the total mmols (from **step 7d**) of fluorescent SAv to the biotinylated HEL every 10 min, until it is completely added.
8. Store the three separate B cell tetramers, the biotinylated HEL, and the biotinylated BSA in a refrigerator in the dark (*see* **Note 6**).
   (a) If the B cell tetramers precipitate, reread **Note 3**.

3.2 Validating and Using the B Cell Tetramers

3.2.1 Validating the B Cell Tetramers

Optional: Use HPLC to see if the biotinylated protein bound to SAv (*see* **Note 7**).

1. Face bleed B6 and MD4 mice into separate 5 mL Eppendorf tubes with ACD-A (*see* **Note 8** and **9**).
2. Use RBC lysis buffer, according to the manufacturer's instructions, to isolate the peripheral white blood cells (WBCs).
3. Wash the WBCs three times with PBS.
4. In a 96-well plate, create wells with the following percentage of MD4 WBCs in B6 WBCs: 100%, 50%, 20%, 10%, 5%, 1%, and 0%. It is best if at least one million cells are plated.
5. Stain each sample with 25 μL of 1:500 Zombie Yellow live/dead viability dye for 15 min at room temperature.
6. Wash the WBCs once with PBS.

7. Stain each sample with 25 μL of an antibody cocktail of 1:50 PE-Dazzle 594 conjugated anti-mouse CD3 antibody, 1:100 BV750 conjugated anti-mouse B220 antibody, and 1:100 of each of the three tetramers for 15 min on ice.
8. Wash the WBCs three times with PBS.
9. Analyze using a flow cytometer. Gate on cells, single cells, live cells, B220+ cells, BSA-tetramer negative cells, and double HEL-tetramer positive cells.

   Expected results: as the percentage of MD4 cells decreases, so should the percentage of HEL-specific B cells.

3.2.2 Using the B Cell Tetramers

1. Design your experiment. For example, 15 B6 recipients are transfused with B6 RBCs, and 15 B6 recipients are transfused with HOD RBCs.
2. On D2, D4, D6, D8, and D10, harvest samples from three mice per group (*see* **Note 10**).
3. Also, obtain peripheral blood from a B6 and an MD4 mouse at each time point.
4. Perform RBC lysis as done above in Subheading 3.2.1.
5. Then follow the staining/analysis protocol in Subheading 3.2.1 above (*see* **Note 11**).

4 Notes

1. Thermo Fisher's sulfo-NHS-LC biotin product is recommended for use. It dissolves more easily in deionized water than some other manufacturer's products.
2. Consider biotinylating extra protein in case B cell tetramer synthesis fails (e.g., precipitation of large aggregates).
3. It is best if there is just one biotin on the protein of interest. Then, the protein can only bind to one SAv. If there are multiple biotins per protein, then the protein can bind to multiple SAv molecules, leading to large aggregates that can precipitate immediately or during storage. If the protein is not expensive (e.g., HEL or BSA), then different quantities of sulfo-NHS-LC biotin can be added to the protein of interest to try to achieve one biotin per protein. A biotin quantification kit can be used to measure the amount of biotin on the protein. Alternatively, enzymatic biotinylation can be used to get exactly one biotin per RBC, however, this requires that the protein of interest have a single AviTag (short peptide sequence). This can be achieved by adding the genetic sequence to the C-terminus, N-terminus, or elsewhere on the genetic sequence of the protein. Then, BirA enzymatically adds a biotin to the AviTag.

4. Sulfo-NHS-LC biotin quickly hydrolyzes—meaning that it must be used soon after it is dissolved in deionized water.
5. Streptavidin can bind to four biotins. So, the mmols of streptavidin should be ¼ the mmols of biotinylated protein. When companies such as Biolegend report the concentration of fluorescent SAv, it often represents the concentration of SAv without the fluorophore. This makes it easier to calculate how much reagent is needed.
6. Consider adding some sodium azide to the reagents to prevent microbial growth. Fluorescent SAv reagents often have some sodium azide in them, but the biotinylated proteins most likely do not. Biolegend stores antibodies in 0.09% sodium azide, so this is a reasonable concentration.
7. Consider using a size exclusion column (SEC) with HPLC to determine if the biotinylated protein binds to the SAv. First, run proteins of known molecular weight (i.e., "standards") on the HPLC column. Then, run the following, (1) each biotinylated protein, (2) each fluorescent streptavidin, and (3) each B cell tetramer. The B cell tetramers should have a larger molecular weight than the biotinylated protein or the fluorescent streptavidin. This equates to a shorter retention time with an SEC.
8. B cells can be examined from multiple tissue types using slight modifications of this protocol. The example included here uses peripheral blood to assess tetramer positive B cells, but samples can include peripheral blood, lymph nodes, spleens, and so forth.
9. The volume of ACD should be ~20% of the estimated total whole blood volume to be collected. The total amount collected will depend on the assay design. We suggest designing the assay and estimating needed cell counts before collecting blood. We typically expect ~one million PBMCs per mL of whole blood collected.
10. Test whether the HEL tetramers bind to 100% MD4 WBCs, but not the BSA tetramer. Neither the HEL tetramers nor the BSA tetramer binds to 100% B6 WBCs.
11. Consider adding additional B cell markers such as CD21, CD23, GL7, and FAS.

Conflict of Interest

This work was funded by NIH P01HL171803, R01 HL165975, R01 HL135575, and R01 HL154034. SRS has received speaker and consultant honoraria from Cerus, Grifols, Novartis, Alexion, and Argenx and has received a research grant from Alexion. No other authors have conflicts of interest.

References

1. Yazdanbakhsh K, Ware RE, Noizat-Pirenne F (2012) Red blood cell alloimmunization in sickle cell disease: pathophysiology, risk factors, and transfusion management. Blood 120(3): 528–537
2. Pirenne F, Floch A, Diop S (2023) Alloimmunisation against red blood cells in sickle cell disease: transfusion challenges in high-income and low-income countries. Lancet Haematol 10(6):e468–e476
3. Arthur CM, Stowell SR (2023) The development and consequences of red blood cell alloimmunization. Annu Rev Pathol 18:537–564
4. Hauser RG et al (2020) The evanescence and persistence of RBC alloantibodies in blood donors. Transfusion 60(4):831–839
5. Tormey CA, Hendrickson JE (2019) Transfusion-related red blood cell alloantibodies: induction and consequences. Blood 133(17):1821–1830
6. Yazdanbakhsh K, Shaz BH, Hillyer CD (2017) Immune regulation of sickle cell alloimmunization. ISBT Sci Ser 12(1):248–253
7. Blenda AV et al (2022) Galectin-9 recognizes and exhibits antimicrobial activity toward microbes expressing blood group-like antigens. J Biol Chem 298(4):101704
8. Jan HM et al (2024) Galectin-4 antimicrobial activity primarily occurs through its C-terminal domain. Mol Cell Proteomics 23(5):100747
9. Wu SC et al (2022) Innate immune Galectin-7 specifically targets microbes that decorate themselves in blood group-like antigens. iScience 25(7):104482
10. Thein SL et al (2020) Hemolytic transfusion reactions in sickle cell disease: underappreciated and potentially fatal. Haematologica 105(3):539–544
11. Waterman HR et al (2016) Transfusion-induced alloimmunization and platelet refractoriness in a mouse model: mechanisms and interventions. Transfusion 56(1):91–100
12. Zerra PE et al (2017) Marginal zone B cells are critical to factor VIII inhibitor formation in mice with hemophilia a. Blood 130(23): 2559–2568
13. Arthur CM et al (2016) CD8+ T cells mediate antibody-independent platelet clearance in mice. Blood 127(14):1823–1827
14. Arthur CM et al (2022) Nonhuman glycans can regulate anti-factor VIII antibody formation in mice. Blood 139(9):1312–1317
15. Covington ML et al (2022) Unmasking delayed hemolytic transfusion reactions in patients with sickle-cell disease: challenges and opportunities for improvement. Transfusion 62(8):1662–1670
16. Habibi A et al (2016) Delayed hemolytic transfusion reaction in adult sickle-cell disease: presentations, outcomes, and treatments of 99 referral center episodes. Am J Hematol 91(10):989–994
17. Narbey D et al (2017) Incidence and predictive score for delayed hemolytic transfusion reaction in adult patients with sickle cell disease. Am J Hematol 92(12):1340–1348
18. Chonat S et al (2019) Challenges in preventing and treating hemolytic complications associated with red blood cell transfusion. Transfus Clin Biol 26(2):130–134
19. Ghosh S et al (2013) Extracellular hemin crisis triggers acute chest syndrome in sickle mice. J Clin Invest 123(11):4809–4820
20. Roumenina LT, Bartolucci P, Pirenne F (2019) The role of complement in post-transfusion hemolysis and hyperhemolysis reaction. Transfus Med Rev 33(4):225–230
21. Poillerat V et al (2020) Hemopexin as an inhibitor of hemolysis-induced complement activation. Front Immunol 11:1684
22. Gerogianni A et al (2022) Heme interferes with complement factor I-dependent regulation by enhancing alternative pathway activation. Front Immunol 13:901876
23. Merle NS et al (2019) Complement activation during intravascular hemolysis: implication for sickle cell disease and hemolytic transfusion reactions. Transfus Clin Biol 26(2):116–124
24. Merle NS et al (2019) P-selectin drives complement attack on endothelium during intravascular hemolysis in TLR-4/heme-dependent manner. Proc Natl Acad Sci USA 116(13): 6280–6285
25. Meuleman MS, Roumenina LT, Grunenwald A (2023) Complement involvement in sickle cell disease. Presse Med 52(4):104205
26. Dumas G et al (2016) Eculizumab salvage therapy for delayed hemolysis transfusion reaction in sickle cell disease patients. Blood 127(8): 1062–1064
27. Chonat S et al (2018) Contribution of alternative complement pathway to delayed hemolytic transfusion reaction in sickle cell disease. Haematologica 103(10):e483–e485
28. Chonat S et al (2025) Complement is activated in patients with acute chest syndrome caused

by sickle cell disease and represents a therapeutic target. Sci Transl Med 17(807):eadl4922
29. Vichinsky EP et al (1990) Alloimmunization in sickle cell anemia and transfusion of racially unmatched blood. N Engl J Med 322(23):1617–1621
30. Chou ST et al (2013) High prevalence of red blood cell alloimmunization in sickle cell disease despite transfusion from Rh-matched minority donors. Blood 122(6):1062–1071
31. Israelyan N et al (2024) RH genotypes and red cell alloimmunization rates in chronically transfused patients with sickle cell disease: a multisite study in the USA. Transfusion 64(3):526–535
32. Wolf J et al (2024) Red cell specifications for blood group matching in patients with haemoglobinopathies: an updated systematic review and clinical practice guideline from the International Collaboration for Transfusion Medicine Guidelines. Br J Haematol
33. Zhong H et al (2014) Hemin controls T cell polarization in sickle cell alloimmunization. J Immunol 193(1):102–110
34. Godefroy E et al (2016) Altered heme-mediated modulation of dendritic cell function in sickle cell alloimmunization. Haematologica 101(9):1028–1038
35. Liu Y et al (2021) Type I interferon is induced by hemolysis and drives antibody-mediated erythrophagocytosis in sickle cell disease. Blood 138(13):1162–1171
36. Vingert B et al (2015) Phenotypic differences of CD4(+) T cells in response to red blood cell immunization in transfused sickle cell disease patients. Eur J Immunol 45(6):1868–1879
37. Evers D et al (2017) Absence of the spleen and the occurrence of primary red cell alloimmunization in humans. Haematologica 102(8):e289–e292
38. Yazdanbakhsh K (2015) Mechanisms of sickle cell alloimmunization. Transfus Clin Biol 22(3):178–181
39. Nakahara H et al (2023) Enhanced IgG immune response to COVID-19 vaccination in patients with sickle cell disease. Br J Haematol 202(5):937–941
40. Zheng Y et al (2023) Proinflammatory state promotes red blood cell alloimmunization in pediatric patients with sickle cell disease. Blood Adv 7(17):4799–4808
41. Stowell SR et al (2013) Alloantibodies to a paternally derived RBC KEL antigen lead to hemolytic disease of the fetus/newborn in a murine model. Blood 122(8):1494–1504
42. Arneja A et al (2016) Interleukin-6 receptor-alpha signaling drives anti-RBC alloantibody production and T-follicular helper cell differentiation in a murine model of red blood cell alloimmunization. Haematologica 101(11):e440–e444
43. Smith NH et al (2012) Generation of transgenic mice with antithetical KEL1 and KEL2 human blood group antigens on red blood cells. Transfusion 52(12):2620–2630
44. Jajosky RP et al (2025) CD47 regulates antigen modulation and red blood cell clearance following an incompatible transfusion. Front Immunol 16:1548548
45. Mener A et al (2018) Complement serves as a switch between CD4+ T cell-independent and -dependent RBC antibody responses. JCI Insight 3(22)
46. Patel SR et al (2018) Recipient priming to one RBC alloantigen directly enhances subsequent alloimmunization in mice. Blood Adv 2(2):105–115
47. Meinderts SM et al (2019) Identification of genetic biomarkers for alloimmunization in sickle cell disease. Br J Haematol 186(6):887–899
48. Jajosky R et al (2023) Prior immunization against an intracellular antigen enhances subsequent red blood cell alloimmunization in mice. Blood 141(21):2642–2653
49. Hendrickson JE et al (2009) The spleen plays a central role in primary humoral alloimmunization to transfused mHEL red blood cells. Transfusion 49(8):1678–1684
50. Hendrickson JE et al (2006) Recipient inflammation affects the frequency and magnitude of immunization to transfused red blood cells. Transfusion 46(9):1526–1536
51. Hendrickson JE et al (2012) Alloimmunization to transfused HOD red blood cells is not increased in mice with sickle cell disease. Transfusion 52(2):231–240
52. Arthur CM et al (2022) Clodronate inhibits alloimmunization against distinct red blood cell alloantigens in mice. Transfusion 62(5):948–953
53. Maier CL et al (2023) Storage differentially impacts alloimmunization to distinct red cell antigens following transfusion in mice. Transfusion 63(3):457–462
54. Arthur CM et al (2017) Antigen density dictates immune responsiveness following red blood cell transfusion. J Immunol 198(7):2671–2680
55. Ryder AB, Zimring JC, Hendrickson JE (2014) Factors influencing RBC alloimmunization: lessons learned from murine models. Transfus Med Hemother 41(6):406–419

56. Mener A et al (2018) Complement component 3 negatively regulates antibody response by modulation of red blood cell antigen. Front Immunol 9:676
57. Couvidou A et al (2023) Marginal zone B cells are responsible for the production of alloantibodies following platelet transfusion in mice. Blood Adv 7(8):1356–1365
58. Kallarakal MA et al (2024) Marginal zone B cells are necessary for the formation of anti-donor IgG after allogeneic sensitization. Transplantation 108(6):1357–1367
59. Zimring JC et al (2005) Nonhemolytic antibody-induced loss of erythrocyte surface antigen. Blood 106(3):1105–1112
60. Zimring JC et al (2007) Nonhemolytic antigen loss from red blood cells requires cooperative binding of multiple antibodies recognizing different epitopes. Blood 110(6):2201–2208
61. Hod EA et al (2008) Cytokine storm in a mouse model of IgG-mediated hemolytic transfusion reactions. Blood 112(3):891–894
62. Liepkalns JS et al (2012) Biphasic clearance of incompatible red blood cells through a novel mechanism requiring neither complement nor Fcgamma receptors in a murine model. Transfusion 52(12):2631–2645
63. Zimring JC, Spitalnik SL (2015) Pathobiology of transfusion reactions. Annu Rev Pathol 10: 83–110
64. Arthur CM et al (2021) Antigen density dictates RBC clearance, but not antigen modulation, following incompatible RBC transfusion in mice. Blood Adv 5(2):527–538
65. Stowell SR et al (2013) Antigen modulation confers protection to red blood cells from antibody through Fcgamma receptor ligation. J Immunol 191(10):5013–5025
66. Girard-Pierce KR et al (2013) A novel role for C3 in antibody-induced red blood cell clearance and antigen modulation. Blood 122(10): 1793–1801
67. Jajosky RP, Covington ML, Liu J, Chai L, Zerra PE, Chonat S, Stowell SR, Arthur CM (2025) CD47 regulates antigen modulation and red blood cell clearance following an incompatible transfusion. Front Immunol 16: 1548548
68. Wabnitz H, Cruz-Leal Y, Lazarus AH (2023) Antigen copy number and antibody dose can determine the outcome of erythrocyte alloimmunization inducing either antibody-mediated immune suppression or enhancement in a murine model. Transfusion 63(4): 696–702
69. Yu H et al (2014) Antibody-mediated immune suppression of erythrocyte alloimmunization can occur independently from red cell clearance or epitope masking in a murine model. J Immunol 193(6):2902–2910
70. Cruz-Leal Y et al (2024) Trogocytosis drives red blood cell antigen loss in association with antibody-mediated immune suppression. Blood 143(9):807–821
71. Qiu A et al (2022) FcgammaRIV is required for IgG2c mediated enhancement of RBC alloimmunization. Front Immunol 13:972723
72. Shinde P et al (2020) IgG subclass determines suppression versus enhancement of humoral alloimmunity to Kell RBC antigens in mice. Front Immunol 11:1516
73. Jash A et al (2021) Antibodies to low-copy number RBC alloantigen convert a tolerogenic stimulus to an immunogenic stimulus in mice. Front Immunol 12:629608
74. Jash A et al (2024) Complement C3 and marginal zone B cells promote IgG-mediated enhancement of RBC alloimmunization in mice. J Clin Invest 134(8)
75. Bernardo L et al (2015) IgG-mediated immune suppression to erythrocytes by polyclonal antibodies can occur in the absence of activating or inhibitory Fcgamma receptors in a full mouse model. J Immunol 195(5): 2224–2230
76. Jajosky RP et al (2023) Antibody-mediated antigen loss switches augmented immunity to antibody-mediated immunosuppression. Blood 142(12):1082–1098
77. Maier CL et al (2018) Antibody-mediated immune suppression by antigen modulation is antigen-specific. Blood Adv 2(21):2986–3000
78. Jajosky RP et al (2024) Dynamics of antibody engagement of red blood cells in vivo and in vitro. Front Immunol 15:1475470
79. Zerra PE et al (2021) Marginal zone B cells mediate a CD4 T-cell-dependent extrafollicular antibody response following RBC transfusion in mice. Blood 138(8):706–721
80. Phelps A et al (2024) Production and use of antigen tetramers to study antigen-specific B cells. Nat Protoc 19(3):727–751

Chapter 18

Determining the Binding Affinity in Monoclonal Antibody-Alloantigen Interactions

Kashyap R. Patel, Ryan P. Jajosky, Victoria M. Vance, Caitlin L. Cepeda, Vivien C. Lee, Sean R. Stowell, and Connie M. Arthur

Abstract

Humoral immunity, a significant facet of the adaptive immune system, neutralizes targets when circulating antigen-specific antibodies recognize a foreign antigen and recruit antibody-dependent effector systems. Antibody-mediated complement deposition and cellular removal through engagement of Fc receptors can mediate intravascular and extravascular hemolysis following an incompatible red blood cell (RBC) transfusion. Efficiency of hemolysis is influenced by the affinity of the antibody-antigen reaction. Therefore, determining the affinities of alloantibodies can be important when investigating the potential consequences of antibody engagement on RBC clearance and possible changes to the target antigen. Here, we describe three techniques, surface plasmon resonance, protein microarray, and flow cytometry, to distinguish affinities of monoclonal antibodies specific to the Hen Egg Lysozyme, Ovalbumin, and Duffy (HOD) fusion model antigen.

Key words Surface plasmon resonance, Protein microarray, Flow cytometry, Binding affinity

1 Introduction

Antibodies are specialized proteins of humoral immunity, capable of recognizing an almost infinite number of antigens through their Fab (Fragment antigen binding) region and engaging distinct immunological effector systems through their Fc (Fragment crystallizable) region. The biological roles of antibodies include neutralization of pathogens and toxins, and recruitment of effector systems, such as complement fixation and antibody-dependent cell mediated cytotoxicity [1, 2]. Structural features of antibodies that govern this function include heavy chain isotype, Fc glycosylation status, and properties of the paratope that dictate its specificity and affinity [3–6]. High antibody-antigen affinity is paramount in the effectiveness of an antibody. B cell activation and differentiation include mechanisms, such as somatic hypermutation, that result in

Sean R. Stowell and Connie M. Arthur (eds.), *Methods in Transfusion Medicine*, Methods in Molecular Biology, vol. 3053, https://doi.org/10.1007/978-1-0716-5376-0_18,

affinity maturation, enhancing the ability of selected antigen-specific B cell clones to engage and respond to the target antigen [7, 8].

Antibodies targeting alloantigens on red blood cells (RBCs) can develop through two primary mechanisms: naturally occurring anti-ABO(H) antibodies form in the first few months of life, while other antibodies often arise from exposure as a result of pregnancy or transfusion [9–11]. While the presence of ABO(H) blood groups and related antigens likely has significant evolutionary implications within host immunity, including the ability of innate immunity to protect against microbes that decorate themselves in blood group-like antigens [12–14], the development of alloantibodies against these antigens can cause significant challenges when seeking to procure compatible blood for transfusion [15–17]. The formation of these antibodies is influenced by a complex interplay of factors, including the recipient's genetic makeup, characteristics of the donor RBCs, and the recipient's inflammatory state at the time of transfusion, which has been outlined in many studies using a variety of clinical and preclinical model systems and overall approaches that illustrate different methods used to study this process [18–34]. Although numerous studies have attempted to elucidate the key pathways responsible for alloantibody development against RBC antigens, including the distinct pathways and overall cells involved in this process [29, 31–39], the ultimate outcome of an incompatible RBC transfusion is likely determined by the antibody's affinity for its target antigen, in addition to its ability to engage antibody effector systems, as illustrated by a wide variety of studies [10, 40–52]. Binding of recipient's antibodies to donor RBC surface alloantigen triggers activation of immune cells and complement proteins, which has been shown in a number of studies to lead to hemolysis of transfused RBCs [9, 24, 35, 47, 50, 53–58]. Antibody-induced hemolysis of transfused RBCs can initiate a cascade effect, leading to hemolysis of the patient's own RBCs. This phenomenon, known as hyperhemolysis, poses a significant risk to life, particularly for individuals with sickle cell disease as documented in a number of studies [16, 59–66].

Antibody response against a large protein alloantigen is likely polyclonal, and discerning their individual affinities is challenging [55]. Nevertheless, high affinity anti-D IgG can clear RhD-positive RBCs comparatively faster than low affinity anti-D IgG [24]. Additionally, common laboratory tests assessing the presence of alloantibodies in recipients rely on high affinity interactions with cell surface antigens [67, 68]. Thus, distinguishing affinities of anti-RBC alloantibodies is important when seeking to understand their overall activity. Following is a brief description of surface plasmon resonance, protein microarray, and flow cytometry techniques and their application in identifying affinity of monoclonal anti-Hen egg lysozyme, Ovalbumin, and Duffy (HOD) alloantibodies [38] (Fig. 1).

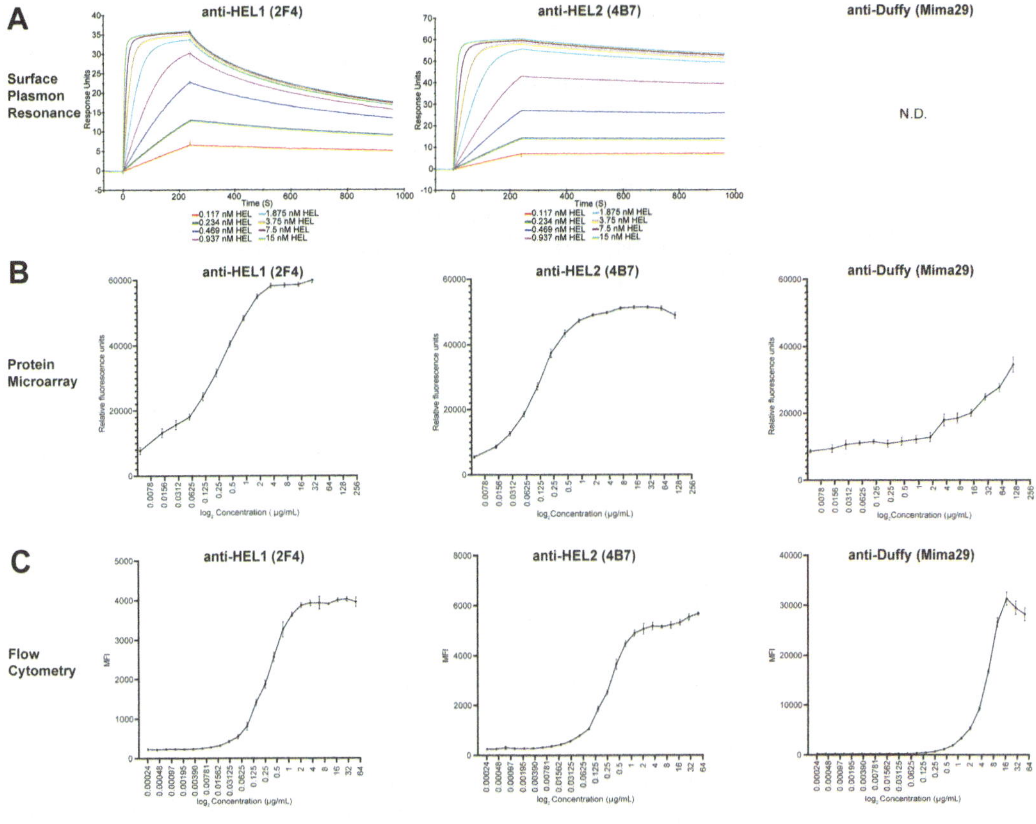

D

	anti-HEL1 (2F4)	anti HEL2 (4B7)	anti-Duffy (Mima29)
SPR	0.0671 nM	0.0211 nM	N. D.
Protein Microarray	1.27 nM	0.626 nM	N. D.
Flow cytometry	1.74 nM	1.81 nM	33.95 nM

Fig. 1 Antibody-antigen binding assay. (**a**) Surface plasmon resonance sensograms showing binding of Hen Egg Lysozyme (HEL) antigen to two mouse monoclonal antibodies, anti-HEL1 IgG1 (2F4) and anti-HEL2 IgG1 (4B7). HEL is injected at increasing concentration over captured anti-HEL antibodies on immobilized anti-mouse IgG. (**b**) Protein microarray binding isotherms generated by incubating mouse monoclonal antibodies, anti-HEL1 IgG1 (2F4), anti-HEL2 IgG1 (4B7), and anti-Duffy IgG2a (Mima29) over printed HEL antigen and Duffy peptide. Relative fluorescence units are plotted against antibody concentration. Binding of Mima29 to Duffy peptide did not reach saturation; therefore, relative K_D (equilibrium dissociation constant) values could not be calculated. (**c**) Flow cytometry binding isotherm produced by staining HOD RBC with 2F4, 4B7 and Mima29. Mean fluorescence intensity is plotted against antibody concentration. (**d**) Calculated absolute K_D values by SPR and relative K_D values by protein microarray and flowcytometry. N. D. = not determined. (Image was adapted from a first version published in *Blood*. Jajosky et al. [38])

Surface Plasmon Resonance (SPR) is a sensitive, well-established technique used to study the kinetics and affinity of antibody-antigen interactions. In brief, photons from incident light reflect off a metal coated surface depending on the amount of plasmons (delocalized oscillating electrons caused by the incidence of light on the metal surface) produced on the surface. The binding of analyte to the immobilized ligand on the metal surface introduces changes in plasmons that alter the angle of light reflection. Signal changes from reflected light are quantified as response units used to calculate binding kinetics [69, 70]. Corresponding binding kinetics data obtained from the produced sensograms are plotted to provide absolute affinity values without the need to label either antigen or antibody with agents to facilitate detection. The main drawback of SPR is the requirement of specialized software and expertise to obtain and analyze SPR data. Additionally, comprehensive analysis requires moderate quantities of antibodies and antigens [71].

Protein microarray is a versatile and sensitive technique to characterize interactions and the overall specificity between proteins and biomolecules [72]. Early protein microarrays were used to identify substrates for protein kinases in yeast; this method has been applied to elucidate many biochemical interactions, including assessment of antibody-antigen affinity and specificity [73–75]. Purified antigens are spotted by contact or non-contact printers at a high density on a chemically impregnated glass slide. After blocking the unoccupied surface, antibodies are incubated at different concentrations. Captured antibodies can be directly labeled or detected using a secondary antibody conjugated with a fluorophore. Fluorescence signal from antigen spots can be quantified and plotted against antibody concentration to establish a binding isotherm that can be used to define the relative affinity of antibody-antigen interactions [72, 76, 77]. A notable benefit of protein microarrays is the lower requirement of sample quantity. Additionally, staining demands less specialized expertise, and printing isolated antigens confers specificity to the assay. Absolute binding affinity values cannot be obtained with this approach; however, estimated relative binding affinities can be compared. Lastly, antigen immobilization can cause changes in conformation which can alter interaction properties.

Flow cytometry is widely implemented in clinical and research laboratories because it can deliver both quantitative and qualitative antibody binding information at single-cell resolution [78]. Flow cytometry is based on probing the cells with antigen-specific antibodies, which can either be directly labeled with a fluorophore or cell bound antibodies detected by fluorescently labeled secondary antibodies, although use of secondary antibodies for antibody detection adds another equilibrium constant that can complicate relative affinity measurements. Stained cell populations are suspended in a compatible buffer and passed through lasers capable of exciting the fluorophore. Emitted signal is proportional to amounts of antibodies bound to the cell [79, 80]. Mean fluorescence intensity from each antibody-RBC pair is plotted against antibody concentrations. Using this approach, relative antibody-antigen affinities are calculated. One advantage of this approach is that antigens are in their native orientation and conformation on the cell surface during staining, allowing the potential influence of cell surface characteristics to be included when assessing antibody affinity. However, absolute affinity values cannot be obtained with flow cytometry.

2 Materials

2.1 Surface Plasmon Resonance (SPR)

2.1.1 Instrument Setup/Priming

1. CM5 chip (Cytiva).
2. Biacore T200 (Cytiva).
3. SPR Running buffer—Phosphate buffered saline without calcium and magnesium with 0.05% Tween 20, pH 7.4 (*see* **Note 1**).

2.1.2 Coupling Anti-mouse Antibody

1. CM5 chip (Cytiva).
2. Anti-mouse antibody (Cytiva, Mouse Antibody Capture Kit).
3. Immobilization buffer, 10 mM Sodium acetate, pH 5.0 (Cytiva, Mouse Antibody Capture Kit).
4. N-Hydroxysuccinimide (NHS) (Cytiva, Amine Coupling Kit).
5. 1-Ethyl-3-(3-dimethylaminopropyl) carbodiimide hydrochloride (EDC) (Cytiva, Amine Coupling Kit).
6. 1 M Ethanolamine hydrochloride-NaOH pH 8.5, 10.5 mL (Cytiva, Amine Coupling Kit).
7. Biacore SPR consumables (Cytiva).

2.1.3 Regeneration Scouting (Fig. 2)

1. CM5 chip with two flow cells coupled to anti-mouse IgG.
2. Anti-HEL1 antibody (2F4) or Anti-HEL2 antibody (4B7).
3. Regeneration buffer 1–1 M NaCl.
4. Regeneration buffer 2–10 mM Glycine, pH 2.5.
5. Regeneration buffer 3–10 mM Glycine, pH 2.
6. Regeneration buffer 4–10 mM Glycine, pH 1.7.
7. Biacore SPR consumables (Cytiva).

2.1.4 Kinetic Analysis

1. CM5 chip with two flow cells coupled to anti-mouse IgG.
2. Anti-HEL1 antibody (2F4) or Anti-HEL2 antibody (4B7).
3. Hen Egg Lysozyme (HEL)—lyophilized powder ≥98% (Sigma-Millipore).
4. Regeneration buffer 4–10 mM Glycine, pH 1.7.
5. Biacore SPR consumables (Cytiva).

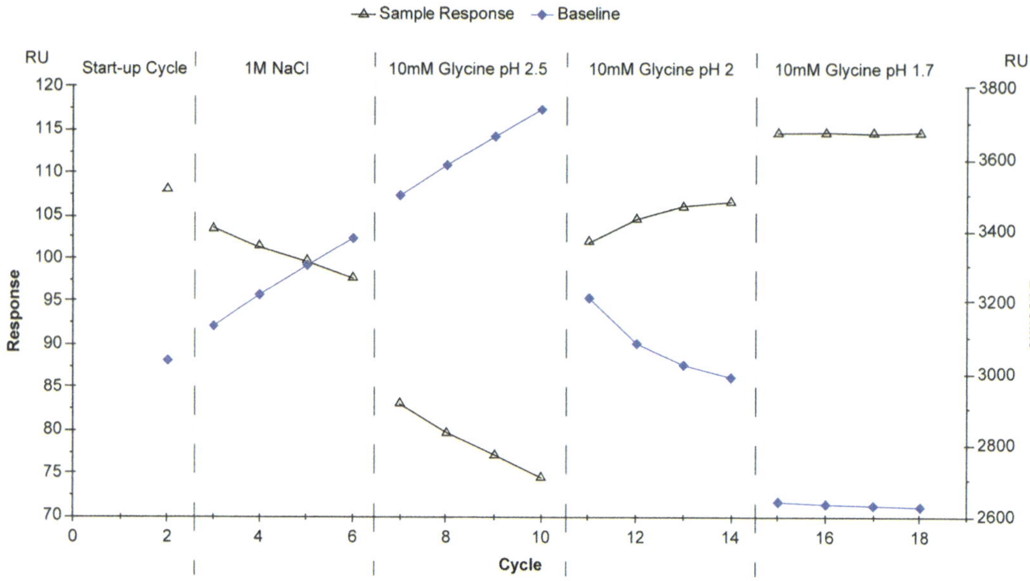

Fig. 2 Regeneration scouting profile. Graph showing changes in baseline (blue diamond) and response unit (white triangle) for repeated four cycles of antibody injections and regeneration by four different regeneration buffers. Selection of optimal buffer conditions is based on observation of stable baseline and response units with each cycle, only noted in 10 mM glycine pH 1.7. (The image was edited from a version exported from T200 control software)

2.2 Protein Microarray

1. Aushon Biosystems 2470 Microarray printer (Quanterix).
2. Nexterion H 3-D Hydrogel-coated slides (Schott Minifab).
3. Hen Egg Lysozyme (HEL)—lyophilized powder ≥98% (Sigma-Millipore).
4. Synthetic Duffy peptide, KRR**VRSKLLLLSTCLAQ-QALDLLLN** RRK (Duffy loop 3 peptide is highlighted by bold text) (*see* **Note 2**).
5. Protein-G—lyophilized powder (Fisher Scientific).
6. Human Serum Albumin—lyophilized powder ≥98% (Sigma-Millipore).
7. Print buffer: 50 mM phosphate buffer, with 100 μg/mL human serum albumin and 0.01% Octyl-β-glucoside, pH 8.0.
8. 185 μm pins for contact printer.
9. 384-well polypropylene plate (BioRad).
10. Anti-HEL1 antibody (2F4), anti-HEL2 antibody (4B7) and anti-Duffy antibody (Mima29).
11. Airtight container with desiccant.
12. 16 wells Grace Bio-Labs ProPlate microarray system (Grace Bio-Labs).

13. Blocking buffer: 25 mM Ethanolamine, 100 mM Phosphate buffer, and 0.05% Tween 20, pH 8.0.
14. Phosphate buffered saline (PBS): Phosphate buffered saline without calcium and magnesium, pH 7.4.
15. PBST: PBS with 0.05% Tween 20, pH 7.4.
16. Anti-mouse IgG conjugated with Alexa Fluor 647 (Jackson Immunoresearch).
17. Deionized water.
18. Microarray scanner (GenePix 4000B) with associated GenePix Pro 7 software.

2.3 Antibody-Antigen Binding by Flow Cytometry

1. FVB HOD mouse (*see* **Note 3**).
2. Sterile 2 mL microcentrifuge tubes.
3. Anticoagulant Citrate Dextrose (ACD-A) Solution.
4. Murine whole blood collection tools based on approved IACUC (Institutional Animal Care and Use Committee) protocol.
5. Phosphate buffered saline (PBS): Phosphate buffered saline without calcium and magnesium, pH 7.4.
6. Centrifuge with adjustable brakes and capable of holding 2 mL tubes and 96-well plate.
7. Anti-HEL1 antibody (2F4), anti-HEL2 antibody (4B7) and anti-Duffy antibody (Mima29).
8. 96-well U-bottom plate.
9. Anti-mouse IgG labeled with Alexa Fluor 647 (Jackson Immunoresearch).
10. Flow cytometer—Cytek Northern Lights cytometer (or other flow cytometer with 635 nm laser).

3 Methods

3.1 Surface Plasmon Resonance (SPR)

3.1.1 Instrument Priming

1. This method describes SPR experiments performed on a Biacore T200 using a CM5 sensor chip.
2. Fill the bottle with running buffer and place it in the buffer tray on the left of the instrument. Connect the tube marked A to the bottle containing running buffer. Empty the waste bottle and place it in the waste tray on the right of the instrument. Connect it to the waste outlet tube. Place a bottle containing 500 mL of water in the waste tray and connect it with tube for water.
3. Remove CM5 chip from 4 °C and let it equilibrate at room temperature for 30 min before removing it from the package.

4. If a dummy chip is already inserted in the instrument, initiate chip ejection. Replace the dummy chip with the new CM5 chip by inserting the new chip with the arrow pointing up and toward the instrument. Manually close the port by gently pushing it in. Select chip type in an insert chip dialog box and click dock chip to initiate chip docking.
5. Set the temperature of the instrument to 25 °C before priming the instrument.
6. Prime the instrument to flush the tubes with running buffer. The CM5 chip surface is ready for coupling after priming concludes.

3.1.2 Coupling Anti-mouse Antibody

1. Anti-mouse antibody immobilization is performed in both reference flow cell and sample flow cell concurrently using the same method and immobilization conditions. Immobilization is performed as per the recommended condition described in the mouse antibody capture kit.
2. Mix the anti-mouse antibody solution by vortexing and briefly centrifuging prior to use. Dilute the antibody to a concentration of 30 μg/mL by adding 5 μL antibody to 162 μL immobilization buffer.
3. Prepare EDC and NHS solutions by adding 10 mL of filter sterilized deionized water to each vial. Dissolve the reagents by gently vortexing the vials.
4. Make single use aliquots of both EDC and NHS and store them at −20 °C. Store ethanolamine at 4 °C.
5. Thaw an aliquot of the EDC and NHS solution and mix it gently to make it homogenous.
6. Select the immobilization, under surface preparation section, as the template in method wizard of T200 control software. The following steps detail input values for each dialog box to complete the experimental setup (*see* **Note 4**).
7. Immobilization setup—select CM5 in the chip type from the dropdown menu and choose the flow cells for immobilization. Choose Amine as the method and enter anti-mouse IgG as the ligand. Set contact time to 420 s and flow rate to 10 μL/min.
8. System preparations—set the analysis and sample compartment temperature at 25 °C. If the instrument is not primed, then check "prime before run" box.
9. Rack position—eject the reagent rack from the sample compartment. Minimal sample volumes for each reagent required to immobilize anti-mouse IgG on CM5 chip surface are indicated. Select an appropriate sample vial depending on volume requirements and pipette the reagents at the base of the vial to prevent air bubbles from getting trapped at the bottom.

10. Clicking on the occupied vial in the rack diagram on the left section of the dialog box will highlight the reagent entered in the table on the right. Cap and load the respective vial in the rack at the designated position according to this diagram. Vial positions can be changed by dragging the occupied vial to an empty position in this dialog box.
11. Load the rack into the sample compartment till it clicks into a locked position.
12. Prepare run—check if all the necessary assay steps are completed and verify if the running buffer is sufficient to finish the immobilization step. Save the template as a method file and start the run. The immobilization procedure will activate the surface with EDC/NHS mixture for 7 min, immobilize the anti-mouse IgG for 7 min, and deactivate the surface for 7 min.
13. After completion, an immobilization sensogram appears on the screen, which can be saved. The immobilization result dialog box contains "response final," which represents immobilization levels on the CM5 sensor chip. A value of over 5000 response units (RU) is expected.
14. Immobilized sensor chips can be stored in a 50 mL tube with wet Kimwipe at 4 °C if required.

3.1.3 Regeneration Scouting

1. Regeneration scouting is important to identify ideal conditions to regenerate (remove all captured analyte and ligand) the immobilized surface. Suboptimal regeneration will reduce surface binding capacity; regeneration with harsh conditions can damage the binding surface, and regeneration with mild conditions will not remove sufficient analyte or ligand.
2. Dilute the anti-HEL1 (2F4) or anti-HEL2 (4B7) antibody at a concentration of 5 μg/mL in running buffer and keep on ice.
3. Insert a CM5 chip with two cells immobilized with anti-mouse IgG by following **steps 4–6** from Subheading 3.1.1. Set the instrument temperature to 25 °C.
4. Select the regeneration scouting, under assay development section, as a template in method wizard of T200 control software. The following steps detail input values for each dialog box to complete experimental setup.
5. Injection sequence—choose the sample flow cell (not the reference flow cell) as flow path for this experiment. Select CM5 in the chip type and check boxes for ligand capture and one regeneration step.
6. Setup—a startup cycle is run by default before testing the first regeneration condition.

7. Injection parameter—write "anti-HEL1 antibody" in the ligand section and input contact time of 60 s with flow rate of 10 μL/min.
8. Experimental parameters—specify flow rate of 30 μL/min in the regeneration parameter section. Select four for the number of conditions and four for the number of cycles. Write out the four regeneration buffers to test in desired order and specify 30 s as the contact time for each (*see* **Note 5**).
9. System preparations—check "prime before run" if the system is not primed and specify analysis temperature of 25 °C.
10. Rack positions—follow **steps 10** and **11** in Subheading 3.1.2 to dispense indicated volume of antibody solution and regeneration buffer 1, 2, 3, and 4 in appropriately sized vials. Specify the rack position for each buffer and install the rack inside the instrument.
11. Prepare run protocol—check if all the assay steps are accurately completed and verify if running buffer is sufficient to finish regeneration scouting. Save the template as a method file and start the run. During the run, regeneration conditions are tested by four consecutive cycles of analyte injection and regeneration with four different buffer conditions.
12. Upon completion, regeneration scouting results are displayed. Evaluate the sample response and baseline level changes between each cycle and select the regeneration condition for kinetic analysis which shows stable levels of sample response and baseline for all four cycles. Regeneration buffer 10 mM glycine, pH 1.7, is ideal for anti-HEL1/2 antibody (*see* **Note 6**).

3.1.4 Kinetic Analysis

1. This section describes methods to determine binding kinetics with multi-cycle analysis (*see* **Note 7**).
2. Spin the anti-HEL1 (2F4) or anti-HEL2 (4B7) antibody stock solution at 10000 × g for 2 min and filter the supernatant using a 0.2-micron nylon syringe filter. Accurately measure antibody concentration and check the antibodies for degradation after filtering (*see* **Note 8**).
3. Dilute anti-HEL1 (2F4) or anti-HEL2 (4B7) antibodies at 2 μg/mL in the running buffer (*see* **Notes 9** and **10**).
4. Dissolve lyophilized Hen Egg Lysozyme (HEL) in running buffer and dilute at concentrations of 15 nM, 7.5 nM, 3.75 nM, 1.875 nM, 0.937 nM, 0.469 nM, 0.234 nM, and 0.117 nM in the running buffer (*see* **Note 11**).
5. Insert a CM5 chip with two cells immobilized with anti-mouse IgG by following **steps 4–6** from Subheading 3.1.1. Set the instrument temperature to 25 °C.

6. Select the kinetics/affinity, under the assay section, as a template in the method wizard of the T200 control software. The following steps detail input values for each dialog box to complete the experimental setup.
7. Injection sequence—select the pair of flow cells with immobilized anti-mouse IgG. Select CM5 as the chip type and check boxes for ligand capture, sample, and regeneration. Select one regeneration step. These steps will be repeated for each cycle of this multi-cycle analysis (*see* **Note 12**).
8. Setup—check the box to run the startup cycle with a running buffer and enter three for the number of cycles.
9. Injection parameters—set contact time of 40 s for ligand capture (diluted antibodies anti-HEL1 (2F4) or anti-HEL2 (4B7)) with a flow rate of 10 μL/min and 0 s as stabilization period. Set contact time of 240 s for the sample (HEL) at a flow rate of 30 μL/min and set dissociation time of 720 s. Set contact time for regeneration solution for 30 s at a flow rate of 30 μL/min with 0 s as stabilization period.
10. Samples—Type in the sample name (HEL) with respective concentration in the sample ID section, molecular weight of 14,600 Da, and respective concentration in nM for each sample dilution (*see* **Note 13**).
11. System preparations—check the prime before running if the system is not primed and set the analysis temperature to 25 °C.
12. Rack position—follow **steps 10** and **11** in Subheading 3.1.2 to dispense the indicated volume of antibody solution, sample, and regeneration buffer 4 in appropriately sized vials. Specify rack position for each vial and install the rack inside the instrument.
13. Prepare run protocol—check if all the assay steps are accurately completed and verify if the running buffer is sufficient to finish the assay. Save the template as a method file and start the run. For each cycle of multi-cycle analysis, the anti-HEL1 or 2 antibody is captured on the surface through immobilized anti-mouse IgG, followed by injection of HEL at specified concentrations and regeneration to remove both captured antibody and HEL.
14. At completion of the run, sensograms from the entire multi-cycle analysis can be opened in the Biocore T200 evaluation software. Signal from blank injections is subtracted from sample injections, and signal from reference flow cell is subtracted from active cell.
15. A 1:1 interaction model is applied to calculate dissociation constants. Values from the association and dissociation sections of the sensogram are extracted, and kinetic parameters are

established. Affinity is calculated from either the kinetic parameters or by plotting a binding isotherm of response units at equilibrium against HEL concentration.

3.2 Protein Microarray

1. The method in this section describes a protein microarray constructed with Aushon Biosystems 2470 Microarray printer (Quanterix) on Nexterion H 3-D Hydrogel-coated slides (*see* **Note 14**).
2. Resuspend lyophilized HEL antigen in PBS and dilute it at a concentration of 300 μg/mL in print buffer to make up to 45 μL final volume.
3. Resuspend the lyophilized Duffy peptide in PBS and dilute it at a concentration of 6000 μg/mL in print buffer to make up to 45 μL final volume (*see* **Note 2**).
4. Dilute Protein-G and Human Serum Albumin at a concentration of 50 μg/mL and 100 μg/mL, respectively, in print buffer to make up to 45 μL final volume (*see* **Note 15**).
5. Load 10 μL of each HEL antigen, Duffy peptide, Protein-G, and Human Serum Albumin in four wells of a 384-well plate according to the sample well positions created by the 2470 microarray printer software after designing the print layout.
6. Print all proteins/peptides in 4 replicates with 185 μm pins in a 16-subarray per slide format. Print 4 slides in total: one for each antibody (anti-HEL1 (2F4), anti-HEL2 (4B7), and anti-Duffy (Mima29)) and one additional slide as a backup in case an experiment needs to be repeated (*see* **Note 16**).
7. Incubate printed slides for 16 h at 4 °C in a closed slide holder. Store the incubated slide in an airtight container with desiccant at −20 °C until staining is performed.
8. Let the slides equilibrate to room temperature before opening the container with desiccant.
9. Wash the slides by submerging them three times in a 50 mL tube containing PBS.
10. Wash the slide once by submerging it in a 50 mL tube containing deionized water.
11. Block slides for 1 h at room temperature by placing them in a 50 mL tube containing blocking buffer.
12. Wash slides twice by submerging them in a 50 mL tube containing PBST.
13. Wash slides twice by submerging them in a 50 mL tube containing PBS.
14. Affix the 16-well ProPlate module on top of the slide and wash each well with 200 μL of PBS.

15. Dilute antibodies anti-HEL1 (2F4), anti-HEL2 (4B7), and anti-Duffy (Mima29) twofold from 150 μg/mL to 0.00915 μg/mL (15 dilutions) in PBST.
16. Aspirate off the PBS with a mild vacuum immediately before adding 100 μL of each antibody dilution per well. Add PBST without antibody to the 16th well.
17. Incubate slides for 2 h at room temperature on a laboratory rocker.
18. Wash each well twice with 200 μL PBST per well to remove unbound antibodies. Aspirate the wash buffer each time immediately before adding the next buffer to prevent slides from drying.
19. Wash each well four times with 200 μL PBS per well. Aspirate the wash buffer each time immediately before adding the next buffer to prevent slides from drying.
20. Dilute anti-mouse IgG conjugated with Alexa Fluor 647 (secondary antibody) at a ratio of 1:200 in PBST.
21. Add 100 μL of secondary antibody per well and stain slides for 1 h at room temperature on a laboratory rocker.
22. Wash each well twice with 200 μL PBST to remove unbound secondary antibodies. Aspirate the wash buffer each time immediately before adding the next buffer to prevent slides from drying.
23. Wash each well four times with 200 μL PBS. Aspirate the wash buffer each time immediately before adding the next buffer to prevent slides from drying.
24. Wash each well twice with 200 μL deionized water. Remove the 16-well ProPlate module gently and let the slide air dry.
25. Use a microarray scanner to acquire the fluorescence image with the 635 nm laser. Use the associated GenePix Pro 7 software to calculate relative fluorescence units for each spot by subtracting the spot fluorescence intensity from the local background intensity.
26. Average the intensity from four replicates and calculate the relative fluorescence intensity by subtracting the signal from the same antigen spots in the 16th well (*see* **Note 17**).
27. Plot the relative fluorescence intensity against concentration. Extract intensity values from HEL antigen spots when stained with anti-HEL1 (2F4) and anti-HEL2 (4B7) antibodies. Extract intensity values from Duffy peptide spots when stained with anti-Duffy (Mima29) antibody.
28. Maximal binding level and relative dissociation constant can be manually calculated from the plotted graphs for each antibody.

A four-parameter logistic (4PL) regression model can be used to fit the antibody-antigen binding curve using graphing software to calculate the K_D values.

3.3 Antibody-Antigen Binding by Flow Cytometry

1. Face bleed an FVB HOD mouse to collect approximately 400 μL whole blood in sterile 2 mL microcentrifuge tubes containing 200 μL of the anticoagulant ACD-A (*see* **Note 18**).
2. Wash the cells by adding 1 mL PBS to the tube and centrifuge at 400 × g for 1 min at room temperature with the brakes set on low.
3. Repeat the washing process two more times, removing the supernatant and re-suspending the pellets in 1.8 mL of PBS each time. After the last wash, remove the supernatant and store packed RBCs on ice.
4. Dilute each of the anti-HEL1 (2F4), anti-HEL2 (4B7), and anti-Duffy (Mima29) antibodies in PBS from 50 μg/mL to 0.00025 μg/mL in a twofold dilution series (24 total dilutions).
5. Add 25 μL of the serially diluted antibodies in triplicate to a 96-well U-bottom plate.
6. Add 1 μL of packed RBCs to each well with the antibody.
7. Incubate the 96-well plate for 15 min at room temperature.
8. Wash the RBCs with 200 μL of PBS per well and centrifuge the plate at 400 × g for 1 min at room temperature with the brakes set on low (*see* **Note 19**).
9. Repeat the washing two more times, decanting the supernatant and re-suspending the pellets in 200 μL of PBS each time.
10. Dilute anti-mouse IgG labeled with Alexa Fluor 647 (secondary antibody) at a ratio of 1:100 in PBS.
11. Stain the RBCs by adding 25 μL of the diluted secondary antibody solution to each well and resuspend the pellet by gentle pipetting.
12. Incubate the well plate in the dark for 15 min at room temperature.
13. Wash the stained RBCs with 200 μL of PBS and centrifuge the 96-well plate at 400 × g for 1 min at RT with the brakes set on low.
14. Repeat the washing two more times, decanting the supernatant and re-suspending the pellets in 200 μL of PBS each time.
15. After the final wash, decant the supernatant and resuspend the pellet in 200 μL PBS.
16. Using the flow cytometer, acquire 50,000 RBC events. Average the fluorescence intensity of three replicates to calculate the mean fluorescence intensity (*see* **Note 20**).

17. Plot the mean fluorescence intensity against concentration and manually calculate the maximal binding level and relative dissociation constant for each antibody. A four-parameter logistic (4PL) regression model can be used to fit the antibody-antigen binding curve using graphing software to calculate the K_D values.

4 Notes

1. Any particulates or aggregates in the buffer will influence results. Filter the SPR running buffer through a 0.2-micron nylon filter. Degas the buffer after filtration by placing the bottle in a bath sonicator for 15 min.
2. A Duffy epitope for Mima29, KRR**VRSKLLLLSTCLAQQALDLLLN** RRK (Bold text represents Duffy loop 3), was synthesized to serve as the Mima29 antigen. This peptide was selected based on a previous publication [81]. Extra lysine residues at each terminal provide a primary amine group for immobilization to Nexterion H slides.
3. Refer to the previous study for background and source of FVB HOD mice [38].
4. Method wizard associated with the Biacore T200 control software contains a method template for several experiments commonly performed on the instrument. These templates can be customized as desired and are ideal for testing preliminary experimental conditions.
5. The recommended repeated cycles of analyte injection and regeneration are five, and the minimum is three. Regeneration testing should be performed from the mildest to the harshest conditions to prevent damage to the immobilized surface.
6. In the graph containing regeneration scouting data, the sample response indicates binding capacity, and baseline response changes indicate regeneration capacity. Decreasing sample response with increasing baseline response implies regeneration conditions are too mild.
7. An assay description for single kinetics is not provided in this chapter. Perform a pilot experiment to determine the disassociation time for HEL when injected with anti-HEL antibody captured on the surface. If more than 10% dissociation does not occur within 10 min after reaching equilibrium, perform a single-cycle kinetic assay to determine binding affinity.
8. Freezing stocks of antibodies could cause precipitation of a fraction of protein molecules. Filtration removes protein aggregates, which can interfere with the assay. Run an SDS-PAGE gel to ascertain that the antibody is intact.

9. Empirically determine the optimal concentration of anti-HEL antibody for the ligand capture step. Typical concentration range is 1 to 10 μg/mL diluted in running buffer. An increase of 500 response units over baseline is sufficient.
10. Required volume of antibody and antigen for the assay is displayed in the "Rack position" section of the kinetic/affinity assay. Therefore, create the method with the intended contact time and flow rates before diluting the antibody and antigen in the running buffer.
11. Test a broader range of HEL concentrations before choosing eight concentration series spanning the K_D value. Initially, try 0.01 to 100× the estimated K_D value.
12. During the ligand capture step of the cycle, the ligand is only applied to the sample cell and not the reference cell.
13. It is recommended to repeat one cycle of the HEL sample with a concentration in the middle of the concentration series to ensure reproducibility. Add two blank injections (running buffer instead of HEL) steps at the beginning and one at the end of the HEL concentration series to establish the baseline for the assay.
14. A different microarray printer (contact or non-contact mode) can be utilized to construct this array. Sixteen replicates of the same array (16 subarrays) are printed per slide. The top and left offset, as well as the distance between each subarray, are discerned from the dimensions of the 16-well Grace Bio-Labs ProPlate microarray system (Grace Bio-Labs Cat# 206862).
15. Diluted Protein-G captures IgG and serves as a positive control. Printing buffer without the addition of antigen serves as a negative control.
16. Desired number of test antibodies and experimental replicates should be considered while deciding the number of slides to be printed.
17. Signal from possible non-specific binding by secondary antibody should be subtracted from the actual signal caused by antibody-antigen binding.
18. Use an appropriate IACUC approved method to collect whole blood from mice.
19. The RBCs will form a visibly packed pellet after centrifugation at the speed and time mentioned in the protocol. If the RBC pellet seems to have dispersed, turn off the brakes on the centrifuge and repeat the centrifugation before decanting the supernatant.
20. Stained RBCs can be gated in side-scatter and/or forward-scatter plots to remove non-specific antibody binding to other cell types. Single cells can be gated to improve the accuracy of the results.

Acknowledgments

This work was funded by NIH P01HL171803, R01 HL165975, R01 HL135575, and R01 HL154034. SRS has received speaker and consultant honoraria from Cerus, Grifols, Novartis, Alexion, and Argenx and has received a research grant from Alexion. No other authors have conflicts of interest.

References

1. Forthal DN (2014) Functions of antibodies. Microbiol Spectrum 2(4):1–17
2. de Taeye SW, Rispens T, Vidarsson G (2019) The ligands for human IgG and their effector functions. Antibodies (Basel) 8(2)
3. Schroeder HW Jr, Cavacini L (2010) Structure and function of immunoglobulins. J Allergy Clin Immunol 125(2 Suppl 2):S41–S52
4. Chiu ML et al (2019) Antibody structure and function: the basis for engineering therapeutics. Antibodies (Basel) 8(4)
5. Vidarsson G, Dekkers G, Rispens T (2014) IgG subclasses and allotypes: from structure to effector functions. Front Immunol 5:520
6. Subedi GP, Barb AW (2015) The structural role of antibody N-glycosylation in receptor interactions. Structure 23(9):1573–1583
7. LeBien TW, Tedder TF (2008) B lymphocytes: how they develop and function. Blood 112(5): 1570–1580
8. Sela-Culang I, Kunik V, Ofran Y (2013) The structural basis of antibody-antigen recognition. Front Immunol 4:302
9. Tormey CA, Hendrickson JE (2019) Transfusion-related red blood cell alloantibodies: induction and consequences. Blood 133(17):1821–1830
10. Stowell SR et al (2013) Alloantibodies to a paternally derived RBC KEL antigen lead to hemolytic disease of the fetus/newborn in a murine model. Blood 122(8):1494–1504
11. Zimring JC, Hudson KE (2016) Cellular immune responses in red blood cell alloimmunization. Hematology Am Soc Hematol Educ Program 2016(1):452–456
12. Jan HM et al (2024) Galectin-4 antimicrobial activity primarily occurs through its C-terminal domain. Mol Cell Proteomics 23(5):100747
13. Wu SC et al (2022) Innate immune Galectin-7 specifically targets microbes that decorate themselves in blood group-like antigens. iScience 25(7):104482
14. Blenda AV et al (2022) Galectin-9 recognizes and exhibits antimicrobial activity toward microbes expressing blood group-like antigens. J Biol Chem 298(4):101704
15. Dean CL et al (2019) Multiple hemolytic transfusion reactions misinterpreted as severe vaso-occlusive crisis in a patient with sickle cell disease. Transfusion 59(2):448–453
16. Chonat S et al (2018) Contribution of alternative complement pathway to delayed hemolytic transfusion reaction in sickle cell disease. Haematologica 103(10):e483–e485
17. Nickel RS et al (2016) Impact of red blood cell alloimmunization on sickle cell disease mortality: a case series. Transfusion 56(1):107–114
18. Pirenne F, Floch A, Diop S (2023) Alloimmunisation against red blood cells in sickle cell disease: transfusion challenges in high-income and low-income countries. Lancet Haematol 10(6):e468–e476
19. Fasano RM et al (2015) Red blood cell alloimmunization is influenced by recipient inflammatory state at time of transfusion in patients with sickle cell disease. Br J Haematol 168(2): 291–300
20. Zheng Y et al (2023) Proinflammatory state promotes red blood cell alloimmunization in pediatric patients with sickle cell disease. Blood Adv 7(17):4799–4808
21. Godefroy E et al (2016) Altered heme-mediated modulation of dendritic cell function in sickle cell alloimmunization. Haematologica 101(9):1028–1038
22. Yazdanbakhsh K, Shaz BH, Hillyer CD (2017) Immune regulation of sickle cell alloimmunization. ISBT Sci Ser 12(1):248–253
23. Pal M et al (2021) Hemolysis inhibits humoral B-cell responses and modulates alloimmunization risk in patients with sickle cell disease. Blood 137(2):269–280
24. Zimring JC, Spitalnik SL (2015) Pathobiology of transfusion reactions. Annu Rev Pathol 10: 83–110

25. Smith NH et al (2012) Generation of transgenic mice with antithetical KEL1 and KEL2 human blood group antigens on red blood cells. Transfusion 52(12):2620–2630
26. Stowell SR et al (2013) Addition of ascorbic acid solution to stored murine red blood cells increases posttransfusion recovery and decreases microparticles and alloimmunization. Transfusion 53(10):2248–2257
27. Stowell SR et al (2014) Transfusion of murine red blood cells expressing the human KEL glycoprotein induces clinically significant alloantibodies. Transfusion 54(1):179–189
28. Calabro S et al (2016) Bridging channel dendritic cells induce immunity to transfused red blood cells. J Exp Med 213(6):887–896
29. Arneja A et al (2016) Interleukin-6 receptor-alpha signaling drives anti-RBC alloantibody production and T-follicular helper cell differentiation in a murine model of red blood cell alloimmunization. Haematologica 101(11): e440–e444
30. Gibb DR et al (2017) Type I IFN is necessary and sufficient for inflammation-induced red blood cell alloimmunization in mice. J Immunol 199(3):1041–1050
31. Arthur CM et al (2017) Antigen density dictates immune responsiveness following red blood cell transfusion. J Immunol 198(7): 2671–2680
32. Thomas TA et al (2023) Reticulocytes in donor blood units enhance red blood cell alloimmunization. Haematologica 108(10):2639–2651
33. Jash A et al (2024) Complement C3 and marginal zone B cells promote IgG-mediated enhancement of RBC alloimmunization in mice. J Clin Invest 134(8)
34. Maier CL et al (2023) Storage differentially impacts alloimmunization to distinct red cell antigens following transfusion in mice. Transfusion 63(3):457–462
35. Shinde P et al (2020) IgG subclass determines suppression versus enhancement of humoral alloimmunity to Kell RBC antigens in mice. Front Immunol 11:1516
36. Jajosky R et al (2023) Prior immunization against an intracellular antigen enhances subsequent red blood cell alloimmunization in mice. Blood 141(21):2642–2653
37. Mener A et al (2018) Complement serves as a switch between CD4+ T cell-independent and -dependent RBC antibody responses. JCI Insight 3(22)
38. Jajosky RP et al (2023) Antibody-mediated antigen loss switches augmented immunity to antibody-mediated immunosuppression. Blood 142(12):1082–1098
39. Arthur CM et al (2022) Clodronate inhibits alloimmunization against distinct red blood cell alloantigens in mice. Transfusion 62(5): 948–953
40. Reverberi R, Reverberi L (2007) Factors affecting the antigen-antibody reaction. Blood Transfus 5(4):227–240
41. Zimring JC et al (2005) Nonhemolytic antibody-induced loss of erythrocyte surface antigen. Blood 106(3):1105–1112
42. Hod EA et al (2008) Cytokine storm in a mouse model of IgG-mediated hemolytic transfusion reactions. Blood 112(3):891–894
43. Zimring JC et al (2007) Nonhemolytic antigen loss from red blood cells requires cooperative binding of multiple antibodies recognizing different epitopes. Blood 110(6):2201–2208
44. Hod EA, Zimring JC, Spitalnik SL (2008) Lessons learned from mouse models of hemolytic transfusion reactions. Curr Opin Hematol 15(6):601–605
45. Hod EA et al (2010) Use of mouse models to study the mechanisms and consequences of RBC clearance. Vox Sang 99(2):99–111
46. Liepkalns JS et al (2012) Biphasic clearance of incompatible red blood cells through a novel mechanism requiring neither complement nor Fcgamma receptors in a murine model. Transfusion 52(12):2631–2645
47. Girard-Pierce KR et al (2013) A novel role for C3 in antibody-induced red blood cell clearance and antigen modulation. Blood 122(10): 1793–1801
48. Stowell SR et al (2012) Initiation and regulation of complement during hemolytic transfusion reactions. Clin Dev Immunol 2012: 307093
49. Liepkalns JS et al (2013) Resistance of a subset of red blood cells to clearance by antibodies in a mouse model of incompatible transfusion. Transfusion 53(6):1319–1327
50. Stowell SR et al (2013) Antigen modulation confers protection to red blood cells from antibody through Fcgamma receptor ligation. J Immunol 191(10):5013–5025
51. Jajosky RP et al (2025) CD47 regulates antigen modulation and red blood cell clearance following an incompatible transfusion. Front Immunol 16:1548548
52. Jajosky RP et al (2024) Dynamics of antibody engagement of red blood cells in vivo and in vitro. Front Immunol 15:1475470
53. Arthur CM, Stowell SR (2023) The development and consequences of red blood cell alloimmunization. Annu Rev Pathol 18:537–564

54. Arthur CM et al (2021) Antigen density dictates RBC clearance, but not antigen modulation, following incompatible RBC transfusion in mice. Blood Adv 5(2):527–538
55. Stowell SR et al (2015) Anti-KEL sera prevents alloimmunization to transfused KEL RBCs in a murine model. Haematologica 100(10):e394–e397
56. Bernardo L et al (2015) IgG-mediated immune suppression to erythrocytes by polyclonal antibodies can occur in the absence of activating or inhibitory Fcgamma receptors in a full mouse model. J Immunol 195(5): 2224–2230
57. Gruber DR et al (2020) Passively transferred IgG enhances humoral immunity to a red blood cell alloantigen in mice. Blood Adv 4(7):1526–1537
58. Jash A et al (2021) Antibodies to low-copy number RBC alloantigen convert a tolerogenic stimulus to an immunogenic stimulus in mice. Front Immunol 12:629608
59. Roumenina LT, Bartolucci P, Pirenne F (2019) The role of complement in post-transfusion hemolysis and hyperhemolysis reaction. Transfus Med Rev 33(4):225–230
60. Meuleman MS, Roumenina LT, Grunenwald A (2023) Complement involvement in sickle cell disease. Presse Med 52(4):104205
61. Merle NS et al (2019) Complement activation during intravascular hemolysis: implication for sickle cell disease and hemolytic transfusion reactions. Transfus Clin Biol 26(2):116–124
62. Thein SL et al (2020) Hemolytic transfusion reactions in sickle cell disease: underappreciated and potentially fatal. Haematologica 105(3):539–544
63. Merle NS et al (2019) P-selectin drives complement attack on endothelium during intravascular hemolysis in TLR-4/heme-dependent manner. Proc Natl Acad Sci USA 116(13): 6280–6285
64. Narbey D et al (2017) Incidence and predictive score for delayed hemolytic transfusion reaction in adult patients with sickle cell disease. Am J Hematol 92(12):1340–1348
65. Dumas G et al (2016) Eculizumab salvage therapy for delayed hemolysis transfusion reaction in sickle cell disease patients. Blood 127(8): 1062–1064
66. Chonat S et al (2025) Complement is activated in patients with acute chest syndrome caused by sickle cell disease and represents a therapeutic target. Sci Transl Med 17(807):eadl4922
67. Sokol RJ et al (1997) Direct Coombs test-negative autoimmune hemolytic anemia and low-affinity IgG class antibodies. Immunohematology 13(4):115–118
68. Parker V, Tormey CA (2017) The direct antiglobulin test: indications, interpretation, and pitfalls. Arch Pathol Lab Med 141(2): 305–310
69. Nguyen HH et al (2015) Surface plasmon resonance: a versatile technique for biosensor applications. Sensors (Basel) 15(5):10481–10510
70. Yesudasu V, Pradhan HS, Pandya RJ (2021) Recent progress in surface plasmon resonance based sensors: a comprehensive review. Heliyon 7(3):e06321
71. Helmerhorst E et al (2012) Real-time and label-free bio-sensing of molecular interactions by surface plasmon resonance: a laboratory medicine perspective. Clin Biochem Rev 33(4):161–173
72. Sutandy FX, et al (2013) Overview of protein microarrays. Curr Protoc Protein Sci Chapter 27(1):Unit 27 1.
73. Berrade L, Garcia AE, Camarero JA (2011) Protein microarrays: novel developments and applications. Pharm Res 28(7):1480–1499
74. Chen, C.S. and H. Zhu, Protein microarrays. BioTechniques, 2006. 40(4): p. 423, 425, 427 passim.
75. Barry R, Soloviev M (2004) Quantitative protein profiling using antibody arrays. Proteomics 4(12):3717–3726
76. Hall DA, Ptacek J, Snyder M (2007) Protein microarray technology. Mech Ageing Dev 128(1):161–167
77. Diez P et al (2012) Data analysis strategies for protein microarrays. Microarrays (Basel) 1(2): 64–83
78. Cossarizza A et al (2019) Guidelines for the use of flow cytometry and cell sorting in immunological studies (second edition). Eur J Immunol 49(10):1457–1973
79. McKinnon KM (2018) Flow cytometry: an overview. Curr Protoc Immunol 120:5 1 1–5 1 11
80. Adan A et al (2017) Flow cytometry: basic principles and applications. Crit Rev Biotechnol 37(2):163–176
81. Wasniowska K et al (2004) The Fya, Fy6 and Fy3 epitopes of the Duffy blood group system recognized by new monoclonal antibodies: identification of a linear Fy3 epitope. Br J Haematol 124(1):118–122

Chapter 19

Modeling the Application of Chimeric Antigen Receptor T Cell Therapy to Eliminate Alloantibodies in Mice

Caroline A. Markmann and Vijay G. Bhoj

Abstract

Chimeric antigen receptor (CAR) T cell therapy has begun to show clinical promise as a strategy for immune-modulation in non-malignant conditions. In a murine model, we have demonstrated the utility of CAR T cells targeting B cells and plasma cells for the elimination of alloantibodies that cause allograft rejection. We describe a method for producing murine CAR T cells, their functional assessment in vitro, as well as their application in an in vivo transplant model. Our methods include a CAR production phase that involves retrovirus production, T cell isolation, activation, transduction and passage, and assessment of CAR expression by flow cytometry. Then, we describe methods for studying CAR T function in vitro using a cytotoxicity assay and in vivo using an islet transplant model.

Key words Alloantibody, Transplant, Immunotherapy, CAR T cell, Retrovirus, B cells, Plasma cells

1 Introduction

Human leukocyte antigens (HLA) are an essential component of our immune system, which, via interaction with T cell receptors and NK cell receptors, enables us to distinguish self from non-self and altered-self [1]. Two features are critical to the role of HLA in host defense: (1) HLA genes have evolved to be highly polymorphic, and (2) each individual expresses multiple HLA molecules such that cells are equipped to display a vast repertoire of foreign peptides to communicate to the immune system. This intrinsic property of the HLA, however, presents the major challenge to organ and tissue transplantation. The polymorphic nature of HLAs combined with the limited availability of organs means that full HLA matching of donors with recipients is not typically feasible. Thus, alloimmunity directed at mismatched HLA, as well as mismatched non-HLA antigens, is inevitable and must be addressed with immunosuppressive therapies. Alloimmunity primarily occurs at the level of T cells

Sean R. Stowell and Connie M. Arthur (eds.), *Methods in Transfusion Medicine*, Methods in Molecular Biology, vol. 3053,
https://doi.org/10.1007/978-1-0716-5376-0_19,

or B cells; here, we specifically address the challenge of humoral alloimmunity.

Humoral alloimmunity, here referring primarily to HLA-directed antibodies, may be pre-existing in transplant candidates or develop de novo in transplant recipients. Patients can develop alloantibodies following exposure to foreign HLA, typically in the settings of blood transfusion, pregnancy, or prior organ or cell transplantation. These sensitization events can lead to the development of high titers of serum donor-specific alloantibodies (DSA) that present a formidable barrier to transplantation due to the risk of hyperacute graft rejection [2]. Measurement of alloantibodies, donor and recipient HLA typing, and the crossmatch form the cornerstone of careful donor-recipient matching to avoid hyperacute rejection due to preformed DSA. Unfortunately, for a subset of patients who are broadly sensitized (i.e., harbor antibodies to most allo-HLA alleles), the inability to find a compatible organ means they experience prolonged wait times and high mortality rates while awaiting a compatible organ [3]. Attempts to eliminate alloantibodies, termed desensitization, have utilized combinations of plasmapheresis, intravenous immunoglobulin (IVIG), Rituximab, and proteasome inhibitors, and additional immunomodulatory agents are in development [4–7]. Currently, however, there is no standard of care approach, reflecting the fact that these strategies have been largely ineffective. In summary, the limitation lies in their inability to deplete the source, allo-specific memory B cells and plasma cells (PCs).

Chimeric antigen receptor (CAR) T cell therapies have emerged as highly effective strategies for target cell elimination. CAR T cells are engineered T cells that have been equipped with a synthetic receptor typically comprising an antibody-derived variable domain(s) as a targeting moiety that is linked to intracellular domains that provide signal 1 and signal 2 (akin to co-stimulation) to T cells. CARs enable redirection of T cells to any target antigen of choice in a pMHC-independent manner. CARTs targeting CD19 (here referred to as CART-19) and B cell maturation antigen (BCMA) (CART-BCMA) were the first to achieve regulatory approval for the treatment of B cell derived and plasma cell malignancies, respectively. These CAR products have demonstrated their remarkable capacity to eliminate malignant B cells and PCs. As expected, they also deplete B cells and/or PCs by virtue of targeting lineage antigens [8–10]. Recognition of this effect has spurred efforts to "re-purpose" B cells and PC-targeted CARTs for the treatment of diseases in which B/PCs play central pathogenic roles. Efforts to deplete autoimmune B cells using CART-19 are well underway, with early clinical results reported over the last few years, and several formal clinical trials for a variety of autoimmune diseases are currently active [11, 12].

Similarly, we have pursued studies to evaluate the utility of B cell/PC-targeted CAR T cells for the eradication of humoral alloimmunity. In this chapter, we discuss our utilization of CAR T cells targeting CD19 and BCMA to eliminate alloantibody producing cells in the context of organ/tissue transplantation. We have previously shown in a syngeneic murine model of allo-sensitization that CAR T cells targeting B cells and long-lived plasma cells can effectively desensitize mice and mitigate hyperacute allograft rejection [9]. We outline our method of mouse CAR T cell production including assays to assess their function as well as an example in vivo application for humoral desensitization.

CAR constructs are usually designed with attention initially paid to the extracellular domain, which is guided by the target antigen of interest. However, the choice of intracellular signaling domains as well as other structural elements (e.g., hinge and transmembrane domains) is an important consideration which could also affect CAR T cell functions such as differentiation, expansion, persistence, and effector activity [13]. A typical CAR would be constructed with a single chain variable fragment (scFv) linked to 4-1BB and/or CD28 intracellular costimulatory domains, followed by the CD3-zeta intracellular domain. Many variations using a wide array of domains, both synthetic and derived from known proteins, have been described [13], but discussion of the variety of options and their implications is beyond the scope of discussion in this chapter, as they are application specific and may need empirical testing.

Production of murine and human CAR T cells using viral vectors follows the same basic principles. However, the protocols we use for each, which are also consistent with those published by others, have significant differences. Thus, the protocol we describe here for the production of murine CAR T cells, which occurs over 6 days, should not be directly applied to human cells. The first step is the design of a CAR construct followed by production of a retroviral plasmid encoding the CAR gene. These steps involve in silico design and basic molecular techniques, which have been simplified by the option to have all hands-on construction performed commercially at a reasonable cost. The CAR gene is inserted into a retroviral plasmid, typically using the Murine Stem Cell Virus (MSCV)-based system; MSCV-based vectors including those with CAR transgenes are available through Addgene. With a CAR-encoding retroviral plasmid in hand, the first step in producing CAR T cells begins with determining the total number of T cells desired for in vitro or in vivo use. This is governed by experimental design and involves back-calculation, based on expected T cell population doublings, to determine the number of T cells used as starting material (Fig. 1). The appropriate number of T cells (CD8+ or bulk T cells) is isolated from spleens and activated using anti-CD3/anti-CD28 beads. At some point, retrovirus must be made to

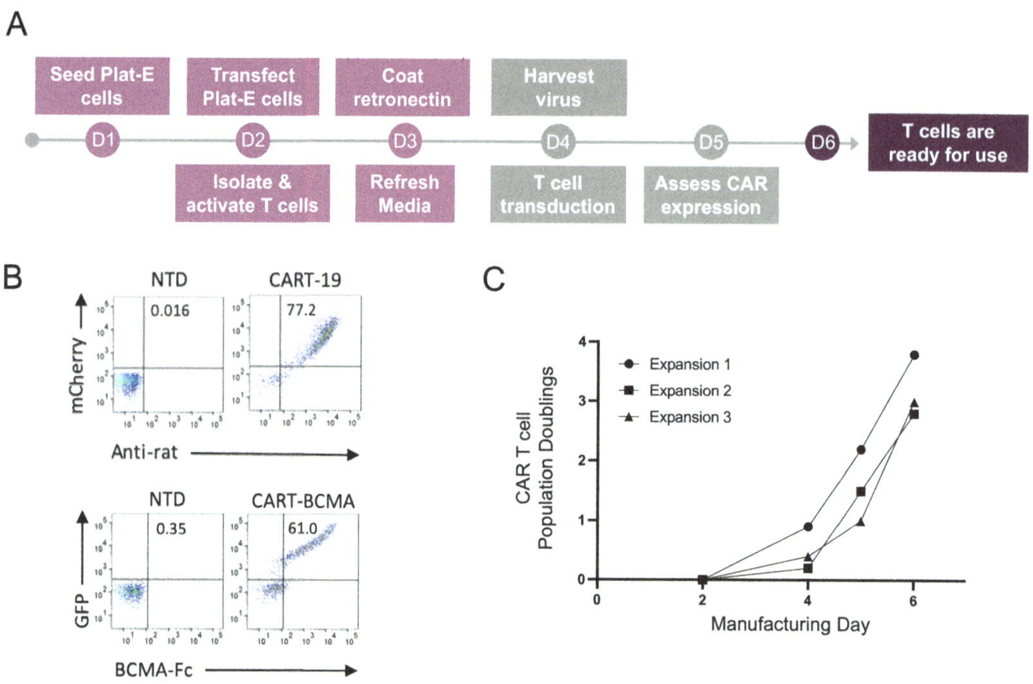

Fig. 1 Murine CAR T cell manufacturing. (**a**) Schema of murine CAR T cell production. (**b**) Flow cytometric evaluation of CAR expression at day 5. CART-19 cells were stained using an anti-rat Vh+Vl antibody that stains the rat 1D3 scFv of the CAR. CART-BCMA cells were stained with BCMA-Fc protein. Both CAR vectors include markers (mCherry or GFP) in bicistronic format with the individual CARs, which is useful for in vivo tracking. (**c**) Examples of three typical CAR T cell expansion curves. NTD—non-transduced T cells (negative control)

transduce the activated T cells for CAR gene transfer; this can be done ahead of time followed by freezing of retrovirus. However, we more commonly make fresh CAR retrovirus in parallel with T cell activation and expansion. Platinum-E cells are used for retrovirus production. Following activation and early during expansion, T cells are transduced via spinoculation with CAR-encoding retrovirus. CAR gene integration is followed by surface expression, which can be detected by flow cytometry 24 h later. Transduction frequency and CAR surface density can vary based on properties of the CAR construct. Using the following protocol, one can routinely achieve a transduction frequency of 60–90%. Following a 5-day manufacturing period, CAR T cells are ready for use (or cryopreservation). We describe assessment of CAR efficacy through in vitro cytotoxicity assays (Fig. 2). There exist several alternative approaches for assessing cytotoxic function, and additional in vitro measures could assess cytokine production and T cell proliferation. Finally, we detail one method for assessing in vivo function in the context of alloimmunity and transplant rejection (Fig. 3).

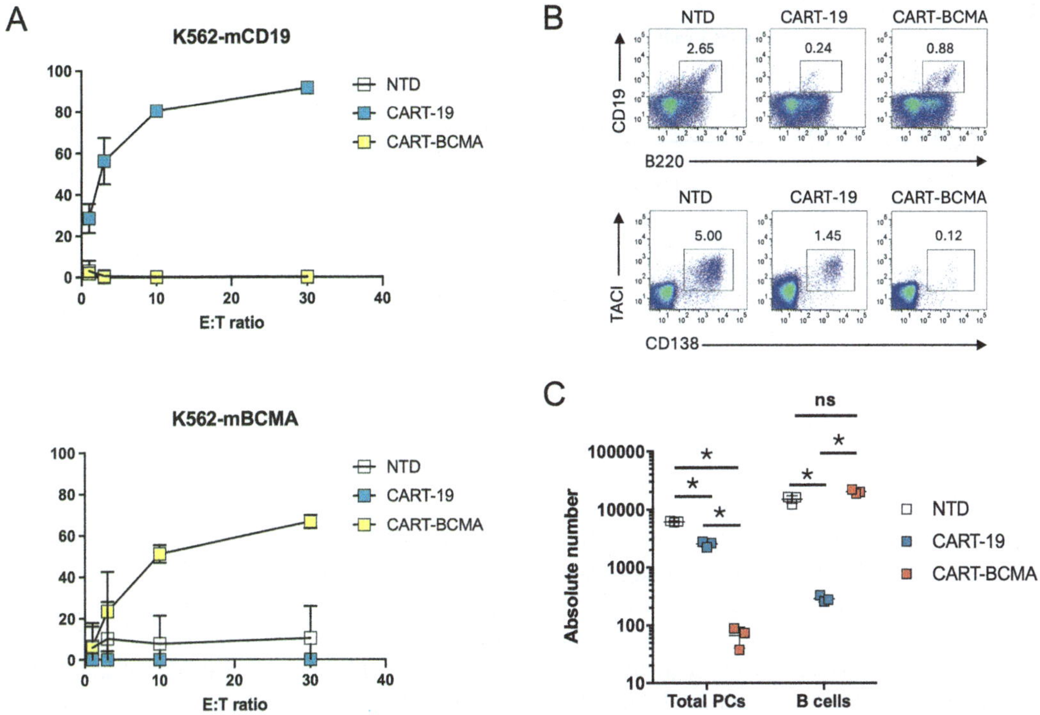

Fig. 2 In vitro assessment of CAR T cytotoxic activity. (**a**) Lysis of antigen-engineered K562 cell lines by CAR T cells after 24 h of co-culture at the indicated effector to target ratios (E:T). K562s were engineered to express click-beetle-green luciferase, allowing the use of luciferin to determine the number of remaining viable cells after co-culture. (**b**, **c**) Analysis of B cells and PCs after 24 h co-culture of splenocytes with indicated CAR T cells at an E:T ratio of 10:1. At the end of co-culture, cells were harvested and stained for B cells and PCs, and analyzed by flow cytometry using absolute counting beads to calculate the number of remaining cells. All error bars indicate mean +/− standard deviation. Statistical comparisons in (**c**) were performed using the Mann-Whitney U test. * $p < 0.05$

Below, we provide a detailed protocol for murine CAR T cell production and in vivo and in vitro methods of assessing CAR T efficacy with relevant references.

2 Materials

2.1 CAR T Production

1. T cell media (TCM) –
   - (a) RPMI 1640 medium (Gibco).
   - (b) 1% GlutaMAX (Gibco).
   - (c) 10% Fetal Bovine Serum (Sigma-Aldrich).
   - (d) 1% HEPES (Gibco).
   - (e) 1% Sodium Pyruvate (Thermo Fisher Scientific).

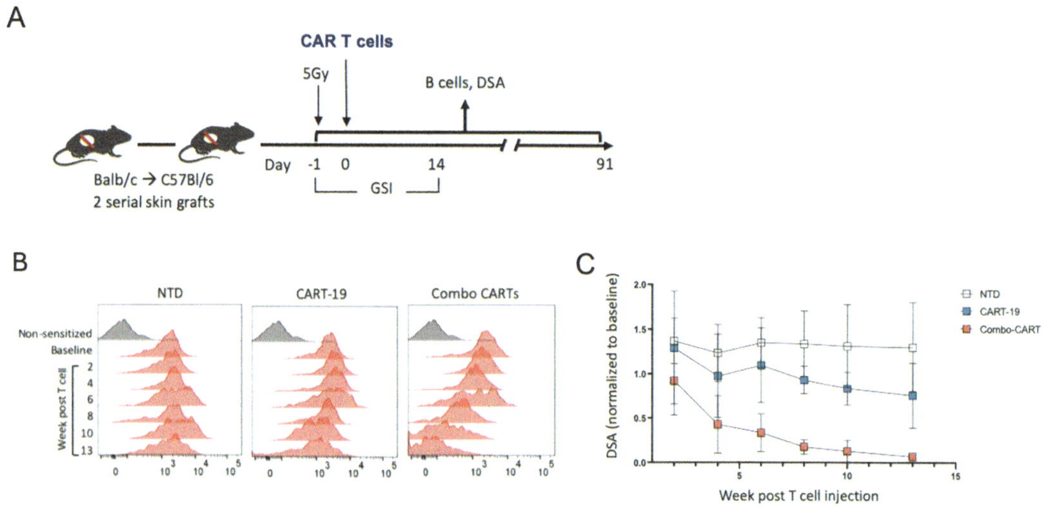

Fig. 3 Combining treatment with CD19 and BCMA targeted CAR T cells to eliminate preformed allo-antibodies in a murine allo-sensitization model. (**a**) Experimental schema indicating two serial skin transplants to induce allo-sensitization, followed by CAR T treatment. Effective expression of BCMA on murine PCs requires treatment with a gamma secretase inhibitor to prevent shedding of BCMA from the surface of PCs. (**b**) Representative flow-crossmatch histograms of mice over the treatment course after treatment with CAR T cells. Histograms shown are from the T cell gate (T cell crossmatch) (**c**) Aggregate T cell flow-crossmatch data. Each mouse is first normalized to their own baseline MFI, and the mean +/− SD is shown for each group

   (f) 1% Non-essential Amino Acids (Thermo Fisher Scientific).
   (g) 1% 55 mM 2-Mercaptoethanol (Gibco).
2. C57BL/6 donor mice (for example).
3. 40uM cell filters.
4. 50 mL conical tubes.
5. 1.5 mL tubes.
6. Round-bottom polystyrene tube compatible with flow cytometer.
7. 5 mL syringe.
8. ACK lysis buffer (Gibco).
9. PBS.
10. STEMCELL mouse CD8+ T cell isolation Kit (Stemcell).
11. Recombinant human IL-2 (R&D Systems).
12. CD3/CD28 beads (Thermo Fisher Scientific).
13. Magnet to wash beads (Thermo Fisher or custom made).
14. Cell culture flasks.
15. CAR retrovirus plasmid.

16. Non-tissue culture treated 6-well cell culture plates (Thermo Fisher).
17. RetroNectin (Takara Bio).
18. Platinum-E (Plat-E) retroviral packaging cell line (Cell Biolabs).
19. Lipofectamine 2000 (Thermo Fisher).
20. Opti-MEM (Invitrogen).
21. DMEM (Gibco).
22. T150 cell culture flask.
23. 10 cm tissue culture dishes.
24. 50 mL conical tubes.
25. 20 mL syringes.
26. 0.45uM filters that fit onto 20 mL syringe.

2.2 Luciferase-Based Cytotoxic Assay

Cell line expressing target with luciferase-based reporter: K562 cells (ATCC), transduced with a lentivirus encoding click-beetle-green luciferase followed by a lentivirus encoding mouse CD19 or BCMA. Antigen positive cells may be FACS sorted to purity.

1. D-Luciferin, Potassium salt (Gold Bio) (15 mg/mL stock).
2. TCM (described above).
3. 96-well flat-bottom black plates.
4. Sodium dodecyl sulfate solution (SDS, Thermo Fisher).
5. Luminometer (e.g., Synergy H4 Microplate Reader, BioTek).

2.3 Flow Cytometry-Based Cytotoxicity Assay Using Primary Cells

1. T cell media (TCM) –
   (a) RPMI 1640 medium (Gibco).
   (b) 1% GlutaMAX (Gibco).
   (c) 10% Fetal Bovine Serum (Sigma-Aldrich).
   (d) 1% HEPES (Gibco).
   (e) 1% Sodium Pyruvate (Thermo Fisher Scientific).
   (f) 1% Non-essential Amino Acids (Thermo Fisher Scientific).
   (g) 1% 55 mM 2-Mercaptoethanol (Gibco).
2. C57BL/6 donor mice (for example).
3. 40uM cell filters.
4. 50 mL conical tubes.
5. 1.5 mL tubes.
6. Round-bottom polystyrene tube compatible with flow cytometer.

7. 5 mL syringe.
8. ACK lysis buffer (Gibco).
9. PBS.
10. STEMCELL mouse CD8+ T cell isolation Kit (Stemcell).
11. Antibodies for flow cytometry staining.
12. Count-brite beads.

2.4 In Vivo Application

1. C57Bl/6 recipient mice.
2. Irradiator for total body irradiation as pre-conditioning (Alternatively, cyclophosphamide can be used).
3. 0.5 mL syringe for injection.
4. Phosphate Buffered Saline.
5. De-beading magnet (Thermo Fisher or custom made).
6. BD Microtainer Blood Collection tubes (Dipotassium-EDTA) (BD Biosciences).
7. FACS Lysing Solution 10× (BD Biosciences).
8. CountBright Absolute Counting Beads (Thermo Fisher).
9. Purified anti-CD16/32 as Fc block (Biolegend).

3 Methods

3.1 CAR T Cell Production

3.1.1 Day 1 Plat-E Cell Preparation

1. Plat-E cells should be passed for at least two passages prior to start of the CAR T production.
2. We culture them in DMEM supplemented with 10% FBS and penicillin/streptomycin (D10F).
3. We pass them by plating 5 × 10^6 in a T150 cell culture flask every 2 days.
4. On day 1 of CAR T cell production, seed 5 × 10^6 Plat-E cells in each 10 cm tissue culture dish in 10 mL of D10F (*see* **Note 1**).

3.1.2 Day 2 Mouse T Cell Isolation and Activation

1. Euthanize 8- to 12-week-old C57BL/6 mouse and harvest spleens using sterile technique into T cell media (TCM).
2. Dissociate spleens through a 40uM filter into 50 mL conical tube using a syringe plunger.
3. Wash filter with 5–10 mL of T cell media.
4. Centrifuge cells (300× *g*, 25 °C, 5 min).
5. Decant and resuspend splenocyte pellet with 3–5 mL ACK lysis buffer for lysis of red blood cells.
6. Incubate for 5 min at room temp (RT).
7. Add 3 volumes of PBS.

8. Centrifuge cells (300× *g*, 25 °C, 5 min).
9. Decant and resuspend well in 4 mL of TCM.
10. Filter through a 40uM filter into a new 50 mL conical tube and rinse filter with an additional 1 mL of TCM into the tube of cells.
11. Count cells using a hemocytometer or an automated instrument, and proceed to T cell isolation.
12. Isolate CD8+ T cells using a mouse CD8+ T cell isolation kit from STEMCELL Technologies, following the manufacturer's protocol.
13. Count isolated CD8+ cells and resuspend to 1 × 10^6/mL in TCM.
14. Determine the number of T cells to start with to ensure enough are available for experiments following expansion (*see* **Notes 2–4**).
15. Take the number of isolated CD8+ T cells required and bring them to a concentration of 1 × 10^6/mL in TCM in a 50 mL tube.
16. Add IL-2 (100 IU/mL final concentration) to the cells.
17. To activate the T cells, add murine T cell activation anti-CD3/anti-CD28 beads (Thermo Fisher Scientific) at a 1:1 T cell to bead ratio.
    (a) Transfer the required number of beads into a sterile 1.5 mL tube.
    (b) Top up the tube with PBS and place it on the magnet to wash.
    (c) After 30–60 s, when the beads are fully adhered to the tube wall, aspirate the supernatant completely.
    (d) Take tube off the magnet and wash with 1 mL of fresh PBS using the magnet 3 more times.
    (e) Resuspend washed beads off the magnet using 1 mL of the cell culture from the 50 mL conical tube, and return the cells + beads to the rest of the cells in the 50 mL tube.
18. Transfer cells to appropriate culture flask and place in 37 ° C incubator (*see* **Note 5**).

3.1.3 Plat-E Transfection for Retrovirus Production

1. Ideally, the Plat-E cells are ~70% confluent in the 10 cm dishes at time of transfection.
2. Gently aspirate media from the transfected Plat-E cells in 10 cm dishes.
3. Gently replace media with 10 mL of fresh D10F.

4. Use Lipofectamine 2000 for the transfection of the CAR plasmid following the manufacturer's instructions (*see* **Note 6**).
   (a) In a 15 mL conical tube ("Mix A"), add 1.5 mL OptiMem.
   (b) Add 14ug of CAR plasmid to "Mix A" tube and pulse vortex to mix.
   (c) In a second 15 mL conical tube ("Mix B"), add 1.5 mL OptiMem.
   (d) Pulse vortex Lipofectamine 2000 tube.
   (e) Add 60 uL of Lipofectamine 2000 to "Mix B" tube and pulse vortex to mix.
   (f) Incubate both tubes for 5 min at room temperature.
   (g) Combine Mix A and Mix B in a single tube and pulse vortex to mix.
   (h) Incubate for 5 min at room temperature.
   (i) Add the mix dropwise to the Plat-E cells.
5. Return cells to 37 °C incubator.

3.1.4 Day 3

1. Gently aspirate media from the transfected Plat-E cells in 10 cm dishes.
2. Gently replace media with 10 mL of fresh TCM.
3. Pre-coat wells of non-TC treated 6-well plate(s) with RetroNectin.
4. Determine the number of wells needed for transduction: Plan to put 2.5–3 $\times$ 10^6 T cells in each well of 6-well plate for transduction.
5. Dilute RetroNectin to 20 ug/mL in PBS and plate 2–2.5 mL/well in the 6-well plate.
6. Place coated plates at 4 °C overnight.

3.1.5 Day 4 T Cell Transduction

1. Prepare RetroNectin plates for transduction.
   (a) Aspirate RetroNectin from wells.
   (b) Wash wells once with 3 mL PBS and aspirate.
   (c) Add 3 mL of 2% BSA in PBS to each well.
   (d) Incubate plates at room temperature while preparing retrovirus supernatants (at least 20 min).
2. Harvest retrovirus containing media from Plat-E cultures and transfer to 50 mL conical tubes.
3. Centrifuge at 900–1000$\times$ *g* for 10 min at 25 °C.
4. Transfer virus supernatant to fresh 50 mL tubes to separate from Plat-E cells and cell debris.

5. Filter supernatant into fresh 50 mL conical using 20 mL syringe fitted with a 0.45 uM filter.
6. Aspirate 2% BSA in PBS from RetroNectin-coated plates.
7. Wash wells once with 5 mL PBS and aspirate.
8. Transfer viral supernatant into wells precoated with RetroNectin (*see* **Note 7**).
9. Centrifuge plates with virus supernatant at 900–1000× *g* for 1 h at 4 °C.
10. While the virus is being spun onto RetroNectin, count the T cells.
11. Seed T cells onto virus spun wells and centrifuge (900–1000× *g*) for 5 mins at 25 °C.
12. 24 h after transduction, count and pass the T cells so they are at a concentration of 0.8e6/mL with the addition of IL-2 (100 IU/mL, R&D Systems).

3.1.6 Day 5

1. Assess CAR T cell expression via flow cytometry with staining reagents specific to each CAR (*see* **Note 8**).
2. 48 h after transduction, CAR T cells are ready for in vitro and in vivo use.

3.2 Luciferase-Based Cytotoxic Assay Using Cell Lines: (See Note 9)

1. Count both target (K562s) and effector (CAR T cells) cells.
2. Calculate total number of effector T cells required based on the number of target cell wells to be tested and account for the effector:target (E:T) ratios (*see* **Note 10**).
3. Calculate total number of target cells required based on the number of T cell groups to be tested (typically 10,000 target cells per well).
4. To set up each condition in triplicate, first plate the T cells in their respective wells.
   (a) Wash the de-beaded T cells and resuspend to 3×10^6/mL in TCM.
   (b) Start with the 30:1 ratio wells, plating 150 uL of T cells/well (in triplicate/target).
   (c) In the 10:1, 3:1, 1:1 ratio wells, add 100 uL of fresh TCM.
   (d) Using a multichannel pipette, mix and transfer 50 uL of cells from the 30:1 wells into the 10:1 wells.
   (e) Similarly, mix the 10:1 wells and serially transfer 50 uL of cells to 3:1 and then 1:1 wells, finally discarding 50 uL from the 1:1 wells. At this point, all wells should have 100 uL of T cells.
5. Next, plate the target cells in the wells containing T cells.

(a) Wash and resuspend each target cell line to 1×10^5/mL in TCM.

(b) Add 100 uL of target cells (10,000 cells) to each respective well containing T cells.

(c) The final co-culture is now a 200 μL volume.

6. As spontaneous lysis controls, set up wells with target cells alone (for each target cell line) and supplement with 100 uL of TCM instead of adding T cells.
7. As maximum lysis controls, set up wells with target cells (for each target cell line) and supplement with 100 μL of 10% SDS diluted in PBS instead of adding T cells.
8. After 4–6 h, add 10 μL of diluted luciferin to each well.

(a) Make a master mix of 1 μL luciferin +9 μL of TCM/well and add 10 μL/well.

9. Incubate plate(s) for 10 min at 37 °C before reading using a luminometer.
10. Plates can be read serially at 24-h intervals.
11. Calculation of lysis:

(a) For each experimental well, calculate % Specific Lysis as follows: 100 × ((spontaneous-experimental)/(spontaneous-maximum).

3.3 Flow Cytometry-Based Cytotoxicity Assay Using Primary Cells

1. Isolate splenocytes to single cell suspension as described above for T cell isolation for CAR T manufacturing.
2. Co-culture splenocytes with CAR T cells at desired effector: target ratios (*see* **Note 11**).
3. After 24 h, stain cells with a viability dye and antibodies against target cell antigens (*see* **Note 12**).
4. Prior to running samples on the flow cytometer, add 5 μL of CountBright beads to samples in order to quantify live target cells remaining in co-cultures.

3.4 In Vivo Application

3.4.1 Preparation of Recipient Mice

1. A day or two prior to injecting CAR T cells, condition recipient mice with either total body irradiation (TBI) (5Gy) or cyclophosphamide (200 mg/kg, intraperitoneal injection) to enhance engraftment of the CAR T cells (*see* **Note 13**).

3.4.2 Cell Preparation for Injection

1. At Day 6 of CAR T manufacturing, harvest cultures and count the cells.
2. Perform calculations to determine how many cells are needed in total based on the CAR positive dose per mouse and the number of mice to be injected in each group. Calculations are based on CAR expression data obtained on day 5 (Subheading 3.1.6) (*see* **Note 14**).

3. Pipette a number of desired cells into a 50 mL conical tube and centrifuge (300× *g*, 5 min, 25 °C).
4. Decant and resuspend cells in 10 mL of PBS and place the tube on a magnet for 1 min to separate cells from the activation beads.
5. While the tube is on the magnet, confirm the separation of beads on the wall of the tube and transfer the cell suspension into a new 50 mL conical tube.
6. Centrifuge the cells (300× *g*, 5 min, 25 °C) and decant.
7. Wash the cell suspension twice more with 20 mL PBS to remove media. If dark color is observed in cell pellets, repeat the de-beading step to remove remaining activation beads.
8. Resuspend the cells in an appropriate volume of PBS for in vivo injection. Generally, volumes injected would be 100–150 uL/ mouse but depend on the route of administration.
9. Hold cells on ice until injection.

3.4.3 Peripheral Blood Analysis by Flow Cytometry

1. At the 2-week post-CAR T infusion timepoint, perform a submandibular vein bleed [14] to collect up to 100 uL of blood into EDTA anticoagulated tubes (*see* **Notes 15–18**).
2. For cell staining, transfer 10 μL of whole blood to a round-bottom polystyrene flow tube.
3. Add titrated antibody cocktail (up to 15 uL in PBS) to the blood and mix gently.
4. Incubate the blood with antibodies for 20 min at room temperature.
5. During the incubation, prepare a master mix of FACS-Lyse Buffer with CountBright beads.
   (a) Mix 45 uL of 10× FACS-Lyse, 5 uL of beads and 400 uL of deionized water / sample.
6. After the 20-min incubation, add 450 uL of the FACS-Lyse + bead mix to each blood tube.
7. Run on a flow cytometer.
8. At a minimum, we use antibodies to CD3, CD4, CD8, B220, and CD19 to assess T and B cell levels. CAR T cells may be identified using the T cell markers combined with the fluorophore in the bicistronic retroviral construct (e.g., GFP, mCherry).
9. Centrifuge the remaining whole blood in the EDTA phlebotomy tube at 3000× *g* for 10 min in a tabletop centrifuge.
10. Harvest plasma and store it in fresh 1.5 mL tubes at −80 °C for subsequent antibody measurement.

3.4.4 Tissue Analysis

1. At defined timepoints or the final experimental endpoint, euthanize mice and harvest tissue for processing and analysis.
2. Spleen, femurs, and lymph nodes (e.g., cervical and/or inguinal) are harvested into complete media on ice.
3. Process tissue into a single cell suspension and RBC lysis as described above for T cell isolation for CAR T cell production.
4. At a minimum, stain cells using CD19, B220, CD138, and TACI to assess B cells and plasma cells.
5. In addition, one may formalin-fix tissues for analysis by immunohistochemistry using antibodies to CD20 or CD138 (*see* **Note 19**).
6. Flow crossmatch for allo-antibody measurement according to **steps 7–22**.
7. Harvest spleen from a naïve donor strain mouse (i.e., same strain as skin donor).
8. Isolate splenocytes as described above.
9. To determine the number of cells needed, calculate 0.5–1 × 10^6 cells/sample to be tested.
10. Resuspend cells in PBS at 0.5–1 × 10^6/45uL in a 15 mL conical tube.
11. Add anti-CD16/32 to cells (10uL/mL).
12. Incubate on ice for 10 min.
13. Pipette 45 μL of cells (0.5–1 × 10^6) of the Fc-blocked donor splenocytes into each well of a 96-well round-bottom plate.
14. Add 3 uL of recipient neat serum to the cells and mix (1/16 final serum dilution).
15. Incubate on ice for 45 min.
16. Add 150 uL of FACS buffer (PBS, 1% BSA)/well and centrifuge (300× *g*, 5 min, 4 °C).
17. Decant quickly by inverting the plate and wash two more times with 200 μL of FACS buffer (PBS, 1% BSA).
18. Add 10 uL of antibody master mix to cell pellets and resuspend well (stain samples with antibodies against CD3, B220, and Igk).
19. Incubate on ice for 30 min.
20. Add 150 uL of FACS buffer (PBS, 1% BSA)/well and centrifuge (300× *g*, 5 min, 4 °C).
21. Decant and resuspend cells in 150 uL/well of 1% paraformaldehyde diluted in PBS.
22. Run on flow cytometer and assess MFI of Igk signal on T cells (CD3 + B220-) and B cells (CD3-B220+) as T and B cell crossmatch, respectively (*see* **Note 20**).

4 Notes

1. The number of 10 cm dishes required depends on the number of constructs to be tested and the number of T cells of each type being made. At least one plate is required for each construct, and numbers can be scaled up according to calculations that follow.
2. To back calculate, we conservatively predict we will achieve 50% transduction efficiency. Therefore, we would plan to make twice the total number of T cells.
3. To account for T cell expansion during culture, we expect ~3 population doublings over 5 days (Fig. 1c). Thus, to make a total of 1.6×10^7 T cells, we would start with about 2×10^6 T cells.
4. For initial expansions until consistency is achieved, it may be worthwhile to make 1.5–2 times the number of cells needed to account for variability and ensure adequacy for planned experiments.
5. To determine the size of the culture flask to use, divide the number of cells by 0.45. Then use the resulting number to determine flask size based on the area of the bottom of the flask. We use the following rules based on the culture plates and flasks we use:
   - If number exceeds 1.9, plate in a well of a 12-well plate,
   - If number exceeds 3.4, plate in a well of a 6-well plate,
   - If number exceeds 9.8, plate in a T25 flask,
   - If number exceeds 25, plate in a T75 flask,
   - If number exceeds 75, plate in a T150 flask.
6. The included protocol is for the transfection of one 10 cm plate and can be scaled accordingly.
7. We typically add 2.5–3 mL of virus supernatant/well of a 6-well plate.
8. For example, for CAR T cells targeting mouse CD19 using the 1D3 scFv derived from a rat antibody, we stain with a goat-anti-Rat reagent. Additionally, if the CAR vector is designed as a bicistronic system that includes a marker such as GFP, assess that signal as well.
9. This method utilizes cell lines engineered to express target antigens of interest and isogenic negative control cells. We typically use K562 cells engineered by lentiviral transduction to express click-beetle-green luciferase as well as relevant target antigens. Cells may be sorted for purity prior to use.

10. We typically use 10,000 target cells per well and use the following effector to target ratios (E:T): 30:1, 10:1, 3:1, 1:1.
11. As shown in Fig. 2, we typically use a single ratio, 10:1.
12. For example, to assess B cells and PCs, we stain co-cultured cells with antibodies against CD19, B220, CD138, TACI, CD3, CD4, and CD8, which enables exclusion of T cells, including CAR T cells.
13. For technical details related to skin transplantation as a method of allo-sensitization, please refer to Cheng et al. [15].
14. Generally, the dose of CAR T cells administered ranges from 1×10^6 to 4×10^6 CAR+ cells per mouse. During the experiment, serial phlebotomy is used to assess circulating B cell levels by flow cytometry.
15. Blood collection is used to assess peripheral B cells and CAR T cells by flow and to harvest plasma for flow-crossmatch analysis.
16. We begin at the 2-week post-CAR T infusion timepoint and sample mice every 2 weeks.
17. PCs are largely undetectable in the periphery and, therefore, we assess their depletion in tissue compartments (spleen, bone marrow, and lymph nodes) when mice are euthanized at pre-specified timepoints or experimental endpoint.
18. In CART-19 treated mice, B cell aplasia is expected to be seen at week 2 and can last for 6–30+ weeks, reflecting the variability of CAR T persistence. CART-BCMA induces PC depletion but has little effect on B cells in our experience. CAR T cells can be identified in small numbers by a decline quickly (by 3–5 weeks) in blood despite evidence of their continued presence and function in tissues.
19. This is a useful method to assess the depth of target cell depletion.
20. We normalize Igk MFI levels to baseline (pre-CART) for each mouse. It is important to test serum samples from multiple timepoints at the same time to avoid batch effects.

Conflicts of Interest

This study was funded by a Career Award for Medical Scientists grant from the Burroughs Wellcome Fund to VGB. VGB has received speaker and consultant honoraria from Alexion. CAM has no conflicts of interest to declare.

References

1. Kenneth Murphy CW (2017) Antigen presentation to T lymphocytes. Janeway's immunobiology. W.W. Norton & Company, New York
2. Hickey MJ, Valenzuela NM, Reed EF (2016) Alloantibody generation and effector function following sensitization to human leukocyte antigen. Front Immunol 7:30. https://doi.org/10.3389/fimmu.2016.00030. Epub 20160204. PubMed PMID: 26870045; PMCID: PMC4740371
3. Schinstock CA, Smith BH, Montgomery RA, Jordan SC, Bentall AJ, Mai M, Khamash HA, Stegall MD (2019) Managing highly sensitized renal transplant candidates in the era of kidney paired donation and the new kidney allocation system: is there still a role for desensitization? Clin Transpl 33(12):e13751. https://doi.org/10.1111/ctr.13751. Epub 20191126. PubMed PMID: 31769104
4. Habal MV (2021) Current desensitization strategies in heart transplantation. Front Immunol 12:702186. https://doi.org/10.3389/fimmu.2021.702186. Epub 20210824. PubMed PMID: 34504489; PMCID: PMC8423343
5. Joher N, Matignon M, Grimbert P (2021) HLA desensitization in solid organ transplantation: anti-CD38 to across the immunological barriers. Front Immunol 12:688301. https://doi.org/10.3389/fimmu.2021.688301. Epub 20210520 PubMed PMID: 34093594; PMCID: PMC8173048
6. Zhao D, Guo Z, Zhao G, Sa R, Zhu L, Chen G (2023) A novel Daratumumab-based regimen for desensitization in highly HLA-Presensitized patients awaiting kidney transplantation. Transpl Int 36:11771. https://doi.org/10.3389/ti.2023.11771. Epub 20230822. PubMed PMID: 37675269; PMCID: PMC10477353
7. Vo A, Ammerman N, Jordan SC (2024) Advances in desensitization for human leukocyte antigen incompatible kidney transplantation. Curr Opin Organ Transplant 29(2): 104–120. https://doi.org/10.1097/MOT.0000000000001131. Epub 20231213. PubMed PMID: 38088373
8. Bhoj VG, Arhontoulis D, Wertheim G, Capobianchi J, Callahan CA, Ellebrecht CT, Obstfeld AE, Lacey SF, Melenhorst JJ, Nazimuddin F, Hwang WT, Maude SL, Wasik MA, Bagg A, Schuster S, Feldman MD, Porter DL, Grupp SA, June CH, Milone MC (2016) Persistence of long-lived plasma cells and humoral immunity in individuals responding to CD19-directed CAR T-cell therapy. Blood 128(3):360–370. https://doi.org/10.1182/blood-2016-01-694356. Epub 20160510. PubMed PMID: 27166358; PMCID: PMC4957161
9. Zhang Z, Markmann C, Yu M, Agarwal D, Rostami S, Wang W, Liu C, Zhao H, Ochoa T, Parvathaneni K, Xu X, Li E, Gonzalez V, Khadka R, Hoffmann J, Knox JJ, Scholler J, Marcellus B, Allman D, Fraietta JA, Samelson-Jones B, Milone MC, Monos D, Garfall AL, Naji A, Bhoj VG (2023) Immunotherapy targeting B cells and long-lived plasma cells effectively eliminates pre-existing donor-specific allo-antibodies. Cell Rep Med 4(12): 101336. https://doi.org/10.1016/j.xcrm.2023.101336. PubMed PMID: 38118406; PMCID: PMC10772570
10. Carpenter RO, Evbuomwan MO, Pittaluga S, Rose JJ, Raffeld M, Yang S, Gress RE, Hakim FT, Kochenderfer JN (2013) B-cell maturation antigen is a promising target for adoptive T-cell therapy of multiple myeloma. Clin Cancer Res 19(8):2048–2060. https://doi.org/10.1158/1078-0432.CCR-12-2422. Epub 20130123. PubMed PMID: 23344265; PMCID: PMC3630268
11. Muller F, Taubmann J, Bucci L, Wilhelm A, Bergmann C, Volkl S, Aigner M, Rothe T, Minopoulou I, Tur C, Knitza J, Kharboutli S, Kretschmann S, Vasova I, Spoerl S, Reimann H, Munoz L, Gerlach RG, Schafer S, Grieshaber-Bouyer R, Korganow AS, Farge-Bancel D, Mougiakakos D, Bozec A, Winkler T, Kronke G, Mackensen A, Schett G (2024) CD19 CAR T-cell therapy in autoimmune disease—a case series with follow-up. N Engl J Med 390(8):687–700. https://doi.org/10.1056/NEJMoa2308917. PubMed PMID: 38381673
12. Oh S, Payne AS (2022) Engineering cell therapies for autoimmune diseases: from preclinical to clinical proof of concept. Immune Netw 22(5):e37. https://doi.org/10.4110/in.2022.22.e37. Epub 20220921. PubMed PMID: 36381961; PMCID: PMC9634148
13. Guedan S, Calderon H, Posey AD Jr, Maus MV (2019) Engineering and Design of Chimeric Antigen Receptors. Mol Ther Methods Clin Dev 12:145–156. https://doi.org/10.1016/j.omtm.2018.12.009. Epub 20181231. PubMed PMID: 30666307; PMCID: PMC6330382

14. Golde WT, Gollobin P, Rodriguez LL (2005) A rapid, simple, and humane method for submandibular bleeding of mice using a lancet. Lab Anim (NY) 34(9):39–43. https://doi.org/10.1038/laban1005-39. PubMed PMID: 16195737

15. Cheng CH, Lee CF, Fryer M, Furtmuller GJ, Oh B, Powell JD, Brandacher G (2017) Murine full-thickness skin transplantation. J Vis Exp 119. https://doi.org/10.3791/55105. Epub 20170102. PubMed PMID: 28117792; PMCID: PMC5408726

Chapter 20

Examination of Class I HLA-Fc Fusion Proteins in Targeting Cognate Antibody-Producing Cells

Ashlee M. Webber, Anushka Bhat, Hongjie Guo, Brian T. Edelson, and Chang Liu

Abstract

Human leukocyte antigen (HLA) alloimmunization poses a significant challenge in various clinical settings, including platelet refractoriness and allogeneic solid-organ and stem cell transplants. We have explored HLA-Fc fusion proteins as a novel therapeutic strategy for suppressing or reversing unwanted HLA alloimmunization. These fusion proteins, combining HLA antigen specificity with Fc-mediated cytotoxicity, show promise in targeting specific antibody-producing B cells. Initial studies using B cell hybridomas demonstrate the feasibility and selectivity of HLA-Fc in killing target cells of cognate specificities. The protocols in this chapter outline the design, production, and evaluation of HLA-Fc proteins, emphasizing their efficacy in vitro and in immunodeficient mouse models. Further research is needed to validate these findings in humanized murine alloimmunization models, potentially providing new therapeutic approaches for managing HLA-sensitized patients in clinical practice.

Key words HLA, HLA-Fc fusion protein, Alloimmunization, Complement-dependent cytotoxicity, Antibody-producing cells

1 Introduction

Alloimmunization to human leukocyte antigens (HLA) creates a critical barrier to life-saving therapies such as platelet transfusions [1], solid-organ transplants [2–4], and hematopoietic stem cell transplants [5, 6]. Approximately 45% of patients awaiting kidney transplants in the United States are HLA-sensitized [7] through previous blood transfusions, pregnancies, or allogeneic transplants. Furthermore, 24.4% of ever-pregnant women are sensitized to HLA [8], which disqualifies them from future blood donation in order to mitigate the risk of transfusion-related acute lung injury. Despite being harmless initially, these anti-HLA antibodies may become problematic later if these women need allogeneic cells or grafts. Preexisting anti-HLA antibodies, if sharing the same

Sean R. Stowell and Connie M. Arthur (eds.), *Methods in Transfusion Medicine*, Methods in Molecular Biology, vol. 3053, https://doi.org/10.1007/978-1-0716-5376-0_20,

specificity as mismatched donor antigens, are called donor-specific antibodies (DSAs) and carry an increased risk for acute or hyperacute antibody-mediated graft rejection (AMR) [9, 10]. De novo alloimmunization to mismatched donor HLA can also occur in the post-transplant setting, especially in patients with insufficient immune suppression or those with increased HLA mismatch load [11]. These de novo DSAs are a leading cause of chronic AMR and shortened graft survival in the era of potent T cell immunosuppression. There have been no FDA-approved therapies for AMR due to preexisting or de novo DSAs [12]. The standard of care remains plasma exchange and intravenous immunoglobulin (IVIG) [13]. Alternatively, treatments may target B cells (e.g., rituximab) [14], plasma cells (e.g., proteasome inhibitors and daratumumab) [15, 16], the complement cascade (e.g., eculizumab) [17], cytokine signaling (e.g., tocilizumab, targeting IL-6) [9, 18, 19], or IgG (e.g., imlifidase) [20]. Despite promising results in some reports, definitive results from randomized clinical trials are not available. Notably, none of the above options targets DSA or DSA-producing cells as the root cause of AMR. Therefore, the toxicity of non-selective immunosuppression may limit their dosing or long-term use.

We recently developed an approach to target antigen-specific antibody-producing cells [21], using HLA-Fc fusion proteins containing a specific class I HLA antigen linked to the Fc region of immunoglobulin, which can dimerize to form an antibody-like molecule (Fig. 1a). The "antigen" portion consists of a single-chain trimer of peptide, human β2 microglobulin, and the extracellular domains of class I HLA. The selected peptide must bind to the HLA with sufficient affinity to stabilize the protein complex. The antigen portion guides the molecule to cognate B cell receptors (BCRs) on the surface of antibody-producing cells, while the Fc can mediate complement-dependent cytotoxicity (CDC) against target cells. The modular design of HLA-Fc enables the incorporation of diverse HLA molecules to target BCRs specific for various donor antigens. Diverse murine and human Fc regions can also be included to test different levels of effector function in murine models and for clinical translation. The investigation of HLA-Fc in treating HLA alloimmunization is at an early stage of development. While our proof-of-concept study using cognate B cell hybridoma cells demonstrated the feasibility and potential of this approach [21], future studies are needed to validate the efficacy of HLA-Fc in HLA-sensitized humanized mice and human subjects.

This chapter will focus on protocols for the design and production of HLA-Fc proteins and their testing using cognate B cell hybridoma cells in vitro and in immunodeficient mice as a model system for initial validation. Evaluation of HLA-Fc in alloimmunization models using HLA transgenic mice is warranted in future studies. The design of single-chain class I HLA as part of the Fc

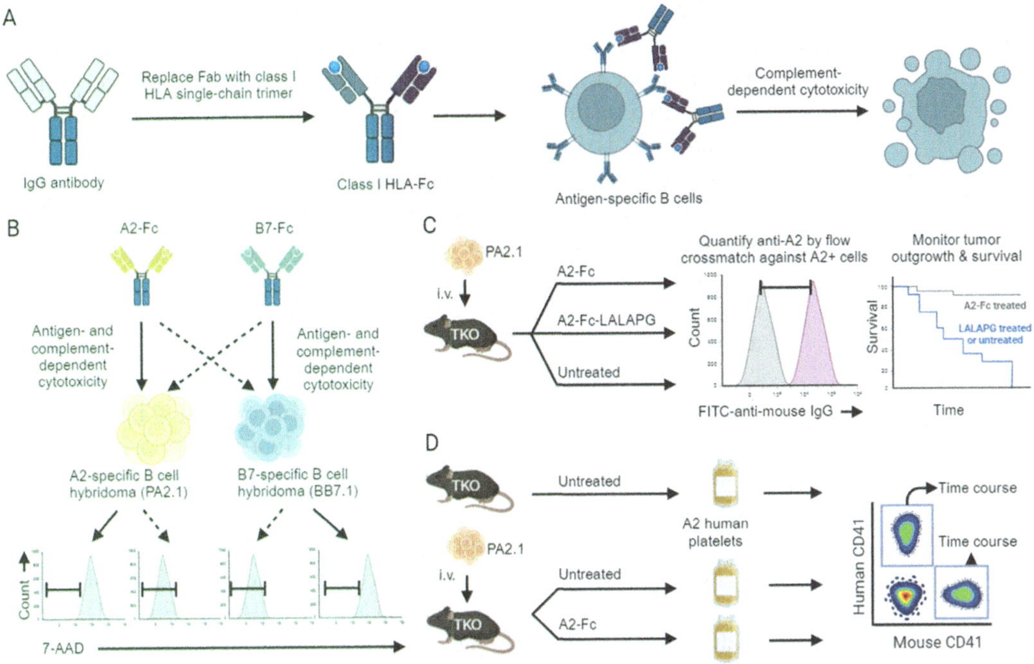

Fig. 1 Schematic of the model system for testing the antigen-specific cytotoxicity effect of HLA-Fc fusion proteins. (**a**) The rationale for HLA-Fc fusion proteins as potential agents for targeting antigen-specific antibody-producing cells for depletion by Fc- and complement-dependent cytotoxicity. (**b**) Measuring complement-dependent cytotoxicity (CDC) of A2-Fc and B7-Fc against B cell hybridoma cells of cognate specificities in vitro, using a flow cytometric CDC assay. The readout of the assay is the percentage of cells killed by HLA-Fc (7-AAD positive), which can be correlated with the concentrations of the fusion protein. Crossover of the HLA-Fc to their non-cognate cells (arrows with broken lines) can serve as a negative control to demonstrate the antigen-selectivity of each HLA-Fc protein. (**c**) Testing the efficacy of HLA-Fc in vivo using immunodeficient TKO mice carrying B cell hybridomas. The mice can be divided into treatment groups, followed by regular peripheral blood collection for antibody assessment by flow cytometric crossmatch against splenocytes from A2+ transgenic mice. The shift in median fluorescence intensity is measured between samples before (gray) and after (purple) the cell transfer and treatment. A2-Fc and A2-Fc-LALAPG were used as an example, with the latter serving as a negative control due to loss-of-function mutations in the Fc region. The cohort is also followed up for hybridoma cell outgrowth and overall survival as an indicator of HLA-Fc's efficacy in vivo. (**d**) An anti-A2 antibody-mediated platelet refractoriness model. TKO mice carrying anti-A2 B cell hybridomas were treated with A2-Fc or untreated and received an infusion of A2+ human platelets. TKO mice not carrying anti-A2 B cell hybridomas were also included as the negative control group. After intravenous injection of platelet-rich plasma, peripheral blood was collected at 10, 60, and 120 min, followed by human and mouse CD41 staining and flow cytometry

fusion protein is based on previous work in the Fremont and Hansen laboratories at Washington University in St. Louis [22–24]. The single-chain class I HLA coding sequences can be designed based on the principles outlined in this protocol. These sequences can be synthesized through commercial vendors and cloned into selected pFUSE-Fc vectors (InvivoGen) in frame with a downstream Fc coding sequence. We expressed the proteins in

Expi293 cells to ensure proper glycosylation of the fusion proteins in a mammalian cell line. Alternative cell lines, such as CHO cells, have not been tested in our hands but should also be acceptable. For in vitro testing of HLA-Fc proteins' efficacy using B cell hybridomas (Fig. 1b), specific B cell hybridomas may be purchased from organizations like ATCC; it is beneficial to include B cell hybridomas of cognate specificity with expected killing by matched HLA-Fc and non-cognate cells as a negative control. We describe a simple flow cytometric assay to quantify CDC mediated by different concentrations of HLA-Fc. HLA-Fc-mediated cytotoxicity can also be tested in vivo using immunodeficient mice that allow engraftment of B cell hybridomas. For this purpose, we used mice deficient in *Rag2*, *Cd47*, and *Il2rg*, abbreviated "TKO." This system allows testing the ability of HLA-Fc to lower cognate anti-HLA antibodies as measured by flow cytometric crossmatch and to deplete target cells in vivo using endogenous complement (Fig. 1c). The in vivo model can be extended to include anti-HLA antibody-mediated platelet refractoriness as a clinically relevant endpoint to evaluate the efficacy of HLA-Fc (Fig. 1d). As an additional tool to characterize anti-HLA antibodies, we also describe the protocol for detecting and identifying anti-HLA antibodies in cell culture supernatants and mouse serum specimens using the single-antigen bead (SAB) assay (One Lambda, West Hills, CA).

2 Materials

2.1 Generation of Constructs for HLA-Fc Proteins

1. pFUSE-mIgG2a-Fc1 vector (InvivoGen; Cat#pfuse-mg2afc1).
2. gBlock gene fragment synthesis (IDT-DNA).
3. Oligonucleotides for cloning, site-directed mutagenesis, and plasmid sequencing (IDT-DNA).
4. One-Shot TOP10 chemically competent *Escherichia coli* (Invitrogen; Cat#C404010).
5. Phusion High-Fidelity PCR Master Mix with HF buffer (NEB; Cat#M0531S).
6. Restriction enzymes (AgeI, NheI, BglII, XhoI) (NEB).
7. Zeocin (Invitrogen; Cat#R25001).
8. LB Lennox Agar Plates with Zeocin-50 (Teknova; Cat#L1038-04).
9. Q5 site-directed mutagenesis kit (NEB; Cat#E0554S).

2.2 Expression and Purification of HLA-Fc Proteins

1. NucleoBond PC 2000 Mega kit (Macherey-Nagel; Cat#740576).
2. Expi293F cells (Gibco; Cat#A14527).

3. Expi293 expression medium (Gibco; Cat#A1435102).
4. OPTI MEM reduced serum medium (Gibco; Cat#31985070).
5. Hype-5 transfection reagent (OZ Biosciences; Cat#HYR10003).
6. HyClone Cell Boost (VWR; Cat#95026-616).
7. Protein A Agarose Resin (50% suspension) (Goldbio; Cat#P-400-100).
8. Sodium Citrate Tribasic Dihydrate (Sigma-Aldrich; Cat#S4641-500G).
9. Tris–HCl buffer, 1 M, pH 8.0 (Corning; Cat#46-031-CM).
10. 10× Phosphate-buffered saline (PBS) (Teknova; Cat#P0195).
11. 30 kDa MWCO Amico® Ultra centrifugal filter tube (Millipore-Sigma; Cat#UFC903008).

2.3 Binding of HLA-Fc to B Cell Hybridomas

1. PA2.1 mouse B cell hybridoma cells (A2/A69-specific, IgG1) (ATCC; Cat#HB-117).
2. BB7.1 mouse B cell hybridoma cells (B7-specific, IgG1) (ATCC; Cat#HB-56).
3. APC-conjugated rat anti-mouse IgG1 (clone M1-14D12) (eBioscience; Cat#17-4015-82).
4. FITC-conjugated rat anti-mouse IgG2a (clone RMG2a-62) (BioLegend; Cat#407106).
5. Rat anti-mouse CD16/32 antibody (TruStain FcX, clone 93) (BioLegend; Cat#100236).
6. 7-AAD viability staining solution (eBioscience; Cat#00699350).
7. Iscove's Modified Dulbecco's Medium (IMDM) 1× (Gibco; Cat#12440046).
8. Hypoxanthine-Thymidine (H.T.) 500× concentrate (ATCC; Cat#71-X).
9. Penicillin-Streptomycin (5000 U/mL) (Gibco; Cat#1540-122).
10. Fetal bovine serum (FBS, heat-inactivated for 30 min at 56 °C) (BioWest; Cat#S1620).
11. Bovine serum albumin (BSA) (Fisher; Cat#BP1600).
12. 1× Phosphate-buffered saline (PBS) (Gibco; Cat#10-010-031).
13. EDTA (Corning; Cat#46-034-CL).
14. Dulbecco's Phosphate-buffered saline (DPBS, Ca-, Mg-) (Gibco; Cat#14190-136).
15. Staining buffer (1× PBS with 0.5% BSA, 2 mM EDTA, and 0.02% sodium azide).

2.4 CDC of HLA-Fc on B Cell Hybridomas

1. PA2.1 mouse B cell hybridoma cells (A2/A69-specific, IgG1) (ATCC; Cat#HB-117).
2. BB7.1 mouse B cell hybridoma cells (B7-specific, IgG1) (ATCC; Cat#HB-56).
3. 7-AAD viability staining solution (eBioscience; Cat#00699350).
4. Iscove's Modified Dulbecco's Medium (IMDM) 1× (Gibco; Cat#12440046).
5. Hypoxanthine-Thymidine (H.T.) 500× concentrate (ATCC; Cat#71-X).
6. Penicillin-Streptomycin (5000 U/mL) (Gibco; Cat#1540-122).
7. Fetal bovine serum (FBS, heat-inactivated 30 min at 56 °C) (BioWest; Cat#S1620).
8. Bovine serum albumin (BSA) (Fisher; Cat#BP1600).
9. 1× Phosphate-buffered saline (PBS) (Gibco; Cat#10-010-031).
10. Dulbecco's Phosphate-buffered saline (DPBS, Ca-, Mg-) (Gibco; Cat#14190-136).
11. Rabbit serum (One Lambda; Cat#CDR-50).
12. Staining buffer (1× PBS with 0.5% BSA, 2 mM EDTA, and 0.02% sodium azide).
13. 7-AAD viability staining solution (eBioscience; Cat#00699350).

2.5 Assessing the Effect of HLA-Fc on B Cell Hybridomas In Vivo

1. B6.129S-$Rag2^{tm1Fwa}$ $Cd47^{tm1Fpl}$ $Il2rg^{tm1wjl}$/J (TKO) mice (Jackson Laboratory; Stock#025730).
2. C57BL/6-$Mcph1^{Tg(HLA\text{-}A2.1)1Enge}$/J mice (Jackson Laboratory; Stock#003475).
3. PA2.1 mouse B cell hybridoma cells (A2/A69-specific, IgG1) (ATCC; Cat#HB-117).
4. APC-conjugated rat anti-mouse CD3 (clone 17A2) (BioLegend; Cat#100236).
5. Rat anti-mouse CD16/32 antibody (TruStain FcX, clone 93) (BioLegend; Cat#100236).
6. Fetal bovine serum (FBS, heat-inactivated 30 min at 56 °C) (BioWest; Cat#S1620).
7. Iscove's Modified Dulbecco's Medium (IMDM) 1× (Gibco; Cat#12440046).
8. I10F medium (Iscove Modified Dulbecco Media with 10% FBS).

9. Staining buffer (1× PBS with 0.5% BSA, 2 mM EDTA, and 0.02% sodium azide).
10. 5 mm lancets.
11. 1 mL tuberculin syringes.
12. 18 G × 1 ½" needles.
13. 27G × ½" needles.
14. 70 μM cell strainers.
15. 5 mL syringes.
16. ACK lysing buffer (Thermo Fisher Scientific; Cat#A1049201).

2.6 Assessing the Effect of HLA-Fc in a Platelet Refractoriness Model

1. PE-conjugated mouse anti-human CD41 (clone HIP8) (BioLegend; Cat#303705).
2. APC-conjugated rat anti-mouse CD41 (clone MWReg30) (BioLegend; Cat#133913).
3. Rat anti-mouse CD16/32 antibody (TruStain FcX, clone 93) (BioLegend; Cat#100236).
4. CountBright™ absolute counting beads (Invitrogen; Cat#C36950).
5. 1 mL tuberculin syringes.
6. 18G × 1 ½ needles.
7. 27G × ½" needles.
8. 5 mm lancets.
9. A2+ human platelet-rich plasma (prepared fresh from A2+ volunteers).

2.7 Single-Antigen Bead Assay

1. PE-conjugated goat anti-mouse IgG (clone Poly4053) (BioLegend; Cat#405307).
2. EDTA (Corning; Cat#46-034-CL).
3. LABScreen Single-Antigen HLA Class I (One Lambda; Cat#LS1A04).

3 Methods

3.1 Generation of Constructs for HLA-Fc Proteins

1. The construct for a single-chain HLA-Fc protein should encode the following components from the 5′ end to the 3′ end (Fig. 2): signal peptide, high-affinity peptide for the specific class I HLA allele in the construct (*see* **Note 1**), linker #1 (GCGASGGGGSGGGGS; *see* **Note 2**), human β2-microglobulin, linker #2 (GGGGS)4, extracellular domains of a class I HLA allele, and Fc from the hinge region to the C-terminal end of the IgG heavy chain.

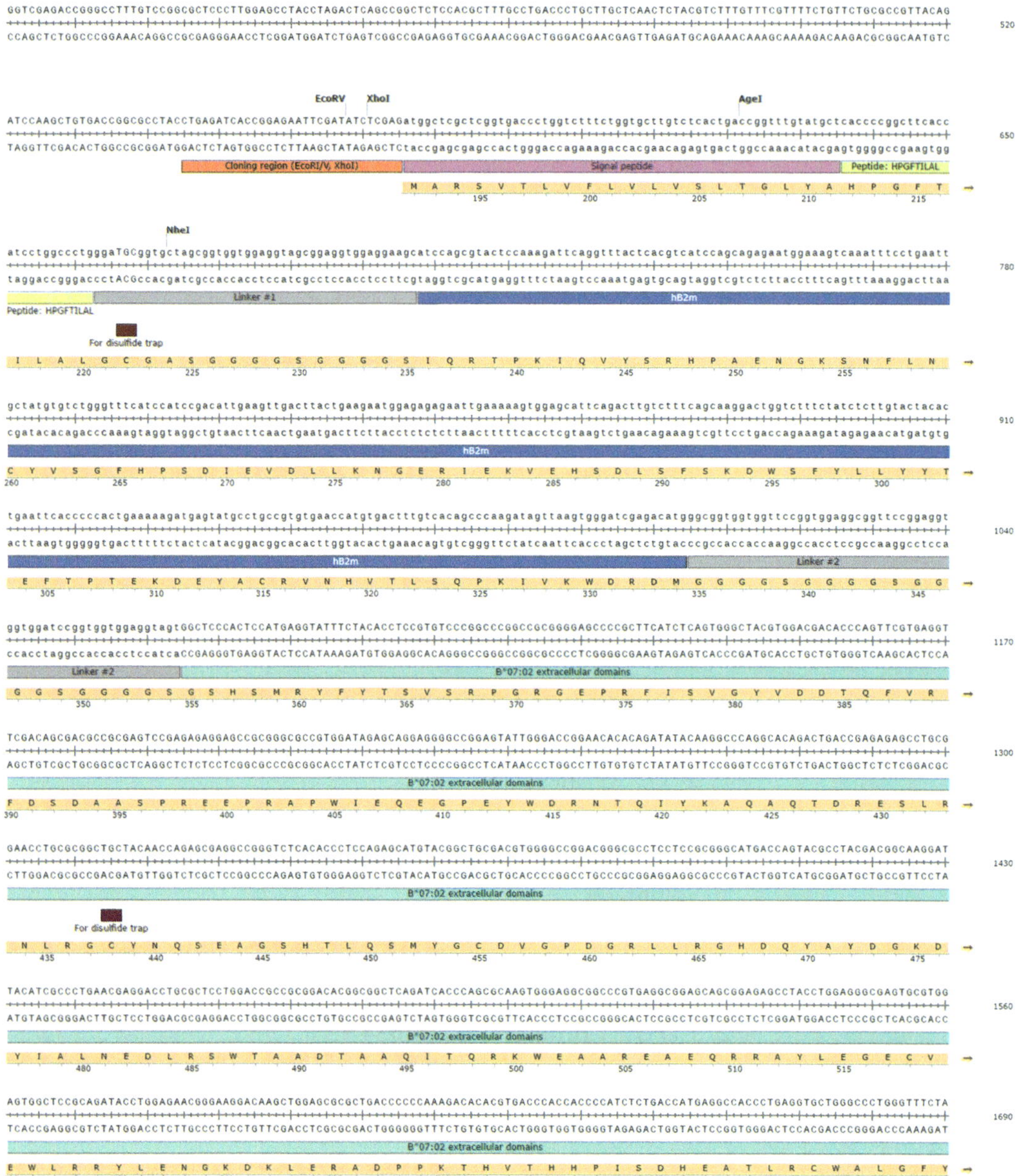

Fig. 2 DNA and protein sequences for B7 (HLA-B*07:02)-Fc (mouse IgG2a) fusion protein in the context of pFUSE-Fc-mIgG2a vector. DNA encoding the B7 single-chain trimer (SCT) was synthesized and cloned between XhoI and BglII sites. The B7-SCT sequence is translated into the following components from the N-terminal end to the C-terminal end: Signal peptide (to be cleaved from the mature protein), peptide bound to the HLA with a high affinity, linker #1, human β2 microglobulin, linker #2, and the extracellular domains of class I HLA. A pair of cysteine residues in linker #1 and the extracellular domains will form a disulfide trap to stabilize the 9-mer peptide in the peptide-binding groove. Downstream of the BglII site is the sequence encoding Fc from mouse IgG2a. Three point mutations (annotated as LALA and PG on the sequence) can be introduced to abolish the function of Fc to create a variant fusion protein for negative control

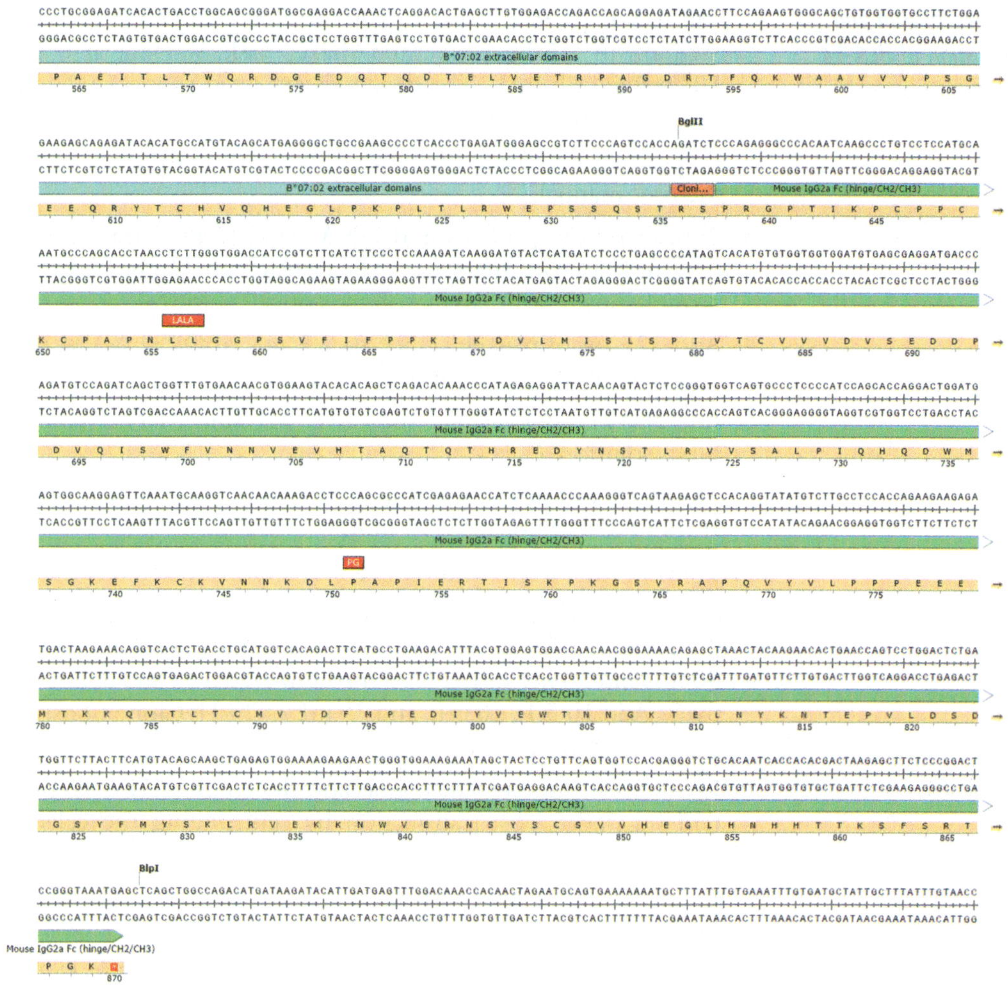

Fig. 2 (continued)

2. Synthesize the DNA encoding the protein sequence from the signal peptide to the end of the α3 domain of class I HLA allele with unique XhoI and BglII restriction sites (with CGGCGG overhangs) at the 5′ and 3′ ends, respectively (IDT-DNA).
3. Digest the synthesized DNA and the pFUSE-Fc vector (*see* **Note 3**) with these two enzymes and ligate the insert into the vector between the XhoI and BglII sites.
4. Generate a negative control HLA-Fc molecule with a non-functional Fc by introducing LALAPG mutations to the Fc [25] using a Q5 site-directed mutagenesis kit following the user manual (NEB; Fig. 2).
5. Sequence the insert and 5′ and 3′ junctions to verify the single-chain HLA sequence and junctional sequences.

3.2 Expression and Purification of HLA-Fc Proteins

1. Culture Expi293F cells in 100 mL of Expi293 expression medium in a 500 mL vented shaker flask, starting at 0.2 × 10^6 viable cells/mL. The density is expected to reach ~1 million cells/mL in 2–3 days.
2. Prepare plasmid using the NucleoBond PC 2000 Mega kit per the user manual.
3. Transfect 125 μg of plasmid DNA using Hype-5 transfection reagent following **steps 4–7**. The transfection can be scaled up proportionally with larger volumes of cell culture.
4. Add 125 μg of plasmid DNA to 2.5 mL of OPTI MEM in a 15 mL conical tube (solution 1).
5. Add 200 μL Hype5 to 2.5 mL OPTI MEM in a 15 mL conical tube (solution 2).
6. Transfer solution 1 to solution 2, invert five times, and incubate at room temperature for 15 min.
7. Transfer the mixed solution (~5 mL total) to the cell culture.
8. Supplement the culture with additional Expi293 medium and 2% HyClone Boost on days 2–4 after the transfection. Add 50 mL and 50 mL of Expi293 medium on days 2 and 3, respectively. Add 10 mL, 20 mL, and 30 mL of 2% HyClone Boost on days 2, 3, and 4, respectively.
9. Harvest the supernatant containing the soluble HLA-Fc protein on day 5 post-transfection by centrifuging the cells at 300 g at 4 °C for 10 min.
10. Filter the supernatant through a 0.2 μm pore-size nylon membrane using a Corning bottle-top vacuum filter system (Millipore-Sigma, CLS430773-12EA). Discard the cell pellet.
11. Follow **steps 12–20** to purify HLA-Fc proteins by protein A chromatography.
12. Add 1 mL of protein A resin to a 20 mL column.
13. Wash with 20 mL binding buffer (2× PBS, pH = 8.0), and drain by gravity.
14. Load filtered supernatant containing HLA-Fc, drain by gravity (this step may take 1–2 h).
15. Wash with 20 mL binding buffer, drain by gravity.
16. Elute HLA-Fc using the elution buffer (100 mM sodium citrate, pH = 5.0). Add 1 mL of elution buffer at a time and collect the flow through in 1.5 mL tubes containing 100 μL of neutralization buffer (1× Tris buffer, pH = 8.0) at room temperature. Repeat for a total of 10 separate elutions.
17. Quantify the protein concentration in each elution using a nanodrop instrument, measuring the absorbance at 280 nm, using a coefficient of 0.71 (Fig. 3).

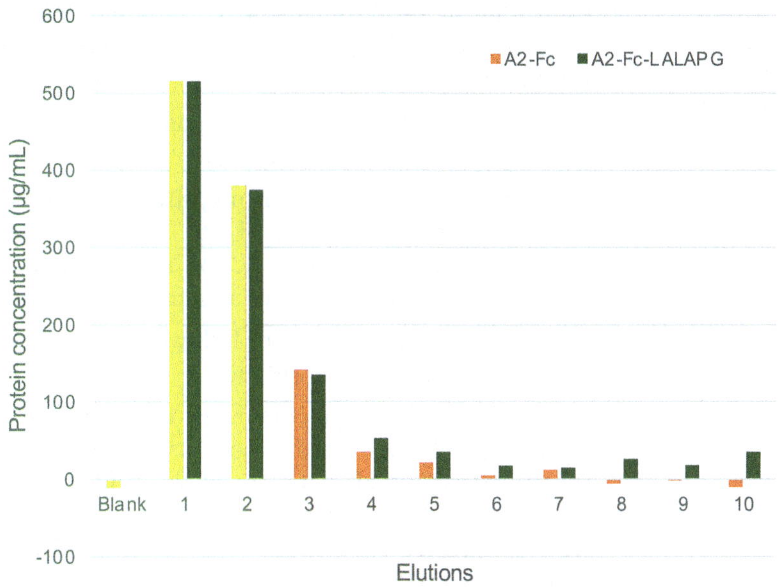

Fig. 3 A2-Fc and A2-Fc-LALAPG protein concentrations in sequential elutions from the protein A column. The protein yield in a representative experiment following the protocol described in Subheading 3.2 is plotted. The first three elutions contain >90% of the proteins extracted from the culture supernatants, ranging from 100–500 μg/mL. These protocols are based largely on our work in the following reference: Webber et al. [21]

18. Combine elutions with sufficient protein concentrations (e.g., > 50 μg/mL).
19. Dialyze the elutions with 1× PBS and concentrate the protein to 1 mg/mL using a 30 kDa MWCO Amico® Ultra centrifugal filter tube.
20. Measure the protein concentration in the concentrate using a nanodrop instrument as above, and adjust the final concentration to 1 mg/mL in 1× PBS.
21. Evaluate the size of the native protein and reduced (use 2-ME for reduction) monomers by SDS-PAGE using standard methods.
22. Snap-freeze the protein preparations in 25–50 μL aliquots and store at −80 °C until thawed for experiments.

3.3 Binding of HLA-Fc to B Cell Hybridomas

1. Culture B cell hybridoma cells in Iscove's Modified Dulbecco's Medium (IMDM; supplemented with 0.1 mM hypoxanthine, 0.016 mM thymidine, 10% FBS, and 1% penicillin) to the exponential growth phase (0.5–1 × 10^6 cells/mL). Alternatively, culture B cell hybridoma cells per instructions from the vendor or source of these cells.
2. Count cells and plate cells at a density of 100,000 cells per well on a V-bottom, 96-well plate.

3. Centrifuge at 1400 rpm and 4 °C for 3 min, flick out supernatant, and wash B cell hybridoma cells in 200 μL ice cold DPBS once.
4. Add 50 μL of staining buffer containing 1:200 TruStain FcX (BioLegend) to block Fc receptors.
5. Add prediluted HLA-Fc (1 mg/mL) at 1:50 in 50 μL of staining buffer to each well for a final concentration of 0.01 mg/mL. Add HLA-Fc of non-cognate specificities, HLA-Fc-LALAPG, or PBS to selected wells as controls.
6. Incubate at 4 °C for 20 min, followed by washing 3 times in 200 μL ice cold staining buffer.
7. After the last wash, stain with individual or mixed fluorochrome-conjugated secondary antibodies specific for the subclasses of HLA-Fc (mIgG2a) and B cell hybridoma cells (IgG1 for PA2.1 and BB7.1 cells). For example, APC-conjugated anti-mouse IgG1 and FITC-conjugated anti-mouse IgG2a, separately and as a cocktail of both at 1: 100 each (*see* **Note 4**).
8. Incubate at 4 °C for 10 min, followed by three washes in 200 μL ice cold staining buffer.
9. After the last wash, resuspend cells in 100 μL staining buffer with 5 μL 7-AAD (1:20).
10. Analyze the sample by flow cytometry to quantify the percentages of unstained, single-positive, and double-positive cells.

3.4 CDC of HLA-Fc on B Cell Hybridomas

1. Culture B cell hybridoma cells in IMDM (supplemented with 0.1 mM hypoxanthine, 0.016 mM thymidine, 10% FBS, and 1% penicillin) to the exponential growth phase (0.5–1 × 10^6 cells/mL).
2. Transfer 10 mL of cultured cells into a 15-mL conical tube and mix by gently pipetting 5 times.
3. Centrifuge at 1000 rpm for 5 min at 4 °C and discard the supernatant.
4. Resuspend in 10 mL DPBS, gently pipette 5 times, centrifuge at 1000 rpm for 5 min at 4 °C, and discard the supernatant.
5. Resuspend cells in 5 mL DPBS, gently pipette 5 times, and invert the tube 10 times. Count cells and adjust the DPBS volume to reach a cell density of 250,000 cells/mL. Transfer all cells to a reservoir.
6. Plate 50,000 cells per well (200 μL of the resuspended cells) on a V-bottom, 96-well plate (*see* **Note 5**).
7. Thaw rabbit serum (fresh complement source) and dilute in DPBS at 1:8 (*see* **Note 6**).

8. Add HLA-Fc protein to the diluted rabbit serum at a concentration of 0.01 mg/mL, followed by 1:2 serial dilutions to a titer up to 8192 in diluted rabbit serum.
9. Pellet B cell hybridoma cells by centrifuging the plate at 1400 rpm and 4 °C for 3 min. Flick out supernatant.
10. Add 45 μL diluted rabbit serum containing serially diluted HLA-Fc or without HLA-Fc to the pelleted cells per well. Incubate at room temperature in the dark for 3 h.
11. Wash cells in 150 μL and then 200 μL ice cold staining buffer, and then resuspend in 100 μL staining buffer containing 5 μL 7-AAD (1:20).
12. Analyze the samples by flow cytometry to quantify the percentage of viable cells.
13. Determine the half-maximal cytotoxic concentration for an HLA-Fc and target cells by nonlinear regression using concentration vs. percent cell survival and a variable slope model in GraphPad.

3.5 Assessing the Effect of HLA-Fc on B Cell Hybridomas In Vivo

1. Collect ~50–100 μL peripheral blood from TKO mice by submandibular technique with a lancet before intravenous injection of B cell hybridomas and weekly after for 7 weeks.
2. Centrifuge peripheral blood at 10,000 rpm for 10 min at room temperature, collect serum, and store at −20 °C.
3. Conduct a tail vein IV injection of TKO mice using an 18G needle to draw up and a 27G needle to deliver 1 million PA2.1 or BB7.1 cells suspended in 300 μL pyrogen-free saline.
4. Immediately conduct intraperitoneal injection of treatment (e.g., 0.4 mg of A2Fc in 0.4 mL PBS) or negative control (e.g., 0.4 mg of A2Fc-LALAPG in 0.4 mL PBS) to TKO mice (Fig. 1c) using an 18G needle to draw up and a 27G needle to deliver the treatment.
5. Quantify the strength of anti-HLA antibodies in serum samples by flow cytometric crossmatch against cognate HLA transgenic splenocytes (e.g., quantify anti-A2 antibodies using A2 transgenic splenocytes; *see* **Note 7**) as described in **steps 6–19**. Alternatively, anti-HLA antibodies can be tested by the SAB assay as described in Subheading 3.7.
6. Euthanize an HLA transgenic mouse and immediately remove the spleen with scissors.
7. Place spleen in a 70 μm cell strainer with 5 mL I10F medium in a petri dish on ice.
8. Mush spleen using the butt of a 5 mL syringe and rinse the strainer with 5 mL I10F.
9. Transfer pass-through into a 50 mL conical tube.

10. Centrifuge the tube at 1400 rpm and 4 °C for 5 min. Pour off supernatant.
11. Resuspend pellet in 5 mL ACK lysing buffer for 2 min at room temperature.
12. Add 8 mL of I10F to stop cell lysis.
13. Centrifuge the tube at 1400 rpm and 4 °C for 5 min. Pour off supernatant.
14. Resuspend the cell pellet in 5 mL of I10F and count cells.
15. Plate 200,000 splenocytes per well in a V-bottom 96-well plate and wash cells once with staining buffer.
16. Add 45 μL of staining buffer containing 1:200 TruStain FcX (BioLegend) to block Fc receptors. Incubate for 5 min at room temperature.
17. Add 5 μL serum to each well (final dilution 1:10) and incubate at room temperature for 10 min.
18. Wash cells in staining buffer twice, pellet cells, and incubate at room temperature for 10 min with a cocktail containing APC-conjugated anti-mouse CD3 (final dilution 1:200) to label T cells and PE-conjugated anti-mouse IgG (final dilution 1:200) to detect antibodies bound to donor T cells.
19. After two more washes with 150 and 200 μL staining buffer, resuspend cells in 100 μL staining buffer, followed by flow cytometric analysis. Gate on the CD3+ lymphocyte population, and report the shift of median fluorescence intensity in the PE channel (ΔMFI) after subtracting the MFI from the prebleed serum samples.
20. Euthanize morbid mice during follow up or surviving mice at the end of 120 days. Perform gross examination of abdominal organs immediately to look for tumors formed by B cell hybridoma cells and collect the liver and spleen for histologic examination.

3.6 Assessing the Effect of HLA-Fc in a Platelet Refractoriness Model

1. Transfer B cell hybridoma cells (e.g., A2-specific PA2.1 cells) into a cohort of TKO mice by tail vein injection at 1 million cells per mouse (*see* Subheading 3.5). Treat half of the cohort right after cell transfer with 0.4 mg of cognate HLA-Fc (e.g., A2-Fc) per mouse via intraperitoneal injection. Leave the other half of the cohort untreated. Include a third group of mice without cell transfer or treatment as negative controls (Fig. 1d).
2. Two weeks after cell transfer, collect 10 mL peripheral blood from a consented human volunteer positive for the cognate HLA (e.g., A2-positive) in an ACD-A tube. Centrifuge the tube at 2000 g at 20 °C for 3 min. Transfer the platelet-rich plasma (PRP) to a 50 mL conical tube (*see* **Note 8**).

3. Transfuse 0.2 mL of PRP per mouse via tail vein injection in all three groups. Record the time of injection.
4. Collect peripheral blood into a heparinized container from each mouse by submandibular bleed at 10, 60, and 120 min after transfusion, alternating the right and left sides of the face with each collection. Immediately transfer 21 μL of blood into a 1.5 mL Eppendorf tube containing 3 μL of ACD-A (1: 8 dilution of ACD-A).
5. Dilute the blood by adding 50 μL of DPBS to the tube, followed by centrifugation at 50 g for 10 min at room temperature.
6. Carefully transfer 50 μL of diluted PRP per sample into a well on a V-bottom 96-well plate. Add 150 μL DPBS and centrifuge at 1942 g at room temperature for 2 min.
7. Discard the supernatant, add 50 μL of staining buffer containing 1:200 TruStain FcX, and incubate at room temperature for 5 min.
8. Add an antibody cocktail of PE-conjugated anti-human CD41 and APC-conjugated anti-mouse CD41 to each well, each antibody with a final dilution of 1:100. Incubate at room temperature in the dark for 10 min.
9. Wash in 150 μL and then 200 μL staining buffer and flick out the supernatant.
10. Resuspend platelets in 100 μL of staining buffer with 20 μL of CountBright™ absolute counting beads, followed by flow cytometric acquisition.
11. Cells in the platelet gate should separate into human CD41+, mouse CD41+, or double-negative populations. Determine human and murine platelet counts per 5000 absolute counting beads and compare the counts directly across different groups. Alternatively, normalize the platelet counts across different experiment cohorts using the average platelet count from the negative control mice as 100% for each time point within each cohort.

3.7 Single-Antigen Bead Assay

1. Make a list of samples to be tested and label a V-bottom 96-well plate accordingly.
2. Vortex LABScreen single-antigen beads to ensure they are well mixed; pipette 2.5 μL of beads per well.
3. Add 20 μL of the supernatant from a class I HLA-specific B cell hybridoma on day 3 of culture with a cell density of approximately 1 million cells/mL. Incubate 20 μL of fresh culture medium with beads in a separate well as the negative control sample, which also provides the background signal for subtraction during analysis.

4. For serum samples from mice with B cell hybridoma grafts, mix 1.25 μL of 6% EDTA in deionized water and 23.75 μL of mouse serum in PCR tubes and then incubate 20 μL of EDTA-treated serum with 2.5 μL of beads per well (*see* **Note 9**). Incubate 20 μL of EDTA-treated serum from before the B cell hybridoma cell transfer with beads in a separate well as the negative control sample, which also provides the background signal for subtraction during analysis.
5. Shake plate in the dark at room temperature for 30 min.
6. While incubating, dilute the wash buffer at 1:10, which can be gently warmed to dissolve salt precipitates prior to use.
7. Dilute PE-conjugated anti-mouse IgG (Poly4053, BioLegend) secondary antibody at 1:100 with diluted wash buffer. Store at 4 °C in the dark until ready to use.
8. Create a sample list for the Luminex data collection software, xPONENT, and for HLA fusion. Build an assay batch in xPONENT using the sample list.
9. After the first incubation, wash the assay plate using 200 μL diluted wash buffer per well, spin the plate for 3 min at 3000 rpm, flick out supernatant, and blot the plate dry on a paper towel.
10. Wash two more times using 200 μL diluted wash buffer per well, flick out supernatant after each wash, and blot the plate dry. Vortex gently to loosen up the beads.
11. Add 100 μL diluted secondary antibody per well, vortex gently, and shake the plate in the dark at room temperature for 30 min.
12. After the second incubation, spin the plate for 3 min at 3000 rpm, flick out the supernatant, and blot the plate dry. Vortex gently.
13. Wash two more times using 200 μL diluted wash buffer per well. Flick out supernatant after each wash and blot the plate dry. Vortex gently.
14. Resuspend beads in 80 μL 1× PBS per well and mix gently with a pipette.
15. Collect data on Luminex using the xPONENT software, followed by data importing and analysis in the fusion software.
16. Record the background normalized mean fluorescence intensity (MFI) values from relevant single-antigen beads in the fusion software as a surrogate for measuring the antibody strength (*see* **Note 10**).

4 Notes

1. The signal peptide guides the fusion protein through the secretory pathway and is expected to be removed from the mature single-chain trimer. The cleavage site between the signal peptide and the high-affinity peptide bound to HLA should be analyzed with bioinformatic tools, such as the SignalP server (default setting for eukaryotic proteins) [26], to ensure a high probability of successful cleavage at the site.
2. Linker #1 consists of three repeating GGGGS units and two mutations at positions 2 and 4 of the linker. The G > C mutation at position 2 enables disulfide trap formation with a cysteine residue in the peptide-binding groove of class I HLA (Fig. 2), which stabilizes the peptide-HLA complex. The G > A mutation at position 4 is the result of a DNA sequence alteration to introduce a NheI restriction site in the linker. This NheI site and the AgeI site in the signal peptide coding region can be used to change the peptide coding sequences between the two restriction sites as needed.
3. InvivoGen offers pFUSE-Fc vectors encoding Fc from a wide range of species (human, mouse, rabbit, and rat) and subclasses. The two most referenced vectors with complement-fixing Fc are pFUSE-hIgG1-Fc and pFUSE-mIgG2a-Fc.
4. Staining HLA-Fc-treated B cell hybridomas with APC-anti-mouse IgG1 and FITC-anti-mouse IgG2a separately and together ensures the detection of any cross reactivity of the two antibodies with other IgG subclasses. These two antibodies showed excellent specificity and no cross reactivity in our experience.
5. It is critical to standardize the number of cells plated per well. An increased cell density may reduce the killing efficacy, likely due to the consumption of complement factors.
6. Undiluted rabbit complement, although adsorbed for antibodies against other species, may increase the background killing in the CDC assay. The dilution factor can be further optimized due to variable susceptibility to CDC among different B cell hybridomas.
7. There is a limited number of HLA transgenic strains available to enable the crossmatch assay described in this chapter. In the absence of suitable HLA transgenic mice with a desired cognate antigen, NIH/3 T3 cells (ATCC; Cat#CRL-1658) are fairly easy to transfect and can be used to express diverse HLA molecules for crossmatch.

8. To minimize platelet clumping, we avoided centrifuging donor platelets at high speeds to remove donor plasma in our study [21]. Mild hemolysis may be noticed in all recipients after transfusion.
9. EDTA treatment is critical to remove complement interference in serum samples tested by the SAB assay [27]. The vendor specified bead volume to use for the SAB assay is 5 μL. Using a smaller bead volume (2.5 μL) allowed us to conserve both this expensive reagent and the limited serum specimens collected from mice. A validation study in our clinical laboratory has shown that bead volumes of 2.5 μL, 3 μL, and 5 μL showed comparable performance in detecting anti-HLA antibodies [28].
10. Background normalized MFI values do not quantify the concentration or affinity of the anti-HLA antibodies detected. However, MFI values can be used as a semiquantitative readout for antibody strength. MFI values from 1 to 15,000 may be considered the linear range of the assay. When >15,000 MFI, the assay may be saturated and may underestimate antibody strengths. The MFI values also suffer from high run-to-run variations [29] and should be interpreted with caution.

Funding Acknowledgment

This work was supported by the Foundation for Barnes-Jewish Hospital (Award Reference Number: 4082; C.L.), a Mallinckrodt-Washington University Challenge Grant from the Edward Mallinckrodt Jr. Foundation (C.L.), and the National Institutes of Health, National Institute of Allergy and Infectious Diseases (AI168706; B.T.E. and C.L.). The authors have no other conflicts of interest to declare that are relevant to the content of this chapter.

References

1. Trial to Reduce Alloimmunization to Platelets Study Group (1997) Leukocyte reduction and ultraviolet B irradiation of platelets to prevent alloimmunization and refractoriness to platelet transfusions. N Engl J Med 337:1861–1869
2. Patel R, Terasaki PI (1969) Significance of the positive crossmatch test in kidney transplantation. N Engl J Med 280:735–739
3. Montgomery RA, Lonze BE, King KE, Kraus ES, Kucirka LM, Locke JE, Warren DS, Simpkins CE, Dagher NN, Singer AL, Zachary AA, Segev DL (2011) Desensitization in HLA-incompatible kidney recipients and survival. N Engl J Med 365:318–326
4. Persaud SP, Duffy B, Phelan DL, Mohanakumar T, Delos Santos R, Gaut JP, Liu C (2017) Accelerated humoral renal allograft rejection due to HLA-C14 mediated allosensitization to HLA-Bw6. Hum Immunol 78: 692–698
5. Spellman S, Bray R, Rosen-Bronson S, Haagenson M, Klein J, Flesch S, Vierra-Green-C, Anasetti C (2010) The detection of donor-directed, HLA-specific alloantibodies in recipients of unrelated hematopoietic cell

transplantation is predictive of graft failure. Blood 115:2704–2708
6. Ciurea SO, Thall PF, Wang X, Wang SA, Hu Y, Cano P, Aung F, Rondon G, Molldrem JJ, Korbling M, Shpall EJ, de Lima M, Champlin RE, Fernandez-Vina M (2011) Donor-specific anti-HLA Abs and graft failure in matched unrelated donor hematopoietic stem cell transplantation. Blood 118:5957–5964
7. National data - OPTN. https://optn.transplant.hrsa.gov/data/view-data-reports/national-data/. Accessed 12 Feb 2022
8. Triulzi DJ, Kleinman S, Kakaiya RM, Busch MP, Norris PJ, Steele WR, Glynn SA, Hillyer CD, Carey P, Gottschall JL, Murphy EL, Rios JA, Ness PM, Wright DJ, Carrick D, Schreiber GB (2009) The effect of previous pregnancy and transfusion on HLA alloimmunization in blood donors: implications for a transfusion-related acute lung injury risk reduction strategy. Transfusion 49:1825–1835
9. Pottebaum AA, Venkatachalam K, Liu C, Brennan DC, Murad H, Malone AF, Alhamad T (2020) Efficacy and safety of tocilizumab in the treatment of acute active antibody-mediated rejection in kidney transplant recipients. Transplant Direct 6:e543
10. Pottebaum AA, January SE, Liu C, Lavine S, Schilling JD, Lavine KJ (2023) Feasibility of interleukin-6 receptor blockade in cardiac antibody-mediated rejection. Transplantation. https://doi.org/10.1097/TP.0000000000004784
11. Wiebe C, Nevins TE, Robiner WN, Thomas W, Matas AJ, Nickerson PW (2015) The synergistic effect of class II HLA epitope-mismatch and nonadherence on acute rejection and graft survival. Am J Transplant 15:2197–2202
12. Velidedeoglu E, Cavaillé-Coll MW, Bala S, Belen OA, Wang Y, Albrecht R (2018) Summary of 2017 FDA public workshop: antibody-mediated rejection in kidney transplantation. Transplantation 102:e257–e264
13. Yamada C, Ramon DS, Cascalho M, Sung RS, Leichtman AB, Samaniego M, Davenport RD (2015) Efficacy of plasmapheresis on donor-specific antibody reduction by HLA specificity in post-kidney transplant recipients. Transfusion 55:727–735
14. Macklin PS, Morris PJ, Knight SR (2017) A systematic review of the use of rituximab for the treatment of antibody-mediated renal transplant rejection. Transplant Rev 31:87–95
15. Woodle ES, Tremblay S, Rossi A, Rojas CC, Alloway R, Roskin K, Allman D, Hildeman D (2020) Plasma cell targeting to prevent antibody-mediated rejection. Am J Transplant 20 Suppl 4:33–41
16. Walsh RC, Brailey P, Girnita A, Alloway RR, Shields AR, Wall GE, Sadaka BH, Cardi M, Tevar A, Govil A, Mogilishetty G, Roy-Chaudhury P, Woodle ES (2011) Early and late acute antibody-mediated rejection differ immunologically and in response to proteasome inhibition. Transplantation 91:1218–1226
17. Marks WH, Mamode N, Montgomery RA, Stegall MD, Ratner LE, Cornell LD, Rowshani AT, Colvin RB, Dain B, Boice JA, Glotz D, C10-001 Study Group (2019) Safety and efficacy of eculizumab in the prevention of antibody-mediated rejection in living-donor kidney transplant recipients requiring desensitization therapy: a randomized trial. Am J Transplant 19:2876–2888
18. January SE, Fester KA, Halverson LP, Witt CA, Byers DE, Vazquez-Guillamet R, Alexander-Brett J, Tague LK, Kreisel D, Gelman A, Puri V, Bahena RN, Takahashi T, Hachem RR, Kulkarni HS (2023) Tocilizumab for antibody-mediated rejection treatment in lung transplantation. J Heart Lung Transplant 42:1353–1357
19. Khairallah P, Robbins-Juarez S, Patel S, Shah V, Toma K, Fernandez H, Dube GK, King K, Mohan S, Husain SA, Morris H, Crew RJ (2022) Tocilizumab for the treatment of chronic antibody mediated rejection in kidney transplant recipients. Clin Transplant 37:e14853
20. Kjellman C, Maldonado AQ, Sjöholm K, Lonze BE, Montgomery RA, Runström A, Lorant T, Desai NM, Legendre C, Lundgren T, von Zur Mühlen B, Vo AA, Olsson H, Jordan SC (2021) Outcomes at 3 years post-transplant in imlifidase-desensitized kidney transplant patients. Am J Transplant. https://doi.org/10.1111/ajt.16754
21. Webber AM, Bradstreet TR, Wang X, Guo H, Nelson CA, Fremont DH, Edelson BT, Liu C (2022) Antigen-guided depletion of anti-HLA antibody-producing cells by HLA-Fc fusion proteins. Blood 140:1803–1815
22. Hansen TH, Connolly JM, Gould KG, Fremont DH (2010) Basic and translational applications of engineered MHC class I proteins. Trends Immunol 31:363–369
23. Hansen T, Yu YYL, Fremont DH (2009) Preparation of stable single-chain trimers engineered with peptide, beta2 microglobulin, and MHC heavy chain. Curr Protoc Immunol Chapter 17:Unit17.5

24. Truscott SM, Wang X, Lybarger L, Biddison WE, McBerry C, Martinko JM, Connolly JM, Linette GP, Fremont DH, Hansen TH, Carreno BM (2008) Human major histocompatibility complex (MHC) class I molecules with disulfide traps secure disease-related antigenic peptides and exclude competitor peptides. J Biol Chem 283:7480–7490
25. Lo M, Kim HS, Tong RK, Bainbridge TW, Vernes J-M, Zhang Y, Lin YL, Chung S, Dennis MS, Zuchero YJY, Watts RJ, Couch JA, Meng YG, Atwal JK, Brezski RJ, Spiess C, Ernst JA (2017) Effector-attenuating substitutions that maintain antibody stability and reduce toxicity in mice. J Biol Chem 292: 3900–3908
26. Petersen TN, Brunak S, von Heijne G, Nielsen H (2011) SignalP 4.0: discriminating signal peptides from transmembrane regions. Nat Methods 8:785–786
27. Liu C, Pang S, Phelan D, Brennan DC, Mohanakumar T (2017) Quantitative evaluation of the impact of ethylenediaminetetraacetic acid pretreatment on single-antigen bead assay. Transplant Direct 3:e194
28. Frick R, Wetter L, Phelan D, Liu C, Tang MS (2023) Evaluation of different microbead volumes in a single antigen bead assay for HLA antibody detection. Am J Clin Pathol 160:S118–S119
29. Reed EF, Rao P, Zhang Z, Gebel H, Bray RA, Guleria I, Lunz J, Mohanakumar T, Nickerson P, Tambur AR, Zeevi A, Heeger PS, Gjertson D (2013) Comprehensive assessment and standardization of solid phase multiplex-bead arrays for the detection of antibodies to HLA. Am J Transplant 13:1859–1870

Chapter 21

Isolation and Characterization of Mesenchymal Stem Cells from Human Umbilical Cord Tissue

Yitian Dai and Avital Mendelson

Abstract

Mesenchymal stem cells (MSCs) were first described over 30 years ago as multipotent stromal cells that can self-renew and differentiate into bone, cartilage, and fat tissues. MSCs have numerous functions, such as modulating the immune system, regulating inflammation, promoting wound healing, improving engraftment following hematopoietic transplant, and providing a supportive microenvironment for hematopoietic stem cells. Human umbilical cord tissue, which is more easily obtained than bone marrow aspirates, contains a population of MSCs. These cells can enhance thrombopoiesis in umbilical cord blood-derived megakaryocytes, leading to the production of platelets with low baseline activation levels. Scaled-up methods to enhance platelet production in vitro while maintaining a low activation state would benefit transfusion medicine and circumvent frequent platelet donor shortages. Here, we outline a protocol to isolate and expand MSCs from human umbilical cord tissue and characterize their cell surface protein expression by flow cytometry, self-renewal potential by colony-forming assay, and tri-lineage differentiation capacity.

Key words Mesenchymal stem cells, Self-renewal, Differentiation, Flow cytometry, Umbilical cord tissue

1 Introduction

Mesenchymal stem cells (MSCs) were first identified by *Friedenstein* et al. 50 years ago as a bone marrow-derived stromal precursor cell that can transfer the hematopoietic microenvironment when transplanted in vivo [1, 2]. These cells were initially described as adherent, spindle-shaped, colony-forming cells when cultured in vitro [2, 3]. This study inspired numerous subsequent investigations to examine additional cell sources, surface markers, differentiation potential, and functional properties in human and murine systems [4–8]. In addition to the bone marrow, MSCs were identified in adipose tissue, synovium, dental pulp, periodontal ligament, umbilical cord tissue, and placenta [9–16]. MSCs were originally found to differentiate into mesodermal tissues such as fat, cartilage,

Sean R. Stowell and Connie M. Arthur (eds.), *Methods in Transfusion Medicine*, Methods in Molecular Biology, vol. 3053, https://doi.org/10.1007/978-1-0716-5376-0_21,

and bone, though recent studies have also identified MSC potential to form cells of additional lineages, such as muscle cells, neurons, epithelial cells, and lung cells [9, 17–20]. While specific cell surface markers to isolate MSCs are still a topic of investigation, human MSCs can be identified based on the positive expression of CD105, CD73, CD44, CD90, CD71, GD2, CD271, and Stro1 along with the lack of expression of CD45, CD34, CD14, CD80, CD86, and CD40 [17].

MSCs have numerous roles in vivo, such as serving as a key niche for hematopoietic stem cell (HSC) regulation, interacting with innate and adaptive immune cells, and performing immunomodulatory functions [9, 17]. Expressing key regulatory factors, MSCs have been found to promote HSC self-renewal, proliferation, and trafficking [21, 22]. Numerous immune-regulating functions have been identified, including the ability to suppress T cell activation and proliferation in vitro [23], induce the formation of regulatory T cells, inhibit B cell proliferation, suppress Natural Killer (NK) cell cytotoxicity against HLA class I positive cells, and disrupt dendritic cell differentiation, maturation, and function [23]. In vivo, infusion of MSCs has been shown to prevent the development of graft versus host disease (GVHD) [24].

While bone marrow-derived MSCs represent the gold standard for cell sources, the invasive nature of their acquisition and limited donor availability hampers their utility [25]. Furthermore, cultured bone marrow-derived MSCs functionally decline with increased passage number [26]. Umbilical cord tissue is normally discarded after birth and could serve as a painless and safe alternative to bone marrow collection [27, 28]. Umbilical cord tissue has two arteries and one vein that are found longitudinal to the length of the cord (Fig. 1). MSCs have previously been isolated from various anatomical parts of the umbilical cord, including Wharton's jelly, arteries, veins, or the umbilical lining [29]. Importantly, umbilical cord-derived MSCs also demonstrate superior self-renewal capability [30] and shorter doubling time compared to bone marrow-derived MSCs, remaining viable after multiple passages [31]. Previously, we found a population of perivascular cells located on the outside of the umbilical arteries express CD51 and CD140a and share numerous properties with bone marrow-derived MSCs [32]. When cultured together with megakaryocyte progenitor cells, these cells could help to expand platelets in vitro and promote the production of platelets with low levels of baseline activation [32] that would be ideal for transfusion [33].

Culturing primary MSCs can be challenging due to low adherence or cell heterogeneity. Here, we describe detailed methods to isolate umbilical cord tissue-derived MSCs from the perivascular region of human umbilical arteries. We describe three methods to further characterize the MSC properties using flow cytometry to assess cell surface marker expression, a colony-forming unit

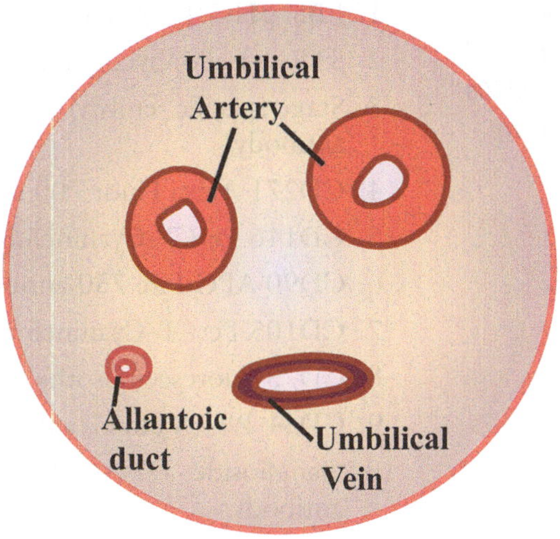

Fig. 1 Human umbilical cord tissue anatomy. Schematic depicting the anatomical structures within a cross-section of a human umbilical cord tissue containing two umbilical arteries, one umbilical vein, and an allantoic duct

fibroblast (CFU-F) assay for assessing clonogenicity, and a differentiation assay to evaluate their potential to form bone, cartilage, and adipose tissue lineages.

2 Materials

2.1 Umbilical Cord Collection and Processing for Culturing Umbilical Cord-Derived MSCs

1. Sterile fine-tip stainless steel forceps.
2. Disposable scalpel with #21 blade.
3. Biosafety cabinet.
4. Phosphate-buffered saline (PBS), pH 7.4 (Gibco).
5. 0.1% Fibronectin solution (Stemcell Technologies).
6. 100 mm tissue culture treated culture dish, sterile (Corning).
7. 24-well tissue culture treated plates, sterile (Corning).
8. Ruler.
9. MEM-α, no phenol red (Gibco).
10. MSC supplement from MesenCult™ Proliferation Kit for human cells (Stemcell Technologies).
11. 10,000 U/mL Penicillin-Streptomycin (Gibco).
12. 200 mM L-Glutamine (Gibco).
13. Fetal bovine serum (FBS) (HyClone).
14. 0.25% Trypsin-EDTA, phenol red (Gibco).
15. Tissue culture incubator.
16. Inverted phase contrast microscope.

2.2 Immuno-phenotyping of Umbilical Cord MSCs by Flow Cytometry

1. PBS, pH 7.4 (Gibco).
2. STRO-1 allophycocyanin (APC) antibody.
3. Stage-specific embryonic antigen-4 (SSEA-4) PE-Cyanine7 antibody.
4. CD271 Alexa Fluor 700 antibody.
5. CD146 PerCP-Cyanine5.5 antibody.
6. CD90 APC-Fire 750 antibody.
7. CD105 PerCP-Cyanine5.5 antibody.
8. CD73 fluorescein isothiocyanate (FITC) antibody.
9. CD44-PE-Cyanine7 antibody.
10. Ganglioside D2 (GD2) fluorescein isothiocyanate (FITC) antibody.
11. PDGFRβ phycoerythrin (PE) antibody.
12. 30% bovine serum albumin (BSA) solution (Sigma).
13. UltraPure™ 0.5 M EDTA, pH 8.0 (Invitrogen).
14. 5 mL round bottom polystyrene tubes, non-sterile (Fisher Scientific).
15. 100 μm reversible cell strainer for 5 mL tubes (Stem Cell Technologies).
16. Hemocytometer for cell counting.
17. LSRFortessa™ Cell Analyzer (BD Biosciences).
18. DAPI (4',6-diamidino-2-phenylindole) solution (1 mg/mL) (Fisher Scientific).

2.3 CFU-Fibroblast (CFU-F) Assay

1. Costar® 12-well clear TC-treated multiple well plates, sterile (Fisher Scientific).
2. MEM-α, no phenol red (Gibco).
3. MSC supplement from MesenCult™ Proliferation Kit for human cells (Stemcell Technologies).
4. 10,000 U/mL Penicillin-Streptomycin (Gibco).
5. 200 mM L-Glutamine (Gibco).
6. Fetal bovine serum (FBS) (HyClone).
7. 0.25% trypsin-EDTA, phenol red (Gibco).
8. PBS, pH 7.4 (Thermo Fisher).
9. 0.4% W/V Giemsa stain solution (Electron Microscopy Science).
10. 4% paraformaldehyde (PFA) in PBS (Boston Bioproducts).

2.4 Tri-Lineage Differentiation Assay

1. MEM-α, no phenol red (Gibco).
2. MSC supplement from MesenCult™ Proliferation Kit for human cells (Stemcell Technologies).
3. 10,000 U/mL Penicillin-Streptomycin (Gibco).
4. 200 mM L-Glutamine (Gibco).
5. Fetal bovine serum (FBS) (HyClone).
6. Human MesenCult™ Osteogenic Differentiation Kit (Stemcell Technologies).
7. Human MesenCult™-ACF Chondrogenic Differentiation Kit (Stemcell Technologies).
8. Human MesenCult™ Adipogenic Differentiation Kit (Stemcell Technologies).
9. 40 mM alizarin-red stain solution, pH 4.1 (Millipore Sigma).
10. Toluidine blue powder (Millipore Sigma).
11. 70% Alcohol.
12. Oil-red-O powder (Millipore Sigma).
13. Methanol (Millipore Sigma).
14. 60% isopropanol (Millipore Sigma).
15. Glacial acetic acid (Millipore Sigma).
16. Hematoxylin solution.
17. PBS, pH 7.4 (Thermo Fisher).
18. 4% or 10% PFA in PBS (Boston Bioproducts).
19. 10% formalin.
20. Sodium chloride.
21. Whatman Grade 1 filter paper.
22. Distilled water (Thermo Fisher).

3 Methods

3.1 Umbilical Cord Collection and Processing (Fig. 2)

1. Autoclave 2 stainless steel forceps. Place them in the culture hood along with a sterile scalpel.
2. Prepare a working solution of fibronectin by diluting 100 μL of 0.1% fibronectin stock solution +4.9 mL of PBS. Sterile filter the solution (*see* **Note 1**).
3. Pipet 200 μL of fibronectin working solution to each well of a 24 well plate. Allow the plate to incubate at room temperature for 40 min to coat the wells (*see* **Note 2**).
4. Aspirate the fibronectin solution and keep the plate covered at 37 °C until ready to use.

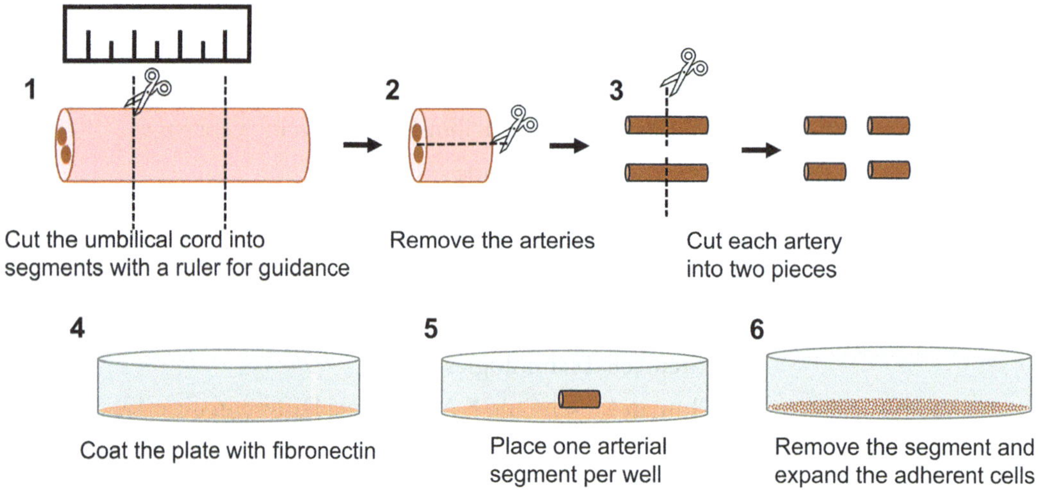

Fig. 2 Methods for isolating human umbilical cord tissue MSCs. Schematic image detailing the 6 steps involved in culturing human umbilical cord tissue-derived MSCs. (1) Cutting the umbilical cord tissue into 1-inch segments using a ruler for guidance. (2) With a shallow incision on the surface of the cord, gently peel the outer layer of tissue and remove the two umbilical cord arteries. (3) Cut each artery into two segments. (4) Coat the bottom of a 24-well tissue culture plate with fibronectin. (5) Place one segment of umbilical artery per well in the 24-well plate. (6) After 3 days, remove the umbilical artery piece and continue to expand the adherent stromal cells

5. Working under a laminar flow cell culture hood, using sterile forceps, transfer the umbilical cord from the delivery bottle to a new 100 mm culture dish containing 5 mL PBS (*see* **Note 3**).
6. Wash the umbilical cord in PBS 2–3 times to remove any attached blood.
7. Using a ruler for guidance, cut the umbilical cord into 1-inch segments using a scalpel and forceps.
8. Transfer the umbilical cord segments to a new 100 mm culture dish containing 5 mL PBS.
9. Make a shallow cut through the top membrane of each segment to expose the umbilical arteries. Gently remove the two umbilical arteries from each segment and transfer them to a new 100 mm culture dish containing 5 mL PBS.
10. Cut each artery again into two equal segments to acquire a total of four arterial segments from each umbilical cord segment.

3.2 Culture of Umbilical Cord-Derived MSCs

1. Prepare 50 mL of human MSC media consisting of α-MEM supplemented with 1% Penicillin-Streptomycin, 1% L-Glutamine, 20% FBS, and 10% Human MSC Supplement. Sterile filter the media.

2. Using sterile forceps, transfer one arterial segment into each well of the fibronectin-coated 24-well plate. Add 1 mL MSC media to each well. Place the plate in a tissue culture incubator at 37 °C with 5% CO_2 (*see* **Note 4**).
3. After 72 h, extract the arterial segment using sterile forceps. Examine adherent cell morphology under a microscope.
4. Allow the adherent cells to proliferate for 14 days. Change the media and replace it with fresh media every 48–72 h.
5. When the cells reach approximately 85% confluence, detach the cells with 300 μL of 0.25% trypsin-EDTA per well and transfer them to 100 mm culture plate for further expansion.

3.3 Immunophenotyping of Umbilical Cord-Derived MSCs by Flow Cytometry

1. Prepare Fluorescence-Activated Cell Sorting (FACS) buffer by combining 489.7 mL PBS with 8.3 mL of 30% BSA solution, and 2 mL of 0.5 M Ethylenediaminetetraacetic acid (EDTA).
2. Prepare DAPI working solution by diluting 1 mg/mL DAPI stock solution 1:20,000 with FACS buffer.
3. Using a non-enzymatic dissociation solution such as Accumax, detach the umbilical cord-derived MSCs from the culture plate (*see* **Note 5**).
4. Aliquot 1×10^5 umbilical cord-derived MSCs to two FACS tubes labeled cocktail 1 and cocktail 2, respectively. Multiple technical replicates are recommended.
5. Prepare two antibody cocktails. Cocktail 1 contains 1 μL of each of the following antibodies: STRO-1 APC, SSEA-4 PE-Cy7, GD2 FITC, CD271 AF700, and CD146 PerCP-Cy5.5 in 95 μL FACS buffer. Cocktail 2 contains 1 μL of CD90 APCFire 750, CD105 PerCP-Cy5.5, CD73 FITC, CD44-PeCy7, and PDGFRβ PE antibody in 95 μL FACS buffer. Vortex to mix. (*see* **Note 6**).
6. Stain the cells for 30 min on ice, covered from light.
7. Add 900 μL FACS buffer. Centrifuge the cells for 5 min at 300× *g*, 4 °C.
8. Remove the supernatant and resuspend the pellet in 200 μL of DAPI working solution.
9. Filter the cell suspensions through 100 μm strainers.
10. Acquire the samples on the LSRFortessa flow cytometer (Fig. 3a) (*see* **Note 7**).

3.4 CFU-Fibroblast (CFU-F) Assay

1. Seed umbilical cord-derived MSCs at a clonal density of 2000 cells per well in a 12-well plate, containing 1 mL of human MSC Media per well (α-MEM supplemented with 1% Penicillin-Streptomycin, 1% L-Glutamine, 20% FBS, and 10% Human MSC Supplement from MesenCult Proliferation Kit).

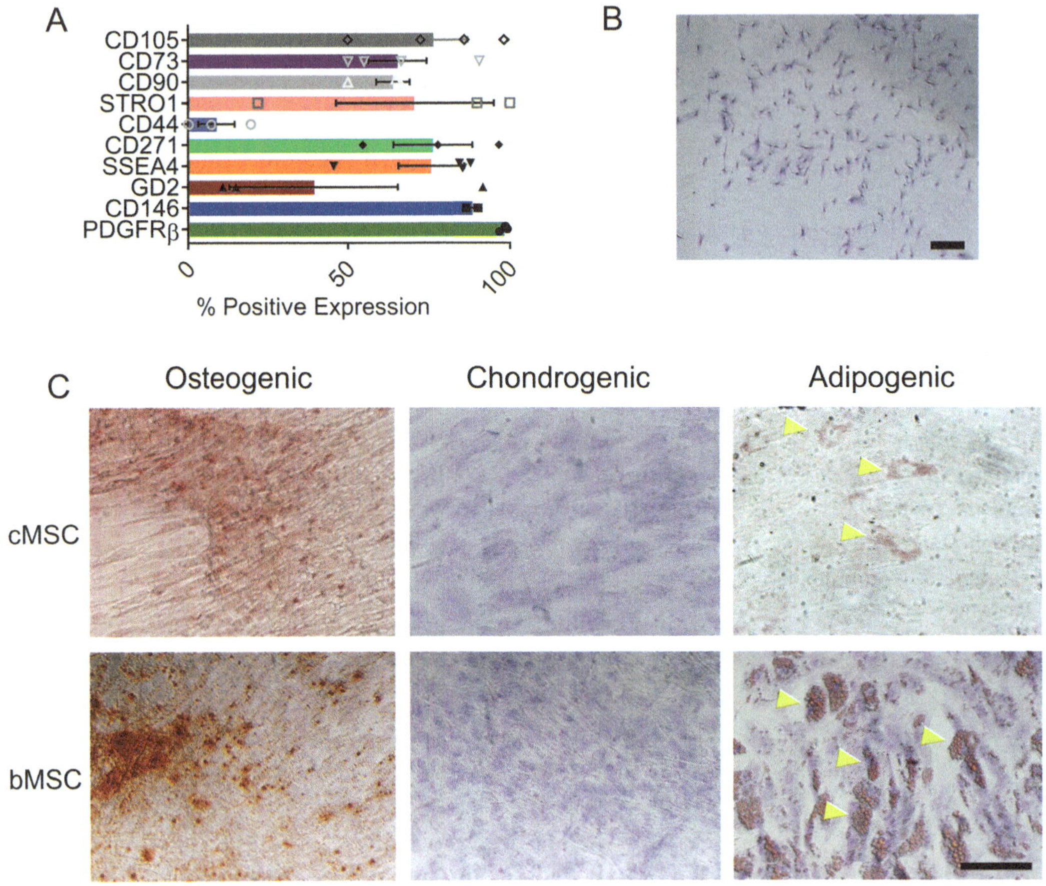

Fig. 3 Phenotypic characterization of umbilical cord-derived MSCs. (**a**) Following expansion, umbilical cord tissue-derived MSCs were assessed by flow cytometry for cell surface marker expression. (**b**) Representative Giemsa-stained colony from a colony-forming unit fibroblast assay performed on umbilical cord-derived MSCs (Scale = 2 mm). Umbilical cord-derived MSCs (cMSCs) were differentiated into adipose, cartilage, and bone lineages. (**c**) Following differentiation, cells are stained with oil-red-O to mark lipid droplets, Toluidine blue to stain cartilage proteoglycans, and alizarin red for calcified bone formation. Differentiated human bone marrow-derived MSCs (bMSCs) are shown for comparison as a positive control. Scale bar = 1 mm. (Data are reproduced from JCI Insight. Mendelson et al. [32]. © the American Society for Clinical Investigation (ASCI))

2. Place the plate in a humidified incubator at 37 °C with 5% CO_2.
3. On day 10, aspirate the media and wash the cells with PBS.
4. Aspirate the PBS and fix the cells with 1 mL of 4% PFA per well for 25 min at room temperature.
5. Dilute the Giemsa stock solution 1:20 with deionized water.
6. Aspirate the PFA solution and wash the cells with 1 mL of PBS per well.
7. Aspirate the PBS and stain the cells with 0.5 mL Giemsa solution per well for 20 min, at room temperature.

8. Aspirate the Giemsa solution and wash the cells with distilled water for 10 min. Allow the plate to air dry.
9. Count the colonies under a microscope (Fig. 3b) (*see* **Note 8**).

3.5 Tri-Lineage Differentiation Assay

3.5.1 Osteogenic Differentiation

1. Seed umbilical cord-derived MSCs at a density of 7.6–15.2 × 10^3 cells/cm^2 in human MSC media (see above) in a 24-well plate as above. Place the plate in a humidified incubator at 37 °C with 5% CO_2.
2. Once the cells reach 75% confluence, replace the old media with an equal volume of osteogenic differentiation media. Replace the media with fresh media every 3–4 days.
3. On day 14, aspirate the media and wash the cells gently with PBS.
4. Fix cells with 10% formaldehyde per well for 15 min at room temperature.
5. Rinse cells with distilled water 3 times for 5 min each.
6. Remove the water and add 1 mL of alizarin-red solution per well. Incubate the cells for 20 min at room temperature.
7. Remove the dye and wash cells with deionized H_2O for 5 min. Repeat the wash 4 times. Keep the cells hydrated in water.
8. Visualize calcium deposits under a microscope (Fig. 3c).

3.5.2 Chondrogenic Differentiation

1. Seed umbilical cord-derived MSCs at a density of 7.6–15.2 × 10^3 cells/cm^2 in human MSC media as above. Place the plate in a humidified incubator at 37 °C with 5% CO_2.
2. Once the cells reach 75% confluence, replace the old media with an equal volume of chondrogenic differentiation media. Replace the media with fresh media every 3–4 days.
3. On day 14, aspirate the media and rinse the cells gently with PBS.
4. Fix cells with 0.5 mL 10% formalin per well for 15 min at room temperature.
5. Make Toluidine blue stock solution by dissolving 1 g of Toluidine blue in 100 mL of 70% alcohol (*see* **Note 9**).
6. Prepare 1% sodium chloride solution by dissolving 0.5 g sodium chloride in 50 mL distilled water. Adjust the pH to 2.3 using glacial acetic acid.
7. Prepare a Toluidine blue working solution by mixing 5 mL Toluidine blue solution with 45 mL 1% sodium chloride, pH 2.3.
8. Rinse cells with distilled water and stain with Toluidine blue working solution for 3 min at room temperature.

9. Wash with distilled water for 1 min. Repeat the wash twice more. Allow the plate to air dry.
10. Visualize the proteoglycan-rich extracellular matrix under a microscope (Fig. 3c).

3.5.3 Adipogenic Differentiation

1. Seed umbilical cord-derived MSCs at a density of 7.6–15.2 × 10^3 cells/cm^2 in human MSC media as above. Place the plate in a humidified incubator at 37 °C with 5% CO_2.
2. Once the cells reach 75% confluence, replace the old media with an equal volume of adipogenic differentiation medium. Replace the media with fresh media every 3–4 days.
3. On day 12, aspirate the media, and rinse the cells gently with PBS.
4. Fix cells with 0.5 mL of 10% formalin per well for 15 min at room temperature.
5. Rinse the cells with tap water for 10 min.
6. Rinse the cells briefly with 60% isopropanol.
7. Prepare oil-red-O stock solution by dissolving 0.5 g of oil-red-O in 100 mL isopropanol with low heat.
8. Prepare oil-red-O working solution by diluting 30 mL of stock solution in 20 mL distilled water. Let the solution stand for 10 min and then filter the solution to remove particles.
9. Stain the cells with 0.5 mL oil-red-O working solution per well for 15 min, at room temperature.
10. Rinse the wells with 60% isopropanol.
11. Stain the nuclei with hematoxylin for 30 s.
12. Rinse the wells with distilled water. Leave the cells in distilled water and visualize lipid droplets under a microscope (Fig. 3c).

4 Notes

1. Other matrix proteins could also be used to coat the culture plate, such as collagen, laminin, gelatin, or poly-D-lysine.
2. The plate can be coated with fibronectin in advance, sealed with parafilm, and stored at 4 °C for up to 1 week.
3. Umbilical cord tissue should be processed within 24 h following birth to maintain cell viability for optimal results. If immediate processing is not feasible, the umbilical cord should be stored at 4 °C to preserve its integrity.
4. Once the umbilical cord segments are placed in culture, do not disturb them for the first 3 days to enhance cell migration and attachment.

5. Check the manufacturer's recommended protocol for optimal dissociation times and volumes to use. If using Accumax, incubate the plate for 8 min at 37 °C. Subsequently, pipet up and down multiple times to dissociate the cells from the plate.
6. Depending on the configuration of your flow cytometer, you can label a single sample with all antibodies in the panel or stain multiple aliquots of cord blood-derived MSCs with smaller combinations of antibodies to phenotype the cells.
7. Make sure to acquire enough events to detect cell surface markers with lower expression. We recommend acquiring at least 60,000 events per sample.
8. Colonies will vary in size and morphology due to the heterogeneous nature of the cells. A transparent grid sheet can be placed under the plate to aid in quantifying the colonies.
9. Alcian blue can be used as opposed to the Toluidine blue chemical stain for measuring anionic glycoconjugates indicative of chondrocyte differentiation.

Conflicts of Interest

The authors have no conflicts of interest to declare that are relevant to the content of this chapter.

Funding

This study was funded by NIH grant P01HL149626.

References

1. Friedenstein AJ et al (1974) Stromal cells responsible for transferring the microenvironment of the hemopoietic tissues. Cloning in vitro and retransplantation in vivo. Transplantation 17(4):331–340
2. Friedenstein AJ et al (1974) Precursors for fibroblasts in different populations of hematopoietic cells as detected by the in vitro colony assay method. Exp Hematol 2(2):83–92
3. Dominici M et al (2006) Minimal criteria for defining multipotent mesenchymal stromal cells. The International Society for Cellular Therapy position statement. Cytotherapy 8(4):315–317
4. Haynesworth SE et al (1992) Characterization of cells with osteogenic potential from human marrow. Bone 13(1):81–88
5. Phinney DG et al (1999) Plastic adherent stromal cells from the bone marrow of commonly used strains of inbred mice: variations in yield, growth, and differentiation. J Cell Biochem 72(4):570–585
6. Peister A et al (2004) Adult stem cells from bone marrow (MSCs) isolated from different strains of inbred mice vary in surface epitopes, rates of proliferation, and differentiation potential. Blood 103(5):1662–1668
7. Sun S et al (2003) Isolation of mouse marrow mesenchymal progenitors by a novel and reliable method. Stem Cells 21(5):527–535
8. Nombela-Arrieta C, Ritz J, Silberstein LE (2011) The elusive nature and function of mesenchymal stem cells. Nat Rev Mol Cell Biol 12(2):126–131

9. Pittenger MF et al (2019) Mesenchymal stem cell perspective: cell biology to clinical progress. NPJ Regener Med 4:22
10. Bianco P, Robey PG, Simmons PJ (2008) Mesenchymal stem cells: revisiting history, concepts, and assays. Cell Stem Cell 2(4):313–319
11. Zuk PA et al (2002) Human adipose tissue is a source of multipotent stem cells. Mol Biol Cell 13(12):4279–4295
12. De Bari C et al (2001) Multipotent mesenchymal stem cells from adult human synovial membrane. Arthritis Rheum 44(8):1928–1942
13. Gronthos S et al (2000) Postnatal human dental pulp stem cells (DPSCs) in vitro and in vivo. Proc Natl Acad Sci USA 97(25):13625–13630
14. Seo BM et al (2004) Investigation of multipotent postnatal stem cells from human periodontal ligament. Lancet 364(9429):149–155
15. In 't Anker PS et al (2004) Isolation of mesenchymal stem cells of fetal or maternal origin from human placenta. Stem Cells 22(7): 1338–1345
16. McElreavey KD et al (1991) Isolation, culture and characterisation of fibroblast-like cells derived from the Wharton's jelly portion of human umbilical cord. Biochem Soc Trans 19(1):29S
17. Uccelli A, Moretta L, Pistoia V (2008) Mesenchymal stem cells in health and disease. Nat Rev Immunol 8(9):726–736
18. Jeon ES et al (2006) Sphingosylphosphorylcholine induces differentiation of human mesenchymal stem cells into smooth-muscle-like cells through a TGF-beta-dependent mechanism. J Cell Sci 119(Pt 23):4994–5005
19. Mareschi K et al (2006) Neural differentiation of human mesenchymal stem cells: evidence for expression of neural markers and eag K+ channel types. Exp Hematol 34(11):1563–1572
20. Paunescu V et al (2007) In vitro differentiation of human mesenchymal stem cells to epithelial lineage. J Cell Mol Med 11(3):502–508
21. Mendelson A, Frenette PS (2014) Hematopoietic stem cell niche maintenance during homeostasis and regeneration. Nat Med 20(8):833–846
22. Mendez-Ferrer S et al (2010) Mesenchymal and haematopoietic stem cells form a unique bone marrow niche. Nature 466(7308): 829–834
23. Nauta AJ, Fibbe WE (2007) Immunomodulatory properties of mesenchymal stromal cells. Blood 110(10):3499–3506
24. Zhang X et al (2023) Mesenchymal stromal cells ameliorate chronic GVHD by boosting thymic regeneration in a CCR9-dependent manner in mice. Blood Adv 7(18):5359–5373
25. Levy O et al (2020) Shattering barriers toward clinically meaningful MSC therapies. Sci Adv 6(30):eaba6884
26. Ganguly P et al (2017) Age-related changes in bone marrow mesenchymal stromal cells: a potential impact on osteoporosis and osteoarthritis development. Cell Transplant 26(9): 1520–1529
27. Semenova E et al (2021) Mesenchymal stromal cells from different parts of umbilical cord: approach to comparison & characteristics. Stem Cell Rev Rep 17(5):1780–1795
28. Mebarki M et al (2021) Human umbilical cord-derived mesenchymal stem/stromal cells: a promising candidate for the development of advanced therapy medicinal products. Stem Cell Res Ther 12(1):152
29. Wang HS et al (2004) Mesenchymal stem cells in the Wharton's jelly of the human umbilical cord. Stem Cells 22(7):1330–1337
30. Sarugaser R et al (2009) Human mesenchymal stem cells self-renew and differentiate according to a deterministic hierarchy. PLoS One 4(8):e6498
31. Mennan C et al (2013) Isolation and characterisation of mesenchymal stem cells from different regions of the human umbilical cord. Biomed Res Int 2013:916136
32. Mendelson A et al (2019) Mesenchymal stromal cells lower platelet activation and assist in platelet formation in vitro. JCI Insight 4(16)
33. Tang A, Mendelson A (2021) Recent lessons learned for ex-vivo platelet production. Curr Opin Hematol 28(6):424–430

Chapter 22

Prolonging the Lifespan of Neutrophils for Granulocyte Transfusion in Neutropenic Mice with Bacterial Pneumonia

Alan Y. Hsu, Yuping Fan, and Hongbo R. Luo

Abstract

Neutrophils act as the first line of defense in our innate immune system, executing essential antimicrobial functions to fight off pathogens. Neutropenia, which can occur due to defects in bone marrow granulopoiesis or treatments such as chemotherapy, significantly increases the risk of infections. To manage complications arising from neutropenia, standard treatments include granulocyte colony-stimulating factor (G-CSF) induction or granulocyte transfusion (GTX), along with standard antibiotic therapies. Here, we present a comprehensive method for inducing neutropenia in mice and using granulocyte transfusion to mitigate acute pneumonic inflammation. However, GTX faces challenges such as the short lifespan of neutrophils and the inability to freeze GTX products. We have previously developed a novel approach, CLON-G treatment, which combines the inhibition of multiple cell death pathways in neutrophils. This treatment extends the lifespan of neutrophils to over 5 days without compromising their essential functions. Our earlier findings suggest a promising strategy for enhancing the efficacy of GTX, improving neutropenia management, and strengthening immune responses against infections. Additionally, we describe a method for transfusing CLON-G-treated neutrophils to enhance host defenses against neutropenia-related complications, as demonstrated in an *Escherichia coli*-induced neutropenic pneumonia model.

Key words Neutropenia, Neutrophil death, Granulocyte transfusion, Mouse models, Pneumonia, Acute lung infection

1 Introduction

Neutrophils, comprising 40%–70% of the total circulating white blood cell count, are terminally differentiated cells crucial to innate immunity, yet with a short lifespan of less than 24 h [1, 2]. To maintain physiological homeostasis, the body produces and removes one billion neutrophils per kilogram of body weight each day in a highly conserved but energetically demanding process [3, 4]. Neutrophils play a pivotal role in the innate immune system as the first responders recruited to infection sites. There, they

Alan Y. Hsu and Yuping Fan have contributed equally to this work.

Sean R. Stowell and Connie M. Arthur (eds.), *Methods in Transfusion Medicine*, Methods in Molecular Biology, vol. 3053,
https://doi.org/10.1007/978-1-0716-5376-0_22,

execute a range of vital functions to combat pathogens, including pathogen phagocytosis, degranulation, release of antimicrobial peptides and reactive oxygen species (ROS), and the formation of neutrophil extracellular traps (NETs) to directly neutralize or confine pathogens [5–7].

Neutropenic infections are a significant concern for individuals undergoing intensive medical treatments such as chemotherapy or stem cell transplantation [8]. These infections arise due to critically low levels of neutrophils due to an array of underlying infections or manipulations. Typically, a healthy adult's blood contains 1500–7000 neutrophils/mm^3; however, neutropenia is defined as an absolute neutrophil count (ANC) below 1500/mm^3 for non-African Americans or 1200/mm^3 for African Americans [9]. The risk of infection increases significantly when ANC falls below 1000/mm^3 and is considered severe when it drops below 500/mm^3. Chemotherapy, commonly used in treating various cancers, often leads to severe neutropenia, making patients highly susceptible to infections. These infections can have detrimental effects, impacting quality of life and may sometimes lead to fatalities [10, 11].

The treatment of infections related to neutropenia has traditionally relied on broad-spectrum antibiotics, granulocyte colony-stimulating factor (G-CSF) treatments to bolster neutrophil production, or granulocyte transfusion with or without G-CSF therapy (approved by the FDA in 1991, which resulted in much higher yields of granulocytes for transfusion) [12]. Granulocyte transfusions are considered one of the earliest forms of cell therapy, as the use of "buffy coat" preparations to treat neutropenic conditions was first documented in 1934 [13]. To study the biology of neutropenia and subsequent granulocyte transfusion, animal models were developed more than 50 years ago, initially in dogs and later in other mammals, including mice [14, 15]. We have previously established a clinically relevant granulocyte transfusion mouse model and investigated how to improve neutrophil transfusion efficacy during neutropenia [16].

However, antibiotic treatment may not always be effective, and G-CSF therapy may not work until bone marrow recovery occurs. Additionally, it can cause side effects such as bone pain, headaches, fatigue, and nausea [17]. Granulocyte transfusion has been considered for severe cases, aiming to combat life-threatening bacterial and fungal infections [18, 19]. Efforts to enhance the immune defenses of the host through neutrophil infusion have been ongoing for years. Studies have indicated that transfusing granulocyte concentrates, obtained with or without G-CSF enhancement, can benefit neutropenic patients with bacterial or fungal infections [20, 21]. Despite progress in obtaining large quantities of neutrophils from healthy donors stimulated with G-CSF, challenges persist in granulocyte transfusion therapy. These challenges include short ex vivo shelf life; rapid in vivo neutrophil death, leading to the need for multiple transfusions, compounded with the inefficiency of transfused neutrophils recruited to the infection sites; and limited pathogen-killing capabilities, which hinder its widespread clinical use in treating neutropenia-related infections [5, 22].

Having dedicated our efforts to exploring the diverse processes underlying neutrophil death and their regulatory pathways, we recently introduced a novel treatment called CLON-G (caspases–lysosomal membrane permeabilization–oxidant–necroptosis inhibition plus granulocyte colony-stimulating factor) [2, 23]. CLON-G comprises Q-VD-oph (pan-caspase inhibitor) [24], Hsp70 (heat shock protein 70), DFO (deferoxamine), NAC (N-acetylcysteine), Nec-1s (necrostatin-1s), and G-CSF (Granulocyte colony-stimulating factor). Neutrophil spontaneous death is mediated by multiple pathways, including apoptosis, necroptosis, and pyroptosis. Q-VD-oph inhibits neutrophil apoptosis by targeting caspase 1, 3, 8, and 9. Neutrophil necroptosis involves a signaling pathway with RIPK1 and MLKL [25], which is inhibited by Nec-1. Hsp70 and DFO prevent lysosomal membrane permeabilization (LMP), a process that can induce neutrophil apoptosis and pyroptosis [26, 27]. Reactive oxygen species (ROS) play crucial roles in neutrophil death by mediating LMP, apoptosis while inhibiting survival signals [28]. NAC acts as an antioxidant, delaying neutrophil death by reducing ROS accumulation. G-CSF activates neutrophil survival signals and inhibits calpain-induced apoptosis [29]. By simultaneously targeting multiple pathways of neutrophil spontaneous death, CLON-G effectively extends neutrophil lifespan to over 5 days without compromising their functions.

Here, we present a murine *Escherichia coli*-induced neutrophilic acute inflammatory pneumonia model to study the role of neutrophils during acute neutropenic lung infection. We demonstrate that CLON-G-treated neutrophils can equally restore immunity as freshly derived cells fit for granulocyte transfusion to combat infections in neutropenic settings.

2 Materials

2.1 Isolating Neutrophils from Mouse Bone Marrow

1. Percoll (Sigma # GE17–0891-02).
2. 10X HBSS (Gibco # 14185052).
3. 15 mL conical tubes.
4. 50 mL conical tubes.
5. Bovine serum albumin (BSA).
6. EDTA.
7. 1X HBSS with no Ca^{2+}/Mg^{2+}, pH 7.4 (Gibco # 14175095).

8. C57BL/6 donor mice (other strains not listed here can also be used).
9. Surgical instruments for mice.
10. Petri dishes.
11. 1 mL syringe.
12. 26G needle.
13. 40 μm strainer.
14. Histopaque 1119 (Sigma # 11191).
15. 20% FBS/RPMI.

2.2 Preparation of CLON-G Components

1. Q-VD-oph (Selleck chem # S7311).
2. Dimethyl sulfoxide (DMSO).
3. microcentrifuge tubes.
4. Hsp70 (Abcam # ab78427).
5. DFO (Sigma # D9533).
6. NAC (Sigma # A9165).
7. RPMI 1640.
8. 15 mL conical tube.
9. 0.2 μm filter.
10. Nec-1s (EMD Millipore # 852391-15-2).
11. G-CSF (Amgen # NEUPOGEN).

2.3 CLON-G Treatment of Neutrophils

1. CLON-G components (*see* Subheadings 2.2 or 3.2).
2. RPMI 1640.
3. 20% FBS/RPMI.
4. Isolated neutrophils (*see* Subheading 3.1).
5. Non-tissue culture-treated 24-well plate.
6. 15 mL conical tube.

2.4 Preparation of E. coli Bacteria for Pneumonia Model

1. *E. coli* (ATCC 19138) bacteria.
2. LB agar plate.
3. Sterile bacterial inoculating loop.
4. LB medium.
5. 15 mL round-bottom tube with cap.
6. Microcentrifuge tube.
7. Saline.

2.5 Preparing CPM-Induced Neutropenic Mice

1. 1 mL syringe.
2. 28G needle.
3. Cyclophosphamide (CPM).
4. Saline.

2.6 Neutrophil Transfusion in E. coli-Induced Neutrophilic Pneumonia

1. Ketamine (Covetrus # 148895).
2. Xylazine (Covetrus # 96406).
3. Hair removal cream.
4. Eye lubricant.
5. Surgical drape.
6. Betadine.
7. 70% ethanol.
8. Surgical instruments for mice.
9. Pre-prepared insulin syringe.
10. Surgical suture.
11. Surgical glue (3 M # 1469SB).
12. Bupivacaine (0.125%) (Meitheal # NDC71288-723-52).
13. Isolated neutrophils (*see* Subheadings 3.1 or 3.3).
14. 28G needle.
15. 31G needle.
16. 0.3 mL insulin syringe.
17. 2% FBS/PBS.
18. Isoflurane (optional).

2.7 Assessing Pneumonic Inflammation

1. Lavage fluid (composed of 0.5 mL of 1000 U heparin and 0.5 g of dextrose in PBS).
2. LB agar plates.
3. Anti-Ly6G antibody (BioLegend # 127613).
4. Anti-Ly6C antibody (BioLegend # 128005).
5. Anti-CD45 antibody (BioLegend # 103114).
6. F4/80 antibody (BioLegend # 123118).
7. 10% formalin (Fisher # SF98-4).

3 Methods

3.1 Isolating Neutrophils from Mouse Bone Marrow

1. Mix Percoll stock with 10X HBSS in a 9:1 ratio to prepare the Percoll mixture, which forms the basis for creating the discontinuous gradient.

2. In 15 mL tubes, prepare 10 mL of 76%, 62%, and 52% density 2.4 mL, 3.8 mL, and 4.8 mL of isolation buffer (0.5% BSA, 15 mM EDTA, in 1X HBSS with no Ca^{2+}/Mg^{2+}, pH 7.4), respectively (*see* **Note 1**).
3. Euthanize C57BL/6 mice (or other strains) and aseptically extract femurs and tibias. Subsequent steps should be performed under sterile conditions.
4. Place the bones in a petri dish containing 3 mL of isolation buffer. Use a 1 mL syringe with a 26G needle to flush out the marrow into a 15 mL tube containing 5 mL of isolation buffer.
5. Filter the marrow through a 40 μm strainer and centrifuge at 400× *g* for 5 min at room temperature (RT). Discard the supernatant and resuspend the pellet in 1 mL of isolation buffer.
6. In a 15 mL tube, layer 2 mL each of 76%, 62%, and 52% Percoll mixtures in the respective order. Place the 1 mL bone marrow cells on top and centrifuge at 1060× *g* for 30 min at RT, with acceleration and breaks set at 3. Repeat for each mouse (*see* **Note 2**).
7. Harvest the lowest (3rd) ring (containing neutrophils) between the 76% and 62% interface. Wash with 5 mL of isolation buffer at 500× *g* for 6 min at RT. Discard the supernatant and resuspend the pellet in 2 mL of isolation buffer (Fig. 1a; *see* **Note 2**).
8. Layer 2 mL of Histopaque-1119 in a 15 mL tube and add the 2 mL neutrophil suspension on top. Centrifuge at 1600× *g* for 30 min at RT, with acceleration and breaks set at 3 to sediment RBCs.
9. Harvest the neutrophils at the interface. Wash with 5 mL of isolation buffer at 500× *g* for 6 min at RT. Discard the supernatant and resuspend the pellet in 20% FBS/RPMI to a concentration of 2 million/mL until ready for use (Fig. 1b).

3.2 Preparation of CLON-G Components

1. Dissolve 50 mg of Q-VD-oph in 973.7 μL of dimethyl sulfoxide (DMSO) to reach a final concentration of 100 mM. Pipette the mixture until clear. Divide into 50 μL aliquots per tube and store at −20 °C.
2. Thaw Hsp70 at 4 °C, centrifuge the vial contents, and dispense into 1 μL aliquots per tube on ice. Store at −80 °C.
3. Dissolve 1 mg of DFO in 7.61 mL of RPMI 1640 to prepare a 200 μM stock solution. Divide into 500 μL aliquots per tube and store at −20 °C.
4. Dissolve 0.1 g of NAC in 2.5 mL of RPMI 1640 in a 15 mL centrifuge tube. Adjust pH to 7–7.4 with NaOH. Add RPMI 1640 to a final volume of 3.06 mL for a 200 mM NAC stock

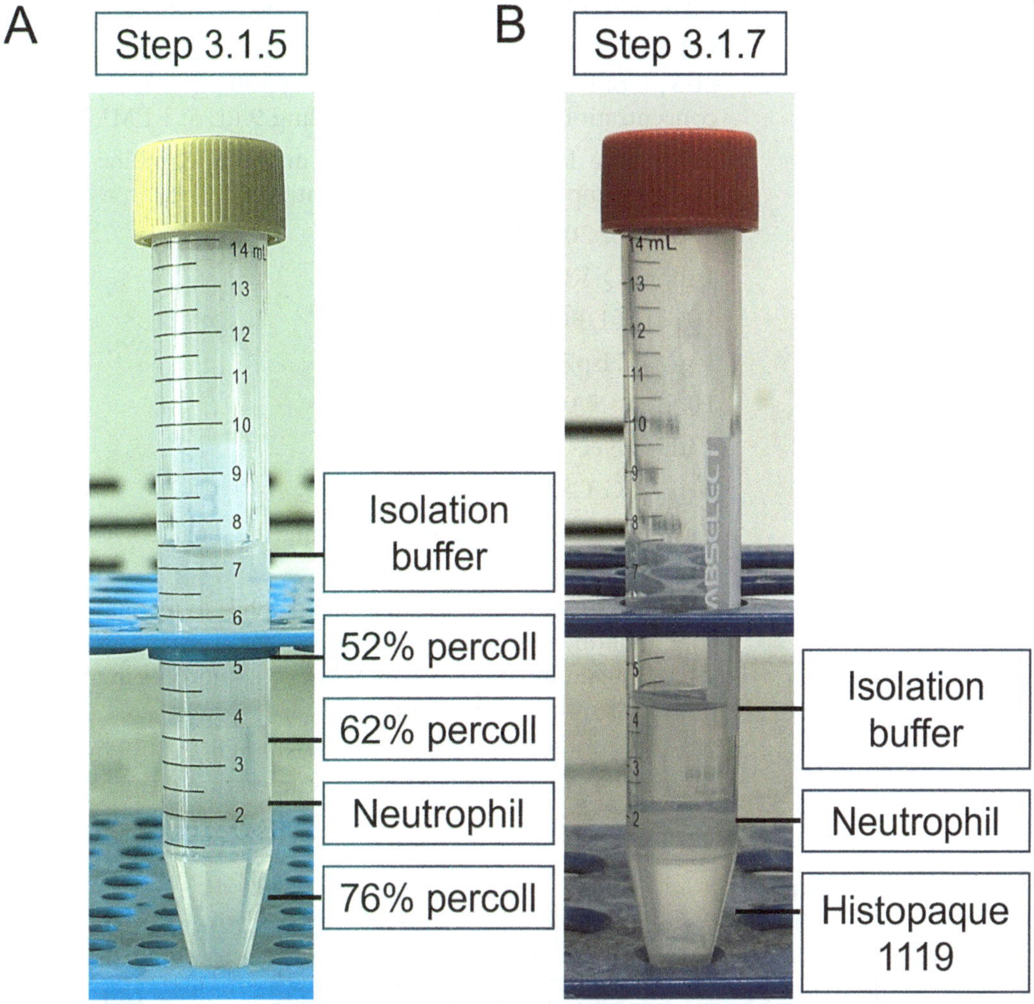

Fig. 1 Schematics of neutrophil isolation. (**a**) Representative results of neutrophil layers after percoll gradient centrifugation. The neutrophils will be in between the 76% and 62% layers. (**b**) After red blood cell sedimentation, neutrophils will be concentrated on the interface of the Histopaque-1119 gradient with the remaining RBCs sedimented on the bottom

solution. Filter with a 0.2 μm filter. Divide into 500 μL aliquots per tube and store at −20 °C (*see* **Note 3**).

5. Dissolve 10 mg of Nec-1s in 1.8 mL of DMSO to achieve a 20 mM concentration. Pipette until clear, divide into 50 μL aliquots per tube, and store at −20 °C, protected from light.
6. Dissolve 250 μg of G-CSF in 1.25 mL of RPMI 1640 to obtain a concentration of 200 μg/mL. Divide into 50 μL aliquots per tube and store at 4 °C.

3.3 CLON-G Treatment of Neutrophils

1. Thaw all CLON-G components from Subheading 3.2 on ice.
2. Dilute 1 μL of Hsp70 to a concentration of 20 μM by adding 606 μL of RPMI 1640. Dilute 1 μL of 200 μg/mL G-CSF to a concentration of 20 μg/mL by adding 9 μL of RPMI 1640.
3. To prepare 1 mL of 2× CLON-G medium, combine the following components in a 15 mL centrifuge tube:

   976 μL of 20% FBS/RPMI

   1 μL of Q-VD-oph (100 mM)

   10 μL of DFO (200 μM)

   1 μL of Hsp70 (20 μM)

   10 μL of NAC (200 mM)

   1 μL of Nec-1s (20 mM)

   1 μL of G-CSF (20 μg/mL).

   Ensure thorough mixing to obtain the final 2× CLON-G medium.
4. Mix 2× CLON-G with isolated neutrophils to a concentration of 1 million/mL and culture in a non-tissue culture-treated 24-well plate for up to 3 days without compromising neutrophilic inflammatory functions (Fig. 2).
5. Harvest cultured neutrophils and wash them in PBS by centrifuging at 4 °C for 5 min at room temperature 3 times.

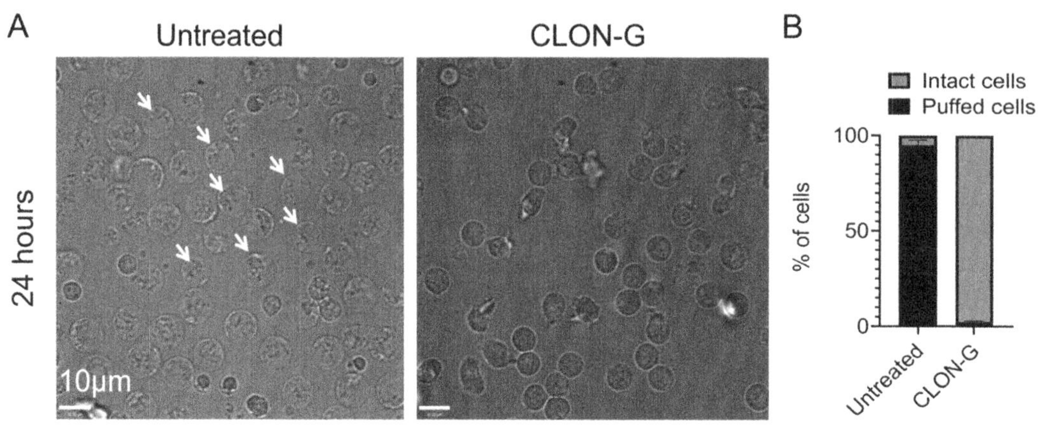

Fig. 2 CLON-G treated neutrophils exhibited a prolonged life span. (**a**) Representative morphological photographs of neutrophils cultured for 24 h. Isolated mouse bone marrow neutrophils were cultured with or without CLON-G-included medium for 24 h and imaged with a 60× light microscope. White arrows indicate puffed cells, which are an indicator of neutrophil cell death. Scale bar = 10 μm. (**b**) Quantification of intact and puffed cell frequency for untreated (UT) and CLON-G treated neutrophils at 24 h of culture. Data were presented as means ± S.D. Puffed cells and intact cells were defined in Am J Hematol. 2017 Aug;92 (8):E156–E159. https:/doi.org/10.1002/ajh.24764. Epub 2017 Jun 9

3.4 Preparation of E. coli Bacteria for the Pneumonia Model

To evaluate the effect of granulocyte transfusion, we utilized an *E. coli* bacterial-induced acute pneumonia model.

1. *E. coli* (ATCC 19138) bacteria are plated using quadrant streaking on an LB agar plate containing no antibiotics and allowed to grow overnight (~16 to 24 h) at 37 °C, two nights prior to the experiment.
2. Single colonies are selected and grown in LB medium overnight (~16 to 24 h) at 37 °C with agitation at approximately 200 rpm.
3. The bacteria are then washed twice with saline at >8000× *g* for 3 min each and resuspended in 1 mL of saline.
4. The bacterial optical density at 600 nm (O.D. 600) is measured, with the calculation of (1 O.D. = 1 × 10^9 CFU), and adjusted to a concentration of 5 × 10^3 CFU/50 μL (1 × 10^5 CFU/mL) in saline. (The same procedure can be followed for other bacteria or stimuli.)
5. Plate the bacteria on an LB agar plate and culture overnight to ensure accuracy of the injected dose.

3.5 Preparing CPM-Induced Neutropenic Mice

1. Mice are treated intraperitoneally with the first dose of 150 mg/kg body weight of cyclophosphamide (CPM) on day 0 and a second dose of 100 mg/kg body weight of CPM on day 3 in a final volume of 500 μL sterile 0.9% saline/dose to deplete neutrophil numbers in mice [30] (*see* **Note 4** and Fig. 3).
2. Other methods such as irradiation or antibody-based depletion can be used as well (*see* **Note 5**).
3. 24 h after the second dose of neutrophil depletion, the mice will be neutropenic and ready for the following experimental procedures.

3.6 Neutrophil Transfusion in E. coli-Induced Neutrophilic Pneumonia

1. Anesthetize the mice using a combination of 100–120 mg/kg ketamine and 10 mg/kg xylazine via intraperitoneal injection (*see* **Note 6**).
2. Once the animal is under anesthesia, remove the hair in the neck region using a hair removal cream and apply eye lubricant to prevent eye dryness (Fig. 4a).
3. After ensuring the mouse is fully anesthetized and unresponsive to toe pinching, place it on a surgical drape. Sterilize the exposed neck region by applying betadine and 70% ethanol 3 times (Fig. 4b).
4. Make a vertical incision in the neck region of the skin (*see* **Note 7**). Identify the line between the sternohyoid/sternothyroid

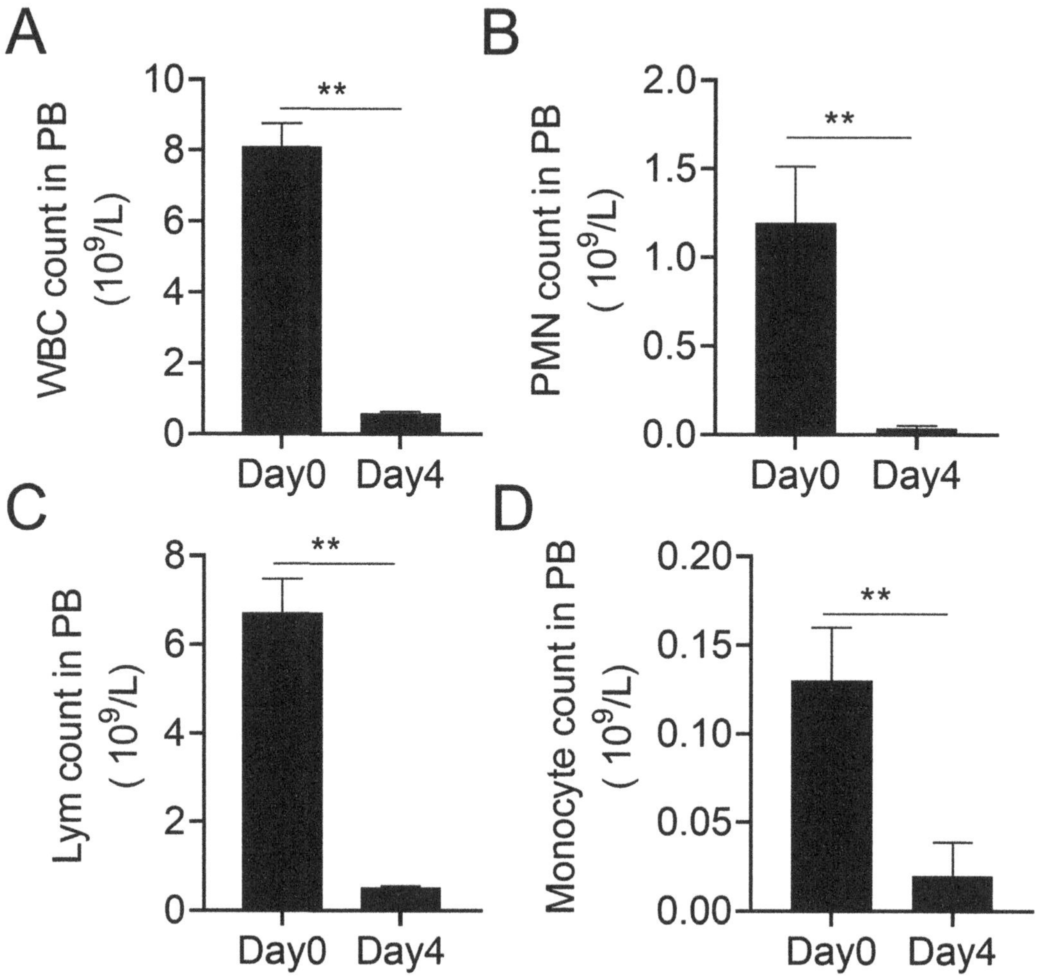

Fig. 3 Cyclophosphamide (CPM) treatment depleted white blood cell counts in the mice's peripheral blood. Peripheral blood of mice after the second CPM treatment was collected and assayed with an automatic blood cell counter. (**a**) White blood cell, (**b**) neutrophil, (**c**) lymphocyte, and (**d**) monocyte counts in the peripheral blood of cyclophosphamide-treated mice significantly declined 18 h post the second injection of cyclophosphamide compared to normal untreated mice. Data were presented as means ± S.D. $^{**}P < 0.05$, $n = 5$

muscles and gently separate them to expose the trachea (*see* **Note 8**).

5. Using a pre-prepared insulin syringe, inject 50 μL of liquid followed by 50 μL of air (Fig. 4c, d; *see* **Note 9**).
6. Securely tie one suture to close the separated muscle.
7. Bring the skin on both sides of the incision together to create a raised area. Apply a drop of glue directly on the incision and hold the skin until the glue dries (Fig. 4e).
8. Administer 100 μL of Bupivacaine (0.125%) subcutaneously, evenly distributed near the surgical site where the hair was removed (*see* **Note 10**).

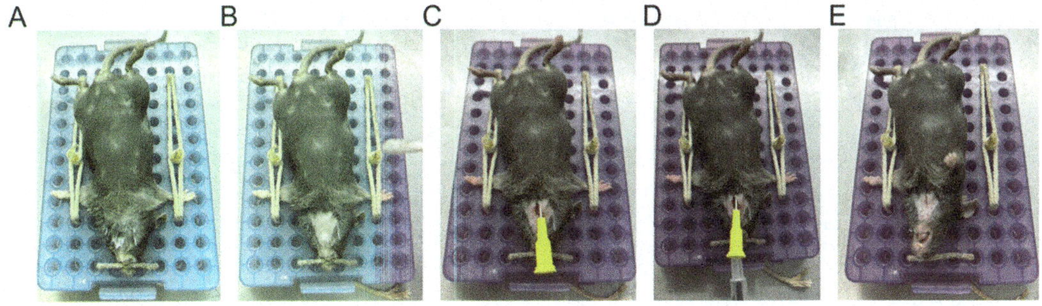

Fig. 4 Representative key steps of the pneumonia induction via intratracheal injection in mice surgical procedure. (**a**) An anesthetized mouse was restrained, and hair removal cream was applied to the neck region. (**b**) Hair was removed by swabbing the neck region followed by regional sterilization with an outward motion beginning at the center. (**c**) An intravenous catheter was placed inside the trachea of the mouse, and then the inner needle was retracted. (**d**) 50 μL of solution containing *E. coli* was intrathecally injected into the mouse. (**e**) The intravenous catheter was removed and the wound was closed with the mouse restraint loosened on one side to allow efficient entry of injected liquid into the lung

9. The mice should regain consciousness within 1–2 h.
10. 5 h post-pneumonia induction; 2~5 million isolated neutrophils (from Subheadings 3.1 or 3.3) can be injected. Retro-orbitally with a 31G needle attached to a 0.3 mL insulin syringe in 100 ~ 300 μL of 2% FBS/PBS (*see* **Note 11**). Take caution not to disrupt the surgical site. Low levels of isoflurane through a nose cone can be used to help sedate the mouse.

3.7 Assessing Pneumonic Inflammation

Acute *E. coli*-induced pneumonic inflammation typically fully resolves within 5 days. In addition to monitoring clinical scores, various quantitative methods can assess inflammation, tissue damage, and neutrophil recruitment in the lungs.

1. Collect bronchoalveolar lavage fluid (BALF) by lavaging the lungs four times with 0.8 mL of lavage fluid (composed of 0.5 mL of 1000 U heparin and 0.5 g of dextrose in PBS), yielding a total of 3.2 mL of fluid (*see* **Note 12**).
2. Centrifuge the BALF at 300× *g* to collect cell pellets for cell quantification and store the supernatant at −80 °C for protein and cytokine measurements.
3. Assessing transfused neutrophil recruitment to the lung by harvesting BALF at 12 h post-transfusion and staining with Ly6G (a neutrophil-specific marker) (Fig. 5a, b).
4. Plate the BALF on LB agar plates with 10^{-1} to 10^{-4} dilution with PBS to assess bacterial load in the BALF as an indicator of host immunity (Fig. 5c, d).
5. Stain the cell pellet with a cocktail of antibodies including Ly6G, Ly6C, CD45, and F4–80 to assess total white blood cell count ($CD45^+$), neutrophil count ($CD45^+/Ly6G^+/$

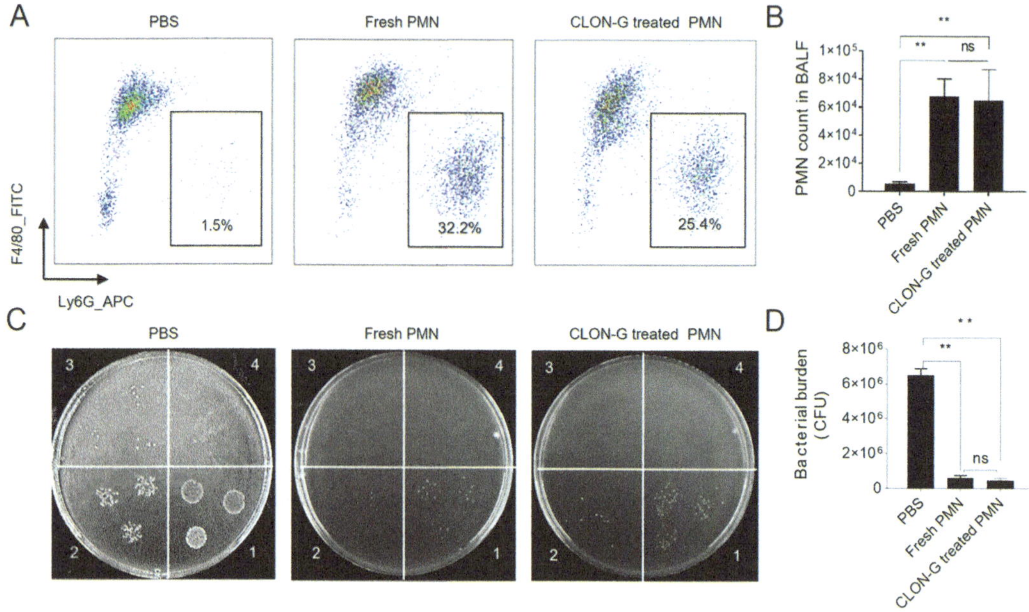

Fig. 5 Representative results of neutrophil transfusion enhancing host immunity toward bacteria clearance. (**a**) Bronchoalveolar lavage fluid (BALF) of transfused mice was collected 12 h post-neutrophil transfusion to assess the effect of neutrophil recruitment after transfusion. Collected BALF was analyzed by Fluorescence-Activated Cell Sorting (FACS) (Ly6G, neutrophil-specific marker; F4/80, macrophage marker). Shown are representative FACS graphs of BALF cells from pneumonic mice with indicated groups. (**b**) Quantification of recruited neutrophil counts in the BALF of infected mice. (**c**) BALF of transfused mice were collected 24 h post-transfusion to assess the effect of neutrophil-mediated bacterial killing. (**a**) Collected BALF was spread on LB plates and cultured overnight to quantify the bacterial load. Representative cultured *E. coli* plates of BALF from transfused mice. Numbers indicated fold dilution (factor of 10) from the original BALF. (**d**) Quantification of Colony Forming Unit (CFU) in the BALF of pneumonic mice with respective treatments. Data were presented as means ± S.D. $^{**}P < 0.05$. $n = 5$. (Adapted from 2021 Jul 28;13(604):eabb1069. © Science Translational Medicine)

Ly6C$^+$), monocyte count (CD45$^+$/Ly6C$^+$), and macrophage count (CD45$^+$/F4–80$^+$) in the alveolar space of the pneumonic mice, providing a measure of inflammation severity (*see* **Note 13**).

6. Additionally, one may harvest whole lungs, fix them in 10% formalin overnight, and section them for histological examination.

4 Notes

1. These volumes are designed for 4 mice, which should be adjusted proportionally.
2. It is crucial that the Percoll gradient for neutrophil purification is freshly prepared with the correct pH and gentle layering, as it

significantly impacts yield and purity. Refer to our previous work [31] for a detailed protocol on neutrophil purification. When removing the gradient, it is advised to aspirate the first two layers first before removing the neutrophil layer to prevent contamination of other cells.

3. The prepared NAC solution should be used within 1 month due to its antioxidant nature, as it rapidly loses potency if kept for prolonged periods of time.
4. Resuspend CPM stock to a concentration of 20 mg/mL and administer at an appropriate volume based on mouse weight.
5. Neutrophils can be depleted using irradiation or α-Ly6G/α-Gr1 antibodies [32–34]. We opted for a CPM-induced neutropenic induction to recapitulate a clinically relevant and consistent phenomenon of patients undergoing chemotherapy who often have hematopoietic defects, including neutropenia.
6. Lean towards a lighter anesthetic dose for neutropenic mice, as they are more sensitive to anesthetics, which could potentially lead to mortality.
7. Use a surgical light to enhance visibility in the surgical area. (Wrap foil around the light source for adjustments if necessary).
8. Apply pressure with swabs if bleeding occurs during surgery until it ceases (~15 s).
9. Inject 50 μL of air before the liquid in the same syringe and administer the injection on mouse inhalation (the chest will rise).
10. Keep the head of the mouse elevated after intratracheal injection to aid liquid entry into the lungs and prevent subsequent choking, which may expel the liquid.
11. During neutrophil transfusion, it is imperative that the cells are placed in 2% FBS/buffer to protect the neutrophils from cell death and damage and at concentrations lower than 5×10^6/300 μL to prevent aggregation in a volume under 300 μL. Additionally, please keep the cells on ice until ready to use and minimize the time the cells are placed on ice. While injecting into the supraorbital vein, scruff the mice in a manner to expose the eye and maintain a moderate but steady rate of injection to prevent leakage and an increased burden on the heart.
12. In the case of excessive red blood cells (RBC) in BALF due to severe inflammation, perform RBC lysis with ACK lysis buffer before cell quantification.
13. Employ Fc blocking before staining to mitigate nonspecific binding [35].

Conflicts of Interest

The authors have no conflicts of interest to declare that are relevant to the content of this chapter.

References

1. Rosales C (2018) Neutrophil: a cell with many roles in inflammation or several cell types? Front Physiol 9:113. https://doi.org/10.3389/fphys.2018.00113
2. Luo HR, Loison F (2008) Constitutive neutrophil apoptosis: mechanisms and regulation. Am J Hematol 83:288–295. https://doi.org/10.1002/ajh.21078
3. Grieshaber-Bouyer R et al (2021) The neutrotime transcriptional signature defines a single continuum of neutrophils across biological compartments. Nat Commun 12:2856. https://doi.org/10.1038/s41467-021-22973-9
4. Hidalgo A, Chilvers ER, Summers C, Koenderman L (2019) The neutrophil life cycle. Trends Immunol 40:584–597. https://doi.org/10.1016/j.it.2019.04.013
5. Kolaczkowska E, Kubes P (2013) Neutrophil recruitment and function in health and inflammation. Nat Rev Immunol 13:159–175. https://doi.org/nri3399. [pii] 10.1038/nri3399
6. Ley K et al (2018) Neutrophils: new insights and open questions. Sci Immunol 3. https://doi.org/10.1126/sciimmunol.aat4579
7. Burn GL, Foti A, Marsman G, Patel DF, Zychlinsky A (2021) The neutrophil. Immunity 54:1377–1391. https://doi.org/10.1016/j.immuni.2021.06.006
8. Viscoli C, Varnier O, Machetti M (2005) Infections in patients with febrile neutropenia: epidemiology, microbiology, and risk stratification. Clin Infect Dis 40(Suppl 4):S240–S245. https://doi.org/10.1086/427329
9. Leung AN et al (1999) Pulmonary infections after bone marrow transplantation: clinical and radiographic findings. Radiology 210:699–710. https://doi.org/10.1148/radiology.210.3.r99mr39699
10. Cameron D (2009) Management of chemotherapy-associated febrile neutropenia. Br J Cancer 101(Suppl 1):S18–S22. https://doi.org/10.1038/sj.bjc.6605272
11. Blayney DW, Schwartzberg L (2022) Chemotherapy-induced neutropenia and emerging agents for prevention and treatment: a review. Cancer Treat Rev 109:102427. https://doi.org/10.1016/j.ctrv.2022.102427
12. Bensinger WI et al (1993) The effects of daily recombinant human granulocyte colony-stimulating factor administration on normal granulocyte donors undergoing leukapheresis. Blood 81:1883–1888
13. Gea-Banacloche J (2017) Granulocyte transfusions: a concise review for practitioners. Cytotherapy 19:1256–1269. https://doi.org/10.1016/j.jcyt.2017.08.012
14. Epstein RB, Zander AR (1977) Granulocyte transfusions in leukopenic dogs. Prog Clin Biol Res 13:227–241
15. Dale DC, Reynolds HY, Pennington JE, Elin RJ, Herzig GP (1976) Experimental pseudomonas pneumonia in leukopenic dogs: comparison of therapy with antibiotics and granulocyte transfusions. Blood 47:869–876
16. Li Y et al (2011) Pretreatment with phosphatase and tensin homolog deleted on chromosome 10 (PTEN) inhibitor SF1670 augments the efficacy of granulocyte transfusion in a clinically relevant mouse model. Blood 117:6702–6713. https://doi.org/10.1182/blood-2010-09-309864
17. Anderlini P, Przepiorka D, Champlin R, Korbling M (1996) Biologic and clinical effects of granulocyte colony-stimulating factor in normal individuals. Blood 88:2819–2825
18. Hubel K, Dale DC, Liles WC (2001) Granulocyte transfusion therapy: update on potential clinical applications. Curr Opin Hematol 8:161–164. https://doi.org/10.1097/00062752-200105000-00006
19. Price TH (2007) Granulocyte transfusion: current status. Semin Hematol 44:15–23. https://doi.org/10.1053/j.seminhematol.2006.09.015
20. Herzig RH, Herzig GP, Graw RG Jr, Bull MI, Ray KK (1977) Successful granulocyte transfusion therapy for gram-negative septicemia. A prospectively randomized controlled study. N Engl J Med 296:701–705. https://doi.org/10.1056/NEJM197703312961301
21. Vogler WR, Winton EF (1977) A controlled study of the efficacy of granulocyte transfusions in patients with neutropenia. Am J Med 63:

548–555. https://doi.org/10.1016/0002-9343(77)90200-5

22. Lahoz-Beneytez J et al (2016) Human neutrophil kinetics: modeling of stable isotope labeling data supports short blood neutrophil half-lives. Blood 127:3431–3438. https://doi.org/10.1182/blood-2016-03-700336
23. Fan Y et al (2021) Targeting multiple cell death pathways extends the shelf life and preserves the function of human and mouse neutrophils for transfusion. Sci Transl Med 13. https://doi.org/10.1126/scitranslmed.abb1069
24. Caserta TM, Smith AN, Gultice AD, Reedy MA, Brown TL (2003) Q-VD-OPh, a broad spectrum caspase inhibitor with potent antiapoptotic properties. Apoptosis 8:345–352. https://doi.org/10.1023/a:1024116916932
25. Wang X, Yousefi S, Simon HU (2018) Necroptosis and neutrophil-associated disorders. Cell Death Dis 9:111. https://doi.org/10.1038/s41419-017-0058-8
26. Loison F et al (2014) Proteinase 3-dependent caspase-3 cleavage modulates neutrophil death and inflammation. J Clin Invest 124:4445–4458. https://doi.org/10.1172/JCI76246
27. Kambara H et al (2018) Gasdermin D exerts anti-inflammatory effects by promoting neutrophil death. Cell Rep 22:2924–2936. https://doi.org/10.1016/j.celrep.2018.02.067
28. Xu Y, Loison F, Luo HR (2010) Neutrophil spontaneous death is mediated by down-regulation of autocrine signaling through GPCR, PI3Kgamma, ROS, and actin. Proc Natl Acad Sci USA 107:2950–2955. https://doi.org/10.1073/pnas.0912717107
29. van Raam BJ, Drewniak A, Groenewold V, van den Berg TK, Kuijpers TW (2008) Granulocyte colony-stimulating factor delays neutrophil apoptosis by inhibition of calpains upstream of caspase-3. Blood 112:2046–2054. https://doi.org/10.1182/blood-2008-04-149575
30. Zuluaga AF et al (2006) Neutropenia induced in outbred mice by a simplified low-dose cyclophosphamide regimen: characterization and applicability to diverse experimental models of infectious diseases. BMC Infect Dis 6:55. https://doi.org/10.1186/1471-2334-6-55
31. Fan Y et al (2023) Neutrophil lifespan extension with CLON-G and an in vitro spontaneous death assay. J Vis Exp. https://doi.org/10.3791/65132
32. Boivin G et al (2020) Durable and controlled depletion of neutrophils in mice. Nat Commun 11:2762. https://doi.org/10.1038/s41467-020-16596-9
33. Olofsen PA et al (2022) Effective, long-term, neutrophil depletion using a murinized anti-Ly-6G 1A8 antibody. Cells 11. https://doi.org/10.3390/cells11213406
34. Bogman MJ, Cornelissen IM, Berden JH, De Jong J, Koene RA (1984) A comparative study of total body irradiation as a method of inducing granulocyte depletion in mice. J Immunol Methods 70:31–38. https://doi.org/10.1016/0022-1759(84)90386-7
35. Andersen MN, Al-Karradi SN, Kragstrup TW, Hokland M (2016) Elimination of erroneous results in flow cytometry caused by antibody binding to Fc receptors on human monocytes and macrophages. Cytometry A 89:1001–1009. https://doi.org/10.1002/cyto.a.22995

Chapter 23

Mouse Models of Transfusion-Related Acute Lung Injury (TRALI)

Simon J. Cleary, Yurim Seo, and Mark R. Looney

Abstract

Transfusion-related acute lung injury (TRALI) is a serious hazard of blood transfusions typically caused by recipient-reactive antibodies in blood products. To model TRALI, we have used MHC class I antibody injections to trigger acute lung injury in mice. Studies using this approach have provided mechanistic insights into TRALI risk factors and pathogenesis. Beyond TRALI, the ability to rapidly provoke acute lung injury with a non-infectious causal agent has also been useful for studying antibody effector mechanisms, inflammatory platelet responses, neutrophil extracellular trap formation, and acute respiratory distress syndrome (ARDS) pathophysiology. Here, we provide a brief overview of mouse TRALI models, a protocol for inducing experimental TRALI, and key considerations for successful experiments.

Key words Transfusion, TRALI, Acute lung injury, ARDS, Alloantibody, Antibody, MHC, Mouse models

1 Introduction

Transfusion-related acute lung injury (TRALI) is a potentially lethal transfusion reaction involving the onset of the acute respiratory distress syndrome (ARDS) during or within 6 h of a transfusion without an apparent alternative cause [1]. Recipient-reactive alloantibodies have been identified as causal agents of TRALI through the analysis of case-associated blood products [2, 3], reduced incidence of TRALI following adoption of a male donor preference for plasma-rich blood products (an intervention that reduced the quantities of alloantibodies given in transfusions) [4–6], and animal studies [7].

Sean R. Stowell and Connie M. Arthur (eds.), *Methods in Transfusion Medicine*, Methods in Molecular Biology, vol. 3053, https://doi.org/10.1007/978-1-0716-5376-0_23,

We have developed mouse models of antibody-mediated TRALI triggered by intravenous injections containing MHC class I antibodies [8–10]. One mouse monoclonal MHC class I antibody, clone 34-1-2S has displayed unique potency at inducing injury in mice expressing multiple cognate antigens [8, 10–12], reflecting clinical findings that only HLA antibodies with particularly strong recipient reactivity are suspected of causing TRALI [13]. Also mirroring findings from human studies linking pre-existing inflammation in transfusion recipients to increased TRALI risk [3, 6, 14], immunologically naïve laboratory mice typically require 'immune priming' for susceptibility to antibody-mediated injury. In our model, intraperitoneal injections containing bacterial LPS are used to prime mice one day before antibody injections [3, 9].

Mouse models using the 34-1-2S antibody have enabled delineation of TRALI pathogenesis. In susceptible recipient mice, intravenously injected 34-1-2S antibody binds to the pulmonary endothelium at sufficient densities to engage in Fc:Fc interactions that trigger excessive complement activation in the lungs [10–12]. This initiating event triggers retention of platelets, neutrophils, and other leukocytes in the lungs, which together release granule contents, reactive oxygen species, and extracellular traps. These responses cause impaired lung microvascular perfusion as well as inflammatory injury to the pulmonary endothelium and a striking pulmonary edema response [8, 9, 15, 16]. Similar mechanisms appear to drive other models of antibody-mediated TRALI using antibodies targeting other MHC antigens, HNA-2 (CD177), HNA-3 (SLC44A2), or CD36 [11, 17–19]. Molecular mediators of non-antibody-mediated TRALI have also been identified in rat and mouse models using "storage lesion"-affected red blood cells and platelets [20–23].

Beyond modeling TRALI, mouse studies involving the use of the 34-1-2S antibody have also become widely used to investigate mechanisms of acute lung inflammation and injury. For example, the rapid onset inflammation in this model has been useful for improving our understanding of platelet-leukocyte interactions [15, 16], circadian rhythmicity in neutrophil responsiveness [24], and mediators suppressing immune responses [25, 26]. Additionally, similarities between antibody-mediated rejection (AbMR) pathogenesis and the mechanisms driving injury in TRALI models mean that models developed for studying TRALI might also be useful for non-surgical studies of mechanisms leading to AbMR in lung transplantation [10, 12].

Here, we describe techniques that we have found useful for modeling TRALI in mice. We provide instructions for approaches enabling precise intravenous injections and notes on determinants of susceptibility that can confound interpretation of experiments if not considered during study design.

2 Materials

2.1 LPS Priming

1. Male BALB/c mice aged 8–16 weeks (Charles River Cat# 028), housed locally for at least 2 weeks (*see* **Notes 1–5**).
2. Balance suitable for mouse body weight measurements (Fisher Cat# S94792F).
3. Sterile phosphate-buffered saline (PBS) (Gibco Cat# 14190).
4. Lipopolysaccharides (LPS) from *Escherichia coli* O55:B5 (Sigma-Aldrich Cat# L2880), reconstituted at 1 mg/mL in PBS and stored in aliquots at −80 °C.
5. Insulin syringes (BD Cat# 329461).

2.2 Anesthesia and Perioperative Care

1. Ketamine hydrochloride 100 mg/mL solution (Zoetis NDC# 54771-2013-1) (*see* **Note 6**).
2. Xylazine 100 mg/mL solution (Akorn NDC# 59399-111-50).
3. Sterile saline (0.9% sodium chloride) solution (Hospira NDC# 00409-4888-20).
4. Insulin syringes (BD Cat# 329461).
5. Thermal support system with heating pad (C2dx Cat# TP700 and Cat# 8002-062-022).
6. Petrolatum eye ointment (Dechra NDC# 17033-211-38).
7. Bupivacaine hydrochloride 0.5% solution (SteriMax Cat# ST-BX113).

2.3 Intravenous Injection

1. Anti-MHC class I clone 34-1-2S (BioXCell Cat# BE0180) and a suitable non-reactive mouse IgG2a isotype control (BioXCell Cat# BE0085) (*see* **Note 7**).
2. Sterile 0.9% sodium chloride (saline) solution (Hospira NDC# 00409–4888-20).
3. A line for jugular injections assembled from a 30G × 1-inch needle (from Covidien Cat# 8881401072), inserted into PE-10 tubing (BD Cat# 427401), inserted into 3 Fr

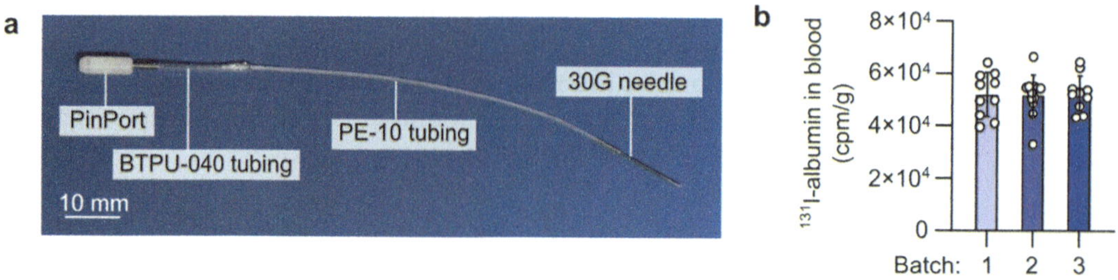

Fig. 1 Precise intravenous injections in anesthetized mice. (**a**) An intravenous catheter assembled from a 22G PinPort™, BTPU-040 tubing, PE-10 tubing, and a 30G 1-inch needle. (**b**) Example data showing consistent levels of i.v. injected ^{131}I-albumin in blood 2 h after injection in 3 batches of mice, with each batch containing mice assigned to groups developing different levels of acute lung injury. Graphs show means and standard errors, batch $n = 10$–11

polyurethane tubing (Instech Cat# BTPU-040), and secured with cyanoacrylate glue, connected to a 22G PinPort (Instech Cat# PNP3F22) (Fig. 1).

4. Ethanol (70% v/v in diH_2O) and sterile water for cleaning the injection line (*see* **Note 8**).
5. Blunted 27G insulin syringes for antibody injections and saline flushes through PinPorts (BD Cat# 329412) (Fig. 1).
6. Paper surgical tape (AMD Ritmed Cat# A5110).
7. Antiseptic swabs pre-saturated with 3.15% (w/v) chlorhexidine gluconate and 70% (v/v) isopropyl alcohol (PDI Healthcare Cat# B10800).
8. Scissors (FST Cat# 14019-13).
9. Curved forceps (FST Cat# 11052-10).
10. Cannulation forceps (World Precision Instruments Cat# 504765).
11. Dissecting microscope and light source.
12. Sterile cotton swab (Henry Schein Cat# 100-9249).
13. Needle holders (FST Cat# 12501-13).
14. Suture, 5-0 with needle (Henry Schein Cat# 101-4148).

3 Methods

3.1 LPS Priming

1. Record body weights of mice.
2. Thaw an aliquot of 1 mg/mL LPS stock in PBS and make a 1: 10 dilution in PBS (e.g., 50 μL LPS stock in 450 μL PBS for 0.1 mg/mL).

3. Load an appropriate volume of the 0.1 mg/mL LPS dilution to yield 0.1 mg/kg body weight (μL dilution = g body weight) into numbered tubes containing 100 μL of PBS.
4. Inject LPS i.p. into mice.

3.2 Anesthesia and Perioperative Care

1. One day after LPS priming, re-weigh mice and anesthetize mice with i.p. injections of 60 mg/kg ketamine and 40 mg/kg xylazine (*see* **Note 6**).
2. Apply eye ointment once mice are immobile and wait 10–15 min for onset of anesthesia.
3. Check for absence of pedal reflex to confirm depth of anesthesia sufficient for surgery. An additional dose of 40 mg/kg ketamine can be given i.p. if necessary.
4. When anesthesia is sufficient, place the mouse in a supine position under the microscope, securing forelimbs with tape.

3.3 Intravenous Injections

1. Prepare injection line (Fig. 1a).
2. One day after LPS priming, re-weigh mice and prepare antibody dilutions in 2 mL tubes so that 150 μL contains the desired dose of antibody (*see* **Note** 7), with 20% excess volume (180 μL) to enable uptake of dose into syringes without introduction of air bubbles (*see* **Note 8**).
3. Use an antiseptic swab to clean the skin and fur overlying the right clavicle of anesthetized mice.
4. Make a small incision (<10 mm) immediately above the right clavicle and gently move muscle and connective tissue aside with forceps to expose the right jugular vein at a site just above where it descends into the thoracic cavity.
5. Irrigate exposed tissue with 3 small drops (~50 μL) of bupivacaine local anesthetic.
6. Ensure the injection tubing is full of sterile saline, detach from the syringe and hold the needle on the tubing with cannulation forceps in the dominant hand.
7. Briefly using forceps held in the non-dominant hand to apply gentle pressure onto the clavicle, insert the needle on the injection tubing into the jugular vein.
8. Switch the non-dominant hand to anchor the injection line at PinPort, release the needle, and use the dominant hand to insert saline syringe into PinPort.
9. Confirm placement of the needle in the vein by injecting a small volume of sterile saline, looking down the microscope to observe entry of saline into the bloodstream, visible as "puffs" of diluted blood (Fig. 1b; also *see* **Notes 9** and **10**).

10. Remove the saline syringe from PinPort and insert the syringe containing the antibody solution.
11. Watching a timer, inject antibody solution over the course of 1 min, recording the time of injection.
12. Flush residual antibody solution through the line into the vein with saline.
13. Use a cotton swab to apply pressure to tissue overlying the vein while removing the needle from the vein.
14. Leave the cotton swab in place for 2–3 min to allow time for hemostasis.
15. Close skin incision with 1 or 2 interrupted sutures.
16. Place animals in a prone position in a cage with heating support and monitor closely.

3.4 Sample Collection and Useful Readouts

1. Key events in pathogenesis such as pulmonary endothelial complement C3 and C4 split product deposition and pulmonary platelet sequestration can be measured by fixing lungs at 5 min after antibody injections (Fig. 2c, d) [10].
2. Susceptible mice have reduced blood oxygen saturation within 5 min of 34-1-2S injections, likely initially a result of lung perfusion deficits [12]. This response is worsened by lung vascular permeability that reaches detectable levels at around 10–15 min after antibody injections (*see* **Note 11**). As key endpoints, we typically make absolute measurements of lung vascular permeability and excess lung water by injecting radiolabeled albumin (Iso-Tex Cat# 7731, 0.008 kBq/mouse) together with antibodies (*see* **Note 12**). For these measurements, blood samples and lungs are then collected at either 2 h post-antibody injections (and ~10 min after overdosing mice with 80 mg/kg ketamine and 40 mg/kg xylazine), or after cessation of respiratory movements (*see* **Note 13**), for quantification of radiotracer distribution and water content (Fig. 3a, b).
3. Depending on susceptibility and antibody dose, some mice die within 2 h of antibody injections (Fig. 3c). By carefully monitoring mice and recording the number of minutes elapsed between injections and cessation of respiratory movements, Kaplan-Meier plots can be constructed for survival analysis (*see* **Note 14**).

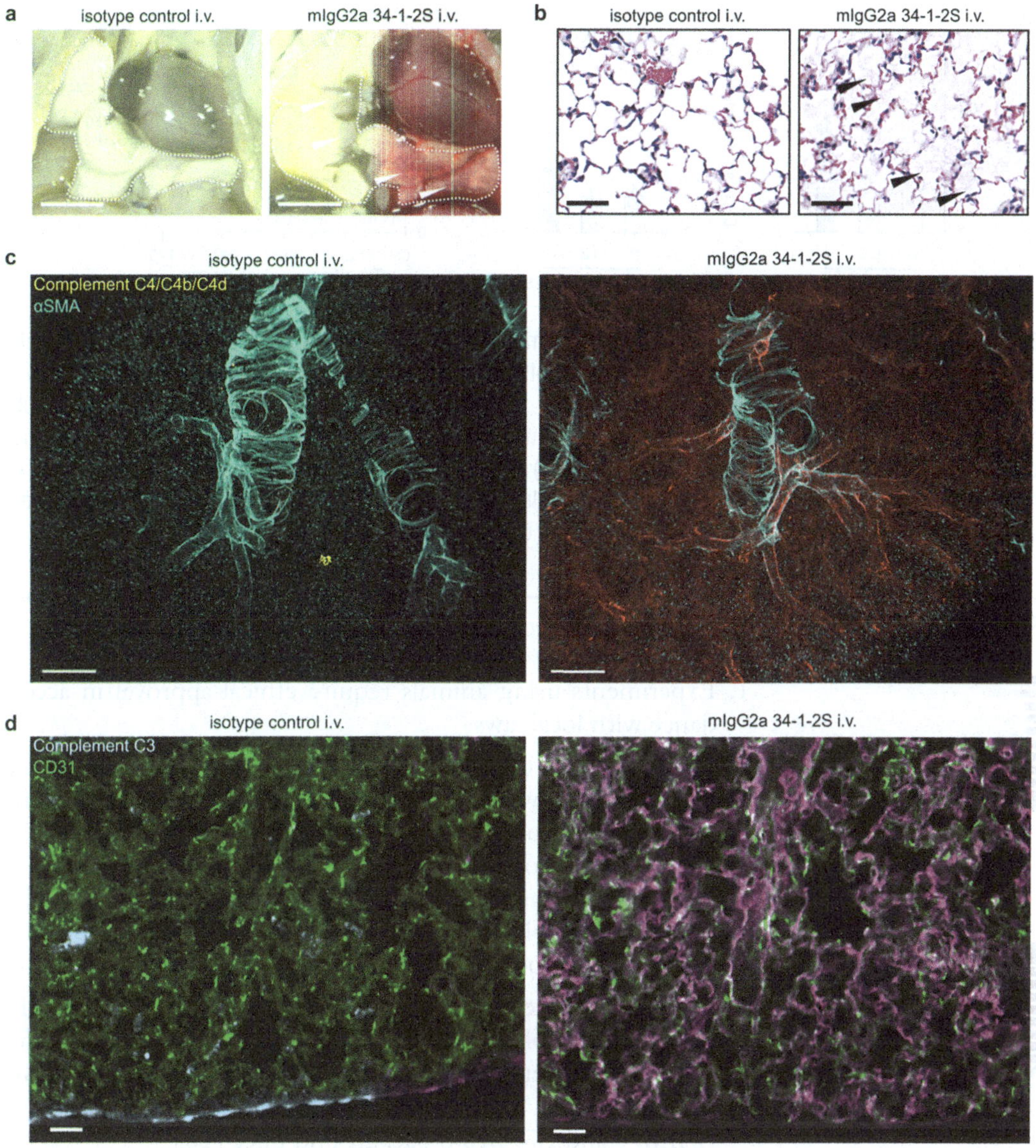

Fig. 2 Experimental TRALI pathology. (**a**) Example gross pathology. Images show lungs in situ after thoracotomy. Lung tissue is outlined with white dotted lines and white arrowheads point to patches of injury. Scale bars: 5 mm. (**b**) Example histopathology. Images show hematoxylin and eosin-stained sections, with black arrowheads pointing to alveolar spaces containing proteinaceous material. Scale bars: 50 μm. (**c**) Immunofluorescence staining for complement C4/C4b/C4d (red) and α-smooth muscle actin (αSMA, cyan) from thick cleared sections of lungs fixed 2 h after antibody injections. Arterioles show strong linear positivity for complement C4 split products after 34-1-2S injections, implicating these vessels as sites of initiation of complement activation. Scale bars: 200 μm. (**d**) Immunofluorescence staining for complement C3 (magenta) and CD31 (green) from thick sections of lungs fixed 5 min after antibody injections. Widespread endothelial complement C3 positivity is seen after 34-1-2S injections. Scale bars: 20 μm. The lungs shown are from LPS-primed B6.*H2*^{d} mice given i.v. injections of mIgG2a 34-1-2S or isotype control. Images are adapted, with permission, from previously published work [10, 12]

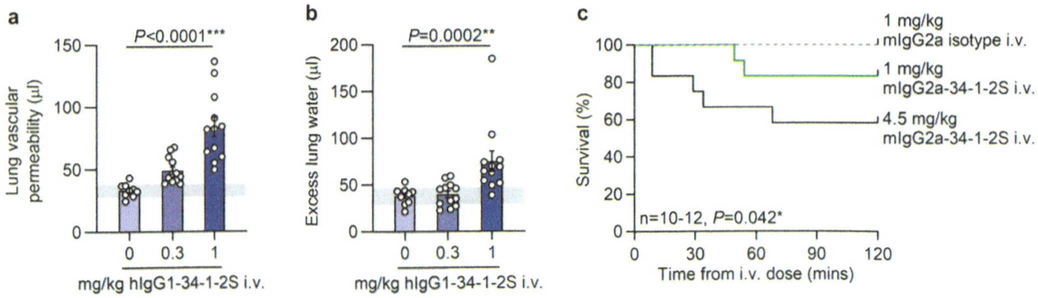

Fig. 3 Dose dependence of acute lung injury and mortality in mouse models of TRALI. (**a**) Lung vascular permeability and (**b**) excess lung water measurements from LPS-primed B6.*H2*^{d} mice given i.v. injections of hIgG1-34-1-2S at indicated doses (mice in group '0' were given 1 mg/kg hIgG1 isotype control i.v.). Graphs show means and standard errors with *P* values for main effects of dose from one-way analysis of variance tests on $\log_{10}$-transformed data, group $n = 9$–12. (**c**) Survival assessment of LPS-primed B6.*H2*^{d} mice given mIgG2a antibody injections as indicated. The *P*-value is from a log-rank (Mantel-Cox) test. (Graphs are adapted, with permission, from previously published datasets [12])

4 Notes

1. Experiments using animals require ethical approval in accordance with local laws.
2. Female mice are not susceptible to 34-1-2S-induced injury, likely due to low levels of complement factors [11]. Housing in specific-pathogen-free facilities appears to render mice relatively resistant to injury caused by 34-1-2S injections, with LPS priming restoring susceptibility [9, 27]. The microbiome and T regulatory lymphocytes appear to exert a powerful suppressive effect in this model [17, 26, 27].
3. As an alternative to BALB/c mice, other mice expressing the H-2^d MHC haplotype are also susceptible and can be useful for studies using genetic modification, including B6.C-*H2*^{d}/bByJ (B6.*H2*^{d}) mice (Jax Cat# 000359) [10] or F1 hybrids of BALB/c and C57BL/6 background mice [28].
4. B6.*H2*^{d} mice can be crossed with the many existing genetically engineered lines on the B6 background to produce B6-congenic mice that express the H-2^d MHC antigens that confer susceptibility within 2 generations, avoiding the 10 or more backcrosses needed to breed a gene carried by B6-background mice to BALB/c congenicity [10]. In our studies, we have bred mice so that they are homozygous carriers of H-2^d antigens.
5. MHC haplotype can be determined by PCR genotyping [29] or by flow cytometry on a small sample of blood leukocytes using antibodies with haplotype specificity, e.g., PE-conjugated anti-H2K^d clone SF1-1.1 (BD Cat# 553566) and FITC-

conjugated anti-H2K^b clone AF6–88.5.5.3 (Thermo Fisher Cat# 11-5958-82). Clone 34-1-2S binds with high affinity to H-2K^d and H-2D^d and with lower affinity to H-2L^d [12, 30]. This antibody also binds with low affinity to H-2K^b expressed by C57BL/6 mice with the H-2^b haplotype but does not readily cause injury in these animals unless they are depleted of T cells and given high doses of 34-1-2S in combination with other antibodies [17]. The hybridoma producing 34-1-2S is available from ATCC (Cat# HB-79), and we have published the sequence of the complementarity determining domains of 34-1-2S to enable recombinant production [12]. Mice with transgenic expression of human FCGR2A have heightened responses to hIgG1-34-1-2S [12, 28].

6. Ketamine is a controlled substance under many jurisdictions, and its use requires appropriate authorization.
7. We use injections containing 1 mg/kg of 34-1-2S in most studies, as this is a subthreshold dose that causes a robust injury response [8, 10, 12] (Fig. 3a, b). For survival analyses of studies with practical group sizes higher than 34-1-2S, doses of 4.5 mg/kg are usually needed (Fig. 3c).
8. Sterilized, pre-assembled injection lines can also be purchased (Instech Cat# C10SS-MTV1826P).
9. Radiolabeled albumin or Evans blue dye can be administered together with antibody injections for measuring vascular permeability.
10. Making injections through a catheter allows confirmation of placement, flushing of 100% of the injected dose into the vein, and a controlled infusion rate (Fig. 1b). Placement can also be confirmed by pulling blood into the tubing, but this can sometimes result in blood clotting and blocking the line. This approach can also be used without surgery by placing the needle in a lateral tail vein. Tail vein injections result in acute lung injury [11], although we have not tested whether using a different injection site alters the extent of pathology.
11. Ketamine/xylazine anesthesia reduces blood oxygen saturation of mice [31], so measurements of gas exchange require provision of supplemental oxygen or alternative anesthetic approaches.
12. We typically make measurements of lung vascular permeability using radiotracers and excess lung water using wet and dry weight ratios of lungs and blood [32] (Fig. 3a, b). Lung vascular permeability can also be measured by injecting Evans blue and quantifying dye absorbance or fluorescence in plasma and extracts of lung homogenates [28, 33] or quantified total protein content of bronchoalveolar lavage fluid [15, 28]. Pulmonary edema has also been measured using lung wet/dry

ratios [27] or imaged using high-definition computed tomography scans [34].

13. Collection of data from mice that do not survive helps to reduce numbers of mice needed for experiments but can increase variance in settings where mice die before substantial pulmonary edema develops (e.g., when giving hFCGR2A transgenic mice injections of hIgG1-34-1-2S) [12].
14. Detection of effects using survival analysis requires high group numbers relative to comparisons of continuous readouts, so mortality should not be the first choice of endpoint for animal studies.

Conflicts of Interest

No other conflicts of interest relevant to this work.

Funding

This study was funded by NIH/NHLBI R35HL161241.

References

1. Vlaar APJ, Toy P, Fung M et al (2019) A consensus redefinition of transfusion-related acute lung injury. Transfusion (Paris) 59: 2465–2476
2. Popovsky MA, Abel MD, Moore SB (1983) Transfusion-related acute lung injury associated with passive transfer of Antileukocyte antibodies. Am Rev Respir Dis 128:185–189
3. Toy P, Gajic O, Bacchetti P et al (2012) Transfusion-related acute lung injury: incidence and risk factors. Blood 119:1757–1767
4. Chapman CE, Stainsby D, Jones H et al (2009) Ten years of hemovigilance reports of transfusion-related acute lung injury in the United Kingdom and the impact of preferential use of male donor plasma. Transfusion (Paris) 49:440–452
5. Toy P, Looney MR, Popovsky M et al (2022) Transfusion-related acute lung injury: 36 years of Progress (1985–2021). Ann Am Thorac Soc 19:705–712
6. Peters AL, Van Stein D, Vlaar APJ (2015) Antibody-mediated transfusion-related acute lung injury; from discovery to prevention. Br J Haematol 170:597–614
7. Looney MR, Matthay MA (2006) Animal models of transfusion-related acute lung injury. Crit Care Med 34:S132
8. Looney MR, Su X, Van Ziffle JA et al (2006) Neutrophils and their Fc gamma receptors are essential in a mouse model of transfusion-related acute lung injury. J Clin Invest 116: 1615–1623
9. Looney MR, Nguyen JX, Hu Y et al (2009) Platelet depletion and aspirin treatment protect mice in a two-event model of transfusion-related acute lung injury. J Clin Invest 119: 3450–3461
10. Cleary SJ, Kwaan N, Tian JJ et al (2020) Complement activation on endothelium initiates antibody-mediated acute lung injury. J Clin Invest 130:5909–5923
11. Strait RT, Hicks W, Barasa N et al (2011) MHC class I-specific antibody binding to non-hematopoietic cells drives complement activation to induce transfusion-related acute lung injury in mice. J Exp Med 208:2525–2544
12. Cleary SJ, Seo Y, Tian JJ et al (2024) IgG hexamers initiate acute lung injury. J Clin Invest 134:178351

13. Kopko PM, Bux J, Toy P (2019) Antibodies associated with TRALI: differences in clinical relevance. Transfusion (Paris) 59:1147–1151
14. Silliman CC (2006) The two-event model of transfusion-related acute lung injury. Crit Care Med 34:S124
15. Hidalgo A, Chang J, Jang J-E et al (2009) Heterotypic interactions enabled by polarized neutrophil microdomains mediate thromboinflammatory injury. Nat Med 15:384–391
16. Caudrillier A, Kessenbrock K, Gilliss BM et al (2012) Platelets induce neutrophil extracellular traps in transfusion-related acute lung injury. J Clin Invest 122:2661–2671
17. Kapur R, Kim M, Aslam R et al (2017) T regulatory cells and dendritic cells protect against transfusion-related acute lung injury via IL-10. Blood 129:2557–2569
18. Bayat B, Nielsen KR, Bein G et al (2021) Transfusion of target antigens to preimmunized recipients: a new mechanism in transfusion-related acute lung injury. Blood Adv 5:3975–3985
19. Bayat B, Tjahjono Y, Sydykov A et al (2013) Anti-human neutrophil antigen-3a induced transfusion-related acute lung injury in mice by direct disturbance of lung endothelial cells. Arterioscler Thromb Vasc Biol 33:2538–2548
20. McVey MJ, Kim M, Tabuchi A et al (2017) Acid sphingomyelinase mediates murine acute lung injury following transfusion of aged platelets. Am J Physiol Lung Cell Mol Physiol 312: L625–L637
21. McVey MJ, Weidenfeld S, Maishan M et al (2021) Platelet extracellular vesicles mediate transfusion-related acute lung injury by imbalancing the sphingolipid rheostat. Blood 137: 690–701
22. Silliman CC, Voelkel NF, Allard JD et al (1998) Plasma and lipids from stored packed red blood cells cause acute lung injury in an animal model. J Clin Invest 101:1458–1467
23. Silliman CC, Bjornsen AJ, Wyman TH et al (2003) Plasma and lipids from stored platelets cause acute lung injury in an animal model. Transfusion (Paris) 43:633–640
24. Adrover JM, Aroca-Crevillén A, Crainiciuc G et al (2020) Programmed 'disarming' of the neutrophil proteome reduces the magnitude of inflammation. Nat Immunol 21:135–144
25. Ortiz-Muñoz G, Mallavia B, Bins A et al (2014) Aspirin-triggered 15-epi-lipoxin A4 regulates neutrophil-platelet aggregation and attenuates acute lung injury in mice. Blood 124:2625–2634
26. He R, Li L, Kong Y et al (2019) Preventing murine transfusion-related acute lung injury by expansion of CD4+ CD25+ FoxP3+ Tregs using IL-2/anti-IL-2 complexes. Transfusion (Paris) 59:534–544
27. Kapur R, Kim M, Rebetz J et al (2018) Gastrointestinal microbiota contributes to the development of murine transfusion-related acute lung injury. Blood Adv 2:1651–1663
28. El Mdawar MB, Maître B, Magnenat S et al (2021) Platelet FcγRIIA-induced serotonin release exacerbates the severity of transfusion-related acute lung injury in mice. Blood Adv 5: 4817–4830
29. Klebs SHG, Hoffmann MW, Musholt PB et al (2003) Detection of H-2 alleles by PCR-RFLP—an alternative to flow cytometry in the screening of transgenic mice. J Immunol Methods 276:197–205
30. Ozato K, Mayer NM, Sachs DH (1982) Monoclonal antibodies to mouse major histocompatibility complex antigens: Iv. A series of hybridoma clones producing anti-H-2d antibodies and an examination of expression of H-2d antigens on the surface of these cells. Transplantation 34:113–120
31. Blevins CE, Celeste NA, Marx JO (2021) Effects of oxygen supplementation on injectable and inhalant anesthesia in C57BL/6 mice. J Am Assoc Lab Anim Sci JAALAS 60:289
32. Lee JS, Su X, Rackley C et al (2011) Priming with endotoxin increases acute lung injury in mice by enhancing the severity of lung endothelial injury. Anat Rec Hoboken NJ 2007 294: 165–172
33. Smith P, Jeffers LA, Koval M (2021) Measurement of lung vessel and epithelial permeability in vivo with Evans Blue. Methods Mol Biol Clifton NJ 2367:137–148
34. Song D, Adrover JM, Felice C et al (2022) PTP1B inhibitors protect against acute lung injury and regulate CXCR4 signaling in neutrophils. JCI Insight 7:e158199

Chapter 24

Methodological Approaches to Study Transfusion-Related Acute Lung Injury (TRALI): From Complement Activation to In Vivo Mouse Model

Farahnaz Rayatdoost and Rick Kapur

Abstract

Transfusion-related acute lung injury (TRALI) is a life-threatening condition, with an increased risk in critically ill patients, characterized by acute non-cardiogenic pulmonary edema occurring within 6 h of blood/blood product transfusion. This chapter provides an overview of comprehensive methodological approaches for studying TRALI, focusing on both in vivo antibody-mediated TRALI and in vitro techniques. Key methodologies covered include assays for measuring the degree of pulmonary edema, bronchoalveolar lavage fluid analysis, neutrophil activation tests, complement system assays, and lung histology and immunohistochemistry. Addressing the challenges of standardizing protocols and replicating human immune responses is crucial for advancing TRALI research and improving diagnostic and therapeutic strategies in transfusion medicine.

Key words Transfusion-related acute lung injury (TRALI), Complement activation, Neutrophil activation, In vivo models, In vitro assays

1 Introduction

Transfusion-related acute lung injury (TRALI) is a critical and life-threatening condition that manifests as acute non-cardiogenic pulmonary edema within 6 h following blood transfusion [1]. TRALI is particularly prevalent in critically ill patients in the intensive care unit. It is categorized into two distinct types: TRALI type I, which occurs without an acute respiratory distress syndrome (ARDS) risk factor, and TRALI type II, which occurs in patients with ARDS risk factors or mild preexisting ARDS [2]. Despite advancements in preventive strategies, TRALI remains a leading cause of transfusion-associated fatalities, without the availability of specific therapies. The pathophysiology has not been fully unraveled, but the underlying clinical condition of the patient (considered as the "first hit") in combination with factors in the transfusion product

Sean R. Stowell and Connie M. Arthur (eds.), *Methods in Transfusion Medicine*, Methods in Molecular Biology, vol. 3053, https://doi.org/10.1007/978-1-0716-5376-0_24,

(considered as the "second hit") is responsible for the initiation of TRALI [1, 3, 4]. The transfusion product may contain antibodies to human leukocyte antigens (HLA) class I or II, or antibodies to human neutrophil antigens (HNA), or non-antibody components such as lipids, which can accumulate during storage of blood products. This is referred to as classical TRALI. Other types of TRALI include TRALI induced by CD36-antibodies (more frequent in the Asian population) [5] and so-called reverse TRALI, in which antibodies are present in the patient and react to the transfusion product, resulting in the development of TRALI [6–8]. Classical TRALI is histopathologically marked by the breakdown of the lung endothelial barrier and the accumulation of pathogenic cells such as neutrophils in the blood vessels of the lungs [9]. This aggregation leads to the release of reactive oxygen species (ROS) from neutrophils, causing significant injury to lung endothelial cells [10]. The pathophysiology of TRALI involves complex mechanisms, characterized by a multicellular immune response, including antibody-mediated activation of leukocytes (including neutrophils) and the pulmonary endothelium through leukocyte- and endothelial-reactive antibodies [11].

An important aspect of TRALI pathophysiology is the involvement of the complement system. Complement activation, whether through the classical, lectin, or alternative pathways, ultimately converges on the cleavage of C5, leading to the production of both C5a and C5b [12]. C5b is involved in the formation of the membrane attack complex (MAC) along with other complement components [13]. This cascade amplifies immune cell recruitment and activation, exacerbating lung injury and inflammation [12]. Despite plausible evidence, studies investigating the role of complement in TRALI prior to 2019 were limited and often presented conflicting findings [12].

Recent systematic studies have provided stronger evidence for the critical role of the complement system in TRALI. These studies show that specific antibodies with a higher ability to activate the complement system through their Fc regions are closely linked to TRALI induction in murine models. This correlation exists even though these antibodies have similar binding affinities to their antigen, similar binding affinities to Fcγ-receptors, and similar Fc glycosylation profiles compared to antibodies that do not induce TRALI [14]. This highlights the significant role of complement activation in the development of TRALI. Additionally, the essential role of complement, particularly C5, in antibody-mediated TRALI has been confirmed in vivo [15]. C5a acts as a potent chemoattractant and activator of neutrophils, which may stimulate the development of neutrophil extracellular traps (NETs), contributing to the inflammatory response and endothelial injury seen in TRALI [15]. In addition, increased complement levels were measured in the plasma of TRALI patients, and a direct correlation between complement activation and NET formation in TRALI patients was observed [15]. These findings suggest that targeting the complement system could be a promising therapeutic approach for managing TRALI [16].

To study TRALI, several mouse models have been developed that closely mimic the human condition. The first hit in these models often involves an inflammatory stimulus, such as lipopolysaccharide (LPS), which primes the immune system. The second hit is the introduction of antibodies or other transfusion-related factors that trigger immune activation and lung injury. In this two-hit model of TRALI, LPS priming is a crucial step for replicating the initial inflammatory state that makes animals susceptible to TRALI. Studies have shown that LPS priming, followed by a secondary insult such as an MHC class I antibody infusion, is necessary to induce TRALI in animal models. For instance, LPS priming was critical in murine models before injecting an MHC I antibody to establish TRALI [12, 17]. However, it's important to note that LPS priming may not be required in untreated barrier-free (BF) mice, as these mice may already be in a mild state of inflammation due to their gut microbiota, which predisposes them to severe lung injury [17]. In contrast, SPF mice have a more sterile environment and different gut flora composition, requiring LPS priming to become susceptible to TRALI [17]. The severity of TRALI varies with animal housing conditions; untreated BF mice suffer from severe antibody-mediated TRALI, whereas SPF and gut flora-depleted BF mice are protected from antibody-mediated TRALI without prior LPS priming. This protection is associated with reduced plasma macrophage inflammatory protein-2 levels (homologue of human IL-8) and decreased pulmonary neutrophil accumulation [17]. In certain models, T-cell depletion (related to depletion of protective T regulatory cells) using CD4 antibodies is performed before TRALI induction [15, 17–19]; however, not all studies perform this [20, 21].

In BALB/c mice, TRALI can be induced using the MHC class I antibody 34-1-2S (IgG2a, anti-H-2K^{d}), whereas the antibody SF1.1.10 (also IgG2a and H-2K^{d} specific) does not trigger TRALI [15]. One of the distinguishing features of the TRALI-inducing antibody 34–1-2S was found to be its ability to potentially activate complement [14]. This 34-1-2S TRALI mouse model is particularly advantageous as it highlights specific immune mechanisms underlying TRALI, which accurately mimics features of human TRALI. Conversely, in C57BL/6 mice, TRALI induction requires a combination of anti-MHC class I antibodies AF6-88.5.5.3 (IgG2a, anti-H-2K^{b}) and a high dose of 34-1-2S, illustrating strain-specific responses and the complexity of TRALI induction, which requires complement activation [14]. An obvious advantage of C57BL/6 mice is that most murine knock-out strains are established on this genetic background, thus enabling studies of specific gene knock-outs [15, 18, 19]. Furthermore, mouse models can involve either anesthetized [22] or awake animals [15]. While anesthesia might influence the development of TRALI, its exact impact has not been systematically studied. Models using awake animals may offer greater translational relevance since patients developing TRALI are not always anesthetized.

Assays to study TRALI encompass various in vivo and in vitro techniques. In vivo assays often include measuring lung wet-to-dry (w/d) weight ratio, a direct and most robust read-out to assess the degree of pulmonary edema, which is the hallmark of acute lung injury. In addition, bronchoalveolar lavage fluid may be evaluated for protein content, cytokines, and cell counts, and furthermore, histopathological examinations of lung tissues can be performed. These assays are essential for assessing the extent of pulmonary edema and the inflammatory response in the lung. Inflammatory and other pathogenic parameters can also be measured in plasma. Complement system assays are critical for understanding the immune responses involved in TRALI. Assays such as C5a ELISA and C1q-C4 complex ELISA measure complement activation levels in plasma samples, revealing the presence of complement components in the pathogenesis of TRALI. Neutrophil activation tests and endothelial cell culture assays (in the presence of specific immune cells) further can clarify the specific pathways through which neutrophils, other immune cells, and complement components interact with the pulmonary endothelium and contribute to the development of TRALI. The MPO-DNA assay detects NETs in plasma, providing insights into the role of NETs in TRALI pathophysiology, which has been previously described [15, 23, 24]. However, these assays can present challenges such as variability in animal responses, difficulties in replicating the complex human immune environment, and the need for precise control of experimental conditions. The genetic background of mouse strains can influence the severity of TRALI, necessitating the careful selection of appropriate models. Replicating the multifaceted interactions between various immune cells and mediators in vitro requires sophisticated experimental setups and meticulous optimization of conditions.

Overcoming these challenges necessitates rigorous standardization of protocols and careful interpretation of results to ensure their applicability to human TRALI. Researchers must consider the limitations of each assay and model, integrating data from multiple approaches to gain a comprehensive understanding of TRALI pathophysiology. Addressing these challenges can improve diagnostic and therapeutic strategies, ultimately enhancing patient care.

2 Materials (*See* Note 1)

2.1 Human Sample Assays

2.1.1 Complement System in Human Plasma Samples

C5a ELISA

1. Pre-coated microwell strips (*see* **Note 2**).
2. Wash buffer (supplied in the kit) (*see* **Note 3**).
3. Stop buffer (supplied in the kit) (*see* **Note 3**).
4. Biotin-conjugated anti-human C5a (supplied in the kit).
5. Streptavidin-HRP (supplied in the kit).
6. TMB substrate solution.

Equipment:

1. Plate reader (BioTek Synergy 2, Winooski, VT) (*see* **Note 4**).
2. Plate shaker.
3. Micropipettes and tips.
4. Multichannel pipette (optional, recommended for efficiency) (*see* **Note 5**).
5. Microcentrifuge tubes.
6. Plate washer (optional, for washing steps).

C1q-C4 Complex ELISA

1. Nunc Maxisorp 96-well plate (Thermo Fisher Scientific).
2. Assay buffer: Phosphate-buffered saline with 1% Tween™ 20 (PBS-T) (*see* **Note 3**).
3. Phosphate-buffered saline (PBS, Ca^{2+}/Mg^{2+} free).
4. High-performance ELISA buffer (HPE).
5. Sulfuric acid (H_2SO_4; 2 M).
6. TMB substrate solution.
7. Ice-cold ammonium sulfate ($(NH_4)_2SO_4$; 2.58 M) (*see* **Note 3**).
8. Sodium chloride (NaCl; 1 M).
9. C4-4 antibody (2 μg/mL in PBS).
10. C1q-85 biotinylated antibody (1:4000 in HPE).
11. Streptavidin poly-HRP.

Equipment:

1. Plate reader (BioTek Synergy 2) (*see* **Note 4**).
2. Centrifuge.
3. Incubator (capable of maintaining room temperature).
4. Micropipettes and tips.
5. Multichannel pipette (optional, recommended for efficiency) (*see* **Note 5**).
6. Microcentrifuge tubes.

7. Plate shaker (optional, for efficient mixing) (*see* **Notes 6** and 7).
8. Plate washer (optional, for washing steps) (*see* **Note 8**).

2.1.2 MPO-DNA ELISA for the Detection of NETs in Plasma

1. Nunc Maxisorp plates (Thermo Fisher Scientific).
2. Coating buffer: Carbonate-bicarbonate buffer (0.05 M, pH 9.6).
3. Phosphate-buffered saline with Tween™ 20 (PBS-T).
4. Phosphate-buffered saline (PBS, Ca^{2+}/Mg^{2+} free).
5. PMN-MPO antibody (Sigma-Aldrich) (*see* **Note 11**).
6. Bovine Serum Albumin (BSA; 1%) in PBS-T (Sigma-Aldrich).
7. EDTA-plasma samples.
8. DNA peroxidase antibody (part of the Cell Death ELISAPLUS kit, Roche Diagnostics GmbH).
9. Incubation buffer (supplied with the Cell Death ELISAPLUS kit, Roche Diagnostics GmbH).
10. TMB substrate solution.
11. Sulfuric acid (H_2SO_4; 2 M).
12. MPO standard (LEGEND MAX Human Myeloperoxidase ELISA Kit, BioLegend Inc).
13. Lambda DNA (Quant-iT PicoGreen dsDNA Assay Kit, Invitrogen).
14. Human native nucleosomes (Merck).

Equipment:

1. Plate reader (BioTek Synergy 2, Winooski, VT) (*see* **Note 4**).
2. Plate shaker (*see* **Note 6**).
3. Incubator (capable of maintaining 4 °C).
4. Micropipettes and tips.
5. Multichannel pipette (optional, recommended for efficiency) (*see* **Note 5**).
6. Microcentrifuge tubes.
7. Plate washer (optional, for washing steps) (*see* **Note 8**).

2.2 Antibody-Mediated Two-Hit TRALI Mouse Model

Animals:

1. Mice strains: C57BL/6 or BALB/c.

Antibodies, chemicals, and biological reagents:

1. Anti-mouse CD4-PE (BD Biosciences) (This is optional and experiment dependent; *see* **Note 9**).
2. Mouse CD4 antibody (BioXCell; Clone: GK1.5) (This is optional and experiment dependent; *see* **Note 9**).

3. Mouse MHC I antibodies (BioXCell; clones: 34-1-2S, AF6.88.5.5.3) (*see* **Note 10**).
4. Isotype antibody for 34-1-2S (BioXCell; Clone: C1.18.4) (*see* **Note 11**).
5. LPS (Sigma-Aldrich; Escherichia coli strain 055:B5).
6. Citrate Phosphate Dextrose (CPD; Sigma-Aldrich).
7. Ethylenediaminetetraacetic acid (EDTA; 0.5 M, ThermoFisher).

Equipment:

1. Scale.
2. Rectal temperature probe.
3. Pre-weighed Eppendorf tubes.
4. Cell strainers (40 μm).
5. Insulin needles.
6. 23G needles.
7. 29G needles.
8. Syringes (1 mL, 5 mL).
9. Tubes (50 mL, 15 mL).
10. Petri dishes (60 mm).

2.2.1 Brochoalveolar Lavage and Total Protein Determination

Reagents and Solutions:

1. PBS (Ca^{2+}/Mg^{2+} free)—Phosphate-Buffered Saline.

Equipment:

1. Tools for mouse dissection (tweezers and scissors).
2. Intradermal tube.
3. Nanodrop 2000 (for protein measurement; Thermo Fisher Scientific).
4. Syringes (1 mL).
5. Collecting tubes (FACS tubes).
6. Razor blade.

2.2.2 Blood and Tissue Processing for Flow Cytometric Analyses

Chemicals:

1. Ammonium chloride (NH_4Cl; Merck).
2. Potassium bicarbonate ($KHCO_3$; Merck).
3. Ethylenediaminetetraacetic acid disodium salt (Na_2EDTA; Merck).
4. Bovine Serum Albumin (BSA; Sigma-Aldrich).
5. Phosphate-Buffered Saline (PBS).

6. Ethylenediaminetetraacetic acid (EDTA; Sigma-Aldrich).
7. Sodium azide (NaN_3; Sigma-Aldrich) (This is optional and experiment dependent; *see* **Note 12**).

Buffers:

1. ACK Lysis Buffer: Used for lysing red blood cells. Prepared with 0.15 M NH_4Cl, 10.0 mM $KHCO_3$, and 0.1 mM Na_2EDTA; adjusted to pH 7.2–7.4.
2. FACS buffer: To make 1 L of FACS buffer, dissolve 5 g BSA (final concentration 0.5%) in 900 mL sterile PBS and 4 mL of EDTA (0.5 M, final concentration 2 mM) plus 0.05% NaN_3, and adjust the volume to 1000 mL with PBS (*see* **Note 12**).
   *Store at 4 °C for up to 1 month.
3. Markers staining fluorophores depending on the purpose of the study and study readouts.

2.2.3 Lung Histology/Immunohistochemistry

1. Histofix (Histolab Products AB).
2. Mayer hematoxylin (Histolab Products AB).
3. Eosin (0.2%; Histolab Products AB).
4. Hydrogen peroxide (H_2O_2 3%; Boster Biological Technology).
5. Citrate buffer pH 6 (Boster Biological Technology).
6. Bovine serum albumin (BSA; 5%; Sigma-Aldrich).
7. Triton-X 100 (0.05%; Sigma-Aldrich Chemie GmbH).
8. PBS (Ca^{2+}/Mg^{2+} free).
9. Specific antibody (depends on the purpose of the study).
10. F(ab')2 donkey anti-rabbit IgG (H + L)-HRP-conjugated secondary antibody (Jackson ImmunoResearch).
11. DAB Chromogenic Substrate kit (Boster Biological Technology).
12. Neo-Mount (Merck KGaA).

Equipment:

1. Microtome.
2. Superfrost Plus slides (Fisher Scientific).
3. Serial baths of xylene and ethanol.
4. Olympus BX60F microscope with SC50 camera.

3 Methods

1. If your ELISA plates are not pre-coated, coat the wells of a 96-well ELISA plate with 100 μL of a capture antibody specific

3.1 Human Sample Assays

3.1.1 Complement System in Human Plasma Samples

C5a ELISA

to human C5a, diluted in coating buffer (e.g., carbonate-bicarbonate buffer, pH 9.6) (*see* **Note 13**).

2. If your plates are pre-coated, you can continue from **step 4**.
3. Incubate the plate overnight at 4 °C.
4. Wash the plate three times with 200 μL of PBS or wash buffer per well (*see* **Note 8**).
5. Remove the wash buffer completely by inverting the plate and tapping it gently on absorbent paper (*see* **Note 14**).
6. Equilibrate all reagents to RT before use.
7. Prepare the standard as suggested by the manufacturer's instructions.
8. Dilute plasma samples if necessary, following a specified dilution factor based on the expected C5a concentration and type of the sample (e.g., plasma, serum, saliva, etc.) (*see* **Note 15**).
9. Add 100 μL of standard or plasma samples to each well (*see* **Notes 16** and **17**).
10. Incubate the plate for 2 h at room temperature on a plate shaker (set to approximately 300 rpm) (*see* **Notes 6** and 7).
11. After incubation, wash the plate five times with 100 μL of wash buffer per well.
12. Ensure complete removal of wash buffer after each wash by gently tapping the plate on absorbent paper.
13. Add 100 μL of the supplied biotin-conjugated anti-human C5a to each well.
14. Incubate the plate for 1 h at room temperature on a plate shaker (set to approximately 300 rpm) (*see* **Notes 6** and 7).
15. Wash the plate five times with 100 μL of wash buffer per well, ensuring thorough removal (*see* **Note 8**).
16. Add 100 μL of the supplied Streptavidin-HRP to each well.
17. Incubate the plate for 1 h at room temperature on a plate shaker (set to approximately 300 rpm) (*see* **Notes 6** and 7).
18. Wash the microwell strips five times with 100 μL of wash buffer per well, ensuring thorough removal (*see* **Note 8**).
19. Add 100 μL of TMB substrate solution to each well.
20. Incubate the plate at room temperature for 4–5 min, monitoring color development closely (*see* **Note 18**).
21. Stop the reaction by adding 100 μL of the supplied stop solution (or H_2SO_4, 5%) to each well as soon as the desired color intensity is achieved.
22. Measure the absorbance at 450 nm with a reference wavelength of 540 nm using a plate reader (BioTek Synergy 2) (*see* **Note 19**).

23. Calculate the mean absorbance value for each standard and sample based on the replicate readings.
24. Generate a standard curve by plotting the standard concentrations on the x-axis and the corresponding mean absorbance values (450 nm) on the y-axis.
25. Use regression analysis to determine the best-fit line for the standard curve. You can use either a log-log transformation or a four-parameter logistic curve fit, depending on your data and the software available.
26. Determine the concentration of the unknown samples by locating their absorbance values on the standard curve.
27. Multiply the concentration obtained from the standard curve by the dilution factor used for the samples to get the final concentration.

C1q-C4 Complex ELISA (*See* **Note 20**)

1. Mix an equal volume of ice-cold 2.58 M ammonium sulfate ($(NH_4)_2SO_4$) with EDTA plasma.
2. Prepare the standard as suggested by the manufacturer's instructions. If the standard preparation involves complex procedures (e.g., serial dilutions, specific incubation times), follow the detailed steps provided by the manufacturer carefully. Ensure that standards are prepared fresh and handled consistently to ensure accuracy.
3. Incubate the mixture on ice for 1 h (*see* **Note 7**).
4. Add 1 mL of 1.29 M ammonium sulfate to the mixture.
5. Centrifuge the mixture at 1300 × g for 30 min at 4 °C (*see* **Note 7**).
6. Dissolve the resulting pellet in a volume of High-Performance ELISA (HPE) buffer with 1 M NaCl, equal to the original plasma volume (*see* **Notes 21** and **22**).
7. Dilute C4-4 antibody to a concentration of 2 μg/mL in PBS.
8. Add 100 μL of the C4-4 antibody solution to each well of the Nunc Maxisorp 96-well plate (*see* **Note 16**).
9. Incubate the plates overnight at room temperature (*see* **Note 7**).
10. Remove the coating solution and wash the plates five times with 200 μL PBS-T per well (*see* **Note 8**).
11. Add 200 μL of High-performance ELISA buffer (HPE) to each well (*see* **Note 22**).
12. Incubate the plates at room temperature for 1 h (*see* **Note 7**).
13. Add 100 μL of standard or the dissolved C1q-C4 complex samples to each well.
14. Incubate the plates at room temperature for 1 h (*see* **Note 7**).

15. Wash the plates five times with 200 μL PBS-T per well.
16. Dilute the C1q-85 biotinylated antibody 1:4000 in HPE (*see* **Note 23**).
17. Add 100 μL of the diluted antibody solution to each well.
18. Incubate the plates at room temperature for 1 h (*see* **Note 7**).
19. Wash the plates five times with 200 μL PBS-T per well (*see* **Note 8**).
20. Prepare the streptavidin poly-HRP solution as per the supplier's instructions.
21. Add 100 μL of the prepared streptavidin poly-HRP solution to each well. Ensure that the streptavidin poly-HRP is prepared fresh and used immediately for best results.
22. Incubate the plates at room temperature for 1 h (*see* **Note 7**).
23. Wash the plates five times with 200 μL PBS-T per well (*see* **Note 8**).
24. Prepare the TMB substrate solution.
25. Add 100 μL of TMB solution to each well.
26. Incubate the plates at room temperature until the desired color development is achieved. Monitor the color development closely and check the plate periodically within the first 4–5 min. If the color change is rapid, be prepared to stop the reaction sooner to avoid overdevelopment.
27. Add 100 μL of 2 M H_2SO_4 to each well to stop the reaction.
28. Measure the absorbance at 450 nm with a reference wavelength of 540 nm using a plate reader (BioTek Synergy 2).
29. Express levels of C1q-C4 complexes in plasma as arbitrary units (AU).
30. Use a standard curve of known concentrations to quantify the complexes, if available.
31. Normalize the results, where 100 AU represents the amount of complexes in a purified C1q sample.

3.1.2 MPO-DNA ELISA for the Detection of NETs in Plasma

Day 1: Plate Coating

1. Prepare the coating buffer (0.05 M carbonate-bicarbonate buffer, pH 9.6).
2. Dilute the PMN-MPO antibody to a concentration of 5 μg/mL in the coating buffer. Ensure that the antibody is fully dissolved and mixed in the coating buffer.
3. Add 100 μL of the anti-PMN-MPO solution to each well of the Nunc Maxisorp plates (*see* **Note 16**).
4. Incubate the plates overnight at 4 °C (*see* **Note 24**).
5. To generate a calibration curve, prepare MPO-nucleosome-DNA complexes by complexing 54 ng of reconstituted

human MPO standard with 1.4 μg of lambda DNA and 1.4 μg of human native nucleosomes (*see* **Note 25**).

6. Incubate this mixture for 30 min at room temperature.
7. After incubation, add 200 μL of PBS to the mixture to prepare a stock standard solution of 100 ng/mL.
8. Further dilute this stock solution to generate a calibration curve with MPO-DNA complex levels ranging from 0.5 to 5 ng/mL of MPO component (*see* **Note 25**).
9. Add 100 μL of these standards to the plates to assess the MPO-DNA complex concentrations in parallel with the samples.

Day 2: Blocking and Sample Addition

1. Remove the coating solution and wash the plates four times with 200 μL PBS-T per well. Washing four times with PBS-T is appropriate for reducing background noise.
2. Prepare the blocking solution (1% BSA in PBS-T).
3. Add 200 μL of blocking solution to each well (*see* **Note 26**).
4. Incubate the plates at room temperature for 30 min. This step reduces non-specific binding in subsequent steps.
5. Remove the blocking solution.
6. Dilute EDTA-plasma samples in PBS at a 1:3 dilution ratio, but it should be adjusted if necessary based on expected concentration ranges (*see* **Note 27**).
7. Add 100 μL of the diluted plasma samples to each well (see **Note 16**).
8. Incubate the plates for 2 h at room temperature on a plate shaker (*see* **Note 6**).
9. Wash the plates four times with 200 μL PBS-T per well. This washing step is necessary to remove unbound components and minimize background noise.
10. Prepare the anti-DNA peroxidase antibody in the supplied incubation buffer from the Cell Death ELISAPLUS kit (Roche Diagnostics GmbH, Mannheim, Germany). Ensure that the antibody is prepared fresh and according to the kit instructions.
11. Add 100 μL of the prepared antibody solution to each well.
12. Incubate the plates for 2 h at room temperature on a plate shaker (*see* **Notes 6** and **7**).
13. Wash the plates four times with 200 μL PBS-T per well.
14. Add 100 μL of TMB solution to each well.
15. Incubate the plates at room temperature until the desired color development is achieved (*see* **Note 18**).

16. Add 100 μL of 2 M H_2SO_4 to each well to stop the reaction.
17. Measure the absorbance at 450 nm with a reference wavelength of 540 nm using a plate reader (BioTek Synergy 2) (*see* **Note 19**).
18. Calculate the mean absorbance value for each standard and sample based on the replicate readings.
19. Plot the standard concentrations (0.5 to 5 ng/mL MPO component) on the x-axis and the corresponding absorbance values on the y-axis to generate a standard curve. Absorbance measurements are taken at 450 nm with a reference wavelength of 630 nm for normalization.
20. Use regression analysis to determine the best-fit line for the standard curve. You can use either a log-log transformation or a four-parameter logistic curve fit, depending on your data and the software available.
21. Determine the concentration of the unknown samples by locating their absorbance values on the standard curve.
22. Multiply the concentration obtained from the standard curve by the dilution factor used for the samples to get the final concentration.

3.2 Antibody-Mediated Two-Hit TRALI Mouse Model (Fig. 1)

Day 1:

1. Weigh the animals and record all relevant details, such as their identification number and any specific observable physical or behavioral conditions (*see* **Note 28**).
2. Measure each animal's body temperature using a rectal temperature probe and record the results. If an animal shows a low body temperature, consider excluding it due to the potential for an underlying condition.
3. Inject each mouse intraperitoneally (IP) with 4.5 mg/kg CD4 antibody diluted in sterile PBS (Ca^{2+}/Mg^{2+} free, ~100 μL) (*see* **Notes 9** and **29**).
4. Inject each mouse IP with 0.1 mg/kg LPS in sterile PBS (Ca^{2+}/Mg^{2+} free) (*see* **Note 30**).

Day 2:

1. Weigh the mice and record their body temperature again (*see* **Note 31**).
2. Inject each mouse with 600 μL of antibody solution: (*see* **Notes 30** and **32**).
   (a) For C57BL/6 mice: 34-1-2s (45 mg/kg)/ AF6-88.5.5.3 (4.5 mg/kg) in PBS (Ca^{2+}/Mg^{2+} free) or control antibody (*see* **Note 10**).
   (b) For BALB/c mice: 34-1-2s (4.5 mg/kg) in PBS (Ca^{2+}/Mg^{2+} free) or control antibody.

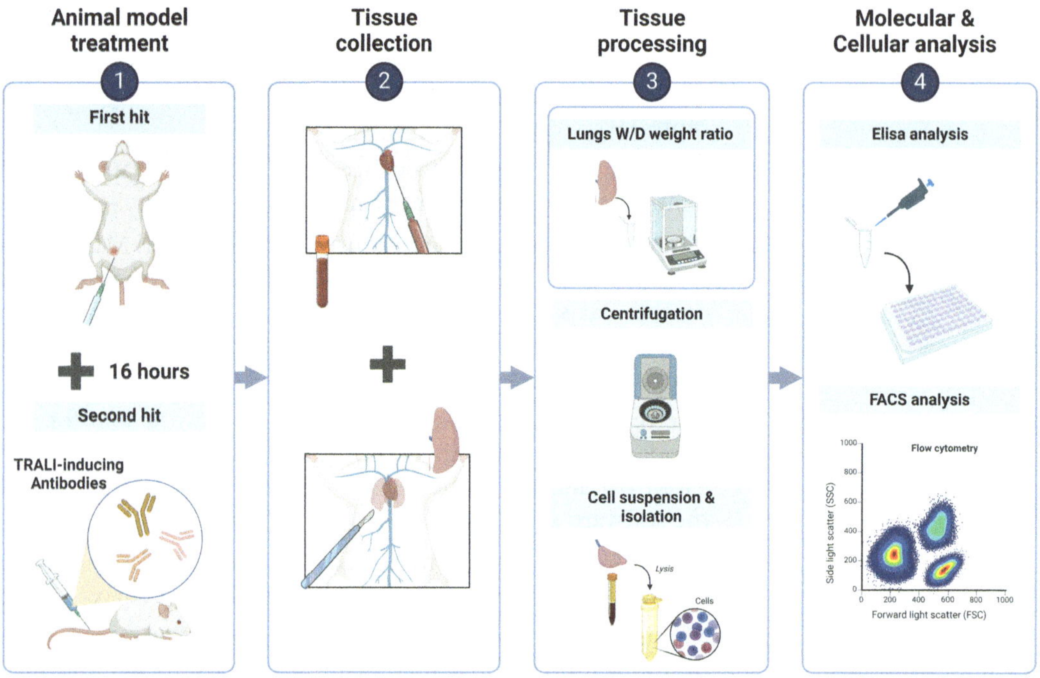

Fig. 1 Workflow for blood and lung sample processing and analysis in TRALI studies. Mice are treated with LPS (and CD4-depleting antibodies) to induce an underlying inflammatory condition, involving intraperitoneal injection followed by a 16-h incubation period to allow the priming phase of the disease model then intravenous injection is performed with specific antibodies to develop TRALI. Blood is collected via cardiac puncture, and lungs are carefully dissected post-mortem. Lungs are processed to determine the lung wet-to-dry weight (W/D) ratio by weighing the lung tissues before and after drying. Blood samples are centrifuged to separate plasma, and lung tissues are prepared into a cell suspension for further analysis. Collected samples undergo various molecular and cellular analyses, including ELISA for measuring complement levels and flow cytometry (FACS) for detailed cellular analysis

3. Measure the body temperature of each mouse every 15 min (*see* **Note 33**).
4. Euthanize the mice that reached the humane endpoint or survived until the end of the experimental time after antibody injection with a ketamine/xylazine solution (*see* **Note 34**).
5. Draw blood from the left ventricle (heart puncture) using a syringe containing CPDA or EDTA (*see* **Note 35**).
6. In case of not proceeding with flow cytometry, transfer the blood to a tube, centrifuge at 2000 × g for 15 min at room temperature without a brake, and collect the plasma.
7. Repeat **step 6** (*see* **Note 17**).
8. Store plasma samples at −80 °C.

9. In case of proceeding with flow cytometry, centrifuge the samples at 300 × g for 4 min at 4 °C.
10. Carefully collect the plasma (upper portion) without disturbing the buffy coat.
11. Centrifuge the collected plasma at 2000 × g for 10 min at 4 °C for the other analysis and store the plasma samples at −80 °C.
12. Dissect the right lung and place it in a pre-weighed tube.
13. Place the tube in an oven to dry for 48 h at 60 °C.
14. Dissect the left lung.
15. Place the left lung in a tube containing 1 mL of formalin for histology.
16. Dissect the spleen to verify CD4 depletion, if applicable.
17. Mash the spleen tissue for flow cytometric analysis, process with ACK buffer, and prepare for CD4 T-cell depletion analysis using flow cytometry (see detailed protocol on Subheading 3.2.3).

3.2.1 Brochoalveolar Lavage Collection (Fig. 2)

1. Euthanize the mouse according to the procedure approved by your Institutional Animal Care and Use Committee (IACUC) (*see* **Note 34**).
2. Place the mouse in a prone position.
3. Remove all skin from the lower part of the thorax up to the neck using tools sterilized with 70% ethanol.

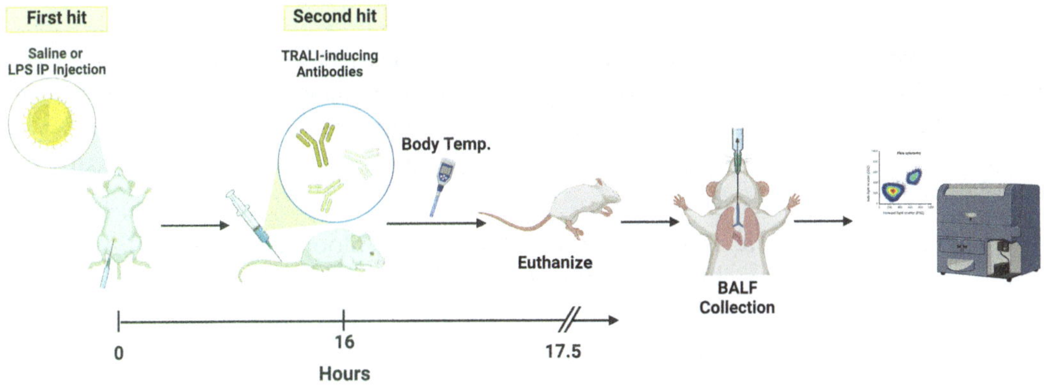

Fig. 2. Procedure for Bronchoalveolar Lavage Fluid (BALF) collection in mice. Mice receive an intraperitoneal injection of either saline or LPS (or CD4-depletion antibodies) at the start (0 h). After 16 h, followed by administration of specific antibodies intraperitoneally, the body temperature is measured according to specific timepoints (e.g., every 15 min). After 90 min (at 17.5 h), the mice are euthanized, and BALF is collected by cannulating the trachea and flushing the lungs with PBS. The collected BALF is then analyzed using flow cytometry to assess cellular and molecular changes

4. Expose the trachea by removing all muscles and tissue around it without damaging or cutting the trachea. Use a small pipette tip to better expose the trachea.
5. Carefully open the thorax to display the lungs and cut the diaphragm. This allows the visualization of the inflation of the lungs and facilitates the inflation process.
6. Cut the trachea halfway with a razor blade and insert the intradermal tube.
7. Inflate the lungs by injecting 1 mL of PBS through the tube with a syringe.
8. Aspirate the PBS back into the syringe and collect it in a FACS tube kept on ice.
9. Repeat the inflation and aspiration steps twice, collecting a total of 3 mL of PBS per mouse (*see* **Notes 36** and **37**).
10. Record the exact amount of PBS recovered to normalize the data (*see* **Note 38**).

3.2.2 Lung W/D Weight Ratio

1. Weigh the tube, including the right lung (from Day 2; **step 12** in Subheading 3.2) (*see* **Note 39**).
2. Place the tube in the oven for 48 h at 60 °C (*see* **Note 40**).
3. After 48 h, weigh the tube again.
4. Calculate the lung W/D weight ratio using this equation and record all the data.

$$\text{Lung W/D weight ratio} = \frac{(\text{Wet tissue weight in tube} - \text{empty tube Weight})}{(\text{Dry Tissue Weight in tube} - \text{empty tube weight})}$$

3.2.3 Blood and Tissue processing for Flow Cytometric Analyses

Blood Collection:

1. Draw blood from the left heart chamber by entering via the apex with the 1 mL syringe containing CPDA or EDTA and transfer the blood to a prepared 1.5 mL Eppendorf tube.
2. Centrifuge the samples at 300 × g for 4 min at 4 °C to pellet the cells.
3. Resuspend the red and white blood cells in 1 mL ACK lysis buffer and transfer to a 15 mL tube, filling up to 14 mL with ACK buffer.
4. Incubate for 5 min with intermittent shaking.
5. Spin down cells at 300 × g for 4 min at 4 °C.
6. Repeat lysis at least twice with FACS buffer.
7. Count cells and make sure to have 1.5 × 10^6 cells in the sample for the FACS staining (*see* **Notes 41–43**).

Lung Tissue Processing

1. Dissect the left lung into two to three pieces (depends on the purpose of the study and availability of the assays).
2. For two-piece samples, use the upper part of the left lung, and for three-piece samples, use the middle part. Place the selected piece in a tube with 1 mL of formalin (specifically, Histofix solution) for fixation.
3. Store at room temperature until proceeding to Subheading 3.2.4.
4. Lower part: Mash in a dish for cytospin analysis.
5. Utilize a sterile pestle to macerate the lower section of the specimen in a petri dish.
6. Carefully pass the macerated sample through a 40 μm cell strainer, collecting the filtrate in a 50 mL tube to ensure removal of debris.
7. Transfer the strained sample into a 15 mL tube containing FACS buffer.
8. Centrifuge the sample at 300 × g for 4 min at 4 °C to pellet the cells.
9. Gently decant the supernatant, being careful not to disturb the cell pellet.
10. Resuspend the pellet in approximately 2 mL of ACK lysing buffer to lyse red blood cells and keep on ice.
11. Add an additional ACK buffer to bring the total volume to 10 mL. Incubate for 5 min on ice, gently inverting.
12. Mix the sample halfway through the incubation at the 3.5-min mark.
13. Repeat the centrifugation at 300 × g for 4 min at 4 °C to pellet the cells post-lysis.
14. Carefully remove the supernatant and resuspend the cell pellet in FACS buffer for a washing step to remove any residual lysing buffer.
15. Centrifuge again at 300 × g for 4 min at 4 °C to pellet the cells.
16. Manually aspirate the supernatant with care to avoid disturbing the cell pellet.
17. Resuspend the final cell pellet in a total volume of 500 μL of FACS buffer.

Spleen Processing

1. Mechanically dissociate the cell culture in the dish to create a homogenous cell suspension suitable for the analysis of CD4 T-cell depletion.
2. Transfer the suspension into a 15 mL conical tube containing FACS buffer.

3. Centrifuge the cell suspension at 300 × g for 4 min at a controlled temperature of 4 °C.
4. Carefully decant the supernatant.
5. Disaggregate the cell pellet using a gentle vortexing technique, ensuring minimal mechanical stress to the cells, then proceed to add in +/−2 mL ACK buffer to the cell pellet.
6. Fill to 5 mL with ACK buffer and incubate the ACK-treated cell suspension on ice for 5 min to allow for optimal lysis conditions.
7. Mix samples after 3.5 min gently.
8. Centrifuge the suspension again under the same conditions: 300 × g for 4 min at 4 °C to pellet the cells.
9. Perform a washing step by resuspending the cell pellet in FACS buffer to remove any remaining ACK buffer residues.
10. Resuspend the final cell pellet in a total volume of 500 μL of FACS buffer.
11. Accurately count the cells and adjust the concentration to 10^6 cells/mL. This ensures that 100 μL of the cell suspension will be suitable for subsequent analysis in flow cytometry.
12. Pipette 100 μL of cell suspension into a suitable tube. Add 1 μL of anti-mouse CD4-PE antibody to the cells for staining purposes.
13. Gently mix the cell-antibody mixture to ensure uniform staining. Incubate the mixture for 20 min on ice, ensuring the tube is adequately covered to protect from light and prevent contamination.
14. Following the incubation period, proceed to analyze the stained cells using a flow cytometer.
15. Adjust the instrument settings as necessary to accurately measure the Mean Fluorescence Intensity (MFI) of the PE (phycoerythrin) signal.

3.2.4 Lung Histology/ Immunohistochemistry (Fig. 3)

1. Fix a segment of the left lung in Histofix (from subheading "Lung Tissue Processing" on Subheading 3.2.3) (*see* **Note 44**).
2. Embed the fixed lung tissue in paraffin and section it into 3 μm thick slices using a microtome.
3. Place the tissue sections on Superfrost Plus slides.
4. Deparaffinize the sections by immersing them in serial baths of xylene and ethanol.
5. Stain the deparaffinized tissue sections with Mayer hematoxylin and 0.2% eosin for hematoxylin and eosin (H&E) staining using the guidelines below;

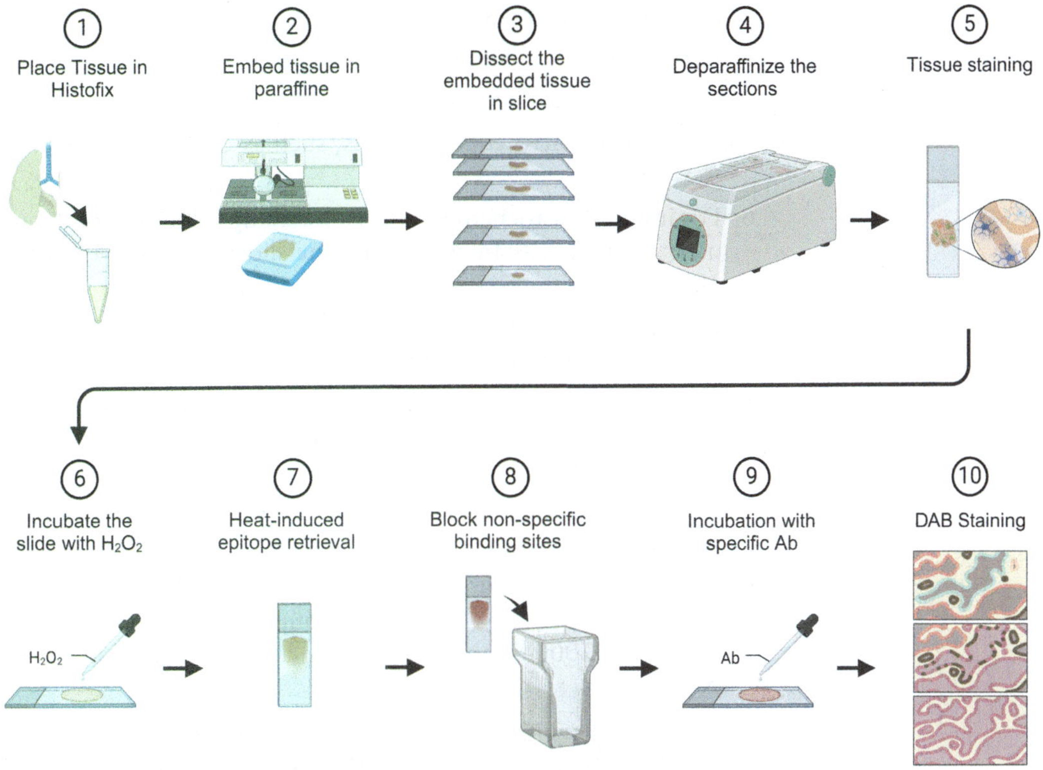

Fig. 3 Lung histology/immunohistochemistry workflow for lung tissue analysis. Lung tissue is first fixed in Histofix to preserve cellular and tissue morphology. The fixed tissue is then embedded in paraffin to provide support for sectioning. The paraffin-embedded tissue is sectioned into thin slices using a microtome. These tissue sections are deparaffinized in serial baths of xylene and ethanol to remove paraffin and prepare the tissue for staining. The sections are stained with Mayer hematoxylin and eosin (H&E) or prepared for immunohistochemistry staining. The slides are incubated with hydrogen peroxide (H_2O_2) to block endogenous peroxidase activity. Heat-induced epitope retrieval is performed by immersing the slides in citrate buffer and heating them, which unmasks antigens for antibody binding. The slides are then incubated in a solution of bovine serum albumin (BSA) and Triton-X 100 to block non-specific binding sites. Subsequently, the slides are incubated with a specific primary antibody overnight at 4 °C. Chromogenic detection can be performed using the DAB substrate kit, followed by counterstaining with Mayer hematoxylin and mounting with Neo-Mount. Finally, the stained slides will be imaged using a microscope

Very relevant:

(a) Accumulation of neutrophils in the alveolar or interstitial space.

(b) Formation of hyaline membranes.

(c) Presence of proteinaceous debris in the alveolar space (such as fibrin strands).

(d) Thickening of the alveolar wall.

(e) Enhanced injury as measured by a standardized histology score.

(f) Somewhat relevant:

(g) Evidence of hemorrhage.

(h) Areas of atelectasis.

(i) Gross macroscopic changes, such as discoloration of the lungs.

6. For immunohistochemistry (IHC) staining, block endogenous peroxidase activity by incubating the slides with 3% H_2O_2 for 10 min.
7. Perform heat-induced epitope retrieval by immersing the slides in citrate buffer pH 6 and heating them.
8. Block non-specific binding sites by incubating the slides in a solution of 5% BSA and 0.05% Triton-X 100 in PBS for 1 h at room temperature (*see* **Note 45**).
9. Incubate the slides with a specific antibody (depends on the purpose of the study) overnight at 4 °C (*see* **Note 46**).
10. Wash the slides with PBS and incubate with F(ab')2 donkey anti-rabbit IgG (H + L)-HRP-conjugated secondary antibodies at a 1:2000 dilution for 45 min at room temperature (*see* **Note 47**).
11. Perform chromogenic detection using the DAB Chromogenic Substrate kit according to the manufacturer's instructions.
12. Counterstain the slides with Mayer hematoxylin (*see* **Note 48**).
13. Mount the slides with Neo-Mount.
14. Image the stained slides using an Olympus BX60F microscope equipped with an SC50 camera.

4 Notes

1. Ensure all materials and reagents are prepared and accessible before starting any assay.
2. Pre-coat microwell strips and other necessary equipment well in advance.
3. Maintain appropriate temperatures for reagents according to the protocol, especially for critical steps such as ELISA and tissue processing.
4. Regularly calibrate and maintain equipment such as plate readers and flow cytometers to ensure accurate measurements.
5. Use multichannel pipettes where possible to ensure uniform reagent addition and improve efficiency.
6. Use a plate shaker set to ~300 rpm during incubations for consistent mixing.

7. Consistent incubation times and conditions across all samples are crucial for reproducibility.
8. Consistent and thorough washing of plates in ELISA is crucial to minimize background noise and improve sensitivity.
9. When utilizing an in vivo model for $CD4^+$ depletion, only these antibodies are required.
10. The AF6.88.5.5.3 antibody should be used with 34-1-2S exclusively when C57BL/6 mice are employed in the TRALI model.
11. Include the isotype control antibody for 34-1-2S only in experimental arms assessing non-specific binding (e.g., background signal controls); it is not required for the standard TRALI model.
12. Use sodium azide in FACS buffer only when staining intracellular targets or to prevent internalization of surface-bound antibodies.
13. If coating the plate, use fresh coating buffer and ensure that the antibody is evenly distributed in each well.
14. A blocking step is not required when using commercially pre-coated ELISA plates, as these are pre-treated to prevent non-specific binding. However, if using manually coated plates (e.g., Nunc Maxisorp), include a blocking step with 1–5% BSA or an appropriate blocking buffer after washing the coated wells to minimize background signal.
15. Accurate antibody preparation and serial dilutions are essential for assay specificity and sensitivity.
16. For statistical robustness, assay each sample in at least two duplicates. Triplicates are recommended when variability is high.
17. Handle plasma samples carefully to avoid degradation and ensure they are within the assay's dynamic range.
18. Monitor color development closely; overdevelopment can saturate readings. Check periodically between 4 and 5 min.
19. Ensure that the plate reader settings are optimized for your specific assay conditions, and consider reading samples in triplicate for accuracy.
20. The C1q-C4 complex ELISA was adapted and modified from Wouters et al., J Immunol Methods, 2005 [25].
21. Ensure complete dissolution of the pellet in the HPE buffer for accurate measurements.
22. The high-salt HPE buffer helps reduce non-specific protein–protein interactions and improves compatibility with downstream ELISA detection. However, it does not replace the

standard blocking step used to prevent non-specific binding to the plate surface.

23. Use freshly prepared and properly diluted antibodies for consistent results.
24. Properly coat plates and incubate overnight at 4 °C to ensure strong binding of the coating antibody.
25. The preparation of the standard and calibration curve was adapted from a method used by Kessenbrock et al. [26], which employed in vitro generated MPO-nucleosome-DNA complexes for quantitative analysis.
26. Perform blocking steps to reduce background noise.
27. Dilute plasma samples appropriately to stay within the assay's dynamic range.
28. Accurate weighing and temperature recording are essential for baseline data.
29. Ensure proper dilution and administration of CD4 antibody and LPS for consistent induction of TRALI.
30. Please consider that the lower doses of LPS or TRALI-inducing antibodies might be possible due to the environmental conditions at the animal facility.
31. Monitor body weight and temperature closely to assess the progression of TRALI.
32. Consistent antibody administration and proper controls (e.g., isotype antibodies) are crucial for comparative analysis.
33. Regular temperature measurement post-antibody injection helps track the progress of the TRALI reaction (lower temperatures may correlate with TRALI development).
34. Ensure proper anesthesia and euthanasia with humane handling during blood collection.
35. Follow precise blood processing protocols to avoid cell loss and ensure accurate plasma and cellular analyses.
36. Perform BALF collection immediately after euthanasia to prevent the degradation of cellular components and proteins in the bronchoalveolar lavage fluid (BALF).
37. Ensure thorough and consistent lavage of the lungs to collect representative samples.
38. Normalize protein concentration data based on recovered PBS volume for accuracy.
39. Accurate weighing and drying procedures are essential for reliable lung water content measurement.
40. Consistent drying conditions (temperature and duration) are critical for reproducibility.

41. Proper blood collection and processing techniques are essential to preserve cell integrity.
42. Thorough cell lysis and washing steps are crucial to obtain a clean cell suspension for flow cytometry.
43. Accurate cell counting and appropriate staining procedures ensure reliable flow cytometric analysis.
44. Proper fixation and sectioning techniques are critical for high-quality histological analysis.
45. Ensure specific and non-specific blocking steps are followed for immunohistochemistry to reduce background staining.
46. Use appropriate staining protocols to highlight key histological features (e.g., neutrophil accumulation, hyaline membranes, and proteinaceous debris).
47. Consistent antibody incubation times and concentrations are crucial for reproducibility.
48. Proper chromogenic detection and counterstaining provide clear visualization of target antigens.

Conflicts of Interest

Rick Kapur has received a research grant from Sanquin (PPOC23-08/L2752). No other conflicts of interest relevant to this work.

References

1. Semple JW, Rebetz J, Kapur R (2019) Transfusion-associated circulatory overload and transfusion-related acute lung injury. Blood. https://doi.org/10.1182/blood-2018-10-860809
2. Vlaar AP, Toy P, Fung M et al (2019) A consensus redefinition of transfusion-related acute lung injury. Transfusion. https://doi.org/10.1111/trf.15311
3. Silliman CC (2006) The two-event model of transfusion-related acute lung injury. Crit Care Med 34. https://doi.org/10.1097/01.CCM.0000214292.62276.8E
4. Silliman CC, Voelkel NF, Allard JD et al (1998) Plasma and lipids from stored packed red blood cells cause acute lung injury in an animal model. J Clin Invest. https://doi.org/10.1172/JCI1841
5. Chen D, Tian K, Xu X et al (2023) Mechanism and intervention of murine transfusion-related acute lung injury caused by anti-Cd36 antibodies. JCI Insight. https://doi.org/10.1172/jci.insight.165142
6. Bayat B, Nielsen KR, Bein G et al (2021) Transfusion of target antigens to preimmunized recipients: a new mechanism in transfusion-related acute lung injury. Blood Adv. https://doi.org/10.1182/bloodadvances.2020003843
7. Jug R, Anani W, Callum J (2021) A possible case of recipient anti-neutrophil and anti-human leukocyte antigen antibody-mediated fatal reverse transfusion-related acute lung injury. Transfusion. https://doi.org/10.1111/trf.16330
8. De Clippel D, Emonds M, Compernolle V (2019) Are we underestimating reverse TRALI? Transfusion. https://doi.org/10.1111/trf.15431
9. Rebetz J, Semple JW, Kapur R (2018) The pathogenic involvement of neutrophils in acute respiratory distress syndrome and transfusion-related acute lung injury. Transfus Med Hemother. https://doi.org/10.1159/000492950

10. Yokoyama A, Sakamoto Y, Jo T et al (2021) Pulmonary disease as a risk factor for transfusion-related acute lung injury. ERJ Open Res 7. https://doi.org/10.1183/23120541.00039-2021
11. Liu Y, Wang R, Song C et al (2023) Crosstalk between neutrophil extracellular traps and immune regulation: insights into pathobiology and therapeutic implications of transfusion-related acute lung injury. Front Immunol. https://doi.org/10.3389/fimmu.2023.1324021
12. Jongerius I, Porcelijn L, Beek AE v et al (2019) The role of complement in transfusion-related acute lung injury. Transfus Med Rev. https://doi.org/10.1016/j.tmrv.2019.09.002
13. Baines AC, Brodsky RA (2017) Complementopathies. Blood Rev. https://doi.org/10.1016/j.blre.2017.02.003
14. van der Laan EAZ, Velden S v d, Bentlage AEH et al (2020) Biological and structural characterization of murine TRALI antibody reveals increased fc-mediated complement activation. Blood Adv. https://doi.org/10.1182/bloodadvances.2020002291
15. Van Der Velden S, Van Osch TLJ, Seghier A et al (2024) Complement activation drives antibody-mediated transfusion-related acute lung injury via macrophage trafficking and formation of NETs. Blood. https://doi.org/10.1182/blood.2023020484
16. Kapur R, Semple JW, Vlaar APJ (2024) The importance of disrupting complement activation in acute lung injury. J Clin Invest 134. https://doi.org/10.1172/JCI182251
17. Kapur R, Kim M, Rebetz J et al (2018) Gastrointestinal microbiota contributes to the development of murine transfusion-related acute lung injury. Blood Adv 2:1651–1663. https://doi.org/10.1182/bloodadvances.2018018903
18. Kapur R, Kasetty G, Rebetz J et al (2019) Osteopontin mediates murine transfusion-related acute lung injury via stimulation of pulmonary neutrophil accumulation. Blood 2019. https://doi.org/10.1182/blood.2019000972
19. Kapur R, Kim M, Aslam R et al (2017) T regulatory cells and dendritic cells protect against transfusion-related acute lung injury via IL-10. Blood. https://doi.org/10.1182/blood-2016-12-758185
20. Cleary SJ, Kwaan N, Tian JJ et al (2020) Complement activation on endothelium initiates antibody-mediated acute lung injury. J Clin Invest. https://doi.org/10.1172/jci138136
21. Kapur R, Kim M, Shanmugabhavananthan S et al (2015) C-reactive protein enhances murine antibody–mediated transfusion-related acute lung injury. Blood. https://doi.org/10.1182/blood-2015-09-672592
22. Gilliss BM, Looney MR (2011) Experimental models of transfusion-related acute lung injury. Transfus Med Rev. https://doi.org/10.1016/j.tmrv.2010.08.002
23. Thomas GM, Carbó C, Curtis BR et al (2012) Extracellular DNA traps are associated with the pathogenesis of TRALI in humans and mice. Blood. https://doi.org/10.1182/blood-2012-01-405183
24. Caudrillier A, Kessenbrock K, Gilliss BM et al (2012) Platelets induce neutrophil extracellular traps in transfusion-related acute lung injury. J Clin Invest. https://doi.org/10.1172/jci61303
25. Wouters D, Wiessenberg HD, Hart M et al (2005) Complexes between C1q and C3 or C4: novel and specific markers for classical complement pathway activation. J Immunol Methods. https://doi.org/10.1016/j.jim.2004.12.018
26. Krinsky N, Sizikov S, Nissim S et al (2023) NETosis induction reflects COVID-19 severity and long COVID: insights from a 2-center patient cohort study in Israel. J Thromb Haemost. https://doi.org/10.1016/j.jtha.2023.02.033

Chapter 25

High-Throughput Metabolomics in Transfusion Medicine

Travis Nemkov, Daniel Stephenson, Julie A. Reisz, and Angelo D'Alessandro

Abstract

Over the past two decades, the introduction of omics technologies to the field of transfusion medicine has contributed to a significant expansion of our understanding of the storage lesion and its impact on transfusion recipients. Hundreds of application papers have leveraged the implementation of novel high-throughput omics techniques, such as the high-throughput metabolomics approach described herein. We will briefly describe how these approaches have been used to learn more about erythrocyte storage biology, chronic and massive transfusion recipient biology, and the development or testing of novel blood products. While this chapter mainly focuses on red blood cell biology, these exact same approaches have been applied to other blood cells (e.g., platelets, white blood cells, and reticulocytes) or biofluids (plasma and serum) and are thus potentially useful to a broad readership of transfusion or hematology experts with an interest in metabolism.

Key words Untargeted metabolomics, Mass spectrometry, Isocratic, Gradient, High-throughput

1 Introduction

Implementation of ultra-high-throughput approaches has been transformative in the field of omics technologies. Over the last two decades, the cost of genome sequencing has decreased from the landmark effort led by J. Craig Venter's team at Celera Genomics, which contributed to sequencing the first human genome at an estimated cost of ~$300 million, to as low as ~$175 per sample as of 2024 using commercial whole-exome sequencing services. As the cost of this technology decreased, personalized medicine initiatives have been launched and are currently thriving around the world.

In recent years, several groups have introduced a similar concept in the field of metabolomics through the development and implementation of multiple orthogonal platforms. High-throughput analytical workflows have evolved significantly, from nuclear magnetic resonance (NMR) to mass spectrometry (MS)-based

Sean R. Stowell and Connie M. Arthur (eds.), *Methods in Transfusion Medicine*, Methods in Molecular Biology, vol. 3053, https://doi.org/10.1007/978-1-0716-5376-0_25,

platforms. This latter approach has progressed from chromatography-assisted resolution of analytes that are subsequently measured by electrospray ionization mass spectrometry (ESI-MS) using targeted, multiple-reaction or parallel-reaction monitoring methods (higher sensitivity and specificity at the expense of diminished metabolome coverage) to flow injection coupled with high-resolution quadrupole-time of flight (qTOF) or quadrupole-Orbitrap-based instruments (higher throughput and coverage at the expense of sensitivity and quantitative capability). Additionally, matrix-assisted laser desorption/ionization (MALDI) offers an alternative chromatography-free method for ionization that decreases acquisition time (sub-30-second) at the expense of limited analyte detection. In the present chapter, we will describe a method developed in our lab [1], which is optimized for the analysis of red blood cells for transfusion medicine focused investigations. These approaches have made the detection and quantification of over 100,000 features and thousands of named metabolites possible in less than 5 min through direct injection, isocratic/gradient-based chromatography, or using in situ imaging approaches. These approaches allow processing of ~450 samples per day and are also compatible with the use of stable isotope-labeled internal standards, which allow for the correction of matrix-dependent ion suppression effects, as well as monitoring the stability of chromatographic peak shape and retention times and the quality of signal intensity at the MS and MS/MS level [2].

Over the past 5 years, we have optimized high-throughput methods for omics applications in transfusion medicine [3–5], with a focus on packed RBCs [6]. First, we have leveraged these approaches to investigate the impact of storage duration on RBC concentrates stored in all currently licensed storage additives, including saline-adenine-glucose mannitol (SAGM), additive solution (AS)-1, 3, 5, phosphate-adenine-glucose-guanosine-saline-mannitol (PAGGSM), and novel alkaline additives, such as AS7, ESOL5, and phosphate-adenine-glucose-guanosine-gluconate-mannitol (PAGGGSM) [7–14]. Then, we focused on alternative processing/storage strategies, such as cryopreservation [15], rejuvenation [16], or hypoxic storage [17–19]. We identified markers of the metabolic storage lesion [20, 21] and correlated storage-induced metabolic changes to the gold standard markers of storage quality as per the FDA and European Council guidelines, i.e., storage hemolysis (in the bag) and post-transfusion recovery (PTR), the percentage of stored RBCs that still circulate 24 h after autologous transfusion [22–31]. Through murine models of blood storage developed by the Zimring lab [32], we leveraged high-throughput metabolomics approaches to investigate the metabolic and genetic determinants of PTR [32], revealing a novel mechanism of ferroptosis (non-apoptotic RBC death by iron-dependent lipid peroxidation) as one of the main drivers of the storage lesion [33]. We leveraged tractable transgenic mouse models to identify the genetic and mechanistic factors contributing to the impaired circulation capacity of stored RBCs [32], including sphingosine kinase 1 (Sphk1) [28], band 3 (SLC4A1) [34, 35], and glucose-6-phosphate dehydrogenase (G6PD) [22, 23, 29, 30, 36–40]. First, we proved that oxidation and fragmentation of the cytosolic N-terminus of SLC4A1 contribute to loss of capacity to activate G6PD and thus the pentose phosphate pathway (PPP) in stored RBCs [41, 42]. We then investigated the effects of genetics on storage quality in 525 outbred mice derived from 46 generations of crosses of 8 genetically diverse founder strains and identified the ferrireductase STEAP3 as a regulator of ferroptosis in mice [32, 33]. Notably, STEAP3 activity is dependent upon NADPH, suggesting that G6PD and the PPP regulate lipid peroxidation cascades, as confirmed by quantitative trait loci analyses in humans and mice [33]. We observed that common *G6PD* polymorphisms impact RBC storage quality (metabolic lesion) and post-transfusion performance [23, 30, 39, 43–45]. Donor sex (G6PD is coded by a gene on chromosome X) was also found to impact the average age of circulating RBCs at the time of donation, which in turn affects the onset, progression, and severity of the storage lesion [46]. Finally, we introduced the concept of the blood donor exposome [47], showing that dietary (alcohol, caffeine consumption [48, 49]) or other exposures (smoking) [50], fatty acid composition of the diet [51], prior infection by flaviviruses [52] or coronaviruses [53, 54], over the counter drugs unrelated to donor deferral [47]) all contribute to modulating RBC metabolism. In so doing, these factors modulate energy and redox metabolism during storage and, ultimately, hemoglobin increments upon transfusion [50, 55, 56]. We concluded that the chronological age of blood (days elapsed since donation) is qualitatively distinct from the metabolic age of the unit (e.g., adenosine triphosphate, carnitine, kynurenine) [57].

In parallel to our focus on the blood donors and products, we set out to elucidate whether the metabolic lesion of stored RBCs would impact the plasma and blood cell metabolism of transfusion recipients. First, we investigated the impact of fresh vs old blood on healthy autologous volunteers [58], prior to moving on to non-healthy, heterologous recipients with a special focus on massively transfused trauma patients [59], pediatric cardiopulmonary bypass patients [60], and sickle cell patients, either receiving standard RBC exchanges [61] or rejuvenated RBC exchanges [62]. From biotinylation studies and single cell oxygenation testing, we showed that the storage lesion impacts RBC oxygen kinetics (transport, intracellular diffusion, and off-loading [16, 63]). These lesions are only partially reversible upon RBC transfusion in healthy autologous recipients [64], whose metabolome is impacted by transfusion (e.g., increased hypoxanthine, plasticizers, and pro-inflammatory oxylipins) [58]. We then developed high-throughput methods to design and test novel storage additives to modulate the metabolic age of stored RBCs [65].

Since high-throughput metabolomics allows testing of blood samples at scale, we leveraged this approach to investigate the genetic and biological underpinnings of the metabolic heterogeneity (and its reproducibility across donation) in over 13,000 blood donors from the Recipient Epidemiology and Donor Evaluation Study (REDS) RBC Omics. Specifically, through this workflow, we have identified metabolic (ATP [31], hypoxanthine [17], carnitine [25], kynurenine [26], HETEs [33], S1P [28]) and genetic factors (including G6PD status) that predict the onset, progression, severity of the storage lesion and transfusion efficacy (in bag hemolysis, PTR, and hemoglobin increments), with the final goal to inform the development of novel Precision Transfusion Medicine [66, 67] strategies based on high-throughput omics, artificial intelligence, and machine learning approaches [66] or lab-on-a-chip approaches [6].

The methods described below are not only applicable to stored blood products or human transfusion biology. Through (in vivo) metabolic tracing [68, 69] in tractable animal models and multiple species of veterinary interest (e.g., rodents, including mice, rats, guinea pigs; porcine or non-human primates, but also cows, donkeys, horses, baboons, macaques, etc.) [69–81] we investigated the role of genetic background across species as a driver of the storage lesion (Zoomics sub-project of the original award) [82–87]; we then tested the impact of transfusion in pre-clinical models [70, 79, 80, 88, 89]. We explored recipient outcomes in massively (e.g., trauma patients) [59, 73, 81, 90] or chronically transfused patients (e.g., sickle cell patients) [43, 61, 91–96]. We then identified novel mechanisms that drive systemic responses to hypoxia and oxidant stress to RBCs in SARS-CoV-2 or post-acute sequelae to Covid-19 [97–105], exercise and blood doping [94, 106–108], high-altitude [109–113], blood cancers [114–136], kidney disease [112, 137–140], neurodegeneration (e.g., Alzheimer's [141–143], Parkinson's [144], multiple sclerosis [145, 146]), hibernation [147–149], pulmonary hypertension [37, 39, 91, 150–159], aging and hematopoiesis [160].

Finally, the methods described herein can be applied to the study of other blood cells than RBCs (platelets [88, 161–167], macrophages [151, 154, 155, 158, 159, 168–175], neutrophils [89, 101, 172], dendritic cells [176–178], lymphocyte [179, 180]) with a focus on (pathological) inflammation [53, 101, 102, 104, 141, 154, 155, 161, 162, 170–175, 177, 178, 181–184] and immunometabolism [89, 154, 158, 159, 171, 185], all systems in which we identified a mechanistic contribution of dysregulated metabolism to clinically relevant phenotypes (e.g., thromboinflammatory complications after trauma and shock in transfusion patients).

2 Materials

Prepare all solutions using the highest quality solvents and reagents. We recommend LC-MS grade solvents, such as Optima™ (Fisher). Solutions can be stored at room temperature unless otherwise stated.

2.1 Preparation of Chromatography Mobile Phases

1. Water.
2. Water containing 0.1% v/v formic acid.
3. Acetonitrile.
4. Acetonitrile containing 0.1% v/v formic acid.
5. Ammonium acetate.
6. Sterile disposable vacuum filtration system (0.22 μm membrane).

2.2 Preparation of Stable Isotope-Labeled Standard Stock Solutions

1. Various compounds and solvents are outlined in Table 1.
2. Concentrated formic acid.
3. Concentrated aqueous ammonium formate.

2.3 Preparation of Metabolite Extraction Solution Containing Stable Isotope-Labeled Standards

1. Water.
2. Acetonitrile.
3. Methanol.
4. Isotype-labeled stock solutions (*see* Subheading 3.2).
5. 1 L glass bottle with cap, preferably new.
6. 1 L glass graduated cylinder, preferably new.

2.4 Metabolite Extraction from Biofluid Samples

1. Bench-top centrifuge capable of 18,213 g with refrigeration to 4 °C.
2. Refrigeration space (4 °C) with power outlet(s) to accommodate vortex(es), often a cold room or chromatography refrigerator.
3. Vortex with foam microcentrifuge tube insert.
4. Extraction solution (*see* Subheading 3.3).
5. Eppendorf tubes.
6. Autosampler vials.
7. Nitrogen blowdown evaporator or vacuum concentrator.

2.5 Metabolite Extraction from Tissue Samples

1. Bead beater (Next Advance, Storm 24).
2. Eppendorf™ Safe-lock tubes, 1.5 mL (catalog no. 022363204).
3. Glass beads, 1.0 mm diameter (NextAdvance SKU GB10).

Table 1
Typical stock concentrations of standards

Compound	Vendor	Product No.	Conc. (mM)
Adenosine	CIL	CLM-3678-0.1	1
Amino acid standard mix	CIL	MSK-A2–1.2	1
Acylcarnitine standard mix	CIL	NSK-B-1	200X[a]
Betaine (*N,N,N*-trimethylglycine) HCl	CDN isotopes	D-3352	0.1–2
Choline	CDN isotopes	D-2464	0.1–2
Citric acid	CIL	DLM-3487-PK	1
N,N-dimethylglycine HCl	CDN isotopes	D-3509	0.1–2
Fumaric acid	CIL	CLM-4454-PK	1
Glucose	CIL	CLM-1396-1	10
Glutathione (reduced)	CIL	CNLM-6245-10	1
α-Ketoglutarate	CIL	CLM-2411-PK	1
Palmitic acid	CIL	CLM-409-0.5	1
Sodium lactate	CIL	CLM-1578-0.5	40
Sphingosine 1-phosphate	Avanti	860659P	1
Succinic acid	CIL	CLM-1571-PK	1
Trimethylamine *N*-oxide	CIL	DLM-4779-1	1
Tryptophan	CIL	NLM-800-0.25	1
Uric acid	CIL	NLM-1697-0.5	1

CIL Cambridge Isotope Laboratories

[a]According to manufacturer instructions, acylcarnitine standards are to be diluted 200-fold into the extraction solution. Concentrations vary for each compound

4. Bench-top centrifuge capable of 18,213 g with refrigeration to 4 °C.
5. Refrigeration space (4 °C) with power outlet(s) to accommodate vortex(es), often a cold room or chromatography refrigerator.
6. Vortex with foam microcentrifuge tube insert.
7. Extraction solution (*see* Subheading 3.3).
8. Autosampler vials.

2.6 Metabolite Extraction from Cell Samples

1. Bench-top centrifuge capable of 18,213 g with refrigeration to 4 °C.
2. Refrigeration space (4 °C) with power outlet(s) to accommodate vortex(es), often a cold room or chromatography refrigerator.

3. Vortex with foam microcentrifuge tube insert.
4. Extraction solution (*see* Subheading 3.3).
5. Eppendorf tubes.
6. Autosampler vials.

2.7 UHPLC-MS Data Acquisition—Isocratic Method

1. Ultra-high-pressure liquid chromatography (UHPLC) system.
2. Analytical column: Kinetex® 1.7 μm C18 100 Å, UHPLC column 150 × 2.1 mm (Phenomenex catalog no. 00F-4475-AN).
3. Guard column: SecurityGuard™ ULTRA cartridge-UHPLC C18 for 2.1 mm ID columns (Phenomenex catalog no. AJ0–8782) with SecurityGuard™ ULTRA holder (catalog no. AJ0-9000).
4. Electrospray ionization (ESI) or heated ESI (HESI) source.
5. Mass spectrometer capable of high-resolution untargeted analysis with MS^1 acquisition. Instrument should be interfaced with a UHPLC system.
6. Mobile phases (*see* Subheading 3.1).

2.8 UHPLC-MS Data Acquisition—Gradient Method

1. Ultra-high-pressure liquid chromatography (UHPLC) system.
2. Analytical column: Kinetex® 1.7 μm C18 100 Å, UHPLC column 150 × 2.1 mm (Phenomenex catalog no. 00F-4475-AN).
3. Guard column: SecurityGuard™ ULTRA cartridge-UHPLC C18 for 2.1 mm ID columns (Phenomenex catalog no. AJ0-8782) with SecurityGuard™ ULTRA holder (catalog no. AJ0-9000).
4. Electrospray ionization (ESI) or heated ESI (HESI) source.
5. Mass spectrometer capable of high-resolution untargeted analysis with MS^1 acquisition. Instrument should be interfaced with a UHPLC system.
6. Mobile phases (*see* Subheading 3.1).

2.9 Data Analysis

1. Data visualization software. We recommend El-Maven (freely available at https://github.com/ElucidataInc/ElMaven) preceded by use of RawConverter (http://fields.scripps.edu/rawconv) to transform Thermo .RAW files into the .mzXML format needed for Maven.
2. Drift and/or batch correction software. We utilize MetaboDrift, an Excel macro add-in (https://github.com/evanscr/MetaboDrift).

3 Methods

3.1 Preparation of Chromatography Mobile Phases

1. Mobile phases for positive ion mode may be used as supplied. Phase A is water with 0.1% formic acid, and phase B is acetonitrile with 0.1% formic acid.
2. Prepare 25 mL of a 2 M stock of ammonium acetate in water. Vacuum filter resulting solution to remove any insoluble material.
3. Prepare 1 L of mobile phase A for negative mode (5% acetonitrile, 95% water, 1 mM ammonium acetate) by first diluting 2 M ammonium acetate (0.5 mL) with water (950 mL), then adding acetonitrile (50 mL). Ensure thorough mixing and complete solubility.
4. Prepare 1 L of mobile phase B for negative mode (95% acetonitrile, 5% water, 0.5 mM ammonium acetate) by first diluting 2 M ammonium acetate (2.5 mL) with water (to the 50 mL mark), then adding acetonitrile to the 1 L mark. Ensure thorough mixing and complete solubility.

3.2 Preparation of Stable Isotope-Labeled Standard Stock Solutions

1. Prepare stock solutions to 1000X the desired final concentration in the extraction solution, which should be within 1–2 orders of magnitude of the typical biological range in the analyzed sample matrix (*see* **Note 1**).
   (a) Weigh and dissolve stock solutions of stable isotope-labeled standards desired for analysis in a solvent according to the chemical nature of the compound and manufacturer instructions. (see Table 1 for various standards).
   (b) Add small volumes (<10 μL) of concentrated formic acid or concentrated aqueous ammonium formate as needed to neutralize pH. Typical stock concentrations (in mM) are given in Table 1.
2. Store stock solutions at −20 °C until use.

3.3 Preparation of Metabolite Extraction Solution Containing Stable Isotope-Labeled Standards

1. Prepare 1 L of extraction solution by adding methanol (0.5 L), acetonitrile (0.3 L), and water (0.2 L) to a clean glass graduated cylinder.
2. Pour into a clean glass bottle, cap, swirl to mix, and cool to subzero temperatures. We recommend overnight storage at −20 °C or when time-restricted, at least 30 min at −80 °C.
3. Unused extraction solution may be stored capped at −20 °C.
4. Remove stable isotope-labeled standard stock solutions from −20 °C and thaw on ice. Ensure that the solution is completely thawed and that no precipitation has occurred due to freeze-thaw. If precipitation has occurred, vortex the solution until the compound has re-dissolved.

5. Pipette stable isotope-labeled standard into pre-cooled extraction solution at desired concentration. We recommend maintaining the total volume of internal standards at or less than 5% of the total extraction solution volume to avoid diluting the organic components and thereby potentially altering extraction efficiency.

3.4 Metabolite Extraction from Biofluid Samples

1. Thaw samples on ice or in the refrigerator. Pre-cool labeled microcentrifuge tubes by immersing them in ice. We utilize 1.7 mL tubes; however, tube size can vary to accommodate the volume of extraction and compatibility with the rotor.
2. Briefly vortex thawed samples to homogenize, then transfer a 20 μL aliquot by micropipette to a labeled and cooled microcentrifuge tube. Remaining volumes may be refrozen and stored at −80 °C.
3. Add chilled extraction solution containing appropriate isotopically labeled standard(s) for absolute quantitation (if applicable to experiment) to each tube. For whole blood and red blood cell samples, add 180 μL of extraction solution so that the extraction ratio is 1:10. For plasma, serum, cell media, and other fluids, add 480 μL of extraction solution so that the extraction ratio is 1:25.
4. Vortex extract samples vigorously for 30 min at 4 °C.
5. Centrifuge for 10 min at 18,213 g (or maximum speed) at 4 °C to pellet insoluble materials such as proteins, nucleic acids, and less polar lipids, and ensure that the resulting supernatant is completely clear. If there are still particulates or cloudiness, transfer supernatants to a new tube and repeat centrifugation.
6. Transfer ~100 μL of extract supernatant into labeled and cooled autosampler vials (*see* **Note 2**).
7. For use as a quality control, prepare a pooled sample of each biological matrix being analyzed by combining 10 μL of each extract supernatant into an autosampler vial. Aliquot size may be adjusted so that the final QC sample volume is sufficient for QC runs at the beginning, middle, and end of the sequence for both positive and negative ion polarity modes, or every 10–20 sample runs, depending on the size of the sample set. Remaining supernatants may be stored at −80 °C (*see* **Note 3**).
8. Prepare a blank sample by adding 100 μL of extraction solution from **step 3** into a new, labeled autosampler vial.
10. Ensure that the sample vials do not contain air bubbles and are kept cold (in the range of −20 °C in the freezer to the LC autosampler at 7 °C) prior to analysis. Perform MS analysis on samples.

3.5 Metabolite Extraction from Tissue Samples

1. Label new 1.5 mL bead-beater-safe tubes (such as Eppendorf™ Safe-lock tubes) and cool on the tube rack immersed in dry ice.
2. Quickly transfer tissue samples from −80 °C freezer to rack on dry ice. Prevent tissue samples from thawing.
3. Transfer tissue to pre-chilled, tared tube. Quickly weigh and record the mass of each tissue to the nearest 0.1 mg, then immediately return the tube to dry ice.
4. Add chilled extraction solution with applicable standard(s) to each tube to obtain a concentration of 15 mg tissue per mL of extraction solution (*see* **Notes 4** and **5**).
5. For powderized tissue: Proceed to **step 6**. For whole pieces of tissue: Add one scoop of glass beads (~50–75 μL of volume) to each sample and bead beat for 5 min at level 4 at 4 °C.
6. Vortex samples vigorously for 30 min at 4 °C.
7. Centrifuge for 10 min at 4 °C at 18,213 g (or maximum speed) to pellet insoluble material (*see* **Note 6**).
8. If extraction was performed at a concentration greater than 15 mg/mL (in **step 4**), dilute an aliquot of supernatant with the same chilled extraction solution used for initial extraction (containing standards if applicable) to obtain a concentration of 15 mg/mL. Then repeat **step 7**.
9. Transfer ~100 μL extract supernatant into labeled and cooled autosampler vials.
10. For use as a quality control, prepare a pooled sample of each biological matrix being analyzed by combining 10 μL of each extract supernatant into an autosampler vial. Aliquot size may be adjusted so that the final QC sample volume is sufficient for QC runs at the beginning, middle, and end of the sequence for both positive and negative ion polarity modes, or every 10–20 sample runs, depending on the size of the sample set. Remaining supernatants may be stored at −80 °C (*see* **Note 3**).
11. Prepare a blank sample by adding 100 μL of extraction solution from **step 4** into a new, labeled autosampler vial.
12. Ensure that the sample vials do not contain air bubbles and are kept cold (in the range of −20 °C in the freezer to the LC autosampler at 7 °C) prior to analysis.
13. Perform MS analysis on samples.

3.6 Metabolite Extraction from Cell Samples

1. Place sample tubes with frozen cells on dry ice.
2. Add ice-cold extraction solution with applicable standard(s) to each tube such that the final extraction concentration is 2×10^6 cells per mL of solution (*see* **Notes 7** and **8**).

3. Ensure the cell pellet is released from the tube into suspension and vortex samples vigorously for 30 min at 4 °C.
4. Centrifuge for 10 min at 18,213 g (or maximum speed) to pellet insoluble material.
5. Transfer ~100 μL extract supernatant into labeled and cooled autosampler vials.
6. For use as a quality control, prepare a pooled sample of each biological matrix being analyzed by combining 10 μL of each extract supernatant into an autosampler vial. Aliquot size may be adjusted so that the final QC sample volume is sufficient for QC runs at the beginning, middle, and end of the sequence for both positive and negative ion polarity modes, or every 10–20 sample runs, depending on the size of the sample set. Remaining supernatants may be stored at −80 °C (*see* **Note 3**).
7. Prepare a blank sample by adding 100 μL of extraction solution from **step 2** into a new, labeled autosampler vial.
8. Ensure that the sample vials do not contain air bubbles and are kept cold (in the range of −20 °C in the freezer to the LC autosampler at 7 °C) prior to analysis.
9. Perform MS analysis on samples.

3.7 UHPLC-MS Data Acquisition—Isocratic Method

1. Prepare an isocratic UHPLC-MS positive ion method with the following chromatography conditions: Flow rate 0.25 mL/min; solvent composition 95% A, 5% B from time zero until 3 min; column temperature 25 °C; sample compartment temperature 7 °C. Utilize a C18 column (method has been optimized for C18 column in Subheading 2.5) with a C18 guard column. Phases for positive mode should be supplemented with 0.1% (v/v) formic acid.
2. The mass spectrometry settings for this method are: resolution 70,000 (Q Exactive) or 60,000 (Q Exactive HF), scan range 65–900 m/z, maximum injection time 200 ms, 2 microscans, automatic gain control (AGC) 3×10^6 ions, ESI source voltage 4.0 kV, capillary temperature 320 °C, and sheath gas 15, auxiliary gas 5, and sweep gas 0 (all nitrogen, measured in arbitrary units). Optimal ESI or HESI gas and voltage parameters may be determined by observing signal intensity as settings are changed.
3. If applicable: Incorporate optimized gas and voltage settings into method.
4. Ensure polarity is set to positive and save method.
5. Prepare a method for negative mode isocratic runs by repeating the above steps with the following changes: Utilize negative ionization solvents supplemented with 1 mM NH_4OAc instead of formic acid, and set solvent composition to 100% A. Save negative mode method.

6. Prepare run sequence starting with several blank runs, 1–2 injections of QC sample, then randomized analytical samples with QC samples inserted every 10–20 runs. End with several blank runs before changing polarities (*see* **Note 9**).
7. Before beginning, ensure stable column back pressure, stable MS background signal, and the absence of air bubbles or leaks in the LC system.

3.8 UHPLC-MS Data Acquisition—Gradient Method

1. Prepare a 5-minute gradient UHPLC-MS positive ion method with the following chromatography conditions: Flow rate 0.45 mL/min; column temperature 45 °C; sample compartment temperature 7 °C. Solvent gradient: 0–0.5 min 5% B, 0.5–1.1 min 5–95% B, 1.1–2.75 min hold at 95% B, 2.75–3 min 95–5% B, 3–5 min hold at 5% B. Utilize a C18 column (method has been optimized for Kinetex C18 column) and a C18 guard column. Phases for positive mode should be supplemented with 0.1% (v/v) formic acid.
2. Add mass spectrometry settings to the gradient UHPLC-MS method: resolution 70,000 (Q Exactive) or 60,000 (Q Exactive HF), scan range 65–900 m/z, maximum injection time 200 ms, microscans 2, automatic gain control (AGC) 3×10^6 ions, source voltage 4.0 kV, capillary temperature 320 °C, and sheath gas 45, auxiliary gas 15, and sweep gas 0 (all nitrogen). Optimal ESI or HESI gas and voltage parameters may be determined by observing signal intensity as settings are changed.
4. If applicable: Incorporate optimized gas and voltage settings into method.
5. Ensure polarity is set to positive and save method.
6. Prepare a method for negative mode 5-minute gradient runs by repeating the above steps with the following changes: Utilize solvents supplemented with 1 mM NH_4OAc (instead of formic acid) to favor negative ionization. Solvent gradient: 0–0.5 min 0% B; 0.5–1.1 min 0–100% B, 1.1–2.75 min hold at 100% B, 2.75–3 min 100–0% B, 3–5 min hold at 0% B. Save negative mode method.
7. Prepare run sequence starting with several blank runs, 1–2 injections of the QC sample, then randomized analytical samples with QC samples inserted every 10–20 runs. End with several blank runs before changing polarities (*see* **Note 9**).
8. Before beginning, ensure stable column back pressure and MS background signal after the column temperature set point has been reached. Ensure also the absence of air bubbles or leaks in the LC system, and then run sequence.

3.9 Data Analysis

1. Quantify metabolite peak areas using the software of choice. We utilize El-Maven, which first requires file conversion from . raw to .mzXML (accomplished using RawConverter), and assign metabolite names using the KEGG or HMDB databases.
2. Utilize QC sample data to assess instrument performance and stability throughout analytical runs. Coefficients of variation (CV) for named metabolites should be <20%. If CV values are above this threshold while other readouts (pump pressure, total signal level, etc.) do not suggest technical issues with instrument performance, consider the use of a batch- or drift-correction software. When needed, we utilize the MetaboDrift normalization algorithms separately on positive and negative ion mode raw peak area data. Once the peak areas are appropriately normalized as needed for each polarity, the data can be merged for subsequent calculations and visualizations.
3. Use the ratio of peak areas for stable isotope-labeled standards and their unlabeled (light) counterparts to determine the absolute values of endogenous metabolites in the extract. Back-calculate the concentrations in the biological samples using the following equations:

For Biofluids:
$[\text{Light}] = (\text{Area}_{\text{light}}/\text{Area}_{\text{heavy}})[\text{Heavy}]*\text{DF}$

where DF is dilution factor- 10 for RBCs and blood, 25 for serum and plasma as described above (*see* **Note 10**).

For Tissues:
$[\text{Light}] = (\text{Area}_{\text{light}}/\text{Area}_{\text{heavy}})[\text{Heavy}]*1/\text{EC}$

where EC is extraction concentration, described here as 15 mg/mL (*see* **Note 11**).

For Cells:
$[\text{Light}] = (\text{Area}_{\text{light}}/\text{Area}_{\text{heavy}})[\text{Heavy}]*1/\text{EC}$

where EC is extraction concentration, described here as 2×10^6 cells/mL (*see* **Note 12**).

4 Notes

1. Experimentally determined reference ranges can be found by searching for the compound of interest in Human Metabolome Database (www.hmdb.ca) and clicking on the "Concentrations" table
2. Please note that, at this step, 100 uL of the extract could be dried down (e.g., under nitrogen flow or SpeedVac) prior to resuspension in an equal volume of pure water (with or without

0.1% formic acid or 10 mM ammonium acetate) or methanol. Though time consuming, this process can be automated in 96-well plate format and ensures significantly improved chromatographic retention of hydrophilic compounds in both the isocratic and gradient-based separations.

3. If/when saved extracts are retrieved for use, spin at max speed for 10 min at 4 °C before aliquoting to AS vial.
4. Tissue extraction method is optimized for 2–20 mg pieces of tissue (wet weight). For powdered tissues, weigh and extract in a similar manner, but skip the bead beating step.
5. If the sample mass is too large to accommodate the volume for 15 mg/mL (e.g., >20 mg), all samples may be extracted at an identical higher concentration and extracts diluted in **step 8** of this section.
6. When centrifuging samples in the presence of glass beads, the supernatant is not often fully clarified. A supernatant aliquot may be transferred to a new tube and respun to ensure complete isolation of insoluble material.
7. The cell extraction concentration of 2×10^6 cells/mL is optimized for average sized eukaryotic cells. Extraction of metabolites from cells with significantly smaller diameters (e.g., T cells, neurons, bacteria) is best performed at higher concentrations.
8. If cell counts are approximated and/or imprecise, the insoluble protein pellet remaining after metabolite extraction may be dissolved in an appropriate chaotrope (e.g., 8 M urea) and quantified by the Bradford or BCA assay for *post-hoc* data normalization.
9. We recommend collecting all data in one polarity mode, then switching to the other to minimize issues with column equilibration. With a sufficient number of blanks to ensure column equilibration when switching modes and solvents, the instrumentation can run continuously under automation.
10. The concentration of the heavy standard utilized here is the final concentration in the extraction. For example, if the extraction solution contains 1 μM of standard and 20 μL of sample is mixed with 180 μL of extraction solution, the resulting concentration of heavy standard would be 0.9 μM.
11. If the concentration of heavy standard is entered in μM units and the concentration of tissue extraction is measured in mg/mL, then the resulting concentration of light (endogenous metabolite) will be in units of μmol of metabolite per mg of tissue.
12. If the concentration of heavy standard is entered in μM units and the concentration of cells in extraction is measured in cells/mL, then the resulting concentration of light (endogenous metabolite) will be in units of μmol of metabolite per cell.

Conflict of Interest

AD and TN are co-founders of Omix Technologies, Inc., and members of the Scientific Advisory Board for Hemanext, Inc. The authors declare that TN and AD are founders of Omix Technologies Inc.

References

1. Nemkov T et al (2019) High-throughput metabolomics: isocratic and gradient mass spectrometry-based methods. Methods Mol Biol 1978:13–26. https://doi.org/10.1007/978-1-4939-9236-2_2
2. Nemkov T, Hansen KC, D'Alessandro A (2017) A three-minute method for high-throughput quantitative metabolomics and quantitative tracing experiments of central carbon and nitrogen pathways. Rapid Commun Mass Spectrom 31(8):663–673. https://doi.org/10.1002/rcm.7834
3. D'Alessandro A et al (2015) An update on red blood cell storage lesions, as gleaned through biochemistry and omics technologies. Transfusion 55(1):205–219. https://doi.org/10.1111/trf.12804
4. Yoshida T, Prudent M, D'Alessandro A (2019) Red blood cell storage lesion: causes and potential clinical consequences. Blood Transfus 17(1):27–52. https://doi.org/10.2450/2019.0217-18
5. Hess JR, D'Alessandro A (2022) Red blood cell metabolism and preservation. In: Rossi's principles of transfusion medicine, pp 143–157
6. Isiksacan Z et al (2023) Assessment of stored red blood cells through lab-on-a-chip technologies for precision transfusion medicine. Proc Natl Acad Sci 120(32):e2115616120. https://doi.org/10.1073/pnas.2115616120
7. D'Alessandro A, Dzieciatkowska M, Hill RC, Hansen KC (2016) Supernatant protein biomarkers of red blood cell storage hemolysis as determined through an absolute quantification proteomics technology. Transfusion 56(6):1329–1339. https://doi.org/10.1111/trf.13483
8. D'Alessandro A et al (2015) Routine storage of red blood cell (RBC) units in additive solution-3: a comprehensive investigation of the RBC metabolome. Transfusion 55(6): 1155–1168. https://doi.org/10.1111/trf.12975
9. D'Alessandro A et al (2018) Metabolic effect of alkaline additives and guanosine/gluconate in storage solutions for red blood cells. Transfusion 58(8):1992–2002. https://doi.org/10.1111/trf.14620
10. D'Alessandro A et al (2015) Red blood cell storage in additive solution-7 preserves energy and redox metabolism: a metabolomics approach. Transfusion 55(12): 2955–2966. https://doi.org/10.1111/trf.13253
11. D'Alessandro A et al (2017) Citrate metabolism in red blood cells stored in additive solution-3. Transfusion 57(2):325–336. https://doi.org/10.1111/trf.13892
12. D'Alessandro A et al (2015) Metabolomics of AS-5 RBC supernatants following routine storage. Vox Sang 108(2):131–140. https://doi.org/10.1111/vox.12193
13. D'Alessandro A, D'Amici GM, Vaglio S, Zolla L (2012) Time-course investigation of SAGM-stored leukocyte-filtered red bood cell concentrates: from metabolism to proteomics. Haematologica 97(1):107–115. https://doi.org/10.3324/haematol.2011.051789
14. D'Alessandro A et al (2018) Metabolic effect of alkaline additives and guanosine/gluconate in storage solutions for red blood cells. Transfusion. https://doi.org/10.1111/trf.14620
15. D'Alessandro A et al (2017) Red blood cell metabolic responses to refrigerated storage, rejuvenation, and frozen storage. Transfusion 57(4):1019–1030. https://doi.org/10.1111/trf.14034
16. Donovan K et al (2022) Stored blood has compromised oxygen unloading kinetics that can be normalized with rejuvenation and predicted from corpuscular side-scatter. Haematologica 107(1):298–302. https://doi.org/10.3324/haematol.2021.279296
17. Nemkov T et al (2018) Hypoxia modulates the purine salvage pathway and decreases red blood cell and supernatant levels of hypoxanthine during refrigerated storage.

Haematologica 103(2):361–372. https://doi.org/10.3324/haematol.2017.178608
18. Nemkov T et al (2017) Metabolism of citrate and other carboxylic acids in erythrocytes as a function of oxygen saturation and refrigerated storage. Front Med (Lausanne) 4:175. https://doi.org/10.3389/fmed.2017.00175
19. D'Alessandro A et al (2020) Hypoxic storage of red blood cells improves metabolism and post-transfusion recovery. Transfusion 60(4): 786–798. https://doi.org/10.1111/trf.15730
20. Paglia G et al (2016) Biomarkers defining the metabolic age of red blood cells during cold storage. Blood 128(13):e43–e50. https://doi.org/10.1182/blood-2016-06-721688
21. D'Alessandro A et al (2017) Omics markers of the red cell storage lesion and metabolic linkage. Blood Transfus 15(2):137–144. https://doi.org/10.2450/2017.0341-16
22. D'Alessandro A et al (2021) Donor sex, age and ethnicity impact stored red blood cell antioxidant metabolism through mechanisms in part explained by glucose 6-phosphate dehydrogenase levels and activity. Haematologica 106(5):1290–1302. https://doi.org/10.3324/haematol.2020.246603
23. Francis RO et al (2020) Donor glucose-6-phosphate dehydrogenase deficiency decreases blood quality for transfusion. J Clin Invest 130(5):2270–2285. https://doi.org/10.1172/jci133530
24. Francis RO et al (2019) Reexamination of the chromium-51-labeled posttransfusion red blood cell recovery method. Transfusion 59(7):2264–2275. https://doi.org/10.1111/trf.15310
25. Nemkov T et al (2024) Genetic regulation of carnitine metabolism controls lipid damage repair and aging RBC hemolysis in vivo and in vitro. Blood. https://doi.org/10.1182/blood.2024023983
26. Nemkov T et al (2024) Regulation of kynurenine metabolism by blood donor genetics and biology impacts red cell hemolysis in vitro and in vivo. Blood 143(5):456–472. https://doi.org/10.1182/blood.2023022052
27. Nemkov T et al (2022) Mirages – REDS explorer: an online portal for longitudinal metabolomics data from the REDS-III RBC Omics Study. Blood 140(Supplement 1): 5713–5714. https://doi.org/10.1182/blood-2022-160274
28. Hay AM et al (2022) S1P has a negative effect on RBC storage quality. Blood Adv. https://doi.org/10.1182/bloodadvances.2022008936
29. Moore A et al (2022) Genome-wide metabolite quantitative trait loci analysis (mQTL) in red blood cells from volunteer blood donors. J Biol Chem 298(12):102706. https://doi.org/10.1016/j.jbc.2022.102706
30. Thomas T et al (2021) Fatty acid desaturase activity in mature red blood cells and implications for blood storage quality. Transfusion 61(6):1867–1883. https://doi.org/10.1111/trf.16402
31. Nemkov T et al (2024) Biological and genetic determinants of glycolysis: phosphofructokinase isoforms boost energy status of stored red blood cells and transfusion outcomes. Cell Metab . 2024 Sep 3;36(9):1979–1997.e13. https://doi.org/10.1016/j.cmet.2024.06.007
32. Howie HL et al (2019) Differences in Steap3 expression are a mechanism of genetic variation of RBC storage and oxidative damage in mice. Blood Adv 3(15):2272–2285. https://doi.org/10.1182/bloodadvances.2019000605
33. D'Alessandro A et al (2025) Ferroptosis regulates hemolysis in stored murine and human red blood cells. Blood; 145(7):765-783. https://doi.org/10.1182/blood.2024026109
34. Issaian A et al (2021) The interactome of the N-terminus of band 3 regulates red blood cell metabolism and storage quality. Haematologica. https://doi.org/10.3324/haematol.2020.278252
35. Rogers SC et al (2021) Quantifying dynamic range in red blood cell energetics: evidence of progressive energy failure during storage. Transfusion 61(5):1586–1599. https://doi.org/10.1111/trf.16395
36. Dziewulska-Cronk K et al (2023) Mechanisms of Primaquine induced hemolysis in a novel humanized murine model of Mediterranean G6PD deficiency. Blood 142:1070. https://doi.org/10.1182/blood-2023-178739
37. Jacob C et al (2022) Mediterranean G6PD variant mitigates expression of DNA methyltransferases and right heart pressure in experimental model of pulmonary hypertension. J Biol Chem. https://doi.org/10.1016/j.jbc.2022.102691
38. Tzounakas VL et al (2022) Red cell proteasome modulation by storage, redox metabolism and transfusion. Blood Transfus 20(1): 27–39. https://doi.org/10.2450/2020.0179-20

39. D'Alessandro A et al (2021) Hematologic and systemic metabolic alterations due to Mediterranean class II G6PD deficiency in mice. JCI. Insight 6(14). https://doi.org/10.1172/jci.insight.147056
40. Wang L et al (2024) Functional effects of an African glucose-6-phosphate dehydrogenase (G6PD) polymorphism (Val68Met) on red blood cell hemolytic propensity and post-transfusion recovery. Transfusion 64(4): 615–626. https://doi.org/10.1111/trf.17756
41. D'Alessandro A et al (2021) Protein-L-isoaspartate O-methyltransferase is required for in vivo control of oxidative damage in red blood cells. Haematologica 106(10): 2726–2739. https://doi.org/10.3324/haematol.2020.266676
42. Reisz JA et al (2018) Methylation of protein aspartates and deamidated asparagines as a function of blood bank storage and oxidative stress in human red blood cells. Transfusion 58(12):2978–2991. https://doi.org/10.1111/trf.14936
43. D'Alessandro A, Xia Y (2020) Erythrocyte adaptive metabolic reprogramming under physiological and pathological hypoxia. Curr Opin Hematol 27(3):155–162. https://doi.org/10.1097/moh.0000000000000574
44. Tzounakas VL et al (2016) Glucose 6-phosphate dehydrogenase deficient subjects may be better "storers" than donors of red blood cells. Free Radic Biol Med 96:152–165. https://doi.org/10.1016/j.freeradbiomed.2016.04.005
45. Tzounakas VL et al (2016) Data on how several physiological parameters of stored red blood cells are similar in glucose 6-phosphate dehydrogenase deficient and sufficient donors. Data Brief 8:618–627. https://doi.org/10.1016/j.dib.2016.06.018
46. Mykhailova O et al (2020) Donor-dependent aging of young and old red blood cell subpopulations: metabolic and functional heterogeneity. Transfusion 60(11):2633–2646. https://doi.org/10.1111/trf.16017
47. Nemkov T, Qadri SM, Sheffield WP, D'Alessandro A (2020) Decoding the metabolic landscape of pathophysiological stress-induced cell death in anucleate red blood cells. Blood Transfus 18(2):130–142. https://doi.org/10.2450/2020.0256-19
48. D'Alessandro A et al (2020) Ethyl glucuronide, a marker of alcohol consumption, correlates with metabolic markers of oxidant stress but not with hemolysis in stored red blood cells from healthy blood donors. Transfusion 60(6):1183–1196. https://doi.org/10.1111/trf.15811
49. D'Alessandro A et al (2020) Stored RBC metabolism as a function of caffeine levels. Transfusion 60(6):1197–1211. https://doi.org/10.1111/trf.15813
50. Stefanoni D et al (2020) Nicotine exposure increases markers of oxidant stress in stored red blood cells from healthy donor volunteers. Transfusion 60(6):1160–1174. https://doi.org/10.1111/trf.15812
51. Kim CY et al (2022) Deuterated linoleic acid attenuates the RBC storage lesion in a mouse model of poor RBC storage. Front Physiol 13:868578. https://doi.org/10.3389/fphys.2022.868578
52. Catala A, Stone M, Busch MP, D'Alessandro A (2022) Reprogramming of red blood cell metabolism in Zika virus-infected donors. Transfusion 62(5):1045–1064. https://doi.org/10.1111/trf.16851
53. Thomas T et al (2020) COVID-19 infection alters kynurenine and fatty acid metabolism, correlating with IL-6 levels and renal status. JCI. Insight 5(14). https://doi.org/10.1172/jci.insight.140327
54. Recktenwald SM et al (2022) Cross-talk between red blood cells and plasma influences blood flow and omics phenotypes in severe COVID-19. medRxiv:2022.2003.2031.22273226. https://doi.org/10.1101/2022.03.31.22273226
55. Roubinian NH et al (2019) Effect of donor, component, and recipient characteristics on hemoglobin increments following red blood cell transfusion. Blood 134(13):1003–1013. https://doi.org/10.1182/blood.2019000773
56. Roubinian NH et al (2022) Donor genetic and nongenetic factors affecting red blood cell transfusion effectiveness. JCI Insight 7(1). https://doi.org/10.1172/jci.insight.152598
57. D'Alessandro A, Zimring JC, Busch M (2019) Chronological storage age and metabolic age of stored red blood cells: are they the same? Transfusion 59(5):1620–1623. https://doi.org/10.1111/trf.15248
58. D'Alessandro A et al (2019) Effects of aged stored autologous red blood cells on human plasma metabolome. Blood Adv 3(6): 884–896. https://doi.org/10.1182/bloodadvances.2018029629
59. LaCroix IS et al (2022) Omics markers of red blood cell transfusion in trauma. Int J Mol Sci 23(22). https://doi.org/10.3390/ijms232213815

60. Swift LM et al (2023) Evidence for the cardiodepressive effects of the plasticizer di-2-ethylhexyl phthalate. Toxicol Sci. 197(1): 79–94.https://doi.org/10.1093/toxsci/kfad105
61. Culp-Hill R et al (2018) Effects of red blood cell (RBC) transfusion on sickle cell disease recipient plasma and RBC metabolism. Transfusion 58(12):2797–2806. https://doi.org/10.1111/trf.14931
62. Gehrke S et al (2018) Metabolomics evaluation of early-storage red blood cell rejuvenation at 4 degrees C and 37 degrees C. Transfusion 58(8):1980–1991. https://doi.org/10.1111/trf.14623
63. Rabcuka J et al (2022) Metabolic reprogramming under hypoxic storage preserves faster oxygen unloading from stored red blood cells. Blood Adv 6(18):5415–5428. https://doi.org/10.1182/bloodadvances.2022007774
64. de Bruin S et al (2022) Storage of red blood cells in alkaline PAGGGM improves metabolism but has no effect on recovery after transfusion. Blood Adv 6(13):3899–3910. https://doi.org/10.1182/bloodadvances.2022006987
65. Nemkov T, Yoshida T, Nikulina M, D'Alessandro A (2022) High-throughput metabolomics platform for the rapid data-driven development of novel additive solutions for blood storage. Front Physiol 13. https://doi.org/10.3389/fphys.2022.833242
66. D'Alessandro A (2023) Red blood cell omics and machine learning in transfusion medicine: singularity is near. Transfus Med Hemother:1–10. https://doi.org/10.1159/000529744
67. D'Alessandro A, Hod EA (2023) Red blood cell storage: from genome to Exposome towards personalized transfusion medicine. Transfus Med Rev 37(4):150750. https://doi.org/10.1016/j.tmrv.2023.150750
68. D'Alessandro A et al (2015) Trauma/hemorrhagic shock instigates aberrant metabolic flux through glycolytic pathways, as revealed by preliminary (13)C-glucose labeling metabolomics. J Transl Med 13:253. https://doi.org/10.1186/s12967-015-0612-z
69. Slaughter AL et al (2016) Glutamine metabolism drives succinate accumulation in plasma and the lung during hemorrhagic shock. J Trauma Acute Care Surg 81(6):1012–1019. https://doi.org/10.1097/ta.0000000000001256
70. Cralley AL et al (2022) Zone 1 REBOA in a combat DCBI swine model does not worsen brain injury. Surgery 172(2):751–758. https://doi.org/10.1016/j.surg.2022.04.055
71. D'Alessandro A et al (2016) Plasma first resuscitation reduces lactate acidosis, enhances redox homeostasis, amino acid and purine catabolism in a rat model of profound hemorrhagic shock. Shock 46(2):173–182. https://doi.org/10.1097/shk.0000000000000588
72. Henriksen HH et al (2020) Metabolic systems analysis of shock-induced Endotheliopathy (SHINE) in trauma: a new research paradigm. Ann Surg 272(6):1140–1148. https://doi.org/10.1097/sla.0000000000003307
73. Nunns GR et al (2020) Succinate activation of SUCNR1 predisposes severely injured patients to neutrophil-mediated ARDS. Ann Surg. https://doi.org/10.1097/sla.0000000000004644
74. Reisz JA et al (2017) Red blood cells in hemorrhagic shock: a critical role for glutaminolysis in fueling alanine transamination in rats. Blood Adv 1(17):1296–1305. https://doi.org/10.1182/bloodadvances.2017007187
75. Slaughter AL et al (2018) The Metabolopathy of tissue injury, hemorrhagic shock, and resuscitation in a rat model. Shock 49(5):580–590. https://doi.org/10.1097/shk.0000000000000948
76. Wiener G et al (2015) Shock releases bile acid inducing platelet inhibition and fibrinolysis. J Surg Res 195(2):390–395. https://doi.org/10.1016/j.jss.2015.01.046
77. Williams AT et al (2020) Transfusion of anaerobically or conventionally stored blood after hemorrhagic shock. Shock 53(3):352–362. https://doi.org/10.1097/shk.0000000000001386
78. Banerjee A et al (2018) Systemic hyperfibrinolysis after trauma: a pilot study of targeted proteomic analysis of superposed mechanisms in patient plasma. J Trauma Acute Care Surg 84(6):929–938. https://doi.org/10.1097/ta.0000000000001878
79. Clendenen N et al (2017) Hemorrhagic shock and tissue injury drive distinct plasma metabolome derangements in swine. J Trauma Acute Care Surg 83(4):635
80. Coleman JR et al (2019) Female platelets have distinct functional activity compared with male platelets: implications in transfusion practice and treatment of trauma-induced coagulopathy. J Trauma Acute Care Surg 87(5):1052–1060. https://doi.org/10.1097/ta.0000000000002398

81. Peltz ED et al (2015) Pathologic metabolism: an exploratory study of the plasma metabolome of critical injury. J Trauma Acute Care Surg 78(4):742–751. https://doi.org/10.1097/ta.0000000000000589
82. Bertolone L et al (2020) ZOOMICS: comparative metabolomics of red blood cells from Old World monkeys and humans. Front Physiol 11:593841. https://doi.org/10.3389/fphys.2020.593841
83. Bertolone L et al (2022) ZOOMICS: comparative metabolomics of red blood cells from Guinea pigs, humans, and non-human primates during refrigerated storage for up to 42 days. Front Physiol 13:845347. https://doi.org/10.3389/fphys.2022.845347
84. Miglio A et al (2022) ZOOMICS: comparative metabolomics of red blood cells from dogs, cows, horses and donkeys during refrigerated storage for up to 42 days. Blood Transfus. https://doi.org/10.2450/2022.0118-22
85. Stefanoni D et al (2020) Red blood cell metabolism in rhesus macaques and humans: comparative biology of blood storage. Haematologica 105(8):2174–2186. https://doi.org/10.3324/haematol.2019.229930
86. Miglio A et al (2024) Effect of leukoreduction on the metabolism of equine packed red blood cells during refrigerated storage. J Vet Intern Med. https://doi.org/10.1111/jvim.17015
87. Miglio A et al (2024) Effect of leukoreduction on the omics phenotypes of canine packed red blood cells during refrigerated storage. J Vet Intern Med. https://doi.org/10.1111/jvim.17031
88. Hadley JB et al (2021) Testosterone, age, and sex affect platelet responsiveness in vitro. J Am Coll Surg 233(5):e208–e209. https://doi.org/10.1016/j.jamcollsurg.2021.08.564
89. Nunns GR et al (2020) Succinate activation of SUCNR1 predisposes severely injured patients to neutrophil-mediated ARDS. Ann Surg. https://doi.org/10.1097/SLA.0000000000004644
90. D'Alessandro A et al (2016) Metabolomics of trauma-associated death: shared and fluid-specific features of human plasma vs lymph. Blood Transfus 14(2):185–194. https://doi.org/10.2450/2016.0208-15
91. Buehler PW et al (2021) Murine models of sickle cell disease and beta-thalassemia demonstrate pulmonary hypertension with distinctive features. Pulm Circ 11(4): 20458940211055996. https://doi.org/10.1177/20458940211055996
92. Gehrke S et al (2019) Metabolic impact of red blood cell exchange with rejuvenated red blood cells in sickle cell patients. Transfusion 59(10):3102–3112. https://doi.org/10.1111/trf.15467
93. Moriconi C et al (2022) Retention of functional mitochondria in mature red blood cells from patients with sickle cell disease. Br J Haematol 198(3):574–586. https://doi.org/10.1111/bjh.18287
94. Nemkov T et al (2022) Plasma levels of acylcarnitines and carboxylic acids correlate with cardiovascular and kidney function in subjects with sickle cell trait. Front Physiol 13: 916197. https://doi.org/10.3389/fphys.2022.916197
95. Song A et al (2022) p97 dysfunction underlies a loss of quality control of damaged membrane proteins and promotes oxidative stress and sickling in sickle cell disease. FASEB J 36(5):e22246. https://doi.org/10.1096/fj.202101500RR
96. Sun K et al (2017) Structural and functional insight of sphingosine 1-phosphate-mediated pathogenic metabolic reprogramming in sickle cell disease. Sci Rep 7(1):15281. https://doi.org/10.1038/s41598-017-13667-8
97. Unali G et al (2023) Interferon-inducible phospholipids govern IFITM3-dependent endosomal antiviral immunity. EMBO J 42(10):e112234. https://doi.org/10.15252/embj.2022112234
98. Setua S et al (2022) Coagulation potential and the integrated omics of extracellular vesicles from COVID-19 positive patient plasma. Sci Rep 12(1):22191. https://doi.org/10.1038/s41598-022-26473-8
99. Recktenwald SM et al (2022) Cross-talk between red blood cells and plasma influences blood flow and omics phenotypes in severe COVID-19. eLife 11:e81316. https://doi.org/10.7554/eLife.81316
100. D'Alessandro A et al (2021) Biological and clinical factors contributing to the metabolic heterogeneity of hospitalized patients with and without COVID-19. Cells 10(9). https://doi.org/10.3390/cells10092293
101. Galbraith MD et al (2021) Seroconversion stages COVID19 into distinct pathophysiological states. elife 10. https://doi.org/10.7554/eLife.65508
102. Sullivan KD et al (2021) The COVIDome explorer researcher portal. Cell Rep 36(7): 109527. https://doi.org/10.1016/j.celrep.2021.109527

103. Thangaraju K et al (2021) The impact of age and BMI on the VWF/ADAMTS13 Axis and simultaneous thrombin and plasmin generation in hospitalized COVID-19 patients. Front Med (Lausanne) 8:817305. https://doi.org/10.3389/fmed.2021.817305
104. D'Alessandro A et al (2020) Serum proteomics in COVID-19 patients: altered coagulation and complement status as a function of IL-6 level. J Proteome Res. https://doi.org/10.1021/acs.jproteome.0c00365
105. Thomas T et al (2020) Evidence for structural protein damage and membrane lipid remodeling in red blood cells from COVID-19 patients. medRxiv. https://doi.org/10.1101/2020.06.29.20142703
106. Nemkov T et al (2021) Acute cycling exercise induces changes in red blood cell deformability and membrane lipid remodeling. Int J Mol Sci 22(2). https://doi.org/10.3390/ijms22020896
107. San-Millan I et al (2020) Metabolomics of endurance capacity in world tour professional cyclists. Front Physiol 11:578. https://doi.org/10.3389/fphys.2020.00578
108. Nemkov T et al (2023) Metabolic signatures of performance in elite world tour professional male cyclists. Sports Med 53(8):1651–1665. https://doi.org/10.1007/s40279-023-01846-9
109. D'Alessandro A et al (2016) AltitudeOmics: red blood cell metabolic adaptation to high altitude hypoxia. J Proteome Res 15(10):3883–3895. https://doi.org/10.1021/acs.jproteome.6b00733
110. Liu H et al (2016) Beneficial role of erythrocyte adenosine A2B receptor-mediated AMP-activated protein kinase activation in high-altitude hypoxia. Circulation 134(5):405–421. https://doi.org/10.1161/CIRCULATIONAHA.116.021311
111. Song A et al (2017) Erythrocytes retain hypoxic adenosine response for faster acclimatization upon re-ascent. Nat Commun 8:14108. https://doi.org/10.1038/ncomms14108
112. Xu P et al (2022) Erythrocyte transglutaminase-2 combats hypoxia and chronic kidney disease by promoting oxygen delivery and carnitine homeostasis. Cell Metab 34(2):299–316.e296. https://doi.org/10.1016/j.cmet.2021.12.019
113. D'Alessandro A et al (2024) Genetic polymorphisms and expression of rhesus blood group RHCE are associated with 2,3-bisphosphoglycerate in humans at high altitude. Proc Natl Acad Sci USA 121(1):e2315930120. https://doi.org/10.1073/pnas.2315930120
114. Adane B et al (2019) The hematopoietic oxidase NOX2 regulates self-renewal of leukemic stem cells. Cell Rep 27(1):238–254.e236. https://doi.org/10.1016/j.celrep.2019.03.009
115. Amaya ML et al (2022) The STAT3-MYC axis promotes survival of leukemia stem cells by regulating SLC1A5 and oxidative phosphorylation. Blood 139(4):584–596. https://doi.org/10.1182/blood.2021013201
116. Gregory MA et al (2016) ATM/G6PD-driven redox metabolism promotes FLT3 inhibitor resistance in acute myeloid leukemia. Proc Natl Acad Sci USA 113(43):E6669–e6678. https://doi.org/10.1073/pnas.1603876113
117. Gregory MA et al (2019) Targeting glutamine metabolism and redox state for leukemia therapy. Clin Cancer Res 25(13):4079–4090. https://doi.org/10.1158/1078-0432.Ccr-18-3223
118. Gregory MA et al (2018) Glutaminase inhibition improves FLT3 inhibitor therapy for acute myeloid leukemia. Exp Hematol 58:52–58. https://doi.org/10.1016/j.exphem.2017.09.007
119. Jones CL et al (2019) Cysteine depletion targets leukemia stem cells through inhibition of electron transport complex II. Blood 134(4):389–394. https://doi.org/10.1182/blood.2019898114
120. Jones CL et al (2018) Inhibition of amino acid metabolism selectively targets human leukemia stem cells. Cancer Cell 34(5):724–740.e724. https://doi.org/10.1016/j.ccell.2018.10.005
121. Jones CL et al (2019) Inhibition of amino acid metabolism selectively targets human leukemia stem cells. Cancer Cell 35(2):333–335. https://doi.org/10.1016/j.ccell.2019.01.013
122. Jones CL et al (2020) Nicotinamide metabolism mediates resistance to Venetoclax in relapsed acute myeloid leukemia stem cells. Cell Stem Cell 27(5):748–764.e744. https://doi.org/10.1016/j.stem.2020.07.021
123. Joshi SK et al (2021) The AML microenvironment catalyzes a stepwise evolution to gilteritinib resistance. Cancer Cell 39(7):999–1014.e1018. https://doi.org/10.1016/j.ccell.2021.06.003
124. Nechiporuk T et al (2019) The TP53 apoptotic network is a primary mediator of resistance to BCL2 inhibition in AML cells. Cancer Discov 9(7):910–925. https://doi.org/10.1158/2159-8290.Cd-19-0125

125. Patel SB et al (2021) Metabolic alterations mediated by STAT3 promotes drug persistence in CML. Leukemia 35(12):3371–3382. https://doi.org/10.1038/s41375-021-01315-0
126. Pei S et al (2016) Rational design of a parthenolide-based drug regimen that selectively eradicates acute myelogenous leukemia stem cells. J Biol Chem 291(48):25280. https://doi.org/10.1074/jbc.A116.750653
127. Pei S et al (2020) Monocytic subclones confer resistance to Venetoclax-based therapy in patients with acute myeloid leukemia. Cancer Discov 10(4):536–551. https://doi.org/10.1158/2159-8290.Cd-19-0710
128. Pollyea DA et al (2018) Venetoclax with azacitidine disrupts energy metabolism and targets leukemia stem cells in patients with acute myeloid leukemia. Nat Med 24(12):1859–1866. https://doi.org/10.1038/s41591-018-0233-1
129. Roma A et al (2022) Glutamine metabolism mediates sensitivity to respiratory complex II inhibition in acute myeloid leukemia. Mol Cancer Res 20(11):1659–1673. https://doi.org/10.1158/1541-7786.Mcr-21-1032
130. Stevens BM et al (2020) Fatty acid metabolism underlies venetoclax resistance in acute myeloid leukemia stem cells. Nat Cancer 1(12):1176–1187. https://doi.org/10.1038/s43018-020-00126-z
131. Stevens BM et al (2018) Characterization and targeting of malignant stem cells in patients with advanced myelodysplastic syndromes. Nat Commun 9(1):3694. https://doi.org/10.1038/s41467-018-05984-x
132. Subedi A et al (2021) Nicotinamide phosphoribosyltransferase inhibitors selectively induce apoptosis of AML stem cells by disrupting lipid homeostasis. Cell Stem Cell 28(10):1851–1867.e1858. https://doi.org/10.1016/j.stem.2021.06.004
133. Tcheng M et al (2021) Very long chain fatty acid metabolism is required in acute myeloid leukemia. Blood 137(25):3518–3532. https://doi.org/10.1182/blood.2020008551
134. Yan D et al (2021) SIRT5 is a DRUGGABLE metabolic vulnerability in acute myeloid leukemia. Blood Cancer Discov 2(3):266–287. https://doi.org/10.1158/2643-3230.Bcd-20-0168
135. Ye H et al (2021) The hepatic microenvironment uniquely protects leukemia cells through induction of growth and survival pathways mediated by LIPG. Cancer Discov 11(2):500–519. https://doi.org/10.1158/2159-8290.Cd-20-0318
136. Zhang C et al (2018) KLF5 controls glutathione metabolism to suppress p190-BCR-ABL + B-cell lymphoblastic leukemia. Oncotarget 9(51):29665–29679. https://doi.org/10.18632/oncotarget.25667
137. Bissinger R et al (2021) Proteinuric chronic kidney disease is associated with altered red blood cell lifespan, deformability and metabolism. Kidney Int 100(6):1227–1239. https://doi.org/10.1016/j.kint.2021.08.024
138. Kalani Roy M et al (2022) Irradiation causes alterations of polyamine, purine, and sulfur metabolism in red blood cells and multiple organs. J Proteome Res 21(2):519–534. https://doi.org/10.1021/acs.jproteome.1c00912
139. Xie T et al (2020) Erythrocyte metabolic reprogramming by sphingosine 1-phosphate in chronic kidney disease and therapies. Circ Res 127(3):360–375. https://doi.org/10.1161/circresaha.119.316298
140. Fox BM et al (2019) Metabolomics assessment reveals oxidative stress and altered energy production in the heart after ischemic acute kidney injury in mice. Kidney Int 95(3):590–610. https://doi.org/10.1016/j.kint.2018.10.020
141. Lonnemann N et al (2020) The NLRP3 inflammasome inhibitor OLT1177 rescues cognitive impairment in a mouse model of Alzheimer's disease. Proc Natl Acad Sci USA 117(50):32145–32154. https://doi.org/10.1073/pnas.2009680117
142. Traxler L et al (2022) Warburg-like metabolic transformation underlies neuronal degeneration in sporadic Alzheimer's disease. Cell Metab 34(9):1248–1263.e1246. https://doi.org/10.1016/j.cmet.2022.07.014
143. Qiang Q et al (2021) Erythrocyte adenosine A2B receptor prevents cognitive and auditory dysfunction by promoting hypoxic and metabolic reprogramming. PLoS Biol 19(6):e3001239. https://doi.org/10.1371/journal.pbio.3001239
144. Anderson CC et al (2021) Maneb alters central carbon metabolism and thiol redox status in a toxicant model of Parkinson's disease. Free Radic Biol Med 162:65–76. https://doi.org/10.1016/j.freeradbiomed.2020.11.028
145. Peruzzotti-Jametti L et al (2024) Mitochondrial complex I activity in microglia sustains neuroinflammation. Nature 628(8006):

195–203. https://doi.org/10.1038/s41586-024-07167-9
146. Leone MA et al (2023) Phase I clinical trial of intracerebroventricular transplantation of allogeneic neural stem cells in people with progressive multiple sclerosis. Cell Stem Cell 30(12):1597–1609.e1598. https://doi.org/10.1016/j.stem.2023.11.001
147. D'Alessandro A et al (2017) Comfortably numb and Back: plasma metabolomics reveals biochemical adaptations in the hibernating 13-lined ground squirrel. J Proteome Res 16(2):958–969. https://doi.org/10.1021/acs.jproteome.6b00884
148. Gehrke S et al (2019) Red blood cell metabolic responses to torpor and arousal in the hibernator Arctic ground squirrel. J Proteome Res 18(4):1827–1841. https://doi.org/10.1021/acs.jproteome.9b00018
149. Rice SA et al (2020) Nitrogen recycling buffers against ammonia toxicity from skeletal muscle breakdown in hibernating arctic ground squirrels. Nat Metab 2(12):1459–1471. https://doi.org/10.1038/s42255-020-00312-4
150. Caruso P et al (2017) Identification of MicroRNA-124 as a major regulator of enhanced endothelial cell glycolysis in pulmonary arterial hypertension via PTBP1 (Polypyrimidine tract binding protein) and pyruvate kinase M2. Circulation 136(25):2451–2467. https://doi.org/10.1161/circulationaha.117.028034
151. D'Alessandro A et al (2018) Hallmarks of pulmonary hypertension: mesenchymal and inflammatory cell metabolic reprogramming. Antioxid Redox Signal 28(3):230–250. https://doi.org/10.1089/ars.2017.7217
152. Graham BB et al (2018) Vascular adaptation of the right ventricle in experimental pulmonary hypertension. Am J Respir Cell Mol Biol 59(4):479–489. https://doi.org/10.1165/rcmb.2018-0095OC
153. Joshi SR et al (2020) Hypoxic activation of glucose-6-phosphate dehydrogenase controls the expression of genes involved in the pathogenesis of pulmonary hypertension through the regulation of DNA methylation. Am J Physiol Lung Cell Mol Physiol 318(4):L773–l786. https://doi.org/10.1152/ajplung.00001.2020
154. Kumar S et al (2021) Complement-containing small extracellular vesicles from adventitial fibroblasts induce pro-inflammatory and metabolic reprogramming in macrophages. JCI Insight. https://doi.org/10.1172/jci.insight.148382
155. Li M et al (2021) Microenvironmental regulation of macrophage transcriptomic and Metabolomic profiles in pulmonary hypertension. Front Immunol 12:640718. https://doi.org/10.3389/fimmu.2021.640718
156. Li M et al (2016) Metabolic reprogramming regulates the proliferative and inflammatory phenotype of adventitial fibroblasts in pulmonary hypertension through the transcriptional corepressor C-terminal binding Protein-1. Circulation 134(15):1105–1121. https://doi.org/10.1161/circulationaha.116.023171
157. Plecitá-Hlavatá L et al (2017) Metabolic reprogramming and redox signaling in pulmonary hypertension. Adv Exp Med Biol 967:241–260. https://doi.org/10.1007/978-3-319-63245-2_14
158. Plecitá-Hlavatá L et al (2016) Constitutive reprogramming of fibroblast mitochondrial metabolism in pulmonary hypertension. Am J Respir Cell Mol Biol 55(1):47–57. https://doi.org/10.1165/rcmb.2015-0142OC
159. Zhang H et al (2017) Metabolic and proliferative state of vascular adventitial fibroblasts in pulmonary hypertension is regulated through a MicroRNA-124/PTBP1 (Polypyrimidine tract binding protein 1)/pyruvate kinase muscle Axis. Circulation 136(25):2468–2485. https://doi.org/10.1161/circulationaha.117.028069
160. Dong S et al (2021) Chaperone-mediated autophagy sustains haematopoietic stem-cell function. Nature 591(7848):117–123. https://doi.org/10.1038/s41586-020-03129-z
161. Cavalli G et al (2017) Interleukin 37 reverses the metabolic cost of inflammation, increases oxidative respiration, and improves exercise tolerance. Proc Natl Acad Sci USA 114(9):2313–2318. https://doi.org/10.1073/pnas.1619011114
162. Davizon-Castillo P et al (2019) TNF-alpha-driven inflammation and mitochondrial dysfunction define the platelet hyperreactivity of aging. Blood 134(9):727–740. https://doi.org/10.1182/blood.2019000200
163. D'Alessandro A et al (2020) Metabolic phenotypes of standard and cold-stored platelets. Transfusion 60(Suppl 3):S96–S106. https://doi.org/10.1111/trf.15651
164. Zhao HW et al (2021) In vitro characterization and Metabolomic analysis of cold-stored platelets. J Proteome Res. https://doi.org/10.1021/acs.jproteome.0c00792
165. Prudent M et al. (2014) Proteome changes in platelets after pathogen inactivation--an

interlaboratory consensus. Transfus Med Rev 28(2):72–83. https://doi.org/10.1016/j.tmrv.2014.02.002

166. D'Alessandro A et al (2021) The impact of donor sex and age on stored platelet metabolism and post-transfusion recovery. Blood Transfus 19(3):216–223. https://doi.org/10.2450/2020.0145-20
167. Hadley JB et al (2022) A pilot study of the metabolic profiles of apheresis platelets modified by donor age and sex and in vitro short-term incubation with sex hormones. Transfusion. https://doi.org/10.1111/trf.17165
168. Catala A et al (2020) Metabolic reprogramming of mouse bone marrow derived macrophages following Erythrophagocytosis. Front Physiol 11:396. https://doi.org/10.3389/fphys.2020.00396
169. El Kasmi KC et al (2018) Macrophage-derived IL-1beta/NF-kappaB signaling mediates parenteral nutrition-associated cholestasis. Nat Commun 9(1):1393. https://doi.org/10.1038/s41467-018-03764-1
170. Friedman JE et al (2018) Pyrroloquinoline quinone prevents developmental programming of microbial dysbiosis and macrophage polarization to attenuate liver fibrosis in offspring of obese mice. Hepatol Commun 2(3):313–328. https://doi.org/10.1002/hep4.1139
171. Janssen WJ et al (2020) Inflammation-induced alternative Pre-mRNA splicing in mouse alveolar macrophages. G3 (Bethesda) 10(2):555–567. https://doi.org/10.1534/g3.119.400935
172. Marchetti C et al (2018) OLT1177, a beta-sulfonyl nitrile compound, safe in humans, inhibits the NLRP3 inflammasome and reverses the metabolic cost of inflammation. Proc Natl Acad Sci USA 115(7):E1530–E1539. https://doi.org/10.1073/pnas.1716095115
173. McCubbrey AL et al (2022) Polyamine import and accumulation causes immunomodulation in macrophages engulfing apoptotic cells. Cell Rep 38(2):110222. https://doi.org/10.1016/j.celrep.2021.110222
174. Mould KJ et al (2017) Cell origin dictates programming of resident versus recruited macrophages during acute lung injury. Am J Respir Cell Mol Biol 57(3):294–306. https://doi.org/10.1165/rcmb.2017-0061OC
175. Soderborg TK et al (2018) The gut microbiota in infants of obese mothers increases inflammation and susceptibility to NAFLD. Nat Commun 9(1):4462. https://doi.org/10.1038/s41467-018-06929-0
176. Thwe PM et al (2017) Cell-intrinsic glycogen metabolism supports early glycolytic reprogramming required for dendritic cell immune responses. Cell Metab 26(3):558–567.e555. https://doi.org/10.1016/j.cmet.2017.08.012
177. Zhang J et al (2021) In situ mapping identifies distinct vascular niches for myelopoiesis. Nature 590(7846):457–462. https://doi.org/10.1038/s41586-021-03201-2
178. Clement CC et al (2021) 3-hydroxy-L-kynurenamine is an immunomodulatory biogenic amine. Nat Commun 12(1):4447. https://doi.org/10.1038/s41467-021-24785-3
179. Champagne DP et al (2016) Fine-tuning of CD8(+) T cell mitochondrial metabolism by the respiratory chain repressor MCJ dictates protection to influenza virus. Immunity 44(6):1299–1311. https://doi.org/10.1016/j.immuni.2016.02.018
180. Klarquist J et al (2018) Clonal expansion of vaccine-elicited T cells is independent of aerobic glycolysis. Sci Immunol 3(27). https://doi.org/10.1126/sciimmunol.aas9822
181. Culp-Hill R et al (2017) Red blood cell metabolism in down syndrome: hints on metabolic derangements in aging. Blood Adv 1(27):2776–2780. https://doi.org/10.1182/bloodadvances.2017011957
182. Hazegh K et al (2021) Blood donor obesity is associated with changes in red blood cell metabolism and susceptibility to hemolysis in cold storage and in response to osmotic and oxidative stress. Transfusion 61(2):435–448. https://doi.org/10.1111/trf.16168
183. Sackheim AM et al (2021) Traumatic brain injury impairs systemic vascular function through disruption of inward-rectifier potassium channels. Function (Oxf) 2(3). https://doi.org/10.1093/function/zqab018
184. van de Wetering C et al (2021) Glutathione-S-transferase P promotes glycolysis in asthma in association with oxidation of pyruvate kinase M2. Redox Biol 47:102160. https://doi.org/10.1016/j.redox.2021.102160
185. McCubbrey AL et al (2022) Polyamine import and accumulation causes immunomodulation in macrophages engulfing apoptotic cells. Cell Rep 38(2):110222

Chapter 26

Assessing the Impact of Intravascular Hemolysis on Erythropoiesis in Sickle Cell Disease

Huan Zhang and Xiuli An

Abstract

Intravascular hemolysis is a hallmark of sickle cell disease (SCD). While it has been well established that the hemolysis-derived products, such as hemoglobin (Hb) and free heme, exert proinflammatory and pro-oxidative effects, contributing to the vascular and tissue damage in SCD, the effects of hemolysis on erythropoiesis have not been studied. We and others have reported that hemolysis in SCD led to upregulation of type I interferon IFNα. We further documented that the ability of Townes sickle mice to increase their erythropoietic capacity to compensate for anemia was impaired. To examine whether the impaired erythropoiesis in SCD is associated with the hemolysis-driven IFNα production and to define the underlying mechanisms, we injected mice with hemin, red cell lysate, or IFNα to mimic the hemolysis status in SCD and then examined erythropoiesis by colony-forming assay, flow cytometric analysis, and western blot. We also examined the effects of hemin and IFNα on erythropoiesis using an in vitro erythroid culture system. We found that intravascular hemolysis inhibited erythropoiesis in SCD through inhibition of erythropoietin (EPO)/erythropoietin receptor (EPOR) signaling via a heme-IFNα-CISH axis. Herein, we describe how to prepare hemin, red cell lysate, and IFNα, and present examples of in vivo and in vitro assays to assess erythropoiesis. Our methods can be applied to study changes in erythropoiesis in other diseases characterized by intravascular hemolysis.

Key words Intravascular hemolysis, Erythropoiesis, Sickle cell disease, Free heme, IFNα, EPO/EPOR

1 Introduction

Sickle cell disease (SCD) is caused by a point mutation in the beta globin gene, which leads to the replacement of glutamic acid with valine in the sixth position of the β globin chain [1]. This mutation causes a rapid decrease in the solubility of hemoglobin (Hb) under hypoxic conditions, resulting in insoluble fibrous crystals, which lead to the generation of sickled red blood cells (RBC) [2, 3]. Clinically, SCD is manifested as chronic hemolytic anemia. Intravascular hemolysis in SCD leads to the release of red cell contents such as Hb and free heme into circulation [4–6]. Physiologically, free heme

Sean R. Stowell and Connie M. Arthur (eds.), *Methods in Transfusion Medicine*, Methods in Molecular Biology, vol. 3053, https://doi.org/10.1007/978-1-0716-5376-0_26,

in plasma is mainly bound by hemopexin (HPX) for clearance via LRP1/CD91-mediated endocytosis of HPX-heme complexes [7, 8]. However, in SCD, a large amount of free heme can cause serious damages [9, 10], including oxidative stress, inflammatory response, cell toxicity, and tissue damage [3–6].

Erythropoiesis is the process by which red blood cells are produced from hematopoietic stem cells. It can be divided into three stages: (1) early-stage erythropoiesis which refers to the process of differentiation of hematopoietic stem and progenitor cells into committed erythroid progenitor burst forming units-erythroid (BFU-E) which then differentiate into colony-forming units-erythroid (CFU-E); (2) Terminal erythroid differentiation that starts from proerythroblasts (Pro) which progressively differentiate into basophilic erythroblasts (Baso), polychromatic erythroblasts (Poly), and Orthochromatic erythroblasts (Ortho), which then undergo enucleation to generate reticulocytes; and (3) Reticulocyte maturation which refers to the process in which polymorphic reticulocytes eventually mature into typical biconcave red blood cells in the bloodstream. The process of erythropoiesis is subject to precise and complex regulation [11–14]. Of note, the hormone erythropoietin (EPO) and its cognate receptor erythropoietin receptor (EPOR) play indispensable roles in erythropoiesis, as evidenced by the findings that deficiency of EPO or EPOR leads to embryonic lethality [15].

In anemia, tissue hypoxia leads to increased production of EPO by the peritubular cells of the kidney [16], which in turn increases the activity of erythropoiesis to compensate for the anemia. We have reported that the erythropoietic activity in the bone marrow of a thalassemia mouse model $Hbb^{th1/th1}$ expanded ~three fold to compensate for the anemia [17]. Similarly, EPO injection also led to a ~2–3-fold increase in Bone Marrow (BM) erythroblasts [18, 19]. These findings indicate that mouse BM can increase its erythropoietic activity by 2–3-fold under erythropoietic stress conditions. Interestingly, we recently found that despite similarly increased EPO levels in Townes sickle mouse and $Hbb^{th3/+}$ thalassemia mice, the elevation of erythropoiesis in the BM of Townes sickle mouse was much lower than that in the $Hbb^{th3/+}$ thalassemia mice [20], indicating impaired erythropoiesis in SCD. Given that intravascular hemolysis is a hallmark of SCD [4], that hemolysis induces IFNα production [20, 21], and that type I interferon inhibits erythropoiesis [22–26], we hypothesized that the impaired erythropoiesis is associated with the intravascular hemolysis and/or hemolysis-driven IFNα production. To test this, we examined the effects of hemin, red cell lysates, or IFNα on erythropoiesis in vitro and in vivo, we found that although hemin had no direct effects on erythroid cells in vitro, injection of hemin or red cell lysate to mice led to suppression erythropoiesis along with inhibition of EPO/EPOR signaling in erythroid cells due to activation of type I interferon signaling pathway. Injection of IFNα into mice also led to suppression of erythropoiesis and inhibition of EPO/EPOR signaling in erythroid cells. Moreover, EPO/EPOR signaling was inhibited and type I interferon signaling was activated in erythroid cells of Townes sickle mice. Together, we have identified defective BM erythropoiesis in a mouse model of SCD along with an impaired response of their BM erythroid progenitors and erythroblasts to EPO. Using various mouse models in conjunction with in vivo and in vitro assays for assessing erythropoiesis, we documented that the impaired erythropoiesis in SCD is due to hemolysis-driven IFNα production. The mouse models we used include C57BL/6 mice and AA mice (control of Townes sickle mice SS). The assays we used include colony-forming assay of erythroid progenitors, flow cytometric analysis of erythroid cells at distinct maturational stages, and detection of EPO/EPOR signal transduction by flow cytometry and Western Blot. Here, we summarize these methods in detail. As intravascular hemolysis is characterized by many diseases, including SCD [4], transfusion reactions [27, 28], various hemolytic anemias such as paroxysmal nocturnal hemoglobinuria [29, 30], pyruvate kinase deficiency [31, 32], G6PD deficiency [33–35], and malaria infection [36, 37], the methods described here have broad applications.

2 Materials

2.1 Preparation and Injection of Hemin, RBC Lysate, and IFNα

1. C57BL/6 mice and AA mice (control of Townes sickle mice SS).
2. 1 mL syringe
3. 1 mL insulin syringe (for retro-orbital injection, ROI)
4. Hemin (sigma)
5. 0.2 mol/L (M) NaOH
6. 1 M HCl
7. Hemin Assay kit (abcam)
8. Mouse IFNα (Miltenyi Biotec)
9. 1× phosphate-buffer saline (PBS), pH 7.4
10. 10× PBS, pH 7.4
11. Ultrapure water

2.2 Preparation of Mouse Bone Marrow (BM) Single Cell Suspension

1. C57BL/6 mice and AA mice (control of Townes sickle mice SS)
2. Isoflurane (or other suitable types of anesthetics)
3. Ophthalmic scissors and tweezers set

4. Buffer I: 1× PBS, pH 7.4 containing 2% Fetal Bovine Serum (FBS) and 2 mM EDTA
5. 20 G needles and 10 mL syringe
6. 70 μm cell strainer
7. Hemocytometer or other kind of cell counter

2.3 Mouse Erythroid Progenitor Colony-Forming Assays

1. Iscove's Modified Dulbecco's (IMDM) medium
2. Fetal Bovine Serum (FBS)
3. Buffer I: 1× PBS, pH 7.4 containing 2% FBS and 2 mM EDTA
4. Methylcellulose medium Methocult M4434, MethoCult M3334, and MethoCult M3234 (STEMCELL Technologies)
5. Rat anti-mouse CD16/CD32 antibody for Fc blocking (BD Biosciences)
6. Biotin-conjugated anti mouse Gr1, CD11b, CD3e, CD45R/B220, and Ter-119 antibodies (BD Biosciences) for depletion of lineage$^+$ cells
7. BV421-conjugated anti-mouse CD16/32, BV605-conjugated anti-mouse CD71, APC-conjugated anti-mouse CD34, APC-conjugated anti-mouse Ly-6A/E (Sca-1), APC-Cyanine7 conjugated anti-mouse CD117 (c-kit), eFluor450-conjugated anti-mouse CD41a, and PerCP-conjugated Streptavidin (BD Biosciences) for analyzing or sorting erythroid progenitors BFU-E and CFU-E
8. Viability marker 7AAD
9. 2.5 mL syringe
10. Extended flat end syringe needles (20G)

2.4 Flow Cytometric Analysis of Mouse BM Terminal Erythropoiesis

1. Buffer I: 1× PBS, pH 7.4 containing 2% FBS and 2 mM EDTA
2. Rat anti-mouse CD16/CD32 antibody for Fc blocking (BD Biosciences)
3. V450-conjugated anti-mouse Ter-119, APC-conjugated anti-mouse CD44, APC-Cy7-conjugated anti-mouse CD45, APC-Cy 7-conjugated anti-mouse CD11b, and APC-Cy7-conjugated anti-mouse Gr1 for analyzing terminal erythropoiesis
4. Viability marker 7AAD

2.5 EPO/EPOR Signal Transduction Detection in Mouse Erythroid Cells

1. Buffer I: 1× PBS, pH 7.4 containing 2% FBS and 2 mM EDTA
2. Rat anti-mouse CD16/CD32 antibody for Fc blocking (BD Biosciences)
3. Biotin-conjugated anti mouse Gr1, CD11b, CD3e, CD45R/B220, and Ter-119 antibodies (BD Biosciences) for depletion of lineage$^+$ cells or enrichment of erythroid cells

4. BV421-conjugated anti-mouse CD16/32, BV605-conjugated anti-mouse CD71, APC-conjugated anti-mouse CD34, APC-conjugated anti-mouse Ly-6A/E (Sca-1), APC-Cyanine7-conjugated anti-mouse CD117 (c-kit), eFluor450-conjugated anti-mouse CD41a, PE-Cy7-conjugated anti-pStat5 antibodies, and PerCP-conjugated Streptavidin (BD Biosciences) for analyzing erythroid progenitors BFU-E and CFU-E
5. V450-conjugated anti-mouse Ter-119, APC-conjugated anti-mouse CD44, APC-Cy7-conjugated anti-mouse CD45, APC-Cy 7-conjugated anti-mouse CD11b, APC-Cy7-conjugated anti-mouse Gr1, and PE-Cy7-conjugated anti-pStat5 antibodies for analyzing terminal erythropoiesis
6. EPO (Stock solution: 10,000 U/mL)
7. RIPA lysis buffer containing protease inhibitors and phosphatase inhibitors
8. BCA protein concentration kit
9. Anti-pSTAT5 and Stat5 antibodies
10. Western blot-related solutions or reagents

2.6 The Effect of Hemin/IFNα on EPO/EPOR Signal Transduction In Vitro

1. Iscove's Modified Dulbecco's (IMDM) medium
2. Fetal Bovine Serum (FBS)
3. Buffer I: 1× PBS, pH 7.4 containing 2% FBS and 2 mM EDTA
4. Hemin solution.
5. Mouse IFNα.

2.7 Isolation of Human CD34+ Hematopoietic Stem/Progenitor Cells (HSPC) from Cord Blood

1. Iscove's Modified Dulbecco's (IMDM) medium
2. Fetal Bovine Serum (FBS)
3. Buffer I: 1× PBS, pH 7.4 containing 2% FBS and 2 mM EDTA
4. Ficoll (1.077 g/mL)
5. Transfer pipette
6. 1.5 mL, 15 mL, and 50 mL tubes
7. Anti-human CD34 microbeads kit (Miltenyi Biotec)
8. MS and LS columns (Miltenyi Biotec)
9. Reagents for complete culture medium: AB serum, AB plasma, insulin, heparin, Holo-transferrin, EPO, stem cell factor (SCF), IL-3, Penicillin, and Streptomycin
10. Reagents for cell treatment: Hemin solution and human IFNα

2.8 Colony-Forming Assays of Cultured Human Erythroid Progenitors

1. StemSpan™ SFEM medium
2. Fetal Bovine Serum (FBS)

3. Methylcellulose medium Methocult H4434 for human BFU-E colony-forming assay, and MethoCult H4330 for human CFU-E colony-forming assay (STEMCELL Technologies)
4. 35 × 10 mm dish
5. 2.5 mL syringe
6. Extended flat end syringe needles (20G)

2.9 Examination of Human Erythroid Differentiation and Enucleation by Flow Cytometry

1. Buffer I: 1× PBS, pH 7.4 containing 2% FBS and 2 mM EDTA
2. Anti-human antibodies and dyes: APC-GPA, PE-CD34, FITC-CD36, PE-Cy7-IL3R, APC-a4 integrin, FITC-Band3, PE-GPA, and Syto16
3. 1× PBS, pH 7.4
4. 5 mM $MgCl_2$
5. Viability marker 7AAD

2.10 Examination of Apoptosis by Flow Cytometry

1. 1× PBS, pH 7.4
2. Annexin V Detection Kit: containing 1× Annexin V binding buffer and APC-Annexin V
3. Viability marker 7AAD

3 Methods

Part 1: The Effect of Hemin, RBC Lysate, and IFNα on Erythropoiesis in Mice

3.1 Preparation and Injection of Hemin, RBC Lysate, or IFNα

3.1.1 Preparation of Hemin

1. Dissolve hemin with 0.2 mol/L (M) NaOH.
2. After hemin is fully dissolved, neutralize the solution to pH 7.2 using 1 M HCl.
3. Determine the concentration of hemin using the hemin assay kit and store it in a −80 °C freezer for future use.
4. Dilute hemin with 1× PBS, pH 7.4 to 7 mM as a stock solution.
5. Inject the mice once at a dose of 70 μmol/kg by ROI using a 1 mL insulin syringe (*see* **Note 1**).
6. Detect erythropoiesis 2 days after hemin injection (*see* **Note 2**).

3.1.2 Preparation of RBC Lysate

1. Anesthetize mice with isoflurane and obtain peripheral blood of wild-type (WT) mice from the heart using a 1 mL syringe.
2. Wash peripheral blood cells three times with 1× PBS, pH 7.4 after each centrifugation at 300× *g* for 5 min.
3. Lyse RBC pellets with ten times the volume of water at room temperature for 30 min.

4. Collect supernatant after centrifugation at 13,000× *g* for 15 min.
5. Add 1/10 volume of 10× PBS, pH 7.4 to adjust its osmotic pressure to physiological level.
6. Inject mice at a dose of 250 μL/mice/day for 3 days by ROI using a 1 mL insulin syringe (*see* **Note 3**).
7. Detect erythropoiesis 1 day after the last injection.

3.1.3 Preparation of Mouse IFNα

1. Dissolve IFNα in 1× PBS, pH 7.4 supplemented with 0.1% BSA to prepare a stock solution at a final concentration of 10^7 U/mL.
2. Dilute mouse IFNα stock solution with 1× PBS, pH 7.4.
3. Inject mice with mouse IFNα at a dose of 10^4 U/mice/day by intraperitoneal (i.p.) injection for 3 days using a 1 mL syringe.
4. Detect erythropoiesis 1 day after the last injection.

3.2 Preparation of Mouse BM Single Cell Suspension

1. Anesthetize mice with isoflurane and then sacrifice them by spinal cord dislocation.
2. Remove the femurs and tibias and keep them in Buffer I.
3. Flush out BM tissues with Buffer I and then gently pass the tissues through 20 G needles 3 to 4 times with a 10 mL syringe.
4. Pass the cells through a 70 μm cell strainer to obtain the BM single cell suspension.
5. Count cell numbers by hemocytometer or cell counter.

3.3 Mouse Erythroid Progenitor Colony-Forming Assays

3.3.1 Preparation of Total BM Cells

1. Suspend 5× 10^5 mouse BM cells in 1 mL IMDM/2% FBS medium.
2. Mix well and add 300 μL suspension to 3 mL methylcellulose medium supplemented with recombinant cytokines (Methocult M4434) for BFU-E colony assay, EPO-only methylcellulose medium (MethoCult M3334), or methylcellulose medium (MethoCult M3334) supplied with different concentrations of EPO (0, 1, 3, or 10 U/mL) for CFU-E colony assay.
3. Vortex thoroughly and stand at room temperature for at least 20 min until no bubbles are visible in the medium.
4. Plate 1.1 mL medium into each 35 × 10 mm dish, spread medium equably by turning the plate gently (*see* **Note 4**).
5. Incubate at 37 °C in a humidified atmosphere with 5% CO_2.
6. Count CFU-E colony number 2 days later and count BFU-E colony number 7 days later.

3.3.2 Flow Cytometric Sorting of BFU-E and CFU-E

1. Suspend mouse BM cells in Buffer I at the concentration of 10^7/100 μL and incubate with rat anti-mouse CD16/CD32 for 15 min on ice for Fc blocking.
2. Incubate the cells with biotin-conjugated anti-mouse lineage antibodies including anti-Gr1, anti-CD11b, anti-CD3e, anti-CD45R/B220, and anti-Ter-119 at 4 °C for 30 min.
3. Wash the cells with Buffer I by centrifugation at 300× *g* for 5 min at 4 °C.
4. Resuspend cells with 36 μL of Buffer I per 10^7 cells and then add 10 μL of Anti-Biotin Microbeads (Miltenyi Biotec).
5. Incubate for 15 min at 4 °C.
6. Wash the cells with Buffer I by centrifugation at 300× *g* for 5 min at 4 °C and then resuspend the cell pellet in 100 μL Buffer I per 10^7 cells.
7. Separate the Lineage$^-$ and Lineage$^+$ cells by magnetic-activated cell separation with MS columns according to the instructions from the manufacturer (Miltenyi Biotec). The flow-through fraction (Lineage$^-$ cells) was collected for further staining.
8. Resuspend Lineage$^-$ cells in Buffer I at the concentration of 1×10^5/35 μL and incubate with rat anti-mouse CD16/CD32 for 15 min on ice for Fc blocking.
9. Stain the cells with flow cytometry antibodies including BV421-conjugated anti-mouse CD16/32, BV605-conjugated anti-mouse CD71, APC-conjugated anti-mouse CD34, APC-conjugated anti-mouse Ly-6A/E (Sca-1), APC-Cyanine7 conjugated anti-mouse CD117 (c-kit), eFluor450-conjugated anti-mouse CD41a, and PerCP-conjugated Streptavidin that can specifically bind to biotin.
10. Incubate at room temperature for 30 min in the dark.
11. Wash the cells with Buffer I by centrifugation at 300× *g* for 5 min, at 4 °C.
12. Resuspend the cells in 200 μL Buffer I and stain them with viability marker 7AAD on ice for 10 min in the dark.
13. Sort BFU-E and CFU-E according to the gating strategy shown in Fig. 1.
14. Sort 2×10^3 mouse BM BFU-E or CFU-E into 1 mL IMDM/2% FBS medium.
15. Conduct a colony-forming assay according to the procedures described in "For total BM cells" in this section.

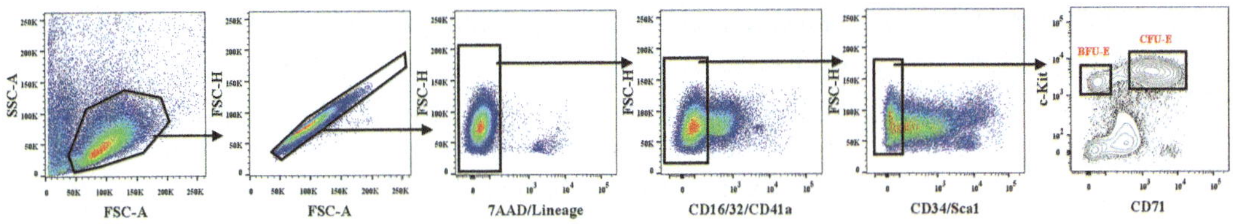

Fig. 1 Flow cytometry analysis of bone marrow (BM) erythroid progenitors. Lineage$^-$ cells are used for analysis. Burst-forming units-erythroid (BFU-E) are defined as Lineage$^-$CD16/32$^-$CD41a$^-$CD34$^-$Sca1$^-$CD71$^-$ cells, and colony-forming units-erythroid (CFU-E) are defined as Lineage$^-$CD16/32$^-$CD41a$^-$CD34$^-$Sca1^{--} CD71^{high} cells.

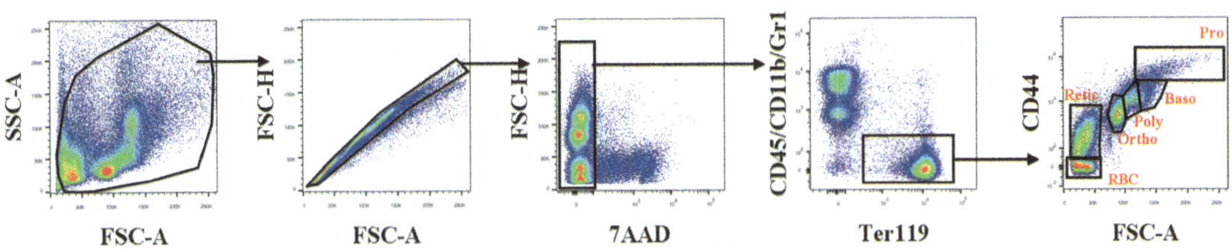

Fig. 2 Flow cytometry analysis of BM terminal differentiated erythroid cells. Total mouse BM cells are used for analysis. Each stage of terminally differentiated erythroid cells is separated in CD45$^-$CD11b$^-$Gr1$^-$Ter119$^+$ cells as labeled in the last panel. Pro proerythroblasts, Baso basophilic erythroblasts, Poly polychromatic erythroblasts, Ortho orthochromatic erythroblasts, Retic reticulocytes, RBC red blood cells

3.4 Flow Cytometric Analysis of Mouse BM Terminal Erythropoiesis

1. Suspend mouse BM cells in Buffer I at the concentration of 10^6/50 μL.
2. Incubate the cells with anti-mouse CD16/CD32 for 15 min on ice.
3. Stain the cells with V450-conjugated anti-mouse Ter-119, APC-conjugated anti-mouse CD44, APC-Cy7-conjugated anti-mouse CD45, APC-Cy7-conjugated anti-mouse CD11b, and APC-Cy7-conjugated anti-mouse Gr1 on ice for 30 min in the dark.
4. Wash the cells with Buffer I by centrifugation at 300× *g* for 5 min at 4 °C.
5. Resuspend the cells in 200 μL Buffer I and stain the cells with the viability marker 7AAD on ice for 10 min in the dark.
6. Detect fluorescence intensity of each antigen on a flow cytometer within 1 h after staining (Fig. 2).

3.5 EPO/EPOR Signal Transduction Detection in Mouse Erythroid Cells

Stat5 is one of the key downstream targets of the EPO/EPOR signaling pathway, which is originally transduced by Janus-tyrosine kinase 2 (Jak2) protein. Here, we show the detection of phosphorylation of Stat5 in erythroid cells after EPO stimulation to reflect the activation of the EPO/EPOR signaling pathway. Phosphorylation of other downstream targets, including JAK2, MAPK/ERK, and PI3K, can also be examined.

3.5.1 Flow Cytometry to Detect Phosphorylation of Stat5

1. Starve enriched Lineage⁻ cells or BM cells for 6 h in Buffer I on ice.
2. Stain the enriched Lineage⁻ cells or BM cells with cell surface antibodies for erythroid progenitors or erythroblast as described above (*see* Subheading 3.3 and 3.4).
3. Stimulate with or without EPO (1 U/mL or other desired concentrations) for 10 min at 37 °C (*see* **Note 5**).
4. Centrifuge at 300× *g* for 5 min and then fix the cells with BD Phosflow™ Fix Buffer I at 37 °C for 10 min.
5. Wash the cells twice with Buffer I by centrifugation at 300× *g* for 5 min at 4 °C.
6. Treat the cells with BD Phosflow™ Perm Buffer III for 30 min on ice.
7. Wash the cells twice with Buffer I by centrifugation at 300× *g* for 5 min at 4 °C.
8. Stain with PE-Cy7-pStat5 at 37 °C for 30 min and detect fluorescence intensity of each antigen on a flow cytometer (*see* **Note 6**).

3.5.2 Western Blot to Detect Phosphorylation of Stat5

1. Enrich erythroid cells by depleting CD11b⁺, Gr1⁺, CD3e⁺, and B220⁺ cells using magnetic activated cell separation (similar to the procedures of lineage⁻ cell enrichment described above in Subheading 3.3).
2. Starve the cells for 6 h in Buffer I on ice.
3. Lyse the starved erythroid cells with RIPA lysis buffer containing protease inhibitors and phosphatase inhibitors.
4. Detect protein concentrations by the BCA protein concentration kit according to the instructions from the manufacturer.
5. Load 25 μg protein for each lane to run western blot.

3.6 The Effect of Hemin/IFNα on EPO/EPOR Signal Transduction In Vitro

1. Suspend mouse BM cells or lineage⁻ cells in IMDM/10% FBS medium.
2. Treat the cells with hemin (0, 10, 20, or 40 μM) or IFNα (0, 10, 100, or 1000 IU/mL).
3. Incubate at 37 °C in a humidified atmosphere with 5% CO_2 for 3 h.
4. Wash the cells twice with Buffer I by centrifugation at 300× g for 5 min at 4 °C.
5. Detect EPO/EPOR signal transduction by flow cytometry or western blot as described in Subheading 3.5.

Part 2: The Effect of Hemin/IFNα on Erythropoiesis of Cultured Human CD34⁺ Cell Derived Erythroid Cells In Vitro

3.7 Isolation of CD34⁺ Hematopoietic Stem/Progenitor Cells (HSPC) from Cord Blood

1. Dilute the cord blood 2.5 times in Buffer I and then carefully add 35 mL to 50 mL tube containing 15 mL Ficoll (1.077 g/mL).
2. Centrifuge at 400× *g* for 30 min with no brake at room temperature (RT).
3. Discard the supernatant and collect the buffy coat with a transfer pipette into a 50 mL tube containing 25 mL Buffer I.
4. Invert the tubes 2–3 times and then centrifuge at 300× *g* for 10 min at RT.
5. Discard the supernatant and pull the pellets into one 50 mL tube containing Buffer I, count the cell number and centrifuge at 200× *g* for 10 min at 4 °C for two times.
6. For each 10^8 cells: Resuspend the cells with 300 μL cold Buffer I, add 100 μL Fc blocking Buffer, and incubate for 5 min on ice, then add 100 μL CD34 microbeads and incubate at 4 °C for at least 30 min.
7. Wash the cells with cold Buffer I at 200× *g* for 10 min at 4 °C.
8. Separate the $CD34^-$ and $CD34^+$ cells by magnetic-activated cell separation with MS columns according to the instructions from the manufacturer (Miltenyi Biotec). Cells binding on the column are $CD34^+$ cells (*see* **Note 7**). Flush down $CD34^+$ cells with 5 mL cold Buffer I.
9. Count the cell number, centrifuge at 300× *g* for 5 min to remove Buffer I, and culture the cells in fresh medium. The formula of the complete medium and the initial culture density of cells are listed in Table 1.
10. Culture the cells at 37 °C in a humidified atmosphere with 5% CO_2.
11. Treat the cells with hemin (0, 10, 20, or 40 μM) or IFNα (0, 10, 100, or 1000 IU/mL) according to the experimental purpose (*see* **Note 8**).

3.8 Colony-Forming Assays of Cultured Human Erythroid Progenitors

1. Suspend cultured Day 6 cells with SFEM at the concentration of 2000 cells/mL.
2. Mix well and add 300 μL to 3 mL methylcellulose medium supplemented with recombinant cytokines (Methocult H4434) for BFU-E colony assay, or EPO-only methylcellulose medium (MethoCult H4330) for CFU-E colony assay.
3. Vortex thoroughly and stand at room temperature for at least 20 min.
4. Plate 1.1 mL medium into each 35 × 10 mm dish, spread medium equably by turning the plate gently.

Table 1
The complete medium and the initial culture density for CD34⁺ cells

Component	Days 0–7	Days 7–11	Days 11–14	Days 15–20
Cell density (10^6/mL)	0.1	0.1	1	5
AB serum	3%	3%	3%	3%
AB plasma	2%	2%	2%	2%
Insulin (μg/mL)	10	10	10	10
Heparin (IU/mL)	3	3	3	3
Transferrin (μg/mL)	200	200	1000	1000
EPO (U/mL)	3	1	1	0
Stem cell factor (ng/mL)	10	10	0	0
IL-3 (ng/mL)	1	0	0	0
Penicillin and Streptomycin	1%, if necessary			
Base medium	IMDM			

5. Incubate at 37 °C in a humidified atmosphere with 5% CO_2.
6. Count CFU-E colony number 7 days later and BFU-E colony number 14 days later.

3.9 Examination of Human Erythroid Differentiation and Enucleation by Flow Cytometry

1. Collect 1×10^5 cells in a 1.5 mL tube and wash one time with Buffer I at 300× *g* for 5 min at 4 °C.
2. Add antibodies or DNA dye to each sample as follows:

   For erythroid progenitor staining:

APC-GPA (1: 50 diluted)	1 μL
PE-CD34	2 μL
FITC-CD36	1 μL
PE-Cy7-IL3R	2 μL

   For erythroblasts staining:

APC-α4 integrin	1.3 μL
FITC-Band3 (1: 10 diluted)	2.5 μL (*see* **Note 9**)
PE-GPA (1: 100 diluted)	1 μL

   For erythroid enucleation:

PBS+ 5 mM $MgCl_2$	30 μL
Syto16 (1: 200 diluted)	0.6 μL

3. Mix well and incubate at room temperature for 15 min, in darkness.
4. Wash the cells with cold Buffer I at 200× *g* for 10 min at 4 °C.

5. Resuspend the cells in 200 μL Buffer I and stain the cells with the viability marker 7AAD on ice for 10 min in the dark.
6. Detect fluorescence intensity of each antigen/dye on a flow cytometer within 1 h after staining.

3.10 Examination of Apoptosis by Flow Cytometry

1. Collect 1×10^5 cells in a 1.5 mL tube and wash one time with 1× Annexin V binding buffer at 300× *g* for 5 min at 4 °C.
2. Resuspend the cells with 25 μL 1× Annexin V binding buffer and add 0.8 μL APC-Annexin V, then incubate at TR for 10 min in the dark.
3. Resuspend the cells in 200 μL 1× Annexin V binding buffer and stain the cells with the viability marker 7AAD on ice for 10 min in the dark.
4. Detect fluorescence intensity of each antigen/dye on a flow cytometer within 1 h after staining.

4 Notes

1. C57BL/6 mice and AA mice have different sensitivity to hemin. We injected 35 μmol/kg hemin into C57BL/6 mice or 70 μmol/kg hemin into AA mice.
2. We detected the influence of hemin on the erythropoiesis of mice at different days following injection. We found that the numbers of erythroblasts in the mouse bone marrow were decreased one day following hemin injection. The decrease in erythroblasts peaked on day 2 and stayed so until day 4, then gradually recovered and returned to a normal level after 8 days. Therefore, we chose to conduct various tests on day 2 after the hemin injection.
3. There are significant differences in the sensitivity of mice with different genetic backgrounds to RBC lysate. We found that erythropoiesis of C57BL/6 mice was significantly inhibited after RBC lysate injection, while AA mice showed no significant changes in erythropoiesis after RBC lysate injection. This indicates that, unlike C57BL/6 mice, AA mice have poor sensitivity to RBC lysate injection. Therefore, researchers need to pay attention to the genetic background of the mice used in RBC lysate injection experiments.
4. According to the protocol we provided, the final number of cells in each dish is 1/10 of the initial number of cells. For example, if 5×10^5 mouse BM cells are added to 1 mL IMDM/2% FBS medium at the beginning, the final number of cells in each dish is 5×10^4.

5. To improve the accuracy of the experiment, we usually use a two-step centrifugation method to remove the supernatant. The first centrifugation removes most of the supernatant, leaving about 50 μL of buffer, and then centrifuges again, carefully discarding all the supernatant. Subsequently, resuspend the cells in 500 μL Buffer I, and add 500 μL Buffer I containing EPO to both the control groups and the experimental groups. Mix well and immediately incubate in 37 °C-water bath.
6. In this step, we always thoroughly remove the supernatant by using a two-step centrifugation method. And when we stain the pStat5 antibody, we always prepare the working solution of the antibody first and then add an equal amount to each group for staining to improve the accuracy of the experiment.
7. In order to improve the purity of the obtained $CD34^{+}$ cells, we often pass through an MS column after passing through an LS column.
8. In this in vitro culture system, during days 0–6, the culture system contains a large number of erythroid progenitor cells. After day 7, the culture system mainly consisted of terminal differentiated erythroid cells. Cells begin to enucleate on day 13 and gradually increase with prolonged culture duration. Therefore, it is possible to choose to add reagents at different cultivation times to detect their effects on erythroid cells at different stages.
9. Considering that Band3 is not a commercial antibody, some research groups also use a combination of CD71, CD105, and GPA [38, 39] or CD36 and GPA [40] to monitor human erythroid cell differentiation.

Conflict of Interest

The authors have no conflicts of interest to declare that are relevant to the content of this chapter.

References

1. Bunn HF (1997) Mechanisms of disease - pathogenesis and treatment of sickle cell disease. N Engl J Med 337(11):762–769
2. Coletta M et al (1982) Kinetics of sickle hemoglobin polymerization in single red-cells. Nature 300(5888):194–197
3. Rees DC, Williams TN, Gladwin MT (2010) Sickle-cell disease. Lancet 376(9757): 2018–2031
4. Kato GJ, Steinberg MH, Gladwin MT (2017) Intravascular hemolysis and the pathophysiology of sickle cell disease. J Clin Invest 127(3):750–760
5. Reiter CD et al (2002) Cell-free hemoglobin limits nitric oxide bioavailability in sickle-cell disease. Nat Med 8(12):1383–1389
6. Gbotosho OT, Kapetanaki MG, Kato GJ (2020) The worst things in life are free: the role of free Heme in sickle cell disease. Front Immunol 11:561917
7. Hrkal Z, Vodrázka Z, Kalousek I (1974) Transfer of heme from ferrihemoglobin and

ferrihemoglobin isolated chains to hemopexin. Eur J Biochem 43(1):73–78
8. Hvidberg V et al (2005) Identification of the receptor scavenging hemopexin-heme complexes. Blood 106(7):2572–2579
9. Oh JY et al (2016) Absorbance and redox based approaches for measuring free heme and free hemoglobin in biological matrices. Redox Biol 9:167–177
10. Thomas AM et al (2019) Complement component C5 and TLR molecule CD14 mediate heme-induced thromboinflammation in human blood. J Immunol 203(6):1571–1578
11. Pastori V et al (2022) Role of nuclear receptors in controlling erythropoiesis. Int J Mol Sci 23(5)
12. Caulier AL, Sankaran VG (2022) Molecular and cellular mechanisms that regulate human erythropoiesis. Blood 139(16):2450–2459
13. Dzierzak E, Philipsen S (2013) Erythropoiesis: development and differentiation. Cold Spring Harb Perspect Med 3(4):a011601
14. Tang P, Wang HQ (2023) Regulation of erythropoiesis: emerging concepts and therapeutic implications. Hematology 28(1)
15. Wu H et al (1995) Generation of committed erythroid BFU-E and CFU-E progenitors does not require erythropoietin or the erythropoietin receptor. Cell 83(1):59–67
16. Semenza GL, Wang GL (1992) A nuclear factor induced by hypoxia via denovo protein-synthesis binds to the human erythropoietin gene enhancer at a site required for transcriptional activation. Mol Cell Biol 12(12): 5447–5454
17. Liu J et al (2013) Quantitative analysis of murine terminal erythroid differentiation in vivo: novel method to study normal and disordered erythropoiesis. Blood 121(8):e43–e49
18. Li W et al (2019) Identification and transcriptome analysis of erythroblastic island macrophages. Blood 134(5):480–491
19. Zhang H et al (2021) EpoR-tdTomato-Cre mice enable identification of EpoR expression in subsets of tissue macrophages and hematopoietic cells. Blood 138(20):1986–1997
20. Han Y et al (2023) Hemolysis-driven IFNα production impairs erythropoiesis by negatively regulating EPO signaling in sickle cell disease. Blood
21. Liu Y et al (2021) Type I interferon is induced by hemolysis and drives antibody-mediated erythrophagocytosis in sickle cell disease. Blood 138:1162
22. Means RT Jr, Krantz SB (1993) Inhibition of human erythroid colony-forming units by tumor necrosis factor requires beta interferon. J Clin Invest 91(2):416–419
23. Yoshida H et al (2005) Lethal anemia caused by interferon-beta produced in mouse embryos carrying undigested DNA. Nat Immunol 6(1): 49–56
24. Cappellini MD et al (2008) In vitro effect of ribavirin and pegylated interferon on erythropoiesis. Blood 112(11):4786
25. Cappellini MD et al (2008) Anemia during pegylated interferon-ribavirin therapy results from both increase suppression of erythroid differentiation and hemolysis. Blood 112(11): 4577–4577
26. Manchinu MF et al (2018) Deficiency in interferon type 1 receptor improves definitive erythropoiesis in Klf1 null mice. Cell Death Differ 25(3):589–599
27. Panch SR, Montemayor-Garcia C, Klein HG (2019) Hemolytic transfusion reactions. N Engl J Med 381(2):150–162
28. Sato T, Goto N, Tasaki T (2019) Hemolytic transfusion reactions. N Engl J Med 381(14): 1396–1397
29. Hill A et al (2017) Paroxysmal nocturnal haemoglobinuria. Nat Rev Dis Prim 3:3
30. Luzzatto L (2020) PNH phenotypes and their genesis. Br J Haematol 189(5):802–805
31. Bianchi P, Fermo E (2020) Molecular heterogeneity of pyruvate kinase deficiency. Haematologica 105(9):2218–2228
32. Helmstädter V et al (1977) Acquired pyruvate kinase deficiency with hemolysis in preleukemia. Acta Haematol 57(6):339–343
33. van Wijk R, van Solinge WW (2005) The energy-less red blood cell is lost: erythrocyte enzyme abnormalities of glycolysis. Blood 106(13):4034–4042
34. Luzzatto L, Ally M, Notaro R (2020) Glucose-6-phosphate dehydrogenase deficiency. Blood 136(11):1225–1240
35. Cappellini MD, Fiorelli G (2008) Glucose-6-phosphate dehydrogenase deficiency. Lancet 371(9606):64–74

36. White NJ (2018) Anaemia and malaria. Malar J 17:17
37. Padua TA, Souza MC (2020) Heme on pulmonary malaria: friend or foe? Front Immunol 11
38. Yan H et al (2021) Comprehensive phenotyping of erythropoiesis in human bone marrow: evaluation of normal and ineffective erythropoiesis. Am J Hematol 96(9):1064–1076
39. Papoin J et al (2024) Phenotypic and proteomic characterization of the human erythroid progenitor continuum reveal dynamic changes in cell cycle and in metabolic pathways. Am J Hematol 99(1):99–112
40. Martell DJ et al (2023) RNA polymerase II pausing temporally coordinates cell cycle progression and erythroid differentiation. Dev Cell 58(20):2112

Chapter 27

Murine Models of Transfusion-Induced Red Blood Cell Alloimmunization

Samata P. Varadkar, Victoria Ortiz, Abraham B. Alton, Brock D. Hughes, Sasikala Muthusamy, Shang-Chuen Wu, William O. Scott, Wenhui Li, Sean R. Stowell, Connie M. Arthur, and Ryan P. Jajosky

Abstract

Blood transfusion, while a life-saving intervention, carries inherent risks ranging from infectious complications to non-infectious hazards, such as transfusion-related acute lung injury, circulatory overload, and hemolytic reactions. While donor screening and pathogen inactivation technologies can significantly reduce infectious risks, preventing non-infectious complications remains challenging due to limited understanding of donor and recipient factors that govern these outcomes. To address this, genetically tractable murine models can be employed to elucidate key biological factors governing immune-mediated complications of transfusion. However, for these models to yield meaningful results, experimental approaches must closely mirror clinical practice. We describe herein methods for obtaining, characterizing, and transfusing red blood cells in murine models, specifically focusing on studying alloimmunization.

Key words Tail vein injection, RBC transfusion, Passive immunization, Antibodies, Intravenous injection, Tail vein bleeding, Lateral tail vein, Mouse restrainer, Intraperitoneal injection

1 Introduction

Preclinical models have been instrumental in advancing our understanding of disease processes for more than a century. These models were initially employed to identify the causative organisms of specific infectious diseases and subsequently expanded to explore host immunity in general [1]. Through preclinical studies, the critical roles of various host immune components in pathogen elimination, including antibodies, complement, phagocytes, T cells, and B cells, were identified and later confirmed as key conserved features of host immunity across mammalian evolution [2–7]. Similar models have provided valuable insights into innate immunity, such as Toll-like receptor signaling and other mechanisms that bridge pathogen exposure to an effective adaptive immune response [8–10]. The

Sean R. Stowell and Connie M. Arthur (eds.), *Methods in Transfusion Medicine*, Methods in Molecular Biology, vol. 3053, https://doi.org/10.1007/978-1-0716-5376-0_27,

knowledge gained from these preclinical studies has shaped our understanding of host immunity, with implications in fundamental biological processes and the advancement of medicine in general [11].

In contrast to many areas of medicine, the origins of transfusion medicine largely bypassed the use of preclinical models. Early attempts to transfer blood between other species and patients resulted in unpredictable outcomes [12]. It was not until the discovery of the immunological basis for blood incompatibility that transfusion became a viable medical procedure [12–17]. The discovery of blood group antigens and corresponding anti-blood group antibodies led to the development of testing methods to predict compatibility between donor red blood cells (RBCs) and recipients [13, 18, 19]. The early success of blood transfusions, made possible by ABO compatibility testing, initially diminished the urgency to investigate the underlying immunological factors that could potentially impede transfusion [19, 20]. However, as blood transfusions have become more common, an increasing number of patients have been shown to develop alloantibodies against various RBC antigens, and transfusion-related complications have become more prominent [12, 14–16, 21, 22]. This can be particularly pronounced in patients who require long-term transfusion therapy [15, 22–26]. For these individuals, such as patients with sickle cell disease (SCD), alloimmunization can result in serious transfusion complications, including both acute and delayed hemolytic transfusion reactions [27–35]. A variety of studies have demonstrated that excessive hemolysis in the setting of transfusion or complications of SCD in general can directly contribute to increased patient morbidity and mortality rates [25, 26, 36, 37].

While blood transfusions initially succeeded despite limited knowledge of immune barriers, organ transplantation often resulted in severe immune-mediated rejection, necessitating the development of models to define the immune mechanisms responsible for transplant incompatibility [38]. The need to understand the underlying immunologic basis for transplant rejection led to significant advancements in our understanding of host immunity, including the discovery of major histocompatibility antigens [7, 38]. Building on this foundation, similar experimental models were developed to study various autoimmune conditions, including experimental autoimmune encephalomyelitis (EAE) for multiple sclerosis [39], the K/BxN serum transfer model for rheumatoid arthritis [40], and the DSS/T cell adoptive transfer model for inflammatory bowel disease and colitis [41, 42]. Discoveries using these models underscore the importance of preclinical models in enhancing our understanding of immune-mediated diseases and have ultimately paved the way for more effective therapeutics [17].

As transfusion-dependent patients live longer [43], coupled with recent data demonstrating more severe complications associated with RBC alloimmunization [25, 29, 36, 44], a greater understanding of the factors that regulate RBC alloantibody development is needed. However, tools available to uncover key features of alloimmunization that may facilitate the identification of targetable immunological nodes responsible for the development of these antibodies have historically not been available. In the last decade, many studies have highlighted the significant advancements that have been made to address limitations in the study of the immunological consequences of not only transfused blood products, but intravenously exposed alloantigens in general [45–52]. These studies, which have benefited from the development of a variety of preclinical models for transfusion medicine, have uncovered unexpected features of the alloimmune response and provided important insight into the development and consequences of RBC alloimmunization [53–55]. Through these models, numerous studies have identified recipient factors, including specific immune populations and pathways, that may regulate alloimmunization [56–60]. Although specific immune pathways exist for different antigens [35, 61, 62], several studies suggest that there may be shared features among these pathways [63]. Identifying and targeting these common nodes could potentially lead to a unified approach for preventing alloimmune responses against a wide range of alloantigens, including other intravenously provided therapeutics [50, 63]. Additional studies have uncovered properties of transfused blood units that appear to impact alloantibody development [64–66], in addition a wide variety of studies that have examined features of RBCs and recipients that dictate incompatible RBC transfusion outcomes [45, 53, 65, 67–71]. In each setting, these models seek to recapitulate key features of blood transfusion used clinically. Herein, we will describe the use of preclinical models to examine alloimmune responses following RBC transfusion.

2 Materials

2.1 Mouse Blood Collection

2.1.1 Submandibular Bleed

1. Biosafety cabinet (BSC), class II A2 or B2.
2. Disinfectant: Make 70% ethanol from ethanol, HPLC/Spectrophotometric Grade, Liquid, ≥99.5%, glass bottle, 200 proof (Sigma-Aldrich, 459828-2L).
3. Paper towels.
4. Mouse blood donors:
   (a) C57BL/6 (B6) mice.
   (b) KEL mice on C57BL/6 background (*see* **Note 1**).

5. Mouse ear puncher, 2 mm diameter.
6. Acid citrate dextrose solution A (ACD-A), sterile 16 × 100 mm 8.5 mL BD Vacutainer® glass whole blood ACD tube (Owens & Minor, 364606).
7. Manual pipette and pipette tips.
8. 1.7 and 5 mL Eppendorf tubes, 50 mL conicals, and tube holders.
9. 5.5 mm sterile animal lancets.
10. Fisherbrand sterile cotton gauze pads, 4 × 4 in (Fisher Scientific, 22-415-469).
11. Empty mouse cage (recovery cage).
12. Marker/Sharpie Permanent Marker, Ultra Fine Tip, Black, Dozen (Staples, 37001).

2.1.2 Retro-Orbital Sinus Bleed

1. Fume hood.
2. Disinfectant: Make 70% ethanol from ethanol, HPLC/Spectrophotometric Grade, Liquid, ≥99.5%, Glass bottle, 200 Proof (Sigma-Aldrich, 459828-2L).
3. Paper towels.
4. Mouse blood donors:
   (a) C57BL/6 (B6) mice.
   (b) KEL mice on C57BL/6 background.
5. Acid citrate dextrose solution A (ACD-A), sterile 16 × 100 mm 8.5 mL BD Vacutainer® glass whole blood ACD tube (Owens & Minor, 364606).
6. Manual pipette and pipette tips.
7. 1.7 and 5 mL Eppendorf tubes, 50 mL conicals, and tube holders.
8. Pivetal® Isoflurane (Patterson Veterinary, 07-893-8441).
9. 1 mL Tuberculin Syringes (MEDLINE INDUSTRIES INC, 309659).
10. Glass staining trough with lid.
11. Surgical tweezers, curved.
12. Fisherbrand sterile cotton gauze pads, 4 x 4 in (Fisher Scientific, 22-415-469).
13. Aluminum foil.
14. Biohazard bag.
15. Marker/Sharpie Permanent Marker, Ultra Fine Tip, Black, Dozen (Staples, 37,001).

2.1.3 Processing Blood for Transfusion

1. Phosphate-buffered saline (PBS), sterile.
2. Motorized serological pipette controller and serological pipettes.
3. Centrifuge.
4. Antibodies for phenotyping the RBCs.
5. Manual pipette and pipette tips.
6. 96-well U bottom plate.
7. Flow cytometer.

2.2 Intraperitoneal Injection

1. Biosafety cabinet (BSC).
2. Disinfectant and paper towels.
3. Mouse recipients (e.g., C57BL/6 mice).
4. Empty mouse cage (recovery cage).
5. Poly(I:C) solution in a 5 mL or 50 mL conical.
   (a) Phosphate-buffered saline, sterile.
6. 1 mL tuberculin syringe, with Luer slip tip, sterile.
7. 30 gauge needles, which are 0.5 inches in length, sterile.
8. Sterile 4″ × 4″ gauze.
9. Sharpie or pen.

2.3 Intravenous Injection or Transfusion into the Lateral Tail Vein

1. Biosafety cabinet (BSC).
2. Disinfectant and paper towels.
3. Mouse recipients (e.g., C57BL/6 mice).
4. Empty mouse cage (recovery cage).
5. RBCs or antibody solution (experimental antibody and isotype control antibody) in a 5 mL Eppendorf or 50 mL conical.
   (a) Phosphate-buffered saline, sterile.
6. Small animal heat lamp, anchored to a support stand using clamps.
7. Mouse ear puncher, 2 mm.
8. 70% ethanol in a spray bottle.
9. Kimwipes.
10. Mouse restrainer and a separate platform to elevate it in the BSC.
11. Magnifying lamp with LED lights.
12. 1 mL tuberculin syringe, with Luer slip tip, sterile.
13. 30 gauge needles, which are 0.5 inches in length, sterile.
14. Sterile 4″ × 4″ gauze.
15. Sharpie or pen.

2.4 Collecting Serum from Alloimmunized Recipients

1. See Materials as used in 2.1.1 Submandibular bleed, except ACD-A is not needed.

2.5 Flow Cytometry Crossmatch to Assess Alloantibody Formation

1. Donor RBCs from C57Bl/6 mice.
2. Donor RBCs from KEL mice on a C57Bl/6 background.
3. 96-well U-bottom plate.
4. 1X Phosphate-buffered saline (PBS).
5. Reagent reservoirs, 50 or 100mL.
6. Allophycocyanin (APC) AffiniPure Goat Anti-Mouse IgG (subclasses 1 + 2a + 2b + 3), Fcγ Fragment. Specific Code: 115–135-164.
7. Fluorescein (FITC) AffiniPure F(ab')$_2$ Fragment Goat Anti-Mouse IgM, μ chain specific. Specific Code: 115–096-075.
8. FACS buffer (0.2% BSA in PBS).
9. 10 μL and 200 μL multichannel pipettes.
10. Centrifuge.
11. Flow cytometer.
12. Ice bucket with ice.

3 Methods

3.1 Mouse Blood Collection

Donor blood for transfusion is collected from a KEL mouse by either submandibular (Subheading 3.1.1) or retro-orbital (Subheading 3.1.2) bleeding. Calculations for appropriate blood volume depend on the number of recipient mice to be transfused (*see* **Notes 2** and **3**).

3.1.1 Submandibular Bleed

1. Calculate how much blood to collect.
2. Sterilize the BSC with a disinfectant and paper towels.
3. Add ACD anticoagulant solution to a blood collection tube (1.7, 5 or 50 mL tube). The volume of ACD should be ~20% of the estimated total whole blood volume to be collected. Use a marker to label the blood collection tube with the blood type.
4. If there are five mice in each cage, use the ear puncher to identify the mice. This can be done by putting one or two holes in the left or right ear and having no holes. These mice can be called L, LL, R, RR, and N.
5. Perform a submandibular bleed of the adult donor mice using a 5.5 mm animal lancet and collect the drops in the tube with ACD. The pointed part of the lancet can be directed downward at the mouse's cheek, midway between the ear and the eye.

6. After the mouse is bled, apply pressure using a sterile gauze pad for a few seconds to stop the bleeding.
7. Place the mouse in the empty mouse cage (i.e., recovery cage).
8. Proceed to bleed additional mice in the same manner.
9. Document which mice were face bled and the date on the cage cards using a marker.

3.1.2 Retro-Orbital Sinus Bleed

1. Calculate how much blood to collect.
2. Clean the fume hood with disinfectant and paper towels.
3. Add ACD anticoagulant solution to a blood collection tube (1.7, 5 or 50 mL tube). The volume of ACD should be ~20% of the estimated total whole blood volume to be collected.
4. Place gauze at the bottom of the glass staining trough.
5. Add 0.3 mL of isoflurane to the gauze in a chamber of ~500 mL.
6. Cover the gauze with aluminum foil.
7. Place a mouse on top of the aluminum foil in the chamber.
8. Watch the mouse as it starts to lose consciousness and breathing slows.
9. Remove the mouse from the chamber and perform a toe pinch to ensure it doesn't respond and has sufficient anesthesia.
10. Scruff the anesthetized mouse and pull the skin such that the eyeball bulges outward.
11. Use the curved tweezer to quickly remove one eyeball.
12. Collect the drops of blood into the ACD solution.
13. Immediately perform cervical dislocation and put the carcass in a biohazard bag.
14. Label the tube of blood accordingly.

3.1.3 Processing Blood for Transfusion

1. Fill the tube of blood with PBS.
2. Centrifuge at 500× *g* for 7 min with break low or off.
3. Carefully remove the supernatant by reverse pipetting.
4. Repeat **steps 1–3** twice for a total of three washes.
5. Phenotype the RBCs using appropriate antibodies. For example, use mouse anti-KEL IgG primary antibodies (MIMA-8 and MIMA-9), followed by APC-conjugated anti-mouse IgG secondary antibody. Then, use a flow cytometer to confirm that the RBCs express KEL.

3.2 Intraperitoneal Injection

1. Sterilize the BSC with a disinfectant and paper towels.
2. Dissolve poly(I:C), also known as PIC, in sterile PBS.

   (a) Each mouse will receive an IP injection of 100 μg poly(I:C) diluted with PBS to 500 μL of total volume or just receive 500uL of PBS.
3. Prepare the syringe and needle with 1 mL of the poly(I:C) solution.
4. Inject the poly(I:C) or PBS.
   (a) Scruff a mouse (*see* **Note 4**).
   (b) Aim the syringe and needle (bevel up) for the right lower quadrant.
   (c) Approach at ~30° angle.
   (d) Slightly insert the needle into the abdomen (*see* **Note 5**).
   (e) Inject the poly(I:C) or PBS.
   (f) Remove the syringe and needle.
5. Return the mouse to the recovery cage.
6. Document the procedure on the cage card.

3.3 Intravenous Injection or Transfusion into the Lateral Tail Vein (See Fig. 1)

1. Sterilize the BSC with a disinfectant and paper towels.
2. Set up the magnifying lamp with LED lights and mouse restrainer.
3. Fill 1 mL syringes with the sterile antibody solution, isotype control antibody, PBS, or RBCs (*see* **Note 6**).
   (a) Often, 100 μg of antibody in 500 μL volume is administered per adult mouse.
4. Warm the recipient mice under the heat lamp for several minutes (*see* **Note 7**).
5. Ear punch the mice.
6. Place a mouse in the restrainer.
   (a) Use the stopper/plug to prevent the mouse from exiting the restrainer. The stopper/plug should be at a position that does not allow the mouse to move around.
   (b) Gently rotate the tail to orient the mouse such that the lateral tail vein is facing upward.
   (c) Disinfect the tail using a Kimwipe soaked in 70% ethanol.
7. Insert the 1 mL syringe with a 30-gauge needle, bevel up, into the distal end of the lateral tail vein (*see* **Note 8**). Inject the antibody solution, isotype control antibody, PBS, or RBCs.
8. If examining incompatible transfusion outcomes following passive administration of an anti-RBC alloantibody, inject the appropriate volume of antibody solution.
9. After successful injection, compress the injection site with a gauze to stop any bleeding.
10. Move the mouse to a recovery cage.

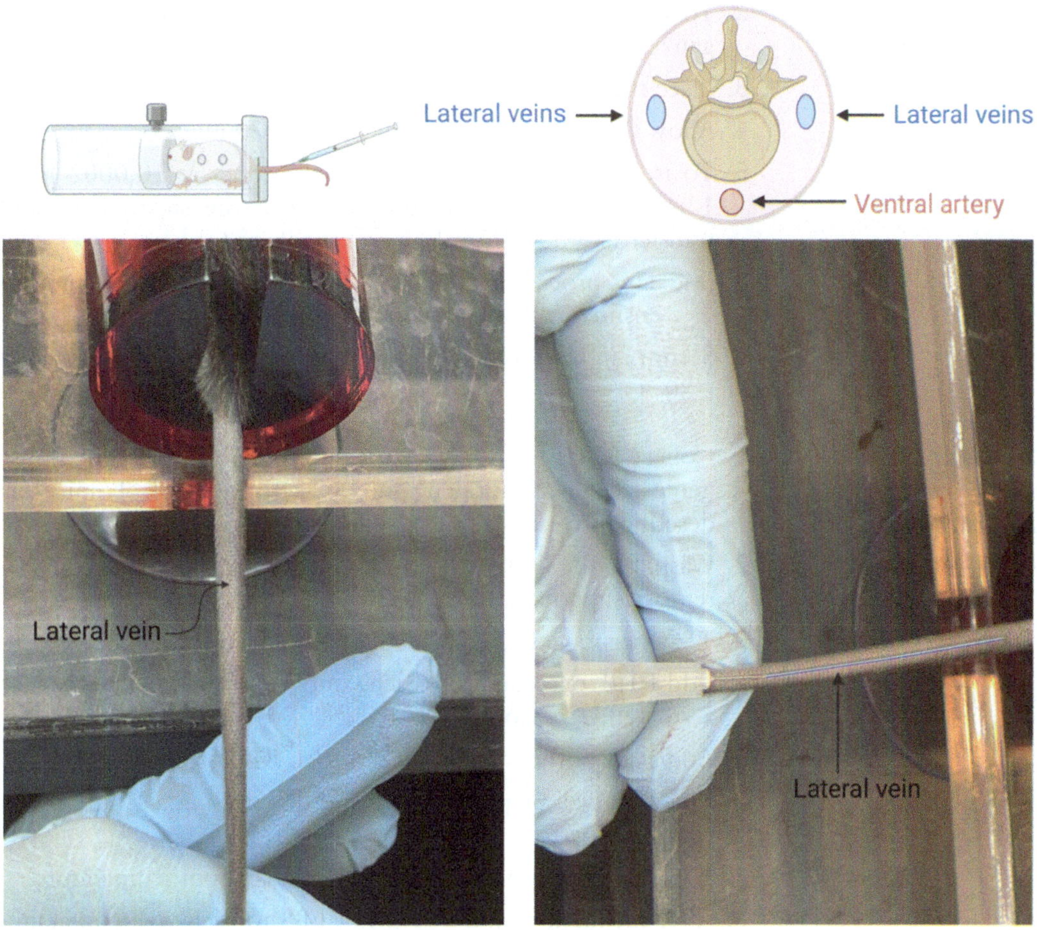

Fig. 1 Intravenous injection into the lateral tail vein of a mouse in a restrainer

11. Continue to passively immunize the remaining mice.
12. Inject the remaining, non-passively immunized recipients with the same volume of PBS.
13. Document the procedure on the mouse cage card.
14. For RBC transfusions in passively immunized recipients and controls, wait at least 30 min for the antibodies to equilibrate. Transfuse the RBCs using the same protocol employed for antibody solution injection.
    (a) 50 μL of packed RBCs diluted in PBS to a total volume of 300 μL is a typical dose for an adult mouse.

3.4 Collecting Serum from Alloimmunized Recipients

1. At defined time points (typically 3 days, 5 days, 7 days, 14 days, 21 days, and 28 days post-transfusion), collect 4–6 drops of whole blood into empty 1.7 mL microcentrifuge tubes via submandibular bleed (refer to Method 3.1.1, but do not use ACD).

2. To stop the bleeding, compress the bleeding site using sterile gauze.
3. Place the mouse in a recovery cage.
4. Allow the blood to clot for at least 20–30 min.
5. To isolate the serum, centrifuge the tubes at 10,000× *g* for 1 min at room temperature. Remove the supernatant and transfer to a new 1.7 mL microcentrifuge tube.
   (a) This process may need to be repeated one more time to ensure no RBCs remain in the serum.
6. Serum can be stored in 1.7 mL microcentrifuge tubes frozen at −80 °C.

3.5 Flow Cytometry Crossmatch to Assess Alloantibody Formation

1. Collect RBCs from mice expressing a high level of the transgenic RBC alloantigen and C57BL/6 control mice as described in Subheading 3.1 (*see* **Notes 9** and **10**).
2. Wash blood 3× with PBS. Use careful reverse pipetting to remove supernatant between washes.
3. Thaw serum collected from alloimmunized recipients.
4. Add 10 μL of serum from each sample into an individual well of a 96-well U-bottom plate on ice.
5. Add 1 μL of the washed packed KEL RBCs to each well.
6. Mix each well by pipetting up and down using a 10 μL multichannel pipette.
7. Incubate the 96-well plate for 15 min at room temperature.
8. After incubation, add 200 μL of PBS to each well containing RBCs, using a 200 μL multichannel pipette.
9. Centrifuge the plate at 500× *g* for 1 min. Once the plate has been spun down, ensure that the pellets are at the bottom of each well and carefully remove the supernatant. The plate can be flicked (rapidly inverted) over a sink to remove the supernatant.
10. Wash the RBCs by repeating **steps 8–9** twice more, for a total of three washes.
11. Prepare secondary antibodies in the FACS buffer solution at a dilution ratio of 1:100 (1 μL APC anti-mouse IgG antibody, 1 μL FITC anti-mouse IgM antibody, and 98 μL FACS buffer).
12. Add 25 μL of prepared secondary antibody solution to each well containing RBCs. Mix by pipetting up and down using a 200 μL multichannel pipette.
13. Incubate the 96-well U-bottom plate for 15 min in the dark at room temperature.

14. Add 200 μL of PBS to each well using a 200 μL multichannel pipette and mix by pipetting up and down.
15. Centrifuge the 96-well U-bottom plate at 500× *g* for 1 min.
16. Once the plate has been spun down, ensure that the pellets are at the bottom of each well and carefully remove the supernatant.
17. Wash the pellets by repeating **steps 14–16** twice for a total of three washes.
18. After the final wash, resuspend each pellet in 200 μL of PBS.
19. Perform flow cytometry.
    (a) Analyze the samples using a flow cytometer.
        (i) Collect 50,000 RBC singlets for each sample.
    (b) Optional: Analyze the data using FlowJo software.
    (c) Export the MFIs for FITC and APC to Microsoft Excel.
    (d) Import the data to GraphPad Prism to create graphs.

4 Notes

1. Several transgenic mouse models are used to study RBC alloimmunization. Although this chapter focuses on the KEL system, other models are also employed, including the HOD system, which involves transgenic expression of a chimeric HEL, OVA, and Duffy antigen, as well as the human glycophorin A (GPA) transgenic model. Additionally, various KEL transgenic founder lines have been described, each exhibiting different levels of KEL expression. Besides using C57BL/6 mice as recipients, studies can also employ knockout or treated mouse models to selectively alter components of the immune system and assess their contributions to alloantibody formation following RBC transfusion.
2. Ensure that experimental protocols and animal procedures performed in these studies are approved by your Institutional Animal Care and Use Committee (IACUC), Institutional Biosafety Committee (IBC), and/or by any other relevant entities. Follow your institution's policies for mouse blood collection (e.g., methods and volumes). When leukoreducing blood, apply blood to the leukoreduction filter prior to exposure to PBS. Effective leukoreduction is assessed by flow cytometry on the final product.
3. To determine how much blood needs to be collected, multiply 50 uL of packed RBCs, the typical dose transfused to mice, by the number of mice that need to be transfused with that blood type. 8–10-week-old male and female B6 mice have a

hematocrit of ~45%, meaning that ~45% of the blood volume is pRBCs. Multiply the amount of pRBCs to be collected by 2.22 to calculate the total volume of whole blood to be collected. Collect more than this amount because some will be lost when processing, when phenotyping, when labeling, and in the dead space of the syringe's needle.

4. Ensure that your hand is entirely behind the mouse so that it cannot push off your hand while performing the IP injection.
5. Insert the needle halfway (approximately 0.25 inches of a 0.5 inch needle) into the mouse to ensure proper intraperitoneal (IP) injection. Inadequate needle depth may result in a subcutaneous injection, which can be identified by a localized fluid bulge under the skin. Note that a PIC injection is not required, though it is sometimes performed to enhance the immune response to the transfused RBCs.
6. When filling the 1 mL syringe with the antibody solution, place the syringe (without a needle) into the solution. Pull the plunger outward to add solution. Invert the syringe, pull the plunger further outward, tap the syringe so that the air goes to the top, and expel the air from the syringe by pushing the plunger inward. Do not pull the plunger so far back that it comes out of the shaft of the syringe. Attach a needle such that the upward bevel aligns with the volume markings on the syringe. Eject the solution to remove air from the dead space of the needle.
7. Do not leave the mice unattended while they are being heated.
8. If there is resistance when injecting the antibody solution, then the needle is not within the lateral tail vein. To rectify this, remove the needle, move closer to the base of the tail, and try again.
9. The volume of blood to collect depends on the number of samples that will be assessed for alloantibodies. 1 μL of RBCs will be needed per sample tested.
10. To determine the appropriate background for binding, this assay can be repeated in parallel using C57BL/6 RBCs instead of KEL RBCs, for at least some of the serum samples.

Conflicts of Interest

This work was funded by NIH P01HL171803, R01 HL165975, R01 HL135575, R01 HL154034, K08HL171877, K99HL169746, and AABB Foundation Early-Career Scientific Research Grants. SRS has received speaker and consultant honoraria from Cerus, Grifols, Novartis, Alexion, and Argenx and has received a research grant from Alexion. Ryan Jajosky is CEO of Biconcavity Inc. No other authors have conflicts of interest.

References

1. Kaufmann SH, Schaible UE (2005) 100th anniversary of Robert Koch's Nobel prize for the discovery of the tubercle bacillus. Trends Microbiol 13(10):469–475
2. Moser M, Leo O (2010) Key concepts in immunology. Vaccine 28(Suppl 3):C2–C13
3. Siggs OM (2014) Dissecting mammalian immunity through mutation. Immunol Cell Biol 92(5):392–399
4. Amit I, Regev A, Hacohen N (2011) Strategies to discover regulatory circuits of the mammalian immune system. Nat Rev Immunol 11(12):873–880
5. Gitlin AD, Nussenzweig MC (2015) Immunology: fifty years of B lymphocytes. Nature 517(7533):139–141
6. Miller JF (2004) Events that led to the discovery of T-cell development and function–a personal recollection. Tissue Antigens 63(6): 509–517
7. Klein J (2001) George Snell's first foray into the unexplored territory of the major histocompatibility complex. Genetics 159(2): 435–439
8. Ozato K, Tsujimura H, Tamura T (2002) Toll-like receptor signaling and regulation of cytokine gene expression in the immune system. BioTechniques Suppl:66–68. 70, 72 passim
9. Kawasaki T, Kawai T (2014) Toll-like receptor signaling pathways. Front Immunol 5:461
10. O'Neill LA, Golenbock D, Bowie AG (2013) The history of toll-like receptors – redefining innate immunity. Nat Rev Immunol 13(6): 453–460
11. Li Y, Baldridge MT (2023) Modelling human immune responses using microbial exposures in rodents. Nat Microbiol 8(3):363–366
12. Zimring JC, Spitalnik SL (2015) Pathobiology of transfusion reactions. Annu Rev Pathol 10: 83–110
13. Storry JR, Olsson ML (2009) The ABO blood group system revisited: a review and update. Immunohematology 25(2):48–59
14. Pirenne F, Pondarre C (2023) Alloimmunization and hyperhemolysis in sickle cell disease. Hematology Am Soc Hematol Educ Program 2023(1):653–659
15. Pirenne F, Floch A, Diop S (2023) Alloimmunisation against red blood cells in sickle cell disease: transfusion challenges in high-income and low-income countries. Lancet Haematol 10(6):e468–e476
16. Pirenne F, Yazdanbakhsh K (2018) How I safely transfuse patients with sickle-cell disease and manage delayed hemolytic transfusion reactions. Blood 131(25):2773–2781
17. Arthur CM, Stowell SR (2023) The development and consequences of red blood cell alloimmunization. Annu Rev Pathol 18:537–564
18. Panch SR, Montemayor-Garcia C, Klein HG (2019) Hemolytic transfusion reactions. N Engl J Med 381(2):150–162
19. Jajosky RP et al (2023) ABO blood group antigens and differential glycan expression: perspective on the evolution of common human enzyme deficiencies. iScience 26(1):105798
20. Joseph A et al (2023) ABO Genotyping finds more A(2) to B kidney transplant opportunities than lectin-based subtyping. Am J Transplant 23(4):512–519
21. Yazdanbakhsh K, Shaz BH, Hillyer CD (2017) Immune regulation of sickle cell alloimmunization. ISBT Sci Ser 12(1):248–253
22. Meuleman MS, Roumenina LT, Grunenwald A (2023) Complement involvement in sickle cell disease. Presse Med 52(4):104205
23. Chang DY et al (2023) The ongoing challenge of RBC alloimmunization in the management of patients with sickle cell disease. Presse Med 52(4):104211
24. Falguiere C et al (2023) Delayed hemolytic transfusion reaction in children with sickle cell disease: first 5-year retrospective study in mainland France. Haematologica 108(3):889–894
25. Viayna E et al (2022) Red cell alloimmunization is associated with increased health care costs, longer hospitalizations, and higher mortality. Blood Adv 6(20):5655–5658
26. Dean CL et al (2019) Multiple hemolytic transfusion reactions misinterpreted as severe vaso-occlusive crisis in a patient with sickle cell disease. Transfusion 59(2):448–453
27. Dumas G et al (2016) Eculizumab salvage therapy for delayed hemolysis transfusion reaction in sickle cell disease patients. Blood 127(8): 1062–1064
28. Chonat S et al (2018) Contribution of alternative complement pathway to delayed hemolytic transfusion reaction in sickle cell disease. Haematologica 103(10):e483–e485
29. Narbey D et al (2017) Incidence and predictive score for delayed hemolytic transfusion reaction in adult patients with sickle cell disease. Am J Hematol 92(12):1340–1348
30. Chonat S et al (2020) Eculizumab for complement mediated thrombotic microangiopathy in

sickle cell disease. Haematologica 105(12): 2887–2891
31. Chou ST, Hendrickson JE (2024) How I treat challenging transfusion cases in sickle cell disease. Blood. https://doi.org/10.1182/blood.2023023648
32. Vichinsky EP et al (1990) Alloimmunization in sickle cell anemia and transfusion of racially unmatched blood. N Engl J Med 322(23): 1617–1621
33. Thein SL et al (2020) Hemolytic transfusion reactions in sickle cell disease: underappreciated and potentially fatal. Haematologica 105(3):539–544
34. Vidler JB et al (2015) Delayed haemolytic transfusion reaction in adults with sickle cell disease: a 5-year experience. Br J Haematol 169(5):746–753
35. Hudson KE et al (2019) Mechanisms of alloimmunization in sickle cell disease. Curr Opin Hematol 26(6):434–441
36. Viayna E, Gehrie EA, Blanchette C (2024) Alloimmunization in myelodysplastic syndrome is associated with higher healthcare costs, longer hospitalizations, and increased mortality. Transfusion 64(9):1640–1647
37. Chonat S et al (2025) Complement is activated in patients with acute chest syndrome caused by sickle cell disease and represents a therapeutic target. Sci Transl Med 17(807):eadl4922
38. Nordham KD, Ninokawa S (2022) The history of organ transplantation. Proceedings (Bayl Univ Med Cent) 35(1):124–128
39. Sabatino JJ Jr et al (2011) High prevalence of low affinity peptide-MHC II tetramer-negative effectors during polyclonal CD4+ T cell responses. J Exp Med 208(1):81–90
40. Christensen AD et al (2016) K/BxN serum-transfer arthritis as a model for human inflammatory arthritis. Front Immunol 7:213
41. Robinson BS et al (2020) Galectin-9 is a novel regulator of epithelial restitution. Am J Pathol 190(8):1657–1666
42. Garcia-Hernandez V et al (2023) Inhibition of soluble stem cell factor promotes intestinal mucosal repair. Inflamm Bowel Dis 29(7): 1133–1144
43. Jiao B et al (2023) Long-term survival with sickle cell disease: a nationwide cohort study of Medicare and Medicaid beneficiaries. Blood Adv 7(13):3276–3283
44. Telen MJ et al (2015) Alloimmunization in sickle cell disease: changing antibody specificities and association with chronic pain and decreased survival. Transfusion 55(6 Pt 2): 1378–1387
45. Hod EA et al (2008) Cytokine storm in a mouse model of IgG-mediated hemolytic transfusion reactions. Blood 112(3):891–894
46. Zimring JC, Hudson KE (2016) Cellular immune responses in red blood cell alloimmunization. Hematology Am Soc Hematol Educ Program 2016(1):452–456
47. Smith NH et al (2012) Generation of transgenic mice with antithetical KEL1 and KEL2 human blood group antigens on red blood cells. Transfusion 52(12):2620–2630
48. Stowell SR et al (2013) Alloantibodies to a paternally derived RBC KEL antigen lead to hemolytic disease of the fetus/newborn in a murine model. Blood 122(8):1494–1504
49. Arthur CM et al (2016) CD8+ T cells mediate antibody-independent platelet clearance in mice. Blood 127(14):1823–1827
50. Zerra PE et al (2017) Marginal zone B cells are critical to factor VIII inhibitor formation in mice with hemophilia A. Blood 130(23): 2559–2568
51. Davenport P et al (2022) Platelet transfusions in a murine model of neonatal polymicrobial sepsis: divergent effects on inflammation and mortality. Transfusion 62(6):1177–1187
52. Arthur CM et al (2022) Nonhuman glycans can regulate anti-factor VIII antibody formation in mice. Blood 139(9):1312–1317
53. Zimring JC et al (2005) Nonhemolytic antibody-induced loss of erythrocyte surface antigen. Blood 106(3):1105–1112
54. Desmarets M et al (2009) Minor histocompatibility antigens on transfused leukoreduced units of red blood cells induce bone marrow transplant rejection in a mouse model. Blood 114(11):2315–2322
55. Smith NH et al (2012) Transfusion in the absence of inflammation induces antigen-specific tolerance to murine RBCs. Blood 119(6):1566–1569
56. Arneja A et al (2016) Interleukin-6 receptor-alpha signaling drives anti-RBC alloantibody production and T-follicular helper cell differentiation in a murine model of red blood cell alloimmunization. Haematologica 101(11): e440–e444
57. Calabro S et al (2016) Bridging channel dendritic cells induce immunity to transfused red blood cells. J Exp Med 213(6):887–896
58. Gibb DR et al (2017) Type I IFN is necessary and sufficient for inflammation-induced red blood cell alloimmunization in mice. J Immunol 199(3):1041–1050
59. Soldatenko A et al (2022) Innate and adaptive immunity to transfused allogeneic RBCs in

mice requires MyD88. J Immunol 208(4): 991–997

60. Jash A et al (2024) Complement C3 and marginal zone B cells promote IgG-mediated enhancement of RBC alloimmunization in mice. J Clin Invest 134(8):e167665
61. Mener A et al (2018) Complement serves as a switch between CD4+ T cell-independent and -dependent RBC antibody responses. JCI Insight 3(22):e121631
62. Shinde P et al (2020) IgG subclass determines suppression versus enhancement of humoral Alloimmunity to Kell RBC antigens in mice. Front Immunol 11:1516
63. Zerra PE et al (2021) Marginal zone B cells mediate a CD4 T-cell-dependent extrafollicular antibody response following RBC transfusion in mice. Blood 138(8):706–721
64. Thomas TA et al (2023) Reticulocytes in donor blood units enhance red blood cell alloimmunization. Haematologica 108(10):2639–2651
65. Jash A et al (2021) Antibodies to low-copy number RBC alloantigen convert a Tolerogenic stimulus to an immunogenic stimulus in mice. Front Immunol 12:629608
66. Jajosky R et al (2023) Prior immunization against an intracellular antigen enhances subsequent red blood cell alloimmunization in mice. Blood 141(21):2642–2653
67. Liepkalns JS et al (2012) Biphasic clearance of incompatible red blood cells through a novel mechanism requiring neither complement nor Fcgamma receptors in a murine model. Transfusion 52(12):2631–2645
68. Arthur CM et al (2021) Antigen density dictates RBC clearance, but not antigen modulation, following incompatible RBC transfusion in mice. Blood Adv 5(2):527–538
69. Escamilla-Rivera V et al (2021) Complement plays a critical role in inflammation-induced Immunoprophylaxis failure in mice. Front Immunol 12:704072
70. Jajosky RP et al (2023) Antibody-mediated antigen loss switches augmented immunity to antibody-mediated immunosuppression. Blood 142(12):1082–1098
71. Girard-Pierce KR et al (2013) A novel role for C3 in antibody-induced red blood cell clearance and antigen modulation. Blood 122(10): 1793–1801

Chapter 28

Establishing, Maintaining, and Cryopreserving In Vitro Cultures of the Asexual Stages of *Babesia divergens*

Divya Beri, Marilis Rodriguez, and Cheryl A. Lobo

Abstract

Human babesiosis is caused by four *Babesia* spp., which are intraerythrocytic Apicomplexan zoonotic parasites that, in the last 50 years, have contributed to establishing the parasitic infection as a significant transfusion-transmitted infectious threat and an escalating public-health problem. Of the four species that infect humans, *B. divergens* was the first to be grown in vitro, via continuous culture in human RBCs. In this chapter, we have comprehensively outlined the basic and necessary tools, protocols, and methodology to successfully grow and study the parasite. Details of in vitro culturing using human serum and Albumax, cryopreservation and thawing, subculturing, maintenance of cultures over extended times, calculation of parasite load using the traditional light microscopy method, and flow cytometry have been elaborated upon. This chapter can serve as standard operating procedures (SOP) for laboratories working on *Babesia* research and those that want to establish in vitro culturing of *B. divergens* field isolates, as well as related parasites.

Key words *Babesia*, Culture, Intra-erythrocytic forms, Flow cytometry, Microscopy, Giemsa

1 Introduction

Human babesiosis is a zoonotic infection caused by *Babesia* parasites transmitted by the bite of ixodid ticks and has distinct geographical distributions based on the presence of their competent natural animal hosts, which include rodents, cattle, and deer. The genus *Babesia* comprises many species of parasites, which are transmitted when the ticks take a blood meal from the vertebrate host (reviewed previously by our research group [1–3]). Parasite infection in its natural hosts, like cattle, results in bovine babesiosis and contributes to a significant economic loss [4]. The severity of human infection is becoming apparent nowadays, whether the disease has been primarily transmitted from a tick bite or secondarily transmitted via a blood transfusion with infected blood [5, 6] or even congenitally during pregnancy [7, 8]. The four identified *Babesia* species definitively confirmed to infect humans so far are

Sean R. Stowell and Connie M. Arthur (eds.), *Methods in Transfusion Medicine*, Methods in Molecular Biology, vol. 3053, https://doi.org/10.1007/978-1-0716-5376-0_28,

B. microti, *B. divergens*, *B. duncani*, and *B. venatorum* [9, 10]. In all species, the general life cycle within humans remains the same; *Babesia* parasites are intracellular obligates that target red blood cells, and the parasite's ability to first recognize and then invade host red blood cells (RBCs) is central to the disease pathology [11, 12].

The study of babesiosis should be considered a priority because *Babesia* is now recognized as a zoonotic parasite with a fast-growing infection rate in humans by transfer from mammalian animal reservoirs. Additionally, *Babesia* represents a potential threat to the blood supply for transfusions since asymptomatic infections in humans, reviewed by us [13], are common, and these can be life-threatening in certain recipients. Transfusion-transmitted babesiosis remains a problem in the US because donor testing is not universal. The spectrum of human babesiosis is broad, ranging from an apparently silent infection to a fulminant, malaria-like disease, resulting occasionally in death. When present, symptoms are typically non-specific and include fever, headache, and myalgia [14, 15]. Human babesiosis is a zoonotic disease; the natural acquisition of human cases is most often the result of interaction with established zoonotic cycles. Emerging diseases are defined as "new, re-emerging or drug-resistant infections whose incidence in humans has increased within the past five decades or whose incidence threatens to increase in the near future." By virtue of the number of human infections since 1970, human babesiosis can be considered an emerging disease [16]. A number of factors have contributed to the "emergence" of human babesiosis, including increased awareness among physicians, changing ecology, and an increased population of immunocompromised individuals, who exhibit severe disease. Human babesiosis has become a significant public-health concern partly because the Ixodes tick has undergone a rapid expansion of its geographic range and the increasing proportion of the population is at risk for complications from *Babesia* infection. The CDC designated babesiosis as a nationally notifiable disease in 2011. The northern part of the US is a babesiosis-endemic area where the incidence has risen to 2000 cases per year in the last decade [17]. Over time, the high-risk areas have expanded due to evolving ecosystems, especially a marked increase in the number and geographic range of white-tailed deer that markedly amplify tick numbers. More recently, climate change is also thought to contribute to the parasite's expanding range [18, 19]. Mortality rates have risen to 30% in susceptible hosts, which include people with a risk factor for severe babesiosis, including extremes in age, lack of a spleen, hemoglobinopathies, cancers, HIV, and use of immunosuppressive therapy [20, 21]. In these patients, babesiosis may be refractory to standard antimicrobial therapy [22] and may result in prolonged illness or death.

Transfusion-transmitted babesiosis remains a problem in the US because donor testing is not universal [23, 24]. Patients are particularly vulnerable if they need a high frequency of transfusion, as this at times requires blood procurement from states where *Babesia* screening is not mandatory. Transfusion recipients are disproportionately at risk of severe or even fatal babesiosis, given their predisposing comorbid risk factors that include extremes of age, cardiorespiratory disease, asplenia, cancer, immunosuppressive therapy, and other immunocompromizing conditions [13].

Research into the causative agents of most diseases, including those caused by parasites, has benefited enormously from the ability to culture forms of the pathogen in vitro. This is exemplified in the case of babesiosis, where understanding the biology and pathogenesis of *Babesia* species like *B. bovis*, *B. divergens*, and now *B. duncani* has accelerated [25–28], in contrast to parasites like B. microti that have not yet been successfully cultivated in vitro. Thus, it is important to detail specific components of the in vitro culture to enable progress in the understanding of host–parasite relationships, parasite biology, and pathophysiology, facilitating new tools for diagnosis, epidemiology, treatment, and prevention of human babesiosis, as well as assisting in developing novel methods to screen blood products.

Parasite blood stage in vitro assays and culture can be divided into four categories, namely: (i) single cycles of growth, which consist of a single maturation cycle from ring to two/four-celled parasite stage without new invasions. Here, parasites are cultured directly from source (animal/human) without the addition of fresh RBCs; (ii) short-term cultures include several cycles of invasion and egress but are not sustainable for a long time. These two are generally the only available routes to obtain host–parasite material when continuous in vitro parasite cultivation has not been successful; (iii) invasion assays, where merozoites are purified and incubated with RBCs from different sources or treated with various enzymes to look for use of specific invasion pathways; (iv) long-term cultures, which should ideally be continuous in vitro propagation once a stable invasion phenotype is obtained. In our laboratory, we have been able to achieve all four types of culture with *B. divergens* [29–32]. Specific protocols for both invasion assays and continuous in vitro culture platforms are detailed below.

2 Materials and Instruments

2.1 In vitro *Culturing, Subculturing, and Maintenance of* B. divergens

1. Albumin sources
   (a) Heat-inactivated pooled A+ or AB+ human serum (matched to the human blood used to grow the parasite) (*see* **Note 1**).
   (b) Albumax II (ThermoFisher Cat # 11021-037) (*see* **Note 2**).
2. RPMI (Gibco; Gibco Catalog # 23400-021) powder.
3. Hypoxanthine (Sigma, Catalog # H9636-5G).
4. 7% sodium bicarbonate solution (Gibco Cat # 25-080-094).
5. 50% hematocrit RBCs (any blood group can be used; we use A+) in 1X RPMI pH 7.2.
6. Sterile culture flasks (T25 and T75 for culture volumes of 7.5–10 mL and 25–30 mL, respectively).
7. Sterile pipettes—plugged and unplugged.
8. Gas cylinder with a mix of 90%N_2/5%O_2/5%CO_2.
9. Microscope slides, Giemsa (VWR Cat # 48311-702), and light microscope.

2.2 . Monitoring Parasitemia Using a Light Microscope

1. Microscope slides.
2. Giemsa (Sigma Cat # GS500).
3. 100% methanol.
4. Light microscope equipped with 100X lens.

2.3 Monitoring Parasitemia Using Flow Cytometry

1. BV421 Mouse Anti-Human CD235a (BD Horizon; Cat # 562938).
2. Vybran DyeCycle™ Green Stain (ThermoFisher Scientific; Cat # V35004).
3. Sterile 1X PBS pH 7.4.
4. Flow tubes (Falcon-A Corning Brand; Fisher Cat # 14-959-5).
5. Flow cytometer equipped with UV, blue, green, and red lasers.

2.4 Purification of Merozoites and Invasion into Washed Human RBCs

1. 5 μm filters (Pall Corporation; Cat # 4199).
2. 1.2 μm filters (Pall Corporation; Cat # 4190).
3. 1 mL BD Luer-Lok tip syringe (Fisher; Cat # 14-823-30).
4. Sterile droppers (VWR; Cat # 73990-096).
5. 50% hematocrit washed human RBCs.
6. Incomplete RPMI.
7. Centrifuge (fixed angle).
8. Polypropylene centrifuge tubes, 15 mL (Fisher; Cat # 14-959-70C).

***2.5 Cryopreservation and Thawing of* B. divergens**

1. Human Serum (80%) in RPMI.
2. DMSO (15%) in RPMI.
3. 50 mL Falcon tube.
4. Fenwal Glycerolyte 57 solution (Fisher catalog # NC2941211).
5. Cryopreservation tubes (Life Technologies Catalog#12-565-167N).
6. 10% serum medium (complete medium) or cRPMI with 0.5% Albumax.
7. 50% hematocrit RBCs.
8. Sterile culture flasks.

3 Methods

3.1 In Vitro *Culturing, Subculturing, and Maintenance of* B. divergens

3.1.1 Maintenance

1. Pre-warm the complete medium at 37 °C for about 30 min before starting.
2. Work in the hood with the laminar flow on and the UV off.
3. Carefully remove the culture flask from the incubator and place it in the hood.
4. Remove the lid.
5. Using a sterile, unplugged pipette attached to the vacuum, remove as much medium as possible by gently lifting the bottom of the flask. Do not aspirate RBCs.
6. Discard the pipette appropriately in the bin labeled "Sharps" and "Biohazard."
7. If required, make a smear using a plugged pipette and stain with Giemsa (as detailed under Subheading 3.3).
8. Stand the flask upright.
9. Add fresh complete RPMI (cRPMI) to maintain appropriate culture volume. Use cRPMI either containing 10% human serum or 0.5% Albumax II (*see* **Note 2**).
10. Using a sterile plugged pipette, gas the culture flask for 30 s (*see* **Note 3**).
11. Securely replace the culture lid.
12. Lay the flask down and return it to the incubator.
13. Return medium and cells to the refrigerator.
14. Clean the hood with 70% ethanol and turn on the UV light.

3.1.2 Maintaining a "Safe" Flask and Maintenance Over a 2-Day Weekend

1. Set the "safe" flask at 0.1% parasitemia, 5% hematocrit on Friday (for a Saturday-Sunday weekend). Set your other flasks as required, but not higher than 1%.

2. Later in the afternoon/evening on Saturday or early Sunday, change the medium for the flasks (*see* **Note 4**).
3. Maintain your "safe" flask at <5% from Mon–Fri and use this flask to seed parasites for the weekend. This ensures propagation of healthy, non-stressed parasites.

3.1.3 Subculturing

1. Pre-warm the complete medium at 37 °C for about 30 min before starting.
2. Determine the parasitemia of the culture that requires subculturing.
3. Using the calculation V1 × C1 = V2 × C2, determine the volume of full culture (RBCs and medium) needed to transfer from the old flask into the new flask:

V1 = volume to transfer	C1 = parasitemia of old culture
V2 = required final volume of new culture.	C2 = required parasitemia of new culture

4. Work in the hood with the laminar flow on and UV off.
5. Add required volume of old culture to new flask.
6. Add the required volume of fresh RBCs to the new flask to maintain 5% hematocrit.
7. Add cRPMI up to the final culture volume required.
8. Using a sterile plugged pipette, gas the culture flask for 30 s^{-1} min, depending on the volume of the flask.
9. Securely replace the culture lid.
10. Lay the flask down and place it in the incubator.
11. Return medium and cells to the refrigerator.
12. If the old culture is to be discarded, add 10–20 mL 10% Clorox to the old flask and mix well, and discard old cells down the sink with plenty of flowing water.
13. Discard the empty flask appropriately in a biohazard labeled bin.
14. Clean the hood with 70% ethanol and turn on the UV light.

3.2 Monitoring Parasitemia Using a Light Microscope

1. Take 50 μL of the full culture into a clean sterile 1.5 mL tube.
2. Spin the sample and remove most of the medium. Resuspend the pellet with ~10–20 μL medium to make the smear.
3. Add ~5 μL of RBC-rich culture to a clean microscope slide at the end nearest to the white end of the slide.
4. Place the narrow edge of a second slide into this sample at a 45° angle and allow the sample to draw across the full width of the slide.

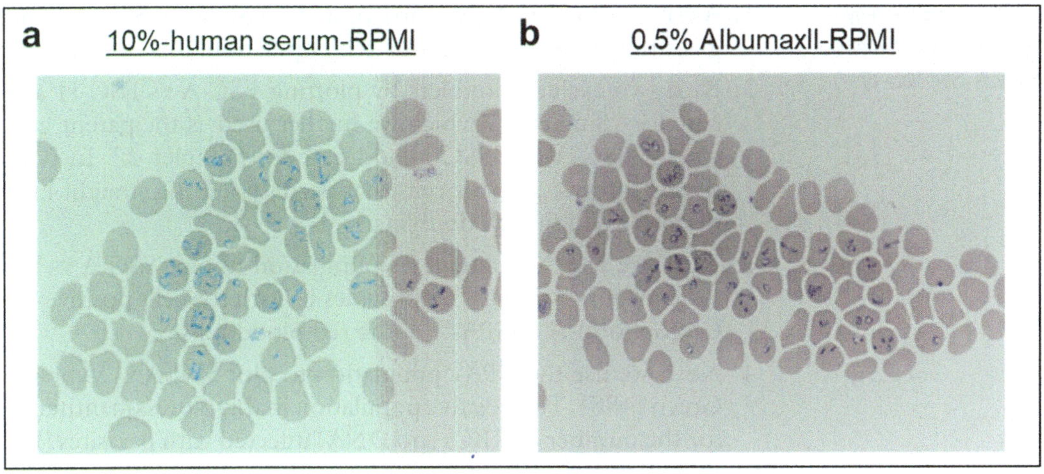

Fig. 1 Representative Giemsa-stained light microscope images of an asynchronous *B. divergens* culture maintained in (**a**) 10% human serum-supplemented RPMI (**b**) 0.5% Albumax-RPMI

5. Firmly and swiftly, pull the second slide along the full length of the first slide, smearing the RBCs at the same time.
6. Allow the slide to air dry for a few minutes.
7. Fix the slide in 100% methanol for 5–10 sec and allow to dry.
8. Prepare a 10% Giemsa mix in distilled water.
9. Overlay the slide with 10% Giemsa and allow it to incubate for 15 mins.
10. Rinse the slide with water and air dry before reading under 100X oil immersion on the microscope (see example images in Fig. 1).
11. To calculate parasitemia, count a minimum of 1000 RBCs to determine parasitemia (= number of parasitized cells/total number of RBCs counted).

3.3 Monitoring Parasitemia Using Flow Cytometry

3.3.1 Flow Cytometry Assay

1. Transfer 5×10^6 cells from a 5% hematocrit culture into a sterile 1.5 mL tube.
2. Prepare the master mix solution containing 1XPBS, 0.5 uL of Vybrant DyeCycle green (10 μM), and 0.5 uL of anti-glycophorin-A (GPA) per 250 uL.
3. Add 250 μL of the solution to each sample.
4. In addition, prepare single stained and unstained controls to run compensation prior to acquiring data for your samples.
5. Incubate at room temperature for 15 min in the dark.
6. Following the 15 min incubation, acquire readings using a flow cytometer for each sample (*see* **Note 5**).
7. Run compensation controls and set appropriate voltages.

3.3.2 Gating Strategy—Detailed Flow Cytometry Analysis (See Note 6)

1. As shown in Fig. 2a, we first plot the FSC-A vs SSC-A. This gives the "intact cells" in our cell population.
2. Next, we exclude doublets by plotting FSC-A vs FSC-H and gate for "Singlet 1," which we further used as the parent gate to plot SSC-A and SSC-H and gate for "Singlet 2." In both these plots, we gate for cells that occur along the straight line, thereby excluding all doublets.
3. Next, we use the "singlet 2" population to plot SSC-A vs the violet channel (405). This provides us with the cells positive for Glycophorin-A ("GPA+")—the red blood cells.
4. Next, we use the GPA+ population to plot SSC-A vs Vybrant-Green (488). The positive population in this plot is quantitative for the number of RBCs (no DNA) infected with parasites (has DNA) and thereby provides us with the parasitemia of the culture being tested.
5. We can further determine the multiplicity of infection using this method and determine the percentage of parasite's sub-populations within the RBC. As shown in Fig. 2a, the "DNA+" cells in SSC-A vs VybrantGreen plot can be further evaluated for their content of DNA and be marked as "1 N,"

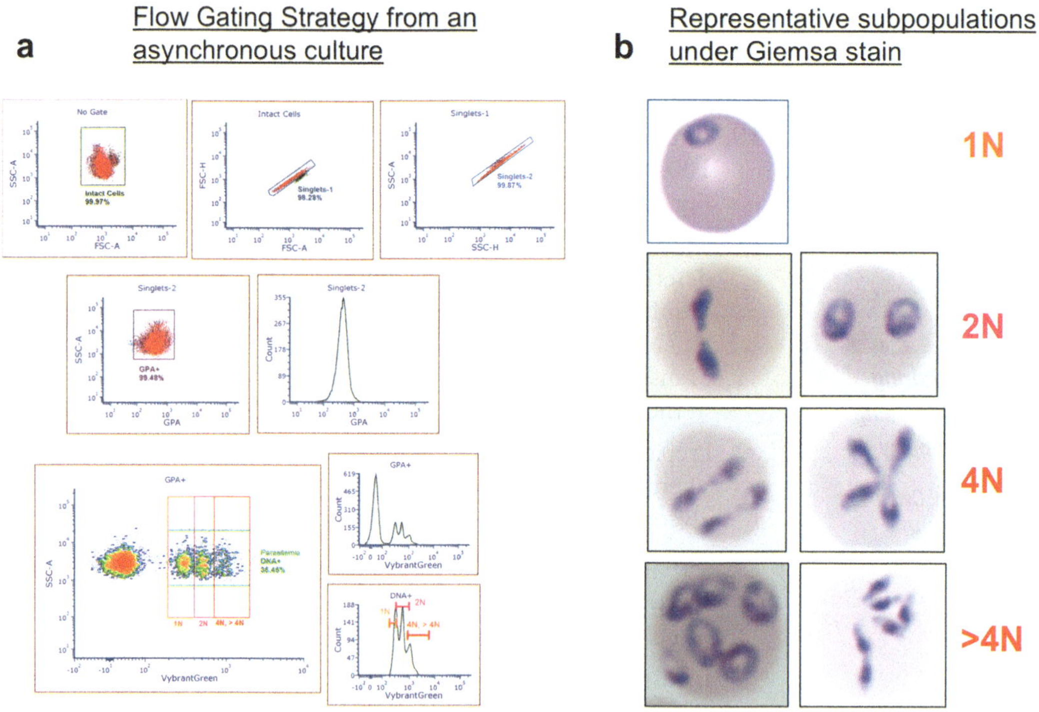

Fig. 2 Flow cytometry and Giemsa staining to monitor parasite culture (**a**) flow cytometry gating strategy to calculate parasitemia (DNA+ population) and characterize sub-populations (1N, 2N, 4N, and gt; 4N) of the parasite residing in the human RBCs. The title of the flow plot shows the parent gate. (**b**) Giemsa-stained microscopic images to show examples of 1N, 2N, 4N, and > 4N sub-populations of in vitro *B. divergens* culture

"2 N," and "4 N, gt;4 N" to quantify RBCs which have one, two, four, or more parasites. This distribution can also be visualized in a histogram, as indicated in Fig. 2b.

3.4 Purification of Merozoites and Invasion into Washed Human RBCs

1. Take a 25 mL culture with an ideal parasitemia of ~30–40% and aspirate overnight supernatant. Spin the culture at 1500 rpm at RT and remove all old medium. Wash once with cRPMI. Resuspend in 5 mL cRPMI (~25% hematocrit).
2. Use a 1 ml syringe with a 5 μm filter attached, deposit the culture, and collect the filtrate in a 15 mL tube (*see* **Note 7**).
3. Take the filtrate from the previous step and filter using a 1 mL syringe with a 1.2 μm filter attached. Collect the filtrate in a new 15 mL tube.
4. Use the filtrate from the previous step and repeat the step using a 1.2 μm filter on a 1 mL syringe and collect the filtrate in a new 15 mL Falcon tube.
5. Centrifuge the filtrate from the previous step at 2500 rpm for 5 min at room temperature. Discard pellet and transfer supernatant to a sterile 13 mL polypropylene centrifuge tube.
6. Centrifuge the 13 mL tube using the Sorvall centrifuge at 10,000 rpm for 5 min. Discard supernatant and resuspend pellet in 2 mL cRPMI (*see* **Note 8**).
7. Count the number of RBCs in each sample of 50% RBCs using a Cellometer or hemocytometer.
8. Take an equal number of RBCs from each sample to ensure that the number of host cells available for invasion is equal across samples. Add cRPMI.
9. To the above mix, add merozoites. Empirically, we have found that adding merozoites from a ~ 35% parasitemia 25 mL 5% hematocrit culture to a 5 mL 5% hematocrit invasion yields invasion parasitemia upwards of 8–10%, while adding half of these merozoites yields an invasion parasitemia of ~2–5%.
10. Keep in a 15 mL or 50 mL Falcon tube at 37 °C for 1 h.
11. At 1 h post-invasion (1hpi), wash the cells with iRPMI twice and resuspend in an appropriate volume of cRPMI. Transfer to a sterile culture flask. Gas and keep in a 37 °C incubator.
12. Calculate parasitemia using Giemsa and flow cytometry. (Representative example shown in Fig. 3).

3.5 Cryopreservation and Thawing of *Babesia divergens*

3.5.1 Cryopreservation of Cultures Maintained in 10% Human Serum

1. Work in the hood with the laminar flow on and the UV light off.
2. Spin down the culture at 2000 rpm for 5 min at room temperature. Aspirate supernatant.
3. Add iRPMI with 80% A+ human serum vol/vol of RBC pellet for cultures maintained in 10% serum.

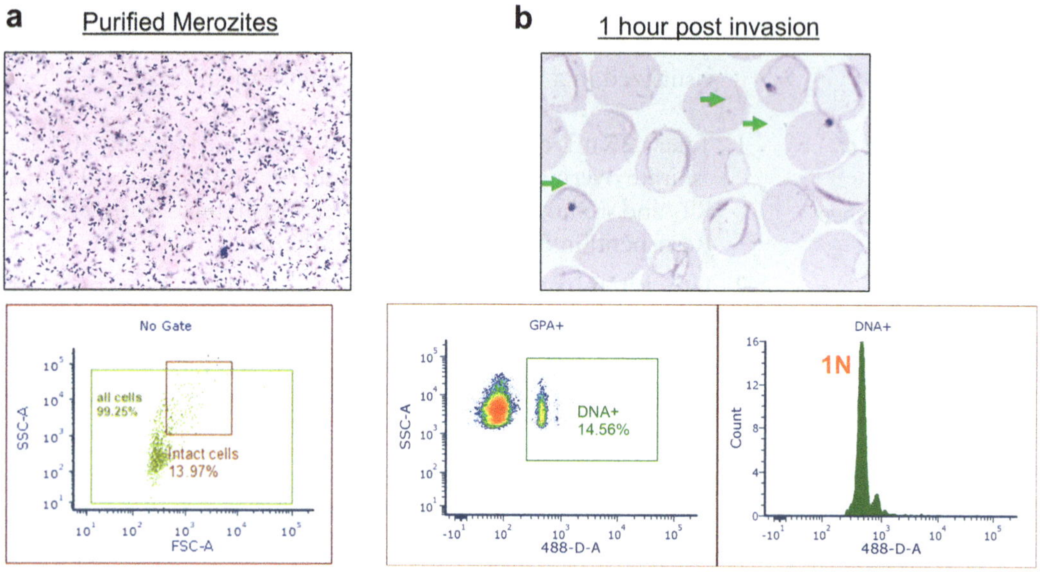

Fig. 3 Representative Giemsa-stained light microscope images and flow cytometry (stained with BV421-GPA and VybrantGreen) plots (**a**) Purified merozoites as seen under the microscope. In flow, these have lower FSC and SSC as compared to intact cells. (**b**) Giemsa-stained microscopic images of merozoites that invade new RBCs at 1 hpi. The flow plot for DNA+ cells shows only the 1 N peak (orange) at 1 hpi

4. Add the 15% DMSO solution vol/vol of total contents from the previous step.
5. Freeze samples at −80 °C for 24 h.
6. Transfer samples from −80 °C to liquid nitrogen tank.

3.5.2 Cryopreservation of Cultures Maintained in 0.5% Albumax

1. Spin down the culture at 2000 rpm for 5 min at room temperature.
2. Aspirate supernatant.
3. Add Glycerolyte solution drop by drop at the edge of the tube vol/vol of the RBC pellet.
4. Transfer to cryopreservation tubes and label them clearly, mentioning the parasite, strain (if known), parasitemia%, media grown in (serum or Albumax), date of cryopreservation, and your name/lab initials.
5. Freeze samples at −80 °C for 24 h.
6. Transfer samples from −80 °C to liquid nitrogen tank.

3.5.3 Thawing from Liquid Nitrogen

1. Pre-warm the complete medium at 37 °C for about 30 min before starting.
2. Work in the hood with the laminar flow on and UV off.
3. Remove samples from storage and thaw in the hand or on the bench.

4. Transfer parasites to a 50 mL Falcon tube.
5. Add 5 mL cRPMI.
6. Add 500 μL 50% hematocrit RBCs and transfer to a T25 culture flask.
7. Gas the culture flask and securely replace the culture lid.
8. Place flask in incubator.
9. Clean the hood with 70% ethanol and turn on the UV light.

4 Notes

1. When using human serum to supplement the media, the blood group of the donor RBCs and serum should match. For example, if using A+ cells, the serum used to grow the parasite should be A+ too to avoid antigen-antibody mismatch. If the blood group of donor cells is not known/cannot be determined, AB+ serum must be used.
2. In our experience, *B. divergens* grows identically in both serum-supplemented and Albumax-supplemented media. However, it does take time (~2–3 weeks) to adapt the parasites to Albumax-cRPMI and grow in the expected pattern if they have been previously grown in human serum-cRPMI. Once adapted, their growth is indistinguishable in the two media.
3. Gassing of cultures is essential to obtaining proper growth patterns for the parasite. The time spent on gassing would depend on the pressure adjusted using the gas knob and on the volume of the culture flask being used, and the exact time needs to be empirically determined.
4. In our hands, in a period of 24 h, the parasite grows 3–4X when the parasitemia is below 10–12%, and about 2X when the parasite is between 12% and 25%, and about 1.5X if the parasite is above 25%. The maximum parasitemia we can achieve in vitro is ~60%. At increased parasite loads, more frequent media changes are necessary to sustain the exponential growth of the parasite.
5. Due to the presence of DMSO in the VybrantGreen, incubations longer than 15–30 min lead to poor separation of sub-populations in flow plots. Therefore, the flow cytometer should be run promptly once staining is performed.
6. Figure 2 shows the gating strategy of a representative example. For the BD Fortessa line of instruments, we use a 405-F laser for GPA and a 488-B laser for VybrantGreen. In each plot, the X and Y-axes represent the flow parameter being evaluated, and the title of each plot shows the respective parent gate being used in that flow plot. Rectangle or polygon gates have been

used to mark the cells belonging to that specific gate. All analyses have been performed in FCS Express De Novo licensed software.

7. If the filter gets clogged, replace the filter rather than pushing the cells through it, as this may cause lysis of cells.
8. The merozoite pellet is a small, whitish-colored pellet. It may be slightly reddish due to host RBC contents sticking to the pellet. Carefully remove the supernatant so that the pellet is not dislodged.

Conflicts of Interest

This study was funded by the National Institutes of Health (NIH), National Heart, Lung, and Blood Institute (Grant P01HL149626 [C.A.L.]), and the NIH, National Institute of Allergy and Infectious Diseases (Grants R61AI187095 [C.A.L.] and K99AI182422 [D.B.]). The authors have no conflicts of interest to declare that are relevant to the content of this chapter.

References

1. Lobo CA, Cursino-Santos JR, Singh M, Rodriguez M (2019) *Babesia* divergens: a drive to survive. Pathogens 8:95
2. Montero E, Gray J, Lobo CA, Gonzalez LM (2022) *Babesia* and Human Babesiosis. Pathogens 11:399
3. Ord RL, Lobo CA (2015) Human Babesiosis: pathogens, prevalence, diagnosis and treatment. Curr Clin Microbiol Rep 2:173–181
4. Almazan C, Scimeca RC, Reichard MV, Mosqueda J (2022) Babesiosis and theileriosis in North America. Pathogens 11:168
5. Levin AE, Krause PJ (2016) Transfusion-transmitted babesiosis: is it time to screen the blood supply? Curr Opin Hematol 23:573–580
6. Villatoro T, Karp JK (2019) Transfusion-transmitted Babesiosis. Arch Pathol Lab Med 143:130–134
7. Saetre K, Godhwani N, Maria M, Patel D, Wang G, Li KI, Wormser GP, Nolan SM (2018) Congenital Babesiosis after maternal infection with Borrelia burgdorferi and *Babesia* microti. J Pediatr Infect Dis Soc 7:e1–e5
8. Tolkacz K, Rodo A, Wdowiarska A, Bajer A, Bednarska M (2021) Impact of *Babesia* microti infection on the initiation and course of pregnancy in BALB/c mice. Parasit Vectors 14:132
9. Kumar A, O'Bryan J, Krause PJ (2021) The global emergence of human babesiosis. Pathogens 10(11):1447
10. Vannier E, Gewurz BE, Krause PJ (2008) Human babesiosis. Infect Dis Clin N Am 22: 469–88, viii–ix
11. Beri D, Singh M, Rodriguez M, Yazdanbakhsh K, Lobo CA (2021) Sickle cell anemia and *Babesia* infection. Pathogens 10: 1435
12. Jalovecka M, Sojka D, Ascencio M, Schnittger L (2019) *Babesia* life cycle – when phylogeny meets biology. Trends Parasitol 35:356–368
13. Lobo CA, Cursino-Santos JR, Alhassan A, Rodrigues M (2013) *Babesia*: an emerging infectious threat in transfusion medicine. PLoS Pathog 9:e1003387
14. Ruebush TK 2nd, Juranek DD, Chisholm ES, Snow PC, Healy GR, Sulzer AJ (1977) Human babesiosis on Nantucket Island. Evidence for self-limited and subclinical infections. N Engl J Med 297:825–827
15. Ruebush TK 2nd, Juranek DD, Spielman A, Piesman J, Healy GR (1981) Epidemiology of human babesiosis on Nantucket Island. Am J Trop Med Hyg 30:937–941
16. Kjemtrup AM, Conrad PA (2000) Human babesiosis: an emerging tick-borne disease. Int J Parasitol 30:1323–1337

17. Lukavska A, Kybicova K (2023) Human babesiosis. Epidemiol Mikrobiol Imunol 72:184–190
18. Drews SJ, Wendel S, Leiby DA, Tonnetti L, Ushiro-Lumb I, O'Brien SF, Lieshout-Krikke RW, Bloch EM, International Society of Blood Transfusion Working Party Parasite S (2023) Climate change and parasitic risk to the blood supply. Transfusion 63:638–645
19. Gray JS, Ogden NH (2021) Ticks, human babesiosis and climate change. Pathogens 10: Article 1430
20. Bloch EM, Day JR, Krause PJ, Kjemtrup A, O'Brien SF, Tobian AAR, Goel R (2022) Epidemiology of hospitalized patients with Babesiosis, United States, 2010–2016. Emerg Infect Dis 28:354–362
21. Bloch EM, Zhu X, Krause PJ, Patel EU, Grabowski MK, Goel R, Auwaerter PG, Tobian AAR (2022) Comparing the epidemiology and health burden of Lyme disease and Babesiosis hospitalizations in the United States. Open forum Infect Dis 9:ofac597
22. Wormser GP, Prasad A, Neuhaus E, Joshi S, Nowakowski J, Nelson J, Mittleman A, Aguero-Rosenfeld M, Topal J, Krause PJ (2010) Emergence of resistance to azithromycin-atovaquone in immunocompromised patients with *Babesia* microti infection. Clin Infect Dis 50:381–386
23. Bloch EM, Busch MP, Corash LM, Dodd R, Hailu B, Kleinman S, O'Brien S, Petersen L, Stramer SL, Katz L (2023) Leveraging donor populations to study the epidemiology and pathogenesis of transfusion-transmitted and emerging infectious diseases. Transfus Med Rev 37:150769
24. Drews SJ, Kjemtrup AM, Krause PJ, Lambert G, Leiby DA, Lewin A, O'Brien SF, Renaud C, Tonnetti L, Bloch EM (2023) Transfusion-transmitted *Babesia* spp.: a changing landscape of epidemiology, regulation, and risk mitigation. J Clin Microbiol 61:e0126822
25. Abraham A, Brasov I, Thekkiniath J, Kilian N, Lawres L, Gao R, DeBus K, He L, Yu X, Zhu G, Graham MM, Liu X, Molestina R, Ben MC (2018) Establishment of a continuous *in vitro* culture of *Babesia* duncani in human erythrocytes reveals unusually high tolerance to recommended therapies. J Biol Chem 293: 19974–19981
26. Alvarez Martinez JA, Figueroa Millan JV, Ueti MW, Rojas-Martinez C (2021) Establishment of *Babesia* bovis *in vitro* culture using medium free of animal products. Pathogens 10:770
27. Brasseur P, Lecoublet S, Kapel N, Favennec L, Ballet JJ (1998) *In vitro* evaluation of drug susceptibilities of *Babesia* divergens isolates. Antimicrob Agents Chemother 42:818–820
28. Jiang W, Wang S, Li D, Zhang Y, Luo W, Zhao J, He L (2023) Continuous *in vitro* culture of *Babesia* duncani in a serum-free medium. Cells 12:482
29. Cursino-Santos JR, Singh M, Pham P, Lobo CA (2017) A novel flow cytometric application discriminates among the effects of chemical inhibitors on various phases of *Babesia* divergens intraerythrocytic cycle. Cytometry A 91: 216–231
30. Cursino-Santos JR, Singh M, Pham P, Rodriguez M, Lobo CA (2016) *Babesia* divergens builds a complex population structure composed of specific ratios of infected cells to ensure a prompt response to changing environmental conditions. Cell Microbiol 18:859–874
31. Montero E, Gonzalez LM, Rodriguez M, Oksov Y, Blackman MJ, Lobo CA (2006) A conserved subtilisin protease identified in *Babesia* divergens merozoites. J Biol Chem 281: 35717–35726
32. Montero E, Rodriguez M, Oksov Y, Lobo CA (2009) *Babesia* divergens apical membrane antigen 1 and its interaction with the human red blood cell. Infect Immun 77:4783–4793

Chapter 29

Building the Toolkits to Examine the Expression and Associated Regulation of RBC Alloantigens

Jun Liu, Xiaoyu Guan, Jue Wang, Ziyang Shen, Daniel Chang, Ling Li, Zhong Liu, and Li Chai

Abstract

The Rh blood group system is the most polymorphic and clinically significant blood group system after ABO. The RhD protein, in particular, encompasses numerous conformation-dependent epitopes that can elicit alloimmune responses, leading to hemolytic disease of the fetus and newborn or hemolytic transfusion reactions. Despite this, traditional serologic methods for RhD typing lack sensitivity and specificity to detect RhD variants like partial D and DEL phenotypes. This chapter describes molecular methods to characterize RhD mRNA expression and identify transcript variants in immortalized leukemic or erythroid cell lines and primary reticulocytes. Conventional PCR and quantitative real-time PCR assays were developed using primers designed against the full-length transcripts of RhD and RhCE and known splicing isoforms of RhD. The relative abundance of RhD isoforms in K562 cells was determined from public RNA-seq databases such as Cancer Cell Line Encyclopedia to guide primer design and template input amounts. The methods detail RNA extraction, cDNA synthesis, PCR amplification, and quantitative real-time PCR quantification protocols, with representative results shown for multiple cell lines that are widely used in research settings. To enable unbiased discovery of novel RhD transcript isoforms, a Nanopore long-read cDNA sequencing approach was established. As an orthogonal method, the flow cytometry assay was optimized to detect the RhD full-length protein on the cell surface. These molecular and cellular approaches complement serologic methods and support the transition to genomics-based approaches for Rh typing. Transcriptome-level data, supported by protein-level validation, can provide insights into the regulation of RhD expression and the functional impact of variants. These protocols can be readily applied to erythroid cell lines for mechanistic studies and extended to other blood group genes.

Key words Rh blood system, RhD variants, RT-PCR, Flow Cytometry, Nanopore sequencing

1 Introduction

The Rh blood group system, which consists of transmembrane proteins RhD and RhCE expressed on the surface of red blood cells, is the most polymorphic human erythrocyte antigen. It is located on chromosome 1 with over ten reported isoforms. Next to ABO, it is the most clinically significant antigen in the practice of

Sean R. Stowell and Connie M. Arthur (eds.), *Methods in Transfusion Medicine*, Methods in Molecular Biology, vol. 3053,
https://doi.org/10.1007/978-1-0716-5376-0_29,

transfusion medicine [1]. Due to its complex polymorphisms, the RhD protein encompasses a collection of conformation-dependent epitopes that can elicit an allo-antigenic immune response. Development of antibodies against erythrocyte antigens through exposure to transfused red blood cells (RBC) or pregnancy, a process called alloimmunization, is a common cause of hemolytic disease of the fetus and newborn (HDFN), which can have devastating sequelae. In addition, accidental re-exposure to the RBCs carrying the RhD antigen in a sensitized individual can cause a life-threatening hemolytic transfusion reaction.

Traditionally, the hospital blood banks use serological methods, which examine the appearance or absence of agglutination in the presence of commercial RhD antibodies and the patients' RBCs to decide if blood donors, recipients, or expectant mothers are positive or negative for RhD [1]. In theory, individuals who are positive for the RhD antigen are not expected to produce alloantibodies. However, these serological methods lack sensitivity and specificity due to the RhD gene locus's inherent complexity, which dictates the complexity of protein conformation and potential alloantigen formation. For example, individuals whose RBCs have an altered form of RhD protein (so-called "partial D") may make an alloantibody against wild-type or common RhD isoforms even though they are indicated as RhD-positive individuals. Depending on which D epitopes are altered, such RBCs are agglutinated by only a proportion of anti-D reagents. Another example is the "RhD DEL phenotype," which constitutes as high as 30% of the population with an initial negative RhD screen in some parts of the world and at least 5% of the US donor pool. These individuals would be typed as negative on routine serology but, in fact, contain weak expression of the RhD antigen that is only detectable through adsorption-elution studies and is capable of eliciting antibody responses in the recipients [2, 3]. Due to the difficulties in typing these individuals, there have been reports of mistyped RhD DEL phenotypes leading to fatal diseases such as HDFN [4].

The RhD blood group variants have significant variations among different ethnic groups. While in most D-negative Caucasians, there is a deletion of the RHD gene, in other populations (notably Japanese and African), the D-negative phenotype is associated with a normal *RHD* sequence, and the reason for the lack of D-antigen expression is not completely understood. In one study, analyses of genes encoding the weak D phenotype showed a normal *RHD* sequence but a severely reduced expression of *RHD* messenger RNA (mRNA), suggesting a defect at the level of transcription or pre-mRNA processing [5, 6]. Recent studies showed that many incidences of DEL phenotypes correlate with changes at the splice site [7–9], but others have reported that the DEL phenotypes, as well as the other weak RhD phenotypes, may have associated genetic changes occurring at additional intronic regions [10]. The sporadic discoveries of intronic mutations have been reported and curated by multiple databases such as the International Society of Blood Transfusion (ISBT), the GenBank database, and the Human RhesusBase inventories, which collectively curated over 700 *RHD* alleles. Which alleles to detect and how to manage allele carriers are recurring questions for immunohematologists and hospital blood bankers. Very few reported cases show a conclusive mechanistic connection between the genetic changes to mRNA or protein expression, making it difficult to rely on these reports to develop clinical genotyping assays and guide clinical management.

Recently, there has been increased interest and effort in using DNA genotyping to facilitate better phenotypic prediction for blood group antigens, including RhD [11, 12]. Although many structural variants and single nucleotide polymorphisms (SNPs) have been shown to affect the expression of the antigen, there is still limited understanding regarding the intronic/non-coding variants and their contributions to RhD expression, and there is limited data on genotype-mRNA-protein-level correlations for even the majority of the non-intronic variants. This is partly due to the general lack of methods to investigate transcript levels and, to some extent, protein-level expression in in vitro models (i.e., using cell lines). To address this void in research tools to study the blood group antigens at the transcript level, we generated RNA-based assays for RhD expression analysis, using cell line models that are amenable to genetic manipulations (i.e., suitable for future mechanistic studies using methods such as Clustered Regularly Interspaced Short Palindromic Repeats (CRISPR)-base editing screens for potential intronic/regulatory elements). We hope to continue expanding the "toolbox" to encompass additional blood group antigens in the long run.

In this chapter, we describe methods to (1) characterize RhD mRNA expression using conventional PCR and quantitative real-time PCR (qPCR) methods, with primers designed against RhD and RhCE full length and the majority of known RhD splicing isoforms; (2) perform Nanopore sequencing to quantify all RhD transcripts; (3) perform flow cytometric analysis to quantify RhD protein expression. These methods are developed and validated using either leukemic/erythroid cell lines or donor-derived reticulocytes. Since RhD and RhCE full-length transcripts share significant homology, it is possible to design primers against RhD full-length transcripts. Still, it is challenging to design RhCE transcripts with 100% specificity. These limitations led to the development of the Nanopore sequencing methodology, which can capture all of the RhD transcript variants [13]. Previously, Nanopore sequencing has been used to successfully characterize alternative splicing of BRCA1 transcripts in breast cancer and to identify novel ELF3 transcript variants in multiple malignancies [14, 15]. Although Nanopore sequencing can directly sequence endogenous mRNAs, we still validated our Nanopore results using the conventional sequencing approach. More specifically, we developed RhD Nanopore sequencing methods using cDNA generated from mRNA (extracted from patient-derived reticulocytes in our method development process), and the results were cross-validated by PCR. Once mRNA is extracted and a cDNA library is generated via reverse transcription, the same methodology can be applied to leukemic/erythroid cell lines. Full-length RhD transcripts from reticulocyte RNA were amplified, sequenced on the Oxford Nanopore platform, and analyzed bioinformatically to identify isoforms and quantify expression levels. The Nanopore sequencing results were also cross-validated by PCR. The general workflow and key considerations for each step are provided below, including library preparation, sequencing on MinION/GridION devices, base calling, read mapping, and isoform detection using tools like FLAIR and SQANTI. Finally, we developed and optimized a flow cytometric method to detect and quantify RhD protein expression on the surface of cell lines. Multiple commercially available RhD primary antibodies and secondary antibodies were compared head-to-head, and methods from published protocols for RhD flow cytometric detection in RhD-expressing leukemic cell lines have been attempted and optimized in an iterative process [16, 17]. We found a monoclonal RhD IgM antisera with optimal performance and identified cell processing conditions and primary/secondary antibody dilutions that minimized background fluorescence. We used reagent human red blood cells known to be positive or negative for the RhD protein as controls during the validation.

In summary, the methods described enable in-depth characterization of RhD mRNA expression and protein expression to study genotype-phenotype correlations and mechanisms underlying RhD diversity. PCR/qPCR assays provide targeted isoform-level quantification, while Nanopore sequencing allows unbiased, full-length isoform discovery and characterization. Flow cytometry can be used to perform protein-level quantification and functional validation of transcriptional regulation. We hope these methods will contribute to transfusion medicine research by providing the basis to investigate the regulatory regions of blood group antigens and support the transition from serological phenotype to sequencing-based DNA genotyping, starting with the RhD antigen. The blood group antigen transcriptomics data will also provide insights into the feasibility of transcript-based, rather than genotype-based, matching for blood group antigens.

2 Materials

2.1 PCR/qPCR Primer Design (see Figs. 1 and 2)

1. Relevant information regarding (q)PCR primers and amplicons is summarized in Table 1.
2. Online RNA-seq data repositories (CCLE and K562 cells only).
3. All primers were designed and validated in-house.

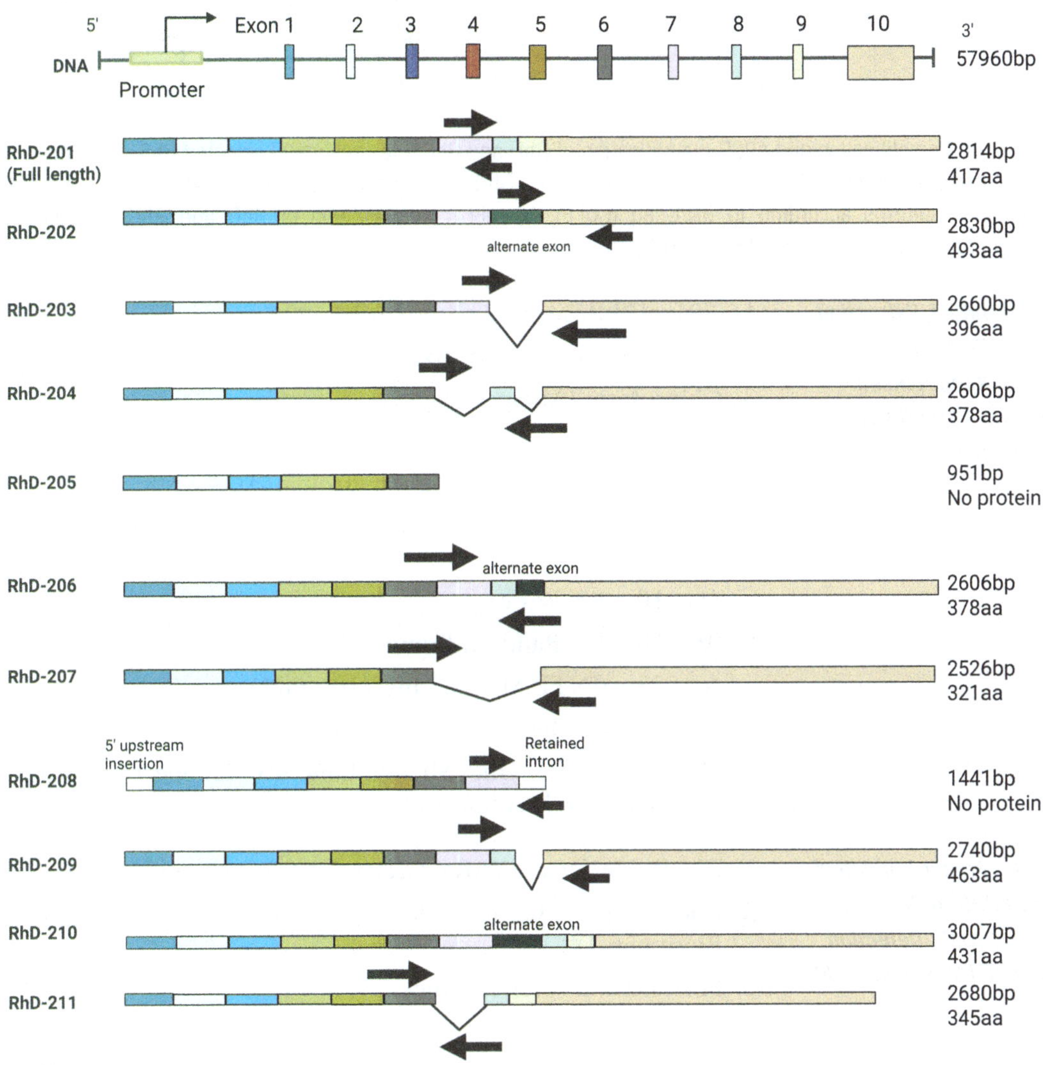

Fig. 1 RhD gene and schematics for various isoforms. RhD is located on chromosome 1p34-p36, with 10 exons and 9 introns. Eleven transcript variants are reported. Transcript names are derived from Ensembl. Primer designs for selected isoforms are indicated by forward and reverse arrows that maximize specificity

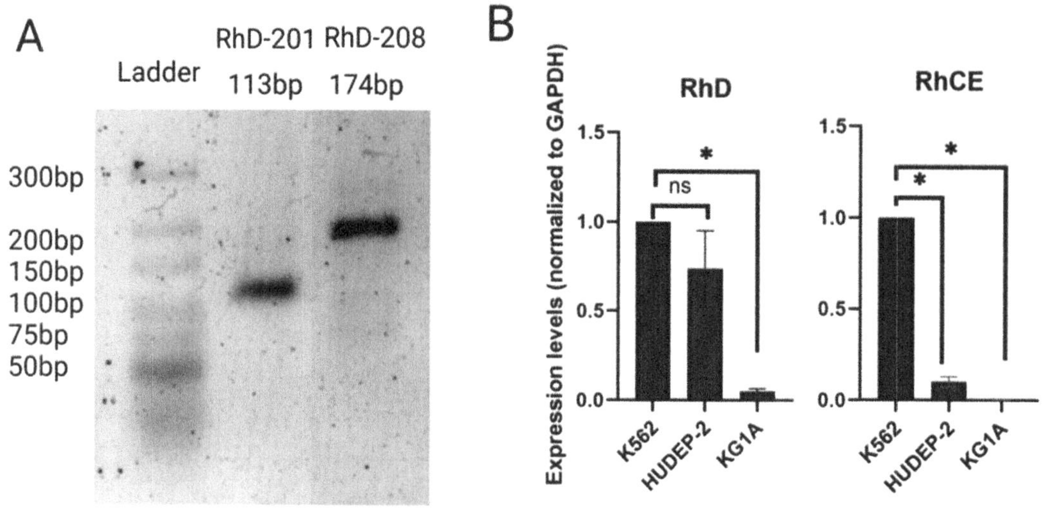

Fig. 2 PCR amplification and qPCR quantification of RhD and RhCE. (**a**) Images of selected RhD transcripts in K562 cells amplified by the traditional PCR methods. RhD-201 and RhD-208 are shown, as they are the dominant isoforms according to RNA-seq (CCLE) (**b**). qPCR amplification of RhD and RhCE full-length transcripts in cell lines (K562, KG1a, HUDEP2)

2.2 mRNA Extraction and cDNA Generation from Immortalized Leukemic/Erythroid Cell Lines

1. TRIzol™ Reagent (Invitrogen™).
2. 1.5 mL RNase-free microcentrifuge tubes.
3. Chloroform (Millipore Sigma).
4. 70% ethanol.
5. PureLink™ RNA Mini Kit (Invitrogen™).
6. High-Capacity cDNA Reverse Transcription Kit (Applied Biosystems™).
   (a) 10× RT Buffer.
   (b) 10× RT Random Primers.
   (c) 25× dNTP Mix, 0.2 mL (100 mM).
   (d) MultiScribe Reverse Transcriptase.
7. NanoDrop One/One^c Microvolume UV-Vis Spectrophotometer (Thermo Scientific™).

2.3 Primer Validation and RhD/RhCE Transcripts Detection in Cell Lines Using PCR

1. iTaq™ Universal SYBR® Green Supermix (Biorad).
2. MicroAmp™ Optical 96-Well Reaction Plate (Applied Biosystems™).
3. Forward and reverse primer.
4. cDNA.
5. MicroAmp™ Optical Adhesive Film (Applied Biosystems™).
6. QuantStudio™ 3 Real-Time PCR System, 96-well, 0.2 mL, laptop (Applied Biosystems™).

Table 1
RhD/RhCE transcripts primer information (*See* Note 1)

RhD variants	Size (bp)	Direction	Primer sequences (5′ to 3′)	RNA-seq (TPM) (CCLE, 2018)
RHD-201	113	Forward Reverse	CCCACAGCTCCATCATGGG GCCAATCATGCCATTGCCGGC	7.1
RHD-202	227	Forward Reverse	TGAAGCAGGTGATGAGGA GGCAACAGTGAGAGGAAG	0
RHD-203	112	Forward Reverse	CCCACAGCTCCATCATGGG AGGAAAATGCCATTGCCGG	0
RHD-204	108	Forward Reverse	CAAGTACCTGCCGGATTG AGCCAAATGAGGAAACTGT	1.04
RHD-206	292	Forward Reverse	CCCACAGCTCCATCATGGG GACCTGGAAGCCAATCCCAC	0.29
RHD-207	53	Forward Reverse	TGGCTGGGCTGATCTCCG CAAATGAGGAAACGGCAGGT	1.72
RhD-208	174	Forward Reverse	CTACATTGTGCTGCTGGT ATATTCACCGAAGCCTACTG	4.21
RhD-209	106	Forward Reverse	GTCTGGTCTCCTGACAGT GCAACAGTGAGAGGAAGTT	0.03
RhCE-201	400	Forward Reverse	CTGCTCTGCTGAGAAGTCCAA TCC ATGCCATTGCCG TTCCAGACAG	5.72

2.4 qPCR Detection of RhD and RhCE Full-Length Transcripts in Cell Lines

1. Platinum™ Taq DNA Polymerase, DNA-free (Invitrogen™).
2. Taq polymerase buffer 10×.
3. Water, nuclease-free.
4. 50 mM MgCl2.
5. 10 μM forward and reverse primer.
6. 10 mM dNTP mix (Invitrogen™).
7. PCR tubes (USA Scientific).
8. MyCycler™ Thermal Cycler (Biorad).
9. Agarose (Fisher Scientific).
10. TBE Buffer.
11. GeneRuler Ultra Low Range DNA Ladder, ready-to-use (Thermo Scientific).

2.5 Nanopore Third-Generation Sequencing of RHD and RHCE Genes (see Fig. 3 for the General Principle of Nanopore Sequencing)

1. T4 DNA Ligase (Rapid) (Vazyme, China).
2. VAHTS™ Universal End preparation Module for llumina V2 (N203-01, N204-01) (Vazyme, China).
3. Qubit® dsDNA HS Assay Kit (Thermo Fisher Company, USA).
4. Ligation Sequencing Kit SQK-LSK109 (ONT, UK).
5. R9 sequencing chip FLO-MIN106 (ONT, UK).
6. Native Barcoding Kit 1-12 (EXP-NBD104) (ONT, UK).
7. Native Barcoding Kit 13-24 (EXP-NBD114) (ONT, UK).
8. Microarray cleaning kit (EXP-WSH004) (ONT, UK).
9. Preparation of 75% (v/v) ethanol.
10. FastStart Universal SYBR Green Master (Roche, USA).
11. AMPure XP Beads (Beckman).
12. DynaMag™ Magnetic Frame.

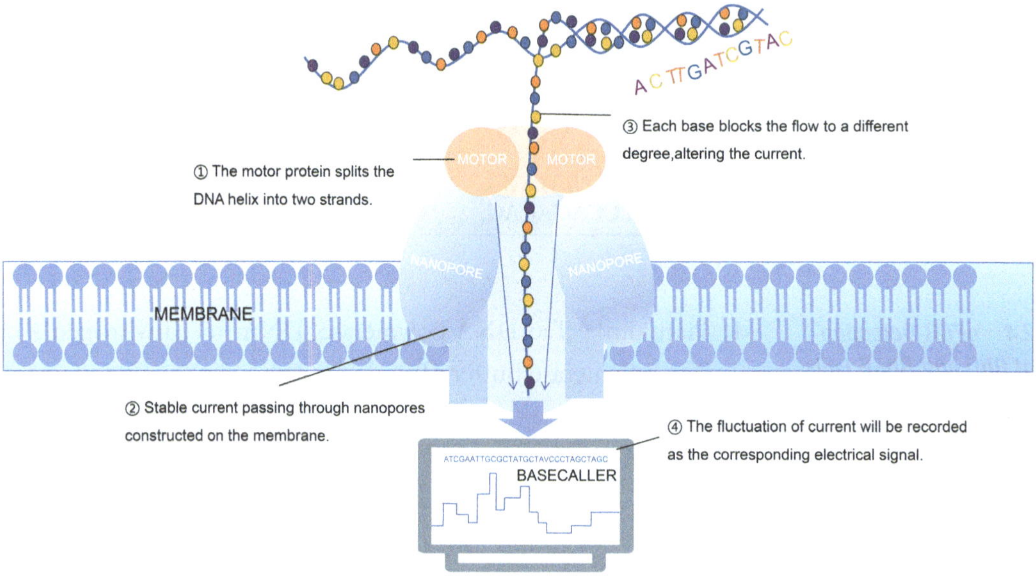

Fig. 3 The principle of Nanopore sequencing. The sequencing principle of Nanopore sequencing technology is a real-time, single-molecule sequencing method based on electrical signals that can directly read double-stranded DNA/RNA molecules. During sequencing, the double-stranded DNA/RNA connects to the motor protein and binds to the Nanopore protein embedded in the membrane to unwind. The motor protein controls the movement of the double-stranded DNA/RNA through the Nanopore, capturing current fluctuation signals during the translocation process. These signals are then converted into recognizable base sequences through algorithmic calculations, completing real-time sequencing

2.6 Nanopore Third-Generation Sequencing of RHD, RHCE Genes: Data Analysis (Fig. 4)

1. Guppy software in the MinKNOW software package.
2. NanoFilt software.
3. NanoPlot software.
4. Ensembl database.
5. Salmon software.

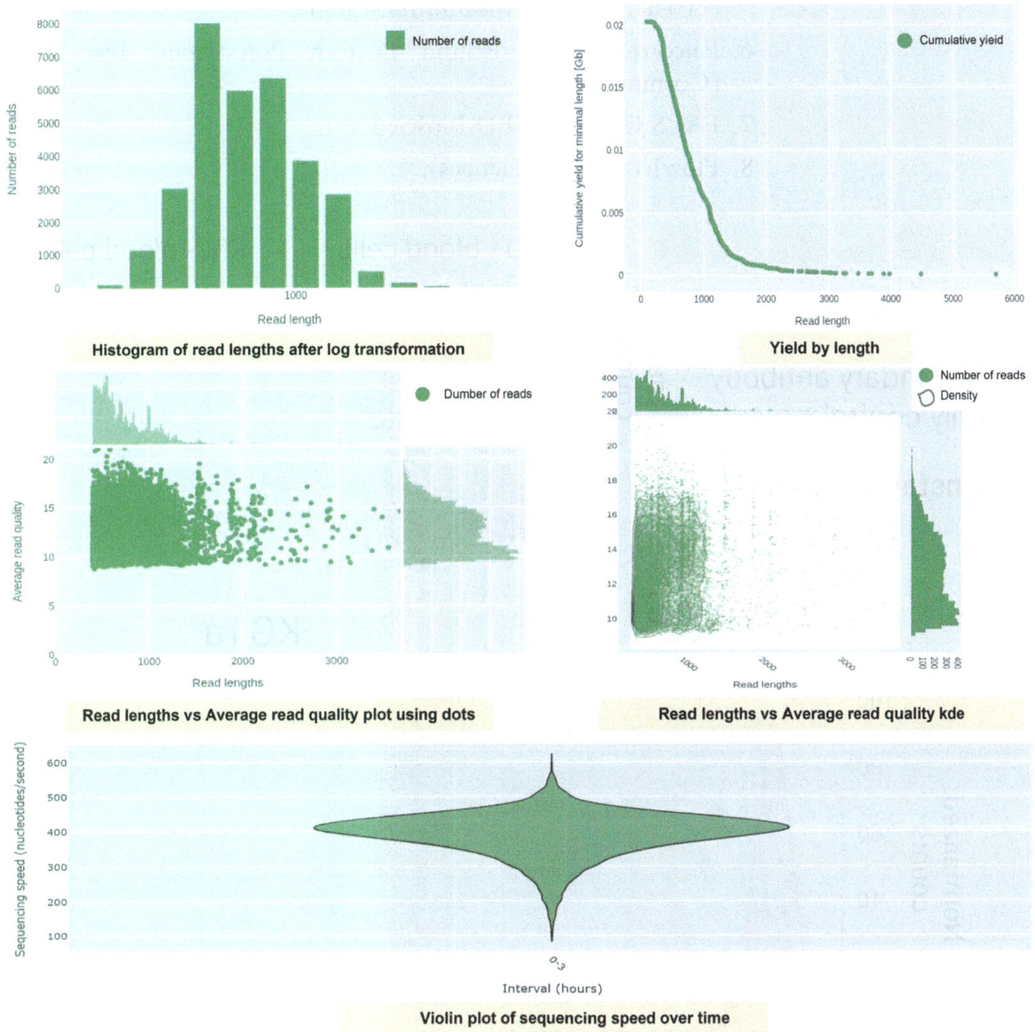

Fig. 4 Nanopore RhD sequencing data QC plot. The raw data format for the Nanopore MinION sequencing machine is FAST5, which stores and organizes a large amount of data. First, the barcodes are split, and the FAST5 data is converted to FASTQ format. Then, the quality control of the output data is performed using NanoPlot software. Representative and organized data are shown here

2.7 Flow Cytometric Detection of RhD Protein on Immortalized Leukemic Cell Lines (Fig. 5)

1. 1.5 mL microcentrifuge tubes.
2. FACS Buffer: PBS + 1% BSA (Biotium) + 5 mM EDTA (American Bioanalytical).
3. Reagent Red Blood Cells Biotestcell® 1 & 2; Biotestcell® 3 (Bio-Rad).
4. Blood Grouping Reagent Anti-D (RH1) Seraclone® Human IgM Monoclonal (BS 226) (Bio-Rad).
5. Alexa Fluor® 488 AffiniPure™ Goat Anti-Human IgG + IgM (H + L) (Jackson ImmunoResearch).
6. Falcon® 5 mL Round Bottom Polystyrene Test Tube (Corning).
7. FACS Cantos II (BD Biosciences).
8. FlowJo (BD Biosciences).

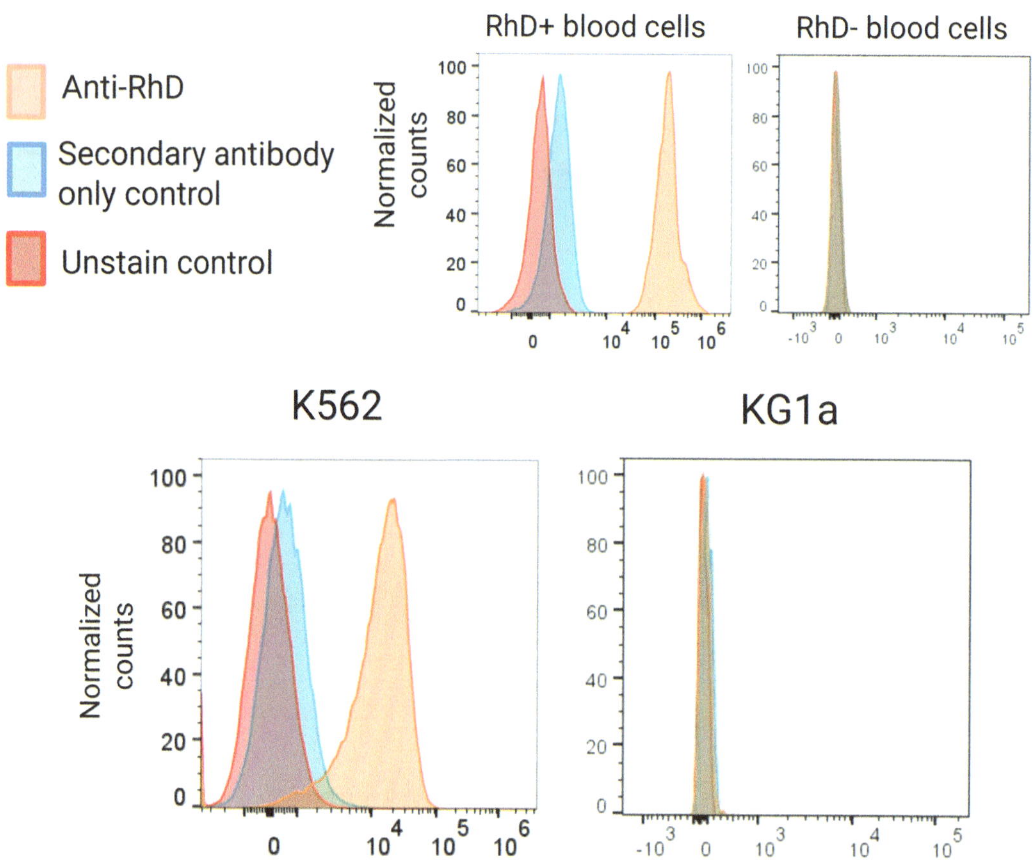

Fig. 5 Representative flow cytometry analysis of RhD expression in K562 and KG1a cells. RhD-positive and RhD-negative blood cells served as positive and negative controls (upper right panels), respectively. A secondary antibody-only control was included to measure background fluorescence (blue). Fresh, unfixed cells were used to minimize background fluorescence. K562 and KG1a cell lines were chosen to demonstrate positive and negative RhD protein expression based on prior qPCR data (lower panels)

3 Methods

3.1 PCR/qPCR Primer Design

1. Obtain mRNA transcripts of RhD and its isoforms through Ensemble (RhD ENSG00000187010) and RhCE (ENSG00000188672) (*see* **Note 1**).
2. Use primer design software (e.g., Primer Premier 5) or manually design primer pairs to target specific isoforms of RhD, following general principles of primer design [18].
3. Design amplicons should be between 80 and 150 bp long, as this gives the best kinetic linearity in a PCR and will improve quantitative amplification.
4. Span the exon-exon junction if possible.
5. To ensure a primer pair doesn't amplify non-RhD/RhCE genes, check all primer pairs by UCSC In-Silico PCR (http://genome.ucsc.edu/cgi-bin/hgPcr?command=start) and with Primer-BLAST (https://www.ncbi.nlm.nih.gov/tools/primer-blast/index.cgi?LINK_LOC=BlastHome).
6. The design of RhCE transcript isoforms is beyond the scope of this chapter but should be performed using similar principles.

3.2 mRNA Extraction and cDNA Generation from Immortalized Leukemic/Erythroid Cell Lines

1. mRNA can be extracted from the appropriate cell line using TRIzol® Reagent with the PureLink® RNA Mini Kit according to the manufacturer's instructions (Publication Number: MAN0000406, pp. 49–52) (*see* **Note 2**).
2. Determine the concentration and purity of the extracted mRNA using the NanoDrop™ One/OneC Microvolume UV-Vis Spectrophotometer according to the manufacturer's instructions.
3. Perform reverse transcription using the High-Capacity cDNA Reverse Transcription Kit according to the manufacturer's instructions (Publication Number: MAN0017977) (1–1.5 μg of RNA is used to generate cDNA, and cDNA is eluted using 30 μL of RNAse-free water per sample).

3.3 Primer Validation and RhD/RhCE Transcript Detection in Cell Lines Using PCR

1. Perform PCR amplification on the cDNA using any desired polymerase mix, such as Platinum™ Taq DNA Polymerase (Publication number: MAN0000925).
2. Carry out the PCR in a thermal cycler in the following conditions: 95 °C for 15 min, and then 30–35 cycles at 95 °C for 30 s, 60 °C for 90 s, and 72 °C for 90 s. Hold at 4 °C. Optimization may be required depending on the specific DNA polymerase used.
3. To visualize RhD isoforms amplified from cDNA, starting cDNA concentrations need to be adjusted based on the relative abundance of each isoform expressed in each cell line (*see* **Note 3**).

4. For agarose gel electrophoresis, prepare a 3–5% agarose gel; in each well, mix the PCR product with an appropriate amount of loading dye, and run the gel at 120 V for 1 h.

3.4 qPCR Detection of RhD and RhCE Full-Length Transcripts in Cell Lines

1. Prepare a reaction mix for each sample. This will require the following:
   (a) Supermix: 10 μL of iTaq™ Universal SYBR® Green Supermix (Biorad).
   (b) Forward and reverse primer: 0.4 μL each.
   (c) Template DNA: varies, but typically <0.5 μL.
   (d) Nuclease-Free Water: to bring the final volume to 20 μL.
   (e) Include non-template controls and housekeeping gene primers such as GAPDH.
   (f) 3 technical replicates per sample.
2. Perform qPCR reactions using thermocycling programs recommended by the SYBR® Green reagent manufacturer's protocol. Note that separate reactions may be carried out due to differing optimal Tm for different primers (*see* Table 1).
3. Obtain and analyze cycle threshold (Ct) values to calculate the relative fold using the 2^-ddCt method. A lower Ct value corresponds to higher mRNA expression [19] (Fig. 2).

3.5 Nanopore Third-Generation Sequencing of RHD and RHCE Genes (see Fig. 3 for the General Principle of Nanopore Sequencing)

1. RNA extraction and generation of a cDNA library based on the standard protocol (described in the previous sections).
2. Calculate the starting amount of DNA product according to the microarray requirements (*see* **Notes 4**), resuspend using nuclease-free water up to 50 μL, flick and mix (do not vortex), and place on ice.
3. Add 15 μL of End-Prep Mix 4 to each well, mix gently by pipetting, then spin down. Perform the PCR reaction: 20 °C/15 min, 65 °C/15 min, and store at 4 °C after completion (*see* **Note 5**).
4. Thaw the native barcodes at room temperature, enough for one barcode per sample. Individually mix the barcodes by pipetting and place them on ice.
5. Add the reagents to the previous end-recovery reaction tube (65 μL remaining) in the following order: 5 μL of Barcode, 25 μL of Rapid Ligation Buffer, and 5 μL of Rapid DNA Ligase for a total of 100 μL in each tube; mix well by pipetting and spin down briefly. Incubate at 20 °C for 20 min.
6. Resuspend the AMPure XP beads by vortexing.
7. Add 100 μL of resuspended AMPure XP beads to the pooled reaction and mix by pipetting. Keep the plate on the magnetic rack until the eluate is clear and colorless.

8. Keep the tube on the magnetic rack and wash the beads with 200 μL of freshly prepared 80% ethanol without disturbing the pellet. Remove the ethanol using a pipette and discard it.
9. Repeat the previous step.
10. Spin down and place the tube back on the magnetic rack. Pipette off any residual ethanol. Allow the pellet to dry for 5 min, but do not dry the pellet to the point of cracking.
11. Remove the tube from the magnetic rack and resuspend the pellet in 26 μL nuclease-free water. Periodically agitate the sample by gently flicking to encourage DNA elution.
12. Pellet the beads on a magnetic rack until the eluate is clear and colorless.
13. Reposition it on the magnetic frame until the liquid clears. Repeat the previous step to ensure that the beads are removed completely.
14. Quantify 1 μL of an eluted sample using a Qubit fluorometer.
15. Calculate the pooling volume, take 1 μL and quantify again with Qubit; add nuclease-free water to dilute the product to 35 μL (100–200 fmol).
16. According to the following reaction system, add reagents to the previous pooling tube in order: 2× Rapid Ligation Buffer 50 μL, T4 DNA Ligase (Rapid) 10 μL, Adapter Mix II 5 μL, and a total volume of 100 μL. Mix well, leave immediately, and place on ice. Incubate at 30 °C for 10 min.
17. Depending on the wash buffer, Long Fragment Buffer (LFB) or Short Fragment Buffer (SFB) used, the clean-up step after adapter ligation is designed to either enrich for DNA fragments of >3 kb or purify all fragments equally.
18. Resuspend the AMPure XP beads by vortexing. Add 50 μL of resuspended AMPure XP beads to the reaction, and mix by pipetting. Incubate for 5 min.
19. Spin down the sample and pellet on the magnetic rack. Keep the tube on the magnet and pipette off the supernatant.
20. Wash the beads by adding either 250 μL LFB or SFB. Flick the beads to resuspend, spin down, then return the tube to the magnetic rack and allow the beads to pellet. Remove the supernatant using a pipette and discard it.
21. Repeat the previous step. Spin down and place the tube back on the magnet. Pipette off any residual supernatant. Allow to dry for 30 s, but do not dry the pellet to the point of cracking.
22. Remove from the magnetic rack and add 15 μL of nuclease-free water. Spin down and incubate for 10 min at 37 °C. Periodically agitate the sample by gently flicking to encourage DNA elution.

23. Pellet the beads on a magnet until the eluate is clear and colorless. Remove and retain 15 μL of eluate containing the DNA library into a clean 1.5 mL EP tube.
24. Quantify 1 μL of the eluted sample using a Qubit fluorometer.
25. Thaw the reagents: Flush Buffer, Sequencing Buffer, Flush Tether, and Loading Beads in advance; lightly vortex; then place the reagents at room temperature; and equilibrate the chip at room temperature for 10–20 min. Place the chip into the sequencer, open the software, and run the initialization of the flow cell for about 10 min. After the initialization, verify the remaining number of wells in the QC.
26. Turn the pipette 90° clockwise to open the priming port. Set a P1000 pipette to 200 μL. Insert the tip into the priming port. Turn the wheel until the dial shows 220–230 μL, or until you can see a small volume of buffer entering the pipette tip.
27. Add 30 μL of thawed and mixed Flush Tether directly to the tube of thawed and mixed Flush Buffer, and mix by vortexing.
28. Load 800 μL of the priming mix into the flow cell via the priming port, avoiding introducing air bubbles. Wait for 5 min. During this time, prepare the library for loading by following the steps below.
29. While the samples are equilibrating, prepare the loading sample by adding the following in order: Sequencing buffer 37.5 μL, loading beads 25.5 μL, and DNA library 12 μL, up to a total volume of 75 μL.
30. Load 200 μL of the priming mix into the flow cell via the priming port (not the SpotON sample port), avoiding the introduction of air bubbles.
31. Add 75 μL of sample to the flow cell via the SpotON sample port in a dropwise fashion. Ensure each drop flows into the port before adding the next.
32. Close the SpotON sample cover, then close the priming port by rotating it counterclockwise, and finally aspirate the liquid out of the line from the waste port (make sure that the priming port and the SpotON sample port are closed).
33. Set the experimental parameters and click Start Sequencing in the software to run the sequencing.
34. After your sequencing experiment is complete, if you would like to reuse the flow cell, please follow the Wash Kit instructions (https://nanoporetech.com/document/flow-cell-wash-kit-exp-wsh004) and store the washed flow cell at 2–8 °C.

3.6 Nanopore Third-Generation Sequencing of RHD and RHCE Genes: Data Analysis (Fig. 4)

1. Sequence analysis and specimen barcode splitting should be performed by Guppy software in the MinKNOW software package, and the data in FAST5 format can then be converted to FASTQ format. The output data are first quality-controlled by using EPI2ME and NanoPlot software.
2. Use NanoFilt software to cut and filter the short fragments and low-quality data in the above FASTQ format file, and set the filtering conditions: sequence length > 550 bp, < 3000 bp, Q score > 7. Finally, use EPI2ME and NanoPlot software again to quality control the filtered, valid data.
3. The measured transcripts were compared with the human reference genome GRCh38 (hg38) from the Ensembl database. Transcripts per million (TPM) of each transcript were quantified using Salmon software.
4. Calculate the percentage of splicing value of each variable splicing according to the TPM of each specimen, using SUPPA software to discover all possible variable splicing events.
5. The "flair align" module of FLAIR software was used to compare the sequences of the three generations of sequencing with the reference genome, and the "flair correct" module was used to correct the cut sites according to the annotation files of the reference genome. The "flair collapse" module clusters and merges the corrected sequences to form a reference sequence of high confidence transcripts from the samples, and "flair quantify" performs expression quantification of isoforms in all samples.
6. "Flair quantify" quantifies the expression of isoforms in all samples and generates expression matrices; "flair diffExp" analyzes the differential expression between groups with specified grouping, and "flair diffSplice" analyzes the differential expression of isoforms in all samples with variable clipping events between groups.

3.7 Flow Cytometric Detection of RhD Protein on Immortalized Leukemic Cell Lines (Fig. 5)

1. Harvest K562 and KG1a cells (1×10^6) and resuspend in microcentrifuge tubes with 100 μL FACS buffer.
2. For reagent red blood cells, aliquot 30 μL of cell suspension into a microcentrifuge tube and resuspend with 1 mL FACS buffer. Centrifuge at 150–300 × g for 5 min and resuspend with 100 μL FACS buffer.
3. Incubate the samples with 20 μL of Blood Grouping Reagent Anti-D (RH1) for 30 min on ice (*see* **Note 6**).
4. Wash the cells by adding 1 mL FACS buffer to resuspend each sample. Centrifuge at 150–300 × g for 5 min at room temperature. Discard the supernatants.

5. Repeat the step above and resuspend samples with 100 μL FACS buffer.
6. Incubate the samples with diluted (1:100) Alexa Fluor® 488 AffiniPure™ Goat Anti-Human IgG + IgM (H + L) for 30 min on ice in the dark.
7. Wash the cells by adding 1 mL FACS buffer to resuspend each sample. Centrifuge at room temperature at 150–300 × g for 5 min. Discard the supernatants.
8. Repeat the step above, resuspend samples with 300 μL of FACS buffer, and transfer all volumes to 5 mL Round Bottom Polystyrene Test Tubes.
9. Run the samples on FACS Cantos II and acquire fluorescence for at least 10,000 events for each sample.
10. Use FlowJo to visualize and analyze the fluorescence data.

4 Notes

1. For RhD 205, we could not design primer pairs because its coding sequence lacks a unique portion, which precludes the design of primers to specifically target its expression. For RhD 210 and 211, RNA-seq data failed to identify transcripts expressed in K562 cells.
2. K562 and KG1a are leukemic cell lines, with K562 derived from human chronic myelogenous leukemia and KG1a from human acute myelogenous leukemia. Each cell line can be cultured in RPMI 1640 with 10% fetal bovine serum. HUDEP cells are immortalized human umbilical cord stem cell lines that can be differentiated into erythroid lineages (including terminal differentiation and enucleation). They are among the most widely used in vitro human erythroid cell line systems since their creation in 2017. HUDEP-2 cells can be cultured in StemSpan base media with supplemental doxycycline, dexamethasone, erythropoietin, and stem cell factor [20]. Other cell lines can be used as well, but the above-mentioned cell lines are selected to represent positive and negative controls for RhD and RhCE full-length transcripts and select splicing variants. See Table 1 for the relative abundance of RhD splicing variants based on online RNA-seq data repositories (CCLE, K562 cells only).
3. For K562 cells, a larger amount of cDNA template (≥100 ng) may be needed for the following isoforms due to low transcript levels: RhD-204, RhD-207, RhD-209, RhD-211.
4. The R9 chip requires 100–200 fmol (or 1 μg) of DNA, which is usually first diluted to the upper limit of the larger value and

can be subsequently adjusted according to the library building results. 1 fmol = fragment size bp × 0.66 × 0.001 (ng) DNA starting amount (μL) = (fragment size bp × 0.66 × 0.001 × number of fmol required by the chip)/ DNA concentration ng/μL.

5. Do not purify after DNA repair and end-prep, and proceed directly to the next step of barcode ligation.
6. Permeabilization and fixation steps are omitted in this flow protocol to reduce background fluorescence from primary and secondary antibodies because RhD is a surface antigen rather than an intracellular antigen.

Conflict of Interest

This study was funded by NIH/NHLBI Grant P01HL095489 and Chengdu Science and Technology Program (Grant No. 2024-YF09-00052-SN) and the Sichuan Science and Technology Program (Grant No. 2025ZDZX0098). The authors have no conflicts of interest to declare that are relevant to the content of this chapter.

References

1. Avent ND, Reid ME (2000) The Rh blood group system: a review. Blood 95:375–387
2. Li Q, Hou L, Guo Z-H et al (2009) Molecular basis of the RHD gene in blood donors with DEL phenotypes in Shanghai. Vox Sang 97: 139–146
3. Wagner FF, Frohmajer A, Flegel WA (2001) RHD positive haplotypes in D negative Europeans. BMC Genet 2:10
4. Turley E, McGowan EC, Hyland CA et al (2018) Severe hemolytic disease of the fetus and newborn due to allo-anti-D in a patient with a partial DEL phenotype arising from the variant allele described as RHD*148+1T (RHD*01EL.31). Transfusion 58:2260–2264
5. Schenkel-Brunner H (2012) Human blood groups: chemical and biochemical basis of antigen specificity. Springer Science & Business Media
6. Rouillac C, Gane P, Cartron J et al (1996) Molecular basis of the altered antigenic expression of RhD in weak D(Du) and RhC/e in RN phenotypes. Blood 87:4853–4861
7. Scott SA, Nagl L, Tilley L et al (2014) The RHD(1227G gt;A) DEL-associated allele is the most prevalent DEL allele in Australian D- blood donors with C+ and/or E+ phenotypes. Transfusion 54:2931–2940
8. Seo MH, Won EJ, Hong YJ et al (2016) An effective diagnostic strategy for accurate detection of RhD variants including Asian DEL type in apparently RhD-negative blood donors in Korea. Vox Sang 111:425–430
9. Kim H, Ko D-H (2019) Reconsidering RhD positive blood transfusion for Asia type DEL patients. Transfus Apher Sci 58:422
10. Ye L, He Y, Gao H et al (2013) Weak D phenotypes caused by intronic mutations in the RHD gene: four novel weak D alleles identified in the Chinese population. Transfusion 53: 1829–1833
11. Lane WJ, Westhoff CM, Gleadall NS et al (2018) Automated typing of red blood cell and platelet antigens: a whole-genome sequencing study. Lancet Haematol 5:e241–e251
12. Lane WJ, Westhoff CM, Uy JM et al (2016) Comprehensive red blood cell and platelet antigen prediction from whole genome sequencing: proof of principle. Transfusion 56:743–754
13. Wang Y, Zhao Y, Bollas A et al (2021) Nanopore sequencing technology, bioinformatics and applications. Nat Biotechnol 39:1348–1365
14. de Jong LC, Cree S, Lattimore V et al (2017) Nanopore sequencing of full-length BRCA1

mRNA transcripts reveals co-occurrence of known exon skipping events. Breast Cancer Res 19:127

15. Boti MA, Adamopoulos PG, Tsiakanikas P, Scorilas A (2021) Nanopore sequencing unveils diverse transcript variants of the epithelial cell-specific transcription factor Elf-3 in human malignancies. Genes 12. https://doi.org/10.3390/genes12060839
16. Kim Y-H, Kim HO, Baek EJ et al (2015) Rh D blood group conversion using transcription activator-like effector nucleases. Nat Commun 6:7451
17. Raud L, Le Tertre M, Vigneron L et al (2021) Missense RHD single nucleotide variants induce weakened D antigen expression by altering splicing and/or protein expression. Transfusion 61:2468–2476
18. (2019) PCR primer design tips. In: Behind the bench. https://www.thermofisher.com/blog/behindthebench/pcr-primer-design-tips/. Accessed 11 Jun 2024
19. Livak KJ, Schmittgen TD (2001) Analysis of relative gene expression data using real-time quantitative PCR and the 2(-Delta Delta C (T)) method. Methods 25:402–408
20. Kurita R, Suda N, Sudo K et al (2013) Establishment of immortalized human erythroid progenitor cell lines able to produce enucleated red blood cells. PLoS One 8:e59890

Chapter 30

Use of Microbial Microarrays to Define Antibody Specificity

Carter J. Stowell, Victoria Ortiz, Caitlin L. Cepeda, Vivien C. Lee, William O. Scott, Connie M. Arthur, Shang-Chuen Wu, and Hau-Ming Jan

Abstract

The formation of alloantibodies against red blood cell (RBC) antigens is the most frequent immune barrier to blood transfusion. Among these antibodies, those that occur naturally within the first few months of life against carbohydrate-based ABO blood group antigens are the most prevalent. Individuals who lack the A or B antigen produce antibodies directed against the corresponding absent antigen. Unlike antibodies that arise following antigen exposure during pregnancy or transfusion, these spontaneously occurring antibodies suggest a role for environmental influences. Early investigations proposed that microbial pathogens bearing carbohydrate motifs resembling blood group antigens could provide such a stimulus. However, characterizing antibody specificities against diverse microbes remains difficult, as each organism often requires unique growth conditions. To address this challenge, glycan microarray technology has been developed, which has enabled high-throughput assessment of antibody binding to a wide variety of microbial carbohydrate determinants, including those mimicking blood group antigens. In this work, we highlight the use of microbial glycan microarrays for defining specificity of antibodies and lectins against microbial mimics of blood group and related antigens.

Key words Immunity, Galectin, Antibody, MGM microarray, Molecular mimicry

1 Introduction

Transfusion of blood products remains one of the most common interventions in hospitalized patients worldwide. The need for transfusion arises in a wide range of clinical contexts, including surgical blood loss, traumatic injury, hematologic disorders, and as critical form of supportive care in oncology [1, 2]. For transfusions to be performed safely, compatibility between donor and recipient blood must be established [3–5]. This requirement stems from the fact that individuals naturally generate antibodies against polymorphic carbohydrate structures expressed on red blood cells (RBCs), most notably the ABO blood group antigens [6–8]. Incompatible transfusions can lead to the rapid opsonization and destruction of donor RBCs, provoking severe inflammatory

Sean R. Stowell and Connie M. Arthur (eds.), *Methods in Transfusion Medicine*, Methods in Molecular Biology, vol. 3053, https://doi.org/10.1007/978-1-0716-5376-0_30,

responses that may culminate in life-threatening hemolytic transfusion reactions [9–13].

In addition to these naturally occurring anti-ABO antibodies, alloimmunization can also occur when individuals are exposed to additional non-self RBC alloantigens that often reflect protein-based polymorphisms expressed on the RBC surface [14–19]. Such antibodies are typically induced following transfusion or during pregnancy as a result of fetomaternal hemorrhage [20–25]. These immune responses are often directed against minor blood group antigens, where the prevalence of these antibodies is much lower than antibodies that naturally arise against ABO antigens [6, 24, 26, 27]. However, despite antigen targets being designated as minor simply to reflect their comparative frequency to ABO blood group antigens, antibodies against these RBC antigens can have major clinical impact if an incompatible transfusion occurs, leading to equally severe hemolytic transfusion reactions and associated complications [9, 28–32].

Although ABO blood group antigens were first described more than a century ago, the immunological mechanisms driving the formation and overall consequences of both naturally occurring anti-ABO antibodies and RBC-induced alloantibodies remain incompletely defined [17, 33–40]. Emerging studies suggest that alloantibody induction after RBC exposure involves the activation of innate-like B cells, as well as innate immune signaling pathways possibly being driven by reticulocytes present in the donated unit that promote antibody production even in the absence of conventional adjuvants [41–50]. Intriguingly, analogous immune mechanisms have been proposed for alloantibody responses against platelet antigens and for inhibitors that develop against therapeutic clotting factors [51–53]. Although antibody-independent mechanisms for platelet clearance have been reported [54], suggesting additional mechanisms may be involved, prior studies examining alloantibody induction raise the possibility that conserved pathways underlie immune responses to intravenously administered biologics [44, 47, 51, 52, 55]. Additional studies have explored mechanisms underlying the consequences of antibody engagement of RBCs in vivo [28–30, 37, 38, 56–59].

In contrast, the spontaneous generation of anti-ABO antibodies may be environmentally driven, although alternative hypotheses certainly exist [33, 60, 61]. A prevailing hypothesis is that antigenic mimicry by microbes plays a central role, as many bacterial species decorate their surfaces with glycan structures that resemble mammalian blood group determinants [62]. Repeated exposure to such cross-reactive microbial glycans during early life may underlie the development of naturally occurring antibodies of direct relevance to both transfusion and transplantation medicine [63]. However, dissecting these interactions requires tools capable of assessing glycan recognition with structural resolution.

To address this, microbial glycan microarrays (MGMs) have been developed that are populated with hundreds of structurally diverse glycans derived from a wide array of microbial species [64–70], similar to strategies employed to define the binding specificity of antibodies and lectins toward mammalian glycan structures, including blood group antigens [71–82]. This high-throughput platform enables simultaneous assessment of antibody and lectin binding against diverse glycan repertoires, thereby providing unique insights into host–microbe interactions that may influence the development of naturally occurring anti-blood group antibodies [65]. We will describe, herein, the use of MGMs to characterize the specificity of antibodies and lectins that target microbial mimics of blood group antigens.

2 Materials

2.1 Culturing and Drying of Bacteria

Special Equipment:

1. Lyophilizer (Labconco).
2. Spectrophotometer (capable of reading OD_{600}).

2.1.1 Medias

1. Luria Bertani (LB) culture media (Fisher).
2. Brain Heart Infusion Media (Bacto, Becton Dickinson, Franklin Lakes, NJ).
3. Hemin, 10 mg/mL (Sigma Aldrich, St. Louis, MO).
4. NADH, 10 mg/mL (Sigma Aldrich).
5. Todd Hewitt Broth (THB) (Bacto, Becton Dickinson, Franklin Lakes, NJ).

2.1.2 Bacteria Cultured in LB Culture Media

1. *E. coli* O86:B7.
2. *S. marcescens* O20.
3. *S. marcescens* control strain (*ATCC#14756*).

2.1.3 Bacteria Cultured in THB

1. *S. agalactiae* A909 (*ATCC#BAA-1138*).

2.2 Preparation of Bacterial Polysaccharides (BPS)

1. Dried bacterial cells (*see* Subheading 2.1 Culturing of bacteria).
2. 90% phenol in water.
3. DNAse, 50 μg/mL.
4. RNAse, 50 μg/mL.
5. Ultracentrifuge machine.
6. 2% acetic acid.
7. Sephadex G-50 column.
8. 0.05 M pyridinium acetate buffer, pH 4.5.

9. Printing buffer: 300 mM phosphate buffer, 0.005% Tween-20, pH 8.4.
10. 96-well microplates.
11. BioMek 1000 printing robot (Beckman/Coulter).

2.3 Printing of the Microbial Glycan Microarray (MGM)

1. Diluted glycan antigens.
2. 384-well microplates.
3. Pipetting robot (BioMek 2000, Beckman Coulter).
4. MicroGrid II (Digilab) microarray printing robot equipped with solid steel Stealth microarray pins (SMP4B, TeleChem).
5. SlideH (Schott/Nexterion) or CodeLink (GE Healthcare) NHS-ester activated microscope slides.
6. Desiccator.
7. Blocking buffer: 50 mM ethanolamine in 50 mM borate buffer.
8. Double distilled water.

2.4 Analysis of Binding to the MGM

1. Sera of humans (*see* **Notes 1** and **4**).
2. Sera of mice, rabbits (*see* **Notes 2** and **4**).
3. Intravenous immunoglobulin (IVIG) (*see* **Notes 3** and **4**).
4. Humidified chamber (*see* **Note 5**).
5. TSM Binding Buffer: Tris buffer/Salts/Metal ions (TSM)—20 mM Tris–HCl, 150 mM sodium chloride, 2 mM calcium chloride, 2 mM magnesium chloride, pH 7.4.
6. Alexa 488-streptavidin (Invitrogen, cat. no. S32354).
7. Goat anti-human IgG, Alexa Fluor 488 (Invitrogen, cat. no. A11013).
8. Goat anti-human IgM, Alexa Fluor 488 (Invitrogen, cat. no. A21215).
9. Goat anti-mouse IgG, Alexa Fluor 633 (Invitrogen, cat. no. A21050).
10. Goat anti-mouse IgM, Alexa Fluor 488 (Invitrogen, cat. no. A21042).
11. Goat anti-rabbit IgG, Alexa Fluor 488 (Invitrogen, cat. no. A11034).
12. Goat anti-human IgG, Alexa Fluor 488 (Invitrogen, cat. no. A21091).
13. Goat anti-mouse IgG, Alexa Fluor 488 (Invitrogen, cat. no. A11001).
14. Microarray scanner (Scan Array Express, PerkinElmer Life Sciences).
15. Imagene software (BioDiscovery) (Fig. 1).

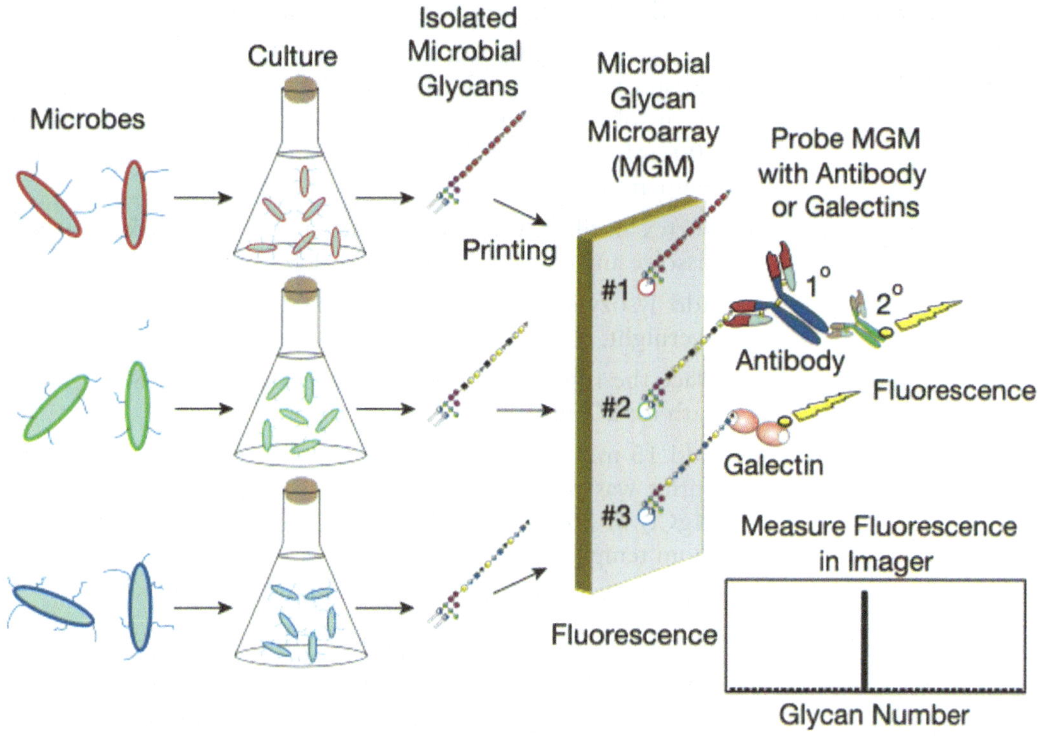

Fig. 1 Illustrates the process of generating microbial glycan microarrays (MGMs). Initially, bacterial cultures undergo amplification, after which individual surface glycans are isolated. These glycans are subsequently attached to slides to generate MGMs, whice can then be probed with various immune factors, such as antibodies in sera. (This research was originally published in Nature Chemical Biology. Stowell et al. [70])

3 Methods

3.1 Culturing and Drying of Bacteria

1. Grow and maintain *E. coli* O86:B7, *S. marcescens* O20, and *S. marcescens* control strain ATCC #14756 in aerobic conditions at 37 °C using LB culture media.
2. Grow and maintain *S. agalactiae* A909 in standard aerobic conditions at 37 °C using Todd Hewitt Broth (THB).
3. Monitor culture growth by OD_{600} and harvest the bacterial cultures between OD_{600} 0.6–0.8 by centrifugation to obtain cell pellets.
4. Wash the cell pellets with PBS to remove residual growth medium components.
5. Lyophilize (freeze-dry) the washed cell pellets to obtain dried bacterial cells.

3.2 Preparation of Bacterial Polysaccharides (BPS)

1. Grind 1 g lyophilized bacteria pellet into a fine powder.
2. Resuspend 1 g of pellet in 5 mL of 50 mM sodium hydrogen phosphate (pH 7) with 5 mM EDTA. This buffer was prepared by dissolving 3.5 g sodium phosphate and 0.93 g EDTA in 500 mL dH_2O. This solution can be preserved at room temperature.
3. Vortex until fully dissolved, then leave on a shaker to help dissolve any clumps that might be left.
4. Add lysozyme and leave on a shaker at room temperature overnight.
5. Place the resuspended pellet with lysozyme in a 37 °C water bath for 20 min.
6. Add 15 mL of 50 mM Na_2HPO_4 with 20 mM $MgCl_2$. This buffer was prepared by dissolving 3.5 g Na_2HPO_4 and 2 g $MgCl_2$ in 500 mL dH_2O. This solution can be preserved at room temperature.
7. Add DNAse and RNAse, both at 50 μg/mL.
8. Incubate in a 37 °C water bath for 1 h.
9. Move to a 60 °C water bath for 1 h.
10. Preheat 90% phenol (18 g phenol +2 g H_2O) to 70 °C (*see* **Note 6**).
11. Mix phenol with bacteria in equal volumes after both are equilibrated to 70 °C.
12. Leave for about 10 min in the water bath.
13. Remove and cool quickly in an ice water bath.
14. Centrifuge at about 3000× g for 40 min.
15. Take the upper (aqueous phase) layer and dialyze against dH_2O until the phenol odor disappears.
16. Dialyze LPS with 4 L changes of dH_2O for 4 days.
17. Recover about 30 mL of dialyzed material (*see* **Note 7**).
18. If bacterial polysaccharides (BPs) are released from lipopolysaccharide (LPS), subject the isolated LPS to mild acid hydrolysis using 2% acetic acid (v/v) to remove the lipid A portion, leaving the inner core, outer core, and O-antigen (BPs).
19. Fractionate the isolated supernatants using a Sephadex G-50 column in 0.05 M pyridinium acetate buffer at pH 4.5.
20. Aliquot the samples and lyophilize for storage.
21. Prior to printing microbial glycans, dissolve lyophilized samples in printing buffer (300 mM phosphate buffer plus 0.005% Tween-20, pH 8.4) to a stock concentration of 1 mg/mL.
22. Dilute the stock solution into 96-well microplates prior to printing by performing twofold serial dilutions using a BioMek 1000 printing robot (Fig. 2).

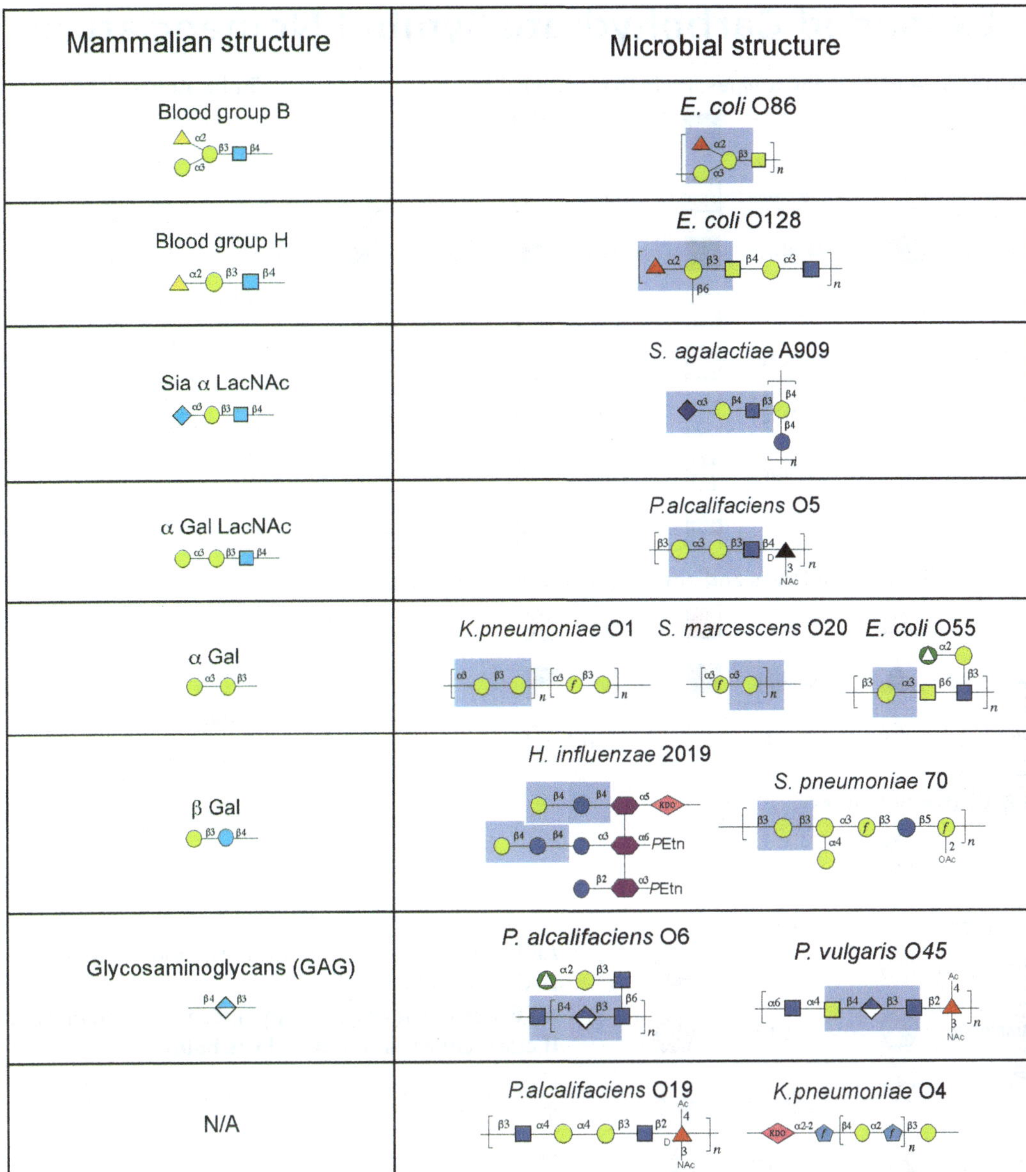

Fig. 2 Schematic representation of mammalian and microbial carbohydrate determinants. Structures of commonly occurring mammalian glycans are shown as indicated with corresponding structures synthesized by the indicated microbial species shown on the right. The carbohydrate symbols used in this figure are defined in the expanded carbohydrate symbol nomenclature shown in Fig. 3. (This research was originally published in Nature Chemical Biology. Stowell et al. [70])

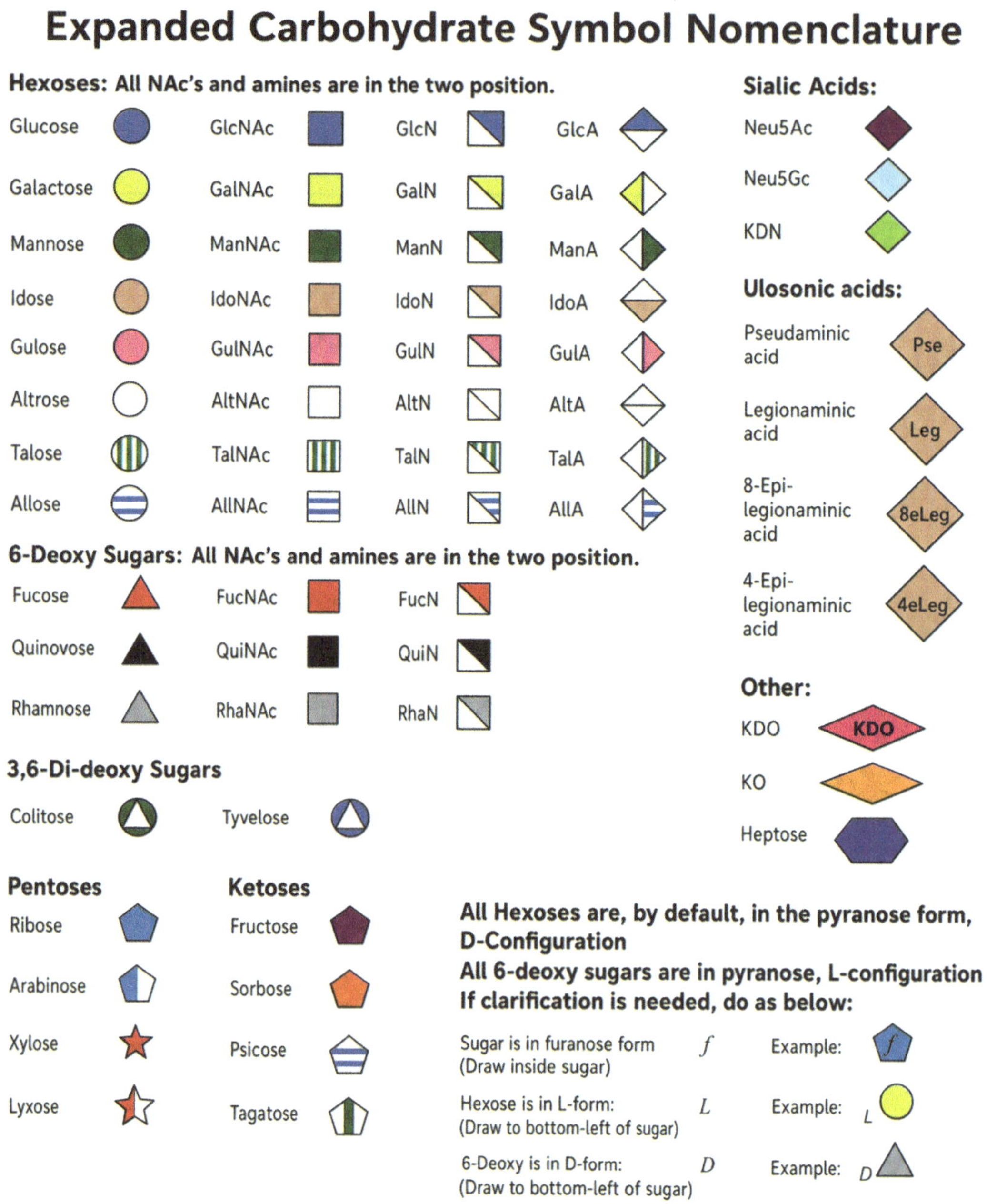

Fig. 3 Symbol nomenclature. (This research was originally published in Nature Chemical Biology. Stowell et al. [70])

3.3 Printing of the Microbial Glycan Microarray (MGM)

1. Deposit 10 μL of diluted glycan antigens into 384-well microplates using a pipetting robot. Then, spot them onto SlideH or CodeLink NHS-ester activated microscope slides with a microarray printing robot equipped with solid steel Stealth microarray pins.
2. Each pin delivers ~1 nL of dissolved sample per spot deposition and six replicate spots of each sample should be imprinted on each array.
3. Print arrays at ~55% relative humidity (RH) and allow 30 min of immobilization at 100% RH before being desiccated at RT. C.
4. After desiccation, immerse the printed arrays in the blocking buffer (50 mM ethanolamine in 50 mM borate buffer) for 1 h on a rotary shaker.
5. Following blocking, rinse slides in ddH_2O and dry by centrifugation prior to incubation/analysis.

3.4 Analysis of Binding to the MGM

1. Printed MGMs were assessed for functionality using sera from humans, mice, and rabbits, as well as IVIG. The sera analyzed on the array represent pooled samples from five individual donors.
2. MGM data were obtained after incubation with pooled normal human sera at a 1:1000 dilution, followed by labeling with anti-IgG and anti-IgM antibodies. Alternatively, the samples were probed with 200 μg/mL IVIG and detected using anti-IgG antibodies, or with pooled normal mouse sera or pooled normal rabbit sera, each at a 1:1000 dilution, applied onto the array surface and incubated for 1 h in a humidified chamber at 25 °C.
3. After 1 h, remove the slide and immerse it in the TSM Binding Buffer.
4. Incubate the slide with species-specific secondary antibodies (Alexa Fluor 488-anti-IgM or Alexa Fluor 647-anti-IgG) targeting primary IgM or IgG, for 1 h at room temperature.
5. After 1 h, remove the slide and immerse it in the TSM Binding Buffer.
6. Detect fluorescence with a microarray scanner.
7. Determine the integrated spot intensities using Imagene software.

4 Notes

1. Normal human sera were obtained from healthy volunteers through venipuncture. Whole blood was collected into sterile serum tubes according to a protocol approved by the Institutional Review Board (IRB).
2. Mouse and rabbit sera were isolated using venipuncture blood-drawing techniques.
3. A IVIG preparation has been examined from Sandoglobulin (CSL Behring, Bern, Switzerland), which underwent extensive dialysis to remove stabilizing components.
4. Isolated sera were then frozen at −80 °C until further use.
5. Prepare the paper towels by saturating them in water and keep them on the site.
6. Please perform the phenol experiment in a fume hood to ensure proper ventilation and to minimize exposure to harmful fumes. Phenol is toxic and can be hazardous to your health if inhaled, so conducting this procedure in a fume hood is essential for maintaining a safe laboratory environment.
7. The purity of LPS was assessed by SDS-PAGE followed by silver staining. Purified LPS samples of 20 μg, 10 μg, 5 μg, and 2.5 μg were subjected to SDS-PAGE. The resulting gel was washed three times with water, shaken in water for 15 min, and then placed in the destaining buffer (ddH_2O:acetic acid:methanol, 5:1:4) overnight at room temperature. The gel was fixed with 0.7% periodic acid in a destaining buffer (0.7 g sodium periodate in 100 mL of destaining buffer) for 30 min, then washed three times with ddH_2O for 15 min each. Staining reagent (115 mL ddH_2O, 2 mL concentrated ammonium hydroxide, 28 mL 0.1 N sodium hydroxide, 5 mL 20% silver nitrate) was prepared and the gel was stained for 10 min, followed by three 10-minute washes with ddH_2O. Developer solution (100 mL ddH_2O, 5 mg citric acid, 50 μL 37% formaldehyde) was applied until bands appeared. The gel was then washed with ddH_2O, and a photograph was taken to record the results.

Conflicts of Interest

This work was funded by NIH P01HL171803, R01 HL165975, R01 HL135575, R01 HL154034, K99HL169746, and AABB Foundation Early-Career Scientific Research Grants. SRS has received speaker and consultant honoraria from Cerus, Grifols, Novartis, Alexion, Argenx, and has received a research grant from Alexion. No other authors have conflicts of interest.

References

1. Metcalf RA et al (2025) Platelet transfusion: 2025 AABB and ICTMG international clinical practice guidelines. JAMA 334(7):606–617
2. Carson JL et al (2021) Transfusion thresholds for guiding red blood cell transfusion. Cochrane Database Syst Rev 12(12): CD002042
3. Li HY, Guo K (2022) Blood group testing. Front Med (Lausanne) 9:827619
4. Fasano RM, Chou ST (2016) Red blood cell antigen genotyping for sickle cell disease, thalassemia, and other transfusion complications. Transfus Med Rev 30(4):197–201
5. Arthur CM, Stowell SR (2023) The development and consequences of red blood cell Alloimmunization. Annu Rev Pathol 18:537–564
6. Reid ME, Lomas-Francis C, Olsson ML (2012) The blood group antigen factsbook, 3rd edn. Elsevier/AP, Amsterdam. xii, 745 pages
7. Storry JR, Olsson ML (2009) The ABO blood group system revisited: a review and update. Immunohematology 25(2):48–59
8. Jajosky RP et al (2023) ABO blood group antigens and differential glycan expression: perspective on the evolution of common human enzyme deficiencies. iScience 26(1):105798
9. Zimring JC, Spitalnik SL (2015) Pathobiology of transfusion reactions. Annu Rev Pathol 10: 83–110
10. Stowell SR et al (2012) Initiation and regulation of complement during hemolytic transfusion reactions. Clin Dev Immunol 2012: 307093
11. Panch SR, Montemayor-Garcia C, Klein HG (2019) Hemolytic transfusion reactions. N Engl J Med 381(2):150–162
12. Chonat S et al (2020) Eculizumab for complement mediated thrombotic microangiopathy in sickle cell disease. Haematologica 105:2887
13. Chonat S et al (2025) Complement is activated in patients with acute chest syndrome caused by sickle cell disease and represents a therapeutic target. Sci Transl Med 17(807):eadl4922
14. Vichinsky EP et al (1990) Alloimmunization in sickle cell anemia and transfusion of racially unmatched blood. N Engl J Med 322(23): 1617–1621
15. Aygun B et al (2002) Clinical significance of RBC alloantibodies and autoantibodies in sickle cell patients who received transfusions. Transfusion 42(1):37–43
16. Klapper E et al (2010) Toward extended phenotype matching: a new operational paradigm for the transfusion service. Transfusion 50(3): 536–546
17. Pirenne F, Floch A, Diop S (2023) Alloimmunisation against red blood cells in sickle cell disease: transfusion challenges in high-income and low-income countries. Lancet Haematol 10(6):e468–e476
18. Chang DY et al (2023) The ongoing challenge of RBC alloimmunization in the management of patients with sickle cell disease. Presse Med 52(4):104211
19. Zimring JC, Hudson KE (2016) Cellular immune responses in red blood cell alloimmunization. Hematology Am Soc Hematol Educ Program 2016(1):452–456
20. Myle AK, Al-Khattabi GH (2021) Hemolytic disease of the newborn: a review of current trends and prospects. Pediatr Health Med Ther 12:491–498
21. Stowell SR et al (2013) Alloantibodies to a paternally derived RBC KEL antigen lead to hemolytic disease of the fetus/newborn in a murine model. Blood 122(8):1494–1504
22. Verweij E et al (2025) Reporting of management and outcomes in the hemolytic disease of the fetus and newborn: a systematic literature review. J Perinatol 45:1513
23. Kilby MD, Bussel JB, Moise KJ Jr (2025) The contemporary management of haemolytic disease of the fetus and newborn. Vox Sang 120(7):644–652
24. Sugrue RP et al (2024) Maternal red blood cell alloimmunization prevalence in the United States. Blood Adv 8(16):4311–4319
25. Webb J, Delaney M (2018) Red blood cell alloimmunization in the pregnant patient. Transfus Med Rev 32(4):213–219
26. Karafin MS et al (2018) Risk factors for red blood cell alloimmunization in the Recipient Epidemiology and Donor Evaluation Study (REDS-III) database. Br J Haematol 181(5): 672–681
27. Fasano RM et al (2019) Impact of red blood cell antigen matching on alloimmunization and transfusion complications in patients with sickle cell disease: a systematic review. Transfus Med Rev 33(1):12–23
28. Hod EA et al (2008) Cytokine storm in a mouse model of IgG-mediated hemolytic transfusion reactions. Blood 112(3):891–894

29. Liepkalns JS et al (2013) Resistance of a subset of red blood cells to clearance by antibodies in a mouse model of incompatible transfusion. Transfusion 53(6):1319–1327
30. Liepkalns JS et al (2012) Biphasic clearance of incompatible red blood cells through a novel mechanism requiring neither complement nor Fcgamma receptors in a murine model. Transfusion 52(12):2631–2645
31. Arthur CM et al (2019) Examining the role of complement in predicting, preventing, and treating hemolytic transfusion reactions. Transfus Med Rev 33(4):217–224
32. Arthur CM et al (2021) Antigen density dictates RBC clearance, but not antigen modulation, following incompatible RBC transfusion in mice. Blood Adv 5(2):527–538
33. Branch DR (2015) Anti-A and anti-B: what are they and where do they come from? Transfusion 55(Suppl 2):S74–S79
34. Yazdanbakhsh K (2016) Immunoregulatory networks in sickle cell alloimmunization. Hematology Am Soc Hematol Educ Program 2016(1):457–461
35. Yazdanbakhsh K, Ware RE, Noizat-Pirenne F (2012) Red blood cell alloimmunization in sickle cell disease: pathophysiology, risk factors, and transfusion management. Blood 120(3): 528–537
36. Bao W et al (2009) Regulatory T-cell status in red cell alloimmunized responder and nonresponder mice. Blood 113(22):5624–5627
37. Jajosky RP et al (2024) Dynamics of antibody engagement of red blood cells in vivo and in vitro. Front Immunol 15:1475470
38. Jajosky RP et al (2025) CD47 regulates antigen modulation and red blood cell clearance following an incompatible transfusion. Front Immunol 16:1548548
39. Mener A et al (2019) Antibody-mediated immunosuppression can result from RBC antigen loss independent of Fcgamma receptors in mice. Transfusion 59(1):371–384
40. Mener A et al (2018) Complement component 3 negatively regulates antibody response by modulation of red blood cell antigen. Front Immunol 9:676
41. Thomas TA et al (2023) Reticulocytes in donor blood units enhance red blood cell alloimmunization. Haematologica 108(10):2639–2651
42. Jash A et al (2024) Complement C3 and marginal zone B cells promote IgG-mediated enhancement of RBC alloimmunization in mice. J Clin Invest 134(8):e167665
43. Jajosky R et al (2023) Prior immunization against an intracellular antigen enhances subsequent red blood cell alloimmunization in mice. Blood 141(21):2642–2653
44. Zerra PE et al (2021) Marginal zone B cells mediate a CD4 T-cell-dependent extrafollicular antibody response following RBC transfusion in mice. Blood 138(8):706–721
45. Mener A et al (2018) Complement serves as a switch between CD4+ T cell-independent and -dependent RBC antibody responses. JCI Insight 3(22):e121631
46. Patel SR et al (2018) Recipient priming to one RBC alloantigen directly enhances subsequent alloimmunization in mice. Blood Adv 2(2): 105–115
47. Patel SR et al (2018) Marginal zone B cells induce alloantibody formation following RBC transfusion. Front Immunol 9:2516
48. Gibb DR et al (2017) Type I IFN is necessary and sufficient for inflammation-induced red blood cell alloimmunization in mice. J Immunol 199(3):1041–1050
49. Gibb DR et al (2017) B cells require Type 1 interferon to produce alloantibodies to transfused KEL-expressing red blood cells in mice. Transfusion 57(11):2595–2608
50. Arthur CM et al (2017) Antigen density dictates immune responsiveness following red blood cell transfusion. J Immunol 198(7): 2671–2680
51. Couvidou A et al (2023) Marginal zone B cells are responsible for the production of alloantibodies following platelet transfusion in mice. Blood Adv 7(8):1356–1365
52. Zerra PE et al (2017) Marginal zone B cells are critical to factor VIII inhibitor formation in mice with hemophilia a. Blood 130(23): 2559–2568
53. Arthur CM et al (2022) Nonhuman glycans can regulate anti-factor VIII antibody formation in mice. Blood 139(9):1312–1317
54. Arthur CM et al (2016) CD8+ T cells mediate antibody-independent platelet clearance in mice. Blood 127(14):1823–1827
55. Arthur CM et al (2022) Clodronate inhibits alloimmunization against distinct red blood cell alloantigens in mice. Transfusion 62(5): 948–953
56. Zimring JC et al (2005) Nonhemolytic antibody-induced loss of erythrocyte surface antigen. Blood 106(3):1105–1112
57. Sullivan HC et al (2017) Daratumumab (anti-CD38) induces loss of CD38 on red blood cells. Blood 129(22):3033–3037
58. Girard-Pierce KR et al (2013) A novel role for C3 in antibody-induced red blood cell clearance and antigen modulation. Blood 122(10): 1793–1801
59. Jajosky RP et al (2023) Antibody-mediated antigen loss switches augmented immunity to

antibody-mediated immunosuppression. Blood 142(12):1082–1098
60. Adam I et al (2025) ABO-A antibody induction in mice is T cell-dependent, estrogen-independent, and modulated by CD22. Am J Transplant 25(6):1180–1192
61. Adam I et al (2023) Sex, T cells, and the microbiome in natural ABO antibody production in mice. Transplantation 107(11):2353–2363
62. Stowell CP, Stowell SR (2019) Biologic roles of the ABH and Lewis histo-blood group antigens part I: infection and immunity. Vox Sang 114(5):426–442
63. Hale RC et al (2024) The role of glycosylation in clinical allergy and immunology. J Allergy Clin Immunol 153(1):55–66
64. Jan HM et al (2024) Galectin-4 antimicrobial activity primarily occurs through its C-terminal domain. Mol Cell Proteomics 23(5):100747
65. Arthur CM, Cummings RD, Stowell SR (2014) Using glycan microarrays to understand immunity. Curr Opin Chem Biol 18: 55–61
66. Blenda AV et al (2022) Galectin-9 recognizes and exhibits antimicrobial activity toward microbes expressing blood group-like antigens. J Biol Chem 298(4):101704
67. Wu SC et al (2022) Innate immune Galectin-7 specifically targets microbes that decorate themselves in blood group-like antigens. iScience 25(7):104482
68. Wu SC et al (2021) The SARS-CoV-2 -receptor-binding domain preferentially recognizes blood group a. Blood Adv 5(5): 1305–1309
69. Wu SC et al (2021) Full-length Galectin-3 is required for high affinity microbial interactions and antimicrobial activity. Front Microbiol 12: 731026
70. Stowell SR et al (2014) Microbial glycan microarrays define key features of host-microbial interactions. Nat Chem Biol 10(6): 470–476
71. Wu SC et al (2023) Blood group A enhances SARS-CoV-2 infection. Blood 142(8): 742–747
72. Liu FT, Stowell SR (2023) The role of galectins in immunity and infection. Nat Rev Immunol 23(8):479–494
73. Luetscher RND et al (2020) Unique repertoire of anti-carbohydrate antibodies in individual human serum. Sci Rep 10(1):15436
74. Rillahan CD, Paulson JC (2011) Glycan microarrays for decoding the glycome. Annu Rev Biochem 80:797–823
75. Stowell SR et al (2008) Galectin-1, -2, and -3 exhibit differential recognition of sialylated glycans and blood group antigens. J Biol Chem 283(15):10109–10123
76. Stowell SR et al (2008) Dimeric Galectin-8-induces phosphatidylserine exposure in leukocytes through polylactosamine recognition by the C-terminal domain. J Biol Chem 283(29): 20547–20559
77. Ho AD et al (2022) An automated approach to assess relative galectin-glycan affinity following glycan microarray analysis. Front Mol Biosci 9: 893185
78. Stowell SR et al (2009) Ligand reduces galectin-1 sensitivity to oxidative inactivation by enhancing dimer formation. J Biol Chem 284(8):4989–4999
79. Tulin EKC et al (2025) Blood group O expression in normal tissues and tumors. FEBS J 292: 5697
80. Jia T et al (2025) Novel click coupling chemistry to explore glycan recognition. ACS Cent Sci 11(5):753–769
81. Stowell SR et al (2008) Differential roles of galectin-1 and galectin-3 in regulating leukocyte viability and cytokine secretion. J Immunol 180(5):3091–3102
82. Stowell SR et al (2010) Innate immune lectins kill bacteria expressing blood group antigen. Nat Med 16(3):295–301

Chapter 31

Production of Induced Pluripotent Stem Cell-Derived Red Blood Cells

Hyun Hyung An, Giulia Pavani, and Stella T. Chou

Abstract

Red blood cell (RBC) transfusion is one of the most common medical treatments, with over 10 million units transfused per year in the United States alone. One complication following transfusion is red cell alloimmunization, the production of antibodies to foreign proteins on donor RBCs. Identifying compatible RBC units for alloimmunized patients may be challenging due to the lack of specific RBC reagents with uncommon or rare RBC antigen phenotypes that are needed to identify the precise antibody target. Human induced pluripotent stem cells (iPSCs) represent a renewable source of cells to generate specialized RBCs by reprogramming rare donor cells or by gene editing iPSCs. These iPSCs can provide an unlimited supply of RBCs with unique antigen expression profiles. Here, we outline protocols to generate developmentally primitive (embryonic) and definitive (fetal) RBCs from iPSCs, and methods to perform antibody identification using iPSC-derived RBCs as reagent cells in gel agglutination assays commonly used by blood banks and reference immunohematology laboratories.

Key words Induced pluripotent stem cells, Hematopoietic progenitor cell, Red blood cell, Red blood cell reagents, Antibody identification

1 Introduction

Red blood cell (RBC) transfusions are a critical therapy for hematologic disorders and the management of trauma, surgery, and cancer. Alloimmunization to donor RBC antigens, which occurs more frequently in heavily transfused populations, including sickle cell disease (SCD) and thalassemia, may lead to the requirement for uncommon or rare RBCs for antibody identification [1–3]. Determination of the precise RBC antibody formed by a patient can be hampered by a lack of reagent RBCs with uncommon or rare antigen phenotypes, which currently rely on donor-derived cells. The inability to complete the antibody identification can delay or prevent adequate pre-transfusion testing to properly select compatible donor RBC units.

Sean R. Stowell and Connie M. Arthur (eds.), *Methods in Transfusion Medicine*, Methods in Molecular Biology, vol. 3053,
https://doi.org/10.1007/978-1-0716-5376-0_31,

Red cells can be produced from embryonic stem cells (ESCs) and induced pluripotent stem cells (iPSCs), which have the capacity for unlimited self-renewal [4]. iPSCs are especially attractive for their ability to be generated from donor somatic cells and can easily be customized by genome engineering to generate rare RBC antigen phenotypes [5–7]. As alloimmunization can lead to difficulty identifying sufficient compatible donor units, iPSC-derived reagent RBCs may facilitate the ability to provide a life-saving transfusion.

iPSCs can be used to generate both primitive and definitive RBCs [4, 6], which refer to the developmental stage of blood formation. Primitive or embryonic hematopoiesis arises from the yolk sac weeks after conception in the human and primarily gives rise to erythroid cells, megakaryocytes, and macrophages. The hematopoietic stem cell (HSC) is first detected within the dorsal aorta of the aorta-gonad-mesonephros region at ~1 month after conception and signifies the definitive wave of hematopoiesis that transitions to the fetal liver and bone marrow [8]. Both differentiation methods require induction to mesoderm, then to hemangioblast and hemogenic endothelium for primitive and definitive programs, respectively, and subsequently to hematopoietic progenitor cells (HPCs). This is achieved either through the formation of embryoid bodies or by monolayer differentiation with or without co-culture with feeder cells to generate HPCs. Subsequent HPC culture with erythroid-specific cytokines facilitates the proliferation and differentiation to mature RBCs. Mature primitive erythroid cells are larger, express embryonic ε-globins and zeta-globins, and remain nucleated, while mature definitive RBCs are smaller, anucleate, and express fetal γ-globin and adult β-globins [4].

2 Materials

2.1 Generation of Primitive Hematopoietic Progenitor Cells (See Table 1)

1. CO_2 incubator.
2. Low O_2 incubator.
3. 6-well plate, tissue culture (TC)-treated (Falcon).
4. 6-well plate, ultra-Low Attachment (Corning).
5. Cell scraper (Sarstedt).
6. TrypLE (Invitrogen).
7. PBS (Corning).
8. ROCK Inhibitor Y-27632 (Cayman Chemical).
9. Growth factor reduced Matrigel (Corning).
10. Collagenase B (Sigma).
11. DNase I (Sigma).
12. Trypsin (Sigma).

Table 1
Primitive hematopoietic progenitor differentiation media

D0 media components	Working concentration	Final concentration
Complete StemPro-34 medium		
Glutamine	100×	1×
Ascorbic Acid (fresh)	5 mg/mL	10 µL/mL
Transferrin	30 mg/mL	5 µL/mL
MTG (fresh)	26 µL/2 mL IMDM	3 µL/mL
hBMP4	25 µg/mL	25 ng/mL
hVEGF	50 µg/mL	50 ng/mL
D2 media components	**Working concentration**	**Final concentration**
Complete StemPro-34 medium		
Glutamine	100×	1×
Ascorbic Acid (fresh)	5 mg/mL	10 µL/mL
Transferrin	30 mg/mL (200×)	5 µL/mL
MTG (fresh)	26 µL/2 mL IMDM	3 µL/mL
hBMP4	25 µg/mL	25 ng/mL
hVEGF	50 µg/mL	50 ng/mL
hSCF	100 µg/mL	50 ng/mL
hTPO	50 µg/mL	50 ng/mL
hFlt3	50 µg/mL	50 ng/mL
hbFGF	100 µg/mL	20 ng/mL
D4, 6 media components	**Working concentration**	**Final concentration**
Complete StemPro-34 medium		
Glutamine	100×	1×
Ascorbic Acid (fresh)	5 mg/mL	10 µL/mL
Transferrin	30 mg/mL (200×)	5 µL/mL
MTG (fresh)	26 µL/2 mL IMDM	3 µL/mL
hVEGF	50 µg/mL	50 ng/mL
hSCF	100 µg/mL	50 ng/mL
hFlt3	50 µg/mL	50 ng/mL
hTPO	50 µg/mL	50 ng/mL
hbFGF	100 µg/mL	20 ng/mL

13. Fetal Bovine Serum, lot tested.
14. Iscove's Modified Dulbecco's Medium (IMDM, Corning).
15. StemPro-34 medium and supplement (Gibco).
16. Penicillin/Streptomycin (Pen/Strep, Invitrogen).
17. L-Glutamine (Invitrogen).
18. Transferrin (Roche).
19. Ascorbic Acid (Sigma).
20. Monothioglycerol (MTG, Sigma).
21. Human bone morphogenic protein 4 (hBMP4, R&D Systems).
22. Human vascular endothelial growth factor (hVEGF, R&D Systems).
23. Human stem cell factor (hSCF, R&D Systems).
24. Human thrombopoietin (hTPO, R&D Systems).
25. Human FMS related receptor tyrosine kinase 3 (hFLT3, R&D Systems).
26. Human basic fibroblast growth factor (hbFGF, R&D Systems).
27. Dimethylsulfoxide (DMSO, Sigma).
28. Phosphate Buffer Saline (PBS).
29. FACS staining buffer (1 L PBS, 0.1% BSA, 0.02% sodium azide, 0.5 mM EDTA).
30. 4% Paraformaldehyde (PFA).
31. Antibodies to monitor differentiation

    SSEA3, FITC, Biolegend 330306 (1:400).
    SSEA4, APC, Biolegend 330408 (1:400).
    Tra1.61, PE, Biolegend 330614 (1:40).
    Tra1.81, APC, Biolegend 330706 (1:20).
    CD31, FITC, BD 558068 (1:100).
    KDR, APC, Biolegend 339910 (1:100).
    CD34, PE, BD 550761 (1:100).
    CD43, FITC, BD 555475 (1:20).
    CD235ab, APC, BD 551336 (1:5000).
    CD41, PE, BD 555467 (1:20).
    CD42, FITC, BD 558818 (1:20).
    CD71; FITC, BD 555536 (1:50).
    CD45, PE, BD555483 (1:20).
    CD18, APC, BD551060 (1:20).

2.2 Generation of Primitive iPSC-Derived Red Blood Cells (See Table 2)

1. Centrifuge.
2. Hemacytometer.
3. IMDM (Corning).
4. AB serum (Millipore Sigma).
5. AB plasma (Sera Care).
6. Pen/Strep (Invitrogen).
7. Holotransferrin (Sigma).
8. Erythropoietin (Epo, AmGen).
9. Human interleukin 3 (hIL-3, Peprotech).
10. hSCF (Peprotech).
11. Insulin (Sigma).
12. Heparin (Sigma).
13. Trypan blue stain.
14. May Grunwald stain.

Table 2
Primitive erythroid differentiation media

Base medium components	Final concentration
IMDM	
Human AB Plasma	2%
Human AB Serum	3%
Pen/Strep	1%

Complete medium components	Working concentration	Phase 1 (HPC recovery) D-1	Phase 2 (Expansion) D0, 3	Phase 3 (Maturation) D6, 9, 12
Base medium	–	9.8 mL	9 mL	9 mL
Holotransferrin	10 mg/mL	0.2 mg/mL	1 mg/mL	1 mg/mL
Heparin	5000 U/mL	3 U/mL	3 U/mL	3 U/mL
Insulin	4 mg/mL (100 U)	10 ug/mL	10 ug/mL	10 ug/mL
Cytokines should be added to the *total culture volume* for each corresponding day of differentiation.				
Epo	10000 U/mL	3 U/mL	3 U/mL	3 U/mL
SCF	100 ng/μL	10 ng/μL	10 ng/μL	–
IL3	50 μg/mL	1 ng/mL	–	–

15. Giemsa stain.
16. Phosphate Buffer Saline (PBS).
17. FACS staining buffer (1 L PBS, 0.1% BSA, 0.02% sodium azide, 0.5 mM EDTA).
18. 4% Paraformaldehyde (PFA).
19. Antibodies to monitor differentiation

    CD235ab, APC, BD 551336 (1:5000).
    CD71; FITC, BD 555536 (1:50).
    CD45, PE, BD555483 (1:20).
    CD18, APC, BD551060 (1:20).

2.3 Generation of Definitive Hematopoietic Progenitor Cells (HPCs) (See Tables 3 and 4)

1. Accutase (Life Tech) A11105-01.
2. 6-well plate, with lid, flat bottom (ultra-low attachment, Corning), 3471.
3. CHIR 99201(Tocris).
4. SB 431542 (Tocris).
5. StemPro 34 (SP34) media + supplement (Thermo Fisher).
6. B27 without Vit A (Thermo Fisher).
7. N2 Supplement (Life Tech).
8. Ham's F12 (Corning, 10-080-CV).
9. IMDM (Corning, 10-016-CV).
10. Pen/Strep (Invitrogen).
11. Glutamax (Invitrogen).
12. Transferrin (Roche, 10 652 202).
13. Collagenase B (Roche, 11 088 831 001).
14. DNase I (Sigma) 1 mg/mL.
15. DMEM/F12 (Invitrogen, 10-092-CV).
16. Fetal Bovine Serum, Lot tested.
17. Bovine Serum Albumin (Sigma, A1470).

Table 3
SFD base media

SFD	For 1 L
IMDM	750 mL
Ham's F12	250 mL
B27 without Vit A	1 vial/L
N2 Supplement	1 vial/L
BSA	0.5%

Table 4
Definitive hematopoietic progenitor differentiation media

Aggregation	Final	Induction 1	Final	Induction 2	Final
SFD		SFD		STEMPRO 34	
Pen/Strep	1×	Pen/Strep	1×	Pen/Strep	1×
Glutamax	1×	Glutamax	1×	Glutamax	1×
Transferrin	150 ug/mL	Transferrin	150 ug/mL	Transferrin	150 ug/mL
Ascorbic Acid	50 ug/mL	Ascorbic Acid	50 ug/mL	Ascorbic Acid	50 ug/mL
MTG	0.04 μL/mL	MTG	0.04 μL/mL	MTG	0.04 μL/mL
BMP4	10 ng/mL	BMP4	10 ng/mL	VEGF	15 ng/mL
		bFGF	5 ng/mL	bFGF	5 ng/mL
		SB431542	6 uM		
		CHIR	3 uM		

Induction 3	Final	Reaggregation	Final	Mainteneance	Final
STEMPRO 34		STEMPRO 34		STEMPRO 34	
Pen/Strep	1×	Pen/Strep	1×	Pen/Strep	1×
Glutamax	1×	Glutamax	1×	Glutamax	1×
Transferrin	150 ug/mL	Transferrin	150 ug/mL	Transferrin	150 ug/mL
Ascorbic Acid	50 ug/mL	Ascorbic Acid	50 ug/mL	Ascorbic Acid	50 ug/mL
MTG	0.04 μL/mL	MTG	0.04 μL/mL	MTG	0.04 μL/mL
VEGF	15 ng/mL	VEGF	5 ng/mL	TPO	30 ng/mL
bFGF	5 ng/mL	TPO	30 ng/mL	IL-3	10 ng/mL
SCF	100 ng/mL	IL-3	10 ng/mL	SCF	100 ng/mL
IGF-1	50 ng/mL	FLT3L	10 ng/mL	IGF-1	25 ng/mL
Retinol	5 uM	SCF	100 ng/mL		
		IGF-1	25 ng/mL		
		bFGF	5 ng/mL		
		BMP4	10 ng/mL		

18. L-ascorbic acid phosphate magnesium salt n-hydrate (Wako).
19. Retinol (Sigma).
20. Monothioglycerol (MTG, Sigma).
21. Human cytokines (R&D Biosystem)

    VEGF, TPO, IL-3, FLT3L, SCF, IGF-1, bFGF, BMP4.

22. Low oxygen incubator.
23. Orbital shaker for incubator.
24. Antibodies for cell sorting

    CD43; MEM-59, FITC (Biolegend).
    CD34; 4H11, PE-Cy7 (Invitrogen).
    CD73; AD2, PE (BD, optional, dilution 1:20).
    CD184; 12G5, APC (BD, optional, dilution 1:100).

25. Antibody for blood progenitors

    CD45; HI30, PB (Biolegend, dilution 1:50).
    CD34; 4H11, PE-Cy7 (Invitrogen, dilution 1:100).

2.4 Generation of Definitive iPSC-Derived Red Blood Cells (See Table 5)

1. SFEMII (StemCell technologies).
2. IMDM (Corning, 10-016-CV).
3. Pen/Strep (Invitrogen).
4. Glutamax (Invitrogen).
5. Human cytokines (R&D Biosystem)
   IL-3, EPO, SCF.
6. Insulin (Sigma).
7. Heparin (Sigma).
8. Octaplas or AB plasma (Sigma).
9. Holotransferrin (Sigma, T0065).
10. Hydrocortisone (Sigma).
11. Antibodies to monitor differentiation

    CD36; APC (Biolegend, dilution 1:100).
    CD71; PE (BD, dilution 1:25).
    CD235a; PB (Biolegend, dilution 1:50).

Table 5
Definitive erythroid differentiation media recipes

M1	Final	M2	Final	M3	Final
SFEMII		SFEMII		IMDM	
Pen/Strep	1×	Pen/Strep	1×	Pen/Strep	1×
Glutamax	1×	Glutamax	1×	Glutamax	1×
Holotransferrin	200 μg/mL	Holotransferrin	200 μg/mL	Holotransferrin	1 mg/mL
SCF	100 ng/mL	SCF	10 ng/mL	Heparin	3 U/mL
IL3	5 ng/mL	EPO	3 U/mL	OCTAPLAS (or AB Plasma)	5%
EPO	3 U/mL			Insulin	10 μg/mL
Hydrocortisone	1 μM			EPO	3 U/mL

2.5 Gel Card Agglutination Assays

1. Buffered & anti-IgG gel cards (Ortho Clinical Diagnostics).
2. Micro Typing Systems 2 diluent (Ortho Clinical Diagnostics).
3. Donor reagent RBCs 0.8% suspension (Ortho Clinical Diagnostics).
4. MTS Workstation (Ortho Clinical Diagnostics).
5. Anti-D (Quotient Biodiagnostics).
6. Anti-C (Immucor).
7. Anti-c (Immucor).
8. Anti-E (Immucor).
9. Anti-e (Immucor).
10. Anti-K (Alba Bioscience).
11. Anti-k (Immucor).
12. Anti-Fya (Ortho Clinical Diagnostics).
13. Anti-Fyb (Ortho Clinical Diagnostics).
14. Anti-Jka (Immucor).
15. Anti-Jkb (Immucor).
16. Anti-M (Biorad).
17. Anti-N (Immucor).
18. Anti-S (Ortho Clinical Diagnostics).
19. Anti-s (Ortho Clinical Diagnostics).
20. 1% ficin solution (Immucor).
21. Phosphate Buffered Saline (PBS).
22. Donor plasma.

3 Methods

3.1 Generation of Primitive Hematopoietic Progenitor Cells

3.1.1 Day-1: Preparing Matrigel Plates

1. Thaw a Matrigel aliquot on ice (~3 h).
2. Place p1000 tips in the −20 °C.
3. When Matrigel is thawed, prepare 6-well plates for Matrigel coating by placing them on ice.
4. Use cold p1000 tips to pipette Matrigel into 1 well of a 6-well TC plate, avoiding bubbles.
5. Once the well is coated, remove excess Matrigel using the cold p1000 and use it to coat the next well. Repeat until all the wells are coated.
6. When all wells are coated, remove excess Matrigel from all the wells and add it back to the original tube. This aliquot can be stored at −20 °C and reused.

7. Incubate Matrigel-coated plates on ice for 30 min.
8. Angle the plate to remove excess Matrigel from the plate.
9. Incubate at 37 °C for at least 1 h prior to plating iPSCs.

3.1.2 Day-1: MEF Depletion of iPSCs

1. To each well of a 6-well plate of iPSCs cultured on MEF feeder cells, add 1 mL/well TrypLE and incubate at room temperature for 3 min.
2. Aspirate off TrypLE and wash 2× with PBS.
3. Add 2 mL hESC medium with ROCK inhibitor (used at 1: 5000 dilution) to each well.
4. Gently scrape iPSCs and resuspend using a p1000.
5. Transfer resuspended iPSCs to Matrigel-coated plates at approximately a 1:1 ratio.
6. Incubate cells overnight at 37 °C, 5% CO_2 (*see* **Note 1**).

3.1.3 Day 0: Embryoid Body (EB) Formation

1. Remove media from 1 well to collect iPSCs for flow cytometry analysis.
   (a) Add 1 mL 0.25% trypsin/EDTA and incubate at room temperature for 5 min.
   (b) Add 1 mL STOP media to inactivate trypsin.
   (c) Pipette iPSCs to a single cell suspension.
   (d) 1× PBS wash and centrifuge iPSCs at 1200 rpm for 5 min.
   (e) Aspirate supernatant and resuspend iPSCs in FACS buffer.
   (f) Stain with SSEA3, SSEA4, Tra1.61, and Tra1.81 for 30 min at 4 °C (Fig. 1).
   (g) Wash iPSCs 1× with PBS and run flow cytometry, or fix cells using 4% PFA and store at 4 °C.
2. To each remaining well, add 1 mL collagenase B with 10 μL/mL DNase I. Incubate at 37 °C for 25 min.
3. Aspirate off collagenase B.
4. Add 1 mL cold trypsin, incubate <1 min at room temp.
5. Aspirate trypsin, then add 1 mL/well STOP media (50% FBS 50% IMDM).
6. Gently scrape iPSCs and pipette up and down using a p1000 until only small cell clusters remain.
7. Add 1 mL IMDM to each well to wash, then harvest cells into a 50 mL conical using 5 mL serological pipette.
8. Centrifuge cells at 250 g for 3 min.
9. Aspirate the supernatant and resuspend cells in Day 0 Media.
10. Plate 2 mL of resuspended cells in low attachment 6-well plates. Incubate at 37 °C, 5% CO_2, 5% O_2.

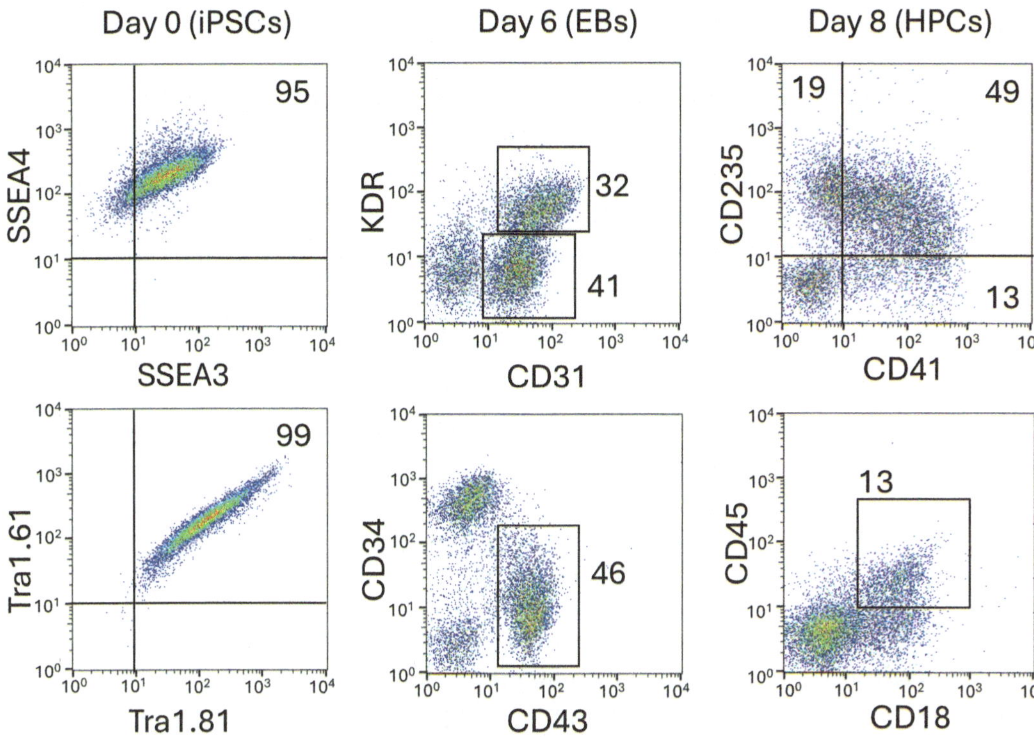

Fig. 1 Flow cytometric analysis of primitive hematopoietic differentiation via embryoid body (EB) culture. Day 0 (D0) iPSCs are SSEA3+ SSEA4+ Tra1.61+ Tra1.81+. Day 6 (D6) EBs contain mesodermal cells (CD31+ KDR +, 32%) and hematopoietic progenitor cells (HPCs, CD31+ KDR- CD43+, 41 and 46%). Day 8 (D8) HPCs released from EBs are multipotent (CD235+ CD41+ CD45- CD18-, 49%). Early lineage commitment of D8 HPCs can be seen based on CD235+ CD41- (erythroid, 19%), CD235- CD41+ (megakaryocyte, 13%), and CD45+ CD18+ (myeloid, 13%)

3.1.4 Days 2, 4, 6: Primitive Hematopoietic Differentiation

1. Gently harvest EBs using 5 mL serological pipette into a 50 mL conical.
2. Wash each well with IMDM to collect all EBs, then add to the 50 mL conical. Keep the low attachment plates.
3. Centrifuge EBs at 150 g for 1 min.
4. Aspirate the supernatant and resuspend cells in fresh differentiation media.
5. Plate 2 mL of EBs back into the same low attachment 6-well plate. Incubate at 37 °C, 5% CO_2, 5% O_2.

3.1.5 Day 6 Only: Flow Cytometry Analysis to Monitor Primitive Hematopoietic Differentiation

1. Centrifuge 1 well of EBs at 150 g for 1 min.
2. Aspirate supernatant and resuspend EBs in 2 mL Collagenase B in serum.

3. Vortex ~30 s to dissociate EBs and incubate at 37 °C for 30 min.
4. Add 4 mL IMDM and pass through a 20 g needle 3×.
5. Centrifuge 330 g for 3 min.
6. Aspirate supernatant and resuspend cells in 1 mL 0.05% trypsin/EDTA.
7. Incubate at room temp for <2 min, vortex intermittently.
8. Add 1 mL STOP media to inactivate trypsin.
9. Add 4 mL IMDM and pass through a 20 g needle 3×.
10. Centrifuge cells at 330 g for 3 min.
11. Aspirate supernatant and resuspend cells in FACS buffer.
12. Stain cells with CD31, KDR, CD34, and CD43 for 30 min at 4 °C (Fig. 1).
13. Wash 1× with PBS and run flow cytometry, or fix cells using 4% PFA and store at 4 °C.

3.1.6 Day 8: Collecting Primitive Hematopoietic Progenitor Cells

1. Harvest EBs and progenitor cells using 5 mL serological pipette into a 50 mL conical.
2. Wash each well with IMDM to collect all EBs and progenitor cells, then add to the 50 mL conical tube. Discard low attachment plates.
3. Centrifuge EBs at 150 g for 1 min.
4. Collect the supernatant (contains progenitor cells but not EBs) using a 5 mL serological pipette, then add to a new 50 mL conical. Contaminating EBs can be further removed by passing the supernatant through a 40 μM cell strainer if needed.
5. Use some of the supernatant for flow cytometry analysis of HPCs.
   (a) 1× PBS wash and centrifuge HPCs at 1200 rpm for 5 min.
   (b) Aspirate supernatant and resuspend HPCs in FACS buffer.
   (c) Stain with CD235ab, CD41, CD42, CD45, and CD18 for 30 min at 4 °C (Fig. 1).
   (d) Wash HPCs 1× with PBS and run flow cytometry, or fix cells using 4% PFA and store at 4 °C.
6. Centrifuge the remaining HPCs at 1200 rpm for 5 min.
7. Aspirate supernatant. Resuspend HPCs in Phase 1 or Phase 2 erythroid differentiation media if cells will be frozen down or used fresh, respectively.

3.2 Generation of Primitive iPSC-Derived Red Blood Cells

3.2.1 Day-1: Starting Primitive Erythroid Differentiation Using Frozen Hematopoietic Progenitor Cells

1. Thaw frozen primitive HPCs by adding cells dropwise onto IMDM wash medium, followed by centrifugation at 1200 rpm for 5 min.
2. Aspirate supernatant and resuspend cell pellet in 1 mL Phase 1 erythroid differentiation media with cytokines (1 ng/mL hIL3, 10 ng/μL hSCF, 3 U/mL Epo). Determine cell count using Trypan Blue.
3. Place cells into a T25 flask for a cell concentration of approximately 100 K cells/mL. Culture at 5% CO_2, 37 °C.

3.2.2 Day 0: Starting Primitive Erythroid Differentiation Using Fresh Progenitor Cells

1. Collect fresh primitive HPCs or frozen HPCs recovered in Phase 1 media overnight by centrifugation at 330 g for 5 min.
2. Aspirate supernatant and resuspend the cell pellet in 1 mL Phase 2 erythroid differentiation media with cytokines (10 ng/μL hSCF and 3 U/mL Epo). Determine cell count using Trypan Blue.
3. Place 500,000 to 1 million cells into a T25 flask for a cell concentration of approximately 100,000 cells/mL. Culture at 5% CO_2, 37 °C for 3 days (*see* **Note 2**).

3.2.3 Day 3: Isolation and Expansion of Primitive Erythroid Progenitors

1. Gently resuspend non-adherent cells by pipetting up and down using a serological pipette and transfer to a new T25 flask. Determine cell count. If desired, perform flow cytometry and cytospin (Fig. 2a, *see* **Notes 3** and **4**).
2. Adjust confluency to 1 million cells/mL by adding complete differentiation media (without cytokines).
3. Add SCF and Epo for the *total culture volume* for a final concentration of 10 ng/μL hSCF and 3 U/mL Epo (*see* **Notes 5** and **6**).

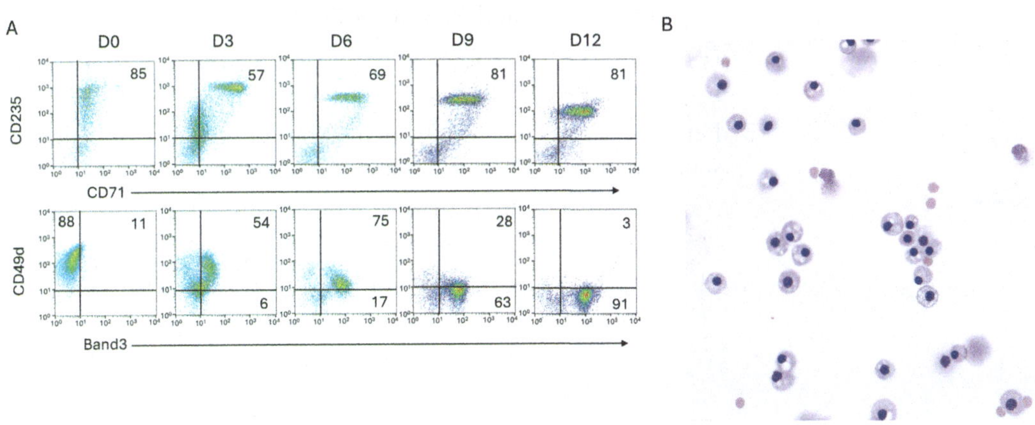

Fig. 2 Primitive erythroid differentiation. (**a**) Flow cytometry analysis during primitive erythroid differentiation (D, day). (**b**) Cytospin of mature primitive erythrocytes on D12 of differentiation (May Grunwald Giemsa). Adult donor RBCs (enucleated) are included for comparison

3.2.4 Day 6: Continued Isolation and Expansion of Primitive Erythroid Progenitors

1. Gently resuspend non-adherent cells by pipetting up and down using a serological pipette and transfer to a new flask. Determine cell count using Trypan Blue. If desired, perform flow cytometry and cytospin (Fig. 2a).
2. Adjust confluency to 1 million cells/mL by adding more Phase 2 differentiation media (without cytokines) on top.
3. Add *Epo only* for the *total culture volume* to a final concentration of 3 U/mL. This method weans the SCF but allows small amounts of remaining SCF in the conditioned media for RBCs to remain healthy in culture.

3.2.5 Day 9: Continued Expansion and Maturation of Primitive Erythroid Progenitors

1. Gently pipet up and down using a serological pipette to resuspend cells and move to a new flask if there are many adherent cells. Determine cell count using Trypan Blue. If desired, perform flow cytometry and cytospin (Fig. 2a).
2. Adjust confluency to 1 million cells/mL by adding more complete differentiation media (without cytokines).
3. Add Epo only for the total culture volume to a final concentration of 3 U/mL.

3.2.6 D12: Primitive Erythroid Cell Maturation Check by Flow Cytometry and Cytospin

1. Gently pipette up and down using a serological pipette to resuspend cells. Determine cell count using Trypan Blue (*see* **Note** 7).
2. Perform flow cytometric analysis of mature RBCs to determine the stage of maturation (Fig. 2a).
   (a) Isolate ~500,000 mature RBCs from culture.
   (b) 1× PBS wash and centrifuge at 330 g for 5 min.
   (c) Aspirate supernatant and resuspend RBCs in FACS buffer.
   (d) Stain mature RBCs with CD235ab, CD71, CD45, CD18, α-integrin4, and Band3 for 30 min at 4 °C.
   (e) Wash 1× with PBS and run flow cytometry, or fix cells using 4% PFA and store at 4 °C.
3. Perform a cytospin followed by May Grunwald and Giemsa staining to determine the stage of maturation (Fig. 2b)
   (a) Isolate 1 million mature RBCs from culture and centrifuge at 330 g for 5 min.
   (b) Aspirate supernatant and resuspend the RBC pellet in 1 mL PBS.
   (c) Centrifuge RBCs at 7600 g for 3 min using a benchtop centrifuge.
   (d) Resuspend pellet in 50 uL PBS.
   (e) Add RBCs to a cytospin funnel.

(f) Centrifuge at 200 rpm for 2 min using low acceleration.

(g) Carefully remove the glass slide from the cytospin funnel and allow spun RBCs to air dry for ~1 min.

(h) Stain with fresh May Grunwald stain for 2 min.

(i) Immediately stain with freshly diluted Giemsa stain (1:20 in water) for 10 min.

(j) Wash slide 3× using water.

(k) Let the slides air dry for ~10 min.

(l) Add 1 drop of cytoseal onto the RBCs and carefully put on the coverslip.

(m) Allow the cytoseal to set for ~10 min and visually confirm that >95% of RBCs are at the orthochromatic erythroblast stage (*see* **Note 8**).

3.3 Generation of Definitive Hematopoietic Progenitor Cells

3.3.1 Day-1: Generation of Embryoid Bodies (EBs)

1. Aspirate media from a 6-well plate of confluent iPSC grown on irradiated mouse embryonic fibroblasts (*see* **Note 9**).
2. Pass iPSC with prewarmed Accutase (1 mL per well, 10–15 min at 37 °C).
3. After cells are detached from the bottom of the plate, pipette up and down to generate a single cell suspension.
4. Transfer cells to a Falcon tube containing IMDM (same volume as Accutase).
5. Centrifuge the cell suspension at 330 g for 3 min.
6. Aspirate supernatant.
7. Resuspend cells in HES10 + ROCKi (1:5000) to achieve a cell concentration of 100,000–300,000 cell/mL.
8. Transfer cells to a 6-well ultra-low attachment plate. Maintain volume between 2.2 mL and 4 mL per well.
9. Place cells on a shaker (80 rpm) in a 5% CO_2, 5% O_2 incubator at 37 °C.

3.3.2 Day 0: bFGF Depletion

1. In the morning (before 11 am), collect cells and centrifuge the cell suspension at 330 × g for 3 min. EBs should be uniform in size (Fig. 3a).
2. Remove at least ¾ of the old media and replace it with HES10.
3. Place cells on a shaker (80 rpm) in a 5% CO_2, 5% O_2 incubator.
4. Six hours later, prepare AGGREGATION MEDIUM, 2 mL per well of EBs.
5. Collect cells from the plate.
6. Centrifuge at 250 × g for 5 min, aspirate, and resuspend in AGGREGATION MEDIUM.

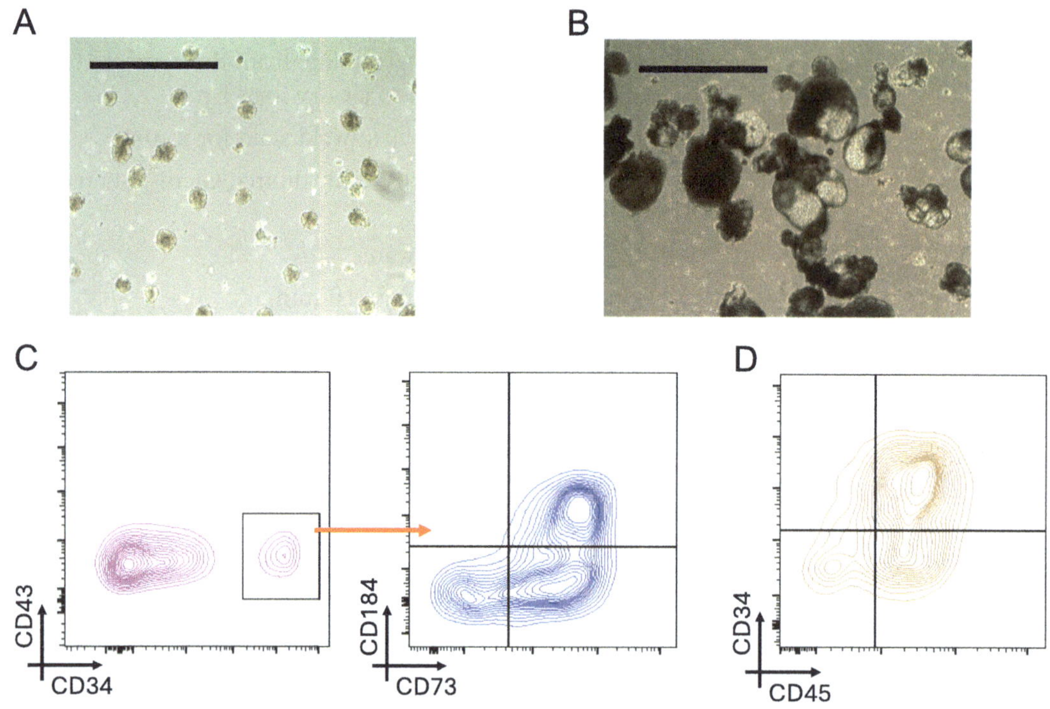

Fig. 3 Representative outcomes of the definitive differentiation protocol. (**a**) EB appearance at Day 0 and (**b**) Day 9, scale bar = 1 mm. (**c**) Flow cytometric analysis at Day 9, CD73 (venous marker) and CD184 (arterial) are detected in the CD34 + CD43- population. (**d**) Flow cytometric analysis for CD43 and CD45 of harvested Day 9 + 8 progenitors

7. Evenly distribute 2 mL of aggregates into each well of a new 6-well ultra-low attachment plate.
8. Incubate for 20 to 24 h under static conditions at 37 °C in a 5% CO_2, 5% O_2 incubator.

3.3.3 Day 1: Feeding Aggregates and Expansion

1. Add 2 mL of AGGREGATION MEDIUM supplemented with 10 ng/mL bFGF to each well. The final concentration of bFGF should be 5 ng/mL.

3.3.4 Day 1.75: Induction

1. Make INDUCTION 1 MEDIUM, 2 mL per well of EBs.
2. Separate the aggregates from the debris by harvesting a maximum of 2 plates into one 50 mL tube and centrifuge at 250 × g for 5 min.
3. After centrifugation, aspirate the supernatant and add INDUCTION 1 MEDIUM. Add aggregates into the same 6-well ultra-low attachment plate at 2 mL per well. Distribute the aggregates evenly.
4. Incubate as above until Day 4 (*see* **Note 10**).

3.3.5 Days 4–8: Induction 2: Specification of Hemogenic Endothelium-Like Cells

1. Transfer EBs from 2 plates into one 50 mL tube.
2. Centrifuge at 150 × g for 5 min. Carefully aspirate the media and add 10 mL of SP34 (without cytokines).
3. Centrifuge and aspirate again. The second wash removes old media and debris.
4. Resuspend the EBs in INDUCTION 2 MEDIA at 2 mL/well and plate into new 6-well ultra-low attachment plates. This medium contains VEGF and FGF at low concentrations necessary for expanding the earliest blood precursors. Incubate at 37 °C in a 5% CO_2, 5% O_2 incubator. The VEGF should promote the growth of "lobules" on the EBs.
5. Feed the cultures on Day 6.5 with the addition of 2 mL of INDUCTION 3 MEDIA.
6. Place cells on the shaker (80 rpm) in a 5% CO_2, 5% O_2 incubator through Day 9.

3.3.6 Day 9: Sterile Sort for Endothelial/Hemogenic Endothelial-like Cells

We recommend starting preparing for the sort early in the morning. The sorter should have a 100 μm nozzle. EBs should have large, transparent lobules (Fig. 3b).

1. Pre-warm trypsin-EDTA and collagenase in the water bath.
2. Harvest cells in 50 mL conical tubes (2 plates/tube), ***keep conditioned media*** (and filter 0.2 μm, put on ice).
3. Centrifuge EBs at 200 × g for 5 min.
4. Aspirate supernatant, add 5 mL Trypsin-EDTA, and incubate at 37 °C for 5 min.
5. Add 5 mL STOP medium: IMDM +50% FBS + 30 μL/mL DNase I.
6. Centrifuge at 250 g for 5 min.
7. Resuspend in 5 mL collagenase +20 μL/mL DNase I.
8. Incubate at 37 °C for 45 min—1 h, mixing every 20–30 min (*see* **Note 11**).
9. Pass through a 20-gauge needle 4–6×, until aggregates are fully dissociated.
10. Add 25 mL IMDM wash (IMDM +5% FBS + 1× P/S).
11. Remove 0.5 mL of cells for cell count and single stains for flow cytometry.
12. Centrifuge at 300 × g for 5 min.
13. Stain with flow cytometry antibodies on ice for 30 min. Prepare unstained and single-stained controls to set sorting gates and compensation (CD34-PeCy7, CD43-FITC).
14. Wash stained cells and control samples with 2 mL of conditioned media.

15. Resuspend cells in 1 mL of media (0.3 mL for controls) and filter through a 70 μm nylon mesh.
16. Prepare collection tubes using cold, filtered, conditioned media.
17. Sort the $CD34^{high+}CD43^{-}$ cells into conditioned media (Fig. 3c).
18. Check post-sort purity for $CD34^{+}$ cells (*see* **Note 12**).
19. Centrifuge sorted cells at 300 × g for 5 min.
20. Resuspend cells in REAGGREGATION MEDIA at a concentration of 240,000 cells/mL.
21. Distribute 50 μL of cell suspension (12,000 cells) in each well of a 96-well U-bottom plate.
22. Incubate overnight at 37 °C in 5% CO_2, 5% O_2.

3.3.7 Day 9 + 1: Generation of Blood Progenitors

1. In the morning, feed with the addition of 100 μL of REAGGREGATION MEDIA.
2. At days 4 to 5 post-sort, progenitors should be budding in the wells. Feed with the addition of 100 μL of maintenance media.

3.3.8 Day 9 + 8–11: Harvest of Hematopoietic Progenitor Cells

1. Harvest HPCs on day 8 post-sort by gently pipetting media up and down.
2. Centrifuge harvested cells at 300 × g for 5 min; while cells are in the centrifuge, feed each well of the plate with 50 μL of maintenance media.
3. After centrifugation, keep the conditioned media and add 150 μL to each well of the plate
4. Incubate at 37 °C in 5% CO_2, 5% O_2.
5. Harvested HPCs can be subsequently cultured in erythroid differentiation media or cryopreserved. HPCs should be $CD34^{+}CD45^{+}$ at this stage (Fig. 3d). Colony-forming assays can also be performed with harvested HPCs.
6. HPC harvest can be repeated at day 11 post-sort (*see* **Note 13**).

3.4 Generation of Definitive iPSC-Derived Red Blood Cells

3.4.1 Day 0

1. Plate definitive HPCs in M1 erythroid media at 50,000 cells/mL:
   50,000 cells/1 mL in M1 + cytokines, in 12-well plate.
   100,000 cells/2 mL in M1 + cytokines, in 6-well plate.
   250,000 cells/5 mL in M1 + cytokines, in T25 flasks (*see* **Note 14**).

3.4.2 Day 2

1. Add 3 volumes of fresh media, transfer to a larger flask if needed (*see* **Note 15**).

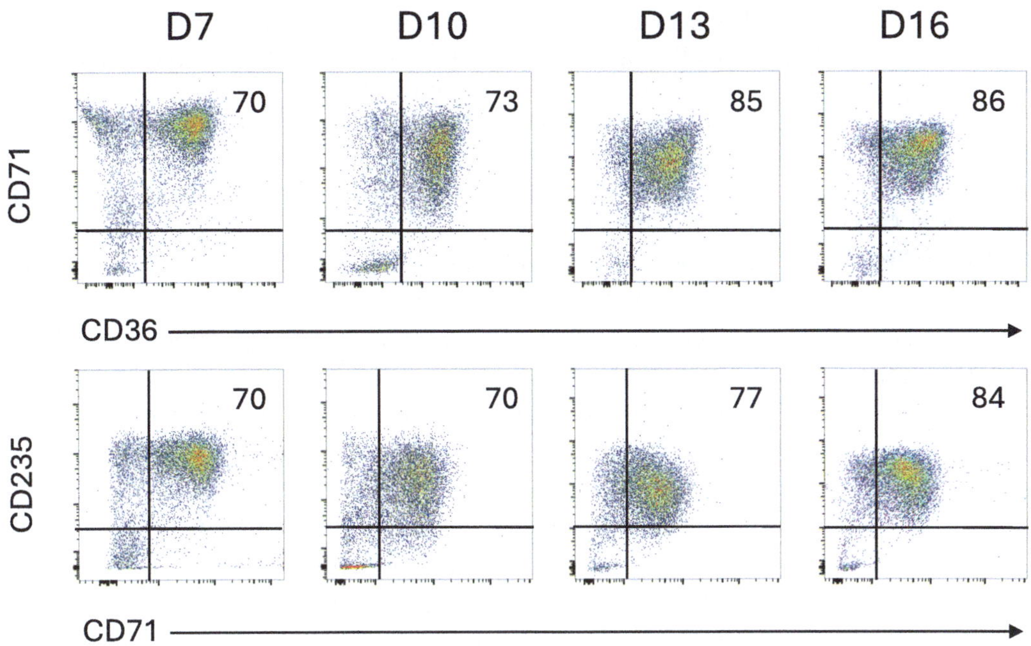

Fig. 4 Maturation kinetics of definitive RBCs. Representative flow cytometry of CD36, CD71, and CD235a expression of definitive erythroblasts during erythroid differentiation on Days 7, 10, 13, and 16

3.4.3 Day 6

1. Count cells, centrifuge at 330 × g for 5 min, and change media to M2. Resuspend cells at 300,000/mL and place them in a new flask. Do not collect attached cells.
2. Check erythroid marker expression (CD71, CD36, CD235ab) by flow cytometry. See Fig. 4 for the kinetics of marker expression.

3.4.4 Day 9

1. Count cells, centrifuge at 330 × g for 5 min, and change at least half of the media to M3. Resuspend cells at 500,000/mL.
2. Check erythroid marker expression (CD71, CD36, CD235ab) by flow cytometry (Fig. 4).

3.4.5 Day 12

1. Count cells, centrifuge at 330 × g for 5 min, and change at least half of the media to M3. Resuspend cells at 500,000/mL.
2. Check erythroid marker expression (CD71, CD36, CD235ab) by flow cytometry (Fig. 4).

3.4.6 Day 15–18

1. Count cells, spin and change half of media to M3. Resuspend cells at 500,000/mL.

   Epo can be removed at this point, and cells can be kept at higher concentrations.

   Increasing plasma to 10% helps with cell survival and maturation.

2. Check erythroid marker expression (CD71, CD36, CD235ab) by flow cytometry and perform cytospin (*see* 3.2.6.3) to determine the stage of maturation (Fig. 4). Day 15 definitive RBCs are generally used in the gel card assay (*see* **Note 16**).

3.5 Gel Card Agglutination Assays with iPSC-Derived Red Blood Cells

3.5.1 Part 1: Testing Compatibility of Mature RBCs with Gel Cards

1. Collect 1~1.5 million mature RBCs by centrifugation at 330 g for 5 min (*see* **Note 17**).
2. Aspirate media and resuspend cells in 1 mL PBS. Transfer cells to a 1.6 mL Eppendorf tube.
3. Centrifuge RBCs at 7600 g for 3 min using a benchtop centrifuge.
4. Carefully aspirate off PBS along with contaminating non-RBCs (if present, these cells will sit on top of the RBC pellet).
5. Resuspend the RBC pellet in 50 μL MTS2 diluent by gently pipetting up and down using a p200 pipette, avoiding bubbles.
6. Pipette resuspended RBCs into the well of the gel column, carefully not to disturb the gel column.
7. Centrifuge gel card on the MTS workstation at 1032 rpm for 10 min.
8. Visually confirm that all RBCs have been spun down to the bottom of the gel column prior to using these RBCs for antigen typing or alloantibody detection (Figs. 5a and 6a).

3.5.2 Part 2: Typing Primitive and Definitive RBCs for RBC Antigen Expression

1. Determine the total number of antigen typings to be performed.
2. Collect 1~1.5 million mature RBCs per antigen typing by centrifugation at 1200 rpm for 5 min.
3. Aspirate media and resuspend cells in 1 mL PBS. Transfer cells to a 1.6 mL Eppendorf tube.
4. Centrifuge RBCs at 9000 rpm for 3 min using a benchtop centrifuge.
5. Carefully aspirate off PBS along with contaminating non-RBCs using a vacuum aspirator without disturbing the RBC pellet (if present, these cells will sit on top of the RBC pellet).
6. Resuspend the RBC pellet in MTS2 diluent so that 50 μL can be used per gel column, avoiding bubbles.
7. Aliquot 50 μL of resuspended RBCs into 1.6 mL Eppendorf tubes, one per gel column.
8. Add 25 μL of typing antibodies onto RBCs and gently pipette up and down to mix.
9. Immediately add the RBC + antibody mixture into the well of the gel column, being careful not to disturb the gel column (*see* **Note 18**).

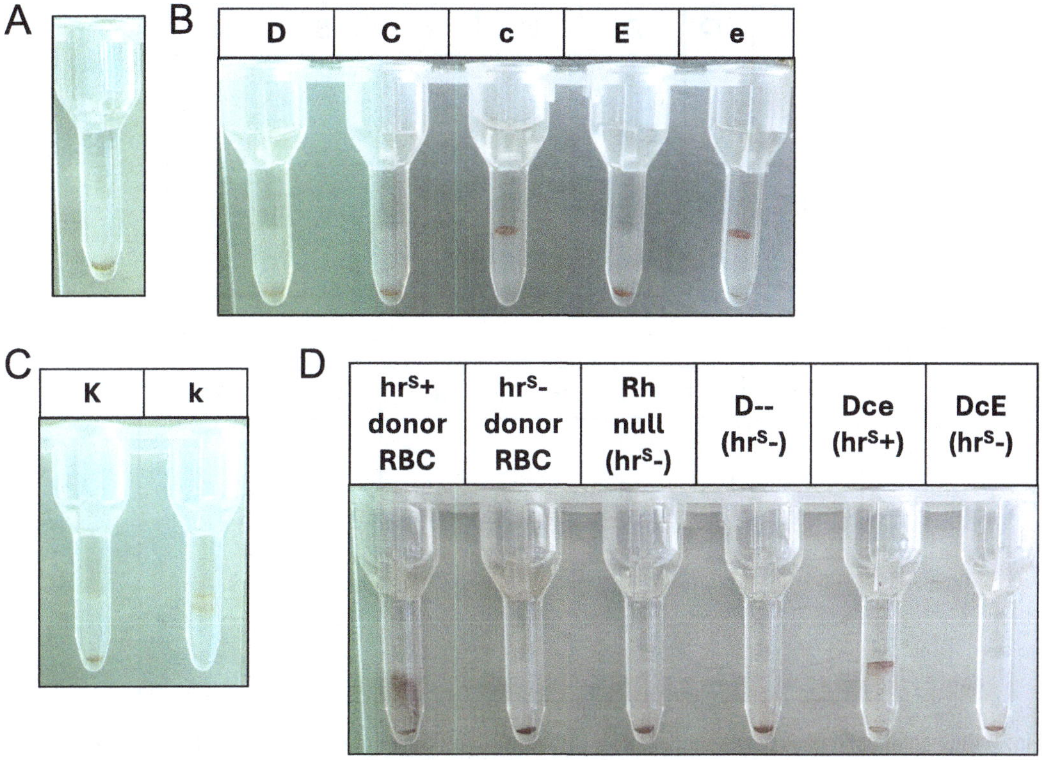

Fig. 5 Gel agglutination assays using primitive RBCs. (**a**) Centrifugation of primitive RBCs on a buffered gel card suggests RBCs are compatible with gel card assay. (**b**) Rh typing using IgM typing antibodies on primitive RBCs that are known to be D-C-c+E-e+ (**c**) Antigen typing for Kell using IgG typing antibodies on K-k + primitive RBCs. (**d**) Antibody identification using ficin-treated primitive RBCs with plasma containing anti-hr^S. Donor RBCs that are hr^S+ and hr^S- are used as positive and negative controls

10. Incubate buffered gel cards and anti-IgG gel cards at 4 °C and 37 °C, respectively, for 30 min to allow RBCs to agglutinate.
11. Centrifuge gel cards on the MTS workstation for 10 min.
12. Visually confirm typing patterns. RBCs positive for each antigen will agglutinate, preventing cells from passing through the gel column. RBCs negative for each antigen will have been spun down to the bottom of the gel column (Figs. 5b, c and 6b, c) (*see* **Note 19**).

3.5.3 Part 3: Using Primitive and Definitive RBCs for Alloantibody Detection in Donor Plasma

1. Determine the total number of gel columns used for alloantibody detection.
2. Collect 1~1.5 million mature RBCs per gel column by centrifugation at 330 g for 5 min.
3. Aspirate off media and resuspend cells in 1 mL PBS. Move cells to a 1.6 mL Eppendorf tube.
4. Centrifuge RBCs at 7600 g for 3 min using a benchtop centrifuge.

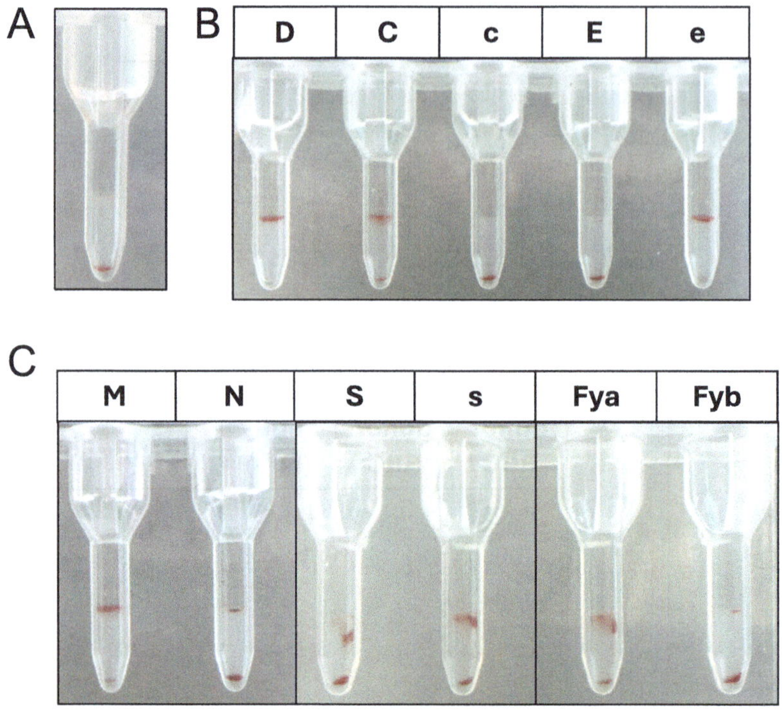

Fig. 6 Gel agglutination assays using definitive RBCs. (**a**) Centrifugation of definitive RBCs on a buffered gel card suggests RBCs are compatible with the gel card assay. (**b**) Rh typing using IgM typing antibodies on definitive RBCs that are known to be D+C+c-E-e+ (**c**) Antigen typing for MNS and Duffy using IgM (M, N) and IgG (S, s, Fya, Fyb) typing antibodies on definitive RBCs with a known phenotype of M+N-S+s+Fya+Fyb-

5. Carefully aspirate off PBS along with contaminating non-RBCs (if present, these cells will sit on top of the RBC pellet) using a vacuum aspirator without disturbing the RBC pellet.
6. If desired, treat RBCs with 0.1% ficin to increase reactivity against Rh antibodies. For ficin treatment, resuspend the RBC pellet in 200 μL PBS.
7. Prepare 200 μL 0.1% ficin solution by diluting 1% ficin with PBS.
8. Add 200 μL 0.1% ficin solution onto RBCs and incubate at 37 °C for 10 min.
9. Wash 3× with 1 mL PBS.
10. Centrifuge ficin-treated RBCs at 7600 g for 3 min using a benchtop centrifuge (*see* **Note 20**).
11. Resuspend the RBC pellet in MTS2 diluent so that 50 μL can be used per gel column, avoiding bubbles.
12. Aliquot 50 μL of resuspended RBCs into 1.6 mL Eppendorf tubes, one per gel column.

13. Add 25 μL of donor plasma onto RBCs and gently pipette up and down to mix.
14. Immediately add the RBC + plasma mixture into the well of the anti-IgG gel column, being careful not to disturb the gel column.
15. Incubate anti-IgG gel cards at 37 °C for 30 min to allow RBCs to agglutinate.
16. Centrifuge gel cards on the MTS workstation at 1032 rpm for 10 min.
17. Visually confirm agglutination patterns. If donor plasma contains antibodies against expressed antigens, RBCs will agglutinate, preventing cells from passing through the gel column (Fig. 5d).

4 Notes

1. Prior to starting EB differentiation, cells should be at least ~75% confluent and maintain distinct colonies. If cells are not ready the next day, continue to culture normally until 75% confluent.
2. If less than 500,000 HPCs are collected for erythroid differentiation, seed cells into a T25 flask with a minimum required volume of 4 mL. In our experience, culturing HPCs in a surface volume smaller than a T25 hinders cell expansion.
3. *Do* not pipette up and down vigorously. Primitive erythroid differentiation often generates adherent macrophage-like cells, which are most prevalent on Day 3 of differentiation. Gentle resuspension maximizes the number of erythroid progenitor cells transferred to the new flask, while minimizing the number of macrophage progenitor cells.
4. Transfer of cells to new flasks every 3 days of erythroid culture allows for removal of non-erythroid cells and is required for Days 3 and 6 of erythroid differentiation. By Day 9, adherent cells should be minimal, and cells may not need to be transferred to new flasks.
5. Adding SCF and Epo for the *adjusted total volume* is required for efficient primitive RBC maturation, as is retention of conditioned media.
6. Robust differentiation of HPCs should yield >1 million cells/mL on Day 3 of culture, but if this confluency is not reached, it is recommended to add 1 mL complete media on top and supplement SCF and Epo for the total volume.
7. Both Day 12 and 13 primitive RBCs can be used for gel card assays. If RBCs are kept in culture until Day 13, adjust the cell

concentration to 1 million cells/mL by adding complete differentiation media without cytokines, and add Epo only for the total culture volume.

8. If the cytospin shows a majority of orthochromatic erythroblasts, it is recommended to use these RBCs for gel card assays. Vacuoles can be present but should be minimal.
9. Prior to starting EB differentiation, cells should be at least ~90% confluent and maintain distinct colonies.
10. Some ESC lines (H1) show higher $CD34^{+}$ yields at Day 9 if the media change to INDUCTION MEDIA2 is performed at Day 3.75 instead of Day 4.
11. Aggregates should still be visible at the end of the collagenase treatment.
12. Only $CD34^{high+}$ $CD43^{-}$ cells are sorted, but expression of endothelial markers CD73 and CD184 within the sorted population can be assessed for quality control of the differentiation (Fig. 3c).
13. If more than 25% of the harvested cells are $CD34^{-}CD45^{+}$, we recommend sorting or magnetic enrichment of $CD34^{+}$ cells.
14. If starting with frozen HPCs, *see* Subheading 3.2.1.
15. *Do not* pipette up and down vigorously. Primitive erythroid differentiation often generates adherent macrophage-like cells, which are most prevalent at the beginning of differentiation. Gentle resuspension maximizes the number of erythroid progenitor cells transferred to the new flask, while minimizing non-erythroid contaminants. By Day 9, adherent cells should be minimal, and cells may not need to be transferred to new flasks.
16. Presence of >10% non-erythroid $CD45^{+}$ cells might affect the performance of RBC in gel card assays. These cells can be removed by magnetic cell depletion.
17. If using definitive RBCs, use 1.5~2 million cells per condition.
18. IgM antibodies (anti-D, anti-C, anti-c, anti-E, anti-e, anti-M, and anti-N) should be used with buffered gel cards, and IgG antibodies (anti-K, anti-k, anti-S, anti-s, anti-Fya, and anti-Fyb) should be used with anti-IgG gel cards. There may be some exceptions depending on the gel card manufacturer or reagent manufacturer.
19. iPSC-derived primitive RBCs do not express Fya, Fyb, Jka, and Jkb, and have weak M, N, S, and s expression that types weakly positive or false negative despite positive antigen genotypes. iPSC-derived definitive RBCs do not express Jka and Jkb.
20. Ficin treatment will cleave MNS and Duffy antigens. If antibodies against these antigens are anticipated, do not treat RBCs with ficin.

Conflicts of Interest

This study was funded by NHLBI HL147879-01 and NHLBI HL169401. Stella Chou has received speaker and consultant honoraria from the American Society of Hematology and Pfizer, Inc.

References

1. Chou ST, Jackson T, Vege S, Smith-Whitley K, Friedman DF, Westhoff CM (2013) High prevalence of red blood cell alloimmunization in sickle cell disease despite transfusion from Rh-matched minority donors. Blood 122(6): 1062–1071. https://doi.org/10.1182/blood-2013-03-490623. Epub 20130530. PubMed PMID: 23723452
2. Linder GE, Chou ST (2021) Red cell transfusion and alloimmunization in sickle cell disease. Haematologica 106(7):1805–1815. https://doi.org/10.3324/haematol.2020.270546. Epub 20210701. PubMed PMID: 33792218; PMCID: PMC8252926
3. Lal A (2020) Challenges in chronic transfusion for patients with thalassemia. Hematology Am Soc Hematol Educ Program 2020(1):160–166. https://doi.org/10.1182/hematology.2020000102. PubMed PMID: 33275743; PMCID: PMC7727587
4. Pavani G, Klein JG, Nations CC, Sussman JH, Tan K, An HH, Abdulmalik O, Thom CS, Gearhart PA, Willett CM, Maguire JA, Chou ST, French DL, Gadue P (2024) Modeling primitive and definitive erythropoiesis with induced pluripotent stem cells. Blood Adv 8(6):1449–1463. https://doi.org/10.1182/bloodadvances.2023011708. PubMed PMID: 38290102; PMCID: PMC10955655
5. Pandey P, Zhang N, Curtis BR, Newman PJ, Denomme GA (2021) Generation of 'designer erythroblasts' lacking one or more blood group systems from CRISPR/Cas9 gene-edited human-induced pluripotent stem cells. J Cell Mol Med 25(19):9340–9349. https://doi.org/10.1111/jcmm.16872. Epub 20210921. PubMed PMID: 34547166; PMCID: PMC8500969
6. An HH, Gagne AL, Maguire JA, Pavani G, Abdulmalik O, Gadue P, French DL, Westhoff CM, Chou ST (2022) The use of pluripotent stem cells to generate diagnostic tools for transfusion medicine. Blood 140(15):1723–1734. https://doi.org/10.1182/blood.2022015883. PubMed PMID: 35977098; PMCID: PMC9707399
7. Gunawardena N, Chou ST (2024) Generation of red blood cells from induced pluripotent stem cells. Curr Opin Hematol 31(3):115–121. https://doi.org/10.1097/MOH.0000000000000810. Epub 20240213. PubMed PMID: 38362913; PMCID: PMC10959681
8. Ditadi A, Sturgeon CM, Keller G (2017) A view of human haematopoietic development from the Petri dish. Nat Rev Mol Cell Biol 18(1):56–67. https://doi.org/10.1038/nrm.2016.127. Epub 20161123. PubMed PMID: 27876786

Chapter 32

Red Blood Cell Storage and Post-transfusion Recovery

Shwatina Jagnarine, Emmalene Kyritsis, Tiffany A. Thomas, and Krystalyn E. Hudson

Abstract

Red blood cell (RBC) transfusion is essential for treating severe anemia, acute blood loss, and RBC production disorders by restoring oxygen-carrying capacity. Ensuring the safety and efficacy of transfused RBCs involves collection, processing, and storage. Despite optimal conditions, stored RBCs experience the "storage lesion," involving biochemical and morphological changes that affect their quality. Post-transfusion recovery (PTR), indicating the survival and functionality of transfused RBCs, is influenced by the storage lesion and varies among donors due to genetic and environmental factors. Although studies in human volunteers have identified factors correlated with PTR, mouse models can be leveraged to establish causative relationships due to the ability to manipulate and control genetic and environmental variables. Herein, using mouse models, we describe how to assess PTR from transfused stored RBC units.

Key words Transfusion, Red blood cell (RBC) storage

1 Introduction

Red blood cell (RBC) transfusion is a critical medical intervention that plays a vital role in treating patients with severe anemia, acute blood loss, and certain medical conditions that impair RBC production. The primary goal of RBC transfusion is to restore adequate oxygen-carrying capacity to tissues, thereby improving patient outcomes and survival rates. Given the life-saving nature of this therapy, the collection, processing, and storage of RBCs are of paramount importance to ensure the safety and efficacy of transfused blood.

RBC collection typically begins with donor recruitment and screening to ensure donor eligibility and the absence of infectious diseases. Once collected, whole blood is processed to separate RBCs from other blood components (e.g., leukocytes), concentrated, and suspended in a preservative solution to extend their shelf life [1–3]. These packed RBC units are stored at refrigerated

Sean R. Stowell and Connie M. Arthur (eds.), *Methods in Transfusion Medicine*, Methods in Molecular Biology, vol. 3053,
https://doi.org/10.1007/978-1-0716-5376-0_32,

temperatures (1–6 °C) to maintain their viability and function [4]. However, even under optimal storage conditions, RBCs undergo biochemical and morphological changes collectively known as the "storage lesion" [5, 6]. This phenomenon includes alterations such as membrane loss, changes in cell shape, depletion of adenosine triphosphate (ATP), and accumulation of metabolic byproducts, all of which can compromise the quality and function of the stored RBCs [7–9].

Post-transfusion quality, particularly post-transfusion recovery (PTR), is a key measure of the efficacy of the transfused RBCs [10]. This refers to the percentage of transfused RBCs that remain in circulation after 24 h, serving as an indicator of their survival and functionality. Various factors, including the severity of the storage lesion, impact this recovery rate. The standard FDA criteria for PTR stipulate that, on average, more than 75% of transfused RBCs should remain in circulation 24 h after transfusion [11]. However, variability in PTR among different human donors is well documented [10]. Genetics, medical conditions, dietary, and/or environmental factors can affect baseline RBC quality, including RBC circulatory lifespan, energy metabolism, and sensitivity to oxidative stress [12–17]; these factors influence the storage capacity of individual donors' cells and collectively dictate the degree of the storage lesion.

Studies in human volunteers have identified factors that correlate with PTR. However, moving from correlative to causative analysis requires the development of robust mouse models, which allow for controlled investigation of RBC storage and PTR [18–20]. The precise manipulation of genetic and environmental variables in mice enables researchers to test specific pathways and factors involved in RBC quality following refrigerated storage. Herein, we describe how to generate a murine RBC unit for storage that can be used to determine PTR, utilizing mouse models to advance our understanding and improve the clinical outcomes of RBC transfusions.

2 Materials

2.1 Red Blood Cell Donor Mice

1. ROSA26-LCB-mCHERRY (mCherry) [18], transgenic mice with mCherry+ RBCs.
2. C57BL/6-Tg (UBC-GFP)30Scha/J (GFP) [21], transgenic mice with GFP+ RBCs.

2.2 Red Blood Cell Collection by Cardiac Puncture

1. Styrofoam block workspace.
2. Bench pad.
3. Push pins.

4. 70% ethanol.
5. Hemostat forceps/clamp.
6. Forceps/Tweezers.
7. Surgical scissors.
8. 1 mL syringe, sterile.
9. CPDA-1 (Citrate, Phosphate, Dextrose, Adenose additive solution, USP; Fresenius Kabi, #4R3611).
10. 25 G × 5/8″ needle (BD Biosciences, #305122).
11. 18 G × 1.5″ needle (Exelint International, #26420).
12. 5 mL Eppendorf tube, sterile (Eppendorf, #0030119487).

2.3 RBC Leukoreduction

1. Sterile 50 mL conical tube (Genesee Scientific, #28-108).
2. Sterile WBC Acrodisc Whole Blood Filtration Device (Pall, #AP-4952).
3. 3 mL sterile luer lock syringe (BD Biosciences, #309657).
4. Tape.
5. 1 mL pipette and filtered tips.
6. 5 mL Eppendorf tubes, sterile (Eppendorf, #0030119487).
7. Centrifuge.

2.4 Blood Bank Generation and Storage

1. 1 mL pipette and filtered tips.
2. 1.5 mL Eppendorf tubes, sterile.
3. Parafilm.
4. Tube rack.
5. 4 °C refrigerator.
6. 75 mm capillary tubes (Fisher Scientific, #22-260950).
7. Capillary tube clay sealant (Fisher Scientific, #02-678).
8. Micro-hematocrit centrifuge (Unico, #UCO-CMH30).
9. Ruler.

2.5 Quantification of RBCs, White Blood Cells, and Platelets by Flow Cytometry

1. 5 mL FACS tubes (Falcon, #352008).
2. Fluorescence activated cell sorting (FACS) buffer: phosphate buffered saline (PBS) supplemented with 0.2 mg/mL bovine serum albumin and 0.9 mg/mL EDTA (ethylenediaminetetraacetic acid).
3. MitoTracker Deep Red (Invitrogen, #M22426); Resuspend MitoTracker in DMSO to prepare a 1 mM stock concentration that can be aliquoted and frozen at −80 °C. Freshly prepare a 1 μM working stock by adding 1 μL into 1 mL of FACS buffer.
4. Vortex.

5. Centrifuge.
6. Anti-mouse CD41a PE-CY7 (Invitrogen, #25-0411-82, Clone eBIoMWReg30).
7. Anti-mouse CD45 BV605 (BD Biosciences, #563053, Clone 30-F11).
8. Anti-mouse Ter119 eF450 (Invitrogen, #48-5921-82, Clone Ter-119).
9. Anti-mouse CD71 FITC (Invitrogen, #11-0711-82, Clone R17217).
10. Dimethyl sulfoxide (DMSO, Sigma-Aldrich, #D2650).
11. CountBright Absolute Counting Beads (ThermoFisher, #C36950).
12. Flow Cytometer and analysis software.

2.6 Transfusion

1. 1 mL pipette and filtered tips.
2. PBS, sterile.
3. 1 mL syringe (BD Biosciences, #306959).
4. 27 ½ G needle (BD Biosciences, #305109).
5. Heat lamp.
6. Mouse restrainer (Braintree Scientific, #TV-150).
7. Gauze.

2.7 Post-transfusion Recovery

1. 96-well deep-well plate (Fisher Scientific, #12566611).
2. ACD (Acid-citrate-dextrose) anticoagulant solution.
3. FACS buffer.
4. 25 G needle (BD Biosciences, #305122).
5. 1 mL pipette and filtered tips.
6. Centrifuge.
7. Flow cytometer and analysis software (FlowJo).

3 Methods

3.1 Red Blood Cell Collection from mCherry Mice by Cardiac Puncture (See Note 1)

1. Prepare surgical workspace by securing a bench pad to a Styrofoam block with push pins.
2. Clean surgical instruments with 70% EtOH and let them dry.
3. Prepare one sterile syringe per mouse: This should be performed in a cell culture hood (i.e., laminar flow hood). Using a 1 mL syringe, draw up 200 μL CPDA-1; attach the 25G needle and, while holding the syringe perpendicular to the ground, tap the syringe with your gloved finger to move the

air bubble to the top. Expel the air and CPDA-1. The dead space of the needle and the syringe will be filled with CPDA-1 (~50 μL).

4. Add CPDA-1 to a 5 mL blood collection tube.
   (a) Calculate the total volume of CPDA-1 required by estimating total RBC collection volume per mouse minus CPDA-1 present in the syringe. The CPDA-1 added should be 14% of the total volume.

   Example: Estimated collection volume of whole blood (650 μL) × 0.14 CPDA-1 − 50 μL CPDA-1 (already present in syringe) = 41 μL CPDA-1 per animal.
5. Anesthetize mouse until unresponsive to the hind toe pinch (*see* **Note 2**).
6. Place the mouse in a supine position on the Styrofoam block workspace.
7. Spray the mouse torso with 70% ethanol.
8. Using forceps and a pair of scissors, lift the skin of the mouse in the center of the abdomen upward, being careful to separate the skin and subcutaneous tissue from the visceral organ. Carefully create a transverse opening in the visceral cavity with scissors (Fig. 1a).
9. Widen the incision by cutting along the central sagittal plane of the mouse abdomen toward the xiphoid process, avoiding abdominal organs and extending along the rib line.
10. Grasp the xiphoid cartilage with forceps and lift to expose the diaphragm (Fig. 1b).
11. Using scissors, cut the diaphragm from left to right being careful to not touch the heart with nonsterile scissors (Fig. 1c).
12. Once the diaphragm is cut, clamp the xiphoid cartilage using the hemostatic forceps and flip backward to expose the heart (Fig. 1d).
13. Use a sterile 18 G needle to gently lift and move the pericardium away from the heart (Fig. 1e).
14. Insert the needle and syringe (primed with CPDA-1) into the right ventricle with the bevel side up (Fig. 1f).
15. Gently pull back on the plunger to initiate blood flow without collapsing the right ventricle, adjusting the needle position by rotating to optimize blood collection.
16. Once blood collection has stalled, remove the needle, and slowly and gently expel the blood into the 5 mL tube with CPDA-1.
17. If more blood was collected than anticipated when calculating the volume of CPDA-1 required, add more CPDA-1 to the blood collection tube so that the final percentage is 14%.

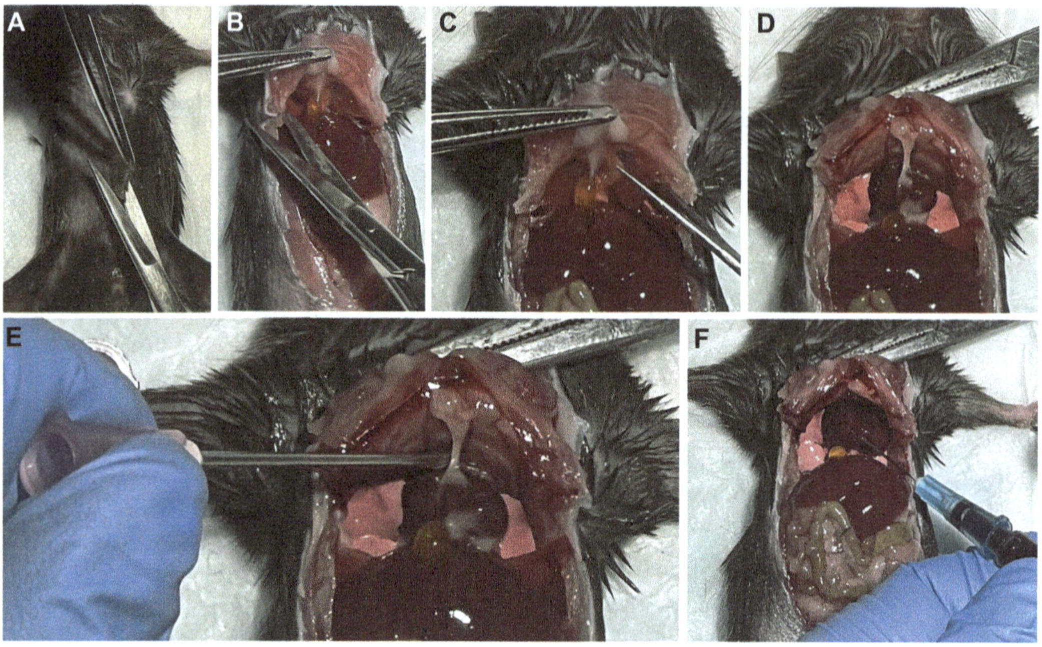

Fig. 1 Red blood cell (RBC) collection by cardiac puncture. Place an anesthetized mouse in dorsal recumbency and (**a**) using forceps and a pair of scissors, lift the abdominal skin and create an opening into the peritoneum. After opening the abdominal cavity up to the xiphoid process. (**b**) Use forceps to grasp the xiphoid cartilage (exposing the diaphragm) and snip the last rib with scissors on both sides. (**c**) While still grasping the xiphoid cartilage, cut the diaphragm around from the prior rib cuts with scissors being careful not to touch the heart then (**d**) clamp the xiphoid cartilage and twist backward to expose the heart. (**e**) Gently lift and move the pericardium away from the heart with a sterile needle. (**f**) Insert the preloaded needle and syringe into the right ventricle, with the bevel side up. Gently pull back on the plunger to initiate blood flow, adjusting the needle position by rotating to optimize blood collection

3.2 RBC Leukoreduction

1. Set aside 6 μL of pre-leukoreduced blood for antibody staining and quantification of cell subsets.
2. In a sterile environment (*see* **Note 3**), remove the lid from a 50 mL conical tube and place a WBC leukoreduction filter on top, securing it in place with tape (Fig. 2a).
3. Attach 3 mL syringe *without* a plunger to the inlet side of the sterile WBC syringe filter.
4. Pipette whole blood in 500 μL aliquots into a 6 mL syringe and allow the blood to filter under gravity (passive flow only). Leukoreduced blood will collect in the 50 mL tube (*see* **Note 4**).

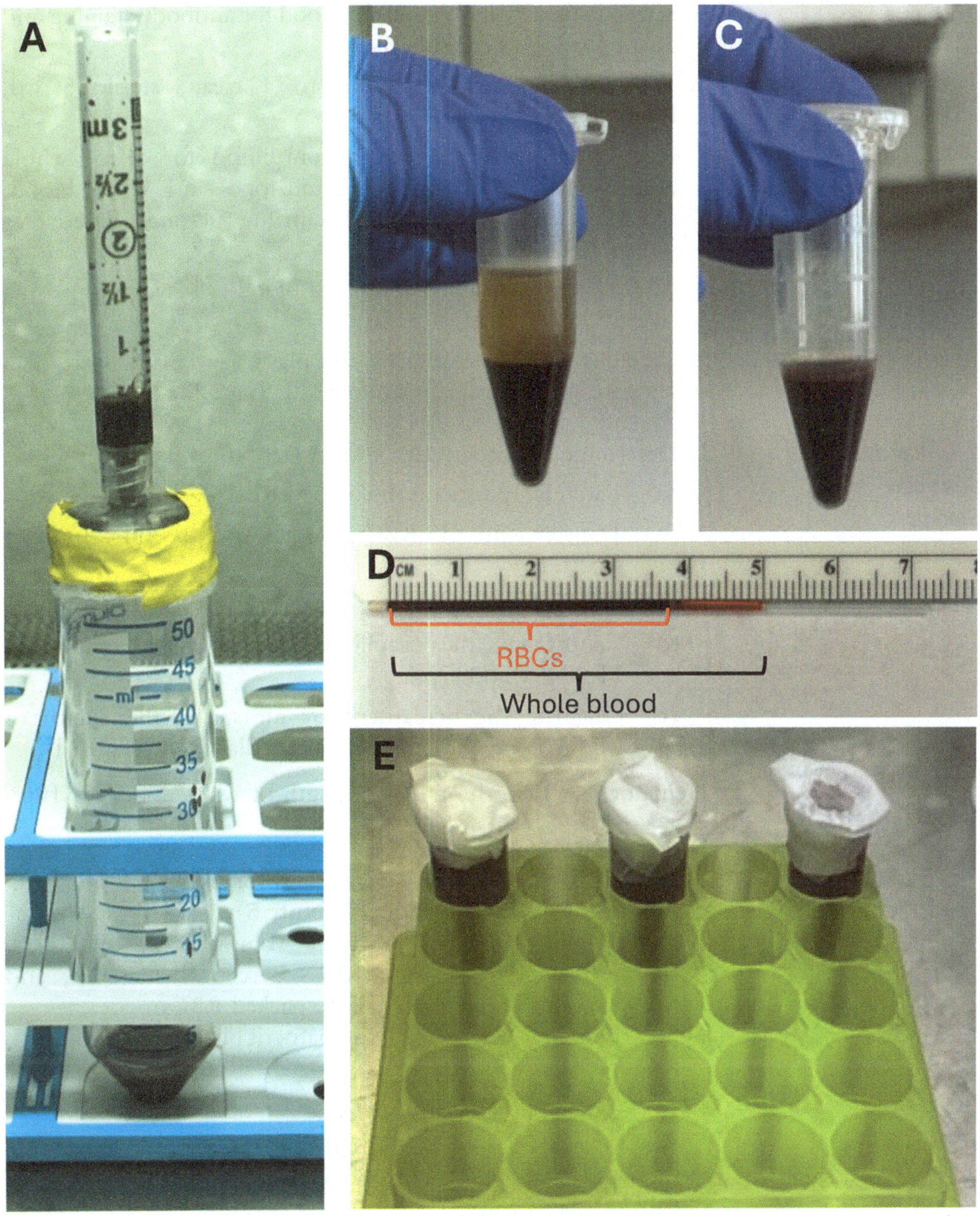

Fig. 2 Generation of leukoreduced RBC blood bank unit. (**a**) A WBC syringe filter is placed atop a sterile 50 mL tube and secured with tape. A sterile syringe (without the plunger) is connected to the top of the filter with a leur lock. Whole blood is gently pipetted into the bottom of the syringe in 500 μL aliquots and allowed to filter, by gravity, into the 50 mL tube. (**b**) Leukoreduced blood is centrifuged to separate plasma and RBCs. (**c**) Plasma is removed from packed RBCs. The RBC volume is determined, and plasma added for a final 60% hematocrit. (**d**) Hematocrit determination with the capillary method, after centrifugation. (**e**) RBC blood bank units, in 1.5 mL tubes, are secured with parafilm, placed in a tube rack, and stored at 4 °C. For this illustration, 3 separate blood banks were generated with storage durations of 1, 6, and 11 days

5. Set aside 6 μL of leukoreduced blood for antibody staining and quantification of cell subsets.
6. Transfer leukoreduced blood to a clean, sterile 5 mL Eppendorf tube.
7. Centrifuge to separate plasma from blood: for <4 mL whole blood, centrifuge at 337 RCF, and for >4 mL whole blood, centrifuge at 427 RCF. Other centrifuge settings: 9 acceleration, 7 brake, 20 °C, 15 min.
8. After centrifugation, a packed red blood cell layer and plasma layer will be evident (Fig. 2b).
9. Carefully pipette to remove the plasma layer and store in a separate sterile 5 mL Eppendorf tube (Fig. 2c).

3.3 Blood Bank Generation and Storage

1. Determine hematocrit by capillary (*see* **Notes 5** and **6**):
   (a) Carefully resuspend the packed RBCs.
   (b) Transfer ~50 μL RBCs into a capillary tube using a pipette.
   (c) Seal both ends of the capillary tube with clay.
   (d) Centrifuge the capillary tube for 5 min at 11,000–12,000 rpm.
   (e) Calculate the hematocrit by measuring the length of whole blood and RBCs in the capillary tube (Fig. 2d).

Hematocrit = (length of RBCs/length of whole blood) × 100

2. Alternatively, using a pipette, determine the volume of packed red blood cells and adjust hematocrit for the final blood bank using the following formula (*see* **Note 5**):

   (b) − (a) = (c), where (a) = volume of packed RBCs, (b) = volume of packed RBCs/percent hematocrit, and (c) = amount of plasma to add to packed RBCs.

   Example: To make a 60% hematocrit blood bank with 2 mL leukoreduced RBCs

   (a) = 2000 μL
   (b) = 2000 μL /0.6 = 3333 μL

   Therefore: 3333 μL − 2000 μL = 1333 μL of plasma to add to packed RBCs
3. Add the calculated plasma back to the packed red blood cells and gently pipette up and down to mix.
4. Transfer the blood to 1.5 mL Eppendorf tubes.
5. Parafilm the lid closed and transfer tubes to 4 °C for storage (Fig. 2e).

3.4 Quantification of RBCs, White Blood Cells, and Platelets by Flow Cytometry

1. Prepare 5 mL FACS tubes with 400 μL FACS buffer for each sample, and necessary controls, to be stained for flow cytometric analysis. Samples:
   (a) One FACS tube containing 2 μL of pre-leukoreduced RBCs (i.e., 1 μL packed RBCs).
   (b) One FACS tube containing 1 μL of post-leukoreduced RBCs.
   (c) FACS tubes of 1 μL of RBCs for control samples (i.e., unstained and fluorescent minus one [FMO] staining controls).
2. MitoTracker staining: Prepare a working solution of 1.25 μL MitoTracker (1 μM working stock) in 100 μL FACS buffer for each sample.
3. Vortex briefly to mix the MitoTracker working solution.
4. Dispense 100 μL per FACS tube, vortex briefly, wrap in foil to protect from light, and incubate at 37 °C for 30 min.
5. Add 4 mL of FACS buffer and centrifuge at 936 RCF for 5 min at 20 °C.
6. Decant supernatant and vortex to resuspend in residual liquid.
7. Antibody surface staining: Prepare an antibody cocktail by adding 100 μL of FACS buffer for every sample to be stained along with the designated antibodies (at the pre-determined dilution):
   (a) CD41 (1:400)
   (b) CD45 (1:400)
   (c) Ter119 (1:100)
   (d) CD71 (1:100)
8. Vortex the antibody cocktail and add 100 μL to each FACS tube and vortex to mix.
9. Incubate for 20 min, protected from light, at room temperature.
10. Add 4 mL of FACS buffer and centrifuge at 936 RCF for 5 min at 20 °C.
11. Decant supernatant and vortex to resuspend in residual liquid.
12. Repeat steps 10–11 for a total of 3 washes.
13. After final wash, decant supernatant, vortex to resuspend in residual liquid and add 1 mL FACS buffer.
14. Vortex CountBright Absolute Counting Beads bottle and add 50 μL to each experimental sample tube.
15. Vortex samples briefly to resuspend.
16. Read samples on a flow cytometer, collecting at least 10,000 events (counting beads alone) or 1000 counting beads when collected in an experimental sample (Fig. 3a).

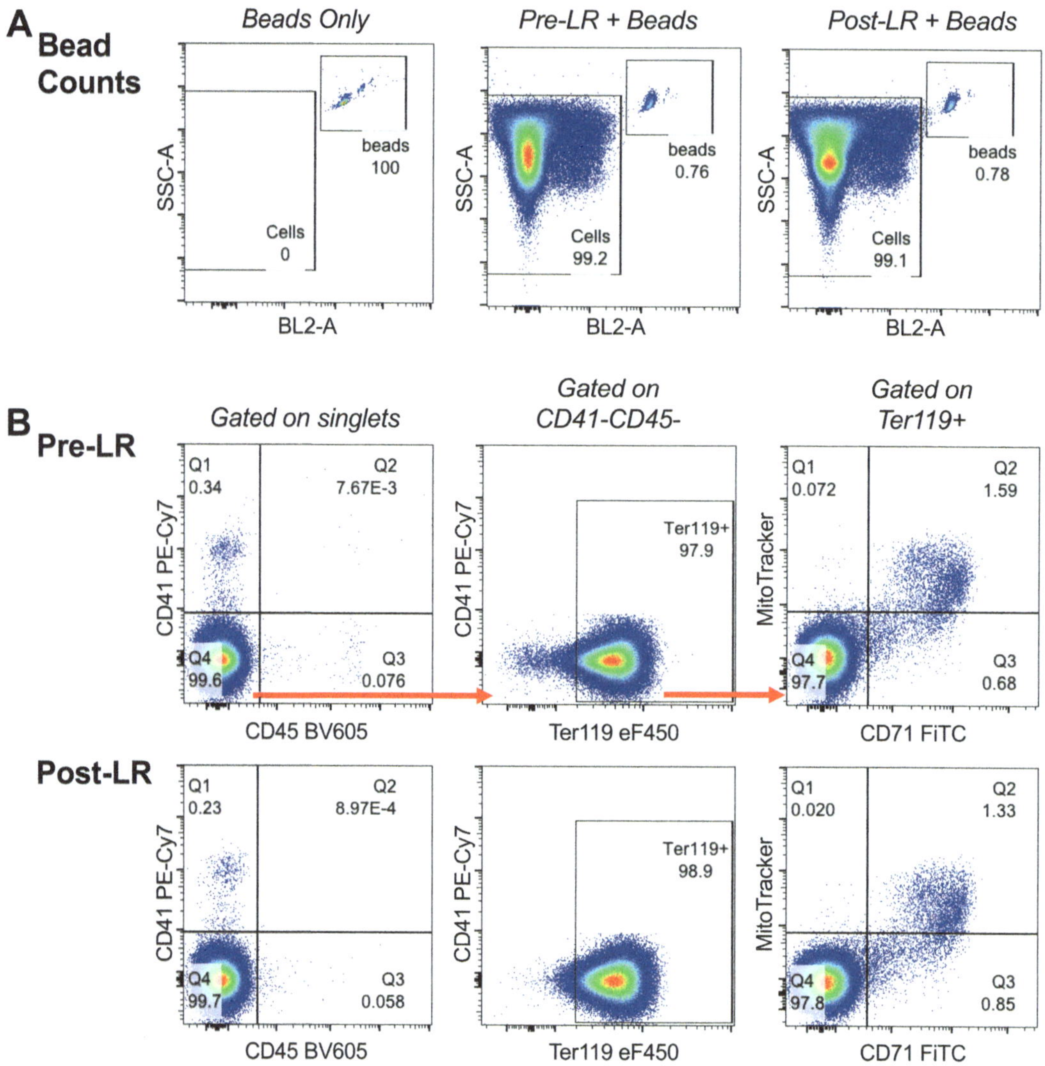

Fig. 3 Quantification of platelets, white blood cells (WBC), and red blood cells (RBC) pre- and post-leukoreduction. CountBright absolute counting beads (50 μL) were added to 1 mL FACS buffer alone or in combination with stained RBCs from pre- and post-leukoreduction samples. (**a**, left) To establish appropriate flow cytometry settings, 10,000 events were collected from bead-only samples, of which 100% fell into the "bead" gate. (**a**, middle and right) In samples containing beads and RBCs, at least 200,000 total events and 1000 beads were collected to determine the cell count, as per the manufacturer's instructions. (**b**) Using the antibody stained RBCs, platelets, WBCs, and RBCs were identified and enumerated in pre- and post-leukoreduced samples. On average, per μL, 100,000 platelets, 10,000 CD45+ WBCs, and 4.7×10^6 RBCs are calculated in pre-leukoreduced samples. Leukoreduction reduces platelets by 30% and WBCs by 35%

17. Using FlowJo (or similar data analysis program), gate on singlets then CD45 v CD41 to visualize white blood cells and platelets, respectively (Fig. 3b).
18. Gating on CD45-CD41- cells, select Ter119+ RBCs and delineate CD71+ reticulocytes from CD71- mature RBCs (*see* **Note 7**).
19. Once WBC, platelets, and RBC subsets are identified, calculate absolute numbers of individual cell populations, per manufacturer's instructions.

3.5 Transfusion

1. To prepare for transfusion, dilute stored blood to 20% hematocrit with sterile PBS.

   Example: For a 3.33 mL leukoreduced RBC unit at 60%, use the formula $C_1V_1 = C_2V_2$ to determine the amount of PBS to add for a final hematocrit of 20%.

   (60% hct)(3333 μL) = (20% hct)(X μL); X = 10,000 μL = final volume

   Additional PBS = 10,000 μL—3333 μL = 6667 μL
2. To control for minor variability in the volume of transfused blood, add 20 μL of freshly-collected RBCs (plasma removed) from GFP+ animals (i.e., "tracer") (as in Subheadings 3.1 and 3.2) for every 167 μL of leukoreduced RBC unit at 60% (i.e., 100 μL packed RBCs) for each blood bank.

   Example: For 3.33 mL leukoreduced RBC unit at 60%, add 400 μL GFP+ RBCs.
3. Mix blood thoroughly by pipetting up and down and save 1 μL to run on the flow cytometer to establish pre-transfusion ratio of mCherry and GFP RBCs.
4. Preload at least one 1 mL syringe with 600 μL of resuspended RBCs, add a 27 ½ G needle, and remove air (as in Subheading 3.1, **step 3**) to ensure no bubbles are infused.
5. For transfusion, heat mice briefly with heat lamp before placing them in a mouse restrainer on their side (*see* **Note 8**).
6. Gently apply pressure with your fingers to the lateral vein at the base of the tail to induce vasodilation.
7. Then, release the pressure, and wrap the tail around the index finger to enable clear visualization of the lateral tail vein.
8. Insert the needle, bevel side up, into the vein and slowly transfuse 500 μL of RBCs.
9. Withdraw the needle and apply gauze to the injection site to stop the bleeding.
10. Transfer the mouse back to housing cage and continue with the next animal.

3.6 Post-transfusion Recovery

1. Prepare a 96 well deep-well plate with 10 μL ACD + 40 μL FACS buffer, one well for each mouse in the experiment.
2. At designated time points, collect 2 μL whole blood by tail prick and add it to one well.
3. Add 800 μL FACS buffer and centrifuge at 936 RCF for 5 min at 20 °C.
4. Decant supernatant, add 1 mL FACS buffer, and pipette up and down to resuspend.
5. Repeat steps 4–5 for a total of 3 washes.
6. After final wash, decant supernatant, add 1 mL FACS buffer, and pipette up and down to resuspend RBCs.
7. Read samples on a flow cytometer, collecting at least 200,000 events to determine the number of mCherry+ and GFP + RBCs.
8. Calculate the post-transfusion recovery by dividing the post-transfusion ratio (Experimental/Tracer) by the pre-transfusion ratio (Experimental/Tracer).

   Example: Data extracted from an RBC blood bank stored 1 day (Fig. 4a)

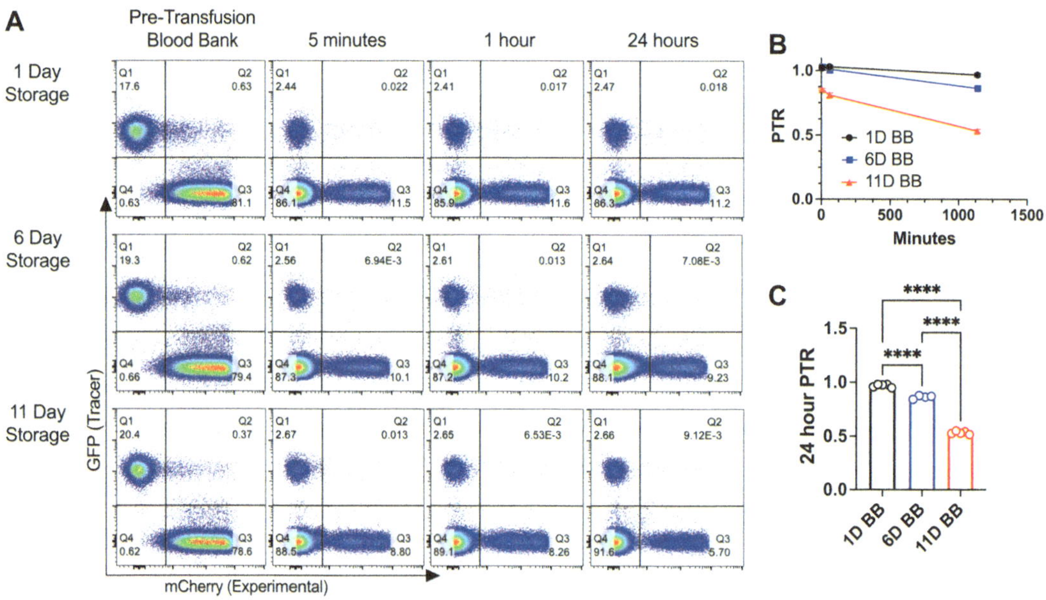

Fig. 4 Post-transfusion recovery of transfused stored RBC blood bank (BB) units. (**a**) Stored (1, 6, or 11 days) mCherry+ RBCs (i.e., experimental) were mixed with freshly collected GFP+ RBCs (i.e., tracer) before transfusion into recipient animals. At designated time points, whole blood from recipients was analyzed for mCherry and GFP RBCs. GFP-mCherry cells are endogenous RBCs (i.e., the recipient mouse's RBCs). (**b**) The post-transfusion recovery of stored mCherry+ RBCs was determined by dividing the post-transfusion ratio of mCherry/GFP by the pre-transfusion ratio of mCherry/GFP. (C) Example showing that longer stored RBCs have lower post-transfusion recovery. Data were analyzed with a one-way ANOVA with multiple comparisons post-test; ****$p < 0.0001$

Time point	# mCherry+ RBCs	# GFP+ RBCs	mCherry/ GFP Ratio	Post-transfusion ratio/pre-transfusion ratio
Pre-transfusion	196,222	42,196	4.65	N/A
5 min	28,593	6026	4.74	1.02
1 h	28,856	6101	4.73	1.02
24 h	26,616	5841	4.56	0.98

9. Post-transfusion recovery can be determined for each time-point and plotted as shown in Fig. 4b, c.

4 Notes

1. RBC identification can be achieved through fluorescence, biotinylation, labeling with lipophilic dyes, or antigen-tracking [18, 21–24].
2. Anesthesia induction and maintenance should be used according to approved institutional animal care and use committee (IACUC) protocol.
3. Leukoreduction and blood unit concentration should be performed sterilely in a cell culture hood. Follow best practices for maintaining sterility throughout this process.
4. WBC leukoreduction filter is validated for 10 mL of whole blood; if more than 10 mL of whole blood requires leukoreduction, split between 2 (or more) filters. On average, the leukoreduction filter retains 0.7 mL of whole blood; account for this potential loss when calculating the number of donors required for the proposed experiment and do not use the plunger to force blood out of the filter.
5. Published literature reports a range of 60–75% hematocrit for blood banks [18, 24]. Individuals should empirically determine which hematocrit is best suited for their studies.
6. Hematocrit determined manually by pipette overestimates hematocrit by ~5–10% depending on the amount of plasma removed.
7. CD71+ reticulocytes can be further subdivided based on presence of mitochondria (i.e., MitoTracker+) [24, 25].
8. RBC transfusion can be performed by tail vein or retro-orbital routes and final transfusate volumes should be adjusted according to the route.

Conflicts of Interest

The authors have no conflicts of interest to declare that are relevant to the content of this chapter.

References

1. Hess JR, Greenwalt TG (2002) Storage of red blood cells: new approaches. Transfus Med Rev 16(4):283–295
2. D'Alessandro A, Culp-Hill R, Reisz JA et al (2019) Heterogeneity of blood processing and storage additives in different centers impacts stored red blood cell metabolism as much as storage time: lessons from REDS-III—omics. Transfusion 59(1):89–100
3. Gamonet C, Desmarets M, Mourey G et al (2020) Processing methods and storage duration impact extracellular vesicle counts in red blood cell units. Blood Adv 4(21):5527–5539
4. Yurkovich JT, Zielinski DC, Yang L et al (2017) Quantitative time-course metabolomics in human red blood cells reveal the temperature dependence of human metabolic networks. J Biol Chem 292(48):19556–19564
5. Yoshida T, Prudent M, D'Alessandro A (2019) Red blood cell storage lesion: causes and potential clinical consequences. Blood Transfus 17(1):27–52
6. Roback JD (2016) Perspectives on the impact of storage duration on blood quality and transfusion outcomes. Vox Sang 111(4):357–364
7. Hess JR (2016) RBC storage lesions. Blood 128(12):1544–1545
8. Pinto RN, Sebastian JA, Parsons MJ et al (2019) Label-free analysis of red blood cell storage lesions using imaging flow cytometry. Cytometry A 95(9):976–984
9. Berezina TL, Zaets SB, Morgan C et al (2002) Influence of storage on red blood cell rheological properties. J Surg Res 102(1):6–12
10. Luten M, Roerdinkholder-Stoelwinder B, Schaap NPM, De Grip WJ, Bos HJ, Bosman GJCGM (2008) Survival of red blood cells after transfusion: a comparison between red cells concentrates of different storage periods. Transfusion 48(7):1478–1485
11. Dumont LJ, AuBuchon JP (2008) Biomedical Excellence for Safer Transfusion C. Evaluation of proposed FDA criteria for the evaluation of radiolabeled red cell recovery trials. Transfusion 48(6):1053–1060
12. Alshalani A, Howell A, Acker JP (2018) Impact of blood manufacturing and donor characteristics on membrane water permeability and in vitro quality parameters during hypothermic storage of red blood cells. Cryobiology 80:30–37
13. Zimring JC (2015) Established and theoretical factors to consider in assessing the red cell storage lesion. Blood 125(14):2185–2190
14. Tzounakas VL, Kriebardis AG, Papassideri IS, Antonelou MH (2016) Donor-variation effect on red blood cell storage lesion: a close relationship emerges. Proteomics – Clin Appl 10(8):791–804
15. Francis RO, D'Alessandro A, Eisenberger A et al (2020) Donor glucose-6-phosphate dehydrogenase deficiency decreases blood quality for transfusion. J Clin Invest 130(5): 2270–2285
16. D'Alessandro A, Fu X, Reisz JA et al (2020) Stored RBC metabolism as a function of caffeine levels. Transfusion 60(6):1197–1211
17. Roubinian NH, Plimier C, Woo JP et al (2019) Effect of donor, component, and recipient characteristics on hemoglobin increments following red blood cell transfusion. Blood 134(13):1003–1013
18. Hay A, Dziewulska K, Gamboni F et al (2023) Hypoxic storage of murine red blood cells improves energy metabolism and post-transfusion recoveries. Blood Transfus 21(1): 50–61
19. Kim CY, Johnson H, Peltier S et al (2022) Deuterated linoleic acid attenuates the RBC storage lesion in a mouse model of poor RBC storage. Front Physiol 13:868578
20. de Karen W, Xiaoyoun F, Larry JD et al (2016) Metabolic pathways that correlate with post-transfusion circulation of stored murine red blood cells. Haematologica 101(5):578–586
21. Schaefer BC, Schaefer ML, Kappler JW, Marrack P, Kedl RM (2001) Observation of antigen-dependent CD8+ T-cell/dendritic cell interactions in vivo. Cell Immunol 214(2):110–122
22. Zimring JC, Cadwell CM, Chadwick TE et al (2007) Nonhemolytic antigen loss from red blood cells requires cooperative binding of multiple antibodies recognizing different epitopes. Blood 110(6):2201–2208

23. Jash A, Usaneerungrueng C, Howie HL et al (2021) Antibodies to low-copy number RBC alloantigen convert a Tolerogenic stimulus to an immunogenic stimulus in mice. Front Immunol 12:629608
24. Thomas TA, Qiu A, Kim CY et al (2023) Reticulocytes in donor blood units enhance red blood cell alloimmunization. Haematologica 108(10):2639–2651
25. Moriconi C, Dzieciatkowska M, Roy M et al (2022) Retention of functional mitochondria in mature red blood cells from patients with sickle cell disease. Br J Haematol 198(3): 574–586

Chapter 33

The Use of Bioengineered Induced Pluripotent Stem Cell-Derived Human Megakaryocytes to Diagnose and Characterize Platelet Allo-, Auto-, and Iso-Immune Disorders

Nanyan Zhang and Peter J. Newman

Abstract

Anti-platelet allo-, auto-, and iso-antibodies, which target platelet surface glycoproteins, play a crucial role in immune-mediated platelet destruction across various clinical scenarios. Whole cell platelet assays—while effective in maintaining the conformation of the offending antigen—are limited in characterizing anti-platelet antibodies due to their lack of specificity. Here, we describe a novel strategy for generating bioengineered HLA class I-negative, "antigen-specific" megakaryocytes (MKs) from induced pluripotent stem cells (iPSCs). These engineered cells can be cryopreserved for later distribution and analysis. Combining bioengineered megakaryocytes with flow cytometry allows for rapid detection and characterization of platelet-specific antibodies present in patient plasma. The enhanced sensitivity and remarkable specificity of this approach hold great promise for diagnosing a variety of immune platelet disorders.

Key words iPSC, Megakaryocyte, Gene editing, Anti-platelet antibody

1 Introduction

Human platelet membrane glycoproteins (GPs) can be immunogenic under certain pathophysiological conditions; the resulting anti-platelet allo-, auto-, or sometimes iso-antibodies often cause increased platelet destruction, leading to thrombocytopenia in patients, and in some cases may impair platelet function.

Human platelet alloantigens (HPAs) are caused by the polymorphisms of platelet membrane glycoproteins. To date, six bi-allelic HPA systems (HPA-1, -2, -3, -4, -5, and -15) as well as 29 single low-frequency antigens have been described on seven platelet glycoproteins, i.e., GPIIb, GPIIIa, GPIbα, GPIbβ, GPIX, GPIa, and CD109 [1]. Almost all the HPAs are caused by single amino acid substitutions encoded by single nucleotide

Sean R. Stowell and Connie M. Arthur (eds.), *Methods in Transfusion Medicine*, Methods in Molecular Biology, vol. 3053, https://doi.org/10.1007/978-1-0716-5376-0_33,

polymorphisms (SNPs) in the corresponding genes. The only exception, HPA-14bw, is caused by an in-frame triplet deletion of a codon in *ITGB3* gene. Anti-platelet *alloantibodies* are induced by exposure to the unmatched HPAs through blood transfusion or during pregnancy. They are responsible for several clinically important alloimmune bleeding disorders, including fetal and neonatal alloimmune thrombocytopenia (FNAIT), post-transfusion purpura (PTP), and multi-platelet transfusion refractoriness (MPTR).

Anti-platelet *autoantibodies* are the antibodies that mistakenly target and attack patients' own platelets in the blood when immune regulation breaks down. Autoantibodies, mainly targeting GPIIb-IIIa, GPIb/IX, GPIa/IIa, and GPV, are the central cause of immune thrombocytopenia (ITP) [2]. Patients with an inherited deficiency of platelet membrane surface GPs, such as Glanzmann's thrombasthenia (GT) and Bernard-Soulier syndrome (BSS) (showing deficiency of GPIIb-IIIa and GPIb/X, respectively), and CD36 (GPIV) negative individuals are capable of developing *isoantibodies* against target proteins during pregnancy or after platelet transfusion.

Serological detection and characterization of platelet-specific antibodies is not only valuable for confirming the clinical diagnosis but may also play a crucial role in guiding treatment decisions and predicting therapeutic responses across various clinical scenarios. Over the past few decades, many creative assays have been developed for detecting platelet-specific antibodies [3]. One such approach involves using intact whole platelets in the platelet immunofluorescence test (PIFT) or similar variants developed by different laboratories [4–7]. These whole-cell assays are simple and sensitive; however, they lack specificity due to the complexity of antigen expression on the platelet surface. In addition to the platelet-specific HPA antigens, platelets also express blood group ABO antigens and HLA class I antigens on the surface. To mitigate interference from anti-A and anti-B antibodies in patient plasma, diagnostic labs often select type O donor platelets. Unfortunately, the presence of anti-HLA class I antibodies—often a result of previous pregnancies or blood transfusions—restricts the widespread use of this method in clinical settings. These anti-HLA antibodies cannot differentiate between anti-platelet-specific antibodies in such cases.

For this reason, antigen capture "GP-specific" assays have gained prominence in clinical diagnostic laboratories worldwide, including the well-known monoclonal antibody immobilization of platelet antigens (MAIPA) [8], modified antigen capture enzyme-linked immunosorbent assay (MACE) [9], and various versions of immunobead assays [10–12]. In this type of assay, the donor platelets are usually first incubated with patient plasma to allow the binding of anti-platelet antibodies and then incubated with a monoclonal antibody targeting a specific platelet GP to allow the capture of GP complex, such as GPIIb-IIIa and GPIb/IX, from the platelet lysate. The formed sandwich immune complexes are attached to a solid phase, either a microtiter plate well or a bead. The patient's GP-specific antibodies are detected with a secondary anti-human IgG and/or IgM. For patients suspected of alloimmune disorders such as FNAIT or PTP, a carefully selected HPA-typed platelet panel helps determine the alloantibody specificity. For anti-platelet auto- and iso-antibody detection, patient antibodies are tested against platelets from several healthy donors, and the presence of the antibody is determined by comparing it with the cut-off value obtained from normal plasma samples. The antigen capture assays show high specificity that circumvents the interference of anti-HLA class I antibodies; however, their sensitivity is relatively low in some clinical contexts. The anti-platelet autoantibodies are only detected in about 50–60% of ITP patients [13]. In a single-center study spanning 12 years and involving over 3000 suspected FNAIT cases, anti-platelet alloantibodies were found in only one-third of cases [14]. The reduced sensitivity of antigen capture assays partly results from the disruption of "labile antigens" during solubilization of platelet glycoproteins with detergent [15, 16]. Additionally, some monoclonal antibodies used to capture the glycoproteins may compete with the binding of patient anti-platelet antibodies, resulting in false negative results.

Recent breakthroughs in CRISPR-mediated genome editing [17] and the in vitro generation of megakaryocytes (MKs) from induced pluripotent stem cells (iPSCs) [18] have opened up exciting possibilities. These innovations allow us to create "antigen-specific" bioengineered MKs that serve as an excellent reagent for testing patient anti-platelet antibodies (Fig. 1) [19–21, 27]. Replacing donor-derived platelets with bioengineered MKs makes the whole-cell assay for anti-platelet antibody detection revive with high sensitivity and extremely high specificity. The flow cytometry-based whole-cell assay provides intact platelet glycoproteins on the surface of real human MKs, which preserves tertiary structure and labile epitopes that sometimes can be disrupted during detergent solubilization. Genetic manipulation to remove the HLA class I antigen from the cell surface ensures the low background binding to human plasma even in the presence of anti-HLA class I antibodies. In this chapter, we demonstrate the genetic conversion of an HPA-1a iPSC founder line to HPA-1b. This strategy can be easily adapted to convert other human platelet antigens (HPAs) and generate allele-specific MKs for detecting anti-platelet alloantibodies. Additionally, we can create GP knockout MKs to determine the specificity of anti-platelet autoantibodies or isoantibodies [27]. In summary, this innovative whole-cell assay system, utilizing bioengineered MKs, holds great promise for diagnosing multiple immune platelet disorders. It combines sensitivity with specificity, paving the way for improved patient care.

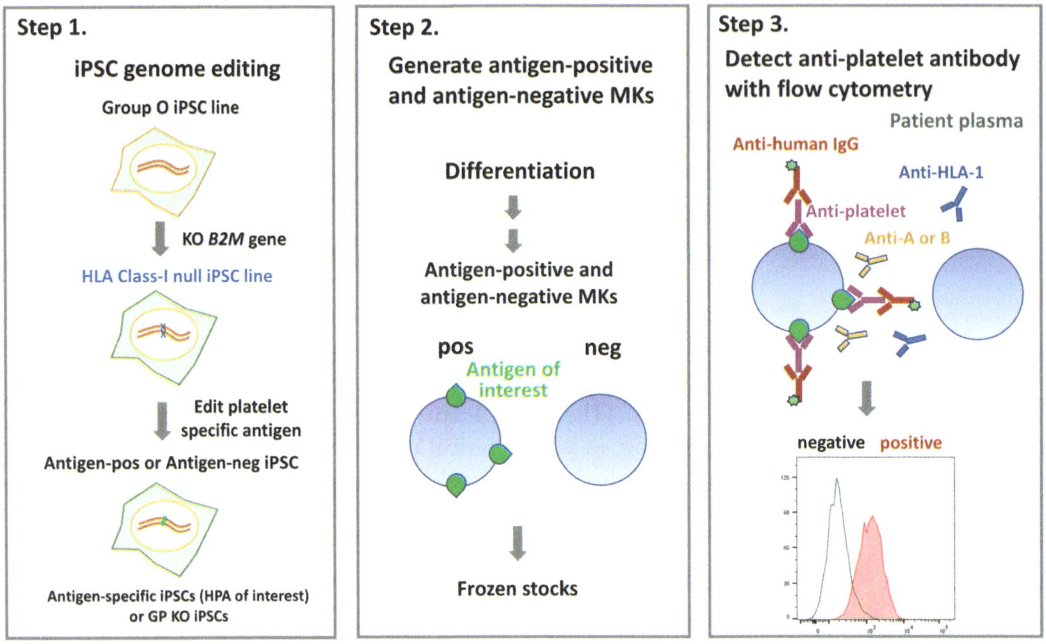

Fig. 1 Schematic overview of generating bioengineered megakaryocytes for whole-cell flowcytometric detection of anti-platelet antibodies from the plasma of patients with immune platelet disorders. iPSC line from a blood group O donor is genetically edited with CRISPR to knockout *B2M* gene. The resulting HLA class I-negative iPSC founder line is further edited, targeting platelet-specific antigens according to different clinical interests. HPA allele-specific cells are used for characterizing anti-platelet alloantibodies. Glycoprotein knockout cells are used for characterizing anti-platelet auto- and iso-antibodies. After differentiation of both antigen-positive and antigen-negative iPSC lines into MKs, the cells can be cryopreserved for later distribution and analysis. The binding of anti-platelet antibodies in patient plasma to antigen-positive MKs can be easily detected using flow cytometry

2 Materials

2.1 Generation of an HLA Class I-Negative iPSC Founder Line

1. PX459 V2.0 plasmid encoding Cas9 (Addgene).
2. Guide oligoes targeting *B2M* gene: Top: 5′- CACCGGAG TAGCGCGAGCACAGCTA -3′, Bottom: 5′- AAAC TAGCTGTGCTCGCGCTACTCC-3′.
3. BbsI (New England Biolabs).
4. Quick ligation kit (New England Biolabs).
5. Endo-free plasmid maxi kit (Qiagen).
6. Blood type O iPSC line (*see* **Note 1**).
7. CO_2 incubator with oxygen control.
8. Tissue culture plates and dishes (24-well, 6-well, 60 mm).
9. DMEM/F12 medium (Thermo Fisher Scientific).

10. Growth factor reduced Matrigel (Corning) diluted with DMEM/F12 medium at 3 mg/mL. Aliquot to 0.5 mL/tube, store aliquoted stocks at −20 °C (*see* **Note 2**).
11. 15 mL Falcon tube.
12. StemFlex Medium (Thermo Fisher Scientific).
13. Phosphate buffered saline (PBS), pH 7.4.
14. ReLeSR (Stemcell Technologies).
15. Amaxa P3 primary cell 4D-Nucleofector kit (Lonza).
16. 4D-Nucleofector X unit (Lonza).
17. ROCK inhibitor Y27632 (StemRD Inc.).
18. Puromycin.
19. Nikon SMZ800N stereo microscope.
20. BD 1 ML tuberculin syringe with 26G needle.
21. 1.5 mL microcentrifuge tubes.
22. Bovine serum albumin (BSA) (Sigma-Aldrich).
23. Fetal bovine serum (FBS) (Thermo Fisher Scientific).
24. Dimethyl sulfoxide (DMSO) (Corning).
25. Fluorescently labeled antibodies: FITC-conjugated anti-human HLA-A, B, C, APC-conjugated anti-human β2-microglobulin (BioLegend).
26. BD FACSCelesta cell analyzer.
27. FlowJo software.

2.2 Conversion of an HPA-1a iPSC Line to HPA-1b

1. General materials for cloning, iPSC culture, and transfection are listed in Subheading 2.1.
2. PX462 V2.0 plasmid encoding Cas9n (D10A nickase mutant) (Addgene).
3. Guide oligoes targeting *ITGB3* gene: Target 1 top: 5′-CACC GTGTCTTACAGGCCCT-GCCTC-3′, Target 1 bottom: 5′-AAACGAGGCAGGGCCTGTAAGACAC -3′, Target 2 top: 5′-CACCGAAGTCCAGCAATCAGAGCTA-3′, Target 2 bottom: 5′-AAACTAGCT-CTGATTGCTGGACTTC-3′.
4. HPA-1b single-stranded oligo-deoxynucleotide (ssODN) repair template: 5′-ACTCGGGCCTCACTCACTGGGAAC TCGATGGATTCTGGGGCACAGTTATCCTTCAGCAGAT TCTCCTTCAGGTCACAGCGAGGTGAGCCGGGTGGCA GGGCCTGTAAGACAGGAGCCCAAAGAGAAGTCCAGC AATCAGAGCTATGCCGACTCTCTACCTCCTGCAGGC CCTACCACTTCC-3′.
5. 1.5 mL microcentrifuge tubes.
6. QuickExtract DNA extraction solution (Epicentre).

7. Nanodrop.
8. Heating block.
9. PCR primers to amplify *ITGB3* fragment: For: 5-′-CGTGGAATTCGGCATCTTACTG-TACAGGCT-3′ and Rev.: 5′-GGCAAGCTTAAGACTTCCTCCTCAGACCT-3′.
10. Herculase II fusion DNA polymerase with dNTPs Combo (Agilent Technologies).
11. Bio-Rad T100 Thermal Cycler.
12. QiaQuick PCR purification kit (Qiagen).
13. Sterile distilled water.
14. NciI with 10× CutSmart buffer (New England Biolabs Inc.).
15. Gel loading dye, purple (6×), no SDS (New England Biolabs Inc.).
16. 100 bp DNA ladder (New England Biolabs Inc.).
17. 2% TBE agarose gel with 0.35 μg/mL ethidium bromide.
18. TBE buffer (Sigma-Aldrich).
19. Agarose gel electrophoresis systems.
20. Gel imaging system with UV.

2.3 Differentiation of iPSCs to MKs

1. General materials for iPSC culture are listed in Subheading 2.1.
2. 100 mm tissue culture dishes.
3. 50 mL Falcon tube.
4. Threefold diluted Matrigel (Growth Factor Reduced, Corning). Mix 10 mL cold Matrigel with 20 mL cold Iscove's Modified Dulbecco's Medium (IMDM, Thermo Fisher Scientific). Aliquot to 1 mL/tube, and store aliquoted stocks at −20 °C.
5. RPMI 1640 medium with HEPES (Thermo Fisher Scientific) supplemented with 2 mM L-glutamine, 50 U/mL penicillin-streptomycin.
6. GSK-3β inhibitor, CHIR99021 (Tocris).
7. StemPro-34 SFM (Thermo Fisher Scientific) supplemented with 2 mM L-glutamine, 50 U/mL penicillin-streptomycin.
8. Serum-free differentiation medium (SFD): a mixture of IMDM (Thermo Fisher Scientific) and Hams F-12 (Corning) at 3:1 ratio with 0.5% N-2 supplement (Thermo Fisher Scientific), 1% B-27 supplement minus vitamin A (Thermo Fisher Scientific), 0.05% BSA, 2 mM L-glutamine, 50 U/mL penicillin-streptomycin.
9. Ascorbic acid (Sigma-Aldrich).
10. 1-Thioglycerol (α-Monothioglycerol, MTG) (Sigma-Aldrich).

11. Growth factors (R&D systems): recombinant human BMP-4 protein, recombinant human VEGF 165 protein, recombinant human FGF basic (146 aa) protein, recombinant human SCF protein, recombinant human Flt-3 ligand/FLT3L protein, and recombinant human thrombopoietin (TPO) protein.
12. XAV939 (Sigma-Aldrich).
13. Corning costar ultra-low attachment 6-well plate.
14. CO_2 incubator.
15. Fluorescently labeled antibodies: Alexa Fluor 488 anti-human/mouse SSEA-3, Alexa Fluor 647 anti-human SSEA-4, PE/Cy7 anti-human CD31, PE anti-human VEGF R2/KDR, FITC anti-human CD41, APC anti-human CD235ab, APC anti-human CD42b (Biolegend).
16. FACSCelesta cell analyzer.
17. FlowJo software.

2.4 Anti-platelet Antibody Testing

1. 15 mL Falcon tube.
2. 1.5 mL microcentrifuge tubes.
3. Iscove's Modified Dulbecco's Medium (IMDM, Thermo Fisher Scientific).
4. Serum-free differentiation medium (SFD) as described in Subheading 2.3.
5. Normal human plasma.
6. Suspected patient plasma.
7. Bovine serum albumin (BSA) (Sigma-Aldrich).
8. Phosphate buffered saline (PBS), pH 7.4, with 1% BSA.
9. PE anti-human IgG (Jackson Immunoresearch).
10. BD FACSCelesta cell analyzer.
11. FlowJo software.

3 Methods

3.1 Generation of an HLA Class I-Negative iPSC Founder Line

1. Insert the annealed oligos targeting the *B2M* gene (Fig. 2a) into the BbsI site of the Cas9 expression plasmids PX459 V2.0 using the Quick ligation kit. For CRISPR design and cloning specifics, refer to the details provided in the reference protocol [17]. Purify PX459 V2.0-B2M plasmid with Endo-Free plasmid maxi kit.
2. Coating tissue culture dishes and plates for iPSC culture. Thaw a vial of 3 mg/mL Matrigel aliquot and dilute with 27 mL of ice-cold DMEM/F12 medium. Add Matrigel solution to tissue culture dishes or plates to cover the entire surface and incubate at 37 °C for 1 h (*see* **Note 2**).

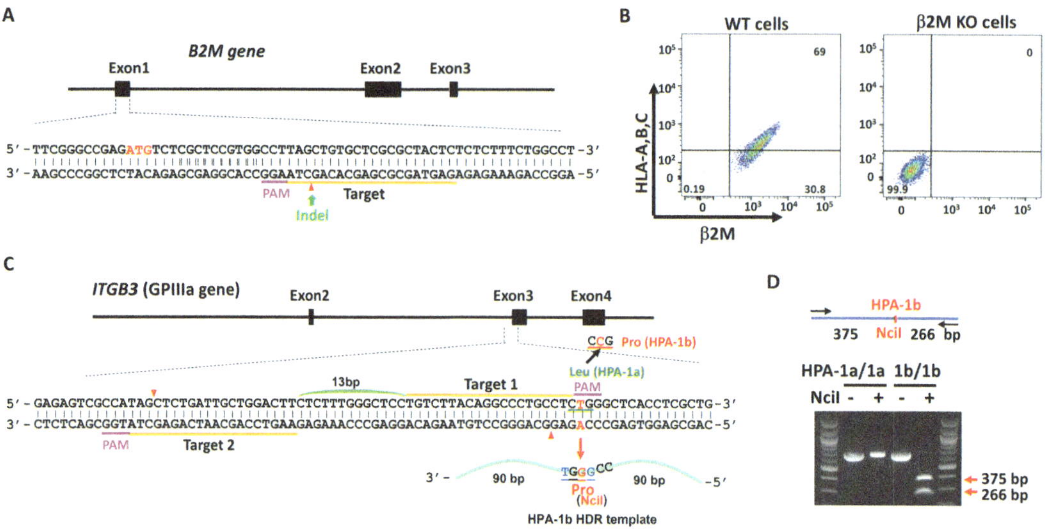

Fig. 2 Genome editing in iPSCs. (**a**) Schematic illustration of the *B2M* locus, showing the location of the gRNA binding site (orange bar) and the protospacer adjacent motifs (PAM) sequence (magenta) necessary to guide Cas9 to its cleavage site (red arrow heads). The ATG start codon for β_2M translation is highlighted in red. The green arrow indicates that an insertion or deletion (Indel) is expected to be introduced into the genome through the non-homologous end joining (NHEJ) DNA repair pathway to cause a frameshift mutation in the *B2M* gene. (**b**) Flow cytometry analysis demonstrating the loss of surface expression of both β_2M and HLA in *B2M* knockout cells. (**c**) Schematic illustration of the *ITGB3* locus, showing the location of the two gRNA binding sites (orange bars) and the PAM sequences (magenta) necessary to guide Cas9n to its cleavage site (red arrow heads). An 181 bp HPA-1b HDR template is designed to introduce the Leu→Pro amino acid polymorphism. The T > C mutation responsible for the HPA-1a/1b polymorphism (highlighted in red) is flanked by 90 nucleotide homology arms and creates an NciI site at the target locus that can be used for genotyping. The HDR template also contains two silent mutations (highlighted in blue) to prevent re-cleavage by Cas9n. (**d**) Genotyping to identify the HPA-1b/1b iPSC clone. Genomic DNA, isolated from iPSCs that had been transfected with px462-Target 1, px462-Target 2, and HPA-1b-ssODN, was PCR amplified and digested with NciI, which differentiates the HPA-1a allelic isoform from HPA-1b. Red arrows indicate the expected fragment sizes of a typical clone that had been converted to HPA-1b. (**a** and **b** are adapted from Ref. [20] **c** and **d** are adapted from Ref. [19] with permission)

3. Thaw a vial of blood type O iPS cells at 37 °C. Transfer the cells to a 15 mL Falcon tube with 2 mL of StemFlex medium and spin at 300 × g for 5 min. Remove supernatant, resuspend cells in 2 mL of StemFlex medium, and plate the cells in Matrigel-coated 60 mm dish.
4. iPSC maintenance. Cells are cultured in Matrigel-coated dishes with StemFlex medium at 37 °C with 4% O_2 and 5% CO_2. Change the culture medium every day or every other day.
5. Passaging cells. Remove culture medium and rinse the cells once with PBS. Add 1 mL of ReLeSR to a 60 mm culture dish and shake gently to allow ReLeSR to cover the entire surface of the culture dish. Remove ReLeSR and keep the culture dish at 37 °C for 6 min. Add 2 mL StemFlex medium

to the dish and shake gently with your hand to detach the cells from the culture dish. Dissociate the cells by pipetting up and down and split the cells at a 1:5 to 1:8 ratio to Matrigel-coated culture dishes. We routinely passage iPSCs twice a week.

6. Preparing cells for transfection. When iPSCs reach 60–80% confluency in culture, pretreat the cells with 10 μM Y27632 in StemFlex medium at 37 °C for 2 h.
7. Wash pretreated iPSCs once with PBS. Treat iPSCs with ReLeSR to detach the cells from culture dishes. Resuspend cells in 2 mL of StemFlex medium gently to get small clumps of 3–5 cells (*see* **Note 3**). Take a small aliquot to break up into single cells for cell counting.
8. Take iPSC suspension containing 5×10^5 cells to a 15 mL Falcon tube, centrifuge at $200 \times g$ for 5 min. Remove supernatant completely.
9. Resuspend the cell pellet in 20 μL of room temperature complete 4D-Nucleofector solution according to the manufacturer's instructions.
10. Resuspend the cells with 1 μg of PX459 V2.0-B2M plasmid.
11. Transfer cell/DNA mixture to NucleoCuvette strips. Start the Nucleofection process using the program CB-150.
12. Add 80 μL of pre-warmed StemFlex medium to the cells, mix gently, and split each transfection into two to four 60 mm Matrigel-coated tissue culture dishes, each containing 2 mL of StemFlex medium with 10 μM Y27632.
13. Prepare a dish of non-transfected cells with a similar cell density as a negative control for puromycin selection.
14. 24-h post-transfection, replace culture medium with fresh StemFlex medium containing 1 μg/mL puromycin.
15. Stop puromycin treatment after 36 to 48 h when the cells in the negative control dish are all killed.
16. Refeed the cells daily with fresh StemFlex medium for 7 to 9 days until distinct colonies become large enough for colony picking.
17. Clonal isolation. Place the culture dish under a stereo microscope to find high-quality cobblestone-like iPSC colonies. Draw a grid of 5 horizontal lines and 5 vertical lines to cut the selected colony into 16 pieces using a 26G needle attached to 1 mL tuberculin syringe. Use a p200 pipette to gently scrape the colony and suck all the detached pieces into the pipette tip. Plate cells directly into a well of a Matrigel-coated 24-well plate containing StemFlex medium with 10 μM Y27632 (*see* **Note 4**).
18. Replace with fresh StemFlex medium on the next day. Feed the cells daily until the cells reach 40–60% confluency.

19. Split the cells with ReLeSR to make replica plates; one contains 70% of cells for clonal genotyping or phenotyping (*see* **Note 5**), and the other contains 30% of cells to keep the clonal line.
20. Feed the cells daily until the cells in the plate for phenotyping reach 50–70% confluency.
21. Detach cells from the plate using ReLeSR. Resuspend the cells with 250 μL StemFlex, collect the cells into 1.5 mL microcentrifuge tubes, and spin at 300 × g for 5 min to remove supernatant.
22. Resuspend cells in 50 μL of PBS with 1% BSA and APC-anti-β 2-microglobulin antibody and FITC-anti-HLA-A,B,C antibody. Incubate at room temperature in the dark for 20 min.
23. Analyze with flow cytometry to identify β2-microglobulin and HLA-A,B,C-negative clones (Fig. 2b).
24. Expand the HLA class I-negative iPSC clones. Freeze down cell aliquots in a freezing solution containing 50% StemFlex medium, 40% FBS, and 10% DMSO. Each >80% confluent 60 mm culture dish can yield 5 frozen vials. Keep cells at −80 °C overnight, then store in liquid nitrogen.

3.2 Conversion of an HPA-1a iPSC Line to HPA-1b

1. Insert the annealed Target 1 and Target 2 oligos targeting the *ITGB3* gene (Fig. 2c) into the BbsI site of the Cas9n expression plasmid PX462 V2.0 (*see* **Note 6**). Purify PX462 V2.0-Target 1 and PX462 V2.0-Target 2 plasmids with Endo-Free plasmid maxi kit.
2. Thaw a vial of HLA Class I-negative iPS cells as described in Subheading 3.1, **step 3**. Maintain cell culture in StemFlex medium.
3. To convert the HPA-1a allele to HPA-1b, an ssODN repair template encoding HPA-1b is co-transfected with CRISPR plasmids (Fig. 2c) (*see* **Note 7**). The DNA mixture containing 0.5 ug of PX462 V2.0-Tartet 1, 0.5ug of PX462 V2.0-Tartet 2, and 40 pmol of the HDR oligonucleotide is transfected into 5×10^5 HLA Class I-negative iPS cells. The transfection, puromycin selection, and clonal isolation procedures are the same as **steps 6–19** in Subheading 3.1.
4. Extract genomic DNA from isolated iPSC clones. When the cells in the 24-well plate for genotyping reach 40–50% confluency, detach the cells with ReLeSR. Resuspend the cells in 200 μL of culture medium and transfer the cells to 1.5 mL microcentrifuge tubes. Spin at 300 × g for 5 min and remove supernatant. Add 40–60 μL of QuickExtract DNA extraction solution to each tube, heat at 65 °C for 6 min, and mix by tapping the tubes gently. Heat at 95 °C for 2 min, mix by tapping. Quick spin to collect evaporated liquid from the cap of the tubes. Measure DNA concentration with a nanodrop.

5. Set up 50 μL PCR reactions using Herculase II Fusion polymerase kit following the manufacturer's protocol to amplify the *ITGB3* gene fragment flanking the HPA-1 site from each clone (Fig. 2d). Each reaction contains 100 ng genomic DNA collected from an isolated clone in **step 4** as template.
6. Run PCR with the following cycling conditions: Initial denature for 3 min at 94 °C, followed by 32 cycles of 30 s denature at 94 °C, 30 s annealing at 59 °C, 30 s extension at 72 °C, with a final extension for 5 min at 72 °C.
7. Purify PCR products with QiaQuick PCR purification kit according to the manufacturer's instructions. Elute the DNA in 35 μL distilled water.
8. HPA-1b conversion introduces an NciI restriction site in the genome, which can be detected by a restriction fragment length polymorphism analysis of the PCR amplicon (Fig. 2d). Set up 20 μL NciI digestion reaction for each clone as follows: 2 μL of 10× CutSmart buffer, 15 μL of purified PCR products in **step** 7, 0.5 μL of NciI, and 2.5 μL of distilled water. Keep the reaction at 37 °C for 1 h.
9. Add 4 μL of gel loading dye to each reaction. Run the digested products on 2% TBE agarose gel.
10. Image the DNA gel under ultraviolet (UV) light to identify the HPA-1b clone (Fig. 2d).
11. Sequence the remaining PCR amplicon in **step 7** from HPA-1b clones using Sanger sequencing to confirm HPA-1b conversion.
12. Expand the HPA-1b iPSC clones. Freeze down cell aliquots as stated in Subheading 3.1, **step 24**.

3.3 Differentiation of iPSCs to MKs

1. Thaw a vial of HPA-1a and HPA-1b iPSCs as described in Subheading 3.1, **step 3**, and maintain cell culture in StemFlex medium. Passage cells to 100 mm tissue culture dishes before splitting cells for differentiation (*see* **Note 8**).
2. Coat 6-well tissue culture plates for iPSC differentiation (*see* **Note 9**). Thaw a tube of threefold diluted Matrigel on ice. Put a prechilled 6-well tissue culture plate on ice, add 1 mL of the diluted Matrigel solution to the first well, and shake the plate gently to allow the Matrigel to cover the surface of the entire well. Transfer the Matrigel from the first well to the second well and repeat the procedure until all the wells on the plate are coated. Remove Matrigel from the last well. Incubate the coated plate in a tissue culture incubator at 37 °C for 20–30 min.
3. When the iPSCs in the 100 mm culture dish reach 70–80% confluency, detach the cells from the culture dish with ReLeSR, resuspend the cells in StemFlex medium gently with a pipette

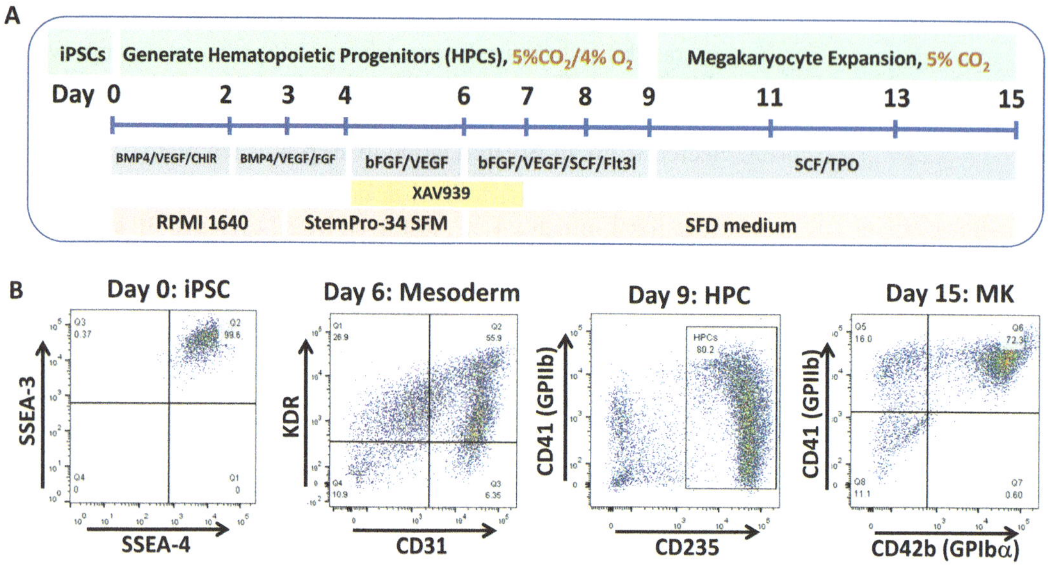

Fig. 3 Ex vivo megakaryocyte production from iPSCs. (**a**) Schematic of the monolayer differentiating protocol for MK generation. (**b**) Flowcytometric analysis to assess cell surface marker expressions at different stages of differentiation. Adherent monolayer cells are analyzed on day 0 and day 6. Non-adherent HPCs emerge from day 7 to day 9; some of them loosely attach to the monolayer adherent cells at the bottom of the culture well. They can be easily separated by gentle pipetting. Only the non-adherent cells in the culture wells are collected and analyzed on day 9. All cells are in suspension from day 9 to day 15

to dissociate cells into small clumps. Split about 2×10^5 cells in 2 mL StemFlex medium into each well of the 6-well plate prepared in **step 2** (*see* **Note 10**).

4. On the next day (Day 0), the cells should reach 40–50% confluency. Sacrifice one well of cells to monitor pluripotency marker SSEA-3 and SSEA-4 expression (Fig. 3a, b) (*see* **Note 11**). High-quality iPSC culture should contain more than 90% SSEA-3 and SSEA-4 double-positive cells.

5. Start differentiation on Day 0 in the afternoon. Rinse iPSCs with 2 mL/well RPMI 1640 medium. Add 4 mL/well RPMI 1640 medium containing 0.4 mM MTG, 50 μg/mL ascorbic acid, 5 ng/mL BMP-4, 50 ng/mL VEGF, and 1 μM CHIR99021 (*see* **Note 12**). Keep the culture at 37 °C with 4% O_2 and 5% CO_2 until HPCs are collected on Day 9.

6. Rinse each well with 2 mL RPMI 1640 medium on Day 2 in the morning. Add 2 mL/well fresh RPMI 1640 medium containing 0.4 mM MTG, 50 μg/mL ascorbic acid, 5 ng/mL BMP-4, 50 ng/mL VEGF, and 20 ng/mL FGF.

7. Rinse each well with 2 mL RPMI 1640 medium on Day 3 in the morning. Add 2 mL/well fresh StemPro-34 SFM containing 0.4 mM MTG, 50 μg/mL ascorbic acid, 5 ng/mL BMP-4, 50 ng/mL VEGF, and 20 ng/mL FGF.

8. Rinse each well with 2 mL PBS on Day 4 in the morning. Add 4 mL/well fresh StemPro-34 SFM containing 0.4 mM MTG, 50 μg/mL ascorbic acid, 15 ng/mL VEGF, 5 ng/mL FGF, and 2 μM XAV939.
9. Rinse each well with 2 mL PBS on Day 6 in the morning. Sacrifice one well of cells to look at mesoderm marker expression (Fig. 3b) (*see* **Note 11**). Add 4 mL/well SFD with 0.4 mM MTG, 50 μg/mL ascorbic acid, 50 ng/mL VEGF, 100 ng/mL FGF, 50 ng/mL SCF, 25 ng/mL FLT3L, and 2 μM XAV939.
10. HPCs emerge on Day 7 in the suspension. Pool culture medium containing HPCs from each well into a 50 mL tube. Add 2 mL HPC medium (SFD with 0.4 mM MTG, 50 μg/mL ascorbic acid, 50 ng/mL VEGF, 100 ng/mL FGF, 50 ng/mL SCF, and 25 ng/mL FLT3L) to each culture well. Spin the pooled culture medium at 300 × g for 5 min, remove supernatant, resuspend the cell pellet in HPC medium (2 mL/well), and add back HPCs to each culture well. Each well contains 4 mL HPC medium in total.
11. More HPCs emerge on Day 8. Repeat Day 7's procedure.
12. Collect HPCs on Day 9. Resuspend the cells in each well by pipetting up and down gently to detach the HPCs that loosely attach to the bottom of the plate. Do not touch the bottom of the plate to disturb or scrape the adherent mesodermal monolayer. Collect all the culture medium with HPCs from each well and combine them into a 50 mL tube. Spin at 300 × g for 5 min, remove 3/4 to 7/8 of supernatant from the top. Resuspend the cells in the remaining medium, count the cells (*see* **Note 13**). Take a small aliquot of cells to stain for HPC surface markers (*see* **Note 11**) (Fig. 3b). A successful differentiation typically yields 0.5×10^6 HPCs/well.
13. Plate $3\text{~}4 \times 10^5$ HPCs/well to Ultra-Low attachment 6-well plate in 4 mL of SFD containing 0.4 mM MTG, 50 μg/mL ascorbic acid, 50 ng/mL SCF, and 50 ng/mL TPO. Move the culture to 37 °C with 5% CO_2 from this step until MKs are produced.
14. Collect all the cells into a 50 mL tube on Day 11, spin at 300 × g for 5 min to remove supernatant. Resuspend cells in 2 mL/well SFD containing 0.4 mM MTG, 50 μg/mL ascorbic acid, 75 ng/mL SCF, and 75 ng/mL TPO, transfer cells back to the original culture plate (2 mL/well).
15. Collect all the cells into a 50 mL tube on Day 13, spin at 300 × g for 5 min to remove supernatant. Resuspend cells in 2 mL/well SFD containing 0.4 mM MTG, 50 μg/mL ascorbic acid, 100 ng/mL SCF, and 100 ng/mL TPO, transfer cells back to the original culture plate (2 mL/well).

16. Count the cells on Day 15. We typically observe 4–8-fold expansion from HPCs. Take a small aliquot of cells to stain for MK surface markers (*see* **Notes 11 and 14**) (Fig. 3b). Freeze down MKs aliquots in freezing solution containing 90% FBS and 10% DMSO. Keep cells at −80 °C overnight, then store in liquid nitrogen.

3.4 Anti-platelet Antibody Testing

1. Thaw a vial of antigen-positive and antigen-negative MKs, e.g., HPA-1a MKs and HPA-1b MKs, at 37 °C. Transfer the cells to a 15 mL Falcon tube with 13 mL IMDM medium. Spin at 300 × g for 5 min to remove supernatant. Resuspend the cells in SFD medium to adjust the cell density to 1×10^6/mL.
2. Aliquot 6×10^5 HPA-1a or HPA-1b MKs into each 1.5 mL microcentrifuge tube (*see* **Note 15**).
3. Spin at 300 × g for 5 min to remove supernatants.
4. Dilute 50 μL of normal human plasma or patient plasma with 50 μL of SFD, split half of the diluted plasma to the tube containing HPA-1a cells, and the remaining half to the HPA-1b cells (*see* **Note 16**). Resuspend the MKs by pipetting gently two to three times.
5. Incubate at room temperature for 30 min.
6. Wash with 1 mL of PBS containing 1%BSA. Invert the tubes several times gently.
7. Spin at 300 × g for 5 min and remove supernatants.
8. Make a master mix of antibodies containing FITC-anti-CD41, APC-anti-CD42b, and PE-anti-human IgG in SFD medium according to the total number of reactions. Distribute 50 μL of antibody mixture to each reaction. Gently resuspend the MKs by pipetting two to three times.
9. Incubate in the dark at room temperature for 20 min.
10. Wash with 1 mL of PBS containing 1%BSA. Invert the tubes gently several times.
11. Spin at 300 × g for 5 min and remove supernatants.
12. Resuspend cells in 250 μL of PBS containing 1%BSA.
13. Analyze samples by flow cytometry. Gate on $CD41^+$ and $CD42b^+$ MKs (Fig. 4b), then analyze the binding of PE-anti-human IgG in this population with FlowJo software (Fig. 4a, c–f) (*see* **Note 17**).

4 Notes

1. iPSCs express the H, but not blood group A or B, antigens on the cell surface when in the undifferentiated state [22]. If necessary, we recommend using genotyping to verify whether

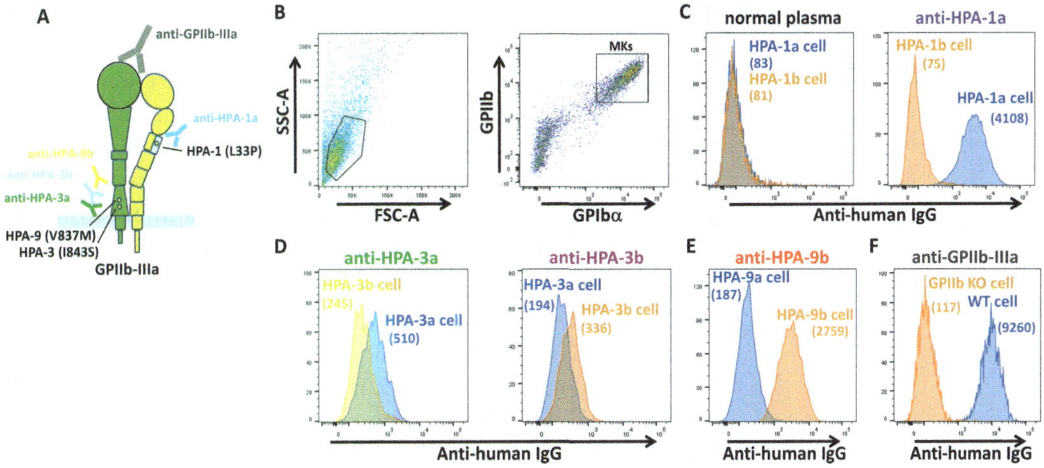

Fig. 4 Whole-cell assay using bioengineered megakaryocytes to detect and characterize anti-platelet antibodies in different clinical conditions. (**a**) Schematic of some anti-platelet antibody binding sites on the GPIIb-IIIa complex on the MK surface. (**b**) Representative flowcytometry gating of GPIIb$^+$/GPIbα$^+$ MKs. (**c**) Reactions of normal human plasma or an anti-HPA-1a alloantibody from an FNAIT patient with HPA-1a (blue) and HPA-1b (orange) allele-specific iPSC-derived MKs in flow cytometric analysis. (**d**) Reactions of an anti-HPA-3a and an anti-HPA-3b FNAIT patient plasma with HPA-3a (blue) and HPA-3b (orange) allele-specific iPSC-derived MKs. These two anti-HPA-3a and -3b alloantibodies were not detectable using standard antigen capture assays (MACE or MAIPA). (**e**) Reactions of an anti-HPA-9b FNAIT patient plasma with HPA-9a (blue) and HPA-9b (orange) allele-specific iPSC-derived MKs. This anti-HPA-9b alloantibody was not detectable using a standard antigen capture assay. (**f**) Reactions of an ITP patient plasma containing anti-GPIIb-IIIa autoantibody with wild type (blue) and GPIIb knockout (orange) iPSC-derived MKs. The numbers in (**c**) to (**f**) indicate the median fluorescence intensities of corresponding peaks. (**d** and **e** are adapted from Ref. [20] with permission)

the iPSC line originates from a type O donor. Additionally, perform genotyping for the targeted HPAs in the selected iPSC founder line. Opting for a founder line with homozygous HPA alleles can streamLine the genome editing process. As an illustrative example, our iPSC line in this protocol is HPA-1a/1a, and we will demonstrate how to convert it to HPA-1b/1b.

2. It is important to keep Matrigel cold at all times. Prechill all cultureware or media coming in contact with Matrigel. Always thaw Matrigel on ice or at 4 °C. The Matrigel-coated dishes for iPSC culture can be used immediately or stored at 4 °C for up to 2 weeks. Remove Matrigel solution right before use.

3. At this stage, we advise against breaking up small cell clumps into single cells. During the transfection process, there are multiple resuspension steps that will further break up the cell clumps. Excessive resuspension can negatively impact cell viability after transfection.

4. For generating gene knockout clones, we typically select 15–20 iPSC colonies for screening. When aiming to create knock-in clones using an HDR repair template, we often screen approximately 50–80 colonies.

5. iPSCs express HLA class I molecules on the cell surface. To screen for HLA class I negative clones, we monitor the HLA class I antigen levels using flow cytometry. When editing platelet-specific antigens, genotyping is essential to identify the target clones. For generating gene knockout clones related to platelet-specific proteins, we recommend using two CRISPR guides paired with WT Cas9 to delete a large fragment from the target gene, facilitating subsequent genotyping.
6. Double-nicking strategy using Cas9n with a pair of guide RNAs (sgRNA) can increase the specificity of genome editing [23]. The two sgRNAs should have an optimal gap of 0–20 base pairs to guide the Cas9 nickase, resulting in a double-strand break with 5′ overhangs. The two guides shown in Fig. 2c targeting the HPA-1 locus meet the requirements for the double-nicking strategy. Alternatively, a single guide paired with WT Cas9 can also create a double-strand break at the target locus. In such a case, insert the annealed Target 1 oligo into the PX459 V2.0 plasmid. Note that Target 2 is too distant from the HPA-1a site and is not suitable for the single-guide strategy.
7. In addition to the target mutation, in this case HPA-1b, silent mutations need to be introduced to the guide recognition sequence and/or the PAM sequence of the HDR repair template to prevent the repaired genome from being repetitively digested by Cas9.
8. After thawing, we recommend culturing cells for at least 2 weeks before initiating differentiation. The differentiation protocol is adapted from Dr. Deborah L. French's group with some modifications [18]. Please refer to their protocol for further details.
9. The Matrigel concentration for iPSC differentiation in Subheading 3.3 is higher than that used for maintaining iPSC culture described in **step 2** of Subheading 3.1. Additionally, the coating procedure for differentiation plates differs. When moving from one well to another for coating, there is always some loss in Matrigel volume. We often use 1 mL of Matrigel solution to coat one 6-well plate, 2 mL for 3 plates, 3 mL for 5 to 6 plates, and 4 mL for 7 to 8 plates. Keep the plate on ice until the last well is coated. Any remaining Matrigel can be stored at −20 °C and reused once. Coated plates for differentiation should be prepared freshly.
10. Avoid breaking cell clumps too small. Small cell aggregates tend to peel off easily during the initial 3 days of differentiation. Seeding density is critical for successful differentiation. Both excessively low and high cell densities can impair the yield of hematopoietic progenitor cell (HPC) production. During

the 9-day differentiation process to generate HPCs, significant cell death occurs in the initial 3 days, followed by dramatic cell proliferation. Each iPSC line exhibits slight variations in proliferation rate; therefore, the seeding density should be adjusted empirically. We typically split iPSCs from a 70–80% confluent 100 mm culture dish to 10 to 13 wells of a 6-well plate.

11. We monitor the cell surface marker expression during the differentiation process (Fig. 3). On Day 0 and Day 6, the adherent cells in a culture well are dissociated with ReLeSR and resuspended in 1 mL PBS. 250~500 μL cells are transferred into a 1.5 mL microcentrifuge tube for immunostaining of corresponding surface markers. Do not start the differentiation if less than 90% of iPSCs are SSEA-3 and SSEA-4 double positive on Day 0. Stop differentiation if there is no KDR and CD31 expression on Day 6. On Day 9 and Day 15, collect 2×10^5 HPCs or MKs in suspension for verifying cell marker expression. For immunostaining, we typically resuspend cells in 50 μL of PBS containing 1% BSA and corresponding fluorescence-labeled antibodies against different cell surface markers. Incubate at room temperature for 20 min, wash with PBS once, and then analyze using flow cytometry.

12. CHIR99021 concentration, typically falling within the range of 0.5–2 μM, should be determined empirically for each lot and each iPSC cell line for efficient HPC production.

13. HPCs can be cryopreserved in 90% FBS and 10% DMSO. After thawing, we incubate them in HPC medium at 37 °C for 2 h to facilitate recovery, then proceed with MK differentiation.

14. The MKs derived from our iPSC founder line exhibit high expression levels of GPIIb, GPIIIa, GPIbα, GPIbβ, GPIX, and relatively high levels of GPIa and CD109. Because all the currently known HPAs are located on these seven glycoproteins, we anticipate that this strategy will be valuable for characterizing most, if not all, anti-HPA alloantibodies when corresponding HPA allele-specific MKs are generated. However, it is essential to note that the surface expression levels of GPIa [24, 25] and CD109 [26] can vary among different donors. Therefore, to ensure accurate testing of alloantibodies against epitopes on these proteins (such as HPA-5 and HPA-15), we recommend evaluating several iPSC lines from diverse donors to select the high expressers for these specific proteins.

15. Cell loss often occurs during antibody incubation and wash steps. Based on our observations, $5{\sim}6 \times 10^5$ cells are optimal for ensuring an adequate number of cells for flow cytometric analysis in most cases. Reducing the cell numbers may result in an insufficient number of cells for final analysis for some patient samples.

16. We typically start with 25 μL of patient plasma mixed with 25 μL of SFD for each reaction in the initial test. The amount of patient plasma can be adjusted based on the initial test result. However, incubating cells with undiluted patient plasma sometimes leads to significant cell death, resulting in an insufficient number of cells for flow cytometric analysis. Occasionally, a gel-like structure may form during incubation with patient plasma. This structure is the fibrin clot, which occurs due to thrombin activation in some patient plasma. To prevent clot formation in such cases, we recommend adding 10 U/mL hirudin during incubation with patient plasma.
17. We routinely gate on $CD41^{+}/CD42b^{+}$ MKs and compare the binding of PE-anti-human IgG to both the antigen-positive and antigen-negative MKs for anti-platelet alloantibody detection (Fig. 4c–e). When one of these MK markers is knocked out for characterizing anti-GPIIb/IIIa or anti-GPIb/IX autoantibody or isoantibody (as shown in Fig. 4f), we either use the remaining single marker to gate the MK population or use GPVI as an alternative MK marker to replace the marker that has been knocked out [27].

Conflicts of Interest

This study was funded by grants R35 HL139937 and P01-HL167668 (to PJN). The authors have no conflicts of interest to declare that are relevant to the content of this chapter.

References

1. Versiti. https://versiti.org/products-services/human-platelet-antigen-hpa-database. Accessed Feb 21
2. Porcelijn L et al (2020) Evolution and utility of antiplatelet autoantibody testing in patients with immune thrombocytopenia. Transfus Med Rev 34(4):258–269. https://doi.org/10.1016/j.tmrv.2020.09.003
3. Porcelijn L, Huiskes E, de Haas M (2020) Progress and development of platelet antibody detection. Transfus Apher Sci 59(1):102705. https://doi.org/10.1016/j.transci.2019.102705
4. von dem Borne AE et al (1978) A simple immunofluorescence test for the detection of platelet antibodies. Br J Haematol 39:195–207
5. Hagenstrom H et al (2000) Quantification of platelet-associated IgG for differential diagnosis of patients with thrombocytopenia. Thromb Haemost 84(5):779–783
6. Schneider W, Schnaidt M (1981) The platelet adhesion immunofluorescence test: a modification of the platelet suspension immunofluorescence test. Blut 43(6):389–392. https://doi.org/10.1007/BF00320318
7. Shibata Y et al (1981) Detection of platelet antibodies by a newly developed mixed agglutination with platelets. Vox Sang 41(1):25–31. https://doi.org/10.1111/j.1423-0410.1981.tb01007.x
8. Kiefel V, Santoso S, Weisheit M, Mueller-Eckhardt C (1987) Monoclonal antibody-specific immobilization of platelet antigens (MAIPA): a new tool for the identification of platelet-reactive antibodies. Blood 70(6):1722–1726
9. Menitove JE et al (1989) Cyclic thrombocytopenia of apparent autoimmune etiology. Blood 73:1561–1569

10. Metzner K et al (2017) Detection and identification of platelet antibodies using a sensitive multiplex assay system-platelet antibody bead array. Transfusion 57(7):1724–1733. https://doi.org/10.1111/trf.14122
11. McMillan R et al (1987) Platelet-associated and plasma anti-glycoprotein autoantibodies in chronic ITP. Blood 70(4):1040–1045
12. Helmberg W, Folsch B, Wagner T, Lanzer G (1997) Detection and differentiation of platelet-specific antibodies by flow cytometry: the bead-mediated platelet assay. Transfusion 37(5):502–506. https://doi.org/10.1046/j.1537-2995.1997.37597293881.x
13. Vrbensky JR et al (2019) The sensitivity and specificity of platelet autoantibody testing in immune thrombocytopenia: a systematic review and meta-analysis of a diagnostic test. J Thrombos Haemostas 17(5):787–794. https://doi.org/10.1111/jth.14419
14. Davoren A, Curtis BR, Aster RH, McFarland JG (2004) Human platelet antigen-specific alloantibodies implicated in 1162 cases of neonatal alloimmune thrombocytopenia. Transfusion 44(8):1220–1225. https://doi.org/10.1111/j.1537-2995.2004.04026.x
15. Harrison CR et al (2003) Severe neonatal alloimmune thrombocytopenia caused by antibodies to human platelet antigen 3a (Bak[a]) detectable only in whole platelet assays. Transfusion 43(10):1398–1402
16. Barba P et al (2010) Post-transfusion purpura caused by anti-HPA-3a antibodies that are only detectable using whole platelets in the platelet immunofluorescence test. Transfus Med 20(3): 200–202. https://doi.org/10.1111/j.1365-3148.2009.00978.x
17. Ran FA et al (2013) Genome engineering using the CRISPR-Cas9 system. Nat Protoc 8(11):2281–2308. https://doi.org/10.1038/nprot.2013.143
18. Mills JA et al (2014) Hematopoietic differentiation of pluripotent stem cells in culture. In: Qu KDBC-K (ed) Methods in molecular biology, vol 1185. Springer Science+Business Media, New York, pp 181–194
19. Zhang N et al (2016) CRISPR/Cas9-mediated conversion of human platelet alloantigen allotypes. Blood 127(6):675–680. https://doi.org/10.1182/blood-2015-10-675751
20. Zhang N et al (2019) Bioengineered iPSC-derived megakaryocytes for the detection of platelet-specific patient alloantibodies. Blood 134(22):e1–e8. https://doi.org/10.1182/blood.2019002225
21. Zhang N, Sullivan MJ, Curtis BR, Newman PJ (2023) O-linked sialic acid residues on platelet membrane glycoprotein IIb mask the human HPA-9b alloepitope. Blood 142(22): 1909–1917. https://doi.org/10.1182/blood.2023021122
22. Ojima T et al (2015) Glycolipid dynamics in generation and differentiation of induced pluripotent stem cells. Sci Rep 5:14988. https://doi.org/10.1038/srep14988
23. Ran FA et al (2013) Double nicking by RNA-guided CRISPR Cas9 for enhanced genome editing specificity. Cell 154(6): 1380–1389. https://doi.org/10.1016/j.cell.2013.08.021
24. Kunicki TJ, Orchekowski R, Annis D, Honda Y (1993) Variability of integrin α2β1 activity on human platelets. Blood 82(9):2693–2703
25. Lagrue-Lak-Hal AH et al (2001) Expression and function of the collagen receptor GPVI during megakaryocyte maturation. JBiolChem 276(18):15316–15325
26. Ertel K, Al-Tawil M, Santoso S, Kroll H (2005) Relevance of the HPA-15 (Gov) polymorphism on CD109 in alloimmune thrombocytopenic syndromes. Transfusion 45(3):366–373. https://doi.org/10.1111/j.1537-2995.2005.04281.x
27. Zhang N, Uzun G, Bakchoul T, Curtis BR, Newman PJ (2026) Differentiating pathogenic from bystander autoantibodies in immune thrombocytopenia using intact glycoprotein-deficient megakaryocytes. Haematologica. https://doi.org/10.3324/haematol.2025.288832

Chapter 34

Defining the Specificity of Blood-Group-Binding Lectins Through Microarray Analysis

Anu Paul, Hau-Ming Jan, Sasikala Muthusamy, Carter J. Stowell, Vivien C. Lee, Victoria Ortiz, William O. Scott, Shang-Chuen Wu, and Connie M. Arthur

Abstract

The assessment of blood group antigens is critical to transfusion medicine practice, as accurately identifying these antigens in both donors and patients is key to ensuring safe transfusions. Although plant lectins have long been used to aid in the identification of many carbohydrate-based blood group antigens, recent research has shown that a family of mammalian proteins known as galectins can also recognize and bind to blood group antigens. However, determining the fine specificity of lectins toward these antigens is challenging because of the structural complexity of the antigens and past limitations in the resources available to characterize their interactions in detail. To overcome this, the Consortium for Functional Glycomics (CFG) developed glycan microarrays composed of chemoenzymatically defined glycans, including a wide range of blood group antigens. This platform enables precise analysis of lectin–antigen interactions and uses additional glycans as controls to refine the specificity of these interactions. We will describe the use of this platform to characterize the specificity and relative affinity of lectins for blood group and related glycans.

Key words CFG glycan array, Galectins, Blood group antigens, Self-like antigens

1 Introduction

Prior to the characterization of the ABO(H) blood group system, the outcomes of blood transfusion were unpredictable [1]. Initial attempts at transfusion yielded inconsistent results; while some recipients tolerated transfusion without apparent complication, others experienced severe, and sometimes fatal, adverse events [1–4]. The seminal discovery by Karl Landsteiner in 1900 of the ABO blood groups and their corresponding antibodies not only represented the first documented example of human polymorphism but also established a mechanistic framework for understanding transfusion incompatibility and predicting transfusion outcomes

Sean R. Stowell and Connie M. Arthur (eds.), *Methods in Transfusion Medicine*, Methods in Molecular Biology, vol. 3053, https://doi.org/10.1007/978-1-0716-5376-0_34,

[5–7]. As a result, routine testing for ABO antigens and their specific antibodies has become standard practice for all transfusion recipients, rendering these the most frequently assessed antigens and polymorphisms in the human population [8–10].

Anti-ABO antibodies typically emerge within the first year of life, independent of prior transfusion or pregnancy, and act as the most common immunological barrier to transfusion and transplantation [11, 12]. Although the precise mechanisms underlying their formation remain incompletely understood, environmental exposure and host-related factors have been proposed as possible contributors to this process [11, 13–15]. The generation of naturally occurring antibodies against ABO and related glycan antigens differs from that of other red blood cell (RBC) alloantibodies, which generally arise only after antigenic exposure through allogeneic transfusion or pregnancy [16–21]. While much remains to be learned about the pathways that govern both naturally arising and exposure-induced alloantibody formation, the establishment of preclinical models for studying alloimmunization in general has driven significant progress in the field, as illustrated by numerous models and overall studies that have begun to elucidate key factors that drive this process [21–31]. Findings from patient studies and these experimental systems have begun to clarify critical immune players and pathways involved, with each study revealing distinct features of this process following exposure to unique alloantigens that collectively suggest that this process is more complicated than previously appreciated [32–40]. Moreover, factors that influence the outcomes of incompatible transfusion, such as antibody engagement, RBC clearance, and the overall consequences of hemolysis, are now being increasingly understood through a similar use of a variety of model systems and parallel clinical studies [41–46].

Despite being recognized for more than a century, the fine structural characteristics of ABO and H antigens remain incompletely defined [3–6]. While the core features of A, B, and H epitopes have long been established, these determinants reside on structurally complex glycan scaffolds attached to glycolipids and glycoproteins of the RBC membrane. Subtle variation in presentation, linkage, and context can modulate the way antibodies and other carbohydrate-binding proteins recognize these structures. This complexity bears direct clinical relevance, as in the distinction between A1 and A2 subgroups, a distinction that has implications for transfusion and transplantation compatibility [47]. Traditional diagnostic tools such as plant-derived lectins can assist in resolving A1 versus A2 [48], but studies have shown that these reagents are imperfect. In the transplant setting, for example, lectin-based discrimination may underestimate compatibility, excluding potential donor–recipient matches [47, 49].

Beyond exogenous plant lectins, mammals produce their own families of lectins with physiologic roles in glycan recognition, including blood group and related antigens [50]. Among these are the galectins, a broadly conserved family of β-galactoside-binding proteins. Each galectin harbors a carbohydrate-recognition domain (CRD) formed by two antiparallel β-sheets folded into a β-sandwich, generating the canonical galectin-binding pocket. Within this CRD, key residues, including histidine, arginine, asparagine, tryptophan, and glutamic acid, form a conserved "carbohydrate-binding cassette" that facilitate recognition of β-galactose moieties [51–55]. Sequence variations outside this conserved cassette are thought to diversify binding specificity across the galectin family and confer differential recognition of more complex glycans, such as the ABO(H) and Lewis antigens [56].

Defining the fine specificity of lectin–glycan interactions has historically been challenging. Early studies inferred binding patterns largely from hemagglutination assays, exploiting the capacity of lectins to crosslink and therefore agglutinate RBCs [57–59]. While useful, such assays are unable to resolve which specific glycan moieties underlie high-affinity recognition, given that the RBC surface displays a heterogeneous and densely glycosylated landscape. To overcome these challenges, high-throughput glycan microarray platforms, such as those developed by the Consortium for Functional Glycomics (CFG), have been applied to systematically assess galectin–glycan interactions, which have provided important insight into the binding specificity of distinct family members and their overall function [50, 60–67]. These arrays display hundreds of well-defined mammalian glycans, including ABO(H), α-Gal, N-acetyllactosamine, and Lewis antigens (A, B, X, Y), allowing direct comparison of binding preferences across multiple galectins [68].

Most prior analyses of galectin binding to glycan arrays have relied on single protein concentrations, which, although informative for outlining overall specificity, offer limited capacity to distinguish subtle differences in affinity. To address this limitation, we have reported an analysis approach of examining multiple human galectins across physiologically relevant concentrations (0.04–10 μM) on glycan arrays, as illustrated in a number of studies [60–62, 69, 70] (Fig. 1). This approach enables not only the accurate identification of preferred glycan ligands but also quantitative estimation of maximal binding (Bmax) and apparent dissociation constants (K_D) [69] (Fig. 2). The ability to resolve these parameters provides a more nuanced understanding of the fine specificity of galectins for blood group and related glycans, thereby advancing both the fundamental biology of lectin–glycan recognition and the development of refined reagents for transfusion and transplantation medicine [71].

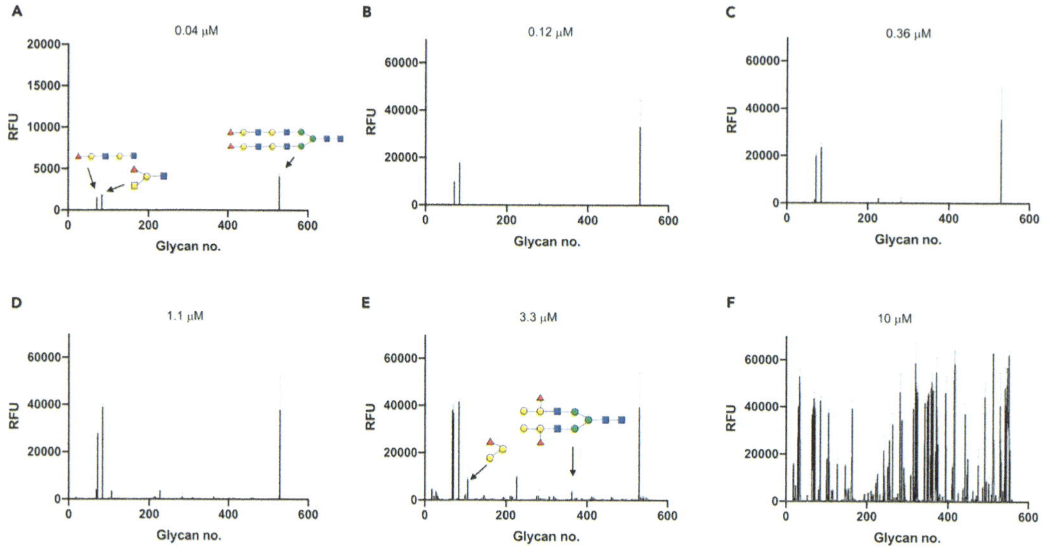

Fig. 1 Galectin-7 (Gal-7) exhibits specific interactions with blood group-containing structures across various concentrations. (**a**–**f**) Data from the Consortium for Functional Glycomics (CFG) glycan microarray, obtained after incubation at the following concentrations of Gal-7: 0.04 (**a**), 0.12 (**b**), 0.36 (**c**), 1.1 (**d**), 3.3 (**e**), and 10 (**f**) μM. RFU stands for relative fluorescence units. Error bars indicate the mean ± SD. (This research was originally published in iScience. Wu et al. [61]. © 2022 The Author(s))

2 Materials

2.1 Preparing Alexa Fluor™ 488 Reagent for Coupling

1. Phosphate-buffered saline (PBS) 1X.
2. Alexa Fluor™ 488 carboxylic acid, succinimidyl ester (Invitrogen) by Thermo Fisher Scientific, A 20100.

2.2 Coupling Galectins with Alexa Fluor 488 for CFG Arrays

1. Recombinantly purified full-length human galectins are stored in an elution buffer containing 14 mM β-mercaptoethanol and 100 mM lactose.
2. PD-10 desalting column, Sephadex™ G-25 M, GE, 17085101.
3. Lactose–Sepharose column for preparing active galectins for glycan array analysis.
4. Lactose.
5. Spectrophotometer.
6. Cuvettes for spectrophotometer.
7. 1.7-mL microcentrifuge tubes.
8. Amicon centrifugal filters.
9. Centrifuge.

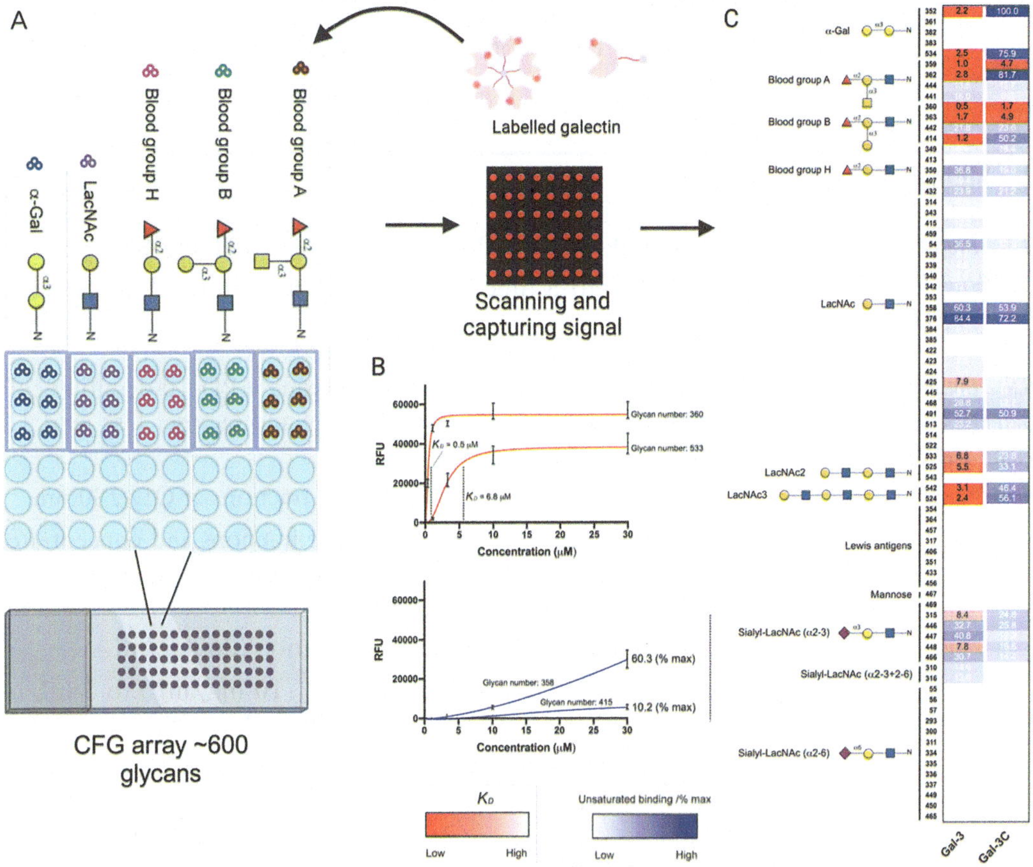

Fig. 2 K_D values for the binding of galectin-3 (Gal-3) and galectin-3C (Gal-3C) to blood group antigens and other mammalian glycans. (**a**) Illustration of the process of using the CFG array. (**b**) Representative binding isotherms were used to determine K_D values and the % maximum binding for unsaturated glycans. (**c**) Blood group antigens are shown with heat maps indicating K_D values (in red) and % maximum binding (in blue). (This research was originally published in *Frontiers in Microbiology* with some modifications. Wu et al.. © 2021 Wu, Ho, Kamili, Wang, Murdock, Cummings, Arthur and Stowell)

2.3 Method for Performing a CFG Glycan Microarray

1. Mammalian glycan array slides provided by the Consortium for Functional Glycomics (CFG).
2. Forceps.
3. Coplin jars.
4. Coverslips to cover the slides after loading galectins.
5. End-over-end rotator shaker.
6. Orbital shaker platform.
7. Blocking buffer: 1% bovine serum albumin (BSA) in 1X PBS with 0.05% Tween-20.
8. Vacuum desiccator.

9. Molecular Devices GenePix 4000B Microarray Scanner.
10. GenePix Pro 7 Software for imaging the slides and analyzing the data.

3 Methods

3.1 Preparing Alexa Fluor™ 488 Reagent for Coupling

1. Add 500 μL of 1X PBS to 5 mg of Alexa Fluor 488.
2. Aliquot into 5 tubes, with 100 μL in each tube, and store at −20 °C.

3.2 Coupling Galectins with Alexa Fluor 488 for CFG Arrays

1. Desalt the recombinant galectins using a PD-10 desalting column to remove 2-mercaptoethanol and lactose. Use cold 1X PBS for wash and elution.
2. Check the absorbance of all eluted fractions at OD 280 nm.
3. Combine the OD 280-nm positive fractions and concentrate. The concentration of the protein used for coupling should be at least 2 mg/mL for optimal results.
4. Add lactose at a 100 mM concentration (36 mg/mL).
5. Add 50 μL of Alexa Fluor 488 dye (10 mg/mL) to 1 mL of galectin (2 mg/mL) solution (*see* **Note 1**).
6. Incubate at room temperature for 1 h on a rotator shaker, avoiding light.
7. After coupling, pass the Alexa Fluor 488-coupled galectin through a PD-10 desalting column to remove any unbound dye and lactose.
8. The collected protein fraction is pooled and passed through 2 mL of lactose–Sepharose column, followed by washing the column with PBS.
9. The bound protein is eluted using 100 mM lactose-containing elution buffer.
10. This fraction contains only the active galectins. Pass this active galectin fraction through a PD-10 desalting column again to remove the lactose.
11. Use the manufacturer's instructions for calculating protein concentration post-labeling.

3.3 Method for Performing a CFG Glycan Microarray

1. Take the slides from the −20 °C freezer and place them in a Coplin jar using forceps.
2. Place the Coplin jar inside the vacuum desiccator. Connect the vacuum and close the valve. Leave the slides in the vacuum for 30 minutes (*see* **Note 2**).

3. Block the slides in blocking buffer containing 1% bovine serum albumin (BSA) in PBST (1X PBS with 0. 05% Tween-20).
4. Prepare PBST, PBS, and distilled water in Coplin jars.
5. Rehydrate the CFG array slide in PBST for 5 minutes.
6. Dilute galectin in blocking buffer to different concentrations: 0.04, 0.12, 0.36, 1.1, 3.3, and 10 μM.
7. Add 200 μL of galectin solution to the slide, and place the microscope cover glass over it.
8. Incubate for 1 h at room temperature, avoiding light.
9. Wash with PBST (4 times).
10. Wash with 1X PBS (4 times).
11. Wash with water (4 times).
12. Spin-dry.
13. Scan the image using GenePix Microarray Scanner at 523 nm (*see* **Note 3**). Save the image as a Tiff file.
14. After acquiring the image, it is aligned to an array map called GenePix Array list file or.gal file that indicates the coordinates of the spots by numbers correlated to the printed material [72].
15. The output file, or GenePix results file (.gpr), contains alignment information for analyzing the data using Microsoft Excel and can be further processed with Prism or GLAD (Glycan Array Dashboard) analysis tools (*see* **Note 4**).

4 Notes

1. Alexa Fluor 647 can also be used for labeling the galectins, followed by array analysis.
2. Exercise caution to ensure that the forceps do not come into contact with the glycan-printed areas, as any inadvertent touch could potentially compromise the integrity of the printed glycans and affect the accuracy of subsequent analyses or experiments.
3. Different scanner machines may have different PMT settings. Use of multiple concentrations of galectin can allow relative K_D values to be obtained.
4. GLAD (Glycan Array Dashboard) is a tool to visualize, analyze, and compare glycan microarray data developed by Dr. Akul Y. Mehta and Dr. Richard D. Cummings.

Conflicts of Interest

This work was funded by NIH P01HL171803, R01 HL165975, R01 HL135575, R01 HL154034, and K99HL169746, and AABB Foundation Early-Career Scientific Research Grants. SRS has received speaker and consultant honoraria from Cerus, Grifols, Novartis, Alexion, and Argenx, and has received a research grant from Alexion. No other authors have conflicts of interest.

References

1. Fastag E, Varon J, Sternbach G (2013) Richard lower: the origins of blood transfusion. J Emerg Med 44(6):1146–1150
2. Marinozzi S, Gazzaniga V, Iorio S (2018) The earliest blood transfusions in 17th-century in Italy (1667–1668). Transfus Med Rev 32(1): 1–5
3. Learoyd P (2012) The history of blood transfusion prior to the 20th century–part 1. Transfus Med 22(5):308–314
4. Hosgood G (1990) Blood transfusion: a historical review. J Am Vet Med Assoc 197(8): 998–1000
5. Bertsch T et al (2019) Karl Landsteiner: the discovery of the ABO blood group system and its value for teaching medical students. Clin Lab 65(6). https://doi.org/10.7754/Clin.Lab.2018.181218
6. Boulton FE (2013) Blood transfusion; additional historical aspects. Part 1. The birth of transfusion immunology. Transfus Med 23(6): 375–381
7. Mohd Noor NH, Siti Asmaa MJ (2024) Karl Landsteiner (1868–1943): a versatile blood scientist. Cureus 16(9):e68903
8. Andic N (2022) Practical solutions for problems in blood grouping and crossmatching. Turk J Haematol 39(1):55–60
9. Alquist CR, Helander L (2021) Transfusion blood Bank (recipient) testing. Clin Lab Med 41(4):599–610
10. Shmookler A et al (2017) Acute hemolytic transfusion reaction caused by a red cell antibody that was missed by Pretransfusion testing using tube method. Lab Med 48(3):258–261
11. Branch DR (2015) Anti-A and anti-B: what are they and where do they come from? Transfusion 55(Suppl 2):S74–S79
12. Arthur CM, Stowell SR (2023) The development and consequences of red blood cell Alloimmunization. Annu Rev Pathol 18:537–564
13. Adam I et al (2025) ABO-A antibody induction in mice is T cell-dependent, estrogen-independent, and modulated by CD22. Am J Transplant 25(6):1180–1192
14. Adam I et al (2023) Sex, T cells, and the microbiome in natural ABO antibody production in mice. Transplantation 107(11):2353–2363
15. Hale RC et al (2024) The role of glycosylation in clinical allergy and immunology. J Allergy Clin Immunol 153(1):55–66
16. Pirenne F, Yazdanbakhsh K (2018) How I safely transfuse patients with sickle-cell disease and manage delayed hemolytic transfusion reactions. Blood 131(25):2773–2781
17. Yazdanbakhsh K, Ware RE, Noizat-Pirenne F (2012) Red blood cell alloimmunization in sickle cell disease: pathophysiology, risk factors, and transfusion management. Blood 120(3): 528–537
18. Zimring JC, Hudson KE (2016) Cellular immune responses in red blood cell alloimmunization. Hematology Am Soc Hematol Educ Program 2016(1):452–456
19. Pirenne F, Floch A, Diop S (2023) Alloimmunisation against red blood cells in sickle cell disease: transfusion challenges in high-income and low-income countries. Lancet Haematol 10(6):e468–e476
20. Chang DY et al (2023) The ongoing challenge of RBC alloimmunization in the management of patients with sickle cell disease. Presse Med 52(4):104211
21. Arthur CM et al (2016) CD8+ T cells mediate antibody-independent platelet clearance in mice. Blood 127(14):1823–1827
22. Desmarets M et al (2009) Minor histocompatibility antigens on transfused leukoreduced units of red blood cells induce bone marrow transplant rejection in a mouse model. Blood 114(11):2315–2322

23. Zimring JC et al (2005) Nonhemolytic antibody-induced loss of erythrocyte surface antigen. Blood 106(3):1105–1112
24. Smith NH et al (2012) Generation of transgenic mice with antithetical KEL1 and KEL2 human blood group antigens on red blood cells. Transfusion 52(12):2620–2630
25. Campbell-Lee SA et al (2006) The production of red blood cell alloantibodies in mice transfused with blood from transgenic Fyb-expressing mice. Transfusion 46(10): 1682–1688
26. Stowell SR et al (2013) Alloantibodies to a paternally derived RBC KEL antigen lead to hemolytic disease of the fetus/newborn in a murine model. Blood 122(8):1494–1504
27. Smith NH et al (2012) Transfusion in the absence of inflammation induces antigen-specific tolerance to murine RBCs. Blood 119(6):1566–1569
28. Couvidou A et al (2023) Marginal zone B cells are responsible for the production of alloantibodies following platelet transfusion in mice. Blood Adv 7(8):1356–1365
29. Jackman RP, Thomas KA (2025) Immune response to platelet transfusions. Curr Opin Hematol 32:357
30. Jackman RP et al (2023) Enhanced alloresponse to platelet transfusion due to immune dysregulation following ablative chemotherapy in mice. Front Immunol 14:1281123
31. Stowell SR et al (2013) Antigen modulation confers protection to red blood cells from antibody through Fcgamma receptor ligation. J Immunol 191(10):5013–5025
32. Thomas TA et al (2023) Reticulocytes in donor blood units enhance red blood cell alloimmunization. Haematologica 108(10):2639–2651
33. Arneja A et al (2016) Interleukin-6 receptor-alpha signaling drives anti-RBC alloantibody production and T-follicular helper cell differentiation in a murine model of red blood cell alloimmunization. Haematologica 101(11): e440–e444
34. Madany E et al (2021) Altered type 1 interferon responses in alloimmunized and nonalloimmunized patients with sickle cell disease. EJHaem 2(4):700–710
35. Gibb DR et al (2017) B cells require Type 1 interferon to produce alloantibodies to transfused KEL-expressing red blood cells in mice. Transfusion 57(11):2595–2608
36. Mener A et al (2018) Complement serves as a switch between CD4+ T cell-independent and -dependent RBC antibody responses. JCI Insight 3(22). https://doi.org/10.1172/jci.insight.121631
37. Jajosky R et al (2023) Prior immunization against an intracellular antigen enhances subsequent red blood cell alloimmunization in mice. Blood 141(21):2642–2653
38. Zerra PE et al (2021) Marginal zone B cells mediate a CD4 T-cell-dependent extrafollicular antibody response following RBC transfusion in mice. Blood 138(8):706–721
39. Patel SR et al (2018) Recipient priming to one RBC alloantigen directly enhances subsequent alloimmunization in mice. Blood Adv 2(2): 105–115
40. Arthur CM et al (2017) Antigen density dictates immune responsiveness following red blood cell transfusion. J Immunol 198(7): 2671–2680
41. Maier CL et al (2018) Antibody-mediated immune suppression by antigen modulation is antigen-specific. Blood Adv 2(21):2986–3000
42. Arthur CM et al (2021) Antigen density dictates RBC clearance, but not antigen modulation, following incompatible RBC transfusion in mice. Blood Adv 5(2):527–538
43. Chonat S et al (2025) Complement is activated in patients with acute chest syndrome caused by sickle cell disease and represents a therapeutic target. Sci Transl Med 17(807):eadl4922
44. Jajosky RP et al (2023) Antibody-mediated antigen loss switches augmented immunity to antibody-mediated immunosuppression. Blood 142(12):1082–1098
45. Mener A et al (2019) Antibody-mediated immunosuppression can result from RBC antigen loss independent of Fcgamma receptors in mice. Transfusion 59(1):371–384
46. Maier CL et al (2023) Storage differentially impacts alloimmunization to distinct red cell antigens following transfusion in mice. Transfusion 63(3):457–462
47. Joseph A et al (2023) ABO Genotyping finds more A(2) to B kidney transplant opportunities than lectin-based subtyping. Am J Transplant 23(4):512–519
48. Garg N et al (2021) Discrepant subtyping of blood type A2 living kidney donors: missed opportunities in kidney transplantation. Clin Transpl 35(10):e14422
49. Bryan CF, Cherikh WS, Sesok-Pizzini DA (2016) A2/A2 B to B renal transplantation: past, present, and future directions. Am J Transplant 16(1):11–20
50. Wu SC et al (2023) Blood group A enhances SARS-CoV-2 infection. Blood 142(8): 742–747
51. Barondes SH et al (1994) Galectins: a family of animal beta-galactoside-binding lectins. Cell 76(4):597–598

52. Yang RY, Rabinovich GA, Liu FT (2008) Galectins: structure, function and therapeutic potential. Expert Rev Mol Med 10:e17
53. Hirabayashi J et al (2002) Oligosaccharide specificity of galectins: a search by frontal affinity chromatography. Biochim Biophys Acta 1572(2–3):232–254
54. Cummings RD, Liu FT (2009) Galectins. In: Essentials of glycobiology. Cold Spring Harbor Laboratory Press, Cold Spring Harbor
55. Diehl RC et al (2024) CH-pi interactions are required for human Galectin-3 function. JACS Au 4(8):3028–3037
56. Feizi T et al (1994) The adhesive specificity of the soluble human lectin, IgE-binding protein, toward lipid-linked oligosaccharides. Presence of the blood group A, B, B-like, and H monosaccharides confers a binding activity to tetrasaccharide (lacto-N-tetraose and lacto-N-neotetraose) backbones. Biochemistry 33(20): 6342–6349
57. de Waard A, Hickman S, Kornfeld S (1976) Isolation and properties of beta-galactoside binding lectins of calf heart and lung. J Biol Chem 251(23):7581–7587
58. Vasta GR (2009) Roles of galectins in infection. Nat Rev Microbiol 7(6):424–438
59. Leffler H, Barondes SH (1986) Specificity of binding of three soluble rat lung lectins to substituted and unsubstituted mammalian beta-galactosides. J Biol Chem 261(22): 10119–10126
60. Jan HM et al (2024) Galectin-4 antimicrobial activity primarily occurs through its C-terminal domain. Mol Cell Proteomics 23(5):100747
61. Wu SC et al (2022) Innate immune Galectin-7 specifically targets microbes that decorate themselves in blood group-like antigens. iScience 25(7):104482
62. Blenda AV et al (2022) Galectin-9 recognizes and exhibits antimicrobial activity toward microbes expressing blood group-like antigens. J Biol Chem 298(4):101704
63. Gao C et al (2019) Glycan microarrays as chemical tools for identifying glycan recognition by immune proteins. Front Chem 7:833
64. Feizi T et al (2003) Carbohydrate microarrays – a new set of technologies at the frontiers of glycomics. Curr Opin Struct Biol 13(5): 637–645
65. Marglous S et al (2024) Serum antibody screening using glycan arrays. Chem Soc Rev 53(5):2603–2642
66. Tran PMH et al (2022) Use of a glycomics array to establish the anti-carbohydrate antibody repertoire in type 1 diabetes. Nat Commun 13(1):6527
67. Kunz PB et al (2025) Development of lamprey-derived antibodies against human blood group antigens. Glycobiology 35: cwaf043
68. Stowell SR et al (2008) Dimeric Galectin-8-induces phosphatidylserine exposure in leukocytes through polylactosamine recognition by the C-terminal domain. J Biol Chem 283(29): 20547–20559
69. Ho AD et al (2022) An automated approach to assess relative galectin-glycan affinity following glycan microarray analysis. Front Mol Biosci 9: 893185
70. Wu SC et al (2023) Whole microbe arrays accurately predict interactions and overall antimicrobial activity of galectin-8 toward distinct strains of Streptococcus pneumoniae. Sci Rep 13(1):5324
71. Arthur CM, Cummings RD, Stowell SR (2014) Using glycan microarrays to understand immunity. Curr Opin Chem Biol 18: 55–61
72. Mehta AY, Heimburg-Molinaro J, Cummings RD (2020) Tools for generating and analyzing glycan microarray data. Beilstein J Org Chem 16:2260–2271

Chapter 35

Characterization of Antigen-Specific CD4$^+$ T Cell Responses to the Transfusion of Red Blood Cells

Jelena Medved, Abhinav Arneja, Alexis Boscia, Emily Burnett, Selby Ireland, Gunnhildur Thorkelsdottir, Arwen Chandler, Benjamin Hester, Catherine Schwarzschild, Conrad Niebuhr, and Chance John Luckey

Abstract

To study the antigen-specific CD4$^+$ T cell responses to transfused red blood cells (RBCs) in vivo, we have utilized the adoptive transfer of naïve RBC-specific CD4$^+$ T cells at low precursor frequencies. Our approach combines the readily available OT-II T cell receptor transgenic mouse, which recognizes ovalbumin, with the Hen egg lysozyme, Ovalbumin, and the human Duffy (HOD) RBC alloimmunization model transgenically expressing a chimeric antigen comprised of hen egg lysozyme, ovalbumin, and human Duffy protein selectively on RBCs. OT-II mice have been crossed to Pep Boy mice to allow for the use of the CD45.1 congenic marker to readily identify antigen-specific cells in a C57/Black6 (C57/B6) CD45.2 background. As both IL-21 and IL-4 are known to support B cell activation, class switching, and differentiation into antibody-secreting plasmablasts, we have further crossed OT-II/CD45.1 mice with mice expressing knock-ins of two separate fluorescent reporters that read out both IL-21 and IL-4 RNA expression. This approach allows for the use of commonly employed multiparameter flow cytometric analysis to characterize the activation, proliferation, and phenotype of RBC antigen-specific T cells, as well as their subsequent cytokine production in response to transfused allogeneic RBCs. Using these approaches, we present examples of antigen-specific T cell responses induced by HOD transfusion in wild-type (WT) C57/B6 recipients.

Key words CD4$^+$ T cells, IL-4, IL-21, Reporter, OT-II, Antigen-specific, HOD, RBC alloimmunization

1 Introduction

Red blood cell (RBC) alloimmunization can be a significant cause of morbidity for those patients who require chronic blood transfusions, and remains a major cause of transfusion-related mortality [1–3]. Despite its clinical impact, our understanding of how transfusions induce immune responses in patients is limited by our lack

Sean R. Stowell and Connie M. Arthur (eds.), *Methods in Transfusion Medicine*, Methods in Molecular Biology, vol. 3053, https://doi.org/10.1007/978-1-0716-5376-0_35,

of access to the relevant immune tissues of patients who are actively undergoing responses to transfusion. We typically only have access to patients' blood, while the cells that initially respond to transfused RBCs and ultimately drive alloantibody production reside in secondary lymphoid organs such as the spleen. Mouse models of alloimmunization allow for the direct interrogation of the cellular and molecular regulators of anti-RBC alloantibody production [4, 5]. These experimentally tractable animal models allow for the in vivo monitoring of key immune cells and their responses to transfused RBCs.

The field of Immunology has focused for decades on antibodies that are generated in response to infections and vaccinations. Most antibodies are produced through a collaborative effort between B cells, which produce the antibodies, and T follicular helper (TFH) cells, a specialized group of CD4$^+$ T cells that instruct B cells when and where to differentiate and make antibodies [6]. We now appreciate that there are multiple different subsets of TFH cells that can be separated based on their location and function [7–9]. After initial naïve T cell activation by dendritic cells [10], a subset of activated T cells (classically referred to as pre-TFH cells) migrates to the T-B border where they can provide initial help to recently activated B cells. These initial T-B cell interactions lead to further B cell activation, and are thought to drive B cell class switching from IgM to IgG [11]. Further T cell help either in extrafollicular areas or in germinal centers then drives B cell differentiation into antibody-secreting plasmablasts. Importantly, there are many diverse molecular events by which TFH cells can signal and provide help to B cells including (1) MHC/peptide–T cell receptor (TCR) signaling, (2) direct cell–cell interactions via co-stimulatory and adhesion molecules, and (3) T cell secretion of cytokines that help drive B cell differentiation [7, 8]. Given the diversity of potential co-stimulatory molecules and cytokines that are known to regulate antibody production, it is important to investigate which of these signals are and which signals are not induced by allogeneic RBC transfusions.

Our mechanistic understanding of the drivers of antibody responses to transfused RBCs has been greatly enhanced by the development of the Hen egg lysozyme, Ovalbumin, and the human Duffy (HOD) mouse model. HOD mice transgenically express a triple fusion construct of Hen egg lysozyme, Ovalbumin, and the human Duffy red cell antigen (HOD red cell antigen selectively on the surface of RBCs [4]. HOD mice can then serve as donors for RBCs where transfusion of these alloantigen-expressing RBCs drives anti-RBC antibody production in C57/B6 mice. Importantly, simple transfusion of fresh HOD RBCs is a poor inducer of anti-RBC IgG, and typically, robust production of anti-RBC IgG requires the exogenous addition of proinflammatory stimuli such as viral mimetics or viral infection at the time of transfusion [12]. We and others have also shown that prolonged refrigerator storage of HOD RBCs (similar to how patient blood is stored) leads to enhancement of anti-HOD IgG production in C57/B6 recipients [13–15]. Importantly, the enhanced IgG induced by prolonged storage is dependent on $CD4^+$ T cells that have been activated by bridging channel dendritic cells [16], suggesting that $CD4^+$ TFH cells play an essential role in driving alloimmunization in response to stored HOD RBC transfusion.

To better understand how $CD4^+$ T cells are activated and respond to stored HOD transfusion, we have taken advantage of the fact that the HOD model allows us to monitor the localization and responses of antigen-specific T cells through the use of congenically marked OT-II T cells [17]. OT-II mice transgenically express a T cell receptor (TCR) specific for chicken ovalbumin (OVA) specifically in their T cells [18]. In the absence of stimulation or infection, the majority of the T cells in OT-II mice remain naïve and express a TCR that is specific for OVA. When OT-II mice are crossed with Pep Boy mice that congenically express the pan-leukocyte maker CD45.1 on a C57/B6 background, naïve $OT\text{-}II^+CD45.1^+$ T cells can then be purified and adoptively transferred into C57/B6 hosts prior to transfusion. The expression of both the congenic marker and the transgenic TCR allows for the facile discrimination of OVA-specific T cells from their endogenous counterparts, and the OVA-specific TCR allows for monitoring anti-HOD-specific $CD4^+$ T cell responses induced by HOD transfusion.

Given the central role that cytokine signaling plays in inducing class switching and B cell differentiation into antibody-secreting plasmablasts, we are interested in better understanding how different T-cell-derived cytokines are induced by transfusion. Two key cytokines that drive both IgG class switching, B cell differentiation, and plasmablast formation are IL-4 and IL-21 [7, 19, 20]. To allow for direct fluorescent detection of IL-4 and IL-21 mRNA expression, OT-II/CD45.1 mice were further crossed with mice in which the fluorescent reporter Katushka was knocked-in to the IL-21 locus, and GFP was knocked-in to the IL-4 locus [21]. Understanding how these cytokines regulate the immune response to transfused RBCs is essential for unraveling the mechanisms behind RBC alloimmunization. This dual-reporter OT-II system provides a powerful tool for tracking and characterizing the expression of these cytokines in antigen-specific $CD4^+$ T cells following RBC transfusion. Collectively, the approaches detailed herein leverage advanced genetic tools and sophisticated, multilocus genetic mouse models to deepen our understanding of $CD4^+$ T cell activation, differentiation, and function in response to transfused RBCs (Fig. 1).

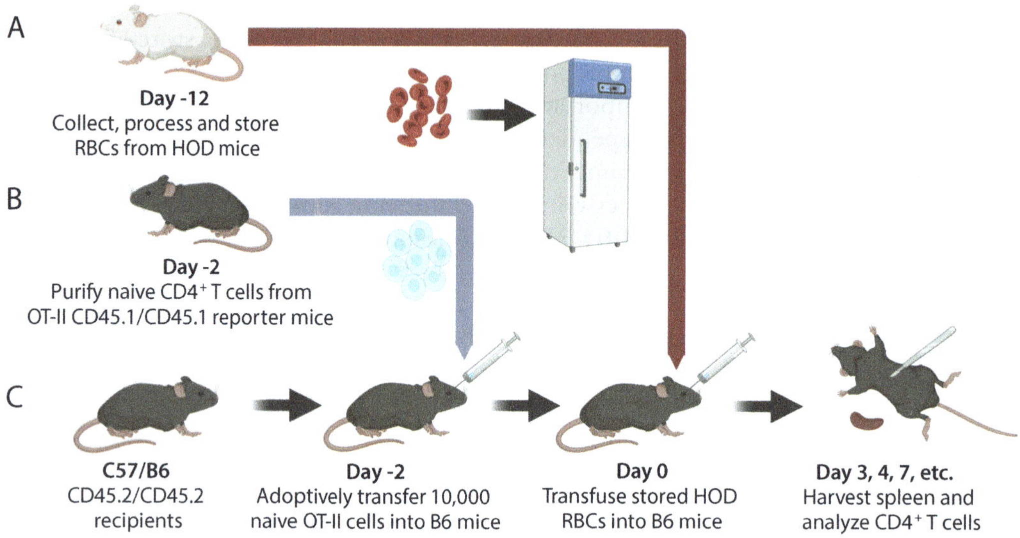

Fig. 1 Experimental approach and timeline. (**a**) Blood from the donor HOD mice is collected, processed, and stored for 12 days. (**b**) Naïve CD45.1 OT-II $CD4^+$ T cells are purified from the spleens of IL-21-Katushka/IL-4-GFP double reporter mice. (**c**) 10,000 $CD4^+$ T cells are transferred into recipient WT C57/B6 mice. Two days after the adoptive transfer, recipient mice receive HOD RBC transfusion. Splenocytes from the recipient mice are harvested at desired time points after transfusion, processed, stained, and analyzed via flow cytometry. (This figure was created with BioRender.com)

2 Materials

2.1 Mice

1. Wild-type (WT) C57BL/6J, Pep Boy, and OT-II mice were purchased from Jackson Laboratories (strain IDs 000664, 019115, and 004194, respectively).
2. HOD mice were described previously [4].
3. IL-21-Katushka/IL-4-GFP double reporter mice were a generous gift from Dr. Joe Craft and were described previously [21, 22].

2.2 Collection of Blood from Donor HOD Mice, Processing, and Storage

1. Anticoagulant citrate phosphate dextrose adenine solution (CPDA-1, Boston BioProducts, IBB-420).
2. 70% ethanol.
3. Two pairs of scissors and two pairs of forceps.
4. 1-mL syringes (BD, 309659), 25G needle (BD, 305122), and 15-mL conical tubes (BD Falcon, 352097).
5. Whole blood cell leukoreduction filter (Pall, AP-4851).
6. 10-mL syringes (BD, 302995) for filter attachment.

2.3 Naïve CD4+ T Cell Purification for Adoptive Transfer

1. Naïve $CD4^+$ T Cell Isolation Kit (Miltenyi Biotec, 130-104-453).
2. $CD4^+$ T Cell Isolation Kit (Miltenyi Biotec, 130-104-454).
3. Petri dishes, 15-mL conical tubes, 50-mL conical tubes (BD Falcon, 352098).
4. 40-μm cell strainers (Falcon, 352340).
5. RBC lysis buffer (Invitrogen, 00-4300-54).
6. Phosphate-buffered saline (PBS), pH 7.4.
7. Sterile PBS (Gibco, 14190-144).
8. MACS buffer: PBS, 0.5% bovine serum albumin (BSA), and 2 mM EDTA.
9. FACS buffer: PBS, 2% heat-inactivated fetal bovine serum (FBS), 0.5% BSA (Sigma, A7906), 0.1% sodium azide (Sigma, S8032).
10. QuadroMACS™ Separator (Miltenyi Biotec, 130-091-051).
11. LS columns for manual magnetic separation of cells (Miltenyi Biotec, 130-042-401).
12. The following antibodies: CD4 APC/Cy7 (BioLegend, 100414), B220 Brilliant Violet 605™ (BioLegend, 103244), CD8 Brilliant Violet 605™ (BioLegend, 100744), CD44 FITC (BioLegend, 103006), and CD62L Brilliant Violet 421™ (BioLegend, 104435).
13. Attune NxT flow cytometer (Thermo Fisher Scientific).
14. Computer software capable of analyzing flow cytometry data, such as FlowJo™ Software (BD).

2.4 Retro-Orbital Injection of CD4+ T Cells or RBCs

1. 1-mL syringes (BD, 309659), blunt needles (BD, 305180), 30G needles (BD, 305106).
2. Isoflurane.

2.5 Collection of Splenocytes from Transfusion Recipients

1. PBS, pH 7.4.
2. 40-μm cell strainers (Falcon, 352340).
3. RBC lysis buffer (Invitrogen, 00-4300-54).
4. FACS buffer: PBS, 2% heat-inactivated FBS, 0.5% BSA (Sigma, A7906), 0.1% sodium azide (Sigma, S8032).

2.6 Staining of Splenocytes for Flow Cytometry

1. PBS, pH 7.4.
2. FACS buffer: PBS, 2% heat-inactivated FBS, 0.5% BSA (Sigma, A7906), 0.1% sodium azide (Sigma, S8032).
3. Zombie Yellow™ Dye (BioLegend, 77168).
4. The following antibodies: Biotin Rat Anti-Mouse CXCR5 (BD Pharmingen, 551960), Biotin Goat Anti-Rat Ig

(BD Pharmingen, 554014), Brilliant Violet 421™ Streptavidin (BioLegend, 405225), CD45.1 PE/Cy7 (BioLegend, 110730), CD45.2 PerCP/Cy5.5 (BioLegend, 109828), CD4 APC/Cy7, APC PD-1 (BioLegend, 135210), B220 Brilliant Violet 605™, and CD8 Brilliant Violet 605™.

5. Attune NxT flow cytometer.
6. FlowJo™ Software.

3 Methods

3.1 Mice

1. All mice should be used at 8–10 weeks of age.
2. IL-21-Katushka/IL-4-GFP double reporter mice are crossed to OT-II and Pep Boy (CD45.1) mice (*see* **Note 1**).

3.2 Collection of Blood from Donor HOD Mice, Processing, and Storage

1. Dissection and cardiac blood collection should be done in a biosafety cabinet to assure aseptic technique (*see* **Note 2**).
2. Sterilize dissection tools by spraying them with 70% ethanol. Air-dry.
3. Prepare 1-mL syringe and 25G needle. Fill the syringe with 50–100 μL CPDA-1 (*see* **Note 3**).
4. Euthanize a HOD mouse. Spray its fur generously with 70% ethanol (*see* **Note 4**).
5. Use the first pair of forceps and scissors to make a midline incision across the abdomen and thorax. Separate the skin to expose the tissue underneath.
6. Use the second pair of forceps and scissors to make a transverse incision across the diaphragm. Cut the ribcage left and right from the sternum while holding the xiphoid process with forceps (Fig. 2a).
7. While still holding the xiphoid process, insert the syringe needle into the right ventricle about 2–3 mm into the heart, ensuring the needle does not penetrate through the back of the right ventricle, right atrium, or septum (Fig. 2b).
8. Slowly draw the blood out (*see* **Notes 5 and 6**).
9. Transfer the collected blood into a 15-mL conical tube, and swirl to thoroughly mix blood and CPDA-1 (*see* **Note 7**).
10. Do not discard the syringe. Refill it with 50–100 μL CPDA-1 (*see* **Note 8**).
11. Repeat **steps 4–10**.
12. Once the desired volume of blood is collected, proceed with leukoreduction (*see* **Notes 9–11**).

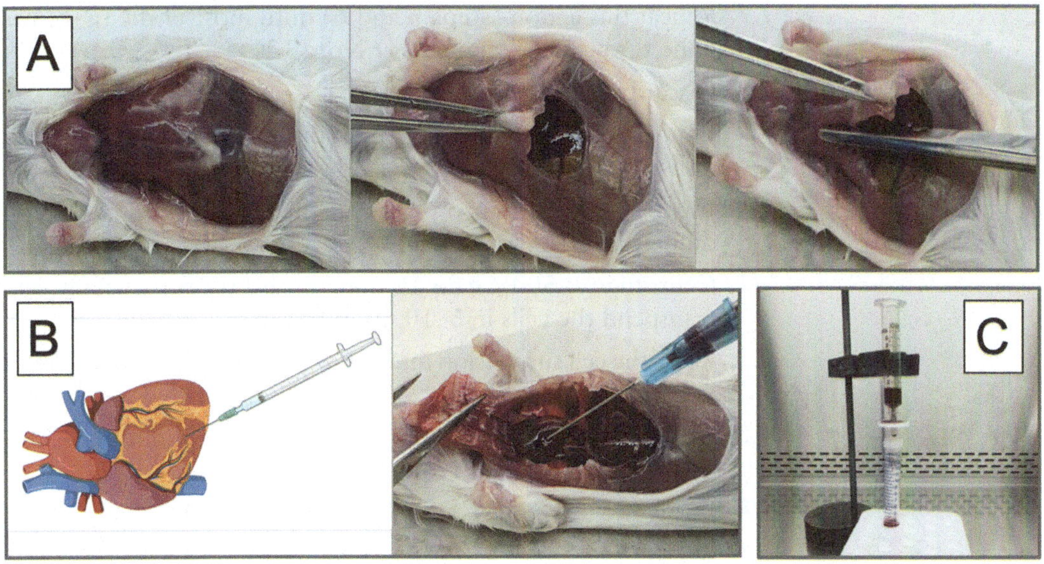

Fig. 2 Blood collection and processing from donor mice. (**a**) Midline incision is made in the skin, and the skin is separated. The ribcage is cut mediolaterally to expose the heart. (**b**) Diagram depicting the point and angle of needle insertion into the heart. The needle is inserted into the right ventricle to collect the blood. (**c**) Leukoreduction filter is attached to a 10-mL syringe, and the collected blood is filtered into a new 15-mL tube

13. Attach a whole blood cell leukoreduction filter to the tip of a 10-mL syringe.
14. Transfer the collected blood and let it drip through the filter. Do not use the syringe plunger to push out the blood left on the filter after filtration (Fig. 2c).
15. Centrifuge the leukoreduced blood at 1200× *g* for 10 min.
16. Adjust the hematocrit level to 75% by pipetting out a portion of the supernatant from the tube.
17. Store the collected blood at 4 °C for 12 days.

3.3 Naïve CD4+ T Cell Purification for Adoptive Transfer

1. All steps should be followed using aseptic technique to ensure sterile conditions.
2. Unless noted differently, all steps should be performed on ice and all reagents should be sterile and kept cold.
3. Euthanize a CD45.1 OT-II double reporter mouse, take out spleen, and put it in a petri dish with cold PBS.
4. Place a cell strainer on top of a 50-mL conical tube. Transfer the spleen to the strainer.
5. To dissociate the splenocytes, press and mash the spleen against the strainer using the flat end of a 3-mL syringe plunger.
6. Add 1 mL of PBS to wash the plunger, and keep the splenocytes from drying out.

7. Repeat this action (**steps 5** and **6**) until most of the tissue has gone through the strainer (*see* **Note 12**).
8. Discard the cell strainer.
9. Centrifuge at 500× *g* for 10 min, discard the supernatant, and resuspend cells in 1 mL of RBC lysis buffer.
10. Incubate for 10 min on ice, and then, add 9 mL of PBS to dilute the RBC lysis buffer.
11. Centrifuge at 500× *g* for 10 min, discard the supernatant, and resuspend the cells in 5–10 mL of PBS.
12. Filter the cell suspension into a new 50-mL conical tube using a new cell strainer.
13. Count the cells, and use the desired number of cells for $CD4^+$ T cell purification (*see* **Note 16**).
14. Purify the naïve $CD4^+$ T cells using Naïve $CD4^+$ T Cell Isolation Kit, according to the manufacturer's instructions (*see* **Notes 13–15**) (Fig. 3a).
15. Collect the cells in 15-mL conical tube and centrifuge at 500× *g* for 10 min.
16. Discard the supernatant, and proceed to $CD4^+$ T cell purification using $CD4^+$ T Cell Isolation Kit, according to the manufacturer's instructions (*see* **Notes 14** and **15**) (Fig. 3a).
17. Take 100–200 μL of the cell suspension, and stain the cells to check cell purity (Fig. 3b).
18. Take the desired number of cells, and transfer them to a new conical tube (*see* **Note 17**).
19. Wash the cells with PBS by centrifuging the tube for 10 min at 500× *g*, discarding the supernatant, and resuspending the pellet in 10 mL of PBS.
20. Centrifuge the cells again for 10 min at 500× *g*, discard the supernatant, and resuspend the pellet in the desired volume of PBS needed for adoptive transfer.
21. Take an aliquot of 200 μL of the cell suspension, and determine the cell count in 100 μL on the Attune NxT flow cytometer.
22. If necessary, adjust the total volume of the cell suspension ensuring the cell number in 100 μL of the cell suspension is as close to 10,000 as possible.
23. Retro-orbitally inject 100 μL of the cell suspension per recipient mouse (see Subheading 3.4).
24. Two days after the adoptive transfer of $CD4^+$ T cells, transfuse WT recipients with 100 μL of stored HOD blood (volume equivalent to 1 unit of packed RBCs in humans) via retro-orbital injection (see Subheading 3.4).

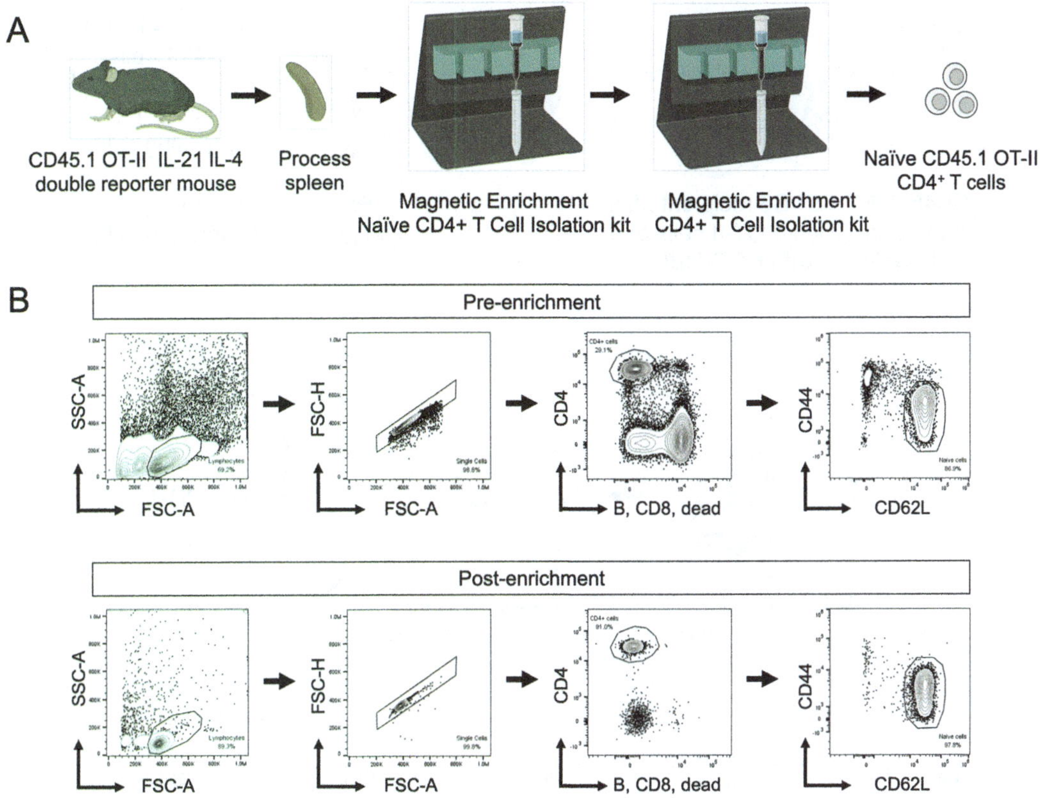

Fig. 3 Naïve $CD4^+$ T cell adoptive transfer into recipient mice. (**a**) Naïve $CD4^+$ T cells are purified from the spleens of CD45.1 OT-II IL-21-Katushka/IL-4-GFP double reporter mice using manual magnetic labeling and separation of cells. Two steps of purification are performed: Naïve $CD4^+$ T Cell Isolation, followed by $CD4^+$ T Cell Isolation. (**b**) Gating strategy for the identification of $CD4^+$ cells and assessment of their purity and naïve state via flow cytometry

3.4 Retro-orbital Injection of $CD4^+$ T Cells or RBCs

1. Anesthetize the recipient mouse.
2. Attach a blunt needle to 1-mL syringe.
3. Pipette the cell suspension up and down slowly to resuspend them avoiding air bubble formation.
4. Replace the blunt needle with 30G needle.
5. Insert needle 2–3 mm into the retro-bulbar space, and inject 100 μL of the cell suspension, as described previously [23].

3.5 Collection of Splenocytes from Transfusion Recipients

1. Euthanize WT recipients 3, 4, and 7 days after transfusion, harvest their spleens, and process them to obtain single-cell suspension (see Subheading 3.3, steps 3 through 13) (Fig. 4a).

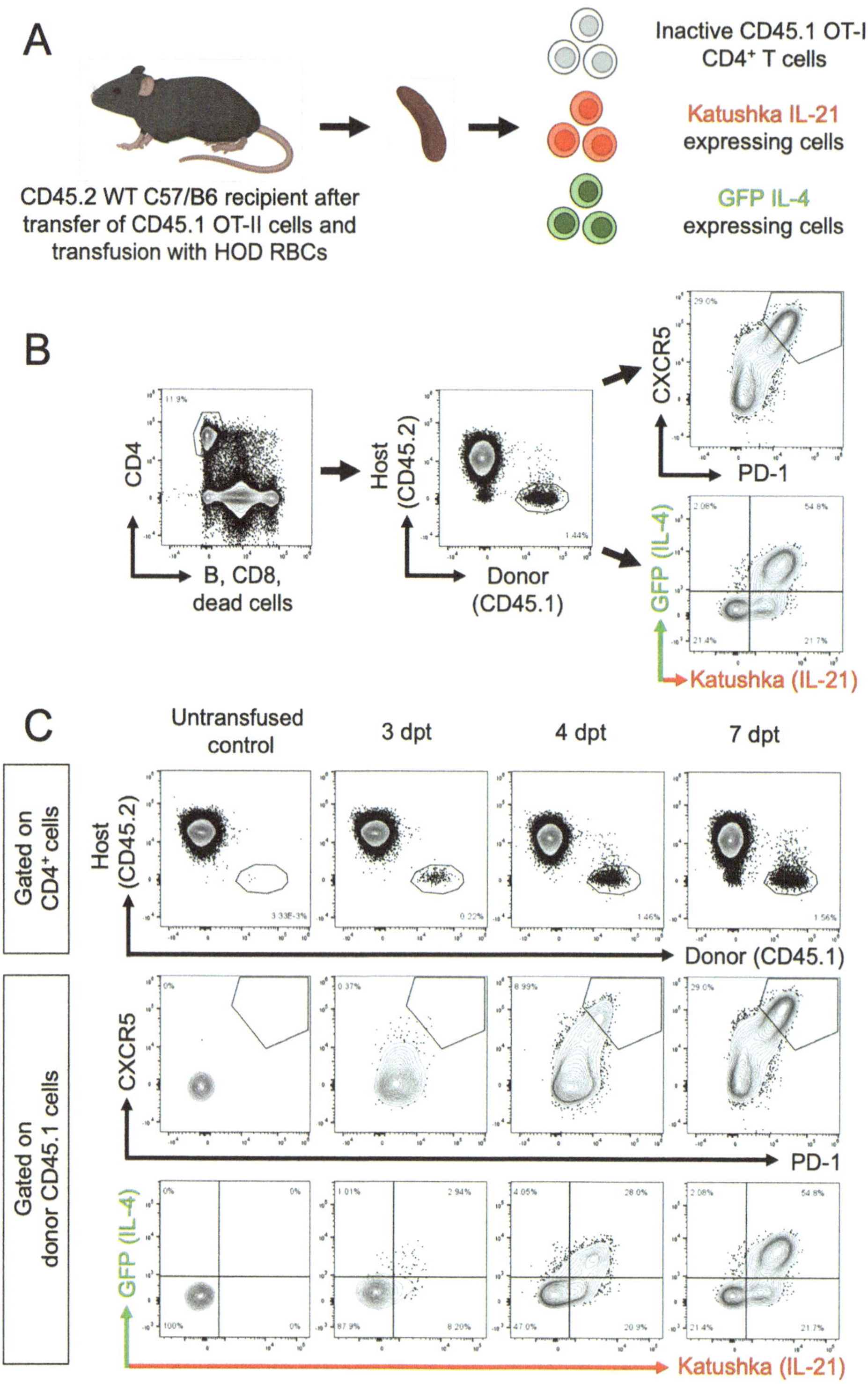

Fig. 4 HOD-specific CD4$^+$ T cell expansion, TFH differentiation, IL-21-Katushka, and IL-4-GFP expression in adoptively transferred CD4$^+$ T cells after transfusion of HOD RBCs. (**a**) Spleens from WT C57/B6 recipient mice are collected and processed. Splenocytes are stained and analyzed using flow cytometry. (**b**) Gating strategy for distinction of host (CD45.2) and donor (CD45.1) CD4$^+$ T cells, identifying CXCR5$^+$ PD-1$^+$ cells, as well as Katushka- and GFP-expressing cells. (**c**) Representative flow plots of CD4$^+$ T cells obtained from untransfused

3.6 Staining of Splenocytes for Flow Cytometry

1. Use ten million splenocytes for staining. All the staining steps are performed in the dark.
2. Stain the splenocytes with the Zombie Yellow™ Dye diluted in PBS for 10 min at 4 °C.
3. Stain the splenocytes with Biotin Rat Anti-Mouse CXCR5 antibody diluted in 10% FBS in PBS for 20 min at 37 °C.
4. Wash the cells twice with FACS buffer.
5. Stain the splenocytes with Biotin Goat Anti-Rat Ig antibody in FACS buffer for 20 min at room temperature.
6. Wash the cells twice with FACS buffer.
7. Subsequently, stain the cells with a master mix containing the following antibodies diluted in FACS buffer: Streptavidin BV421, PD-1 APC, CD45.1 PE/Cy7, CD45.2 PerCP/Cy5.5, CD4 APC/Cy7, B220 BV605, and CD8 BV605 for 20 min at room temperature.
8. Wash splenocytes 3 times with FACS buffer, resuspend them in FACS buffer, and analyze using an Attune NxT flow cytometer and FlowJo Software (*see* **Notes 18–20**) (Fig. 4b).

4 Notes

1. To allow ready detection of fluorescent reporters, we have found that the IL-4-GFP knock-in gene can be heterozygous, while the IL-21-Katushka knock-in gene needs to be homozygous. It should be noted that both reporters are knocked-in just after the stop codons of both genes to avoid disruption of cis-regulatory elements in the 3' UTR and the polyadenylation signal, and their presence appears to not disrupt normal IL-4 and IL-21 expression.
2. While others have done blood collection from donor mice using either terminal retro-orbital bleed or cardiac blood collection by puncturing the heart without opening the thoracic cavity [24], we have found that using these non-sterile techniques occasionally results in bacterial contamination. To minimize the risk of contamination, we prefer to collect blood in the sterile field after surgically opening the thoracic cavity.
3. When filling the syringe with CPDA-1, consider that the needle itself holds roughly 100 μL liquid.

Fig. 4 (continued) controls or splenocytes collected 3, 4, and 7 days after transfusion. The percentage of donor HOD-specific $CD4^+$ T cells increases over time, as well as the expression level of TFH-specific markers CXCR5 and PD-1, Katushka, and GFP expression

4. In order to yield the largest volume of blood possible, it is important that mice are euthanized one by one and that cardiac blood is collected within 5 min of death. It is helpful if the mouse is placed in a chamber already saturated with CO_2.
5. When the endocardial tissue blocks the blood draw, rotate the syringe in your hand to release the tissue from the needle tip.
6. Each mouse typically yields 500–1000 μL of blood, females and younger mice yielding less blood.
7. Consider putting 100–200 μL of CPDA-1 in the 15-mL conical tube before adding collected blood. This step is optional.
8. This step is to ensure no CPDA-1 is lost in the needle, and the final CPDA-1 percentage is 20%.
9. Estimate the total volume of blood that needs to be collected ahead of time. This is determined empirically. Assume 1 mL loss of volume in the leukoreduction filter. Assume the percentage of packed RBCs after filtration will be less than 40% due to 20% CPDA-1 mixed with the collected cardiac blood. For example, for the transfusion of 20 mice, the total volume of blood mixed with CPDA-1 should typically be 6 mL.
10. The total volume of collected blood should not exceed 8 mL due to leukoreduction filter capacity. If more than 8 mL of blood needs to be collected, split it between 2 leukoreduction filters.
11. Aliquot desired volume of CPDA-1 into 1.7-mL sterile tube ensuring the final CPDA percentage is 20%. For example, if 6 mL of cardiac blood needs to be collected, aliquot 1200 μL of CPDA-1. At the end of cardiac collection, total blood volume, which consists of collected blood and CPDA-1, should be 6 mL.
12. It is expected for some connective tissue to remain on the strainer.
13. Naïve $CD4^+$ T cell Isolation Kit should be used before $CD4^+$ T cell Isolation Kit. Counterintuitively, isolating naïve $CD4^+$ T cells before total $CD4^+$ T cells yields the best results in terms of $CD4^+$ T cell purity.
14. To achieve optimal $CD4^+$ T cell purity in the shortest possible time using manual magnetic separation, LS columns are recommended.
15. If the purity is lower than expected after $CD4^+$ T cell isolation, consider incubating splenocytes with the biotin–antibody cocktail and microbeads at room temperature instead of in the refrigerator (for reference, see the manufacturer's instructions included in the Naïve $CD4^+$ or $CD4^+$ T Cell Isolation kits).

16. The number of splenocytes that should be used for $CD4^+$ T cell purification is determined empirically and depends on the number of recipient mice. For example, ten million total splenocytes typically yield 500,000 cells containing 90–96% of $CD4^+$ T cells.
17. When adjusting the cell number and volume for the injection of enriched $CD4^+$ T cells, assume that there is 25% loss of cells after each centrifugation step.
18. As soon as the staining procedure is completed, proceed with the analysis on the flow cytometer. Delaying the analysis might interfere with the reporter expression.
19. It is necessary for the cells to be run live. Fixing the cells prior to analysis diminishes reporter expression.
20. Pre-TFH and TFH cells are commonly identified by their relative expression of CXCR5 and PD-1, with pre-TFH cells expressing intermediate levels of PD-1 and CXCR5, while germinal center-localized TFH cells express the highest expression of CXCR5 and PD-1.

Acknowledgments

This work has been supported by grants to Chance John Luckey from National Institutes of Health (NIH) (R01 HL134691 and P01 HL132819). Some of the graphic illustrations and all of Fig. 1 were created with BioRender.com.

Conflicts of Interest This study was funded by the NIH grant R01HL134691. The authors have no conflicts of interest to declare that are relevant to the content of this chapter.

References

1. Arthur CM, Stowell SR (2023) The development and consequences of red blood cell alloimmunization. Annu Rev Pathol Mech Dis 18:537–564. https://doi.org/10.1146/annurev-pathol-042320-110411
2. Rollins MR, Chou ST (2022) Adverse events of red blood cell transfusions in patients with sickle cell disease. Transfus Apher Sci 61: 103557. https://doi.org/10.1016/j.transci.2022.103557
3. Tormey CA, Hendrickson JE (2019) Transfusion-related red blood cell alloantibodies: induction and consequences. Blood 133: 1821–1830. https://doi.org/10.1182/blood-2018-08-833962
4. Desmarets M, Cadwell CM, Peterson KR, Neades R, Zimring JC (2009) Minor histocompatibility antigens on transfused leukoreduced units of red blood cells induce bone marrow transplant rejection in a mouse model. Blood 114:2315–2322. https://doi.org/10.1182/blood-2009-04-214387
5. Stowell SR, Girard-Pierce KR, Smith NH, Henry KL, Arthur CM, Zimring JC, Hendrickson JE (2013) Transfusion of murine red blood cells expressing the human KEL glycoprotein induces clinically significant alloantibodies. Transfusion. https://doi.org/10.1111/trf.12217

6. Crotty S (2019) T follicular helper cell biology: a decade of discovery and diseases. Immunity 50:1132–1148. https://doi.org/10.1016/j.immuni.2019.04.011
7. Eisenbarth SC, Baumjohann D, Craft J, Fazilleau N, Ma CS, Tangye SG, Vinuesa CG, Linterman MA (2021) CD4+ T cells that help B cells—a proposal for uniform nomenclature. Trends Immunol 42:658–669. https://doi.org/10.1016/j.it.2021.06.003
8. Wellford SA, Schwartzberg PL (2024) Help me help you: emerging concepts in T follicular helper cell differentiation, identity, and function. Curr Opin Immunol 87:102421. https://doi.org/10.1016/j.coi.2024.102421
9. Seth A, Craft J (2019) Spatial and functional heterogeneity of follicular helper T cells in autoimmunity. Curr Opin Immunol 61:1–9. https://doi.org/10.1016/j.coi.2019.06.005
10. Yin X, Chen S, Eisenbarth SC (2021) Dendritic cell regulation of T helper cells. Annu Rev Immunol 39:759–790. https://doi.org/10.1146/annurev-immunol-101819-025146
11. Roco JA, Mesin L, Binder SC, Nefzger C, Gonzalez-Figueroa P, Canete PF, Ellyard J, Shen Q, Robert PA, Cappello J et al (2019) Class-switch recombination occurs infrequently in germinal centers. Immunity 51: 337–350.e7. https://doi.org/10.1016/j.immuni.2019.07.001
12. Zimring JC, Hendrickson JE (2008) The role of inflammation in alloimmunization to antigens on transfused red blood cells. Curr Opin Hematol 15:631–635. https://doi.org/10.1097/MOH.0b013e328313695e
13. Medved J, Knott BM, Tarrah SN, Li AN, Shah N, Moscovich TC, Boscia AR, Salazar JE, Santhanakrishnan M, Hendrickson JE et al (2021) The lysophospholipid-binding molecule CD1D is not required for the alloimmunization response to fresh or stored RBCs in mice despite RBC storage driving alterations in lysophospholipids. Transfusion. https://doi.org/10.1111/trf.16554
14. Hendrickson JE, Hod EA, Spitalnik SL, Hillyer CD, Zimring JC (2010) Storage of murine red blood cells enhances alloantibody responses to an erythroid-specific model antigen. Transfusion 50:642–648. https://doi.org/10.1111/j.1537-2995.2009.02481.x
15. Maier CL, Jajosky RP, Patel SR, Verkerke HP, Fuller MD, Allen JW, Zerra PE, Fasano RM, Chonat S, Josephson CD et al (2023) Storage differentially impacts alloimmunization to distinct red cell antigens following transfusion in mice. Transfusion 63:457–462. https://doi.org/10.1111/trf.17251
16. Calabro S, Gallman A, Gowthaman U, Liu D, Chen P, Liu J, Krishnaswamy JK, Nascimento MSL, Xu L, Patel SR et al (2016) Bridging channel dendritic cells induce immunity to transfused red blood cells. J Exp Med 213: 887–896. https://doi.org/10.1084/jem.20151720
17. Arneja A, Salazar JE, Jiang W, Hendrickson JE, Zimring JC, Luckey CJ (2016) Interleukin-6 receptor-alpha signaling drives anti-RBC alloantibody production and T follicular helper cell differentiation in a murine model of red blood cell alloimmunization. Haematologica. https://doi.org/10.3324/haematol.2016.149278
18. Barnden MJ, Allison J, Heath WR, Carbone FR (1998) Defective TCR expression in transgenic mice constructed using cDNA-based alpha- and beta-chain genes under the control of heterologous regulatory elements. Immunol Cell Biol 76:34–40. https://doi.org/10.1046/j.1440-1711.1998.00709.x
19. Ettinger R, Kuchen S, Lipsky PE (2008) The role of IL-21 in regulating B-cell function in health and disease. Immunol Rev 223:60–86. https://doi.org/10.1111/j.1600-065X.2008.00631.x
20. Bélanger S, Crotty S (2016) Dances with cytokines, featuring TFH cells, IL-21, IL-4 and B cells. Nat Immunol 17:1135–1136. https://doi.org/10.1038/ni.3561
21. Weinstein JS, Herman EI, Lainez B, Licona-Limón P, Esplugues E, Flavell R, Craft J (2016) TFH cells progressively differentiate to regulate the germinal center response. Nat Immunol 17:1197–1205. https://doi.org/10.1038/ni.3554
22. Shulman Z, Gitlin AD, Weinstein JS, Lainez B, Esplugues E, Flavell RA, Craft JE, Nussenzweig MC (2014) Dynamic signaling by T follicular helper cells during germinal center B cell selection. Science 345:1058–1062. https://doi.org/10.1126/science.1257861
23. Yardeni T, Eckhaus M, Morris HD, Huizing M, Hoogstraten-Miller S (2011) Retro-orbital injections in mice. Lab Anim 40:155–160. https://doi.org/10.1038/laban0511-155
24. Retro Orbital, Tail and Intra-cardiac Blood Collection in Rodents (Video) | JoVE https://www.jove.com/v/10246/retro-orbital-tail-and-intra-cardiac-blood-collection-in-rodents

Chapter 36

Defining the Role of Dendritic Cells in Red Blood Cell Alloimmunization

Matthew R. Thakur, Emily M. Flowers, Stephanie C. Eisenbarth, and Adam Williams

Abstract

Storage of red blood cells (RBCs) increases the incidence of alloimmunization following transfusion. Mouse transfusion models have revealed the central role that splenic dendritic cells (DCs) play in storage-dependent RBC alloimmunization. The use of flow cytometry, immunofluorescence imaging, and T-cell proliferation assays combined with various genetically modified mouse strains has provided a detailed understanding of the processes by which DCs instruct the generation of alloantibodies. We and others have established a sequence of events in which transfused stored RBCs are taken up by splenic DCs, resulting in their activation and subsequent migration into T-cell zones. Once there, DCs drive MHCII-dependent T-cell activation and eventually alloantibody production. Herein, we described various methods that allow for the investigation of DC function in the context of alloimmunization.

Key words Dendritic Cells, Alloimmunization, Transfusion, Adaptive Immunity, Innate Activation, DC Migration, T Cell Priming

1 Introduction

Red blood cell (RBC) transfusion is one of the most practiced clinical procedures and is especially important for patients with sickle cell anemia or beta thalassemia who require chronic transfusions. Occasionally, transfusion recipients can generate allogeneic immune responses against transfused blood, even when the blood is appropriately sterile and ABO type matched. This antibody response, termed alloimmunization, can have potentially fatal consequences if the patient is transfused again with the same allogeneic blood, leading to an acute hemolytic transfusion reaction. Importantly, alloimmunization is more prevalent within populations requiring frequent transfusion. RBC alloimmunization occurs in 3–10% of the general population and up to 50% of chronically transfused patients [1–4]. There are currently no therapeutic

Sean R. Stowell and Connie M. Arthur (eds.), *Methods in Transfusion Medicine*, Methods in Molecular Biology, vol. 3053, https://doi.org/10.1007/978-1-0716-5376-0_36,

interventions to prevent RBC alloimmunization due to transfusion, other than screening blood units to minimize the potential for alloreactivity before transfusion. This can delay transfusion for chronically transfused groups. Given the large number of transfusions occurring every year in the United States and their potentially fatal consequences, thorough investigations into the mechanisms that regulate alloimmunization are greatly needed.

In the United States, on average, it is estimated that blood units are stored for 18 days before transfusion [5]. Using mouse models, we and others have shown that transfusion of stored but not fresh blood results in dendritic cell (DC) activation and alloantibody production. During storage, blood units accumulate a variety of metabolic and oxidative changes collectively referred to as the storage lesion [6]. These molecular changes include the release of various damage-associated molecular patterns (DAMPs), which have the potential to activate DCs and other innate immune cells. DAMP activation occurs through pattern recognition receptors (PRRs) on immune cells, which detect molecular moieties indicative of cellular damage or pathogens [7].

DCs are the bridge between innate and adaptive immunity and are required for alloantibody responses. Dendritic cells can be divided into multiple subsets, including plasmacytoid DCs (pDCs), conventional DCs (cDCs), monocyte-derived DCs (moDCs), and Langerhans cells [8]. pDCs are known to be potent producers of type I interferons, which are required for alloimmunization in some mouse models [9]. cDCs can be further subdivided into type 1 (cDC1s) and type 2 (cDC2s). In mice, cDC1s and cDC2s are differentiated by the former's expression of XCR1 and preference for priming $CD8^+$ T cells and the latter's expression of 33D1 and preference for priming $CD4^+$ T cells. While cDC1 and cDC2 populations are both activated during allogeneic transfusion, only cDC2s are required for alloantibody generation [10]. So far, moDCs and Langerhans cells have not been implicated in alloimmunization. To connect innate sensing and adaptive immune activation, DCs possess many innate PRRs, which allow them to sense and respond to inflammatory signals. They also possess several phagocytic and endosomal receptors, allowing them to acquire antigens for MHC processing. In the spleen, where alloimmunization occurs, murine pDCs and cDCs can be found in blood-exposed regions such as the bridging channel, allowing them direct access to transfused RBCs.

We have used multiple analytical techniques to investigate the role that DCs play in alloimmunization (Fig. 1). After transfusion with immunostimulatory stored blood, flow cytometry analysis of splenocytes can be used to measure innate activation of DCs by quantifying the level of costimulatory molecules on their surface. We and others have observed that transfusion of immunostimulatory RBCs activates DCs, as evident by an increase in costimulatory

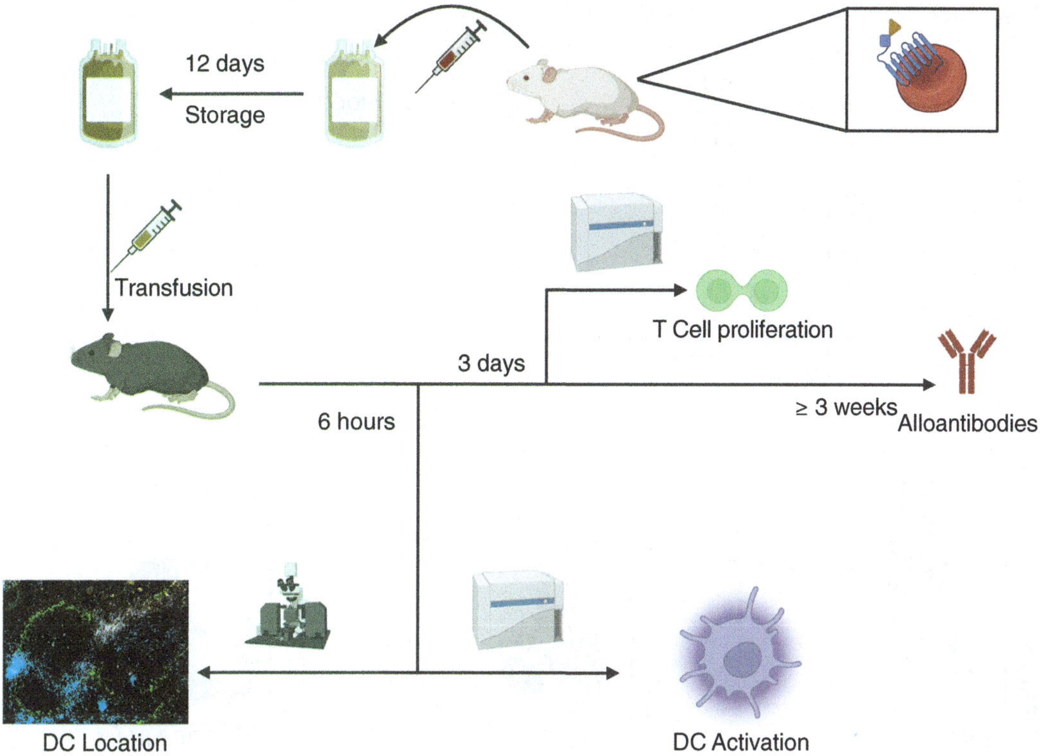

Fig. 1 Graphical overview of methods. Blood is collected from transgenic HOD mice, possessing a model foreign antigen, and stored for 12 days before transfusion into C57BL/6 recipients. The recipient response can be measured at 6 h for DC activation and migration, at 3 days for T-cell activation, or at 3 weeks for alloantibody responses. (Created with BioRender.com under agreement number AL272Q6XAZ)

surface molecules such as CD86, while transfusion of non-immunostimulatory blood does not (Fig. 2) [11]. Transfusion of fluorescently labeled RBCs can be analyzed by flow cytometry to measure the uptake of RBCs by different cell subsets. Using this method, we have observed that DCs uptake fluorescently labeled RBCs [10]. Immunofluorescence staining of splenic sections can also be done to observe the localization of DCs after transfusion (Fig. 3). Consistent with what is known about DCs, we have observed that DCs migrate into the T-cell zone of the spleen following transfusion with stored blood [12]. Activation of cDC2s with LPS 1 h prior to transfusion causes the DCs to migrate into T-cell zones and out of blood-exposed regions and prevents alloimmunization [10]. In these systems, T-cell activation by DCs can be measured both in vivo and in vitro by measuring the proliferation of CFSE-labeled T cells. Serum antibodies specific to foreign antigens on transfused RBCs can be measured from recipients 3 weeks after transfusion as an indicator of alloimmunization (Fig. 4).

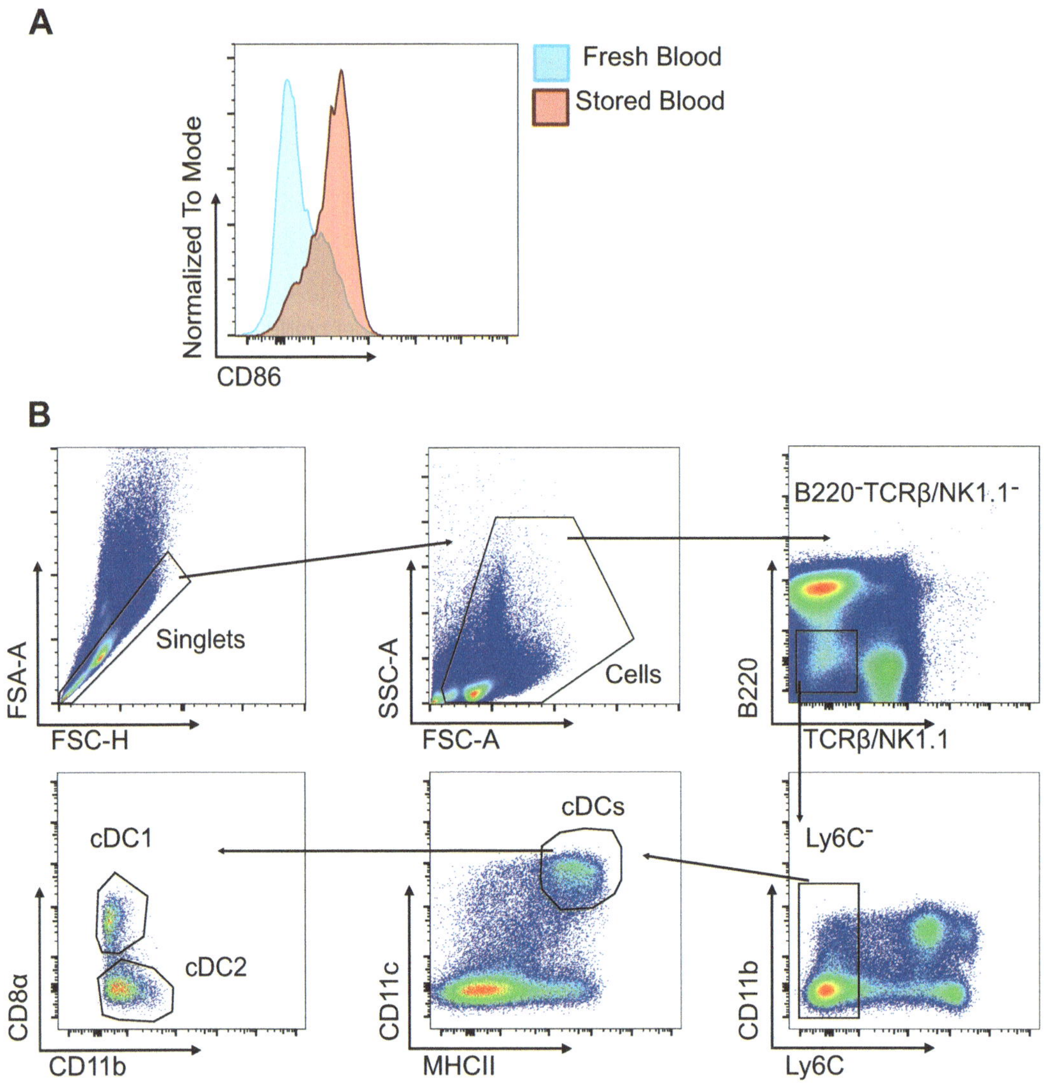

Fig. 2 (**a**) Representative histogram of DC activation 6 h post-transfusion with stored blood. (**b**) Flow cytometry gating for **a**

To support mechanistic studies, numerous genetically modified mouse strains are available that lack specific DC subsets or have differently impaired DC function. These strains, when used in combination with the methods described herein, can provide great insight into the role that DCs play in adaptive immune responses in the spleen. For example, mice which lack the ability to generate cDC2s fail to develop alloantibody responses following transfusion [10]. In addition, the use of mice in which DC migration is genetically impaired led to the discovery that DC migration is necessary for mice to develop antibodies to immunostimulatory blood [12]. Herein, we describe the methodology for these techniques.

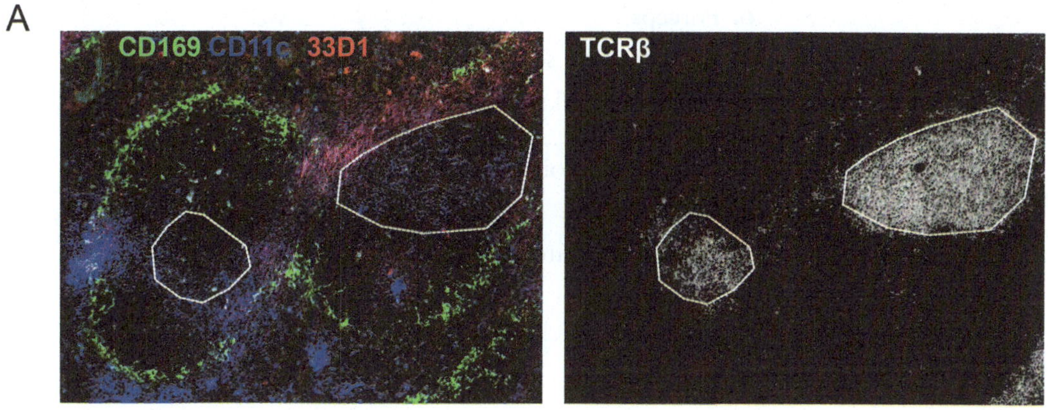

Fig. 3 Representative image of immunofluorescence staining of a spleen 6 h post-transfusion with stored blood using OCT preservation methods

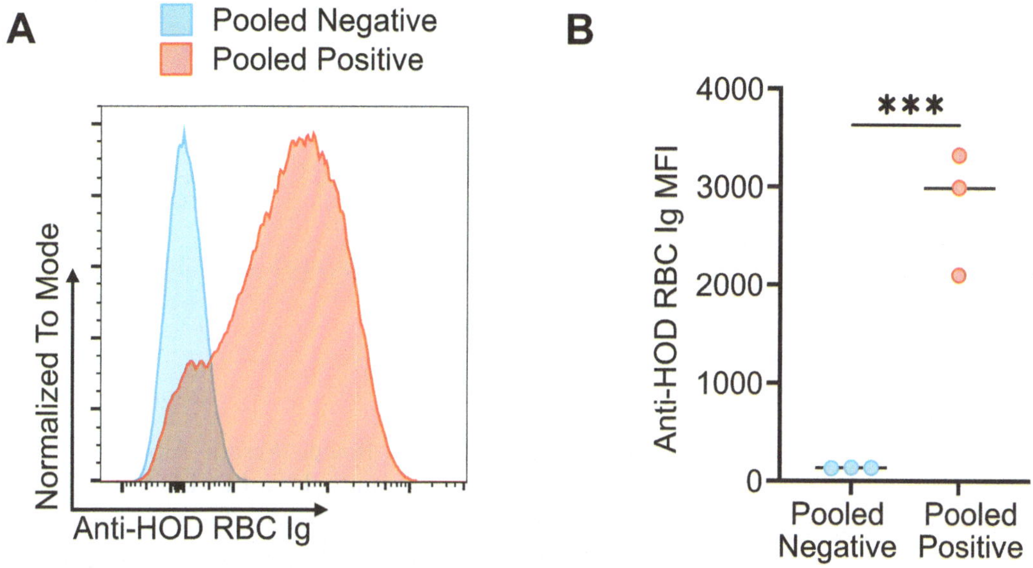

Fig. 4 Representative histogram of HOD-specific antibody levels 3 weeks post-transfusion with stored blood. Pooled positive and pooled negatives from standardization in subheading "Optional: Standardization of the Crossmatch Assay to Allow Qualitative Comparison between Experiments" are shown. (**a**) Mean fluorescence intensity (MFI) values for **a**

2 Materials

2.1 Materials for the Collection, Storage, and Transfusion of Blood

2.1.1 Sterile Blood Collection

1. CPDA-1 solution (Jorgensen Laboratories).
2. 3 mL syringes.
3. 22-gauge needles.
4. 70% EtOH.
5. Isoflurane (Covetrus).

6. Forceps.
7. 2× dissection scissors.
8. 50 mL conical vial.

2.1.2 Blood Leukoreduction and Storage

1. Leukoreduction filter (Pall).
2. 5 mL syringe.
3. Zipocrit hematocrit capillary tubes (Drummond).
4. Microfuge.
5. Clay.
6. Parafilm wax.
7. Eppendorf tubes.

2.1.3 Transfusion

1. 50 mL conical vial.
2. 1 mL syringe.
3. 22–24-gauge needles.
4. 26–27-gauge needles.
5. Isoflurane (Covetrus).
6. Propylene glycol (Sigma).

2.2 Methods for General Analyses of DC Function and Activation

2.2.1 Flow Cytometry Analysis of Spleen

1. Isoflurane (Covetrus).
2. Forceps.
3. Dissection scissors.
4. Eppendorf tubes.
5. FACS buffer
   (a) PBS (Gibco) with 2% Bovine Serum Albumin (BSA) (Fisher Bioreagents) and 1 mM EDTA (Quality Biological).
   (b) Allow BSA to dissolve (usually takes a few minutes) then sterile filter and store at 4 °C.
6. 100 um mesh (Fisher Brand).
7. DAPI (Sigma).
8. FACS tubes.
9. Razor blades (do not need to be sterile).
10. RBC lysis buffer (Biolegend).
11. For CD86 staining we use the following clone: GL-1 (Biolegend).

2.2.2 Cryopreserved Immunofluorescence Analysis of Spleen

1. PBS (Gibco).
2. Sucrose (Sigma).
3. Tissue-Tek Cryomold (15 mm × 15 mm × 5 mm).

4. OCT (Fisher Healthcare).
5. Washing Solution (~50 μL per section).
   (a) 100 mL 1× PBS (Gibco).
   (b) 1 g Bovine Serum Albumin (BSA) (Fisher Bioreagents) → Final Solution Concentration 1%.
   (c) 100 μL Tween 20 (MP biomedicals) → Final Solution Concentration 0.1%.
6. Blocking Solution (~50 μL per Section)
   (a) 4.5 mL Washing Solution.
   (b) 500 μL Rat Serum → Final Solution Concentration 10%.
7. PAP Pen.
8. ProLong Gold Antifade (with or without DAPI).
9. Fisher Tissue Path Superfrost Plus Gold Microscope Slides.
10. Square Cover Slips 18 mm × 18 mm.
11. Kimwipes.
12. Forceps.
13. 1.3% PFA (Azer Scientific).

2.2.3 FFPE Immunofluorescence Analysis of Spleen

1. Coplin jars for rehydration.
2. 10% formalin (Fisher Chemical).
3. CitriSolv (Decon Laboratories).
4. Paraffin (Paraplast X-tra, Lecia Biosystems).
5. Cassette (Fischer Healthcare).
6. Hot plate.
7. Forceps.
8. Base mold.
9. Histology grade EtOH—dilute in MilliQ water as needed.
10. IHC Antigen retrieval (AR) solution (Invitrogen).
11. Washing Solution (*see* Subheading 2.2.2, **item 5**).
12. Blocking Solution (*see* Subheading 2.2.2, **item 6**).
13. PAP Pen.
14. ProLong Gold Antifade.
15. Square Cover Slips 18 mm × 18 mm.
16. Fisher Tissue Path Superfrost Plus Gold Microscope Slides.

2.2.4 In Vivo RBC-Uptake Measurements

1. *See* Subheadings 2.1 and 2.2 for materials.
2. GFP-UBC mice.

2.3 Materials for Investigating the Role of DCs in T-Cell Activation

2.3.1 In Vitro T-Cell Proliferation

1. 70 um mesh (Fisher Brand).
2. Pan DC Isolation Kit (Miltenyi Biotec).
3. PBS (Gibco).
4. Glutaraldehyde (Sigma Aldrich).
5. Glycine (Sigma).
6. DC media (RPMI) (ATCC) with: 10% FBS (Gibco), 1% L-glutamine (Gibco), 1% sodium pyruvate (Gibco), 1% MEM-NEAA (Gibco), 1% pen/strep (Gibco), 55 μM 2-mercaptoethanol (Corning).
7. OTI/OTII mice.
8. EasySep Mouse CD4$^+$ T-cell isolation kit (StemCell).
9. FACS buffer (*see* Subheading 2.2.1, **item 5** for recipe).
10. Forceps.
11. Syringe (any kind).
12. 100 um mesh (Fisher Brand).
13. EasySep Mouse CD4$^+$ T-cell isolation kit.
14. CFSE working solution.
    (a) 5 μL CFSE (Invitrogen) + 10 mL PBS (Gibco).
15. FBS (Gibco).
16. RPMI complete medium (500 mL high glucose RPMI (ATCC) with: 10% FBS (Gibco), 1% Pen/Strep (Gibco), 1% L-Glutamine (Gibco), 10 mM HEPES (Gibco), 1 mM Sodium Pyruvate (Gibco), 0.05 mM beta-Mercaptoethanol (Gibco)).
17. Hemacytometer (Hausser Scientific).

2.3.2 In Vivo T-Cell Proliferation

See Subheadings 2.1, 2.2.1, and 2.3.1 for reagents.

2.4 Materials for Investigating the Role of DCs in Alloimmunization

2.4.1 Measurement of the Alloimmune Antibody Response by Crossmatch

1. 3 mL syringe with 26–27-gauge needles.
2. FACS buffer (*see* Subheading 2.2.1, **item 5** for recipe).
3. Anti-Ig antibody (we use a goat anti-mouse antibody from BD Pharmingen, catalog number: 550826).

3 Methods

3.1 Methods for the Collection, Storage, and Transfusion of Blood

These procedures have been developed to mimic the clinical methodologies for the collection, storage, and handling of human blood. Blood is collected sterilely and leukoreduced to remove white blood cells (as is done clinically). Blood is handled according to clinical guidelines and stored in a medical-grade refrigerator.

3.1.1 Sterile Blood Collection

1. Draw ~300 μL of anticoagulant citrate-phosphate-dextrose-adenine (CPDA-1) solution into 3 mL syringes—will need 1 needle for every 2 mice.
2. Spray down operating area with 70% EtOH.
3. Euthanize mouse with 100% isoflurane (*see* **Notes 1** and **2**).
4. Quickly place mouse on its back, and liberally coat its abdomen with EtOH.
5. Using sterilized forceps and scissors, cut open abdomen but not ribcage.
6. Using fresh sterilized scissors, cut open ribcage until the heart is visible, being careful not to cut the heart.
7. Insert CPDA loaded needle into the right atrium of the beating heart and draw blood until the liver turns lighter pink/gray (*see* **Note 3**).
8. Combine blood from all mice into one sterile 50 mL conical vial at room temperature, making sure that CPDA remains at least at 13% by volume (*see* **Note 4**).
9. Immediately proceed to Subheading 3.1.2.

3.1.2 Blood Leukoreduction and Storage

1. Perform all steps at room temperature.
2. In a biosafety cabinet, sterilely filter blood using a syringe and leukoreduction filter by removing the syringe plunger, attaching the filter, placing onto a blood collection tube, and loading the blood into the open syringe.
3. Allow the blood to drip through the filter. Do not use the syringe plunger to apply pressure (*see* **Note 5**).
4. After filtration is complete, centrifuge blood at 750 × g for 5 mins.
5. The blood should separate into 2 phases; remove as much of the upper CPDA + plasma layer as possible, until only a thin film remains (*see* **Note 6**).
6. Mix the blood and the remaining CPDA + plasma and follow **steps** 7–**9** to measure the adjusted hematocrit.
7. Collect mixed blood in a capillary tube and block the bottom end of the tube with clay.
8. Using a hematocrit microfuge, spin the capillary tube for 2 min.
9. Determine the hematocrit using the hematocrit graph.
10. Repeat **steps 5–9**, adding or removing CPDA + plasma as needed until hematocrit reads 60–70% (*see* **Note 7**).

11. Aliquot blood into sterile 700 μL Eppendorf tubes, and seal with parafilm. Minimal air space should be left in the tube.
12. Store at 4 °C (*see* **Note 8**).

3.1.3 Transfusion

1. Perform all steps at room temperature.
2. Remove HOD blood from tubes and combine in a 50 mL conical vial, being careful to avoid the generation of bubbles. Do not adjust hematocrit before transfusion.
3. Before the RBCs can settle, draw up HOD blood into 1 mL syringes (*see* **Notes 9** and **10**).
4. Anesthetize mouse (*see* **Note 11**).
5. Retro-orbitally (RO) inject 150–200 μL of HOD blood per mouse.
6. Monitor recovery and keep mouse warm until it wakes up from anesthesia (*see* **Note 12**).
7. After transfusion, use the recipient mice in the assays in Subheadings 3.2, 3.3, and 3.4 as described below (*see* **Note 13**).

3.2 Methods for General Analyses of DC Function and Activation

To analyze DC activation, one can perform flow cytometry on the splenocytes of transfused mice. DC activation can be evaluated by measuring upregulation of the activation marker CD86. We have observed that activation increases from 1 to 6 h after transfusion and decreases thereafter (Fig. 2).

3.2.1 Flow Cytometry Analysis of Spleen

1. 6 h post-transfusion, euthanize a mouse with 100% isoflurane as described in Subheading 3.1.
2. Remove the spleen through the left flank and immediately place it in cold FACS buffer (*see* materials for recipe) on ice.
3. Dissociate the spleen by finely chopping with a razor, then resuspend in 2 mL of FACS buffer and filter through 100 um mesh (*see* **Notes 14–16**).
4. Centrifuge at 700 × g for 3 min to pellet cells (slower can work if needed) and pour off supernatant.
5. Resuspend one sample at a time in 500 μL of cold (4 °C or on ice) RBC lysis buffer (*see* materials Subheading 2.2.1) (*see* **Note 17**).
6. Incubate for approximately 2 min on ice and then neutralize with 2 mL of FACS buffer (*see* **Note 17**).
7. Centrifuge at 700 × g for 3 min at 4 °C to pellet cells (slower can work if needed) and pour off supernatant.
8. Resuspend in 1 mL FACS buffer and filter again through mesh.

Table 1
Antibodies tested for use in DC investigations using flow cytometry of splenocytes

Target	Clone	Dilution
CD11c	N418	1:200
MHCII	M5/114.15.2	1:800
B220	RA3-6B2	1:300
CD11b	M1/70	1:400
CD86	GL-1	1:200
33D1	33D1	1:200

9. Cells can now be aliquoted into a 96-well plate or tubes for staining.
10. Stain with desired flow cytometry antibodies in FACS buffer. Antibodies and dilutions may vary, but an example panel is presented in Table 1:
11. * Optional step: Prior to washing steps DAPI live/dead stain can be included: add DAPI at 1 ug/mL in FACS buffer and incubate cells for 5 min at 4 °C in the dark.
12. Wash cells: add 150 μL of FACS buffer, resuspend cells, spin at 700 × g for 3 mins, and then decant the supernatant.
13. Wash twice more (3 times total).
14. Resuspend cells in 150 μL of FACS buffer and transfer to FACS tubes.
15. Add 150 μL of FACS buffer.
16. Analyze samples by flow cytometry.

3.2.2 Cryopreserved Immunofluorescence Analysis of Spleen

One of the primary functions of splenic DCs is to help activate naïve T cells, and to do this, they must migrate to the T-cell zones of the splenic white pulp. We have used immunofluorescence to observe DC movement, which is apparent 6 h after transfusion (Fig. 3). We have had more success using cryopreservation to prepare spleen sections, but formalin fixation and paraffin embedding (FFPE) can be used as well.

1. Harvest the spleen as in Subheading 3.2.1, except collect the spleen in cold PBS. Keep at 4 °C throughout.
2. Cut the spleen in half along the transverse axis (shorter axis).
3. Fix with ~1.3% PFA for 4–6 h (*see* **Note 18**).

4. To dehydrate and cryoprotect tissue, transfer to sequential solutions of sucrose diluted in PBS:
   (a) 10% sucrose in PBS for at least 1 h.
   (b) 20% sucrose in PBS for at least 1 h.
   (c) 30% sucrose in PBS for at least 1 h (overnight if possible).
5. Mount tissue in a cryomold with optimal cutting temperature (OCT) compound over a bed of dry ice as follows:
   (a) Dry the spleen with a Kimwipe and put some OCT in the mold.
   (b) Put the cut face of the tissue facing down in the mold so that it will be trimmed during sectioning (*see* **Note 19**).
   (c) Freeze over dry ice or liquid nitrogen (*see* **Note 20**).
6. Store mounted tissue at −80 °C until further processing.
7. Using a cryostat, cut into 5 mm sections and place on glass microscope slides at −19 °C.
8. Keep slides in −80 °C freezer until ready to stain; preferably cut slides within one week of use.
9. Remove slides from −80 °C freezer and warm to room temperature for approximately 15 min.
10. Rehydrate slides by submerging in a PBS bath for 20 min at room temperature (*see* **Note 21**).
11. Dry slide slightly and draw circles around tissue with PAP pen.
12. Block with 50 μL Blocking Solution (see materials for recipe) for 20 min in a humidified chamber (*see* **Note 22**).
13. Tap slides while above absorbent pads to remove Blocking Solution.
14. Add 50 μL of primary antibodies mixed in Washing Solution (see materials for recipe) per tissue section.
15. Cover slides in humidified chamber and incubate for 1 h at room temperature.
16. Tap off antibody solution as before and wash 3 times with 50 μL of Washing Solution for 10 min each. Alternatively, wash 3 times in separate baths of Washing Solution using Coplin jars or other staining jars for 10 min each.
17. Tap slide dry or blot with a cotton bud (without touching the tissue) and add 50 μL of secondary antibodies mixed in Washing Solution.
18. Cover slides in humidified chamber and incubate for 1 h at room temperature.
19. Tap off antibody solution as before and wash 3 times with 50 μL of Washing Solution for 10 min each.

20. If needed, add tertiary antibodies and wash as with primary and secondary antibodies.
21. Wash slides by submerging in a dark, covered PBS bath on a shaker for 10 min at room temperature.
22. Remove slides from the PBS bath and tap/blot off any excess PBS as above.
23. Allow slides to dry slightly in a dark chamber and then add 1 drop of ProLong Gold Antifade to each tissue section (*see* **Note 23**).
24. Place cover slip onto antifade such that no air bubbles are created (*see* **Note 24**).
25. Store prepared slides in 4 °C fridge in the dark until imaging (*see* **Note 25**).

3.2.3 FFPE Immunofluorescence Analysis of Spleen

FFPE immunofluorescence can be used to observe the same migration of DCs as seen with OCT immunofluorescence. FFPE has additional advantages for use in spatial transcriptomic analyses but requires different antibodies and handling procedures.

1. Remove spleen as in Subheading 3.2.1 and keep cold (4 °C).
2. Bisect the spleen along the transverse axis to increase the rate of fixation.
3. Fix spleen in 4 °C 10% neutral buffered formalin (or 4% paraformaldehyde) as soon as possible (*see* **Notes 26** and **27**).
4. After fixation for 12–24 h at 4 °C, replace formalin with 70% EtOH by washing 2 times with an equal volume of EtOH, then storing the tissue fully submerged in 70% EtOH.
5. Store at 4 °C until further processing (*see* **Note 28**).
6. Dehydrate the spleen prior to clearing and paraffin embedding:
   (a) Place spleens into a cassette. Then, place the cassette into a beaker filled with 70% EtOH at room temperature. Use a sufficient volume of alcohol to fully submerge the cassettes.
   (b) After 15 min, replace the 70% EtOH with 80% EtOH.
   (c) After 15 min, replace the 80% EtOH with 95% EtOH.
   (d) After 15 min, replace the 95% EtOH with 100% EtOH.
   (e) Wash with 100% EtOH 2 more times at 15-min intervals.
7. After the final 15-min interval, replace the 100% EtOH with CitriSolv solution.
8. Wash 2 times with CitriSolv at 15-min intervals.
9. Place the tissue cassettes into a bath of 60 °C paraffin—this is generally accomplished in a tissue embedding machine's

warming chamber. However, if that is not available, paraffin can be melted in a water bath for the embedding steps.

10. After 1 h, move the tissue to a fresh 60 °C paraffin bath.
11. To embed the tissue with an embedding machine:
    (a) Place a base mold under a paraffin dispenser tap.
    (b) Remove the cassette from the paraffin tank, temporarily place on hot plate, and open.
    (c) Dispense a small amount of paraffin into the base mold, enough to cover the base of the dimple.
    (d) Using hot forceps, transfer spleens into the dimple of base mold and orient as necessary.
    (e) Remove the base mold from the hot plate and place on a room temperature surface for 10–30 s to allow paraffin to harden just enough to set the spleens in place inside the dimple.
    (f) Place cassette on top of base mold without the lid.
    (g) Dispense paraffin until both base mold and cassette are covered. Optionally, set the base mold on top of the hot plate briefly (for approximately 5 s—no more) to let the previously hardened paraffin layer at the bottom mix with the fresh paraffin layer on top.
    (h) Leave mold with cassette on top of a cold plate or at room temperature to solidify. After thoroughly cooling, remove the block from the base mold—if the block does not readily release from the mold, place the block and mold at −20 °C overnight.
12. Section tissue as follows:
    (a) Place the paraffin block at −20 °C overnight—cold blocks generally section more cleanly.
    (b) Cut 5–7 micrometer sections with a microtome.
    (c) Use charged slides for better adhesion if tissue is prone to detaching while staining.
    (d) Dry the section overnight in a ventilated area (drying oven, 37 °C warm room, or benchtop). Ensure the slides are fully dry before storing at room temperature for future staining.
13. When ready to stain tissue sections, begin by heating antigen retrieval (AR) reagents (*see* **step 17**).
14. Bake slides at 60 °C for 30 min to adhere tissue sections onto the slide more securely.

15. Deparaffinize spleen sections by washing in a Coplin jar filled with the following:
    - (a) 2 washes in CitriSolv for 5 min each.
    - (b) 1 wash in 100% EtOH for 5 min.
    - (c) 2 washes in 95% EtOH for 5 min each.
16. Leave spleens in PBS to rehydrate pending antigen retrieval, and exchange PBS after antigen retrieval if the slides are placed back in the Coplin jar to remain hydrated.
17. Perform AR:
    - (a) Heat Coplin jars of DI water and AR solution to 99 °C prior to antigen retrieval.
    - (b) Dip slides in preheated DI water for 10 s (Note: for spatial transcriptomics this needs to be DEPC water).
    - (c) Submerge in 99 °C AR solution for 15 min.
    - (d) Return to PBS Coplin jar with fresh PBS.
18. Block with 10% FBS or rat serum in Washing Solution (Blocking Solution, see materials for recipe).
    - (a) Circle sections with a PAP pen.
    - (b) Apply a 10% serum solution and incubate at 4 °C for 45 min.
19. Stain:
    - (a) Tap Blocking Solution off slides, but do not rinse.
    - (b) Apply 50 μL of Primary antibodies in Washing Solution for each tissue section and incubate in the dark at 4 °C for 45 min.
    - (c) Tap stains off the slides.
    - (d) Wash 2 times with Washing Solution, 5 min each at 4 °C.
    - (e) Wash in a PBS bath for 5 min at 4 °C.
    - (f) Apply Secondary antibodies in Washing Solution with 50 μL per section and incubate in the dark at 4 °C for 45 min.
    - (g) Wash as above (two 5-min washes in Washing Solution, one 5-min wash in PBS bath at 4 °C).
20. Remove excess PBS without allowing the tissue to dry.
21. Apply 1 drop of desired mounting media (*see* **Note 29**).
22. Apply coverslip on top of the slide.
23. Store slides lying flat in the dark pending imaging. Store at 4 °C if not imaging within a few hours.
24. We have found that certain antibodies work best with FFPE sections, and others work best with OCT sections. Below is a table of which antibodies we have found to work with each method (*see* **Note 30**) (*see* Table 2).

Table 2
Antibodies tested for use in cryopreserved and FFPE splenic biopsies

Antigen	Clone	Fluorophore or biotin	Cryosection Fresh Spleen	FFPE Spleen
CD11c	A20	AF647	Yes	No
CD169	MCA847F	FITC	Yes	No
TCR beta	H57-597	APC	Yes	No
CD19	60MP31	–	Untested	No
aSMA	1A4	AF488	Yes	Yes
B220	RA3-6B2	BV421	Yes	Yes
CD3	17A2	AF647	Yes	Yes
CD79b	EPR6861	AF594	Yes	Yes
XCR1	ZET	AF647	Yes	No
BCL6	K112-91	–	Untested	No
BLIMP1	5E7.	–	Untested	No
kappa LC	RMK-45	–	Untested	No
CD138	300506	–	Untested	No
CD20	L26	efluor 615	Untested	Yes
PCNA	PC10	Biotin	Yes	Yes
33D1	33D1	AF647	Yes	No

3.2.4 *In Vivo RBC-Uptake Measurements*

DCs must first phagocytose RBCs to become activated and present RBC antigens to T cells. Transfusion on GFP-labeled RBCs into mice allows for flow cytometric detection of RBC phagocytosis by DCs. Generally, around 10–20% of DCs in the spleen will be GFP positive 30 min post-transfusion. At later time points only limited GFP signal is detectable, potentially due to its degradation following uptake by phagocytic cells.

1. This protocol uses RBCs from mice that express GFP under the control of the human ubiquitin C promoter (*see* Table 3).
2. Collect and leukoreduce RBCs from these GFP mice as in Subheadings 3.1.1 and 3.1.2.
3. Transfuse GFP blood into non-GFP expressing recipients as in Subheading 3.1.3.
4. After 30 min, harvest spleens as in Subheading 3.2.1.
5. Prepare cells for and perform flow cytometry as in Subheading 3.2.1, leaving the GFP channel open.

Table 3
Mouse strains useful for investigating the role of dendritic cells in alloimmunization

Mouse strain	Effect	Insights into DC function	Additional notes
Zbtb46-DTR bone marrow chimera—Jackson Labs Strain #019506	Eliminates cDCs upon addition of DT.	Allows the acute ablation of cDCs.	Injection of Diphtheria toxin (DT) into Zbtb46-DTR mice is lethal. Bone marrow from Zbtb46-DTR donor mice needs to be injected into lethally irradiated B6 recipients. For transient DC depletion in Zbtb46-DTR bone marrow chimeric mice inject DT intraperitoneally (IP) on day 0 followed by a second dose on day 2 [note: each batch of DT must be titrated].
CD11c-DTR Jackson Labs Strain #004509	Eliminates $CD11c^+$ cells on addition of DT (which includes DCs).	Allows the acute ablation of DCs. Ablation of a more broad DC population than with Zbtb46-DTR.	For transient DC depletion inject DT IP on day 0 followed by a second dose on day 2 [note: each batch of DT must be titrated].
Dock8$^{fl/fl}$ conditional knockout [13]	Impairs migration of cDC2s.	Can investigate the migration of cDC2s specifically.	Must be crossed to a relevant cre such as a CD11c cre (Jackson Labs Strain #008068).
Myd88$^{-/-}$ Jackson Labs Strain #009088	Eliminates most TLR canonical signaling (except TLR3).	Can observe the effect of TLR signaling in DCs and other cells.	
Trif$^{-/-}$ Jackson Labs Strain #005037	Eliminates TLR3 signaling.	Can observe the effect of TLR3 signaling in DCs and other cells.	
Batf3$^{-/-}$ Jackson Labs Strain #013755	Eliminates cDC1s.	Can observe the function of cDC1s in alloimmunization.	
Irf4$^{fl/fl}$ conditional knockout Jackson Labs Strain #009380	Eliminates cDC2s.	Can observe the function of cDC2s in alloimmunization.	Must be crossed to a relevant cre such as a CD11c cre (Jackson Labs Strain #008068).
Ccr7$^{-/-}$ Jackson Labs Strain #006621	Eliminates DC migration.	Can determine the requirement of DC migration into secondary lymphoid follicles during alloimmunization.	Caveats include altered secondary lymphoid structure.

(continued)

Table 3 (continued)

Mouse strain	Effect	Insights into DC function	Additional notes
GFP-UBC Jackson Labs Strain #004353	GFP labels all cells (including erythrocytes).	Can transfuse into recipients to observe cell populations which phagocytose RBCs.	Importantly, the HOD antigen is not required for 6 h activation of DCs.
OTI Jackson Labs Strain #003831	All $CD8^+$ T cells are OVA specific.	Can isolate $CD8^+$ T cells and test the ability for DCs to induce proliferation in vivo and in vitro.	
OTII Jackson Labs Strain #0041944	All $CD4^+$ T cells are OVA specific.	Can isolate $CD4^+$ T cells and test the ability for DCs to induce proliferation in vivo and in vitro.	

3.3 Methods for Investigating the Role of DCs in T-Cell Activation

3.3.1 In Vitro T-Cell Proliferation

To measure the ability of DCs to activate T-cells post-transfusion, we have isolated DCs 6 h after transfusion from the spleens of recipient mice and cultured them with T cells ex vivo. The HOD antigen contains OVA, which provides a T-cell epitope that the DCs can present. We can therefore measure the activation of OVA specific OT-I/OT-II T cells. Activation is measured by the dilution of CFSE which occurs by the proliferation of T cells, an indication of activation.

1. Collect HOD blood, leukoreduce, and transfuse as in Subheading 3.1.
2. 8 h after transfusion, sacrifice the mouse and quickly remove the spleen as in Subheading 3.2.1 (*see* **Note 31**).
3. Process the spleen as described in Subheading 3.2.1.
4. Purify DCs by using CD11c MACS microbeads following the manufacturer's protocols.
5. Wash once with PBS to remove BSA. Flick the pellet to thoroughly resuspend it in the remaining volume before re-suspending at 5×10^6 cells/mL in ice cold 0.025% glutaraldehyde.
6. Incubate at 4 °C for 3 min.
7. Stop the reaction with an equal volume of 0.2 M glycine and incubate at room temperature for 10 min.
8. Spin down the DCs at $375 \times g$ for 5 min at room temperature, remove supernatant, and add DC media (see materials for recipe).
9. Repeat **step 8** twice more (*see* **Note 32**).

10. Purify OT-I and/or OT-II T cells from OT-I and/or OT-II transgenic mice (*see* Table 3):
    (a) Sacrifice OT-I/OT-II mice and harvest spleens.
    (b) Under sterile conditions, pick up the spleen with sterile tweezers and put it in a 70 um cell filter that is lightly wetted with FACS buffer (with EDTA) and push it through the filter with the back of a syringe.
    (c) Rinse the filter with FACS buffer and grind the residue some more with the back of the syringe and rinse again to maximize cell number, pour it into tubes through a nylon filter.
    (d) Add 2 mL of 4 °C RBC lysis buffer, incubate for 1 min at 4 °C, and then quench with 2 mL of 4 °C FACS buffer.
    (e) Spin cells at 375 × g for 5 min at room temperature, discard the supernatant, and resuspend the cells in 1 mL of FACS buffer.
    (f) Filter cells again through a sterile cell filter.
    (g) Count the cells using a hemocytometer.
    (h) Use the EasySep Mouse $CD4^+$ T-cell isolation kit and follow the directions in the kit to isolate T cells (EasySep buffer = FACS buffer with EDTA) (*see* **Note 33**).
11. CFSE label the OT-I and/or OT-II T cells:
    (a) Count cells.
    (b) Wash cells once by filling the tube with PBS and centrifuging at 375 × g for 5 min at room temperature.
    (c) Resuspend the cell pellet in 10 mL of warm or room temperature PBS (*see* **Note 34**).
    (d) Prepare 10 mL of CFSE working solution by adding 5 μL stock (4 mM) into 10 mL of warm PBS.
    (e) Add 10 mL of CFSE working solution into 10 mL of cell suspension and mix quickly (*see* **Note 35**).
    (f) Incubate mixture for 5 min in a 37 °C water bath in the dark.
    (g) Add 10 mL of pure, cold (4 °C) FBS.
    (h) Spin down cells in centrifuge at 375 × g for 5 min at room temperature.
    (i) Add 10 mL 10% RPMI complete media (see materials for recipe), then centrifuge at 1500 rpm for 5 min at room temperature and decant the supernatant.

(j) Add 10 mL 10% RPMI complete media, then centrifuge at 375 × g for 5 min at room temperature and decant the supernatant.

(k) Resuspend cells in RPMI complete media at the desired concentration (*see* **Notes 36** and **37**).

12. Add the T cells to wells containing DCs and incubate for 72 h at 37 °C in an incubator with 5% CO_2.
13. Remove the cells from the plates and perform flow cytometry as in Subheading 3.2.1, **steps 7–16**. Stain for CD4, CD8, and measure CFSE dilution levels to observe T-cell proliferation.

3.3.2 In Vivo T-Cell Proliferation

The activation of T cells can also be measured in vivo. Because of the T-cell OVA epitope expressed on the surface of HOD RBCs, OVA specific OT-I/OT-II mice can be adoptively transferred to measure T-cell activation similar to the in vitro methods. Again, CFSE dilution indicates T-cell proliferation/activation.

1. Purify OT-I and OT-II T cells from OT-I and OT-II mice and CFSE label as in Subheading 3.3.1.
2. Perform adoptive transfer of these T cells by intravenous infusion into recipient mice.

   (a) We inject 1 × 10^6 cells per mouse by injecting 200 μL RO of a 5 × 10^6 cells/mL solution in PBS.

3. 24 h later, transfuse recipient mice as in Subheading 3.1.
4. 3 days after transfusion, harvest spleens as in Subheading 3.2.1.

   Isolate cells and stain spleens for flow cytometry using anti-CD4 and anti-CD8 antibodies, and measure CFSE dilution levels to observe T-cell proliferation.

3.4 Methods for Investigating the Role of DCs in Alloimmunization

3.4.1 Measurement of the Alloimmune Antibody Response by Crossmatch

To measure the adaptive immune responses of transfused mice, we use a clinically derived crossmatch assay (Fig. 4). This measures the antibodies that can bind to the HOD antigen in the serum of recipients (*see* Table 3), which provides a measurement of the adaptive response. We have found that antibody levels reach a maximum at around 3 weeks after transfusion and then plateau after that.

Crossmatch Procedure

1. Transfuse mice as in Subheading 3.1.
2. 3 weeks after transfusion, collect sera from recipient mice via cardiac puncture (*see* **Notes 38** and **39**).
3. Spin the sera at 1500 × g for 5 min at room temperature to pellet the RBCs.
4. Collect the sera above the pelleted RBCs.

   (a) Sera can be stored at −20 °C.

5. Collect fresh HOD blood from HOD mice sterilely as in Subheading 3.1.1 (*see* **Note 40**).
6. Dilute the fresh HOD blood 2:10 in FACS buffer.
7. Dispense 10 μL of diluted HOD blood into the well of a 96-well plate, with 1 well per sample.
8. Add 3.3 μL of sera from the sample to each well.
9. Mix the samples by vortexing for 5 s.
10. Incubate for 30 min at room temperature.
11. Wash 3 times with 150 μL of FACS buffer at room temperature. Spin at 750 × g for each wash.
12. Add APC-conjugated anti-Ig antibody at 1:100 in 100 μL of FACS buffer to each well and mix gently by pipetting (*see* **Note 41**).
13. Incubate for 30 min at room temperature.
14. Wash 3 times with 150 μL of FACS buffer at room temperature. Spin at 750 × g for each wash.
15. Resuspend RBCs in 50 μL of FACS buffer, dilute as needed (see below), and run on a flow cytometer (*see* **Note 42**).
16. Higher fluorescence of the anti-Ig antibody indicates more alloimmunization (*see* **Note 43**).

Optional: Standardization of the Crossmatch Assay to Allow Qualitative Comparison between Experiments

1. Create a pooled positive sera from transfused wild-type mice. There is significant variability in antibody titer, so 10+ mice from different transfusions is preferable.
2. Select a geometric mean for the pooled positive that will be used in every experiment:
   (a) Stain 3 wells of RBCs with the pooled positive sera as described above (3 technical replicates). Stain 1 well with negative sera from a naïve mouse, or a pooled negative.
   (b) Run pooled positive RBCs on your preferred cytometer and observe the histogram of stained RBCs. If your cytometer software allows, show sample statistics and display the geometric mean of the sample.
   (c) Adjust the voltage of your staining channel until you reach the desired geometric mean for a positive sample.
   (d) The pooled positive's geometric mean should be in the middle of where you expect a positive sample to be, as the pooled positive is an average of many mice with higher and lower titers.
   (e) Run the RBCs with naïve/pooled negative sera and confirm that there is good separation between the geometric means of the positive and negative samples.

(f) Confirm that all three technical replicates of the pooled positive have similar geometric means. If there is variability, repeat staining and correct for any inaccuracies in pipetting or mixing.

(g) Record the desired geometric mean for future reference.

3. For each experiment, stain one well of RBCs with the pooled positive sera.
4. Before acquiring samples, run the RBCs stained with pooled positive and adjust the cytometer voltage to give the desired geometric mean.
5. Store the pooled positive in small aliquots at −20 °C.

Mouse Strains for Investigating the Role of DCs in Alloimmunization

Different knockout mouse strains and bone marrow chimeras can be used to investigate DC subsets, DC migration, and the mechanisms of DC activation. Crossing of knockouts and generation of mixed bone marrow chimeras could be used to further investigate the simultaneous effects of these factors.

4 Notes

1. Note, do not use CO_2, as this will acidify the blood and cause the heart to fully stop beating by the time death is confirmed.
2. After the moment of death, there are approximately 5 min to collect blood before the heart stops beating.
3. For mice aged 8–12 weeks, males generally give up to 1 mL of blood, and females generally give up to 700 μL.
4. Given the significant sample loss during leukoreduction (described below) we normally process a minimum of 5 mL of blood.
5. It is normal to lose about 1 mL of blood to the filter.
6. When in doubt, remove more CPDA + plasma.
7. If hematocrit is too high, dilute with the appropriate amount of CPDA. If too low, spin again and remove more CPDA + plasma.
8. Storage longer than specified results in loss of intact RBCs and does not accurately model clinical transfusion.
   (a) Wild-type B6 blood should be stored 14 days before transfusion for optimal DC activation.
   (b) HOD-FVB blood should be stored 12 days before transfusion for optimal alloantibody response.
9. Use needle gauge sizes 22–24 to slowly draw up blood and minimize shearing RBCs.

10. Change needles and use needle gauge sizes 26–27 for transfusion.
11. We have found that using isoflurane as an anesthetic agent is more effective than ketamine, as ketamine appears to cause diminished DC activation at 6 h.
12. It is normal for the mouse to have red/brown urine in the hours after transfusion with stored blood.
13. Mice do not experience negative effects from transfusion and may be analyzed at any future time points as needed.
14. Processing the spleen with a razor results in better DC recovery than grinding the tissue between slides.
15. Keep the spleen and cells cold during this process.
16. This process does not need to be sterile unless splenocytes are needed for culture.
17. Work in small batches to prevent cells from sitting in RBC lysis buffer for longer than 2 min.
18. We frequently omit this fixing step because we have found that the background staining with the MOMA antibody decreases drastically with no fixation. Instead, we directly proceed to the sucrose dehydration of the fresh tissue.
19. If the spleen is too large, this orientation may leave some tissue above the level of the mold—either layer a bubble of OCT over the tissue or cut the spleen into quarters, retaining the orientation when the spleen is frozen.
20. Tissue can also be frozen over a bath of 2-methylbutane (isopentane) in liquid nitrogen. The colder temperatures result in more rapid freezing and minimize the risk of forming large ice crystals. However, overly rapid cooling will result in the block cracking. Rapid freezing over 2-methylbutane in liquid nitrogen must be used for fresh tissues (including spleens) that have not been dehydrated in sucrose.
21. Do not let the tissue dry and avoid exposing the samples to light, as both will diminish the quality and quantity of the fluorescence.
22. A humidified chamber can be made by spraying paper towels with water and putting some in the bottom of a closed chamber.
23. If DAPI staining is desired it can be included within the ProLong Gold Antifade, but it is not necessary to observe DC location.
24. It may be helpful to use forceps and lower the coverslip slowly after placing one edge on the antifade mounting medium.
25. Image within 1 week of staining for peak fluorescence.

26. The volume of fixative should be 10–20 times the volume of tissue. For this protocol one mouse spleen can typically be fixed in 1 mL of fixative. Increase fixative volume if unsure.
27. Cardiac perfusion with formalin is not necessary if the spleen is kept cold and placed in cold fixative immediately after dissection. If the spleen is not kept cold hemolysis will occur soon after dissection.
28. Over-fixation can diminish or abolish staining. If validated stains are not working, extend wash times after fixation—allow fixed tissue to sit in EtOH washes for 30–60 min for each wash. This prevents continued fixation while the tissue is stored. Time in fixative may also be shortened. Formalin penetrates tissue at approximately 1 mm/h, meaning mouse spleens may be fixed by immersion for 6 h or less.
29. ProLong Gold or ProLong Glass is recommended to preserve fluorescent signal.
30. Differences may arise with different antigen retrieval methods (*see* Table 2).
31. From this point on everything must be sterile.
32. Alternatively, store the pellet in a small volume at 4 °C and complete the washes before use.
33. We routinely get 2–3 $\times$ 10^6 naïve T cells from one OT-II mouse. Lymph nodes can also be included to increase yields.
34. We stain at 5 $\times$ 10^6 cells per mL.
35. Add solution drop by drop during vortex mixing. This is critical for getting uniform labeling.
36. For in vitro experiments, we plate varying ratios of DCs/T cells in each well (1:1–1:10 DCs/T cell ratio).
37. For in vivo experiments (described in 3.3.2), make a solution with 5 $\times$ 10^6 T cells/mL.
38. Sera does not need to be sterile.
39. Alloantibody levels can be measured prior to 3 weeks, but peak at 3 weeks and maintain that titer for multiple weeks [10].
40. There is no need to leukoreduce this blood (skip Subheading 3.1.2).
41. The assay works for detecting specific isotypes. If desired, replace anti-Ig in this step with a secondary antibody specific for the desired mouse isotype (i.e., anti-IgM or anti-IgG).
42. RBCs are extremely abundant and must be diluted before analysis by flow cytometry. We have found that diluting samples 1:5 (i.e., add 200 μL per sample) before acquisition works well, but higher dilutions may be required.

43. We generally include a negative control sample containing sera pooled from naïve mice and a positive control sample containing sera pooled from mice which have significant antibody responses. These control sera serve as a reference to set the voltages to produce similar fluorescence intensities across experiments, increasing reproducibility (described in greater detail in subheading "Optional: Standardization of the Crossmatch Assay to Allow Qualitative Comparison between Experiments").

Conflicts of Interest

This study was funded in part by the NIH R01HL172760 (S.C.E and A.W). The authors have no conflicts of interest to declare that are relevant to the content of this chapter.

References

1. Tormey CA, Fisk J, Stack G (2008) Red blood cell alloantibody frequency, specificity, and properties in a population of male military veterans. Transfusion (Paris) 48:2069–2076
2. Heddle NM et al (1995) A prospective study to determine the frequency and clinical significance of alloimmunization post-transfusion. Br J Haematol 91:1000–1005
3. Vichinsky EP et al (1990) Alloimmunization in sickle cell anemia and transfusion of racially unmatched blood. N Engl J Med 322:1617–1621
4. Tormey CA, Stack G (2009) The characterization and classification of concurrent blood group antibodies. Transfusion (Paris) 49: 2709–2718
5. Roback JD (2016) Perspectives on the impact of storage duration on blood quality and transfusion outcomes. Vox Sang 111:357–364
6. Tinmouth A, Fergusson D, Yee IC, Hébert PC, ABLE Investigators and the Canadian Critical Care Trials Group (2006) Clinical consequences of red cell storage in the critically ill. Transfusion (Paris) 46:2014–2027
7. Lewis SM, Williams A, Eisenbarth SC (2019) Structure and function of the immune system in the spleen. Sci Immunol 4:eaau6085
8. Yin X, Chen S, Eisenbarth SC (2021) Dendritic cell regulation of T helper cells. Annu Rev Immunol 39:759–790
9. Gibb DR et al (2017) Type I IFN is necessary and sufficient for inflammation-induced red blood cell alloimmunization in mice. J Immunol 199:1041–1050
10. Calabro S et al (2016) Bridging channel dendritic cells induce immunity to transfused red blood cells. J Exp Med 213:887–896
11. Soldatenko A et al (2022) Innate and adaptive immunity to transfused allogeneic RBCs in mice requires MyD88. J Immunol 208:991–997
12. Calabro S et al (2016) Differential intrasplenic migration of dendritic cell subsets tailors adaptive immunity. Cell Rep 16:2472–2485
13. Krishnaswamy JK et al (2017) Migratory CD11b+ conventional dendritic cells induce T follicular helper cell–dependent antibody responses. Sci Immunol 2:eaam9169

Chapter 37

Examination of the Immunological Role of Toll-Like Receptor 9 on Red Blood Cells

Emily A. Oatman, Layal Sayegh, and Nilam S. Mangalmurti

Abstract

Red blood cells (RBCs) were historically regarded as immunologically inert; however, current research has revealed their active participation in the innate immune response through the expression of various surface immune receptors. Notably, the nucleic-acid-sensing receptor toll-like receptor 9 (TLR9) enables RBCs to sequester and scavenge cell-free DNA under basal conditions and to deliver DNA during inflammatory states. Consequently, the presence of TLR9 on RBCs endows them with distinct immune functions. Novel techniques were developed to study the immunological function of red blood cells. This paper delineates the methodologies for detecting TLR9 on mammalian RBCs (murine, human, chimpanzee, and bat) and isolating and preparing murine RBCs for transfusion, as well as for binding CpG DNA oligodeoxynucleotides to RBCs for both in vitro and in vivo studies. These methodologies are crucial for evaluating the contributions of RBCs to the immune response.

Key words Red blood cells, Toll-like receptor 9, Sepsis, Transfusion

1 Introduction

Although red blood cells (RBCs) are the most abundant cell type in the human body [1], they have historically been viewed as passive oxygen carriers, lacking any immunological function. Recently, it has been established that the RBCs play a role in several immune functions [2, 3]. The expression of various surface receptors, including the Duffy antigen receptor for chemokines (DARC, ACKR1), complement receptor 1 (CR1), and the most recently discovered toll-like receptor 9 (TLR9), allows RBCs to actively engage in the innate immune response. Expression of these receptors on RBCs is likely an evolutionarily conserved mechanism, as other mammalian species' RBCs retain these immunomodulatory receptors [2].

Toll-like receptors belong to the class of pattern recognition receptors, which are essential for initiating the innate immune

Sean R. Stowell and Connie M. Arthur (eds.), *Methods in Transfusion Medicine*, Methods in Molecular Biology, vol. 3053, https://doi.org/10.1007/978-1-0716-5376-0_37,

response to pathogen-associated molecular patterns (PAMPs). In addition to sensing PAMPs, these receptors are also able to bind damage-associated molecular patterns (DAMPs) that are elevated during inflammatory or disease states. A subset of these TLRs functions to detect nucleic acids, specifically TLR3 and TLR7-9 [4]. The nucleic acid-sensing TLRs are typically located within the endosome, where they are concealed from activation by self-derived extracellular nucleic acids [5–7]. Specifically, TLR9 detects unmethylated CpG-containing DNA motifs, initiating inflammatory downstream signaling [8]. While mammalian DNA is usually methylated, microbial and mitochondrial DNA are rich in immunostimulatory unmethylated CpG motifs, allowing for the detection of pathogen DNA and mitochondrial DNA (a prototypic DAMP) by TLR9 [9].

Although not previously known to be on erythrocytes, we recently discovered the presence of TLR9 on the surface of mammalian RBCs [10, 11]. This orientation allows for sequestration of extracellular DNA in circulation during basal conditions and inflammatory states. Importantly, RBC TLR9 does not initiate downstream intracellular signaling within the RBC itself but participates in the immune response in an alternative manner by either clearing extracellular DNA or by delivering it to organs to induce downstream signaling and immune activation. The capture of CpG DNA by RBC TLR9 may offer significant advantages to the host because RBC-nucleic acid-binding leads to accelerated erythrophagocytosis and DNA delivery to immune cells, enabling RBCs to function as one of the earliest messengers to trigger critical inflammatory responses essential for host defense. Under basal conditions, RBCs sequester synthetic CpG [12]. However, during inflammatory states when CpG DNA is in excess, its binding by RBCs leads to accelerated RBC senescence characterized by morphologic alterations of the RBC membrane, loss of the marker of self (CD47), and enhanced erythrophagocytosis [10]. These findings suggest that RBCs function as a physiologic rheostat, maintaining homeostasis by scavenging low levels of cell-free CpG DNA under basal conditions but triggering erythrophagocytosis when excess DNA is present, thus delivering DNA to immune cells.

In vitro, DNA binding to RBCs results in accelerated senescence marked by altered RBC morphology and loss of the CD47 antiphagocytic epitope. In vivo, CpG-treated RBCs undergo accelerated erythrophagocytosis that is dependent on RBC-TLR9 [10, 13]. Moreover, infusion of CpG-treated RBCs into naïve mice elicited an interferon-dependent inflammatory response in the spleen. In a reductionist model of CpG-delivery and clinically relevant murine models of polymicrobial sepsis, deletion of RBC-TLR9 resulted in attenuated plasma and spleen inflammatory cytokine production, signifying the critical role of cf-DNA binding and delivery by RBCs in the host inflammatory response [10].

To ascertain the immunological role of TLRs on RBCs, we utilized in vitro and in vivo models, including a mouse model of RBC transfusion. Here, we will provide the methodology for preparing murine RBCs for transfusion, DNA loading RBCs, and a protocol for evaluating erythrophagocytosis. We also describe the methods for detecting TLR9 on human, chimpanzee, murine, and bat RBCs. Utilizing these techniques, we were able to gain insight and understanding into the functional immunological role of TLR9 on RBCs.

2 Materials

2.1 Acquisition of Red Blood Cells

2.1.1 Human and Chimpanzee Red Blood Cells

1. EDTA tubes (Human samples).
2. ACD collection tubes (Chimpanzee samples, BD Biosciences).
3. Swinging bucket centrifuge.

Leukoreduction Filter Isolation

4. Phosphate buffered saline (PBS), pH 8.0.
5. Leukoreduction filters (Acrodisc White Blood Cell Syringe Filter, Pall Medical).

Magnetic Cell Isolation

6. Leibovitz L-15 media.
7. CD235a (Glycophorin A) MICROBEADS, human (Miltenyi Biotec, 130-050-501).
8. LS columns (Miltenyi Biotec, 130-042-401).
9. MidiMACS separator (Miltenyi Biotec, 130-042-302).
10. MACS MULTISTAND (Miltenyi Biotec, 130-042-303).
11. Phosphate buffered saline (PBS), pH 8.0.
12. Hemacytometer.

Ensuring the Purity of Red Blood Cell Isolation

13. Anti-human-CD41 antibody (APC, 150 ug/mL, Clone A2A9/6, BioLegend).
14. Anti-human CD235a (Glycophorin A) antibody (PE, 0.5 mg/mL, BioLegend).
15. FACS buffer (PBS + 2% fetal bovine serum (FBS)).

2.1.2 Murine Red Blood Cells

1. Heparinized 1 mL syringe and 25G needle.
2. Ketamine/Xylazine cocktail (80/10 mg/kg).
3. WT BL6 mice, TLR9KO mice (TLR9 KO mice were produced by S. Akira and provided by E. Behrens (Children's Hospital of Philadelphia)). Mice lacking TLR9 in the erythroid

compartment are generated by crossing ErGFPcre mice (a gift from U. Klingmüller, German Cancer Research Center) and TLR9 KO Conditional (TLR9 flx obtained from the European Mutant Mouse Archive) [14], erythroid TLR9 deleted mice (Ery$^{tlr9-/-}$).

4. 70% Ethanol.
5. Swinging bucket centrifuge.

Leukoreduction Filter Isolation

6. Phosphate buffered saline (PBS), pH 8.0.
7. Leukoreduction filters (Acrodisc white blood cell syringe filter, Pall Medical).

Magnetic Cell Isolation

8. Leibovitz L-15 media.
9. Anti-Ter119 MicroBeads, mouse (Miltenyi Biotec, 130-049-901).
10. LS columns (Miltenyi Biotec, 130-042-401).
11. MidiMACS separator (Miltenyi Biotec, 130-042-302).
12. MACS MULTISTAND (Miltenyi Biotec, 130-042-303).
13. Phosphate buffered saline (PBS), pH 8.0.
14. Hemocytometer.

Ensuring Purity of Red Blood Cell Isolation

15. Anti-mouse CD41 antibody (APC, 0.5 mg/mL, BioLegend).
16. Anti-mouse Ter119 antibody (PE, 0.2 mg/mL, BioLegend).
17. FACS buffer (PBS + 2% FBS).

2.1.3 Bat Red Blood Cells

1. EDTA microcontainers.
2. Swinging bucket centrifuge.
3. Phosphate buffered saline (PBS), pH 8.0.
4. Hemacytometer.

2.2 Red Blood Cell TLR9 Detection with Flow Cytometry

2.2.1 Human Red Blood Cells

1. FACS Buffer (PBS + 2%FBS).

Surface TLR9 Detection

2. TLR9 antibody (FITC, 1ug, Clone 5G5, Abcam).

Intracellular TLR9 Detection

3. 0.05% Glutaraldehyde, EM Grade (Polysciences) in PBS.
4. 0.1% Triton-X 100 in PBS.

5. Anti-human TLR9 antibody (FITC, 10 ug/mL, Clone 26C593.2, Abcam).
6. Anti-human glycophorin A antibody (PE, 10 ug/mL, BioLegend).
7. Anti-human CD41 antibody (APC, 10 ug/mL, BioLegend).
8. Flow cytometer.
9. FlowJo Software (FlowJo, LLC).

2.2.2 Murine Red Blood Cells (Surface TLR9 Detection)

1. FACS buffer (PBS + 2%FBS).
2. TLR9 antibody (FITC, 5ug, Clone 5G5, Abcam).
3. Flow cytometer.
4. FlowJo Software (FlowJo, LLC).

2.3 Red Blood Cell TLR9 Detection with Immunofluorescent Imaging

1. Phosphate buffered saline (PBS), pH 8.0.
2. PKH Membrane Labeling Kit (MIDI26-1KT, Sigma aldrich).
3. 0.05% Glutaraldehyde, EM Grade (Polysciences) in PBS.

2.3.1 Human Red Blood Cells

Surface TLR9 detection

4. TLR9 antibody (20 ug/mL, Clone 5G5, Abcam).

Intracellular TLR9 detection

5. 0.1% Triton-X 100 in PBS.
6. TLR9 antibody (10 ug/mL, ab187148, Abcam).
7. TLR9 antibody (10 ug/mL, Clone 26C593.2, Abcam).
8. Dylight 488 anti-mouse secondary antibody.
9. Dylight 594 anti-rabbit secondary antibody.
10. Charged slides.
11. Fluoromount G (Invitrogen).
12. Confocal microscope.
13. ImageJ software.

2.3.2 Chimpanzee Red Blood Cells (Intracellular Detection)

1. PKH 26 or PKH 67 Membrane Labeling Kits (MIDI26-1KT or MIDI67-1KT, Sigma Aldrich).
2. Surface TLR9 and CD47 co-detection.
3. CD47 antibody (10 ug/mL, Clone 2D3, eBioscience).
4. TLR9 antibody (10 ug/mL, ab187148, Abcam).

Intracellular TLR9 Detection

5. 0.05% Glutaraldehyde, EM Grade (Polysciences) in PBS.
6. 0.1% Triton-X 100 in PBS.

7. TLR9 antibody (5 μg/mL, 26C593.2, Novus Biologicals).
8. Dylight 488 anti-mouse secondary antibody.
9. Dylight 594 anti-rabbit secondary antibody.
10. Charged Slides.
11. Fluoromount G (Invitrogen).
12. Confocal Microscope.
13. ImageJ Software.

2.3.3 Murine Red Blood Cells

1. PBS + 1% Bovine Serum Albumin (BSA) + 5% Goat serum.
2. FACS buffer (PBS + 2% FBS).

Intracellular TLR9 Detection

3. 0.05% Glutaraldehyde, EM Grade (Polysciences) in PBS.
4. 0.1% Triton-X 100 in PBS.
5. TLR9 antibody (5 ug/mL, ab27154, Abcam).
6. Ter119 antibody (5 ug/mL, Clone ter119, Biolegend).
7. Alexa Fluor 488 goat anti-mouse (Jackson ImmunoResearch).
8. Alexa Fluor 555 goat anti-rabbit (Invitrogen).
9. Fluoromount G (Invitrogen).
10. Charged slides.
11. Confocal Microscope.
12. ImageJ Software.

2.3.4 Bat Red Blood Cells (Intracellular Detection)

1. PBS-T (PBS + 0.05% Tween-20).
2. 0.05% Glutaraldehyde, EM Grade (Polysciences) in PBS.
3. 0.1% Triton-X 100 in PBS.
4. PBS-T + 1% BSA.
5. TLR9 antibody (1:200, Clone 26C593.2, Abcam).
6. Alexa Fluor 488 goat anti-mouse (Jackson ImmunoResearch).
7. Fluoromount G (Invitrogen).
8. Charged Slides.

2.4 Synthetic DNA Binding to Red Blood Cells

2.4.1 Human Red Blood Cells

1. Incubator.
2. FACS buffer (PBS+2%FBS).
3. Binding studies.
4. FITC labeled CpG DNA (ODN2006, 10, 100 pmol per 250,000 cells, IDT).
5. Flow cytometer.
6. CpG DNA (ODN2006, 40,400 pmol per 1×10^6 cells, IDT).

7. CpG DNA representing sequences from *Plasmodium falciparum* (2000 pmol per 1×10^6 cells).
8. TLR9 antibody (FITC, 5ug, Clone 5G5, Abcam).
9. CD47 (APC, 0.5ug, CC2C6, Biolegend) or CD47 (APC, 1ug, Clone 2D3, eBiosciences).
10. Flow cytometer.
11. FlowJo Software (FlowJo, LLC).

2.4.2 Murine Red Blood Cells

1. Phosphate buffered saline (PBS), pH 8.0.
2. Incubator.
3. FACS buffer (PBS + 2% FBS).
4. Binding Studies.
5. FITC Labeled CpG DNA (Invivogen).
6. CpG Pre-Treatment Studies.
7. CpG DNA (ODN1826, 40 or 400 pmol per 1×10^6 cells, IDT).
8. CD47 antibody (PE, 1ug, Clone miap301, Biolegend).
9. Flow cytometer.
10. FlowJo Software (FlowJo, LLC).

2.5 Erythrophagocytosis In Vivo Murine Studies

1. PKH 26 or PKH 67 Membrane Labeling Kits (MIDI26-1KT or MIDI67-1KT, Sigma Aldrich).
2. Dulbecco's Modified Eagle Medium (DMEM).
3. DMEM with 10% Fetal Bovine Serum (FBS).
4. DMEM with 5% FBS.
5. Phosphate buffered saline (PBS), pH 8.0.
6. DNA Lo-Bind tubes.
7. 25 nM CpG (ODN1826, IDT).
8. 25G needle.
9. Mouse restrainer.
10. 70 uM mesh cell filter (Falcon).
11. Scale.
12. ACK RBC lysis solution (Thermo Fisher).
13. Live/Dead Fixable Violet Dead Cell Stain Kit (L34955, Invitrogen).
14. Fc Block (CD16/32, Clone 93, 14-0161-82, Invitrogen).
15. F4/80 (Alexa Fluor 700, Clone BM8, 123130, BioLegend).
16. CD45 (Allophycocyanin (APC), Clone 30-F11, 103112, BioLegend).

17. CD3 (Brilliant violet 711, Clone 145-2C11, 100349, BioLegend).
18. FACS buffer (PBS + 2% FBS).
19. Flow Cytometer.
20. FlowJo Software (FlowJo, LLC).

2.6 Transfusion of CpG DNA Loaded RBCs In Vivo Murine Studies

1. 150 uM 1826 CpG DNA (15,000 pmol per 1×10^9 cells, IDT).
2. Incubator.
3. 25G needle.
4. Mouse restrainer.
5. Phosphate buffer saline (PBS), pH 8.0.
6. DuoSet enzyme-linked immunosorbent assay (ELISA) Assays-IFNγ, IL6, (R&D systems).
7. Formalin.
8. Paraffin.
9. Heparinized syringe and needle, 25G needle with 1 mL syringe.
10. Ketamine/Xylazine cocktail (80/10 mg/kg).
11. WT BL6 mice, TLR9KO mice (Akira), erythroid $TLR9^{-/-}$ mice.
12. 70% ethanol.
13. Swinging bucket centrifuge.

2.7 CpG DNA on RBCs Detection In Vivo

1. PKH 26 or PKH 67 Membrane Labeling Kits (MIDI26-1KT or MIDI67-1KT, Sigma Aldrich).
2. 50 ug/mouse of AF647-labeled CpG DNA (ODN1826, IDT).
3. Mouse restrainer.
4. 25G needle and syringe.
5. Heparinized 25G needle and 1 mL syringe and needle.
6. Ketamine/Xylazine cocktail (80/10 mg/kg).
7. WT BL6 mice, TLR9KO mice (Akira), erythroid $TLR9^{-/-}$ mice.
8. 70% ethanol.
9. RPMI media.
10. 70 um filters (Falcon).
11. Flow cytometer.
12. Leibovitz L-15 media.

13. Anti-Ter119 MicroBeads, mouse (Miltenyi Biotec, 130-049-901).
14. LS columns (Miltenyi Biotec, 130-042-401).
15. MidiMACS Separator (Miltenyi Biotec, 130-042-302).
16. MACS MultiStand (Miltenyi Biotec, 130-042-303).
17. Phosphate buffered saline (PBS), pH 8.0.

3 Methods

3.1 Acquisition of Red Blood Cells

3.1.1 Human and Chimpanzee Red Blood Cells

1. Obtain whole blood from healthy human donors in EDTA tubes or from chimpanzees in ACD tubes. Centrifuge the sample for 10 min at 1500 g with a deceleration of 6. Aspirate the plasma and buffy coat, then proceed to isolation using leukoreduction filters or magnetic cell isolation.

Leukoreduction Filter Isolation *If using magnetic cell isolation, skip to **Step 4**.

2. Resuspend the remaining cell pellet in PBS. Pre-moisten a leukoreduction filter with PBS in a 15 mL conical tube, followed by the resuspended cell pellet, and rinse again with PBS to flush out the remaining cells in the filter (*see* **Note 1**).
3. Following leukoreduction, centrifuge the solution at 800 g for 5 min with a deceleration of 6 and aspirate supernatant. Resuspend the final cell solution in PBS and serially dilute it for manual cell counting using a hemacytometer.

Magnetic Cell Isolation *If using leukoreduction filter isolation, skip to **Step 10**.

4. After spinning and aspirating, take 30 uL of the packed cell pellet to 70 uL of Leibovitz L-15 media and 15 uL of anti-GPA beads, mix well, and incubate at 4 °C for 15 min (*see* **Note 2**).
5. Following incubation, wash the solution with 1 mL of Leibovitz L-15 media, then centrifuge at 300 g for 5 min and remove the supernatant. Resuspend cells in 500 uL of Leibovitz L-15 media.
6. Place the LS column in the MidiMACS separator attached to the MACS MultiStand, and rinse the column with 3 mL of Leibovitz L-15 media. Once the media passes through the column fully, place the 500 uL of resuspended cells into the column. Rinse the column two times with 3 mL of Leibovitz L-15 media.
7. After washing the column twice, remove the LS column from the separator and collect cells by pipetting 5 mL of Leibovitz L-15 media into the column and flushing with the plunger into a 15 mL conical tube.

8. Once collected, spin down cells at 800 g for 5 min with a deceleration of 6, remove the supernatant, and wash cells with 5 mL of PBS.
9. After washing, remove supernatant, washing, remove the supernatant, and resuspend in 1 mL of PBS. Serially dilute the cell solution and proceed to manual cell counting using a hemacytometer.

Testing Purity of Isolation

10. Following RBC isolation, take 1×10^6 cells and wash one time with FACS buffer (PBS + 2%FBS). Incubate cells with anti-human-CD41 antibody (150 ug/mL, Clone A2A9/6, BioLegend) and anti-human CD235a (Glycophorin A) antibody (0.5 mg/mL, BioLegend).
11. Wash cells three times with FACS buffer, then resuspend in 400 uL of FACS buffer and proceed to flow cytometry.

3.1.2 Murine Red Blood Cells

1. Euthanize mice with an intraperitoneal injection of ketamine/xylazine (80/10 mg/kg).
2. Once mice are at a surgical plane of anesthesia, place them in the supine position, clean the chest with 70% ethanol, and perform cardiac puncture with a heparinized 25G needle and 1 mL syringe to collect whole blood.
3. Remove the needle prior to placing whole blood in a tube on ice until processing.
4. Centrifuge whole blood at 1500 g for 10 min with a deceleration of 6 (slow deceleration).
5. After spinning, aspirate the plasma and buffy coat, then proceed to leukoreduction filter isolation or magnetic cell isolation.

Leukoreduction Filter Isolation* If using magnetic cell isolation, skip to **Step 10**.

6. Resuspend the remaining cell pellet in PBS.
7. Pre-moisten a leukoreduction filter with PBS in a 15 mL conical tube, followed by the resuspended cell pellet, and rinse again with PBS to flush out the remaining cells in the filter (*see* **Note 1**).
8. Following leukoreduction, centrifuge the solution at 800 g for 5 min with a deceleration of 6 and aspirate the supernatant.
9. Resuspend the final cell solution in PBS and serially dilute it for manual cell counting using a hemacytometer.

Magnetic Cell Isolation *If using leukoreduction filter isolation, skip to **Step 20**.

10. After spinning and aspirating, take 30 uL of the packed cell pellet to 70 uL of Leibovitz L-15 media and 15 uL of anti-Ter119 beads, mix well, and incubate at 4 °C for 15 min (*see* **Note 2**).
11. Following incubation, wash the solution with 1 mL of L-15 media, then centrifuge at 300 g for 5 min to remove the supernatant.
12. Resuspend cells in 500 uL of Leibovitz L-15 media.
13. Place the LS column in the MidiMACS separator attached to the MACS MultiStand, and rinse the column with 3 mL of Leibovitz L-15 media.
14. Once the media passes through the column fully, place the 500 uL of resuspended cells into the column and allow them to fully pass through the column.
15. Once the cell solution passes through the column, rinse two times with 3 mL of Leibovitz L-15 media, allowing the solution to fully pass through the column each wash.
16. After washing the column twice, remove the LS column from the separator and collect cells by pipetting 5 mL of L-15 media into the column and flushing with the plunger into a 15 mL conical tube.
17. Once collected, spin down cells at 800 g for 5 min with a deceleration of 6, remove supernatant, and wash cells with 5 mL of PBS.
18. After washing, aspirate the supernatant and resuspend in 1 mL of PBS.
19. Serially dilute the cell solution and proceed to manual cell counting using a hemacytometer.

Testing Purity of Red Blood Cell Isolation

20. Following RBC isolation, take 1×10^6 cells and wash one time with FACS buffer (PBS+2%FBS). Incubate cells with anti-mouse CD41 antibody (0.5 mg/mL, BioLegend) and anti-mouse Ter119 antibody (0.2 mg/mL, BioLegend).
21. Wash cells three times with FACS buffer, then resuspend in 400 uL of FACS buffer and proceed to flow cytometry.

3.1.3 Bat Red Blood Cells

1. Collect blood from bats into EDTA microcontainers. Then centrifuge whole blood at 800 g for 5 min, aspirate plasma and buffy coat, then resuspend the cell pellet in 1 mL of PBS for washing.
2. Centrifuge the cells again and remove supernatant as well as a small amount of the packed red blood cells at the top of the pellet. Resuspend in PBS, then serially dilute and count cells using a hemacytometer.

3.2 Red Blood Cell TLR9 Detection with Flow Cytometry

3.2.1 Human Red Blood Cells

1. Follow the leukoreduction protocol above to obtain 1×10^6 isolated RBCs.
2. Wash cells one time with PBS (*see* **Note 3**).

Red Blood Cell Surface TLR9 Detection (Fig. 1)

3. Incubate isolated RBCs in FITC-TLR9 (1 ug, Clone 5G5, Abcam), PE-Glycophorin A, and APC-CD41 (10 ug/mL, BioLegend) antibodies in FACS buffer for 1 h at room temperature.

Red Blood Cell Intracellular TLR9 Detection

4. Fix RBCs using 0.05% EM grade glutaraldehyde for 15 min at room temperature. Following fixation, wash the cells two times using FACS buffer (PBS + 2% FBS).
5. Permeabilize the cells with 0.1% Triton-X 100 for 15 min at room temperature. Wash cells with FACS buffer two times and proceed to staining.
6. Incubate RBCs with mouse monoclonal TLR9 antibody (IgG1,k, 10 ug/mL, Abcam), PE-Glycophorin A, and APC-CD41 (10 ug/mL, BioLegend) for 1 h at room temperature.
7. Following incubation, wash RBCs two times with FACS buffer. Resuspend cells in 400 uL of FACS buffer and proceed to FACS acquisition.

3.2.2 Murine Red Blood Cells (Surface TLR9 Detection) (Fig. 1)

1. Obtain 1×10^6 murine RBCs utilizing the leukoreduction protocol listed above.
2. Wash RBCs one time with PBS (*see* **Note 3**).
3. Incubate RBCs with monoclonal TLR9 antibody (5 ug, Clone 5G5, Abcam) for 1 h at room temperature.

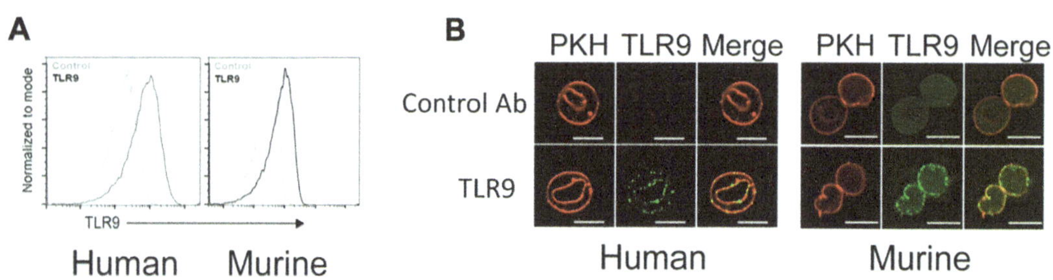

Fig. 1 TLR9 is expressed on the surface of RBCs. (**a**) Flow cytometry of TLR9 expression on nonpermeabilized RBCs is shown. (**b**) Confocal images show TLR9 (green) and PKH 26 (red) in red blood cells (RBCs). Scale bars, 5 μm (Fig. 1a and b, originally published in Lam, Sc Trans Med 2021)

4. Following incubation, wash cells two times with FACS buffer (PBS + 2% FBS), then resuspend in 400 uL of FACS buffer and proceed to FACS acquisition and analysis.

3.3 Red Blood Cell TLR9 Detection with Immunofluorescent Imaging

3.3.1 Human Red Blood Cells

1. Isolate healthy human RBCs either by leukoreduction or magnetic cell isolation as described previously and count to a 1×10^5 concentration.
2. Wash RBCs one time with PBS prior to proceeding with staining.
3. Stain RBCs with PKH membrane dye (PKH MIDI 2601KT, Sigma Aldrich). Label RBCs with either PKH 26 or PKH 67 dye according to the conjugation of TLR9 staining. Stain RBCs with 4 uL PKH dye for 5 min following the manufacturer's protocol.
4. After incubation, stop staining by adding excess Dulbecco's Modified Eagle Medium (DMEM) with 10% fetal bovine serum (FBS) and incubate for 1 min.
5. Centrifuge cells at 800 g for 5 min with a deceleration of 6, then wash two times with DMEM +5% FBS.
6. Resuspend the stained cells in PBS.

Red Blood Cell Surface TLR9 Detection (Fig. 1).

7. Wash cells with PBS, then incubate with TLR9 antibody (10 ug/mL, Clone 5G5, Abcam) overnight at 4 °C (*see* **Note 4**).

Red Blood Cell Intracellular TLR9 and CD47 Co-Detection

8. If staining for TLR9 colocalization with CD47, fix cells with 0.05% glutaraldehyde for 15 min, followed by permeabilization with 0.1% Triton-X in PBS for 15 min (*see* **Note 5**).
9. Wash and incubate in the following antibody solution overnight at 4 °C: CD47 (10 ug/mL, Clone 2D3 eBioscience) and TLR9 (10 ug/mL, ab187148, Abcam).
10. Following incubation, wash cells three times with FACS buffer (2% FBS in PBS). Incubate with Dylight 488 anti-mouse antibody and Dylight 594 anti-rabbit antibody solutions at a 1:200 dilution in FACS buffer for 30 min at 4 °C.
11. Following secondary incubation, wash cells three times with FACS buffer.
12. Mount cells with Fluoromount G on charged slides, allow to dry. Acquire images using a confocal microscope.

3.3.2 Chimpanzee Red Blood Cells (Intracellular TLR9 Detection).

1. Isolate 1×10^5 chimpanzee RBCs as described above. Label RBCs with either PKH 26 or PKH 67 dye as described previously with human RBCs.
2. Fix the cells with 0.05% EM grade glutaraldehyde for 15 min at room temperature (*see* **Note 5**).
3. Wash the cells two times with FACS buffer (PBS + 2% FBS).
4. Permeabilize cells with 0.1% Triton-X in PBS for 15 min at room temperature, then wash cells with FACS buffer.
5. Incubate RBCs with mouse anti-TLR9 antibody (5 μg/mL, 26C593.2, Novus Biologicals) overnight at 4 °C (*see* **Note 6**).

3.3.3 Murine Red Blood Cells (Intracellular Detection)

1. Isolate RBCs using leukoreduction or bead isolation to a concentration of 2.5×10^5 cells per staining reaction, wash cells one time with PBS prior to fixation.
2. Fix the cells with 0.05% EM grade glutaraldehyde for 15 min at room temperature.
3. Wash the cells two times with FACS buffer (PBS + 2% FBS) (*see* **Note 5**).
4. Permeabilize cells with 0.1% Triton-X in PBS for 15 min at room temperature, then wash cells once with FACS buffer.
5. Block cells in PBS + 1%BSA + 5% goat serum for 1 h at room temperature.
6. Incubate cells overnight at 4 °C in TLR9 (5ug/ml, ab37154, Abcam) and Ter119 (5 ug/mL, clone Ter-119, BioLegend) antibodies.
7. Wash cells three times using FACS buffer, then incubate for 1 h at room temperature in the following antibodies diluted to 1: 500 concentrations in PBS + 2% FBS: Alexa Fluor 488 goat anti-mouse (Jackson ImmunoResearch) and Alexa Fluor 555 goat anti-rabbit (Invitrogen).
8. Mount cells onto charged slides using Fluoromount G and allow to dry, then proceed to microscopy.

3.3.4 Bat Red Blood Cells (Intracellular Detection)

1. Obtain 1×10^6 RBCs as written previously. Fix the cells with 0.05% EM grade glutaraldehyde in PBS for 15 min at room temperature. Wash the cells two times with PBS-T (PBS + 0.05% Tween 20). (*see* **Note 5**).
2. Permeabilize cells with 0.1% Triton-X in PBS for 15 min at room temperature, then wash cells twice with PBS-T.
3. Block cells with PBS-T with 1% BSA added for 1 h at room temperature, then pellet the cells at 800 g for 5 min with a deceleration of 6 and remove supernatant.

4. Resuspend the cell pellet in TLR9 (Clone 26C593.2, Abcam) antibody diluted at 1:200 in PBS-T, and incubate overnight at 4 °C (*see* **Note 6**).
5. Following overnight incubation, wash cells three times in PBS-T. After the final wash, incubate in secondary antibody solution diluted in PBS-T for 1 h at room temperature. Then wash three times in PBS-T.
6. Resuspend the cell pellet in 10 uL of PBS, and mount 5 uL of the RBC pellet with 5 uL of Fluorogold G on a charged slide, then seal with a coverslip.

3.4 Synthetic DNA Binding to RBCs

3.4.1 Human RBC DNA Binding (Fig. 2)

1. Isolate RBCs as described above and obtain 250,000 cells for binding studies. Wash cells one time with PBS prior to incubation.
2. Incubate cells with 100 nM or 1uM fluorescein isothiocyanate (FITC) -labeled CpG (ODN2006, 10, 100 pmol per 250,000 cells) for 2 or 4 h with gentle agitation at 37 °C.
3. Following incubation, wash with FACS buffer (PBS + 2% FBS) two times. Resuspend cells in 400 uL of FACS buffer and proceed to FACS acquisition and analysis.
4. Masking of the CD47 antiphagocytic epitope.
5. Incubate one million isolated RBCs for 2 h with gentle shaking at 37 °C with one of the following: 400 nM, 4uM CpG DNA (40, 400 pmol per 10^6 cells, IDT) or 20 uM synthetic CpG DNA representing sequences from *Plasmodium falciparum* (2000 pmol per 1×10^6 cells) or CpG 2006.
6. After DNA binding, wash cells with PBS and proceed to antibody staining. Incubate RBCs with the following antibodies at room temperature for 1 h: mouse monoclonal against CD47

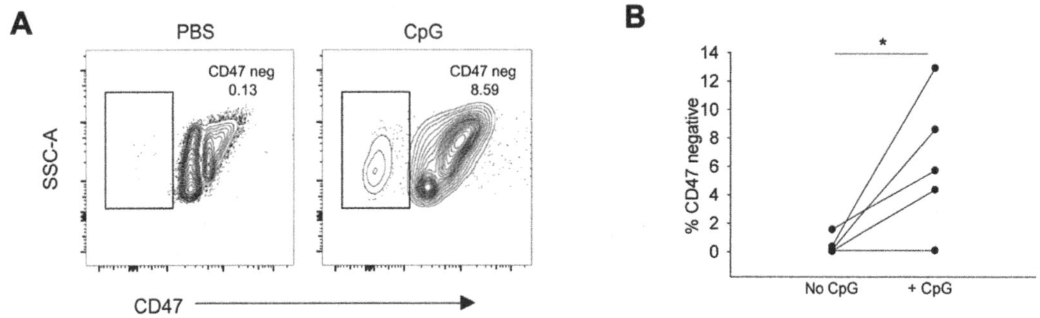

Fig. 2 CpG binding by RBCs leads loss of CD47 detection. (**a** and **b**) Representative results (**a**) and quantification from five donors (**b**) are shown for CD47 detection (with antibody clone CC2C6) on human RBCs after incubation with CpG (10 μg/mL). Data were analyzed by a paired t-test. SSC-A, side scatter area. $^*P < 0.05$ (Fig. 3A and B, originally published in Lam, Sc Trans Med 2021)

(0.5 ug, CC2C6, BioLegend, detects the antiphagocytic epitope) or CD47 (1 ug, Clone 2D3, eBiosciences, detects the "damage" epitope) (*see* **Note 7**).

7. Wash cells twice with FACS buffer, resuspend in 400 uL FACS buffer, then proceed to FACS analysis.

3.4.2 Murine RBC DNA Binding and Masking of the CD47 Antiphagocytic Epitope

1. Obtain 1 × 10^6 murine RBCs using the isolation protocol above. Wash RBCs with PBS prior to DNA binding.
2. Incubate RBCs with either 400 nM or 4uM CpG DNA (ODN1826, 40 or 400 pmol per 1 × 10^6 cells, IDT) for 2 h at t 37 °C with gentle agitation.
3. Wash RBCs two times with PBS following incubation. After washing, incubate cells with phycoerythrin (PE) CD47 (1ug, Clone miap301, BioLegend) diluted in FACS buffer (PBS + 2% FBS) for 45 min at room temperature.
4. Wash cells two times with FACS buffer, then resuspend in 400 uL FACS buffer and proceed to FACS acquisition.

3.5 Erythrophagocytosis In Vivo-Murine Studies

1. Cardiac puncture and process RBCs from WT and TLR9KO mice as described above.
2. Label RBCs with either PKH 26 or PKH 67 dye. For labeling, 2 × 10^9 RBCs are stained with 4 uL PKH dye for 5 min following the manufacturer's protocol and as described in the section "RBC TLR9 Detection with Immunofluorescent Imaging."
3. Suspend either WT or TLR9 KO RBCs as 1 × 10^8 cells per 200 uL solution in DNA lo-bind tubes. Add either PBS or 25 nM CpG (ODN1826, IDT) to the RBC mixture and immediately transfuse the solution to WT or TLR9 KO mice through a tail vein injection using a 25G needle.
4. At 1 h post-transfusion, euthanize mice with ketamine/xylazine (80/10 mg/kg), then harvest and weigh their spleens. Mince the spleens and pass through a 70 um nylon mesh filter to create a single-cell suspension. Once in a single-cell suspension, lyse RBCs using ACK buffer (Thermo Fisher) to obtain only white blood cells (WBCs) in the solution.
5. WBCs are then stained for 30 min at 4 °C with following solutions: Live/Dead Fixable viability violet stain (Invitrogen) diluted at 1:1000 in PBS, Fc block (1:100, CD16/32, clone 93, Invitrogen), and antibody cocktail against F4/80 (Alexa Fluor 700, BM8, BioLegend), CD45 (Allophycocyanin (APC), 30-F11, BioLegend), and CD3 (Brilliant Violet 711, 145-2C11, BioLegend) at 1:200 dilution in FACS buffer (PBS + 2% FBS). Spin the stained cells at 800 g for 5 min with a deceleration of 6 and wash three times with FACS buffer.

6. Proceed to FACS analysis with cells suspended in 500 uL of FACS buffer and gather at least 10,000 events. Analyze data using FlowJo software.

3.6 Transfusion of CpG DNA Loaded RBCs In Vivo Murine Studies

1. Obtain RBCs from WT mice as described previously. Incubate 1×10^9 cells with 150uM of CpG DNA (ODN1826, 15,000 pmol per 1×10^9 cells, synthesized by IDT) for 2 h at 37 °C with gentle agitation. Spin RBCs at 800 g for 5 min with a deceleration of 6 and wash once with PBS.
2. Inject either PBS, RBCs, or CpG-treated RBCs into the recipient mouse's tail vein with a 25G needle. Six-hours post injection, euthanize mice with ketamine/xylazine (80/10 mg/kg) solution, then obtain whole blood using cardiac puncture.
3. Centrifuge whole blood at 10,000 rpm for 5 min and save the plasma for enzyme linked immunosorbent assay (ELISA) per manufacturer's instructions (DuoSet ELISA Assays, R&D Systems).

3.7 CpG DNA on WT and TLR9KO RBCs Detection In Vivo

1. Isolate RBCs from WT or TLR9KO mice, then label one with PKH26 and the other with PKH67.
2. Combine 1×10^8 of WT and TLR9KO RBCs in a 200 uL suspension, then inject this via the tail vein. Immediately following RBC transfusion, inject 50 ug/mouse of class B Alexa 647 CpG DNA (IDT) (*see* **Note 8**).
3. One hour post-transfusion, sacrifice mice with ketamine/xylazine and collect whole blood using cardiac puncture, and place on ice until processing.
4. Dissect the spleen and place it in RPMI media on ice until processing.

Whole blood processing

5. Bead isolate RBCs from the blood using MACS separation as described previously.
6. Once isolated, manually count the RBCs and suspend in 2% BSA in PBS at a concentration of 1×10^7 cells/mL. Add 100 ul of this cell suspension to flow cytometry tubes and proceed to FACS analysis.
7. Analyze the concentration of fluorescently labeled CpG on RBCs and interpret data using FlowJo software.

Spleen processing

8. Mince the spleens and pass them through 70 um filters into a 50 mL conical tube. Rinse the filter two times with 5 mL of RPMI media.

9. Centrifuge splenocytes at 1500 rpm for 5 min, then remove supernatant and wash once in Leibowitz L-15 media. Following washing, pellet cells by spinning at 800 g for 5 min with a deceleration of 6, and remove supernatant.
10. Take 30 uL of packed splenocytes and add to 70 uL of Leibovitz L-15 media with 15 uL of anti-Ter119 beads. Mix well and incubate for 15 min at 4 °C.
11. Following incubation, wash the solution with 1 mL of Leibovitz L-15 media, then centrifuge at 300 g for 5 min and remove the supernatant. Resuspend cells in 500 uL of L-15 media.
12. Place the LS column in the MACS magnetic separator and rinse it with 3 mL of L-15 media. Once the media passes through the column fully, place the 500 uL of resuspended cells into the column. Rinse the column two times with 3 mL of Leibovitz L-15 media.
13. After washing the column twice, remove it from the magnetic separator and collect cells by pipetting 5 mL of L-15 media into the column and flushing it with the plunger into a 15 mL conical tube.
14. Once collected, spin down cells at 800 g for 5 min with a deceleration of 6, remove the supernatant, and then resuspend in 1 mL of FACS buffer (PBS + 2% FBS).
15. Manually count the RBCs and suspend them in 2% BSA in PBS at a concentration of 1e7 cells/mL.
16. Add 100 uL of this cell suspension to have 1e6 cells per tube for flow cytometry and proceed to FACS analysis.
17. Analyze the concentration of fluorescently labeled CpG on RBCs and interpret data using FlowJo software.

4 Notes

1. When using leukoreduction filters to obtain murine RBCs, if flushing with PBS, the cells cannot be stored and used later. If stored after a PBS flush, they are sensitive to hemolysis. Use the RBCs the same day if using leukoreduction filters and using a PBS flush.
2. When performing magnetic cell separation, be sure to gently mix MicroBeads before use, as beads will settle at the bottom of the container.
3. When handling RBCs, do not vortex as they are sensitive and will lyse. Gently mix by running the flow tube containing cells against the flow tube rack.

4. The TLR9 antibody 5G5 clone works best on fresh RBCs; do not fix cells until after incubation with this antibody, as aldehyde fixation will limit detection with the 5G5 clone.
5. Glutaraldehyde fixation yielded the best detection of TLR9 on the RBCs; do not use paraformaldehyde.
6. The TLR9 antibody Clone 26C593.2 works best on fixed and permeabilized cells; detection using this antibody is dependent on permeabilized cells.
7. Use of the CD47 (Clone CC2C6) antibody to stain RBCs leads to aggregates.
8. Ensure CpG DNA used is class B, containing a phosphorothioated backbone.

Conflict of Interest

The authors have no conflicts of interest to declare that are relevant to the content of this chapter.

References

1. Bianconi E, Piovesan A, Facchin F, Beraudi A, Casadei R, Frabetti F et al (2013) An estimation of the number of cells in the human body. Ann Hum Biol 40(6):463–471. https://doi.org/10.3109/03014460.2013.807878
2. Anderson HL, Brodsky IE, Mangalmurti NS (2018) The evolving erythrocyte: red blood cells as modulators of innate immunity. J Immunol 201(5):1343–1351. https://doi.org/10.4049/jimmunol.1800565
3. Dobkin J, Mangalmurti NS (2022) Immunomodulatory roles of red blood cells. Curr Opin Hematol 29(6):306–309. https://doi.org/10.1097/moh.0000000000000734
4. Roers A, Hiller B, Hornung V (2016) Recognition of endogenous nucleic acids by the innate immune system. Immunity 44(4):739–754. https://doi.org/10.1016/j.immuni.2016.04.002
5. Blasius AL, Beutler B (2010) Intracellular toll-like receptors. Immunity 32(3):305–315. https://doi.org/10.1016/j.immuni.2010.03.012
6. Ewald SE, Lee BL, Lau L, Wickliffe KE, Shi GP, Chapman HA et al (2008) The ectodomain of toll-like receptor 9 is cleaved to generate a functional receptor. Nature 456(7222):658–662. https://doi.org/10.1038/nature07405
7. Mouchess ML, Arpaia N, Souza G, Barbalat R, Ewald SE, Lau L et al (2011) Transmembrane mutations in toll-like receptor 9 bypass the requirement for ectodomain proteolysis and induce fatal inflammation. Immunity 35(5):721–732. https://doi.org/10.1016/j.immuni.2011.10.009
8. Ohto U, Shibata T, Tanji H, Ishida H, Krayukhina E, Uchiyama S et al (2015) Structural basis of CpG and inhibitory DNA recognition by toll-like receptor 9. Nature 520(7549):702–705. https://doi.org/10.1038/nature14138
9. Hemmi H, Takeuchi O, Kawai T, Kaisho T, Sato S, Sanjo H et al (2000) A Toll-like receptor recognizes bacterial DNA. Nature 408:740–745. https://doi.org/10.1038/35047123
10. Lam LKM, Murphy S, Kokkinaki D, Venosa A, Sherrill-Mix S, Casu C et al (2021) DNA binding to TLR9 expressed by red blood cells promotes innate immune activation and anemia. Sci Transl Med 13(616):eabj1008. https://doi.org/10.1126/scitranslmed.abj1008
11. Lam LKM, Dobkin J, Eckart KA, Gereg I, DiSalvo A, Nolder A et al (2022) Bat red blood cells express nucleic acid-sensing receptors and bind RNA and DNA. Immunohorizons 6(5):299–306. https://doi.org/10.4049/immunohorizons.2200013

12. Hotz MJ, Qing D, Shashaty MGS, Zhang P, Faust H, Sondheimer N et al (2018) Red blood cells homeostatically bind mitochondrial DNA through TLR9 to maintain quiescence and to prevent lung injury. Am J Respir Crit Care Med 197(4):470–480. https://doi.org/10.1164/rccm.201706-1161OC
13. He Y, Cheng C, Liu Y, Chen FM, Chen Y, Yang C et al (2024) Intravenous senescent erythrocyte vaccination modulates adaptive immunity and splenic complement production. ACS Nano 18(1):470–482. https://doi.org/10.1021/acsnano.3c07943
14. Heinrich AC, Pelanda R, Klingmüller U (2004) A mouse model for visualization and conditional mutations in the erythroid lineage. Blood 104(3):659–666. https://doi.org/10.1182/blood-2003-05-1442

Chapter 38

Examining Inflammatory Effects of Reticulocyte Erythrophagocytosis in Human Macrophage Cultures

Rosario Hernández-Armengol, Kausik Paul, Che-Yu Chang, June Young Lee, Krystalyn E. Hudson, and David R. Gibb

Abstract

Red blood cell (RBC) interaction with phagocytes in the spleen and liver may trigger or attenuate inflammatory responses that could influence innate and adaptive immune responses to RBC antigens. Such interactions are particularly relevant in patients with sickle cell disease (SCD), who have elevated rates of auto- and alloimmunity against RBC antigens. Many phagocyte-expressed pattern recognition receptors (PRRs) are intracellular and recognize nucleic acids. Reticulocytes and recently described mature RBCs abnormally retaining mitochondria have nucleic acids and, upon erythrophagocytosis, can access PRRs and affect inflammatory cytokine production. Here, we describe co-culture experiments of human macrophages and RBC subsets from patients with or without SCD to enable examination of erythrophagocytosis-induced inflammatory cytokine responses.

Key words Sickle cell disease (SCD), Erythrophagocytosis, Reticulocyte, RBC opsonization, Type 1 interferons (IFNα/β)

1 Introduction

Sickle cell disease (SCD) is a chronic inflammatory disease characterized by hemolysis, leukocytosis, endothelial damage, oxidative stress, and enhanced RBC clearance [1]. While RBC transfusion is a critical therapy for many patients with SCD, such patients have the highest rate of transfusion-induced RBC alloimmunization, which can mediate potentially fatal hemolytic events [2]. Inflammatory pathways in spleen innate immune cells, including dendritic cells and macrophages, have been implicated in promoting alloimmunization in patients [2–5] and pre-clinical transfusion models [6–9]. While many inflammatory pathways are elevated in patients with SCD, one pathway implicated in alloimmunization in pre-clinical models is the production of proinflammatory type 1 interferons (IFNα/β) [10–14], which were discovered for their

Sean R. Stowell and Connie M. Arthur (eds.), *Methods in Transfusion Medicine*, Methods in Molecular Biology, vol. 3053, https://doi.org/10.1007/978-1-0716-5376-0_38,

critical role in anti-viral immunity [15]. Multiple studies have recently demonstrated elevated IFNα/β activation in patients with SCD [16–19]. However, mechanisms of IFNα/β production, including the ligands, receptors, and pathways that induce IFNα/β in SCD, remain poorly understood.

Nearly all IFNα/β-inducing receptors are intracellular receptors that bind nucleic acids. Thus, IFNα/β is induced following transport of cell-free nucleic acids or phagocytosis of RNA/DNA-containing cells or vesicles [20]. In patients with SCD, erythrophagocytes, including spleen red pulp macrophages, consume sickled RBCs at an accelerated rate, contributing to a reduced RBC lifespan of 10–20 days [21]. Anti-RBC allo- and autoantibodies, elevated in patients with SCD [22], can further increase extravascular hemolysis. Many lines of evidence indicate that erythrophagocytosis of mature RBCs is generally immunosuppressive [23, 24]. However, reticulocytes containing mitochondria and RNA are elevated in patients with SCD [25], and reticulocyte transfusion has recently been implicated in RBC alloimmunization [26]. It was also reported that erythrophagocytosis of mitochondrial-containing RBCs induces IFNα/β activity in patients with lupus [27].

Thus, we generated methods to test the hypothesis that erythrophagocytosis of reticulocytes and/or recently described mitochondrial-containing mature SCD RBCs [28–30], may induce IFNα/β production and signaling in innate immune cells of patients with SCD. Here, we describe ex vivo erythrophagocytosis experiments utilizing co-cultures of monocyte-derived macrophages from healthy platelet donors with RBCs and reticulocytes from patients with SCD. Such experiments can have informative read-outs including efficiency of erythrophagocytosis, inflammatory cytokine production, macrophage activation and polarization, RNA sequencing, and targeted transcriptional profiling. Similar experiments can also be performed with monocyte cell lines that can be differentiated into macrophages (i.e., Phorbol-12-myristate-13-acetate (PMA)-induced THP1 cells) or with monocyte-derived macrophages from patients with SCD. THP1-Dual cells (Invivogen) can also be used to report both NFκB and IFNα/β activation. There are also many tools that can be utilized to examine the role of erythrophagocytosis, such as FcγR blockade, chemical inhibition of phagocytosis, hemopexin chelation of heme, inhibitors of FcγR signaling (i.e., Syk inhibition), and inhibitors of specific pathways leading to production of IFNα/β or other inflammatory cytokines, which are not specifically described here. Finally, while the methods were developed to examine IFNα/β production and IFNα/β stimulated gene (ISG) expression, they can be generally applied to other pathways altered in SCD.

Purpose Examine effects of antibody-mediated erythrophagocytosis on macrophage inflammatory cytokine responses (i.e., IFNα/β and ISG expression). Prepare co-cultures of RBCs and reticulocytes from patients with or without SCD and human monocyte-derived macrophages.

2 Materials

2.1 Peripheral Blood Mononuclear Cell (PBMC) Isolation from Leukocyte Reduction System (LRS) Cone by Ficoll-Paque Density Gradient Centrifugation

1. LRS cone from a platelet donor.
2. Ficoll-Paque Premium sterile solution (density 1.077 g/mL) (e.g., Cytiva)
   (a) Shelf life is 6 months after opening.
3. Sterile Phosphate Buffered Saline (PBS) without Ca/Mg *or Phosphate Buffered Saline (PBS) without Ca/Mg + EDTA 1mM,* pH 7.4.
4. Sterile 10 mL syringe with a 23G × ¾ (0.6 mm × 1 9mm) needle (e.g., BD PrecisionGlide™ Needle).
5. Sterile conical centrifuge tubes, 15 mL and 50 mL.
6. Disposable plastic pipettes in 5 mL, 10 mL, and 25 mL graduations.
7. Sterile Ammonium-Chloride-Potassium (ACK) lysing buffer (e.g., Quality Biological).
8. Automated cell counter device or cell counting chamber (Hemocytometer).

2.2 Monocyte Isolation Using EasySep™ Human Monocyte Enrichment Kit without CD16 Depletion

1. PBMC suspension in the recommended medium.
2. Sterile 5 mL Polystyrene round-bottom tubes (12 × 75 mm style) with cap (e.g., Falcon®).
3. EasySep™ Human Monocyte Enrichment Kit without CD16 Depletion (Stemcells™ Technologies).
4. EasySep™ Buffer (Stemcells™ Technologies).
5. EasySep™ Magnet (Stemcells™ Technologies).

2.3 Monocyte Cell Culture Preparation for Differentiation into Human Macrophages

1. Recombinant Human GM-CSF lyophilized (10 μg), (e.g., Gibco™).
2. Macrophage SFM (serum-free media) 1X, with L-Glutamine (e.g., Gibco™).
3. Penicillin/Streptomycin (P/S) (e.g., Gibco™).
4. Sterile cell culture plates with flat bottom (12-well or 96-well plate).

2.4 Red Blood Cells (RBC) Separation from a Sample of a Healthy Donor by Ficoll-Paque Density Gradient Centrifugation

1. Blood sample from a healthy donor in an EDTA-containing purple top tube.
2. Ficoll-Paque Premium sterile solution (density 1.077 g/mL) (e.g., Cytiva).
3. Sterile Phosphate Buffered Saline (PBS) without Ca/Mg *or Phosphate Buffered Saline (PBS) without Ca/Mg + EDTA 1 mM,* pH 7.4.
4. Sterile conical centrifuge tubes, 15 mL and 50 mL.
5. Disposable plastic pipettes in 5 mL, 10 mL, and 25 mL graduations.
6. Automated cell counter device or cell counting chamber (Hemocytometer).

2.5 RBC and Reticulocyte Enrichment by Percoll Density Gradient Centrifugation, Sample from a Patient with Sickle Cell Disease (SCD)

1. Blood sample in an EDTA-containing purple top tube from a patient with SCD.
2. Percoll sterile solution (density 1.130 g/mL) (e.g., Cytiva).
3. Sterile 5 mL Polystyrene round-bottom tube (12 x 75 mm style) with cap (e.g., Falcon®).
4. Sterile Phosphate Buffered Saline (PBS) without Ca/Mg *or Phosphate Buffered Saline (PBS) without Ca/Mg + EDTA 1 mM,* pH 7.4.
5. Sterile Dulbecco's Phosphate Buffered Saline (DPBS) 10X without Ca/Mg (Corning).
6. Sterile cell culture media RPMI 1640, 1X with L-glutamine and 25 nM HEPES (e.g., Corning, Gibco™, Thermo Scientific).
7. Sterile conical centrifuge tubes, 15 mL and 50 mL.
8. Disposable plastic pipettes in 5 mL, 10 mL, and 25 mL graduations.
9. Automated cell counter device or cell counting chamber (Hemocytometer).

2.6 Flow Cytometry Staining for Cell Sorting of RBCs and Reticulocytes from Patients with SCD (for 50 μL of Reticulocyte-Enriched Cells)

1. Reticulocyte-enriched cell suspension (50 μL) in sterile flow cytometry staining buffer (FACS buffer, see **Step 5**).
2. MitoTracker™ Deep Red Dye for Mitochondria Labeling (e.g., Invitrogen™).
3. Sterile 5 mL Polystyrene round-bottom tube (12 × 75 mm style) with cap (e.g., Falcon®).
4. Sterile 5 mL Polystyrene round-bottom tube (12 × 75 mm style) with cell-strainer cap (e.g., Falcon®).
5. Sterile FACS buffer (500 mL of PBS without Ca/Mg, pH 7.4/ 0.1 g bovine serum albumin (BSA)/0.45 g EDTA).

6. FACS antibodies: PE anti-human CD45 Antibody (clone: HI30), FITC anti-human CD41 Antibody (clone: HIP8), APC/Cyanine7 anti-human CD71 Antibody (clone: CY1G4) (Biolegend®).
7. UltraComp eBeads Compensation Beads (Invitrogen).
8. Flow cytometer.
9. Fluorescence activated cell sorter.
10. Flow cytometric analysis software (i.e., FlowJo).

2.7 RBC Opsonization with Anti-RBC Antibodies

1. RBCs and reticulocyte suspensions in PBS.
2. Sterile Phosphate Buffered Saline (PBS) without Ca/Mg *or Phosphate Buffered Saline (PBS) without Ca/Mg + EDTA 1 mM,* pH 7.4.
3. Anti-D (anti-RH1, monoclonal-polyclonal blend) opsonizing antibody (e.g., BioClone®, Ortho-Clinical Diagnostics).
4. Water bath warmed at 37 °C.
5. cRPMI: Sterile RPMI 1640 media supplemented with: HEPES 1%/Non-Essential Amino Acids Solution (NEAA) 1%/L-Glutamine 1%/Sodium Pyruvate (NaPyr) 1%/Penicillin/Streptomycin 1% / Heat Inactivated Fetal Bovine Serum (FBS) 10% (e.g., Gibco™).

2.8 CFSE Cell Staining (Modified for RBCs) for Flow Cytometry Analysis of Erythrophagocytosis

1. RBC and reticulocyte suspensions in PBS.
2. Sterile Phosphate Buffered Saline (PBS) without Ca/Mg *or Phosphate Buffered Saline (PBS) without Ca/Mg + EDTA 1 mM,* pH 7.4.
3. Dimethyl sulfoxide (DMSO) (e.g., Sigma-Aldrich).
4. CellTrace™ CFSE Cell Proliferation Kit (Invitrogen™).
5. Water bath warmed at 37 °C.
6. cRPMI (*see* Subheading 2.7, **item 5**).

2.9 Co-culture of Macrophages with Reticulocytes and Mature RBCs

1. RBC suspension in complete RPMI (cRPMI, *see* Subheading 2.7, **item 5**).
2. Sterile cell culture plates with flat bottom (12-well or 96-well plate).
3. cRPMI: (*see* Subheading 2.7, **item 5**).
4. Human IFNβ (1ug/mL, Invivogen).

2.10 Flow Cytometry for Erythrophagocytosis Analysis After Co-culture

1. Macrophages collected from co-culture plates.
2. Trypsin-EDTA (0.25%), phenol red (e.g., Gibco™).

Table 1
Antibody concentrations used to evaluate macrophages for erythrophagocytosis of CFSE+ opsonized and non-opsonized RBCs and reticulocytes

Human FACS antibodies	2x concentration
hCD14 BV421	1:100
hCD64 BV785	1:100
hCD86 BV510 (optional activation marker)	1:100
hCD38 APC (optional ISG)	1:200
hSiglec-1 PerCP/Cy 5.5 (optional ISG)	1:50
GPA PE/Cy7 (CD235a)	1:1000
Zombie NIR	1:500

The 2x concentrate will be diluted to 1x following the addition of 50 μL antibody mixture to 50 μL containing Human TruStain FcX™ (Fc Receptor Blocking Solution) and Super Bright Complete Staining Buffer. ISG, IFNα/β stimulated gene

3. Sterile Phosphate Buffered Saline (PBS) without Ca/Mg *or Phosphate Buffered Saline (PBS) without Ca/Mg + EDTA 1 mM*, pH 7.4.
4. FACS Buffer.
5. Human TruStain FcX™ (Fc Receptor Blocking Solution), (Biolegend®).
6. Super Bright Complete Staining Buffer (e.g., eBioscience™, Invitrogen).
7. Flow cytometer (i.e., Cytek® Northern Lights™ System flow cytometer, Cytek Biosciences, Inc., CA).
8. Cell surface marker antibodies and antibodies targeting proteins of interest (See Table 1).

3 Methods

3.1 PBMC Isolation from LRS Cone by Ficoll-Paque Density Gradient Centrifugation

1. Collect the LRS cone from the platelet donor.
2. Clean both ends of the cone with ethanol (see Fig. 1a).
3. Place an inverted cone on a 50 mL tube under a biosafety cabinet.
4. Cut the bottom tubing with sterile scissors (autoclaved). Cut the top tubing. Allow blood to drip into the tube (see Fig. 1a).
5. Insert a 10 mL syringe with a 23G needle into the top tubing.
6. Push 10 mL of air into the syringe, followed by 10 mL of sterile PBS into the top tubing. Allow PBS to drip into the tube (see Fig. 1a).

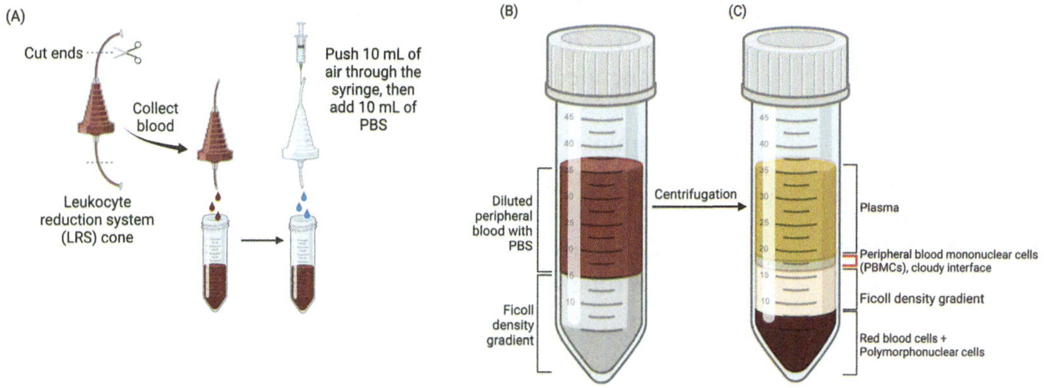

Fig. 1 Isolation of peripheral blood mononuclear cells (PBMCs) from leukocyte reduction system cones. (**a**) A leukocyte reduction system (LRS) cone of a healthy platelet donor. Dotted lines mark the pinched-off flexible tubes, which have to be opened using scissors to transfer the blood product into a 50 mL tube. (**b**) The diluted blood product was carefully overlaid onto a Ficoll-Paque density gradient separation medium (clear phase). Phases should be completely separated without mixing. (**c**) After centrifugation of the tube prepared as shown in (**b**), erythrocytes and granulocytes build a pellet at the bottom of the tube, while PBMCs are contained in the interphase (gray interface marked with red bracket) between Ficoll-Paque density gradient separation medium and the plasma. The interphase is collected in order to isolate PBMCs. (Created with BioRender.com)

7. Fill tube to 50 mL with sterile PBS and centrifuge at 800× *g* for 10 min at 4 °C.
8. Remove supernatant and resuspend in sterile PBS to 4x volume of packed RBCs (pRBCs).
9. Add a 1:1 ratio of Ficoll-Paque Premium to a sterile 50 mL conical tube (= the total blood/PBS volume from **Step 8**) (*see* **Note 1**).
10. Overlay blood in a careful and slow manner over Ficoll in the 50 mL sterile tube without disturbing the interface (see Fig. 1b).
11. Centrifuge samples at 400× *g* for 15 min at room temperature. Be sure to use breakoff (Brake: 0; Acceleration: 5).
12. Remove the PBMC layer (cloudy interface between the plasma and Ficoll-Paque layers) into 15 mL conical tubes (see Fig. 1c).
13. Optional: If the PBMC interface has some RBCs, remove them by adding 5 mL of RBCs lysis buffer (ACK). Mix well and incubate for 3–5 min at RT.
    (a) Add 5 mL of sterile PBS, mix well, and spin down at 350× *g* for 5 min at 4 °C and remove the lysate.
14. Wash cells by filling tubes with 10 mL of sterile PBS and centrifuge at 350× *g* for 5 min at 4 °C.
15. Resuspend the PBMCs in 1 mL of EasySep Buffer for the monocyte isolation.

16. Count PBMCs with a cell counter device (adjust the cell size from 7 to 20 μm) or a hemocytometer. A 1:100 dilution is recommended for counting PBMCs.

3.2 Monocyte Isolation Using EasySep™ Human Monocyte Enrichment Kit Without CD16 Depletion

1. In a laminar flow biosafety cabinet, prepare a sample at the indicated cell concentration in the kit within the volume range: 5×10^7 cells/mL in EasySep Buffer.
2. Add sample to a sterile 5 mL (12 × 75 mm) polystyrene round-bottom tube with cap.
3. Add 50 μL/mL of Enrichment Cocktail to the sample.
4. Mix and incubate at 2–8 °C for 10 min.
5. Vortex Magnetic Particles for 30 s.
6. Add 50 μL/mL of Magnetic Particles to the sample.
7. Mix and incubate at 2–8 °C for 5 min.
8. Add recommended medium (EasySep Buffer) to top up the sample to 2.5 mL. Mix by gently pipetting up and down 2–3 times.
9. Place the tube (without lid) into the magnet and incubate for 2.5 min at RT.
10. Pick up the magnet, and in one continuous motion, invert the magnet and tube, pouring the enriched cell suspension into a new 5 mL sterile tube (isolated cells are ready for use) (*see* **Note 2**).
11. Spin down the cells at 350× *g* for 5 min at 4 °C and remove the EasySep Buffer.
12. Resuspend the cells in Macrophage SFM cell culture media.
13. Count the isolated monocytes with a cell counter device (adjust the cell size from 7 to 20 μm) or a hemocytometer.

3.3 Monocyte Cell Culture Preparation for Differentiation into Human Macrophages

1. Place the desired number of cells according to the experiment:
   (a) For FACS staining: 1.5–2 × 10^6 cells/well in 1 mL in 12-well plate for cell culture.
   (b) For qPCR analysis: 0.2 × 10^6 cells/well in 0.2 mL in 96-well plate for cell culture.
2. Culture the monocytes for 5 days in prewarmed Macrophage SFM + P/S (1:1000 dilution) + 50 ng/mL GM-CSF cell culture media (*see* **Note 3**).
3. Replace with fresh prewarmed cell culture media on day 3.
4. If desired, macrophages can be primed on day 5 with IFN-gamma (10–25 ng/mL) +/− LPS (100 ng/mL) in fresh Macrophage SFM media (+GM-CSF) for 48 h prior to use.

3.4 RBC Separation from Sample of Healthy Donor by Ficoll-Plaque Density Gradient Centrifugation

1. Collect the blood sample from the healthy donor in a 4 mL EDTA purple top tube.
2. Transfer the blood sample to a 50 mL tube.
3. Fill tube to 50 mL with sterile PBS and centrifuge at 800× *g* for 10 min at 4 °C.
4. Remove supernatant and resuspend cells in sterile PBS to 4x volume of pRBCs.
5. Add a 1:1 ratio of Ficoll-Paque Premium to a sterile 50 mL conical tube (= the total blood + PBS volume in **Step 4**) (*see* **Note 1**).
6. Overlay blood in a careful and slow manner over the Ficoll in a 50 mL sterile tube without disturbing the interface (see Fig. 1b).
7. Centrifuge samples at 400 × g for 15 min at room temperature. Be sure to use breakoff (Brake: 0; Acceleration: 5).
8. Remove and discard the plasma, PBMC, and Ficoll-Paque layers.
9. Transfer 50 μL of the RBC layer (in the bottom of the tube) into appropriately labeled 15 mL conical tubes.
10. Wash cells 3 times by filling tubes with 10 mL of sterile PBS and centrifuge at 350× *g* for 5 min at 4 °C.
11. Remove all the PBS after the final wash step.
12. Transfer 20 μL of the pRBCs to 980 μL of sterile PBS (stock for work in the next steps) (*see* **Note 4**).
13. Count RBCs with a cell counter device (adjust the cell size from 3 to 8 μm) or with a hemocytometer.

3.5 RBC and Reticulocyte Enrichment by Percoll Density Gradient Centrifugation, Sample from Patient with Sickle Cell Disease (SCD)

1. Collect the blood sample from a patient with SCD in a 4 mL EDTA purple top tube (*see* **Note 5**).
2. Transfer the sample to a sterile 5 mL (12 × 75 mm) polystyrene round-bottom tube with cap.
3. Spin down whole blood at 150× *g* for 10 min at 4 °C.
4. Remove the plasma and add the same volume removed with PBS and store at 4 °C or keep on ice (see Fig. 2a) (*see* **Note 6**).
5. Prepare a Percoll gradient with the following specifications: 1 tube with Percoll gradient at 75% and 1 tube with Percoll gradient at 45% (see Table 2).
6. Add the first 6 mL of the Percoll gradient at 75% in a new 15 mL tube, then add 2.4 mL of Percoll gradient at 45% slowly without disturbing the interface.

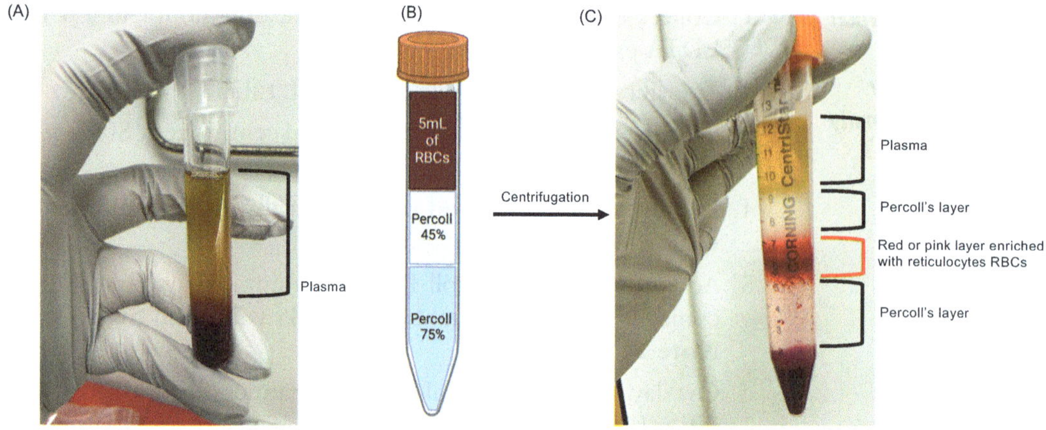

Fig. 2 Enrichment of reticulocytes for fluorescence activated cell sorting. (**a**) A sample from a patient with SCD is centrifuged to remove plasma. (**b**) Diluted RBCs are added above 75% and 45% Percoll layers. (**c**) Following centrifugation without a break, the light red layer is collected and labeled for cell sorting

Table 2
Percoll gradient calculations for reticulocyte enrichment

Percoll gradient at 75%	Percoll gradient at 45%
Percoll: 5.25 mL	Percoll: 1.35 mL
Sterile DPBS 10X: 700 μL	Sterile DPBS 10X: 300 μL
DMEM or RPMI media: 1.05 mL	Sterile MiliQ H_2O: 1.35 mL
Final volume: 7 mL	Final volume: 3 mL
Volume used: 6 mL	**Volume used: 2.4 mL**

7. Overlay blood over Percoll gradient in a careful and slow manner in the tube without disturbing the interface (see Fig. 2b).
8. Spin down at 250× *g* for 30 min at 4 °C. Be sure to use breakoff (Brake: 0; Acceleration: 10).
9. Remove the pink or red layer (reticulocyte-enriched) between the two Percoll layers (see Fig. 2c).
10. Wash the cells with 10 mL of sterile PBS.
11. Centrifuge at 1000× *g* for 5 min at 4 °C.
12. Remove the PBS.
13. Collect the reticulocyte-enriched RBCs (approximately 50 μL) *see* **Note 7**.

3.6 Flow Cytometry Staining for Cell Sorting of RBCs and Reticulocytes from Patients with SCD (for 50 µL of Reticulocyte-Enriched RBCs from Subheading 3.5)

1. Dilute the MitoTRACKER (MT) at 1:1000 with sterile FACS buffer.
2. Transfer the 50 µL of reticulocyte-enriched RBCs to a sterile 5 mL Polystyrene round-bottom tube (12 × 75 mm style) with cap.
3. Prepare FACS staining with the following specifications: 62.55 µL of MT + 50 µL reticulocyte-enriched RBCs +3.9 mL of FACS buffer.
4. Prepare 2 tubes for controls:
   (a) Tube pre-enrichment: 1 µL of whole blood from SCD donor (before the Percoll gradient) + 400 µL FACS buffer +1.25 µL of MT.
   (b) Tube post-enrichment: 1 µL of reticulocyte-enriched RBCs from SCD donor (after the Percoll gradient) + 400 µL FACS buffer +1.25 µL of MT.
5. Incubate the RBC/MT from **Steps 3** to **4** for 30 min, in a water bath at 37 °C, protected from the light with foil, and mix or invert the tube every 10–15 min.
6. Spin down the RBCs at 350× *g* for 5 min at 4 °C and remove supernatant.
7. For the 50 µL reticulocyte-enriched RBCs, create the antibody cocktail with the following concentrations, in a final volume of 4 mL. Alternatively, add antibodies directly to 3.9 mL of RBCs/FACS buffer. Anti-CD41: 30 µL, anti-CD45: 30 µL, anti-CD71: 60 µL (Table 3).
8. Resuspend the 2 control tubes **from 4.a to 4.b** with 400 µL (4.1) or 500 µL (4.2) of FACS buffer. Remove 100 µL from the post-enrichment sample (4.2) to use for the MT single color control for FACS sorting. Stain remaining cells by adding 1 µL anti-CD41 + 1 µL anti-CD45 + 2 µL anti-CD71.
9. Incubate samples from **Steps** 7 to **8** for 30 min in the dark on ice or in 4 °C refrigerator.

Table 3
Antibody concentrations used for FACS sorting mature RBCs and reticulocytes

Human FACS antibodies	1x concentration	Volume (uL)
hCD41 FITC	1:400	30
hCD45 PE	1:400	30
hCD71 APC/Cy7	1:200	60
Final volume	–	**120/sample**

10. Spin down at 350× *g* for 5 min at 4 °C and remove the supernatant. Resuspend the 50 μL reticulocyte-enriched RBC sample in 1 mL of FACS buffer.
11. Transfer the 1 mL of cells from **Step 10** to another sterile cytometry tube with a filter in the cap (blue cap). Wash the original tube with PBS to ensure all cells are transferred.
    (a) Prior to transferring the cells, wet the filter by adding 500 μL of FACS buffer.
12. Fill to 4 mL with FACS buffer. Further dilution in 2 tubes may be needed if the sample is too dense for cell sorting.
13. Add 500 μL of FACS buffer to the FACS collection tubes before sorting the reticulocytes and mature RBCs.
14. For compensation controls, make unstained cells with 1 μl of RBCs from the original patient tube and 2 mL of FACS buffer. Prepare single color compensation controls by staining one drop of compensation beads with 1 μL of anti-CD41, anti-CD45, or anti-CD71.
15. Prior to sorting, calculate the number of RBCs needed for the experiment: A 1:2 ratio of Macrophages:RBCs/reticulocytes for culture is recommended.

    Example: For flow cytometry: (12-well plate) 3×10^6 RBCs/well.

    For qPCR: (96-well plate) 0.4×10^6/well.
16. Sort reticulocytes: $CD41^-CD45^-CD71^+MitoTracker^+$ and mature RBCs: $CD41^-CD45^-CD71^-MitoTracker^-$ (Fig. 3). Also sort mitochondrial-containing mature RBCs if desired, Mito+ RBCs: $CD41^-CD45^-CD71^-MitoTracker^+$. *See* **Note 8**.

3.7 RBC Opsonization with Anti-RBC Antibodies

1. Count the reticulocytes and mature cells collected from cell sorting.

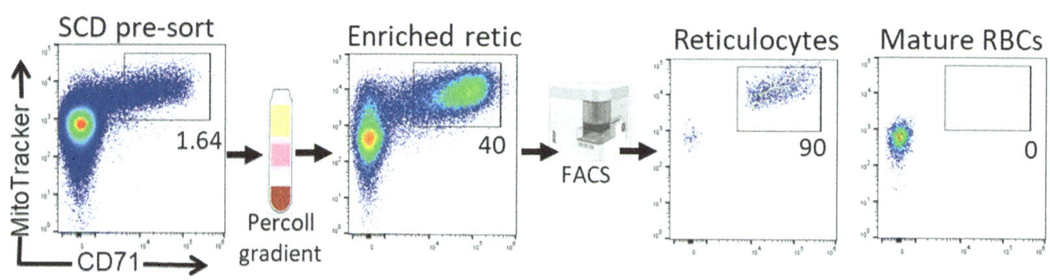

Fig. 3 Reticulocyte and RBC isolation. Representative flow cytometric analysis of RBCs from patients with SCD. Reticulocytes ($mitoTracker^+$ $CD71^+$) were enriched by a Percoll gradient prior to fluorescence activated cell sorting of mature RBCs and reticulocytes. Numbers on plots indicate the percent of $CD45^-$ $CD41^-$ cells (non-WBC, non-platelet) in the gate

2. Opsonize healthy donor RBCs and sorted mature RBCs and reticulocytes from a patient with anti-D RH1 antibody: *See* **Note 9**.
   - Use the RH1 antibody in a dilution of 1:20 in a final volume of 200 μL (adequate for a maximum amount of 10×10^6 RBCs). Incubate for 1 h. at 37 °C (mixing every 20 min).
   - In parallel, incubate the non-opsonized RBCs in the same conditions (1 h. at 37 °C (mixing every 20 min)).
   - *Optional step: As a control to avoid Fc receptor signaling, erythrophagocytosis can be enhanced by heating RBCs rather than opsonization. Heat RBCs at 50 °C for 20 min, then rest for >15 min.

3a. For downstream analysis other than erythrophagocytosis by flow cytometry:
   1. Centrifuge cells for 5 min at 300× *g* and resuspend the cell pellet in 1 mL PBS.
   2. Wash x3 to remove excess RH1 antibody.
   3. Resuspend in cRPMI media.

3b. For erythrophagocytosis by flow cytometry analysis, proceed to Subheading 3.8. Washing to remove excess RH1 antibody is not needed.

3.8 CFSE Cell Staining (Modified for RBCs) for Flow Cytometry Analysis of Erythrophagocytosis (See Note 10)

1. Add 18 μL DMSO to a vial of CellTrace CFSE staining solution = stock solution.
2. Dilute 0.9 μL CFSE stock solution into 1 mL of PBS (warmed to 37 °C) for a 5 μM staining solution.
3. Centrifuge cells (opsonized and non-opsonized RBCs and reticulocytes) for 5 minutes at 300× *g* and carefully remove supernatant.
4. Add 100 μL of CellTrace CFSE staining solution (from **step 2** above).
5. Incubate cells for 20 min in a 37 °C water bath.
6. Add 1 mL cRPMI.
7. Incubate cells for 5 min.
8. Centrifuge cells for 5 min at 300× *g* and resuspend the cell pellet in 1 mL PBS.
9. Wash x3.
10. Resuspend in cRPMI media.
11. Resuspend in volume so that 50 μL RBCs = 0.4×10^6 RBCs, for qPCR.
12. For FACS, resuspend in volume so that 50 μL RBCs = 3×10^6 RBCs.

3.9 Co-culture of Macrophages with Reticulocytes and Mature RBCs (Fig. 4)

1. For downstream flow cytometry, add 3×10^6 RBCs per well in 12-well plate in 1 mL cRPMI (CFSE stained cells).

   *For positive control of ISGs, add 10 ng/mL IFNβ (dilution 1:100 of 1 μg/mL = 10 μL).

2. For qPCR, add 0.4×10^6 RBCs per well in 96-well plate in 200 μL cRPMI (no CFSE staining cells). For positive control, add 2 μL of IFNβ.
3. Co-culture for 3, 12, or 18 h.
4. For 96-well plate (i.e., qPCR, transcriptomics, cytokine analysis), collect supernatant, and gently wash macrophages 1x with PBS.
5. For 96-well qPCR plate, add RLT buffer containing β-mercaptoethanol at a 100:1 ratio (200 uL/well) and store at −80 °C for future qPCR analysis.

3.10 Flow Cytometry for Erythrophagocytosis Analysis After Co-culture

1. Remove the media from each well of the co-culture plate to a tube.
2. To remove RBCs from supernatants, spin down in a microcentrifuge at 640× *g* for 5 min.
3. Collect the supernatant and storage for future analysis.
4. To collect macrophages, add 1 mL of trypsin + EDTA 0.25% per well; incubate 15 min at 37 °C with CO_2.
5. Remove the cells into the FACS tube (non-sterile).
6. Add 1 mL of cRPMI and spin down at 350× *g* for 5 min at 4 °C.
7. Discard the supernatant and wash once with FACS buffer.
8. Incubate the cells with TruStain Fc Block (1:100) and Brilliant Stain Buffer (1:10) + FACS buffer for a total of 50 μL per tube and incubate for 10 min on ice or refrigerator, in the dark.

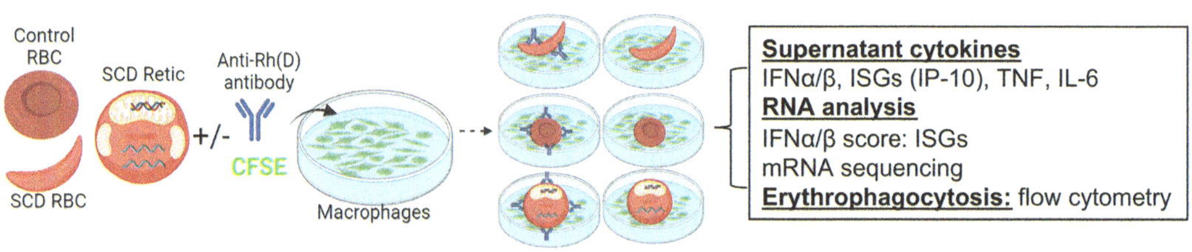

Fig. 4 Experimental schematic for RBC-induced IFNα/β activity. Flow cytometric sorted mature RBCs and reticulocytes (CD71+ MitoTracker+) from patients with SCD and leukoreduced RBCs from control subjects were or were not opsonized with anti-RBC antibodies (anti-Rh(D)). RBCs used for flow cytometric erythrophagocytosis analysis were labeled with CFSE. RBCs and reticulocytes were incubated with human monocyte-derived macrophages

9. Add 50 μL per tube of Ab cocktail (2x concentration) with FACS buffer (Table 1):
10. Incubate for 30 min on ice or in a refrigerator, in the dark.
11. Add 500 μL of FACS buffer and spin down 350× *g* for 5 min, discard the supernatant.
12. Add 300 μL to each tube and analyze by flow cytometry. *See* **Notes 11** and **12**.

4 Notes

1. May need to use 2 tubes if blood volume is >12 mL.
2. Leave the magnet and tube inverted for 2–3 s, then return upright. Do not shake or blot off any drops that may remain hanging from the mouth of the tube.
3. Filter the media with a sterile filter before use with the cells. Due to the lack of serum, the P/S concentration is tenfold less than that used in most complete media.
4. If necessary, make another dilution of 1:10 from work's stock and count the cells.
5. If possible, collect samples from patients with SCD with a high reticulocyte count and/or an elevated Hemoglobin S. If collecting from a patient on regular RBC exchange, collect the sample immediately prior to the RBC exchange procedure.
6. RBC volume will vary. If the blood sample is >5 mL, 2X 15 mL tubes will be needed for the isolation by Percoll density gradient.
7. If cells are left overnight, resuspend the RBCs in 15 mL of cRPMI and store at 4 °C until use.
8. The frequency of Mito+ RBCs may be reduced in reticulocyte-enriched samples.
9. If opsonizing with anti-D RH1, samples must be collected from an Rh(D)+ donor. Rh(D)– donors can serve as controls. Alternatively, anti-GPA (CD235a) or polyclonal rabbit anti-RBC antibodies can be used, regardless of Rh(D) typing.
10. For downstream analysis other than flow cytometry (i.e., qPCR, RNA sequencing), cells do not need to be stained with CFSE.
11. While erythrophagocytosis can be analyzed at any culture time point, the maximal signal is at ≤3 h.
12. For erythrophagocytosis analysis, GPA+ (CD235+) RBCs should be gated out to remove non-phagocytosed CFSE + RBCs.

Conflict of Interest Statement

This study was funded by the National Institute of Health [grant number R01 HL165169]. The authors have no conflicts of interest to declare that are relevant to the content of this chapter.

References

1. Hebbel RP, Osarogiagbon R, Kaul D (2004) The endothelial biology of sickle cell disease: inflammation and a chronic vasculopathy. Microcirculation 11(2):129–151. Epub 2004/07/29
2. Karafin MS, Westlake M, Hauser RG, Tormey CA, Norris PJ, Roubinian NH, Wu Y, Triulzi DJ, Kleinman S, Hendrickson JE, Epidemiology NR, Donor Evaluation S III (2018) Risk factors for red blood cell alloimmunization in the Recipient Epidemiology and Donor Evaluation Study (REDS-III) database. Br J Haematol. 181(5):672–681. https://doi.org/10.1111/bjh.15182. Epub 2018/04/21. PubMed PMID: 29675950; PMCID: PMC5991618
3. Papay P, Hackner K, Vogelsang H, Novacek G, Primas C, Reinisch W, Eser A, Mikulits A, Mayr WR, Kormoczi GF (2012) High risk of transfusion-induced alloimmunization of patients with inflammatory bowel disease. Am J Med 125(7):717 e1–717 e8. https://doi.org/10.1016/j.amjmed.2011.11.028
4. Ryder AB, Hendrickson JE, Tormey CA (2015) Chronic inflammatory autoimmune disorders are a risk factor for red blood cell alloimmunization. Br J Haematol. https://doi.org/10.1111/bjh.13781
5. Ramsey G, Smietana SJ (1995) Multiple or uncommon red cell alloantibodies in women: association with autoimmune disease. Transfusion 35(7):582–586
6. Ryder AB, Zimring JC, Hendrickson JE (2014) Factors influencing RBC alloimmunization: lessons learned from murine models. Transfus Med Hemother 41(6):406–419. https://doi.org/10.1159/000368995. PubMed PMID: 25670928; PMCID: PMC4280453
7. Bao W, Yu J, Heck S, Yazdanbakhsh K (2009) Regulatory T-cell status in red cell alloimmunized responder and nonresponder mice. Blood 113(22):5624–5627. Epub 2009/04/02. https://doi.org/10.1182/blood-2008-12-193748
8. Yu J, Heck S, Yazdanbakhsh K (2007) Prevention of red cell alloimmunization by CD25 regulatory T cells in mouse models. Am J Hematol 82(8):691–696
9. Arneja A, Salazar JE, Jiang W, Hendrickson JE, Zimring JC, Luckey CJ (2016) Interleukin-6 receptor-alpha signaling drives anti-RBC alloantibody production and T-follicular helper cell differentiation in a murine model of red blood cell alloimmunization. Haematologica 101(11):e440–e4e4. https://doi.org/10.3324/haematol.2016.149278
10. Gibb DR, Liu J, Natarajan P, Santhanakrishnan M, Madrid DJ, Eisenbarth SC, Zimring JC, Iwasaki A, Hendrickson JE (2017) Type I IFN Is Necessary and Sufficient for Inflammation-Induced Red Blood Cell Alloimmunization in Mice. J Immunol. 199(3):1041–1050. https://doi.org/10.4049/jimmunol.1700401. Epub 2017/06/21. PubMed PMID: 28630094; PMCID: PMC5568771
11. Gibb DR, Liu J, Santhanakrishnan M, Natarajan P, Madrid DJ, Patel S, Eisenbarth SC, Tormey CA, Stowell SR, Iwasaki A, Hendrickson JE (2017) B cells require Type 1 interferon to produce alloantibodies to transfused KEL-expressing red blood cells in mice. Transfusion 57(11):2595–2608. https://doi.org/10.1111/trf.14288. Epub 2017/08/25. PubMed PMID: 28836263; PMCID: PMC5745367
12. Lee JYME, El Kadi N, Pandya S, Ng K, Yamashita M, Jefferies CA, Gibb DR (2020) Type 1 interferon gene signature promotes RBC alloimmunizaiton in a lupus mouse model. Front Immunol 11. https://doi.org/10.3389/fimmu.2020.584254
13. Liu D, Gibb DR, Escamilla-Rivera V, Liu J, Santhanakrishnan M, Shi Z, Xu L, Eisenbarth SC, Hendrickson JE (2019) Type 1 IFN signaling critically regulates influenza-induced alloimmunization to transfused KEL RBCs in a murine model. Transfusion 59(10):3243–3252. https://doi.org/10.1111/trf.15482. Epub 2019/08/14. PubMed PMID: 31403208; PMCID: PMC6785373
14. Paul K, Hernandez-Armengol R, Lee JY, Chang CY, Shibata T, Yamashita M,

Jefferies C, Gibb DR (2024) Distinct RBC alloantibody responses in type 1 interferon-dependent and -independent lupus mouse models. Front Immunol 14:ARTN 1304086. https://doi.org/10.3389/fimmu.2023.1304086.
PubMed PMID: WOS:001152156600001

15. Isaacs A, Lindenmann J (1957) Virus interference. I. The interferon. Proc R Soc Lond B Biol Sci 147(927):258–267. Epub 1957/09/12. https://doi.org/10.1098/rspb.1957.0048
16. Hermand P, Azouzi S, Gautier EF, Guillonneau F, Bondet V, Duffy D, Dechavanne S, Tharaux PL, Mayeux P, Le Van Kim C, Koehl B (2020. Epub 2020/03/07) The proteome of neutrophils in sickle cell disease reveals an unexpected activation of interferon alpha signaling pathway. Haematologica. https://doi.org/10.3324/haematol.2019.238295
17. Hounkpe BW, Fiusa MM, Colella MP, da Costa LN, Benatti RO, Saad ST, Costa FF, dos Santos MN, De Paula EV (2015) Role of innate immunity-triggered pathways in the pathogenesis of Sickle Cell Disease: a meta-analysis of gene expression studies. Sci Rep. 5: 17822. https://doi.org/10.1038/srep17822. Epub 2015/12/10. PubMed PMID: 26648000; PMCID: PMC4673434
18. Liu Y, Pal M, Bao W, Shi PA, Lobo CA, An X, Manwani D, Zhong H, Yazdanbakhsh K (2021) Type I interferon is induced by hemolysis and drives antibody-mediated erythrophagocytosis in sickle cell disease. Blood. 138(13): 1162–1171. https://doi.org/10.1182/blood.2021011629. Epub 2021/06/25. PubMed PMID: 34166491; PMCID: PMC8570059
19. Madany E, Lee J, Halprin C, Seo J, Baca N, Majlessipour F, Hendrickson JE, Pepkowitz SH, Hayes C, Klapper E, Gibb DR (2021) Altered type 1 interferon responses in alloimmunized and nonalloimmunized patients with sickle cell disease. E J Haem 2(4):700–710. https://doi.org/10.1002/jha2.270. Epub 2022/02/08. PubMed PMID: 35128535; PMCID: PMC8813163
20. McNab F, Mayer-Barber K, Sher A, Wack A, O'Garra A (2015) Type I interferons in infectious disease. Nat Rev Immunol 15(2): 87–103. https://doi.org/10.1038/nri3787
21. Kanter J, Kruse-Jarres R (2013) Management of sickle cell disease from childhood through adulthood. Blood Rev 27(6):279–287. Epub 2013/10/08. https://doi.org/10.1016/j.blre.2013.09.001
22. Nickel RS, Horan JT, Fasano RM, Meyer E, Josephson CD, Winkler AM, Yee ME, Kean LS, Hendrickson JE (2015) Immunophenotypic parameters and RBC alloimmunization in children with sickle cell disease on chronic transfusion. Am J Hematol 90(12): 1135–1141. Epub 2015/09/12. https://doi.org/10.1002/ajh.24188
23. Pfefferlé M, Dubach IL, Buzzi RM, Düerst E, Schulthess-Lutz N, Baselgia L, Hansen K, Imhof L, Koernig S, Le Roy D, Roger T, Humar R, Schaer DJ, Vallelian F (2023) Antibody-induced erythrophagocyte reprogramming of Kupffer cells prevents anti-CD40 cancer immunotherapy-associated liver toxicity. J Immunother Cancer 11(1):ARTN e005718. https://doi.org/10.1136/jitc-2022-005718.
PubMed PMID: WOS:000907632800001
24. Olonisakin TF, Suber T, Gonzalez-Ferrer S, Xiong ZY, Peñaloza HF, van der Geest R, Xiong YT, Osei-Hwedieh DO, Tejero J, Rosengart MR, Mars WM, Van Tyne D, Perlegas A, Brashears S, Kim-Shapiro DB, Gladwin MT, Bachman MA, Hod EA, St Croix C, Tyurina YY, Kagan VE, Mallampalli RK, Ray A, Ray P, Lee JS (2021) Stressed erythrophagocytosis induces immunosuppression during sepsis through heme-mediated STAT1 dysregulation. J Clin Invest 131(1): ARTN e137468. https://doi.org/10.1172/JCI137468.
PubMed PMID: WOS:000607625100001
25. Lee E, Choi HS, Hwang JH, Hoh JK, Cho YH, Baek EJ (2014) The RNA in reticulocytes is not just debris: it is necessary for the final stages of erythrocyte formation. Blood Cells Mol Dis 53(1–2):1–10. Epub 2014/03/07. https://doi.org/10.1016/j.bcmd.2014.02.009
26. Thomas TA, Qiu A, Kim CY, Gordy DE, Miller A, Tredicine M, Dzieciatkowska M, Dei Zotti F, Hod EA, D'Alessandro A, Zimring JC, Spitalnik SL, Hudson KE (2023) Reticulocytes in donor blood units enhance red blood cell alloimmunization. Haematologica. 108(10): 2639–2651. https://doi.org/10.3324/haematol.2023.282815. Epub 2023/04/20. PubMed PMID: 37078267; PMCID: PMC10543191
27. Caielli S, Cardenas J, de Jesus AA, Baisch J, Walters L, Blanck JP, Balasubramanian P, Stagnar C, Ohouo M, Hong S, Nassi L, Stewart K, Fuller J, Gu J, Banchereau JF, Wright T, Goldbach-Mansky R, Pascual V (2021) Erythroid mitochondrial retention triggers myeloid-dependent type I interferon in human SLE. Cell. 184(17):4464–79 e19. https://doi.org/10.1016/j.cell.2021.07.021.

Epub 2021/08/14. PubMed PMID: 34384544; PMCID: PMC8380737

28. Moriconi C, Dzieciatkowska M, Roy M, D'Alessandro A, Roingeard P, Lee JY, Gibb DR, Tredicine M, McGill MA, Qiu AN, La Carpia F, Francis RO, Hod EA, Thomas T, Picard M, Akpan IJ, Luckey CJ, Zimring JC, Spitalnik SL, Hudson KE (2022) Retention of functional mitochondria in mature red blood cells from patients with sickle cell disease. Brit J Haematol 198(3):574–586. https://doi.org/10.1111/bjh.18287. PubMed PMID: WOS:000807005700001

29. Jagadeeswaran R, Vazquez BA, Thiruppathi M, Ganesh BB, Ibanez V, Cui S, Engel JD, Diamond AM, Molokie RE, DeSimone J, Lavelle D, Rivers A (2017) Pharmacological inhibition of LSD1 and mTOR reduces mitochondrial retention and associated ROS levels in the red blood cells of sickle cell disease. Exp Hematol. 50:46–52. https://doi.org/10.1016/j.exphem.2017.02.003. Epub 2017/02/28. PubMed PMID: 28238805; PMCID: PMC6263958

30. Martino S, Arlet JB, Odievre MH, Jullien V, Moras M, Hattab C, Lefebvre T, Gouya L, Ostuni MA, Lefevre SD, Le Van Kim C (2021) Deficient mitophagy pathways in sickle cell disease. Br J Haematol 193(5):988–993. Epub 2021/03/24. https://doi.org/10.1111/bjh.17416

Chapter 39

Anemia and Transfusion in Preclinical Models of Neonatology

Mary Vallecillo-Zuniga, Samata P. Varadkar, Carter J. Stowell, Wenhui Li, Luke L. Westhoff, Sean R. Stowell, and Connie M. Arthur

Abstract

Anemia is one of the most common complications observed in preterm infants. Red blood cell (RBC) transfusion is a standard therapy for treating neonatal anemia, but it is not without risk. Several studies suggest that while transfusion may reverse anemia, it can also cause inflammation and impaired barrier function in the developing intestine, potentially leading to necrotizing enterocolitis. However, the features of the developing immune system in a preterm infant, along with the characteristics of the transfused RBC unit that contribute to neonatal complications, have been difficult to define using correlative clinical studies alone. To overcome this limitation, a phlebotomy-induced anemia model has been developed that allows for determining critical factors related to the pathology of anemia and the impact of various treatment options. This protocol defines the model of phlebotomy-induced anemia in murine pups for studying anemia and transfusion-associated gut injury and inflammation.

Key words Phlebotomy-induced anemia, Transfusion, Tissue collection, Tissue processing, Flow cytometry, Sysmex, Immunohistochemistry

1 Introduction

Anemia is a hematological condition characterized by impaired function or decreased quantity of red blood cells (RBC). It can occur acutely, as a result of hemorrhagic complications associated with trauma, or it can manifest gradually in chronic conditions that necessitate ongoing transfusion support to maintain stable hemoglobin (Hb) levels [1–4}. Transfusion itself is one of the first examples of personalized medicine, where allogeneic differences between donor and recipient must be honored to ensure compatibility [8], thereby reducing the likelihood of immune-mediated complications. While these differences likely have important implications in infectious disease [5–7], a variety of studies have demonstrated that the development of alloantibodies against RBC

Sean R. Stowell and Connie M. Arthur (eds.), *Methods in Transfusion Medicine*, Methods in Molecular Biology, vol. 3053,
https://doi.org/10.1007/978-1-0716-5376-0_39,

alloantigens can severely complicate transfusion safety and directly contribute to morbidity and mortality of transfusion recipients [9–13]. Many studies have sought to define the role of various immune cells, innate immune factors, distinct immune pathways, and RBC features that may influence the development of immune responses against blood group antigens [14–32]; however, much remains to be learned regarding the governing principles that regulate the development and consequences of RBC alloimmunization [33–38].

In contrast to most patients with anemia requiring transfusion, preterm infants are less likely to develop alloantibodies following transfusion, yet they remain at risk for other types of immune-mediated transfusion complications. This is especially apparent in very low birth weight (VLBW) infants [39]. The most severely anemic newborns (Hb concentration below 7 g/dL), including VLBW infants (weighing less than 1500 g), frequently receive RBC transfusions to increase hemoglobin levels and improve tissue oxygenation [40, 41]. However, this practice has been associated with adverse effects including systemic inflammatory responses, possible gut injury, and the development of severe complications such as necrotizing enterocolitis (NEC) [42, 43].

NEC is a severe gastrointestinal inflammatory disorder and is the principal cause of death in preterm VLBW newborns in the United States [44, 45]. This devastating disease affects premature infants and is associated with intestinal inflammation and bacterial invasion, leading to gut injury and necrosis [46]. Although the exact mechanisms by which anemia influences the development of NEC are not yet well understood, studies in murine models suggest neonatal anemia increases newborns' susceptibility to intestinal inflammation and injury by promoting inflammatory macrophage activation, increased intestinal permeability, and hypoxia of gut tissue [47]. Although NEC remains incompletely understood, studies identify NEC as a multifactorial disease. Current research has shown evidence of a connection between anemia, transfusion, and NEC-associated symptoms [48, 49]. Data from more than 600 VLBW infants showed an elevated percentage of NEC among babies with severe anemia [50]. Data also demonstrates the increased likelihood of NEC within 48 h after RBC transfusion [40]. These results, among others, shed light on connections between anemia, transfusion, and NEC.

Despite clinical studies demonstrating an association between anemia, transfusion, and NEC, the underlying basis for this association remains to be fully elucidated. This is, in part, due to a historical lack of animal models capable of recapitulating key features of neonatal anemia which could possibly uncover key features of anemia and transfusion on intestinal injury in the developing neonate. Preclinical models have been developed that have provided important insight through a number of studies into

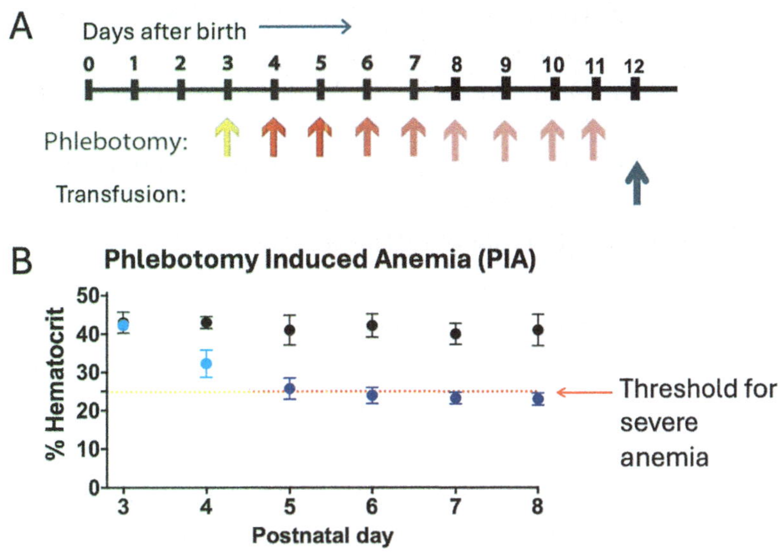

Fig. 1 Phlebotomy-Induced Anemia (PIA). (**a**) Schematic of protocol for induction of PIA. (**b**) Hematocrit of neonates with (blue) or without (black) phlebotomy on days 3–8 after birth P3-P8). The red line indicates the threshold for anemia (25%). (This research was originally published in Transfusion. Arthur et al. [47])

other adverse consequences of transfusion and other therapeutics [16, 18, 19, 33, 51–61], including alloimmunization against various transfused blood products and even related therapeutics [23, 24, 37, 38, 51, 52, 54, 55, 62–66], However, similar studies are only beginning to emerge within the area of neonatal transfusion [67]. These types of studies are especially important as developmental differences in neonatal recipients and adult blood donors may impact transfusion outcomes. As a result, studies specifically tailored to address these unique variables are needed if the distinct features of neonatal transfusion are to be defined [47]. This chapter explains the preclinical phlebotomy-induced anemia (PIA) model in neonatal pups through timed phlebotomy [47] (Fig. 1), as well as the protocols for retro-orbital transfusion and tissue processing post-transfusion. This method holds promise in providing more insight into the etiology behind transfusion-related intestinal injury in susceptible anemic neonates requiring transfusion.

2 Materials

2.1 Phlebotomy-Induced Anemia (PIA) (P3-P11)

1. Jax Mice Pup Appearance by Age chart—JAX Mice Pup Appearance by Age (nih.gov).
2. Animal Weighing Scale (Kent Scientific Corporation—Stainless Steel Digital Animal Weighing Scale (4000 g Capacity), Catalog: SCL-4000).

3. Weigh boat (e.g., VWR—Ward's® Standard Weighing Boats, Catalog# 470306–942).
4. Oppen Identification Marker (Braintree Scientific, KN-297 -V-6).
5. GOLDENROD LANCET 3MM 1000/CS (Fisher Scientific, NC0024199).
6. CTAD anticoagulant solution.
7. Heparinized hematocrit tubes.
8. Micropipettor and tips.
9. Gauze.
10. Sealing clay for hematocrit tubes.
11. Microcentrifuge tubes.
12. Hematocrit tube centrifuge, gel card reader, or Sysmex analyzer.

2.2 Blood Collection for Transfusion

1. Adult donor mice.
2. 5 mm sterile lancet (Fisher Scientific, NC9467425).
3. Citrate-phosphate-dextrose solution with adenine (CPDA).
4. Phosphate Buffered Saline (PBS) (Cytiva, SH30256.02).
5. Centrifuge-compatible tube for collection.
6. Pipettor.
7. Centrifuge.

2.3 Retro-orbital Transfusion in P12 Neonates

1. 30 G BD™ Needle 1/2 in. single use, sterile (Owens & Minor, 305106).
2. Sterile Phosphate Buffered Saline (PBS) (Cytiva, SH30256.02).
3. Animal Weighing Scale (Kent Scientific Corporation—Stainless Steel Digital Animal Weighing Scale (4000 g Capacity), Catalog: SCL-4000).
4. Weigh boat (e.g., VWR—Ward's® Standard Weighing Boats, Catalog# 470306–942).
5. 1 mL Tuberculin Syringes (MEDLINE INDUSTRIES INC, 309659).
6. Pivetal® Isoflurane (Control substance VI) (Patterson Veterinary, 07-893-8441).
7. Breathing Circuits and Accessories, VetEquip®, Complete Dual Procedure Non-Rebreathing Circuit (Fisher Scientific, 921400).
8. Fisherbrand Gauze Sponges; Nonsterile; 4x4 in.; 12-ply; 2000/CS (Fisher Scientific, 1376152).

9. Fisherbrand aluminum Foil (Fisher Scientific, 01-213-100).
10. Heating mat (if needed).

2.4 Blood Collection for Serum/Plasma and Neonatal Mouse Sacrifice

1. KIMBLE® Heparinized Micro-Hematocrit Capillary Tubes; Color Red; ID 1.1 mm; Length 75 mm; 90 expansion soda lime glass (VWR, 14705-003).
2. Axygen® MaxyClear 1.7 mL Polypropylene Snap Cap Microcentrifuge Tubes, Nonsterile, Bulk Bag, Clear (Corning, MCT-175-C).
3. K2 EDTA plasma collection tubes MiniCollect® TUBE 0.25/ 0.5 mL K2E K2EDTA, Lavender Cap (VWR, 76343-512).
4. CPDA.
5. 16x100 mm 8.5 mL BD Vacutainer® glass whole blood ACD tube (Owens & Minor, 364606).
6. Phosphate Buffered Saline (PBS) (Cytiva, SH30256.02).
7. Pivetal® Isoflurane (Control substance VI) (Patterson Veterinary, 07-893-8441).
8. Breathing Circuits and Accessories, VetEquip®, Complete Dual Procedure Non-Rebreathing Circuit (Fisher Scientific, 921400).
9. Razor blades (VWR, 55411-050).
10. Scissors (Braintree Scientific, Catalog# SCT-I 528).
11. Micro-Tissue Forceps (Braintree Scientific, SKU: FC14).
12. Make 70% Ethanol from Ethanol, HPLC/Spectrophotometric Grade, Liquid, ≥99.5%, Glass bottle, 200 Proof (Sigma-Aldrich, 459828-2L).

2.5 Harvesting Spleens and Isolation of Splenocytes

1. Easystrainer™ Cell Sieves, Greiner Bio-One, EASYstrainer™ Cell Sieves, 70 μm, Color = Blue, Sterility = Sterile (Greiner Bio-One, 542070).
2. RBC Lysis Buffer (10X) (BioLegend, 420302).
3. Falcon 15 mL Polystyrene Centrifuge Tube, Conical Bottom, with Dome Seal Screw Cap, Sterile, 50/Bag, 500/Case (Fisher Scientific, 05-527-90).
4. 96-well counting plate.
5. Gibco Trypan Blue Solution, 0.4% (Thermo Fisher Scientific, 15-250-061).
6. Phosphate Buffered Saline (PBS) (Cytiva, SH30256.02).
7. Hemocytometer Hausser Scientific Bright-Line Counting Chamber (Fisher Scientific, 02-671-51B).
8. Standard growth media (SGM).

2.6 Harvesting Intestines for Immunohistochemistry

1. Scissors (Braintree Scientific, Catalog# SCT-I 528).
2. Std Pattern Dressing Forceps (Braintree Scientific, Catalog# FC 100 2).
3. Phosphate Buffered Saline (PBS) (Cytiva, SH30256.02).
4. Methyl-Carnoy's.
5. Protocol 10% Buffered Formalin, Fisher Diagnostics (Fisher Scientific, 23-245684).
6. Make 70% Ethanol from Ethanol, HPLC/Spectrophotometric Grade, Liquid, ≥99.5%, Glass bottle, 200 Proof (Sigma-Aldrich, 459828-2L).
7. H&E stains.
8. Alcian blue solution for microscopy, Packaging = Plastic Bottle, Size = 500 mL (Sigma-Aldrich, 1016470500).
9. FISH stains.
10. Falcon 15 mL Polystyrene Centrifuge Tube, Conical Bottom, with Dome Seal Screw Cap, Sterile, 50/Bag, 500/Case (Fisher Scientific, 05-527-90).
11. Set up for paraffin embedding.
12. Tissue slicer.

2.7 Tissue collection (Intestines) and Immune Cell Isolation

1. Hanks' Balanced Salt solution, HBSS Modified, with phenol red, without calcium, without magnesium, liquid (Sigma-Aldrich, 55021C-1000ML).
2. 5% Fetal Bovine Serum (R&D Systems, S11550) (Boston Bio-Products, BM-150).
3. EDTA (0.5 M, pH 8.0), autoclaved (Boston BioProducts, BM-150).
4. 50 mL Fisherbrand™ Easy Reader™ Conical Polypropylene Centrifuge Tubes (FisherScientific, 05-539-13).
5. Orbital shaker with temperature control Fisherbrand™ Incubating Microplate Shakers (FisherScientific, 02-217-760).
6. Easystrainer™ Cell Sieves, Greiner Bio-One, EASYstrainer™ Cell Sieves, 70 μm, Color = Blue, Sterility = Sterile (Greiner Bio-One, 542070).
7. RPMI 1640 Complete Medium, with 2 mM L-Glut and 10% FBS, RPMI 1640 Complete Medium, with 2 mM L-Glut and 10% FBS (EMD Millipore, SLM-240-B).
8. Collagenase from Clostridium histolyticum, release of rat epididymal adipocytes and hepatocytes, Type VIII, 0.5–5.0 FALGPA units/mg solid, ≥125 CDU/mg solid (Sigma-Aldrich, C2139-500MG).

2.8 Splenocyte and Gut Cell Staining

1. Costar 96 Well Clear Round Bottom Tissue Culture-Treated Microplate with Lid, Sterile, Individually Wrapped, 50/case (Fisher Scientific, 3799).
2. Phosphate Buffered Saline (PBS) (Cytiva, SH30256.02).
3. LIVE/DEAD™ Fixable Blue Dead Cell Stain Kit, for UV excitation (ThermoFisher, Catalog# L34962).
4. TruStain FcX™ (anti-mouse CD16/32) Antibody (Biolegend, Catalog# 101320).
5. Selected fluorescently tagged primary antibodies (*see* **Note 1**).
6. Flow Cytometer.
7. QC beads.

3 Method

3.1 Phlebotomy-Induced Anemia (PIA) (P3-P11)

1. Identify the age of pups (*see* **Note 2**). Induction of phlebotomy-induced anemia should begin on post-natal day 3 (P3) (*see* **Note 3**).
2. To calculate the appropriate volume for phlebotomy, measure the weight of the pups on a weighing balance using a weigh boat to keep the pups in one area. Note the weight in grams and calculate the collection volume of 5.25 μLof whole blood per gram of weight.
3. Use a 3 mm (about 0.12 in) lancet to puncture the submandibular vein. Collect the calculated volume of whole blood (5.25 μL/g) using a micropipettor or pre-marked heparinized tube. Use collected blood to determine hematocrit using a hematocrit card reader (**Step 1.5**) or Sysmex analyzer (**Step 1.6**) (*see* **Note 4**).
4. In parallel, to account for stress, perform a needle stick in the neck of control pups without drawing blood.
5. To determine hematocrit by plate reader, plug the hematocrit tube containing blood with clay and spin for 5 min at 10,000 rpm, followed by analysis of hematocrit with a card reader.
6. *For Sysmex analysis of blood for the hemotocrit (HCT%), hemoglobin, and the differential count*: collect and dilute 20 μL of blood in 180 μL of CTAD (1:10 diluted) (*see* **Note 5**).
7. Repeat **Steps 1.2–1.6** every day until the desired hematocrit is achieved (<25%). This normally occurs by P7-P8.
8. Once the desired hematocrit threshold is achieved, continue bleeds with a decreased volume of 3.5 μL/g to maintain anemia through the desired experimental duration.

3.2 Blood Collection for Transfusion

1. Sterilize the Biosafety cabinet with disinfectant (70% ethanol) and paper towels.
2. The collection tube should have sterile CPDA (Citrate-phosphate-dextrose solution with adenine: anticoagulant) in an amount which is equivalent to 14–20% of the total volume of blood to be collected (*see* **Note 6).**
3. Collect blood from an adult donor mouse by submandibular bleed using a 5 mm sterile lancet.
4. Mix blood thoroughly with the CPDA to avoid clots (*see* **Note** 7).
5. Add sterile PBS and centrifuge the tube at 500 rcf (g) for 5 min at 4 °C with the brakes off.
6. Carefully remove supernatant by reverse pipetting.
7. Repeat **Steps 5** and **6** twice more.
8. Before transfusing, reconstitute the blood with PBS to its original hematocrit (~50%).

3.3 Retro-orbital Transfusion of P12 Neonates

1. Use a 30-gauge needle for retro-orbital transfusions in neonates. Use separate needles for PBS and blood transfusions.
2. Weigh the pups and calculate the amount of blood/PBS to be transfused for each pup, using 20 μL blood or PBS per gram of body weight.
3. Fill the 1 mL TB syringes with the fluid to be transfused (PBS/ blood) and remove any air from the syringe.
4. Prepare the isoflurane chamber (cotton gauze on bottom, foil on top), add 0.5 mL of isoflurane to the gauze in a chamber of ~250 mL.
5. Place the pup on the aluminum foil in the isoflurane chamber. Close the chamber and monitor the pup for sedation.
6. Remove the pup from the isoflurane chamber when breathing has slowed by ~50%.
7. Open the sealed eyes by slowly stretching the eyelids apart, using the transfusion needle tip to gently break through the connective tissue. Be gentle and make sure not to poke or injure the eye.
8. Make sure the neonate is still completely under anesthesia (if not, place the pup back in the isoflurane chamber to achieve sedation) (*see* **Note 8**).
9. To complete retro-orbital transfusion into the retro-orbital sinus behind the eyeball, from the corner of the eye socket, carefully and slowly insert the needle into the cavity behind the eyeball. Place the bevel of the needle downwards away from the eyeball to ensure there is no injury to the eyeball. Do not go

too deep, just until the bevel is completely in, then slowly transfuse the pup. Slowly remove the needle and monitor the pup for recovery from anesthesia (*see* **Note 9**).

10. Keep the pup warm by holding it in your hand and/or using a heating mat until completely recovered.
11. Note the time of transfusion to allow for accurately timed sample collection post-transfusion. Hematocrit change following transfusion can be assessed at the time of sacrifice, following the steps outlined in Subheading 3.1.

3.4 Blood Collection for Serum/Plasma and Neonatal mouse Sacrifice

1. At desired timepoint(s) (depending on the experimental design), collect blood by submandibular bleed using a 3 mm lancet and heparin-coated capillary tubes (*see* Subheading 3.1) (*see* **Note 10**).
2. Transfer blood into a microcentrifuge tube for serum or into a plasma collection tube containing EDTA (*see* **Note 11**).
3. At the experiment endpoint, follow **Steps 1** and **2** outlined above to perform a submandibular bleed to collect the maximum blood volume possible for serum or plasma. This bleed will be terminal, and the pup should be sacrificed immediately after collection (*see* **Note 12**).
4. *Serum collection*—Spin the microcentrifuge tube containing the collected blood at 1000 g for 10 min. Collect the supernatant. Freeze it or directly use it for cytokine assays.
5. *Plasma collection*—Spin the collection tube with blood at 500 g for 5 min with soft braking or brakes off. Collect the supernatant (plasma) and freeze or use directly for desired assays.
6. Immediately following plasma collection, add 200 μL of PBS to the pellet of blood cells and reconstitute the whole blood.
7. Sedate the pup with isoflurane as described and verify sedation by toe pinch before decapitating the pup using a razor blade (*see* **Note 13**).

3.5 Harvesting Spleens and Isolation of Splenocytes

1. Immediately following sacrifice, spray the abdomen with 70% ethanol. Pinch the skin near the abdomen and make small incisions to open the abdominal cavity.
2. Harvest the spleen (pink to red mass of bean-shaped tissue in the upper abdominal cavity behind the stomach).
3. Prepare a single cell suspension from the spleen by forcing it through a 70 μm mesh filter, washing the filter with PBS (*see* **Note 14**).
4. Centrifuge for 10 min at 500× *g*.
5. Pour off the supernatant and flick the pellet into suspension (the pellets should be blood red at this point).

6. Suspend the cells in RBC lysis buffer (2 mL/spleen) and incubate at room temperature for 5 min.
7. Add PBS to make up a final volume of 15–20 mL (volume can be adjusted), and centrifuge for 10 min at 500× *g*.
8. Pour off the supernatant and flick the pellet into suspension (the pellet should be white at this point with just a small layer of red on top).
9. Suspend the cells in 10 mL of PBS and mix well.
10. Repeat this wash 2 additional times.
11. Take 20 μLof each sample and place in a 96-well counting plate before centrifuging the tubes on the final wash.
12. Add 20 μL trypan blue and 160 μL PBS to each of the 20 μLcell specimens.
13. Place 10 μL of each stained sample in a hemocytometer and count the number of viable cells in one 4x4 unit of squares.
14. The number of your count equals the total number of cells you have $\times 10^6$. For example, if you get a count of 86, you have 86 million cells in the corresponding tube.
15. Pour off the supernatant, flick the pellet into suspension, and suspend the cells in PBS at a concentration of 20 million cells per mL.
16. Calculate the amount of SGM by dividing the cell number by 20. For example, if you have 86 million cells, 86/20 = 4.3 mL of PBS.
17. Perform staining for flow cytometry (Subheading 3.8).

3.6 Harvesting Intestines and Processing Them for Immunohistochemistry

1. Maintaining moisture is critical for sample integrity. Use PBS to moisten as needed.
2. Make an incision on the intestine close to the distal end of the intestine (end of the colon).
3. Slowly start pulling out the intestine while getting rid of the fat tissue layer (mesentery), using standard dressing or tissue forceps (*see* **Note 15**).
4. Once you have a clean and intact (if possible) intestine, spread it into a straight line onto a piece of aluminum foil with a small amount of PBS to keep the cells hydrated.
5. Carefully collect stool pellets from the colon using forceps to push the pellets slowly one at a time. Put the stool pellets in a microcentrifuge tube and freeze them over dry ice.
6. Note the details of the neonatal pup and take a picture of it against a scale to measure the gut length.

7. For H&E staining, fix the tissue in 1:10 formalin for 24 h. Wash with PBS twice and store in 70% ethanol for paraffin embedding (*see* **Note 16**).

3.7 Tissue Collection (Intestines) and Immune Cell Isolation

1. Harvest the intestines (follow Subheading 3.6, **steps 1–4**). Cut open the intestines longitudinally and wash the fecal content by suspending the tissue in HBSS +5% FBS and swirling it around gently.
2. Wash the intact tissue 3–4 times with HBSS +5% FBS.
3. Perform washes by cutting tissue into 1.5 cm pieces and transferring them into a 50 mL conical tube with 10 mL HBSS, 5% FBS, and 40 μL of 0.5 M EDTA (pH 8). Tightly cap the tube.
4. Place the tube horizontally for 20 min in a 37 ° C orbital shaker at 250 rpm.
5. Collect the tissue using a 70-μm mesh filter. Put it back into 10 mL HBSS, 5% FBS, and 40 μL of 0.5 M EDTA (pH 8). Tightly cap the tube. Repeat Steps 3.8.4 and 3.8.5 two to three times.
6. Collect the tissue in a 70 μm mesh filter. Wash the tissue with HBSS and remove any remaining media by gently placing a corner of a Kim wipe at the edge of the filter. Using sharp scissors, mince the tissue.
7. Place the minced tissue in a 15 mL tube with 6 mL of RPMI complete and 0.5 mg/mL of Type VIII collagenase. Place the tube in a 37 °C orbital shaker at 150 rpm for exactly 10 min (*see* **Note 17**).
8. Collect the single cell suspension by passing the liquid through a mesh filter.
9. Spin down the supernatant at 500× *g* for 10 min to obtain the cell pellet for downstream analysis (*see* **Note 18**).
10. If desired, count the cells as described in Subheading 3.5.

3.8 Splenocyte and Gut Cell Staining

1. Prepare the stain mix by diluting the desired antibodies according to manufacturer recommendations.
2. Add 50 μL of each resuspended sample to a 96-well plate and wash 3x with 200 μL PBS, centrifuging at 500× *g* for 2 min.
3. After the final wash, add 50 μL of Live/Dead Blue stain (diluted 1:400 in PBS) and incubate for 15 min in the dark at room temperature (*see* **Note 19**).
4. After the incubation is complete, add 200 μL of PBS to each well and centrifuge at 500× *g* for 2 min.
5. Carefully remove the supernatant and add 25 μL of Fc block (1: 100). Incubate for 10 min in the dark at room temperature.

6. Add 25 μL of stain (2x Master Mix (MM)—2x MM should have 1x Fc block) to each sample.
7. Incubate the samples in the dark at on ice for 30 min.
8. Following the incubation, add 200 μL PBS and centrifuge at 500× *g* for 2 min.
9. Remove the supernatant by carefully pipetting and wash 1–2 more times with PBS.
10. After the final wash, resuspend the pellet in 200 μL FACS or PBS and analyze by flow cytometry.

4 Notes

1. We have not included specific antibodies for staining in this protocol, but the protocol included should be appropriate for most surface staining antibodies.
2. We typically use number markings on the pup's belly as they seem least likely to be cleaned off. Markings must be refreshed every day; they will not usually last multiple days. You can also use toe clips (before the pup turns 7 days old) if you are not trying to study immune and physiological responses to injury.
3. Identify and note the age of the mice neonates by referring to the Jax Mice Pup Appearance by Age chart—JAX Mice Pup Appearance by Age (nih.gov).
4. Heparanized tubes must be marked for the appropriate volume using sterile PBS prior to bleeding. If using a micropipettor, it is essential that the tip be coated with anticoagulant prior to use. This can be accomplished by simply pipetting up and down in the tube containing the anticoagulant used for collection. If planning to use a Sysmex analyzer to monitor blood hematocrit, then using the micropipette method is recommended to allow for accurate collection and immediate dilution into an anticoagulant to prevent clotting that can interfere with accurate Sysmex measurements.
5. Avoiding clots is critical for accurate measurements. Coat a 20 μL pipette tip with CTAD (1:10 diluted) by pipetting it in and out a few times. Place the pipette near you. Perform submandibular venipuncture and pipette 20 μL of blood. Mix that blood thoroughly with 180 μL of CTAD (1:10 diluted). Collect the remaining amount of blood using another pipette set to the required values to collect the remaining blood.
6. Example: to collect 1 mL of blood, add 140–200 μL CPDA (14%–20% of the total volume of blood to be collected) to a 5 mL sterile tube and collect 800–860 μL of FVB.HOD mice blood, respectively.

7. Thoroughly mix the blood with CPDA to reduce the chances of clot formation, as the blood will be used to transfuse neonates.
8. Also, monitor the pup closely for regular and continuous breathing and take care not to occlude airways at any point during the transfusion process.
9. Make sure to hold the pup gently and not to block its air supply or put excess pressure on the neck or head.
10. Volume collected may vary, but for non-terminal bleeds, collect the minimum volume necessary for your planned assay. Consider the percent of blood, the percent of the total blood volume taken with each bleed, and avoid taking amounts that may significantly affect the pups' physiology while the experiment is ongoing. Always follow institutional IACUC guidelines.
11. Choice of serum or plasma collection is dependent on the desired downstream assay.
12. This bleed may also be performed by retro-orbital bleed using a heparinized capillary tube, with the pup sedated by isoflurane.
13. Verify appropriate sacrifice techniques based on age and IACUC guidelines at your institution.
14. Use the flat end of a plunger of a syringe to mash the spleen and pass it through the mesh filter. Be sure to collect all tissue from the underside of the strainer.
15. Use the most suitable forceps available to make sure that there is no puncture, damage, or breakage of the intestine. Gently peel away fat and connective tissue.
16. It is recommended to place tissue into an appropriate orientation within a cassette before formalin fixation, as tissue is less pliable after.
17. Extending the incubation at this step may result in lower cell viability.
18. Given the low cell yield from neonatal guts, we have omitted the Percoll gradient from this protocol; however, this step can be added back in to more completely remove non-immune gut cells. With the omission of the gradient step, it is critical to include CD45 in the flow cytometry stain as a pan-leukocyte marker.
19. Live/Dead Blue is used as an example viability stain, but a different choice may be more appropriate depending on the panel of antibodies being utilized for cell staining.

Conflict of Interest Statement

This work was funded by NIH P01HL171803, R01 HL165975, R01 HL135575, and R01 HL154034. SRS has received speaker and consultant honoraria from Cerus, Grifols, Novartis, Alexion, and Argenx and has received a research grant from Alexion. No other authors have conflicts of interest.

References

1. Chou ST, Hendrickson JE (2024) How I treat challenging transfusion cases in sickle cell disease. Blood
2. Lal A et al (2021) The transfusion management of beta thalassemia in the United States. Transfusion 61(10):3027–3039
3. Butwick AJ, Goodnough LT (2015) Transfusion and coagulation management in major obstetric hemorrhage. Curr Opin Anaesthesiol 28(3):275–284
4. Jajosky RP et al (2023) ABO blood group antigens and differential glycan expression: perspective on the evolution of common human enzyme deficiencies. iScience 26(1):105798
5. Wu SC et al (2023) Blood group a enhances SARS-CoV-2 infection. Blood 142(8): 742–747
6. Jan HM et al (2024) Galectin-4 antimicrobial activity primarily occurs through its C-terminal domain. Mol Cell Proteomics 23(5):100747
7. Wu SC et al (2022) Innate immune Galectin-7 specifically targets microbes that decorate themselves in blood group-like antigens. iScience 25(7):104482
8. Zimring JC, Spitalnik SL (2015) Pathobiology of transfusion reactions. Annu Rev Pathol 10: 83–110
9. Viayna E, Gehrie EA, Blanchette C (2024) Alloimmunization in myelodysplastic syndrome is associated with higher healthcare costs, longer hospitalizations, and increased mortality. Transfusion 64(9):1640–1647
10. Viayna E et al (2022) Red cell alloimmunization is associated with increased health care costs, longer hospitalizations, and higher mortality. Blood Adv 6(20):5655–5658
11. Telen MJ et al (2015) Alloimmunization in sickle cell disease: changing antibody specificities and association with chronic pain and decreased survival. Transfusion 55(6 Pt 2): 1378–1387
12. Dean CL et al (2019) Multiple hemolytic transfusion reactions misinterpreted as severe vaso-occlusive crisis in a patient with sickle cell disease. Transfusion 59(2):448–453
13. Chonat S et al (2025) Complement is activated in patients with acute chest syndrome caused by sickle cell disease and represents a therapeutic target. Sci Transl Med 17(807):eadl4922
14. Zimring JC et al (2005) Nonhemolytic antibody-induced loss of erythrocyte surface antigen. Blood 106(3):1105–1112
15. Shinde P et al (2020) IgG subclass determines suppression versus enhancement of humoral alloimmunity to Kell RBC antigens in mice. Front Immunol 11:1516
16. Jash A et al (2021) Antibodies to low-copy number RBC alloantigen convert a tolerogenic stimulus to an immunogenic stimulus in mice. Front Immunol 12:629608
17. Arneja A et al (2016) Interleukin-6 receptor-alpha signaling drives anti-RBC alloantibody production and T-follicular helper cell differentiation in a murine model of red blood cell alloimmunization. Haematologica 101(11): e440–e444
18. Thomas TA et al (2023) Reticulocytes in donor blood units enhance red blood cell alloimmunization. Haematologica 108(10):2639–2651
19. Jash A et al (2024) Complement C3 and marginal zone B cells promote IgG-mediated enhancement of RBC alloimmunization in mice. J Clin Invest 134(8)
20. Pal M et al (2021) Hemolysis inhibits humoral B-cell responses and modulates alloimmunization risk in patients with sickle cell disease. Blood 137(2):269–280
21. Godefroy E et al (2015) TIGIT-positive circulating follicular helper T cells display robust B-cell help functions: potential role in sickle cell alloimmunization. Haematologica 100(11):1415–1425
22. Godefroy E et al (2016) Altered heme-mediated modulation of dendritic cell function in sickle cell alloimmunization. Haematologica 101(9):1028–1038

23. Jajosky RP et al (2023) Antibody-mediated antigen loss switches augmented immunity to antibody-mediated immunosuppression. Blood 142(12):1082–1098
24. Zerra PE et al (2021) Marginal zone B cells mediate a CD4 T-cell-dependent extrafollicular antibody response following RBC transfusion in mice. Blood 138(8):706–721
25. Zhi H et al (2021) Preclinical evaluation of immunotherapeutic regimens for fetal/neonatal alloimmune thrombocytopenia. Blood Adv 5(18):3552–3562
26. Newman DK, Newman PJ (2024) Antigen-specific immunotherapy for platelet alloimmune disorders. Hum Immunol 85(6):111172
27. Zhi H et al (2022) Prophylactic administration of HPA-1a-specific antibodies prevents fetal/neonatal alloimmune thrombocytopenia in mice. Blood 140(20):2146–2153
28. Xu X et al (2021) Successful prenatal therapy for anti-CD36-mediated severe FNAIT by deglycosylated antibodies in a novel murine model. Blood 138(18):1757–1767
29. Vadasz B et al (2015) Platelets and platelet alloantigens: lessons from human patients and animal models of fetal and neonatal alloimmune thrombocytopenia. Genes Dis 2(2):173–185
30. Li C et al (2013) Co-stimulation with LPS or Poly I:C markedly enhances the anti-platelet immune response and severity of fetal and neonatal alloimmune thrombocytopenia. Thromb Haemost 110(6):1250–1258
31. Li C et al (2011) The maternal immune response to fetal platelet GPIbalpha causes frequent miscarriage in mice that can be prevented by intravenous IgG and anti-FcRn therapies. J Clin Invest 121(11):4537–4547
32. Chen P et al (2010) Animal model of fetal and neonatal immune thrombocytopenia: role of neonatal Fc receptor in the pathogenesis and therapy. Blood 116(18):3660–3668
33. Hudson KE et al (2019) Mechanisms of alloimmunization in sickle cell disease. Curr Opin Hematol 26(6):434–441
34. Yazdanbakhsh K, Shaz BH, Hillyer CD (2017) Immune regulation of sickle cell alloimmunization. ISBT Sci Ser 12(1):248–253
35. Arthur CM, Stowell SR (2023) The development and consequences of red blood cell alloimmunization. Annu Rev Pathol 18:537–564
36. Jajosky RP et al (2025) CD47 regulates antigen modulation and red blood cell clearance following an incompatible transfusion. Front Immunol 16:1548548
37. Jajosky R et al (2023) Prior immunization against an intracellular antigen enhances subsequent red blood cell alloimmunization in mice. Blood 141(21):2642–2653
38. Maier CL et al (2018) Antibody-mediated immune suppression by antigen modulation is antigen-specific. Blood Adv 2(21):2986–3000
39. Aher S, Malwatkar K, Kadam S (2008) Neonatal anemia. Semin Fetal Neonatal Med 13(4): 239–247
40. Colombatti R, Sainati L, Trevisanuto D (2016) Anemia and transfusion in the neonate. Semin Fetal Neonatal Med 21(1):2–9
41. MohanKumar K et al (2019) A murine neonatal model of necrotizing enterocolitis caused by anemia and red blood cell transfusions. Nat Commun 10(1):3494
42. Lee EY et al (2020) Effect of red blood cell transfusion on short-term outcomes in very low birth weight infants. Clin Exp Pediatr 63(2):56–62
43. Zerra PE, Josephson CD (2021) Transfusion in neonatal patients: review of evidence-based guidelines. Clin Lab Med 41(1):15–34
44. Wolf MF et al (2023) Trends and racial and geographic differences in infant mortality in the United States due to necrotizing enterocolitis, 1999 to 2020. JAMA Netw Open 6(3): e231511
45. Zozaya C et al (2020) Incidence, treatment, and outcome trends of necrotizing enterocolitis in preterm infants: a multicenter cohort study. Front Pediatr 8:188
46. Neu J (2020) Necrotizing enterocolitis: the future. Neonatology 117(2):240–244
47. Arthur CM et al (2019) Anemia induces gut inflammation and injury in an animal model of preterm infants. Transfusion 59(4):1233–1245
48. Khashu M et al (2022) Current understanding of transfusion-associated necrotizing enterocolitis: review of clinical and experimental studies and a call for more definitive evidence. Newborn (Clarksville) 1(1):201–208
49. Rose AT, Saroha V, Patel RM (2020) Transfusion-related gut injury and necrotizing enterocolitis. Clin Perinatol 47(2):399–412
50. Patel RM et al (2016) Association of red blood cell transfusion, anemia, and necrotizing enterocolitis in very low-birth-weight infants. JAMA 315(9):889–897
51. Desmarets M et al (2009) Minor histocompatibility antigens on transfused leukoreduced units of red blood cells induce bone marrow transplant rejection in a mouse model. Blood 114(11):2315–2322

52. Smith NH et al (2012) Generation of transgenic mice with antithetical KEL1 and KEL2 human blood group antigens on red blood cells. Transfusion 52(12):2620–2630
53. Zimring JC, Hudson KE (2016) Cellular immune responses in red blood cell alloimmunization. Hematol Am Soc Hematol Educ Program 2016(1):452–456
54. Smith NH et al (2012) Transfusion in the absence of inflammation induces antigen-specific tolerance to murine RBCs. Blood 119(6):1566–1569
55. Stowell SR et al (2013) Alloantibodies to a paternally derived RBC KEL antigen lead to hemolytic disease of the fetus/newborn in a murine model. Blood 122(8):1494–1504
56. Yu H et al (2014) Antibody-mediated immune suppression of erythrocyte alloimmunization can occur independently from red cell clearance or epitope masking in a murine model. J Immunol 193(6):2902–2910
57. Liepkalns JS et al (2012) Biphasic clearance of incompatible red blood cells through a novel mechanism requiring neither complement nor Fcgamma receptors in a murine model. Transfusion 52(12):2631–2645
58. Liepkalns JS et al (2013) Resistance of a subset of red blood cells to clearance by antibodies in a mouse model of incompatible transfusion. Transfusion 53(6):1319–1327
59. Qiu A et al (2022) FcgammaRIV is required for IgG2c mediated enhancement of RBC alloimmunization. Front Immunol 13:972723
60. Girard-Pierce KR et al (2013) A novel role for C3 in antibody-induced red blood cell clearance and antigen modulation. Blood 122(10): 1793–1801
61. Stowell SR et al (2015) Anti-KEL sera prevents alloimmunization to transfused KEL RBCs in a murine model. Haematologica 100(10):e394–e397
62. Soldatenko A et al (2022) Innate and adaptive immunity to transfused allogeneic RBCs in mice requires MyD88. J Immunol 208(4): 991–997
63. Gruber DR et al (2020) Passively transferred IgG enhances humoral immunity to a red blood cell alloantigen in mice. Blood Adv 4(7):1526–1537
64. Zerra PE et al (2017) Marginal zone B cells are critical to factor VIII inhibitor formation in mice with hemophilia a. Blood 130(23): 2559–2568
65. Mener A et al (2018) Complement serves as a switch between CD4+ T cell-independent and -dependent RBC antibody responses. JCI Insight 3(22)
66. Arthur CM et al (2022) Nonhuman glycans can regulate anti-factor VIII antibody formation in mice. Blood 139(9):1312–1317
67. Davenport P et al (2022) Platelet transfusions in a murine model of neonatal polymicrobial sepsis: divergent effects on inflammation and mortality. Transfusion 62(6):1177–1187

Chapter 40

Expression and Characterization of Blood Group Binding Lectins

Hsien-Ya Lin, Shang-Chuen Wu, Hau-Ming Jan, Anu Paul, Victoria Ortiz, Courtney A. Winters, Carter J. Stowell, Vivien C. Lee, and Connie M. Arthur

Abstract

Carbohydrate-binding proteins, often called lectins, possess the unique ability to engage other macromolecules through recognition of carbohydrate structures. Among lectins, galectins have emerged as unique mammalian lectins that can possess high specificity for human carbohydrate-based blood group antigens. As such, galectins can differentiate red blood cells (RBCs) based on the blood group status of an individual. The ability of galectins to engage glycans can be studied by a wide variety of approaches. We describe herein the production of galectins and the characterization of galectin glycanbinding affinity using isothermal titration calorimetry (ITC).

Key words Galectin, Blood group antigens, Galectin purification, Isothermal titration calorimetry, Binding affinity

1 Introduction

The use of lectins dates back to 1888 when ricin, a protein found in the seeds of the castor plant (*Ricinus communis*), was discovered to cause the clumping of red blood cells (RBCs) from various species [1]. In 1902, Karl Landsteiner's group showed that extracts of various seeds had several types of hemagglutinating activity on RBCs from many different animals [2], similar to the ability of serum to distinguish human A, B, and O blood groups based on differential agglutination (Fig. 1) [3]. In 1954, plant extracts, including those from lima beans, were shown to react with red blood cells of distinct blood types [4, 5]. More specifically, these studies demonstrated that lima bean extract possessed the ability to clump blood group A RBCs but had no effect on type B or O blood agglutination. Boyd and Shapleigh coined the term "lectin" to describe these proteins, derived from the Latin word "legere", meaning to gather or select.

Sean R. Stowell and Connie M. Arthur (eds.), *Methods in Transfusion Medicine*, Methods in Molecular Biology, vol. 3053, https://doi.org/10.1007/978-1-0716-5376-0_40,

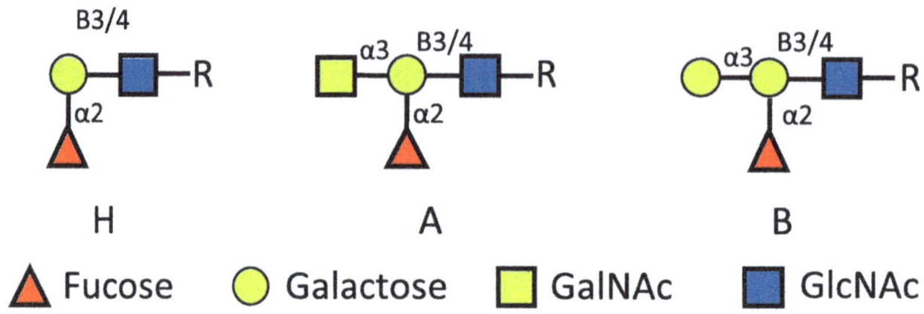

Fig. 1 Glycan structures of blood group antigens A, B, and H

Numerous studies have demonstrated that lectins constitute an evolutionarily conserved class of proteins. They are widely distributed in plants, fungi, animals, insects, and microbes [6–8], having many functions, where their ability to modulate glycoconjugate function can impact a wide variety of cellular processes [9]. Due to the high local concentration of the glycan determinants that often decorate a cell surface and the predominant oligomeric nature of lectins, lectin-glycoconjugate interactions are often multivalent in nature [10, 11]. Lectins are often grouped by specificity depending on the monosaccharide(s) for which they show the highest affinity and their distinct preference for α- or β anomers of the sugar. This characteristic makes it possible to differentiate between subtypes within the same blood group.

Lectins are grouped by specificity according to the monosaccharide(s) or oligosaccharide(s) for which they exhibit the highest affinity. Among lectins with binding specificities toward blood group antigens, *Dolichos biflorus* agglutinin (DBA) has been shown to preferentially bind to the A1 subtype of red blood cells, which is characterized by a higher density and distinct qualitative features of the A antigens on the RBC surface. This property allows DBA to distinguish between the blood subgroups A1 and A2, which is an important consideration when resolving discrepancies in blood typing and the potential ability to transplant across traditional ABO(H) blood group barriers. Despite this specificity, it should be noted that distinguishing A1 and A2 using DBA alone can be incomplete, and additional strategies are being developed to more accurately define A1 versus A2 blood group status [12, 13].

In addition to ABO(H) blood group antigens (Fig. 1), RBCs can be populated with other blood group polymorphisms, including the I and i antigens, the P antigens, and Lewis structures, each of which can often be the target of autoantibodies or alloantibodies. Unlike anti-carbohydrate antibodies directed against ABO (H) RBC alloantigens, which often, but do not always, form spontaneously in the first few months of life, patients can become alloimmunized against a wide variety of platelet, clotting factor, and other RBC alloantigens that can complicate pregnancy outcomes and make the procurement of compatible RBCs for transfusion difficult, which has been studied using a number of models that illustrate both distinct and common pathways involved in this process [14–18]. Indeed, a variety of studies have demonstrated that patients who have become alloimmunized experience higher morbidity and mortality [19, 20]. While a variety of preclinical and clinical studies are beginning to uncover key features of the antigens, transfused blood products and recipientcellular and innate immune factors that regulate the development and overall consequences of RBC alloimmunization [21–32], much still needs to be learned regarding the development of alloantibodies against blood group antigens and the factors that regulate the subsequent consequences of hemolysis in chronically transfused patient populations (although a number of studies have begun to uncover this and illustrate the importance of developing different model systems and overall approaches to study this) [33–39].

In addition to the use of lectins to differentiate blood group status as clinical tools to increase the safety of blood transfusion and transplantation, recent studies have demonstrated that some host lectins likewise possess high proclivity for carbohydrate-based blood group polymorphisms [40–45]. Among these, galectins in particular have not only been shown to bind blood group antigens, but also an entire array of glycan determinants [45] (Fig. 2). These interactions have been shown to facilitate the ability of galectin to regulate a wide variety of host processes, from autophagy to key features of host immunity [7, 46]. Galectins also possess the ability to engage microbial glycans, where recognition of microbes appears to provide a mechanism to protect the host against microbes that utilize molecular mimicry [7, 41, 43, 47, 48].

While there are a variety of methods, including biolayer interferometry (BLI) or surface plasmon resonance (SPR), X-ray

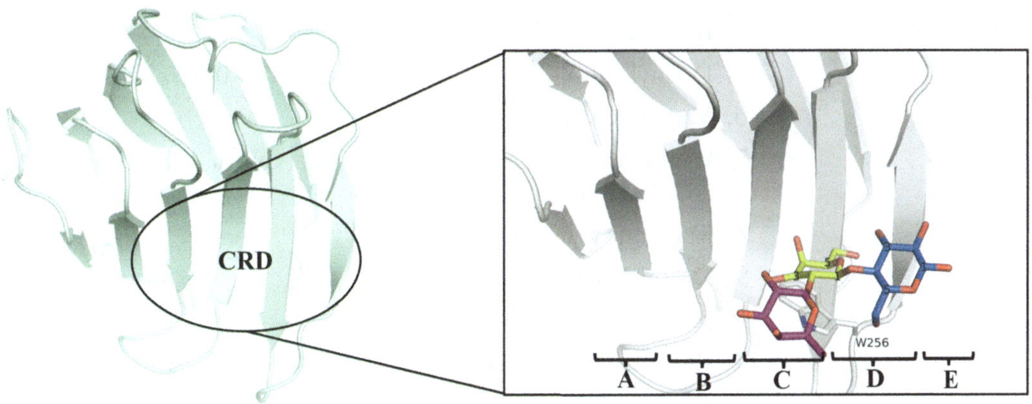

Fig. 2 The structure of human galectin-4's C-terminal CRD in complex with blood group H type II (PDB code: 4YM1). The illustration depicts the glycan binding area and the subsites A-E. The protein is represented as a cartoon, blood group H type II as sticks, with fucose in magenta, galactose in yellow, and glucose in marine

crystallography, and nuclear magnetic resonance (NMR) to characterize galectin interactions with glycan determinants [49–51], we will describe herein the use of isothermal titration calorimetry (ITC). ITC quantifies the association constant (K_a), enthalpy (ΔH), and stoichiometry (N) of galectin-ligand binding. By employing the following thermodynamic equations, the entropy (ΔS) and Gibbs free energy (ΔG) can be calculated

$$\Delta G = \Delta H - T\Delta S$$

$$\Delta G = -RT \ln Ka$$

where R is the gas constant with a value of 8.314 J K^{-1} mol^{-1}, and T is the temperature of the reaction in Kelvin [49, 52]. These thermodynamic properties represent the average of the micro-reactions. Examining the parameters obtained with different ligands reveals differences in energy contributions and interactions with the surrounding solution. Another advantage of this approach is that it can directly monitor the heat change that occurs during the binding process, eliminating the need for further chemical labeling of the protein or ligand. As such, ITC is a robust and informative technique that provides a deep understanding of the thermodynamics of protein interactions, which is crucial for applications in drug design, protein engineering, and understanding biological processes at a molecular level.

2 Materials

2.1 Preparation of the Lactosyl-Sepharose Column

2.1.1 Preparation of Lactosyl-Sepharose Beads

1. Sepharose™ gel filtration base matrix (Cytiva, CAT No. 17012001, Sepharose 4B).
2. Sodium carbonate (Na_2CO_3).
3. Glass beakers (2 L).
4. Buchner funnel.
5. Divinyl sulfone, 98% purity (VWR 77-77-0) (*see* **Note 1**).
6. Magnetic stirrer.
7. Whatman qualitative filter paper (Cytiva, 150 mm, CAT No. 1540-150).
8. Magnetic Stir Bar.
9. Double-distilled water.
10. pH meter.
11. Phosphate buffered saline (PBS).
12. Fume hood.
13. Sodium azide (CAS 26628-22-8).
14. D-Lactose monohydrate, ACS certified grade.

15. Spatula to transfer the gel.
16. β-Mercaptoethanol (Sigma Aldrich M3148) (*see* **Note 2**).
17. Buffers:

(a) Buffer A: 2 L, 0.5 M Na_2CO_3, pH 11.0.
(b) Buffer B: 10% (w/v) lactose in 100 mL Buffer A.
(c) Column storage buffer: PBS with 14 mM β-mercaptoethanol and 0.02 (w/v) sodium azide.

2.1.2 Packing of the Lactosyl-Sepharose Chromatography Column

1. Coupled Lactosyl-Sepharose (50% (v/v) in PBS).
2. Econo-Column® chromatography columns, 1.5 × 50 cm (Bio-Rad, CAT No.7370717).
3. Iron stands for attaching the Econo-column.
4. Tubing for passing solutions to the chromatography column.
5. 3-prong dual adjustable clamps to connect the column to the stand.
6. Sand, white quartz, 50–70 mesh particle size.
7. Wash buffer: PBS with 14 mM β-mercaptoethanol.

2.2 Expression of recombinant Human Galectin-3

1. LB broth powder (RPI Research Products International L24060).
2. 50 mL conical sterile centrifuge tubes (6 tubes).
3. 2 L Erlenmeyer conical flasks (6 flasks).
4. Double-distilled water.
5. Laboratory autoclave.
6. Fisherbrand™ aluminum foil 24 × 25 ft. (01-213-100).
7. Indicator Tape, autoclave steam sterilization, 3/4″ × 165′ (VWR 10153-150).
8. Ampicillin-sodium salt (Sigma Aldrich A9518).
9. Glycerol stocks of BL21(DE3) transformed with the galectin-3 expressing plasmid stored at −80 °C.
10. Six 20 mL LB-ampicillin media in 50 mL sterile conical centrifuge tubes.
11. Disposable inoculating loops (Fisher Scientific 22-363-605).
12. Six 1 L LB broths in 2 L flasks.
13. Isopropyl β-D-1-thiogalactopyranoside (IPTG) (Fisher BioReagents BP1755100). Prepare 1 M IPTG in double-distilled water and sterilize using a 0.22 μm filter.
14. Shaking incubator for bacterial growth (set at a temperature range of 16–37 °C).
15. Spectrophotometer for measuring OD at 600 nm.

2.3 Purification of recombinant Human Galectin-3

2.3.1 Processing of Bacterial Pellets

1. Centrifuge (Sorvall RC5B Plus).
2. Sorvall plastic centrifuge bottles with a capacity of 1 L.
3. PBS.
4. β-Mercaptoethanol.
5. Pierce™ protease inhibitor tablets, EDTA-free (ThermoFisher Scientific A32965).
6. Lysozyme from chicken egg white, lyophilized powder (Sigma Aldrich L6876). Dissolve in sterile double-distilled water to a stock concentration of 100 mg/mL and store at −20 °C.
7. Ribonuclease A from bovine pancreas (Sigma Aldrich R4875). Dissolve in sterile double-distilled water to a stock concentration of 10 mg/mL and store at −20 °C.
8. DNase I, lyophilized powder from bovine pancreas (Sigma Aldrich 11284932001). Dissolve in sterile double-distilled water to a stock concentration of 10 mg/mL and store at −20 °C.
9. Sonicator (Fisher Scientific Model FB120).
10. Beckman centrifuge.
11. JA-25.50 fixed-angle rotor and Nalgene™ Oak Ridge high-speed PPCO centrifuge tubes with sealing caps.

2.3.2 Purification of Human Galectin-3 Using a Lactosyl-Sepharose Column

1. Lactosyl-Sepharose column.
2. 1.5 mL vials.
3. 1 L PBS with 14 mM β-mercaptoethanol.
4. 100 mL PBS with 14 mM β-mercaptoethanol and 100 mM lactose.
5. Amicon® ultra centrifugal filters, 10 kDa MWCO (Millipore, UFC901024).
6. Spectrophotometer for measuring OD at 280 nm.
7. PBS with 0.02% (w/v) sodium azide and 14 mM β-mercaptoethanol.
8. SurePAGE™, Bis-Tris, 10 x 8, 4–20%, 12 wells (GenScript, M00656).
9. Tris-MOPS-SDS Running Buffer Powder (GenScript, M00138).

2.3.3 Purification of Human Galectin-3 Using a Ni^{2+}-Column

1. HisTrap excel (Cytiva, 17371206).
2. ÄKTA go™ systems (Cytiva).
3. Imidazole (Sigma Aldrich, 1202).
4. Sodium chloride (NaCl).
5. Tris(hydroxymethyl)aminomethane hydrochloride (Tris–HCl).

6. Corning® bottle-top vacuum filter system, pore size 0.22 μm (Millipore, CLS430517).
7. Buffers (Filtered through a 0.22 μm filter):
   (a) A buffer: 150 mM NaCl, 20 mM Tris–HCl, pH 8.0.
   (b) B buffer: 150 mM NaCl, 20 mM Tris–HCl, pH 8.0, 300 mM imidazole.
8. Double-distilled water.
9. Millex-HV Filter, 0.45 μm, PVDF, 13 mm, non-sterile (Millipore, SLHVX13NK).

2.4 Preparation of Galectin for Thermodynamic Study

2.4.1 Removal of Lactose from Purified Galectin Solution Using PD-10 Desalting Column

1. Disposable PD-10 desalting columns (Cytiva, 17085101).
2. 1.5 mL vials.
3. Spectrophotometer for measuring OD at 280 nm.
4. Iron stand to connect the PD10 desalting column.
5. 150 mM NaCl, 20 mM Tris–HCl, pH 8.0.
6. Amicon® ultra centrifugal filters, 10 kDa MWCO (Millipore, UFC901024).

2.4.2 Removal of Lactose from Purified Galectin Solution by Dialysis

1. Dialysis tubing, flat width 1.0 in., length 6–8 in., MWCO 8000 Da.
2. 200 μL gel loading tips.
3. 150 mM NaCl, 20 mM Tris–HCl, pH 8.0.
4. Magnetic stirrer and magnetic bars.
5. Large volume beakers.
6. 2 L conical flasks.

2.5 ITC Procedure

1. MicroCal iTC200 (Malvern).
2. Purified human galectin-3.
3. Thiodigalactose (TDG).
4. Origin software (OriginLab Corporation).
5. 0.2 mL PCR Tubes (Fisher Scientific, 14222262).
6. Double-distilled water.
7. Methanol.

3 Methods

3.1 Preparation of the Lactosyl-Sepharose Column

3.1.1 Preparation of Lactosyl-Sepharose Beads

1. Place a Whatman qualitative filter paper on the Buchner funnel and gently pour double-distilled water over it to ensure the paper adheres firmly to the funnel. This step prevents any leakage of Sepharose gel during the coupling procedure.

2. Add 100 mL of Sepharose 4B to the Buchner funnel and wash with buffer A (0.5 M Na_2CO_3) until the pH reaches 11.
3. Drain the gel into a beaker using a spatula and resuspend it in 100 mL of buffer A.
4. Place the beaker on a magnetic stirrer plate and add a stir bar inside.
5. Slowly add 10 mL of divinyl sulfone (in 2 mL aliquots over 10–15 min) to the gel while gently stirring.
6. The mixture will turn grayish brown. Any undissolved drops of divinyl sulfone will dissolve eventually.
7. Allow the gel mixture to stir slowly on the magnetic stirrer plate for up to 70 min at 23 °C.
8. Transfer the gel mixture to the Buchner funnel and wash with 300 mL of buffer A (0.5 M Na_2CO_3).
9. Drain the gel mixture into a beaker.
10. Resuspend the gel mixture in 100 mL of buffer B (10% lactose in 100 mL buffer A).
11. Place the beaker on a magnetic stirrer plate and add a stir bar.
12. Stir the mixture gently to facilitate the coupling reaction.
13. Allow the reaction to proceed for 15 h or overnight.
14. Transfer the gel to a Buchner funnel lined with a fresh Whatman filter paper, as done previously.
15. Wash the gel with 300 mL of buffer A (0.5 M Na_2CO_3).
16. Wash the gel with 300 mL of distilled water.
17. Wash the gel with 300 mL of PBS.
18. If not used immediately, store the gel in column storage buffer at 4 °C.

3.1.2 Packing of the Lactosyl-Sepharose Chromatography Column

1. Pour sand into the column to create a 6–8 cm layer at the bottom (*see* **Note 3**).
2. Add 60 mL of coupled Lactosyl-Sepharose (50% (v/v) in PBS) into the Econo-column.
3. Attach the adaptor to the top of the column.
4. Wash the column with 10 column volumes of PBS containing 14 mM β-mercaptoethanol to remove the storage buffer.

3.2 Expression of Recombinant Human Galectin-3

1. Prepare 6x 1 L flasks and 1x 200 mL flask of LB media according to manufacturer guidelines and autoclave.
2. Prepare an ampicillin stock solution of 100 mg/mL and pass it through a 0.22 μm filter. The solution can be aliquoted into 1.5 mL vials and stored at −20 °C until use.

3. To prepare LB-ampicillin media, dissolve ampicillin solution into each autoclaved LB broth to a final concentration of 100 μg/mL (1:1000 dilution of stock ampicillin solution).
4. Use disposable inoculating loops to pick some bacteria from the glycerol stock and individually inoculate them into 200 mL LB-ampicillin media. Incubate at 37 °C with shaking at 250 rpm overnight.
5. Transfer 20 mL of the overnight culture into each of the six 1 L LB broth flasks. Incubate at 37 °C with shaking at 250 rpm for approximately 1.5–2.5 h until the OD_{600} value is between 0.6 and 0.8.
6. Add 0.5 mL of 1 M IPTG (final concentration 0.5 mM IPTG) and incubate at 16 °C with shaking at 250 rpm for 20–24 h.

3.3 Purification of Human Galectin-3 (See Note 4)

3.3.1 Processing Bacterial Pellets

1. Pour the bacterial culture into Sorvall plastic centrifuge bottles and centrifuge at 5500 rpm, 4 °C for 30 min. Discard the supernatant and collect the pellet.
2. Prepare the lysis buffer: Add 2 protease inhibitor tablets, 60 μL of 100 μg/mL lysozyme, 60 μL of 10 μg/mL ribonuclease A, and 60 μl of 10 μg/mL DNase I into 60 mL PBS with 14 mM β-mercaptoethanol (*see* **Note 2**).
3. Resuspend the pellet in the lysis buffer.
4. Sonicate the cell suspension on ice at 60% amplitude (sonication intensity setting) for 15 min with 10 s ON and 10 s OFF intervals.
5. Transfer the lysate to Nalgene™ Oak Ridge high-speed PPCO centrifuge tubes and centrifuge using a JA-25.50 fixed-angle rotor at 18000 rpm, 4 °C for 30 min twice.
6. Collect the supernatant and discard the pellet.
7. Continue purification of galectin-3 from collected supernatant using methods outlined in Subheading 3.3.2 *OR* Subheading 3.3.3. Choose one of these methods; do not complete both.

3.3.2 Purification of Human Galectin-3 Using a Lactosyl-Sepharose Column

1. Pre-equilibrate the Lactosyl-Sepharose column with PBS containing 14 mM β-mercaptoethanol.
2. Load the supernatant onto the Lactosyl-Sepharose column (*see* **Note 5**).
3. Wash the column with PBS containing 14 mM β-mercaptoethanol until the OD_{280} approaches zero.
4. Elute the galectin protein using PBS with 14 mM β-mercaptoethanol and 100 mM lactose. Collect 1 mL fractions.
5. Monitor protein elution via OD_{280} readings and verify purity by SurePAGE™.
6. Concentrate the protein solution at 4 °C using Amicon® Ultra centrifugal filters, 10 kDa MWCO (*see* **Note 6**).

3.3.3 Purification of Human Galectin-3 Using a Ni^{2+}-Column

1. Turn on the ÄKTA go™ system and connect it to the computer control interface. Place the "A," "B," and "sample" tubing in double-distilled water. In "manual run," select "pump wash."
2. At a flow rate of 2 mL/min, connect the HisTrap Excel column to the system, ensuring no air enters the tubing or column. Allow the column to be washed with five column volumes of water.
3. Place the "A" and "sample" tubing in the prepared A buffer (150 mM NaCl, 20 mM Tris, pH 8.0). Place the "B" tubing in the B buffer (150 mM NaCl, 20 mM Tris, pH 8.0, 300 mM imidazole). In "manual run," select "pump wash."
4. Wash the column with five column volumes of A buffer at a flow rate of 2 mL/min to ensure the column is fully equilibrated with A buffer.
5. Place the "sample" tubing into the centrifuged supernatant and load the sample onto the column at a flow rate of 1 mL/min.
6. Wash the column with ten column volumes of A buffer at a flow rate of 2 mL/min.
7. Elute bound proteins with a 25 column volume linear gradient from 0% to 50% B buffer at a flow rate of 2 mL/min, collecting 1 mL fractions.
8. Further elute with five column volumes of 100% B buffer using a step gradient at a flow rate of 2 mL/min, collecting 1 mL fractions.
9. Analyze the collected fractions by SurePAGE™, based on peaks observed at OD_{280} to confirm protein purity.
10. Concentrate the protein fractions at 4 °C using Amicon® Ultra centrifugal filters, 10 kDa MWCO.

3.4 Preparation of Galectin for Thermodynamic Study (See Note 7)

3.4.1 Removal of Lactose from Purified Galectin Solution Using PD-10 Desalting Column

1. Wash the column with five column volumes of 150 mM NaCl, 20 mM Tris, pH 8.0.
2. After washing the column with the buffer, load 0.5–2 mL of protein onto the column.
3. Collect the flow-through in 1.5 mL Eppendorf tubes, with each fraction being 0.5 mL.
4. Continue washing the column with 150 mM NaCl, 20 mM Tris, pH 8.0.
5. Collect up to 10 fractions.
6. Measure the OD at 280 nm using a spectrophotometer.
7. Pool the fractions with positive OD readings.
8. Concentrate the protein at 4 °C using an Amicon® Ultra centrifugal filter, 10 kDa MWCO. The desalted galectin can then be used for biochemical studies.

3.4.2 Removal of Lactose from Purified Galectin Solution by Dialysis

1. Soak and wash the appropriate dialysis tubing with deionized ultrapure water to remove any contaminants or impurities.
2. After washing, tie one end of the dialysis tubing. Using a 200 μL gel loading tip, pour the purified galectin-3 into the tubing. When the tube is 75% full, tie it off as close to the galectin-3 eluent level as possible to limit the dilution of galectin-3 during dialysis.
3. Place the dialysis bag containing galectin-3 into a 2 L flask filled with buffer (150 mM NaCl, 20 mM Tris–HCl, pH 8.0) and set it on a magnetic stirrer. Dialyze the secured galectin-3-filled dialysis bag at 4 °C. Change the buffer every 4 h until the lactose concentration reaches a sub-nanomolar level (*see* **Note 8**).
4. After dialysis is complete, use a 200 μl gel loading tip to pour out the galectin-3 and determine its concentration.

3.5 ITC Procedure (Fig. 3)

3.5.1 Evaluate Protein and Ligand Concentrations Before ITC

1. Open the MicroCal iTC200 software and select the "Experimental Design" tab.
2. For the initial evaluation of concentration conditions, select either the "minimum protein" or "high-speed" mode for the experiment.
3. Enter the predicted dissociation constants (K_d) value based on reference literature or other methods of measuring K_d. Set the N value to 1 because galectin-3 has only one CRD, meaning theoretically one galectin can bind to one TDG molecule. Estimate the ΔH to be around −10 kcal/mole based on previous galectin and disaccharide binding experiments. Set the temperature to 25 °C.
4. Click "update experiment curve."
5. Make sure that the "Total Heat" and "C Value" fields on the right side of the window are green. If they are red, adjust the concentrations in the "cell" or "syringe" fields as predicted by the software.

3.5.2 ITC Study for Human Galectin-3 and TDG

1. Thoroughly clean the ITC cell and syringe with distilled water, completely remove the water, and dry the cell chamber with nitrogen gas.
2. Switch to the "Advanced Experimental Design" tab in the MicroCal iTC200 software. Since the first titration point often has a larger error and will be removed later, the volume of the first injection can be halved.
3. Fill both the cell and syringe with 150 mM NaCl, 20 mM Tris, pH 8.0. Place the long needle of the syringe properly inside the cell. Ensure that all processes avoid air bubbles, then press "run." This is a buffer-to-buffer control experiment to check if the cell chamber and syringe are clean. A flat baseline with no endothermic or exothermic activity should be obtained.

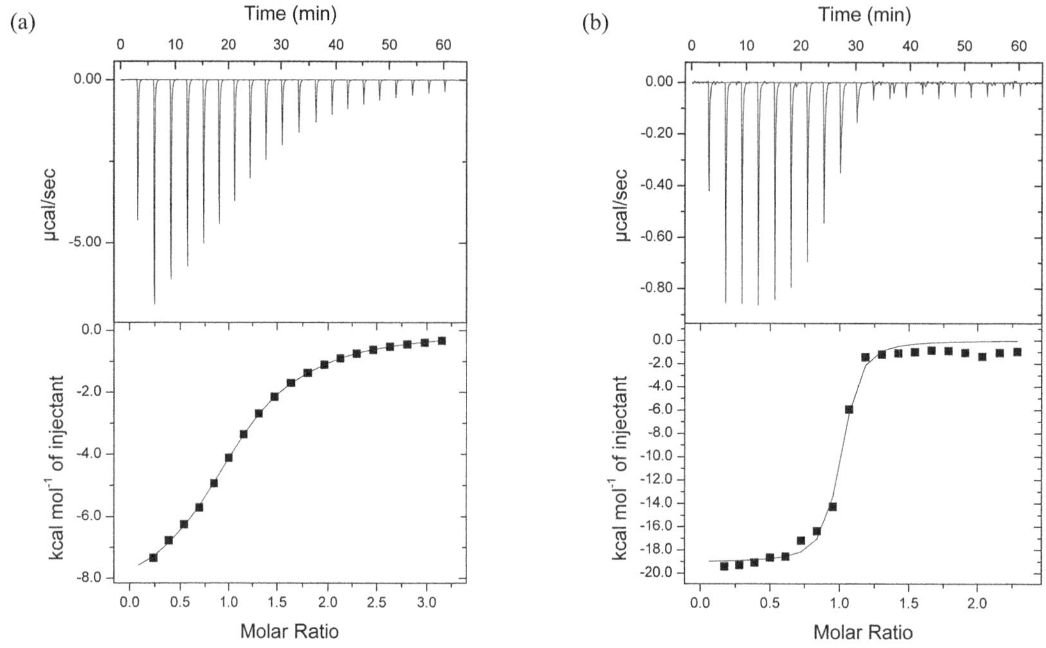

Fig. 3 Plots of the isothermal titration of human galectin-3 with (**a**) TDG and (**b**) TD139 (galectin-3 inhibitor). Experiments were conducted at 298 K in 150 mM NaCl, 20 mM Tris–HCl buffer. Due to the K_d of TDG for galectin-3 being 75 µM and ΔH approximately −9.4 kcal/mol, a higher concentration is required to reach the saturation curve for titration. The initial concentration of galectin-3 was 500 µM, while TDG was 7.5 mM. In contrast, TD139 has a ΔH of −18.2 kcal/mol and a K_d of 0.068 µM, indicating it not only releases more heat but also has a K_d 1000 times better than TDG. Therefore, the initial concentration of galectin-3 needed was only 10 µM, and TD139 was 100 µM. (This research was originally published in Frontiers in Microbiology with some modifications. Wu et al. © 2021 Wu, Ho, Kamili, Wang, Murdock, Cummings, Arthur, and Stowell

4. Clean the cell and syringe thoroughly with 150 mM NaCl and 20 mM Tris pH 8.0 (at least three complete washes) and dry with nitrogen gas.
5. Adjust the concentration of purified galectin-3 with 150 mM NaCl, 20 mM Tris, pH 8.0, based on the "experiment design." Fill the cell with the required volume of galectin-3 after degassing, ensuring no air bubbles are trapped in the cell.
6. Fill the syringe with 150 mM NaCl, 20 mM Tris, pH 8.0. Place the long needle of the syringe properly inside the cell. Press "run." This is a buffer-to-galectin-3 titration control to check if galectin-3 undergoes any conformational changes that result in endothermic or exothermic reactions during dilution.
7. Clean the cell and syringe thoroughly with 150 mM NaCl and 20 mM Tris pH 8.0 (at least three complete washes) and dry with nitrogen gas.
8. Fill the cell with 150 mM NaCl, 20 mM Tris, pH 8.0, and fill the syringe with ligands at the desired concentrations. Place the

long needle of the syringe properly inside the cell. Press "run." This is a TDG-to-buffer control to check for any endothermic or exothermic reactions during ligand dilution.

9. Clean the cell and syringe thoroughly with 150 mM NaCl, 20 mM Tris pH 8.0 (at least three complete washes), and dry with nitrogen gas.
10. Fill the cell with galectin-3 and the syringe with TDG. Place the long needle of the syringe properly inside the cell. Press "run." Monitor the quality of the ITC profile and the baseline. The run should be stopped if the profile quality is not good.
11. Continue injections until saturation (*see* **Note 9**).
12. After the experiment, import the data into Origin software. Subtract the heat obtained from buffer-to-buffer, buffer-to-galectin-3, and TDG-to-buffer experiments from the galectin-TDG data. Click the "One Set of Sites" button.
13. Clean the cell and syringe thoroughly with 150 mM NaCl and 20 mM Tris pH 8.0 (at least three complete washes).
14. Clean the cell and syringe thoroughly with distilled water (at least three complete washes).
15. Rinse the cell and syringe with methanol and dry with nitrogen gas (*see* **Note 10**).

4 Notes

1. Divinyl sulfone is a toxic reagent. Store and use it in a fume hood and avoid contact with skin.
2. Always use a fume hood while working with β-mercaptoethanol. When the galectin does not contain solvent-exposed cysteines, such as in galectin-3, β-mercaptoethanol is not necessarily required. Please note, when using a Ni^{2+}-column, the maximum concentration of β-mercaptoethanol typically should not exceed 5 mM.
3. The purpose of packing sand in the column is to make subsequent pipetting and handling of the column easier.
4. Purification of galectin-3 can be achieved using either a Lactosyl-Sepharose column or by adding a His tag to the N-terminal sequence of galectin-3 to enable Ni^{2+} binding. Each method has its advantages and disadvantages. Using a Lactosyl-Sepharose column ensures that the purified protein retains its carbohydrate-binding activity. However, to avoid interference with the binding of other ligands, additional steps are required to completely remove any residual lactose bound to galectin-3 after purification. Galectin and lactose do not form covalent bonds, so lactose can be displaced by other

ligands with higher binding affinities, which might mitigate the impact. Nonetheless, since ITC measures the total heat change from all association and dissociation events in the system, it is essential to ensure that the CRD of galectin is unoccupied. Complete removal of lactose can be time consuming and difficult. In contrast, while purification of galectin-3 using a Ni^{2+}-column can eliminate this concern entirely, this method does not ensure active galectin-3 binding activity.

5. This step must maintain the sample at 4 °C, so it needs to be performed in a cold room.
6. Concentration = OD at 280 nm/Extinction coefficient × Path length × Molecular weight × Dilution factor.
7. This section describes methods to remove lactose from the galectin that was collected by affinity chromatography (using a Lactosyl-Sepharose column). This is necessary only if galectin was purified using a Lactosyl-Sepharose column. When using a Lactosyl-Sepharose column to purify galectin-3, it is essential to remove lactose before conducting ITC experiments. Two methods for removing lactose are provided below: the PD-10 desalting column and dialysis. Although the PD-10 column can quickly remove excess lactose, it sometimes fails to completely remove lactose bound to galectin, which can interfere with subsequent experiments. Therefore, the more time-consuming dialysis method can be used in addition to or as an alternative.
8. Calculate the residual lactose concentration in the tubing using the following formula: (initial lactose concentration of the galectin-3 sample in the tubing) × (volume of the galectin-3 sample in the tubing) = (C) × (volume of the buffer in which the tubing is being dialyzed), where C represents the final lactose concentration of the galectin-3 sample in the tubing. The number of buffer changes required will depend on the volume of galectin-3 in the dialysis tubing and the volume of buffer used. Typically, 6–8 changes are needed.
9. If the heat absorption/release approaches the baseline in the final three to four titration injections, it can be regarded as having reached saturation. If the titration curve does not reach saturation, update the values of ΔH, K_d, etc. in the "Experimental Design" tab with current data. Re-evaluate the concentrations to be employed until a saturation curve is produced. After determining the concentration, use the "high quality" option to increase the number of titration points, resulting in more precise ΔH, N, and K_a readings. Lactose and other ligands with galectin binding affinities in the mM range may require a very high concentration to achieve a saturation curve.

However, binding in the mM range is close to ITC's detection limit; it is recommended that you employ alternative biophysical approaches to confirm K_d before proceeding.

10. Please ensure that the machine is fully cleaned after each use, leaving no residues of salts, proteins, or ligands to alter the next usage's results.

Conflict of Interest Statement

This work was funded by NIH P01HL171803, R01 HL165975, R01 HL135575, and R01 HL154034. SRS has received speaker and consultant honoraria from Cerus, Grifols, Novartis, Alexion, and Argenx and has received a research grant from Alexion. No other authors have conflicts of interest.

References

1. Stillmark H (1888) Über Ricin ein giftiges Ferment aus den Samen von Ricinus communis L. und einige anderen Euphorbiaceen. University of Dorpat, Dorpat
2. Ehrlich P (1891) Experimentelle untersuchungen über immunität. I Ueber ricin. Dtsch Med Wochenschr 17(32):976–979
3. Landsteiner K, Raubitschek H (1907) Observations on hemolysis and hemagglutination. C Bakt:45
4. Boyd WC (1963) The lectins: their present status. Vox Sang 8(1):1–32
5. Boyd WC, Shapleigh E (1954) Specific precipitating activity of plant agglutinins (lectins). Science 119(3091):419
6. Hu D, Tateno H, Hirabayashi J (2015) Lectin engineering, a molecular evolutionary approach to expanding the lectin utilities. Molecules 20(5):7637–7656
7. Liu FT, Stowell SR (2023) The role of galectins in immunity and infection. Nat Rev Immunol 23(8):479–494
8. Lam SK, Ng TB (2011) Lectins: production and practical applications. Appl Microbiol Biotechnol 89(1):45–55
9. Zhang Y, Gao Y, Yong Y (2022) Lectin-mediated coimmobilization of cascade glycoenzymes. Methods Mol Biol 2487:189–195
10. Martinez-Bailen M, Rojo J, Ramos-Soriano J (2023) Multivalent glycosystems for human lectins. Chem Soc Rev 52(2):536–572
11. Dam TK, Brewer CF (2010) Lectins as pattern recognition molecules: the effects of epitope density in innate immunity. Glycobiology 20(3):270–279
12. Jajosky RP et al (2023) ABO blood group antigens and differential glycan expression: perspective on the evolution of common human enzyme deficiencies. iScience 26(1):105798
13. Joseph A et al (2023) ABO genotyping finds more A(2) to B kidney transplant opportunities than lectin-based subtyping. Am J Transplant 23(4):512–519
14. Maier CL et al (2018) Antibody-mediated immune suppression by antigen modulation is antigen-specific. Blood Adv 2(21):2986–3000
15. Mener A et al (2018) Complement serves as a switch between CD4+ T cell-independent and -dependent RBC antibody responses. JCI Insight 3(22)
16. Patel SR et al (2018) Marginal zone B cells induce alloantibody formation following RBC transfusion. Front Immunol 9:2516
17. Zerra PE et al (2017) Marginal zone B cells are critical to factor VIII inhibitor formation in mice with hemophilia A. Blood 130(23): 2559–2568
18. Arthur CM et al (2022) Nonhuman glycans can regulate anti-factor VIII antibody formation in mice. Blood 139(9):1312–1317
19. Thein SL et al (2020) Hemolytic transfusion reactions in sickle cell disease: underappreciated and potentially fatal. Haematologica 105(3):539–544
20. Thein SL et al (2020) Hemolytic transfusion reactions in sickle cell disease:

underappreciated and potentially fatal. Haematologica 105:539
21. Arthur CM et al (2021) Antigen density dictates RBC clearance, but not antigen modulation, following incompatible RBC transfusion in mice. Blood Adv 5(2):527–538
22. Jajosky R et al (2023) Prior immunization against an intracellular antigen enhances subsequent red blood cell alloimmunization in mice. Blood 141(21):2642–2653
23. Zimring JC, Hudson KE (2016) Cellular immune responses in red blood cell alloimmunization. Hematol Am Soc Hematol Educ Program 2016(1):452–456
24. Hudson KE et al (2019) Mechanisms of alloimmunization in sickle cell disease. Curr Opin Hematol 26(6):434–441
25. Jajosky RP et al (2023) Antibody-mediated antigen loss switches augmented immunity to antibody-mediated immunosuppression. Blood 142(12):1082–1098
26. Jash A et al (2021) Antibodies to low-copy number RBC alloantigen convert a tolerogenic stimulus to an immunogenic stimulus in mice. Front Immunol 12:629608
27. Arthur CM et al (2022) Clodronate inhibits alloimmunization against distinct red blood cell alloantigens in mice. Transfusion 62(5): 948–953
28. Stowell SR et al (2013) Alloantibodies to a paternally derived RBC KEL antigen lead to hemolytic disease of the fetus/newborn in a murine model. Blood 122(8):1494–1504
29. Stowell SR et al (2013) Antigen modulation confers protection to red blood cells from antibody through Fcgamma receptor ligation. J Immunol 191(10):5013–5025
30. Jajosky RP et al (2025) CD47 regulates antigen modulation and red blood cell clearance following an incompatible transfusion. Front Immunol 16:1548548
31. Jajosky RP et al (2024) Dynamics of antibody engagement of red blood cells in vivo and in vitro. Front Immunol 15:1475470
32. Gruber DR et al (2020) Passively transferred IgG enhances humoral immunity to a red blood cell alloantigen in mice. Blood Adv 4(7):1526–1537
33. Bird GW (1952) Relationship of the blood sub-groups A1, A2 and A1B, A2B to haemagglutinins present in the seeds of Dolichos biflorus. Nature 170(4329):674
34. Chonat S et al (2025) Complement is activated in patients with acute chest syndrome caused by sickle cell disease and represents a therapeutic target. Sci Transl Med 17(807):eadl4922
35. Vidler JB et al (2015) Delayed haemolytic transfusion reaction in adults with sickle cell disease: a 5-year experience. Br J Haematol 169(5):746–753
36. Gardner K et al (2015) How we treat delayed haemolytic transfusion reactions in patients with sickle cell disease. Br J Haematol 170(6): 745–756
37. Habibi A et al (2016) Delayed hemolytic transfusion reaction in adult sickle-cell disease: presentations, outcomes, and treatments of 99 referral center episodes. Am J Hematol 91(10):989–994
38. Noizat-Pirenne F et al (2015) The use of rituximab to prevent severe delayed haemolytic transfusion reaction in immunized patients with sickle cell disease. Vox Sang 108(3): 262–267
39. Dumas G et al (2016) Eculizumab salvage therapy for delayed hemolysis transfusion reaction in sickle cell disease patients. Blood 127(8): 1062–1064
40. Stowell SR et al (2008) Dimeric Galectin-8-induces phosphatidylserine exposure in leukocytes through polylactosamine recognition by the C-terminal domain. J Biol Chem 283(29): 20547–20559
41. Blenda AV et al (2022) Galectin-9 recognizes and exhibits antimicrobial activity toward microbes expressing blood group-like antigens. J Biol Chem 298(4):101704
42. Wu SC et al (2022) Innate immune Galectin-7 specifically targets microbes that decorate themselves in blood group-like antigens. iScience 25(7):104482
43. Jan HM et al (2024) Galectin-4 antimicrobial activity primarily occurs through its C-terminal domain. Mol Cell Proteomics 23(5):100747
44. Ho AD et al (2022) An automated approach to assess relative galectin-glycan affinity following glycan microarray analysis. Front Mol Biosci 9: 893185
45. Arthur CM et al (2024) ABO blood groups and galectins: implications in transfusion medicine and innate immunity. Semin Immunol 74–75:101892
46. Liu D, Zhu H, Li C (2023) Galectins and galectin-mediated autophagy regulation: new insights into targeted cancer therapy. Biomark Res 11(1):22
47. Mishra A et al (2019) Structure-function and application of plant lectins in disease biology and immunity. Food Chem Toxicol 134: 110827
48. Swaminathan GJ et al (1999) Selective recognition of mannose by the human eosinophil

Charcot-Leyden crystal protein (galectin-10): a crystallographic study at 1.8 A resolution. Biochemistry 38(42):13837–13843
49. Hsieh TJ et al (2016) Dual thio-digalactoside-binding modes of human galectins as the structural basis for the design of potent and selective inhibitors. Sci Rep 6:29457
50. Chan YC et al (2018) Dissecting the structure-activity relationship of galectin-ligand interactions. Int J Mol Sci 19(2)
51. Hsieh TJ et al (2015) Structural basis underlying the binding preference of human Galectins-1, -3 and -7 for Galbeta1-3/4GlcNAc. PLoS One 10(5):e0125946
52. Brewer CF (2002) Thermodynamic binding studies of galectin-1, -3 and -7. Glycoconj J 19(7–9):459–465

Chapter 41

Acute Incompatible Red Blood Cell Transfusion in Mice

Ryan P. Jajosky, Brock D. Hughes, Caitlin L. Cepeda, Sasikala Muthusamy, Andre J. H. Wittig, Wenhui Li, Samata P. Varadkar, Shang-Chuen Wu, William O. Scott, Carter J. Stowell, Sadie Larson, Katelyn Sturgis, Connie M. Arthur, and Sean R. Stowell

Abstract

Alloantibodies, which can arise naturally in early life or after exposure to allogeneic red blood cells (RBCs), can pose a significant risk to blood transfusion. When patients with alloantibodies receive incompatible RBCs, they may experience potentially fatal hemolytic transfusion reactions (HTRs). Transfusion services work to prevent such reactions by identifying compatible blood; however, complications can still occur, especially in patients with complex alloantibody profiles. Given the consequences of these reactions clinically, various preclinical models have been developed to study incompatible RBC transfusions and their consequences. These models provide valuable insights into the mechanisms of HTRs and suggest potential preventive strategies. We will describe key considerations when using preclinical models to study the overall consequences of incompatible RBC transfusions, using the KEL model as an example.

Key words Incompatible, Transfusion, Red blood cells, Preclinical models, Antigen modulation

1 Introduction

Red blood cell (RBC) transfusion is employed across a broad spectrum of patient populations. It is utilized in the management of acute hemorrhage as well as in chronic conditions characterized by impaired production or shortened lifespan of RBCs [1–3]. These latter cases often require long-term transfusion support. While allogeneic differences between donors and recipients likely evolved to provide protection against infectious disease and certainly have implications in host immune function, including the interactions between a number of innate immune factors that engage microbes decorated in blood group antigens [4–8], these differences can result in immune barriers to transfusion. As a result, compatibility testing for blood transfusions is essential to reduce the likelihood of immune-mediated transfusion complications

Sean R. Stowell and Connie M. Arthur (eds.), *Methods in Transfusion Medicine*, Methods in Molecular Biology, vol. 3053, https://doi.org/10.1007/978-1-0716-5376-0_41,

[4, 9–11]. This process involves examining both ABO(H) antigens and the presence of various alloantibodies against other RBC alloantigens that can cause incompatibility prior to transfusion.

While alloimmunization can impact the efficacy of other therapeutics, such as platelet transfusions or other intravenous therapies [12–14], incompatible RBC transfusion is particularly life-threatening [15–17]. These reactions can be very severe in patients with sickle cell disease and can lead to hyperhemolysis, a process shown in numerous studies to lead to hemolysis of a patient's own RBCs [16, 18–24]. Unlike cases of incompatible platelet transfusion, incompatible RBC transfusions can result in the release of free heme, which several studies have now shown can lead to significant immune activation through toll-like receptor engagement and complement activation [25–28]. While several studies have shown that complement inhibition holds promise in treating delayed hemolytic transfusion reactions [29–32], additional studies are needed to establish the efficacy of this approach in managing such severe immunological responses to incompatible blood transfusions [29, 33–35].

Not all incompatible RBC transfusions result in a HTR [36]. Prior studies suggest that the probability of an HTR may be influenced by various characteristics of both the target antigen and the antibody involved [9, 17]. These factors include the quantity, arrangement, and lateral mobility of alloantigens and other regulators of cellular sensitivity to phagocytosis (e.g., CD47), which can significantly impact the overall outcome of antibody engagement with respect to RBC removal [37–40]. A number of studies have demonstrated that the specific isotypes and subclass composition of IgG antibodies can also play a critical role in determining whether complement activation occurs, Fc receptors are engaged, a combination of both processes takes place, or neither is involved [41–46]. Recently, a variety of studies suggest that when antibodies bind to RBCs, it can lead to the removal of antigens from the cell surface [47], potentially decreasing the RBC's susceptibility to further antibody-mediated removal [39, 48–51].

The varied outcomes of antibody engagement can result in intravascular hemolysis, extravascular hemolysis, or both [9, 17, 52]. When intravascular hemolysis occurs, free hemoglobin is released into the plasma, which can overwhelm haptoglobin's binding capacity and result in hemoglobinemia and hemoglobinuria. The breakdown of free hemoglobin into heme can saturate hemopexin, while released hemoglobin and arginase can also deplete nitric oxide (NO), causing vasoconstriction and pulmonary hypertension. In contrast, increases in cytokine levels, endothelial activation, and possible injury may lead to disseminated intravascular coagulation (DIC), acute kidney injury (AKI), and, when severe, multiorgan failure [17]. Free heme can also activate complement, exacerbating inflammation, vascular injury, and multiorgan failure.

Several studies suggest that inhibiting complement activation may not only prevent antibody-induced complement activation from directly inducing hemolysis but may also reduce the impact of heme-induced complement activation and attendant sequelae.

Given the clinical implications of incompatible RBC transfusions, studies have sought to develop several preclinical models to investigate key regulators and consequences of RBC incompatibility. These models, which commonly express antigens like HEL, glycophorin A (GPA), KEL, and a chimeric antigen of HEL, OVA, and Duffy (HOD), have been used in numerous studies to gain insight into the immune populations, innate immune factors, and signaling pathways that govern RBC alloantibody development and incompatible transfusion outcomes [53–62]. Studies using these models have uncovered a wide range of potential consequences, from tolerance induction to CD4 T cell-independent IgG antibody formation [60, 61, 63]. This variability suggests the involvement of distinct cytokines, innate immune signaling pathways, and B and T cells in alloantibody development [64–67]. Furthermore, use of these models and related clinical studies have shown through a number of studies that the effects of antibody engagement can differ, with some antibodies inducing complement activation, others engaging Fc receptors, and some functioning independently of both [36, 38, 39, 46, 52, 68, 69]. This chapter describes the methods used to examine incompatible RBC transfusions in murine models, with a particular focus on the KEL system as an example.

2 Materials

2.1 Collecting B6 Control and Antigen-Positive Mouse RBCs

2.1.1 Mouse Blood Collection—Submandibular Bleed

1. Biosafety cabinet (BSC), class II A2 or B2.
2. Disinfectant; Make 70% ethanol from ethanol, HPLC/Spectrophotometric Grade, Liquid, ≥99.5%, Glass bottle, 200 Proof (Sigma-Aldrich, 459828-2L).
3. Paper towels.
4. Mouse blood donors:
   (a) C57BL/6 (B6) mice.
   (b) Mice with an antigen on their RBCs that B6 recipients would perceive as foreign (e.g., B6.KEL mice).
5. Mouse ear puncher, 2 mm diameter.
6. Acid citrate dextrose solution A (ACD-A), sterile 16x100 mm 8.5 mL BD Vacutainer® glass whole blood ACD tube (Owens & Minor, 364606).
7. Manual pipette and pipette tips.

8. 1.7 and 5 mL Eppendorf tubes, 50 mL conicals, and tube holders.
9. 3 and 5 mm sterile animal lancets.
10. Fisherbrand sterile cotton gauze pads, 4 × 4 in (Fisher Scientific, 22-415-469).
11. Empty mouse cage (recovery cage).
12. Marker/Sharpie Permanent Marker, Ultra Fine Tip, Black, Dozen (Staples, 37001).

2.1.2 Mouse Blood Collection—Retro-orbital Sinus Bleed

1. Fume hood.
2. Disinfectant; Make 70% ethanol from ethanol, HPLC/Spectrophotometric Grade, Liquid, ≥99.5%, Glass bottle, 200 Proof (Sigma-Aldrich, 459828-2L).
3. Paper towels.
4. Mouse blood donors:
   (a) C57BL/6 (B6) mice.
   (b) Mice with an antigen on their RBCs that B6 recipients would perceive as foreign (e.g., B6.KEL mice).
5. Acid citrate dextrose solution A (ACD-A), sterile 16 × 100 mm 8.5 mL BD Vacutainer® glass whole blood ACD tube (Owens & Minor, 364606).
6. Manual pipette and pipette tips.
7. 1.7 and 5 mL Eppendorf tubes, 50 mL conicals, and tube holders.
8. Pivetal® Isoflurane (Control substance VI) (Patterson Veterinary, 07-893-8441).
9. 1 mL Tuberculin Syringes (MEDLINE INDUSTRIES INC, 309659).
10. Glass staining trough with lid.
11. Surgical tweezers, curved.
12. Fisherbrand sterile cotton gauze pads, 4 × 4 in (Fisher Scientific, 22-415-469).
13. Aluminum foil.
14. Biohazard bag.
15. Marker/Sharpie Permanent Marker, Ultra Fine Tip, Black, Dozen (Staples, 37001).

2.1.3 Washing and Quantifying Collected Blood

1. Sterile serologic pipettes and an electronic pipettor, or sterile pipette tips and manual pipettes.
2. Phosphate buffered saline (PBS): 0.0067 M PO_4, without magnesium or calcium, pH 7.4, sterile.

3. Centrifuges for 5 mL or 50 mL conical tubes and 1.7 mL Eppendorf tubes.
4. Blood sample.
5. 1.7 and 5 mL Eppendorf tubes, 50 mL conicals, and tube holders.
6. Manual pipette and pipette tips.
7. Optional: Hematology analyzer.

2.2 Phenotyping the Donor B6 Control and Transgenic Antigen-Positive RBCs

1. 96-well, U-bottom plate Costar 96 Well Clear Round Bottom Tissue Culture-Treated Microplate with Lid, Sterile, Individually Wrapped, 50/case (Fisher Scientific, 3799).
2. Washed RBCs with the alloantigen (e.g., KEL RBCs) and without (e.g., B6 RBCs).
3. 1.7 mL Eppendorf tubes.
4. Antibodies:
   (a) Primary antibodies against the model RBC antigen of interest (*see* **Note 1**).
   (b) Fluorescently labeled secondary detection antibodies.
   (c) e.g., APC anti-mouse IgG.
5. Phosphate buffered saline (PBS): 0.0067 M PO_4, without magnesium or calcium, pH 7.4 phosphate buffered saline (PBS) (Cytiva, SH30256.02).
6. Sterile pipette tips and manual pipettes, including a multichannel pipette.
7. Reagent reservoirs.
8. Timer.
9. Flow cytometer.

2.3 Fluorescent Labeling of the RBCs

1. Washed RBCs with the alloantigen (e.g., HOD RBCs or KEL RBCs) and without (e.g., B6 RBCs).
2. 50 mL Fisherbrand™ Easy Reader™ Conical Polypropylene Centrifuge Tubes (FisherScientific, 05-539-13).
3. Fluorescent label.
   (a) chloromethylbenzamido 1,1′-dioctadecyl-3,3,3′,3′-tetramethylindocarbocyanine perchlorate (DiI).
   (b) 3,3′-dihexadecyloxacarbocyanine perchlorate (DiO).
4. Dimethyl sulfoxide (DMSO), sterile.
5. Phosphate buffered saline (PBS): 0.0067 M PO4, without magnesium or calcium, pH 7.4 phosphate buffered saline (PBS) (Cytiva, SH30256.02).
6. 37 °C warm water bath.
7. Timer.

8. Flow cytometer.
9. 96-well, U-bottom plate Costar 96 Well Clear Round Bottom Tissue Culture-Treated Microplate with Lid, Sterile, Individually Wrapped, 50/case (Fisher Scientific, 3799).

2.4 Passive Immunization and RBC Transfusion

1. Biosafety cabinet (BSC Level II).
2. Disinfectant and paper towels.
3. Sterile 50 mL tubes.
4. Manual pipette and pipette tips.
5. 2″ × 2″ sterile gauze.
6. Sterile phosphate buffered saline (PBS): 0.0067 M PO4, without magnesium or calcium, pH 7.4.
7. Antigen-specific polyclonal or monoclonal antibody (*see* **Note 1**).
8. Prepared RBCs for transfusion (*see* Subheadings 3.1, 3.2, and 3.3).
9. Mouse restrainer (for use during mouse tail vein injections).
10. 1 mL Tuberculin syringe, sterile.
11. 30 gauge, 0.5″ needles, sterile.

2.5 Collecting Post-transfusion Specimens (Plasma, Serum, Urine, Organs)

1. Disinfectant and paper towels.
2. Experimental mice (e.g., transfused mice).
3. Empty mouse cage (recovery cage).
4. Small animal heat lamp, anchored to a support stand using clamps.
5. 70% ethanol in a squirt bottle.
6. Kimwipes.
7. Mouse restrainer (for use during mouse tail vein bleeds).
8. Razor blade.
9. Sterile "4 × 4" gauze.
10. 96-well U-bottom plate.
11. ACD-A.
12. Manual pipette and pipette tips.
13. Heparinized microhematocrit capillary tubes.
    (a) Optional: rubber bulb attachment.
14. Sharpie or pen.
15. Parafilm.
16. Tape.
17. Eppendorf tubes and tube rack.

18. 10% neutral buffered formalin.
19. Mouse autopsy supplies.
    (a) Isoflurane and chamber.
    (b) 1 mL Tuberculin syringe.
    (c) Dissection board.
    (d) Autopsy pins.
    (e) 70% ethanol spray bottle.
    (f) Scissors.
    (g) Forceps.
    (h) Biohazard bag.

2.6 Obtaining Mouse Serum

1. 1.7 mL Eppendorf tubes and tube rack.
2. Micropipettor and tips.
3. Centrifuge.

2.7 Measuring Survival of Transfused RBCs, Performing DATs, IATs, and Complement Stains

1. 96-well U-bottom plate.
2. Phosphate buffered saline (PBS): 0.0067 M PO_4, without magnesium or calcium, pH 7.4 Reservoir.
3. Manual pipette, multi-channel pipette, and pipette tips.
4. RBC antigen-specific monoclonal or polyclonal antibody (*see* **Note 1**).
5. Fluorescently labeled secondary detection antibody.
    (a) e.g., APC anti-mouse IgG (Jackson Immunoresearch).
6. Biotinylated anti-C3 antibodies.
7. Biotinylated anti-C3b antibodies.
8. APC streptavidin (for detection of biotinylated anti-C3 or C3b antibody).
9. Flow cytometer.
10. APC anti-mouse TER-119.

2.8 Analyzing the Serum and Urine

1. Kit for quantifying free hemoglobin, such as one using Drabkin's Reagent.
2. Spectrophotometer (e.g., NanoDrop).

3 Methods

3.1 Collecting B6 Control and Antigen-Positive RBCs

1. Design the experiment to allow for the calculation of the amount of donor blood needed:
    (a) One group of mice should be passively immunized with 50 μL of B6 serum, and another group should receive

50 μL of polyclonal or monoclonal antibody specific to the antigen of interest in the utilized mouse model.
   - (b) Recipient mice will receive 50 μL of packed antigen-positive RBCs and 50 μL of B6 RBCs.
2. Calculate how much blood to collect (*see* **Note 2**).
3. Proceed with the collection of donor RBCs by either submandibular (**step 1**) or retro-orbital bleed (**Step 2**) (*see* **Note 3**).
4. Following the collection of whole blood (regardless of collection method), proceed to **Step 3** to complete blood processing.

3.1.1 Mouse Blood Collection—Submandibular Bleed

1. Sterilize the BSC with a disinfectant and paper towels.
2. Add ACD anticoagulant solution to a blood collection tube (5 or 50 mL tube). The volume of ACD should be ~20% of the estimated total whole blood volume to be collected.
3. Perform a submandibular bleed of the adult donor mice using a 5 mm animal lancet and collect the drops in the tube with ACD (*see* **Notes 4** and **5**).
4. After the mouse is bled, apply pressure using a sterile gauze pad for a few seconds to stop the bleeding.
5. Place the mouse in the empty mouse cage (i.e., recovery cage).
6. Proceed to bleed additional mice in the same manner, keeping the blood from antigen-positive mice separate from the blood collected from B6 mice.
7. Document which mice were face bled and the date on the cage slips using a pen.
8. Label each tube of blood accordingly and keep blood collected from different mouse strains separate at all times.

3.1.2 Mouse Blood Collection—Retro-orbital Sinus Bleed

1. Clean the fume hood with disinfectant and paper towels.
2. Add ACD anticoagulant solution to a blood collection tube (1.7, 5, or 50 mL tube). The volume of ACD should be ~20% of the estimated total whole blood volume to be collected.
3. Place gauze at the bottom of the glass staining trough.
4. Add 0.3 mL of isoflurane to the gauze in a chamber of ~250 mL.
5. Cover the gauze with aluminum foil.
6. Place a mouse on top of the aluminum foil in the chamber.
7. Watch the mouse as it starts to lose consciousness and slows its breathing significantly for several seconds.
8. Remove the mouse from the chamber.

9. Scruff the anesthetized mouse and pull the skin such that the eyeball bulges outward.
10. Use the curved tweezers to quickly remove one eyeball.
11. Collect the drops of blood into the ACD solution.
12. Immediately perform cervical dislocation and put the carcass in a biohazard bag (*see* **Note 6**).
13. Label the tube of blood accordingly and keep blood collected from different mouse strains separate at all times.

3.1.3 Washing and Quantifying Collected Blood

1. To the tube with collected blood, add at least 10x volume of PBS.
2. Centrifuge at 500× *g* for 7–10 min with a break, low or off.
3. Carefully remove supernatant by reverse pipetting.
4. Repeat **Steps 1–3** twice more for a total of three washes.
5. After the final wash, remove the supernatant. The pelleted RBCs are considered packed RBCs (pRBCs). 50uL of packed RBCs is considered equivalent to one unit of RBCs.
6. Use reverse pipetting to measure the volume of pRBCs.
7. *Optional—Alternatively, the RBC count can be obtained using a hematology analyzer. Dilute the packed RBCs to a desired concentration, such as 50% hematocrit, and evaluate using a hematology analyzer. The RBC count is the number of RBCs per microliter.

3.2 Phenotyping the Donor B6 Control and Transgenic Antigen-Positive RBCs (See Note 7)

1. On the lid of the 96-well plate, or a piece of paper with a 96-well plate graph, write down what each well will contain in terms of RBCs, primary antibodies, and secondary antibodies.
2. In a 1.7 mL Eppendorf, create 60 μL of a 1:100 dilution of primary antibody (specific to the RBC alloantigen of interest) solution.
3. Pipette 25uL of the antibody solution into each well of a 96-well plate for 2 wells.
4. Pipette 25uL of PBS solution in each well of a 96-well plate, for 2 different wells.
5. Pipette 1 uL of packed B6 RBCs into the PBS solution and into the antibody solution.
   (a) Repeat this step for the antigen-positive RBCs (e.g., KEL2N RBCs).
6. Mix the RBCs with solutions by either pipetting or vortexing the plate.
7. Incubate for 15 min at room temperature (25 °C).

8. Wash 3 times:
   (a) Add 200 uL of PBS to each well, using a multi-channel pipette.
   (b) Centrifuge at 500 g for 1 min at 4 °C to pellet the RBCs.
   (c) Flick (rapidly invert) the plate over a sink to toss out the supernatant. The pelleted RBCs will remain in the wells. Alternatively, reverse pipette the supernatant to take it into the pipette tip and then discard it.
   (d) Repeat **Steps a–c** two more times.
9. In a 1.7 mL Eppendorf, create 120 uL of a 1:100 dilution of secondary antibody (e.g., anti-mouse IgG APC).
10. Pipette 25 uL of antibody solution into each of the 4 wells.
11. Repeat **Steps** 7 and **8**.
12. Add 200 uL of PBS to each well and analyze using a flow cytometer.
13. Gate on RBCs and then singlets, and collect 50,000 singlet events.

    Expected Results: The antigen-positive RBCs should express the antigen of interest (APC positivity), while the controls should be negative.

3.3 Fluorescent Labeling of RBCs [66] (See Note 8)

Label B6 RBCs with DiO and antigen-positive RBCs with DiI

1. In a 50 mL conical, suspend 1 mL of washed, packed B6 RBCs in 4mLs of sterile PBS (This reaction can be scaled up or down as needed.)
2. In a separate 50 mL conical, suspend 1 mL of packed alloantigen-positive RBCs in 4 mLs of sterile PBS.
3. Dissolve the DiI and DiO according to the manufacturer's instructions (which may require DMSO).
4. Make sure the RBC suspensions are homogeneous and that the RBCs have not settled to the bottom of the conical. If the suspensions are not homogeneous, then swirl the conicals.
5. In a different 50 mL conical, dissolve ~15 uL of DiO in 5 mLs of sterile PBS and mix well (*see* **Note 9**).
6. Quickly pour the DiO solution onto the B6 RBCs and immediately mix well by gently inverting the tube.
7. In a different 50 mL conical, dissolve 100 uL of DiI in 5 mLs of sterile PBS and mix well.
8. Quickly pour the DiI solution onto the antigen-positive RBCs (e.g., KEL RBCs) and immediately mix well by gently inverting the tube.

9. Incubate both conicals for 30 min in the dark in a 37 °C water bath, and manually swirl the tubes every 10 min.
10. Wash the RBC solutions three times.
11. Analyze unstained B6 RBCs, DiO B6 RBCs, unstained antigen-positive RBCs, and DiI antigen-positive RBCs in separate wells of a 96-well U-bottom plate with flow cytometry to ensure that they are adequately labeled.
12. The concentration of DiI and DiO may need to be adjusted depending on your results.

    Expected Results: 90% of the B6 and antigen-positive RBCs should be labeled with fluorescent lipophilic dyes.

3.4 Passive Immunization and RBC Transfusion

3.4.1 Passive Immunization

1. Prepare 50 mL conical tube containing sterile PBS to be used for control injections.
2. Prepare 50 mL conical tube containing the antibody solution to be used for passive immunization. Each mouse will receive primary antigen-specific antibody diluted to a total volume of 500 μL per mouse in sterile PBS. Calculate enough for at least 3 extra mice (*see* **Note 10**).
3. Sterilize the BSC with a disinfectant and paper towels.
4. Set up the mouse restrainer.
5. Fill 1 mL syringes with sterile antibody solution or PBS.
6. Warm recipient mice under a heat lamp for several minutes (*see* **Note 11**).
7. Ear punch mouse (to allow for identification through the remaining procedure) and place it in the mouse restrainer.
8. Insert the appropriately filled syringe with a 30-gauge needle, bevel up, into the distal end of the lateral tail vein and inject the appropriate antibody solution.
9. Wait at least 30 min after passive immunization before proceeding with transfusion.

3.4.2 RBC Transfusion

1. Prepare RBCs for transfusion.
   (a) Calculate for each mouse to receive a lateral tail vein injection with a predetermined amount of DiO B6 RBCs and DiI antigen-positive RBCs diluted to ~33% hematocrit.
      (i) Preparation Example: For 10 recipient mice to receive 50 μL DiO B6 and 50 μL DiI KEL2N RBCs, mix 500 μL of packed DiO B6 RBCs with 500 μL of packed DiI KEL2N RBCs and 2 mL of sterile PBS. Inject 300 μL per mouse.
   (b) Always calculate for additional mice to account for blood loss during the transfusion procedure.

2. Fill syringes with prepared (mixed) RBCs.
3. Follow the tail vein injection procedure as described in Subheading 3.4.1 to transfuse each mouse recipient. Accurately note the time of each transfusion to allow for accurate post-transfusion sample collection.

3.5 Collecting Post-transfusion Specimens (Plasma, Serum, Urine)

1. At 10 min, perform a submandibular bleed to collect 5–8 drops into an empty 1.7 mL Eppendorf for serum collection, and immediately use a heparinized microhematocrit capillary tube to remove ~20uL of whole blood and place this into a 96-well plate with ACD-A (*see* **Note 12**).
2. At 1 h, perform a tail bleed to collect ~20uL of whole blood in a heparinized microhematocrit capillary tube and place this into a 96-well plate with ACD-A.
   (a) Sterilize the BSC with a disinfectant and paper towels.
   (b) Add 20 μL of ACD-A to each well of a 96-well U-bottom plate that will have blood added to it.
   (c) Optional: Warm the mice under the heat lamp. This will dilate the tail vein and enable larger volumes of blood to be collected rapidly. Do not leave the mice unattended.
   (d) Place a mouse in the restrainer as done previously for lateral tail vein injections (Subheading 3.4).
   (e) Disinfect the tail using a Kimwipe soaked in 70% ethanol.
   (f) Use a razor blade to create a small incision and quickly use a heparinized capillary tube to collect ~20 μL of the blood that pools from the lateral tail vein incision (*see* **Note 13**).
   (g) To stop the bleeding, compress the bleeding site using sterile gauze.
   (h) Place the mouse in a recovery cage.
   (i) Eject the blood from the capillary tube into a well of a 96-well plate containing ACD-A, which will serve as the "source plate" from which you will pull RBCs for all staining (*see* **Notes 14–16**).
3. At 2 h, tape a 4 × 4″ area of parafilm onto the lab bench top. Then, scruff a mouse over the parafilm so that when it urinates, the urine can be collected using a pipette and placed into a 1.7 mL Eppendorf tube.
4. Also, at 2 h, perform a submandibular bleed to collect 6–8 drops of blood into an empty 1.7 mL Eppendorf for serum collection, and immediately use a heparinized microhematocrit capillary tube to remove ~20uL of whole blood and place this into a 96-well plate with ACD-A.

5. At 24 h, perform a tail bleed to collect ~20uL of whole blood and place this into a 96-well plate with ACD-A (see **Step 2** above).
6. After the 24 h tail bleed has been performed, the mouse can be euthanized using isoflurane, followed by cervical dislocation.
7. *Optional: Perform a mouse autopsy to harvest the appropriate organs, such as the kidneys (*see* **Note 17**)
   (a) Place the mouse on its back and pin its paws to the autopsy board.
   (b) Spray the mouse's chest and abdominal fur with 70% ethanol.
   (c) Use forceps and scissors to open the abdominal cavity.
   (d) Dissect out the kidneys.
   (e) Place them into a tissue cassette labeled with the mouse's experimental group.
   (f) Add the cassette to 10% neutral buffered formalin, which is at least 10x the specimen volume.
   (g) These specimens can be further processed and analyzed (*see* **Note 17**).

3.6 Obtaining Mouse Serum

1. For the samples collected by submandibular bleed at 10 min and 2 hr. post-transfusion, harvest the serum.
   (a) Allow the blood to clot for at least 20–30 min at room temperature.
   (b) To isolate the serum, centrifuge the tubes at 10,000× *g* for 4 min at room temperature. Remove the supernatant and transfer to a new sterile 1.7 mL microcentrifuge tube.
   (c) Repeat this process one more time to ensure no RBCs remain in the serum.
2. Freeze serum until needed.

3.7 Measuring Survival of Transfused RBCs, Performing DATs, IATs, and Complement Stains

3.7.1 Measuring Transfused RBC Clearance

1. After obtaining the post-transfusion blood samples, centrifuge the 96-well plate at 500× *g* for 1 min.
2. Add 200 μL PBS per well to a new 96-well plate and then add 1 μL of packed RBCs into each well (*see* **Note 16**).
3. Analyze using a flow cytometer.
   (a) Gate on the RBCs using SSC-H vs FSC-H, then gate on singlets using FSC-A vs FSC-H, and finally plot DiO vs DiI.
   (b) Collect 50,000 RBC singlets (*see* **Note 18**).
   (c) Show the statistics for the percentage of singlets which are DiO B6 RBCs and DiI Ag + RBCs.

(i) Divide the % DiI antigen-positive RBCs by the % DiO B6 RBCs for each sample.

(ii) Divide each ratio by the mean ratio at the 10-min time point for 5 IC group mice. This will set the 10-min IC group survival to 100% (*see* **Note 19**).

Expected Results: B6 RBCs, which will lack your antigen of interest, won't be cleared by the antigen-specific antibodies, while the antigen-positive RBCs should show a meaningful increase in clearance. Notable clearance is not expected in mice that received PBS only or a non-antigen-specific antibody.

3.7.2 Measuring IgG on the RBC Surface (Direct Antiglobulin Test, DAT)

This will allow for assessment of antigen-specific antibody in circulation in the transfused mice to the RBC antigen on the transfused RBCs.

1. Add 200 μL PBS to each well of the source plate and centrifuge plate at 500× *g* for 1 min.
2. Remove supernatant by careful reverse pipetting.
3. Repeat **Steps 1** and **2** twice more for a total of 3 washes.
4. Create a 1:100 dilution of APC anti-mouse IgG.
5. Add 25 μL of staining solution to the appropriate wells of the 96-well plate. Consider adding the antibody solution to a reservoir and then using a multi-channel pipette to distribute the antibody solution to the wells.
6. Use a multi-channel pipette to add 1 μL of pRBCs into the antibody solution.
7. Incubate for 15 min at room temperature.
8. Wash x 3 with PBS.
9. Use a flow cytometer to acquire 2000 DiI (antigen-positive) RBC singlets and then show the statistics for the mean fluorescence intensity (MFI) of APC anti-mouse IgG.
10. Plot the data for the PBS group and the antigen-specific antibody group.

Expected Results: The DAT for the PBS only group should have a very low background MFI. In contrast, the DAT for the group that was passively immunized with antigen-specific antibody. This group should have a high MFI, which should decline over time as antigen modulation continues.

3.7.3 Antigen Quantification Via Flow Cytometry (Indirect Antiglobulin Test, IAT)

1. Ensure the whole blood has been washed three times.
2. Make a solution containing an appropriate dilution of antigen-specific primary antibody (*see* **Notes 20** and **21**).

3. Make a separate solution containing a 1:25 dilution of APC anti-TER-119.
4. Add 25 μL of each staining solution to the appropriate wells of a 96-well plate. Do not measure multiple antigen levels in the same well.
5. Use a multi-channel pipette to add 1 μL of packed RBCs into each antibody solution.
6. Incubate for 15 min at room temperature.
7. Wash x 3 with PBS.
8. For samples stained with APC anti-TER-119 (or any other directly labeled antibody), you can add 200 μL and proceed directly to analysis using a flow cytometer.
9. For samples stained with unlabeled antigen-specific primary antibody, after the final wash, add 25 μL of a 1:100 dilution of APC anti-mouse IgG.
10. Incubate for 15 min at room temperature, protected from light.
11. Wash x 3 with PBS and fill all wells with 200 μL PBS after the final wash, and proceed to analysis by flow cytometry.
12. Using the flow cytometer, acquire 2000 DiI antigen-positive RBC singlets and show the statistics for the MFI of APC.
13. For a specific time point, divide each mouse's APC MFI by the mean APC MFI for the mice in the PBS only group at that time point. This will set antigen levels to 100% for each PBS control group timepoint and enable you to determine if the experimental antibodies are causing antigen modulation (*see* **Note 22**).

    Expected Results: The RBC antigen level of interest should be high in the PBS only group and lower in the passively immunized group due to antigen modulation. Antigen levels should continue to decline over each consecutive time point as antigen modulation continues.

3.7.4 Measuring C3 and C3b Deposition on RBCs

1. Ensure the whole blood (source plate) has been washed three times.
2. Make a solution containing a 1:100 dilution of biotinylated anti-C3.
3. Add 25 μL of the solution into a 96-well plate to stain all samples.
4. Make a separate solution containing a 1:100 dilution of biotinylated anti-C3b.
5. Add 25 μL of the solution into a 96-well plate to stain all samples.

6. Use a multi-channel pipette to add 1 μL of post-transfusion pRBCs into the antibody solutions.
7. Incubate for 15 min at room temperature.
8. Wash x 3 with PBS.
9. Add 25 μL of APC streptavidin.
10. Incubate for 15 min at room temperature.
11. Wash x 3 with PBS.
12. Using the flow cytometer, acquire 2000 DiI antigen-positive RBC singlets and show the statistics for the MFI of APC.

Expected Results: Expected results for complement fixation are highly dependent on the model utilized (*see* **Note 23**).

3.8 Analyzing the Serum and Urine

1. Photograph all 1.7 mL Eppendorf tubes that contain the serum in one image for visual assessment of hemolysis.
   (a) Use a white background.
   (b) Ensure that the tubes are clearly labeled.
2. Measure the hemoglobin in the serum using a hemoglobin quantification kit or by measuring the absorbance at 414 nm.
3. Photograph all 1.7 mL Eppendorf tubes which contain the urine in one image.
   (a) Use a white background.
   (b) Ensure that the tubes are clearly labeled.
4. Measure the hemoglobin in the urine using a hemoglobin quantification kit or by measuring the absorbance at 414 nm.

4 Notes

1. Primary antibody should be either a polyclonal or a monoclonal antibody produced to match the transgenic antigen expressed in the mouse model utilized. Examples include KEL, HOD, and GPA models outlined briefly in Subheading 1 of this chapter. We recommend reference to current literature to identify appropriate antibody clones for your chosen mouse model (REFs).
2. Multiply 50 uL of packed RBCs, the typical dose transfused to mice, by the number of mice that need to be transfused with that blood type. 8–10-week-old male and female B6 mice have a hematocrit of ~45%, meaning that ~45% of the blood volume is pRBCs. Multiply the amount of pRBCs to be collected by 2.22 to calculate the total volume of whole blood to be collected. Collect more than this amount because some will be lost when processing, when phenotyping, when labeling, and in the dead space of the syringe's needle.

3. Ensure that experimental protocols and animal procedures performed in these studies are approved by your Institutional Animal Care and Use Committee (IACUC), Institutional Biosafety Committee (IBC), and/or any other relevant entities. Follow your institution's policies for mouse blood collection (e.g., methods and volumes).
4. For a submandibular bleed (i.e., face bleed), the mouse should be suspended far enough above the tube so that it does not contaminate it, bite it, or try to grasp the tube, which may knock it over. Using a cube rack that holds four 50 mL conicals is wise because it is heavy enough to prevent the tube from getting knocked over if the mouse grasps onto it.
5. As submandibular bleeds are not necessarily a terminal procedure, mice should always be identified prior to performing any bleeds so that the volume and frequency of blood collection can be monitored to not exceed safety guidelines for the donor mouse. Appropriate IACUC-approved guidelines should be followed for the institution in which the procedure is being performed. We typically identify mice by distinct ear punches.
6. It is critical that the mouse never regain consciousness during or after this retro-orbital sinus bleed procedure (particularly once the eye has been removed). If the mouse appears to be regaining consciousness during the bleed, halt the bleed and repeat exposure to isoflurane as needed to ensure adequate sedation.
7. Transgenic mice expressing specific alloantigen on RBCs are typically phenotyped instead of genotyped to ensure normal alloantigen expression patterns. Phenotyping can be done separately from the actual experiment, but it is always recommended, and phenotyping of the exact blood that is transfused is the best practice. Importantly, if the HOD mouse model is being utilized, it is important to note that B6.HOD mice often have a small subset of RBCs which lack HOD expression. This subset may be 10% of RBCs, but it can be greater. If not accounted for, this subset may affect the interpretation of results when assessing antigen modulation. Additionally, if antigen expression is too low, then RBCs from that donor may not be appropriate to use for this procedure. If the percentage of RBCs lacking HOD expression is very high, then these mice can be euthanized. FVB.HOD mice are less likely to have a subset of RBCs lacking HOD expression. Alternatively, ROSA26-HOD mice, on a C57BL/6 background, were recently generated, which have a very small percentage of RBCs lacking HOD expression [70].

8. This protocol describes the use of lipophilic dyes to label RBCs. However, other dyes, such as CFSE, can be used. This dye reacts with free amines on and within RBCs.
9. The volume of DiO and DiI added to each solution may need to be adjusted based on your individual needs. It is also difficult to get the MFI of the DiO and DiI-labeled RBCs to be identical.
10. The amount of antigen-specific primary antibody needed will vary depending on the mouse model system being utilized. Review relevant literature for recommended antibody concentrations or titrate to optimize empirically.
11. Do not leave mice unattended during this step. Ensure all mouse handling is compliant with institutional IACUC requirements.
12. The time points which are used for specimen collection may vary based on the mouse model. Sometimes intravascular hemolysis will happen so quickly that plasma and urine will show evidence of hemolysis at the 10 min time point.
13. If the injection site starts to bleed, then blood can be collected. Otherwise, carefully use a razor blade to make a small and superficial cut into the lateral tail vein. Sometimes the injection site will spontaneously bleed or will spontaneously bleed when the tail is wiped with a Kimwipe, rubbed with a capillary tube, or after the mouse is warmed using a heat lamp. In these situations, the mouse tail vein does not need to be cut using a razor blade. However, if there is minimal bleeding, a razor blade may be used to make a cut to obtain larger volumes of blood.
14. Eject the whole blood into a 96-well plate containing 20 μL of ACD-A. This plate will be known as the "source plate" from which you will pull blood for all further assays. After washing (which will occur further down in the protocol), this plate should be stored in a cold, dark location. Additionally, the supernatant should be removed when packed RBCs are being pulled from the plate for the various indicated stains in this protocol. When stored (not actively being used), the RBCs should be covered in sufficient saline buffer to prevent the samples from drying out. With appropriate storage, RBCs from this plate should be relatively stable and can be used for staining for up to a day (and possibly longer) without variable results.
15. The blood can be ejected either by ejecting air into the capillary tube using a pipette with an attached tip or a rubber bulb attachment.

16. Before washing the RBCs, 1 μL of packed RBCs should be taken for measuring RBC clearance. This is included in Subheading 3.6 of this protocol. Afterward, the RBCs can be washed three times. This step is included in Subheading 3.7 of this protocol but may be completed as soon as the sample for measuring RBC clearance has been removed. Because there is a large volume of RBCs in each well, the plate cannot be flicked (inverted) after centrifugation when washing. Use a multi-channel pipette to reverse pipette the supernatant and then discard it.
17. We do not provide any additional processing guidelines in this protocol, but if desired, organ harvest followed by histological analysis for evidence of hemolysis can provide complementary information regarding the HTR severity.
18. Ideally, the 50,000 RBC singlets will yield at least 2000 DiI antigen-positive RBCs. If not, increase the number of RBC singlets that are collected (e.g., 100,000). Failure to collect sufficient DiI antigen-positive RBC events can hinder accurate data analysis.
19. There is a different approach to normalizing RBC survival that can be used if the time points are prior to D3, when alloantibodies can start forming. Instead of setting only the 10-min PBS control group mean to 100% survival, each PBS control group time point can be set to 100% survival.
20. While the appropriate dilution may vary depending on the antibody and model antigen system being used, we have found that between 1:50 and 1:200 will usually produce optimal staining for most antibody antigen combinations commonly used within the field.
21. In some cases, multiple antibodies could be used to assess antigen levels. For example, as the HOD antigen contains multiple antigen components (HEL, OVA, and Duffy) in the same chimeric antigen, other primary antibodies besides the common anti-HEL antibodies commonly used in literature (e.g., anti-OVA antibodies or anti-Duffy antibodies) can be used to measure antigen levels. However, it is important to remember that if antibody targeting an epitope other than the epitope targeted through passive immunization, then when using standard staining practice (primary detection antibody followed by fluorescent secondary antibody) the secondary detection antibodies will bind to the passively immunized antibody (i.e., the anti-HEL antibodies given to the mouse by passive immunization) along with the primary antibody used for staining (i.e., anti-OVA or anti-Duffy primary antibodies) and confound the results. To avoid this, antibodies used for staining can be biotinylated using sulfo-NHS-LC-biotin

(according to the manufacturer's protocol) to eliminate the need for secondary reagents. When using this approach, the unbound biotin can be removed using a biotin removal column. Therefore, in this example, APC streptavidin can be used to detect the binding of biotinylated anti-OVA or anti-Duffy antibodies to HOD RBCs.

22. Be careful when trying to measure antigen levels at later than day 3 post-transfusion. This is because mouse alloantibodies can start to form against the RBC antigens, and this endogenous antibody will bind to transfused RBCs and may modulate antigen levels in the PBS control group.
23. Some models of RBC transfusion, the KEL model in particular, may exhibit more significant complement deposition than others.

Conflict of Interest Statement

This work was funded by NIH P01HL171803, R01 HL165975, R01 HL135575, R01 HL154034, K08HL171877, K99HL169746, and AABB Foundation Early-Career Scientific Research Grants. SRS has received speaker and consultant honoraria from Cerus, Grifols, Novartis, Alexion, and Argenx and has received a research grant from Alexion. Ryan Jajosky is CEO of Biconcavity Inc. No other authors have conflicts of interest.

References

1. Chou ST, Hendrickson JE (2024. Epub 20240510) How i treat challenging transfusion cases in sickle cell disease. Blood. https://doi.org/10.1182/blood.2023023648
2. Lal A, Wong T, Keel S, Pagano M, Chung J, Kamdar A et al (2021) The transfusion management of beta thalassemia in the United States. Transfusion. 61(10):3027–3039. https://doi.org/10.1111/trf.16640. Epub 20210828. PubMed PMID: 34453453; PubMed Central PMCID: PMCPMC9292563
3. Butwick AJ, Goodnough LT (2015) Transfusion and coagulation management in major obstetric hemorrhage. Curr Opin Anaesthesiol 28(3):275–284. https://doi.org/10.1097/ACO.0000000000000180. PubMed PMID: 25812005; PubMed Central PMCID: PMCPMC4567035
4. Jajosky RP, Wu SC, Zheng L, Jajosky AN, Jajosky PG, Josephson CD et al (2023) ABO blood group antigens and differential glycan expression: perspective on the evolution of common human enzyme deficiencies. iScience 26(1):105798. https://doi.org/10.1016/j.isci.2022.105798. Epub 20221214. PubMed PMID: 36691627; PubMed Central PMCID: PMCPMC9860303
5. Jan HM, Wu SC, Stowell CJ, Vallecillo-Zuniga ML, Paul A, Patel KR et al (2024) Galectin-4 antimicrobial activity primarily occurs through its C-terminal domain. Mol Cell Proteomics 23(5):100747. https://doi.org/10.1016/j.mcpro.2024.100747. Epub 20240313. PubMed PMID: 38490531; PubMed Central PMCID: PMCPMC11097083
6. Wu SC, Kamili NA, Dias-Baruffi M, Josephson CD, Rathgeber MF, Yeung MY et al (2022) Innate immune Galectin-7 specifically targets microbes that decorate themselves in blood group-like antigens. iScience. 25(7):104482. https://doi.org/10.1016/j.isci.2022.104482. Epub 20220530. PubMed PMID: 35754739; PubMed Central PMCID: PMCPMC9218387

7. Blenda AV, Kamili NA, Wu SC, Abel WF, Ayona D, Gerner-Smidt C et al (2022) Galectin-9 recognizes and exhibits antimicrobial activity toward microbes expressing blood group-like antigens. J Biol Chem 298(4): 101704. https://doi.org/10.1016/j.jbc.2022.101704. Epub 20220209. PubMed PMID: 35148986; PubMed Central PMCID: PMCPMC9019251
8. Storry JR, Olsson ML (2009) The ABO blood group system revisited: a review and update. Immunohematology 25(2):48–59
9. Panch SR, Montemayor-Garcia C, Klein HG (2019) Hemolytic transfusion reactions. N Engl J Med 381(2):150–162. https://doi.org/10.1056/NEJMra1802338
10. Pirenne F, Yazdanbakhsh K (2018) How I safely transfuse patients with sickle-cell disease and manage delayed hemolytic transfusion reactions. Blood. 131(25):2773–2781. https://doi.org/10.1182/blood-2018-02-785964. Epub 20180503. PubMed PMID: 29724898; PubMed Central PMCID: PMCPMC6014354
11. Arthur CM, Stowell SR (2023) The development and consequences of red blood cell alloimmunization. Annu Rev Pathol. 18:537–564. https://doi.org/10.1146/annurev-pathol-042320-110411. Epub 20221109. PubMed PMID: 36351365; PubMed Central PMCID: PMCPMC10414795
12. Zerra PE, Cox C, Baldwin WH, Patel SR, Arthur CM, Lollar P et al (2017) Marginal zone B cells are critical to factor VIII inhibitor formation in mice with hemophilia A. Blood. 130(23):2559–2568. https://doi.org/10.1182/blood-2017-05-782912. Epub 2017/10/06. PubMed PMID: 28978569; PubMed Central PMCID: PMCPMC5721282
13. Arthur CM, Patel SR, Sullivan HC, Winkler AM, Tormey CA, Hendrickson JE et al (2016) CD8+ T cells mediate antibody-independent platelet clearance in mice. Blood. 127(14):1823–1827. https://doi.org/10.1182/blood-2015-10-673426. Epub 2016/01/21. PubMed PMID: 26787734; PubMed Central PMCID: PMCPMC4825415
14. Arthur CM, Zerra PE, Shin S, Wang J, Song X, Doering CB et al (2022) Nonhuman glycans can regulate anti-factor VIII antibody formation in mice. Blood 139(9):1312–1317. https://doi.org/10.1182/blood.2020009210. PubMed PMID: 34019619; PubMed Central PMCID: PMCPMC8900271
15. Yazdanbakhsh K, Shaz BH, Hillyer CD (2017) Immune regulation of sickle cell alloimmunization. ISBT Sci Ser. 12(1):248–253. https://doi.org/10.1111/voxs.12296. Epub 20161115. PubMed PMID: 28261322; PubMed Central PMCID: PMCPMC5330297
16. Pirenne F, Floch A, Diop S (2023) Alloimmunisation against red blood cells in sickle cell disease: transfusion challenges in high-income and low-income countries. Lancet Haematol. 10(6):e468–ee76. Epub 20230413. https://doi.org/10.1016/S2352-3026(23)00066-2
17. Zimring JC, Spitalnik SL (2015) Pathobiology of transfusion reactions. Annu Rev Pathol 10: 83–110. https://doi.org/10.1146/annurev-pathol-012414-040318
18. Narbey D, Habibi A, Chadebech P, Mekontso-Dessap A, Khellaf M, Lelievre JD et al (2017) Incidence and predictive score for delayed hemolytic transfusion reaction in adult patients with sickle cell disease. Am J Hematol 92(12): 1340–1348. Epub 2017/09/20. https://doi.org/10.1002/ajh.24908
19. Chonat S, Jones JA, Patel SR, Briones WM, Schoettler ML, Maarouf M et al (2025) Complement is activated in patients with acute chest syndrome caused by sickle cell disease and represents a therapeutic target. Sci Transl Med 17(807):eadl4922. Epub 20250716. https://doi.org/10.1126/scitranslmed.adl4922
20. Thein SL, Pirenne F, Fasano RM, Habibi A, Bartolucci P, Chonat S, et al. Hemolytic transfusion reactions in sickle cell disease: underappreciated and potentially fatal. Haematologica. 2020;105(3):539–544. doi:https://doi.org/10.3324/haematol.2019.224709. Epub 2020/02/08. PubMed PMID: 32029505; PubMed Central PMCID: PMCPMC7049330
21. Chou ST, Alsawas M, Fasano RM, Field JJ, Hendrickson JE, Howard J et al (2020) American Society of Hematology 2020 guidelines for sickle cell disease: transfusion support. Blood Adv. 4(2):327–355. https://doi.org/10.1182/bloodadvances.2019001143. Epub 2020/01/28. PubMed PMID: 31985807; PubMed Central PMCID: PMCPMC6988392
22. Vidler JB, Gardner K, Amenyah K, Mijovic A, Thein SL (2015) Delayed haemolytic transfusion reaction in adults with sickle cell disease: a 5-year experience. Br J Haematol 169(5): 746–753. Epub 2015/03/11. https://doi.org/10.1111/bjh.13339
23. Gardner K, Hoppe C, Mijovic A, Thein SL (2015) How we treat delayed haemolytic transfusion reactions in patients with sickle cell disease. Br J Haematol. 170(6):745–756. Epub 20150513. https://doi.org/10.1111/bjh.13494

24. Mekontso Dessap A, Pirenne F, Razazi K, Moutereau S, Abid S, Brun-Buisson C et al (2016) A diagnostic nomogram for delayed hemolytic transfusion reaction in sickle cell disease. Am J Hematol 91(12):1181–1184. Epub 2016/08/19. https://doi.org/10.1002/ajh.24537
25. Falguiere C, Allali S, Khazem B, Kamdem A, Arnaud C, Belloy M et al (2023) Delayed hemolytic transfusion reaction in children with sickle cell disease: first 5-year retrospective study in mainland France. Haematologica. 108(3):889–894. https://doi.org/10.3324/haematol.2022.281050. Epub 20230301. PubMed PMID: 36325889; PubMed Central PMCID: PMCPMC9973478
26. Meuleman MS, Roumenina LT, Grunenwald A (2023) Complement involvement in sickle cell disease. Presse Med 52(4):104205. Epub 20231114. https://doi.org/10.1016/j.lpm.2023.104205
27. Ghosh S, Adisa OA, Chappa P, Tan F, Jackson KA, Archer DR et al (2013) Extracellular hemin crisis triggers acute chest syndrome in sickle mice. J Clin Invest 123(11):4809–4820. https://doi.org/10.1172/JCI64578. PubMed PMID: 24084741; PubMed Central PMCID: PMCPMC3809772
28. Thomas AM, Gerogianni A, MB MA, Floisand Y, Lau C, Espevik T et al (2019) Complement component C5 and TLR molecule CD14 mediate heme-induced thromboinflammation in human blood. J Immunol. 203(6):1571–1578. https://doi.org/10.4049/jimmunol.1900047. Epub 20190814. PubMed PMID: 31413105; PubMed Central PMCID: PMCPMC6731449
29. Merle NS, Boudhabhay I, Leon J, Fremeaux-Bacchi V, Roumenina LT (2019) Complement activation during intravascular hemolysis: implication for sickle cell disease and hemolytic transfusion reactions. Transfus Clin Biol. 26(2):116–124. Epub 20190222. https://doi.org/10.1016/j.tracli.2019.02.008
30. Chonat S, Graciaa S, Shin HS, Newton JG, Quarmyne MO, Boudreaux J et al (2020) Eculizumab for complement mediated thrombotic microangiopathy in sickle cell disease. Haematologica. 105(12):2887–2891. https://doi.org/10.3324/haematol.2020.262006. Epub 20201201. PubMed PMID: 33256394; PubMed Central PMCID: PMCPMC7716365
31. Floch A, Morel A, Zanchetta-Balint F, Cordonnier-Jourdin C, Allali S, Grall M et al (2020. Epub 2020/07/04) Anti-C5 antibody treatment for delayed hemolytic transfusion reactions in sickle cell disease. Haematologica. https://doi.org/10.3324/haematol.2020.253856
32. Pirenne F, Bartolucci P, Habibi A (2017) Management of delayed hemolytic transfusion reaction in sickle cell disease: prevention, diagnosis, treatment. Transfus Clin Biol 24(3):227–231. Epub 2017/07/04. https://doi.org/10.1016/j.tracli.2017.05.016
33. Godefroy E, Liu Y, Shi P, Mitchell WB, Cohen D, Chou ST et al (2016) Altered heme-mediated modulation of dendritic cell function in sickle cell alloimmunization. Haematologica. 101(9):1028–1038. https://doi.org/10.3324/haematol.2016.147181. Epub 20160526. PubMed PMID: 27229712; PubMed Central PMCID: PMCPMC5060019
34. Merle NS, Paule R, Leon J, Daugan M, Robe-Rybkine T, Poillerat V et al (2019) P-selectin drives complement attack on endothelium during intravascular hemolysis in TLR-4/heme-dependent manner. Proc Natl Acad Sci U S A. 116(13):6280–6285. https://doi.org/10.1073/pnas.1814797116. Epub 20190308. PubMed PMID: 30850533; PubMed Central PMCID: PMCPMC6442544
35. Noizat-Pirenne F, Habibi A, Mekontso-Dessap A, Razazi K, Chadebech P, Mahevas M et al (2015) The use of rituximab to prevent severe delayed haemolytic transfusion reaction in immunized patients with sickle cell disease. Vox Sang 108(3):262–267. Epub 2014/12/20. https://doi.org/10.1111/vox.12217
36. Zimring JC, Hair GA, Chadwick TE, Deshpande SS, Anderson KM, Hillyer CD et al (2005) Nonhemolytic antibody-induced loss of erythrocyte surface antigen. Blood 106(3):1105–1112. Epub 2005/04/16. https://doi.org/10.1182/blood-2005-03-1040
37. Liepkalns JS, Hod EA, Stowell SR, Cadwell CM, Spitalnik SL, Zimring JC (2012) Biphasic clearance of incompatible red blood cells through a novel mechanism requiring neither complement nor Fcgamma receptors in a murine model. Transfusion 52(12):2631–2645. Epub 2012/04/17. https://doi.org/10.1111/j.1537-2995.2012.03647.x
38. Stowell SR, Winkler AM, Maier CL, Arthur CM, Smith NH, Girard-Pierce KR et al (2012) Initiation and regulation of complement during hemolytic transfusion reactions. Clin Dev Immunol. 2012:307093. https://doi.org/10.1155/2012/307093. Epub 2012/11/03. PubMed PMID: 23118779; PubMed Central PMCID: PMCPMC3479954
39. Girard-Pierce KR, Stowell SR, Smith NH, Arthur CM, Sullivan HC, Hendrickson JE

et al (2013) A novel role for C3 in antibody-induced red blood cell clearance and antigen modulation. Blood. 122(10):1793–1801. https://doi.org/10.1182/blood-2013-06-508952. Epub 2013/07/24. PubMed PMID: 23878139; PubMed Central PMCID: PMCPMC3765059

40. Jajosky RP, Covington ML, Liu J, Chai L, Zerra PE, Chonat S, Stowell SR, Arthur CM (2025) CD47 regulates antigen modulation and red blood cell clearance following an incompatible transfusion. Front Immunol. 16: 1548548
41. Shinde P, Howie HL, Stegmann TC, Hay AM, Waterman HR, Szittner Z et al (2020) IgG subclass determines suppression versus enhancement of humoral alloimmunity to Kell RBC antigens in mice. Front Immunol. 11: 1516. https://doi.org/10.3389/fimmu.2020.01516. Epub 20200716. PubMed PMID: 32765523; PubMed Central PMCID: PMCPMC7378678
42. Jash A, Usaneerungrueng C, Howie HL, Qiu A, Luckey CJ, Zimring JC et al (2021) Antibodies to low-copy number RBC alloantigen convert a tolerogenic stimulus to an immunogenic stimulus in mice. Front Immunol. 12: 629608. https://doi.org/10.3389/fimmu.2021.629608. Epub 20210312. PubMed PMID: 33777014; PubMed Central PMCID: PMCPMC7994621
43. Jajosky RP, Patel KR, Allen JWL, Zerra PE, Chonat S, Ayona D et al (2023) Antibody-mediated antigen loss switches augmented immunity to antibody-mediated immunosuppression. Blood 142(12):1082–1098. https://doi.org/10.1182/blood.2022018591. PubMed PMID: 37363865; PubMed Central PMCID: PMCPMC10541552
44. Maier CL, Mener A, Patel SR, Jajosky RP, Bennett AL, Arthur CM et al (2018) Antibody-mediated immune suppression by antigen modulation is antigen-specific. Blood Adv 2(21):2986–3000. https://doi.org/10.1182/bloodadvances.2018018408. PubMed PMID: 30413434; PubMed Central PMCID: PMCPMC6234375
45. Jajosky RP, Ayona D, Mener A, Stowell SR, Arthur CM (2024) Dynamics of antibody engagement of red blood cells in vivo and in vitro. Front Immunol. 15:1475470. https://doi.org/10.3389/fimmu.2024.1475470. Epub 20241128. PubMed PMID: 39669570; PubMed Central PMCID: PMCPMC11634868
46. Mener A, Patel SR, Arthur CM, Stowell SR (2019) Antibody-mediated immunosuppression can result from RBC antigen loss independent of Fcgamma receptors in mice. Transfusion 59(1):371–384. Epub 2018/11/27. https://doi.org/10.1111/trf.14939
47. Stowell SR, Liepkalns JS, Hendrickson JE, Girard-Pierce KR, Smith NH, Arthur CM et al (2013) Antigen modulation confers protection to red blood cells from antibody through Fcgamma receptor ligation. J Immunol 191(10):5013–5025. https://doi.org/10.4049/jimmunol.1300885
48. Sullivan HC, Gerner-Smidt C, Nooka AK, Arthur CM, Thompson L, Mener A et al (2017) Daratumumab (anti-CD38) induces loss of CD38 on red blood cells. Blood 129(22):3033–3037. https://doi.org/10.1182/blood-2016-11-749432. PubMed PMID: 28373263; PubMed Central PMCID: PMC5454337
49. Sullivan HC, Arthur CM, Thompson L, Patel SR, Stowell SR, Hendrickson JE et al (2018) Anti-RhD reduces levels of detectable RhD antigen following anti-RhD infusion. Transfusion 58(2):542–544. Epub 2018/02/08. https://doi.org/10.1111/trf.14452
50. Arthur CM, Allen JWL, Verkerke H, Yoo J, Jajosky RP, Girard-Pierce K et al (2021) Antigen density dictates RBC clearance, but not antigen modulation, following incompatible RBC transfusion in mice. Blood Adv 5(2): 527–538. https://doi.org/10.1182/bloodadvances.2020002695. PubMed PMID: 33496748; PubMed Central PMCID: PMCPMC7839377
51. Jajosky RP, Covington ML, Liu J, Chai L, Zerra PE, Chonat S et al (2025) CD47 regulates antigen modulation and red blood cell clearance following an incompatible transfusion. Front Immunol. 16:1548548. https://doi.org/10.3389/fimmu.2025.1548548. Epub 20250404. PubMed PMID: 40255405; PubMed Central PMCID: PMCPMC12006802
52. Liepkalns JS, Cadwell CM, Stowell SR, Hod EA, Spitalnik SL, Zimring JC (2013) Resistance of a subset of red blood cells to clearance by antibodies in a mouse model of incompatible transfusion. Transfusion 53(6): 1319–1327. Epub 2012/10/05. https://doi.org/10.1111/j.1537-2995.2012.03910.x
53. Desmarets M, Cadwell CM, Peterson KR, Neades R, Zimring JC (2009) Minor histocompatibility antigens on transfused leukoreduced units of red blood cells induce bone marrow transplant rejection in a mouse model. Blood. 114(11):2315–2322. https://doi.org/10.1182/blood-2009-04-214387. Epub 20090612. PubMed PMID: 19525479;

PubMed Central PMCID: PMCPMC2745850

54. Smith NH, Henry KL, Cadwell CM, Bennett A, Hendrickson JE, Frame T et al (2012) Generation of transgenic mice with antithetical KEL1 and KEL2 human blood group antigens on red blood cells. Transfusion 52(12):2620–2630. https://doi.org/10.1111/j.1537-2995.2012.03641.x. PubMed PMID: 22494154; PubMed Central PMCID: PMC3580151
55. Smith NH, Hod EA, Spitalnik SL, Zimring JC, Hendrickson JE (2012) Transfusion in the absence of inflammation induces antigen-specific tolerance to murine RBCs. Blood. 119(6):1566–1569. https://doi.org/10.1182/blood-2011-09-382655. Epub 20111110. PubMed PMID: 22077064; PubMed Central PMCID: PMCPMC3286217
56. Stowell SR, Girard-Pierce KR, Smith NH, Henry KL, Arthur CM, Zimring JC et al (2014) Transfusion of murine red blood cells expressing the human KEL glycoprotein induces clinically significant alloantibodies. Transfusion. 54(1):179–189. https://doi.org/10.1111/trf.12217. Epub 2013/04/30. PubMed PMID: 23621760; PubMed Central PMCID: PMCPMC3732531
57. Hendrickson JE, Hod EA, Spitalnik SL, Hillyer CD, Zimring JC (2010) Storage of murine red blood cells enhances alloantibody responses to an erythroid-specific model antigen. Transfusion. 50(3):642–648. https://doi.org/10.1111/j.1537-2995.2009.02481.x. Epub 2009/11/13. PubMed PMID: 19906034; PubMed Central PMCID: PMCPMC3568949
58. Hendrickson JE, Hod EA, Perry JR, Ghosh S, Chappa P, Adisa O et al (2012) Alloimmunization to transfused HOD red blood cells is not increased in mice with sickle cell disease. Transfusion. 52(2):231–240. https://doi.org/10.1111/j.1537-2995.2011.03255.x. Epub 2011/07/28. PubMed PMID: 21790627; PubMed Central PMCID: PMCPMC3218203
59. Patel SR, Bennett A, Girard-Pierce K, Maier CL, Chonat S, Arthur CM et al (2018) Recipient priming to one RBC alloantigen directly enhances subsequent alloimmunization in mice. Blood Adv. 2(2):105–115. https://doi.org/10.1182/bloodadvances.2017010124. Epub 2018/01/25. PubMed PMID: 29365318; PubMed Central PMCID: PMCPMC5787868
60. Mener A, Patel SR, Arthur CM, Chonat S, Wieland A, Santhanakrishnan M et al (2018) Complement serves as a switch between CD4+ T cell-independent and -dependent RBC antibody responses. JCI Insight. 3(22) Epub 2018/11/16. https://doi.org/10.1172/jci.insight.121631
61. Mener A, Arthur CM, Patel SR, Liu J, Hendrickson JE, Stowell SR (2018) Complement component 3 negatively regulates antibody response by modulation of red blood cell antigen. Front Immunol. 9:676. https://doi.org/10.3389/fimmu.2018.00676. Epub 2018/06/27. PubMed PMID: 29942300; PubMed Central PMCID: PMCPMC6004516
62. Gibb DR, Liu J, Santhanakrishnan M, Natarajan P, Madrid DJ, Patel S et al (2017) B cells require Type 1 interferon to produce alloantibodies to transfused KEL-expressing red blood cells in mice. Transfusion. 57(11): 2595–2608. https://doi.org/10.1111/trf.14288. Epub 2017/08/25. PubMed PMID: 28836263; PubMed Central PMCID: PMCPMC5745367
63. Arthur CM, Patel SR, Smith NH, Bennett A, Kamili NA, Mener A et al (2017) Antigen density dictates immune responsiveness following red blood cell transfusion. J Immunol 198(7): 2671–2680. https://doi.org/10.4049/jimmunol.1601736. Epub 20170301. PubMed PMID: 28250159; PubMed Central PMCID: PMCPMC5777137
64. Jajosky R, Patel SR, Wu SC, Patel K, Covington M, Vallecillo-Zuniga M et al (2023) Prior immunization against an intracellular antigen enhances subsequent red blood cell alloimmunization in mice. Blood 141(21):2642–2653. https://doi.org/10.1182/blood.2022016588. PubMed PMID: 36638335; PubMed Central PMCID: PMCPMC10356576
65. Arneja A, Salazar JE, Jiang W, Hendrickson JE, Zimring JC, Luckey CJ (2016) Interleukin-6 receptor-alpha signaling drives anti-RBC alloantibody production and T-follicular helper cell differentiation in a murine model of red blood cell alloimmunization. Haematologica. 101(11):e440–e4e4. https://doi.org/10.3324/haematol.2016.149278. Epub 20160804. PubMed PMID: 27662015; PubMed Central PMCID: PMCPMC5394864
66. Patel SR, Gibb DR, Girard-Pierce K, Zhou X, Rodrigues LC, Arthur CM et al (2018) Marginal zone B cells induce alloantibody formation following RBC transfusion. Front Immunol. 9:2516. https://doi.org/10.3389/fimmu.2018.02516. Epub 20181116. PubMed PMID: 30505302; PubMed Central PMCID: PMCPMC6250814

67. Zerra PE, Patel SR, Jajosky RP, Arthur CM, McCoy JW, Allen JWL et al (2021) Marginal zone B cells mediate a CD4 T-cell-dependent extrafollicular antibody response following RBC transfusion in mice. Blood 138(8): 706–721. https://doi.org/10.1182/blood.2020009376. PubMed PMID: 33876205; PubMed Central PMCID: PMCPMC8394907
68. Yu H, Stowell SR, Bernardo L, Hendrickson JE, Zimring JC, Amash A et al (2014) Antibody-mediated immune suppression of erythrocyte alloimmunization can occur independently from red cell clearance or epitope masking in a murine model. J Immunol 193(6):2902–2910. Epub 2014/08/15. https://doi.org/10.4049/jimmunol.1302287
69. Hod EA, Cadwell CM, Liepkalns JS, Zimring JC, Sokol SA, Schirmer DA et al (2008) Cytokine storm in a mouse model of IgG-mediated hemolytic transfusion reactions. Blood. 112(3):891–894. https://doi.org/10.1182/blood-2008-01-132092. Epub 2008/05/17. PubMed PMID: 18483395; PubMed Central PMCID: PMCPMC2481546
70. Jash A, Hay AM, Collins JB, Heo J, Luckey CJ, Hudson KE et al (2023) The role of RBC antigen transgene integration sites on RBC biology in mice. Transfusion 63(1):239–248. Epub 20221127. https://doi.org/10.1111/trf.17197

Chapter 42

In Vitro Phagocytosis Assays

Yeniley Ruiz Noa, Melika Loriamini, Selena Cen, Tik Nga Tong, Lindsay K. Hillis, Gurleen Sandhu, Clemence Salou, Beth Binnington, and Donald R. Branch

Abstract

We have used an in vitro phagocytosis assay called the monocyte monolayer assay (MMA) for over 40 years to assess the potential clinical significance of antibodies to red blood cells. This assay uses human monocytes, not macrophages, but has been a reliable predictor of hemolysis outcomes in the face of auto- or alloantibodies. However, this assay can be slightly modified to be used with phagocytic cells other than monocytes and with different animals' phagocytes. Indeed, we have been working on using human macrophages in this assay as well as mouse monocyte-macrophages. Thus, we now use the acronym MOMA to mean MOnocyte-Macrophage Assay. Herein, we present detailed methods for performing in vitro phagocytosis assays that use human monocytes, cultured macrophages (MOMA), M1 or M2 macrophages, mouse PBMCs, or the mouse macrophage cell line, RAW 264.7.

Key words Phagocytosis, Monocyte monolayer assay, MMA, M1 macrophages, M2 macrophages, Mouse macrophages

1 Introduction

Since the 1970s, transfusion medicine scientists have been searching for a non-invasive means to determine the potential clinical significance of auto- and alloantibodies [1]. In the early 1980s, investigators reported the first in vitro assays for quantifying phagocytosis of antibody-opsonized red blood cells (RBCs) and suggested these assays could be used to determine the potential for a clinically significant antibody [1–11]. One group named their assay the monocyte-macrophage assay (MMA) [3, 5]. Later, the acronym's meaning was changed to the "monocyte monolayer assay" [11], as the assay used monocytes as the source of phagocytes exclusively. In the years that followed, the MMA, with minor modifications [12–17], has been used to successfully predict outcomes of transfused donor blood in the face of recipient

Sean R. Stowell and Connie M. Arthur (eds.), *Methods in Transfusion Medicine*, Methods in Molecular Biology, vol. 3053, https://doi.org/10.1007/978-1-0716-5376-0_42,

alloantibodies [18–24]. Thus, the MMA has become a useful tool in transfusion medicine to aid in the selection of donor blood that would result in the least adverse events, e.g., hemolysis [25]. During this period, much has been learned when using an MMA to improve outcomes and provide successful predictions of the potential for hemolysis of a given antibody [1, 11, 12, 14, 15, 18, 21, 22, 24]. The MMA is not only a proven assay to predict auto- and alloantibody potential for clinical significance, but it has also become an in vitro assay for the evaluation of treatment strategies that inhibit phagocytosis and studies of Fc receptor usage [25–31].

Recently, we have used the basic approach of the monocyte monolayer assay to study phagocytosis using human and mouse macrophages. Because we now are using an assay that uses a macrophage cell line or macrophages that are derived from peripheral blood monocytes, we have begun to use a slightly different acronym to our original description of the MMA. To distinguish our monocyte-derived macrophage assay from the monocyte monolayer assay, we are using the acronym MOMA.

Using peripheral blood mononuclear cells (PBMCs) from different sources, we have previously shown that whole blood in acid-citrate-dextrose (ACD) kept at room temperature for up to 36–48 h is ideal for the MMA and is our preferred choice for performing an autologous MMA. We have now shown that buffy coats in citrate-phosphate-dextrose (CPD) anticoagulant can be used within 24 h of procurement but that the buffy coat left for one more day, 48 h after procurement, stored at room temperature provides the best conditions for the MMA having little background "junk" and platelet contamination, and still gives a phagocytic index similar to using the buffy coat PBMCs after 24 h (Fig. 1). This is our preferred source for PBMCs when doing an allogeneic MMA and M-MA assay. Indeed, we have now used PBMC-derived monocytes from 2-day-old buffy coats, cultured and polarized to inflammatory (M1) and anti-inflammatory (M2) macrophages, in a MOMA. We find that phagocytosis of antibody-opsonized RBCs is greater when using M2 compared to M1 macrophages (Fig. 2). We have preliminary evidence that this difference in phagocytosis between M1 and M2 is likely due to differences in Fc receptor expression between the two macrophages. We have found that the MMA can be performed using mouse PBMCs or a mouse macrophage cell line, RAW 264.7. Using mouse PBMCs from two different mouse strains gives minimal phagocytosis using antibodies to mouse RBC antigens such as TER-119, band 3, or KEL (Fig. 3). Using RAW 264.7 macrophages results in a higher phagocytic index. We would recommend that when trying to inhibit phagocytosis by mouse monocyte-macrophages, the sheep RBC/anti-sheep RBC system be used with RAW 264.7 macrophages, as phagocytosis is more robust than when using antibodies to mouse RBC antigens (Fig. 3).

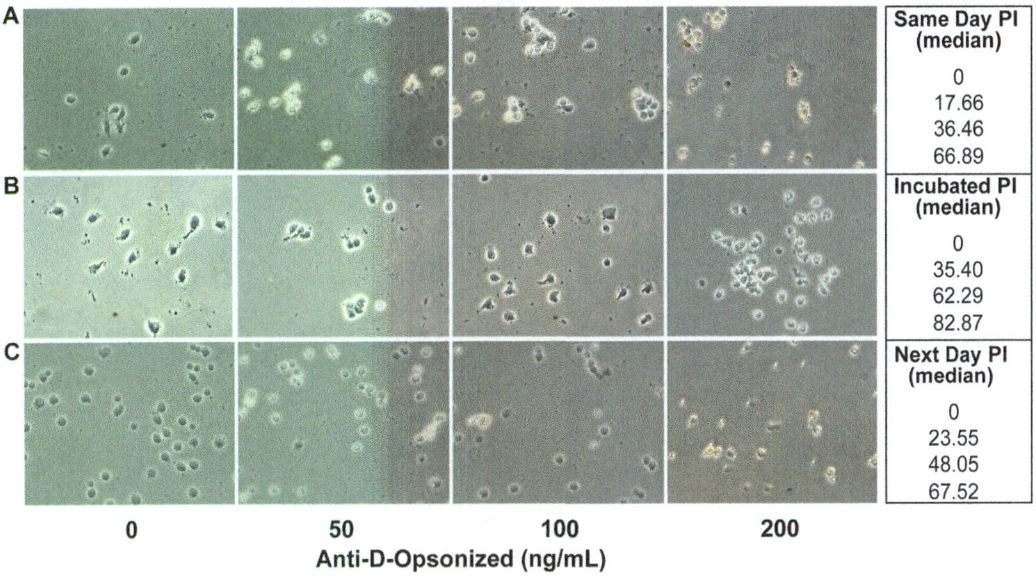

Fig. 1 Monocyte assay(MMA) showing monocyte phagocytosis using buffy coat PBMCs and different amounts of anti-D to opsonize RBCs, performed at different time points post collection of PBMCs from buffy coats. Photos and phagocytic indices (PI) were obtained using peripheral blood mononuclear cell-derived monocytes from the same buffy coat. (**a**) PBMCs from 24 hr. old buffy coat. (**b**) PBMCs from 24 h. old buffy coat that had been incubated overnight in chamber slides, and (**c**) PBMCs tested after 48 h of storage of the buffy coat. Results show the concentrations of anti-D (WinRho) used for the phagocytosis—left to right, 0, 50, 100, 200 ng/mL—used to opsonize the R2R2 RBCs. *Notes*: Optimal is storage of buffy coat for 48 h at room temperature, as it results in a clearer background with less platelet contamination

Other investigators continue to look for approaches to maximize the use of the MMA and to make it more user-friendly. Some are beginning to use the human macrophage cell line THP-1 [32, 33]. Some have utilized a flow-based approach with RBC dyes and THP-1 cells [32, 34, 35]. The methods for doing in vitro phagocytosis assays with peripheral blood-derived monocytes, human cultured macrophages, and macrophage cell lines is an important development for the study of auto- and alloantibody-mediated phagocytosis, use of Fcγ receptors, and potential for clinical significance of these antibodies in immune cytopenias, including immune thrombocytopenia (ITP) and allo- and autoimmune hemolytic anemias. Indeed, the MMA and MOMA are powerful in vitro tools to study phagocytosis, not just for Fcγ receptor-mediated phagocytosis but for other mechanisms of phagocytosis, e.g., mannose receptor-mediated, phosphatidylserine (PS)-mediated, and the role of the "don't eat me" signal provided by CD47 on RBCs. Herein, we describe, in detail, current in vitro phagocytosis assay methods developed in our laboratory. We also briefly describe future potential methods and improvements that may come to fruition and replace or enhance these assays.

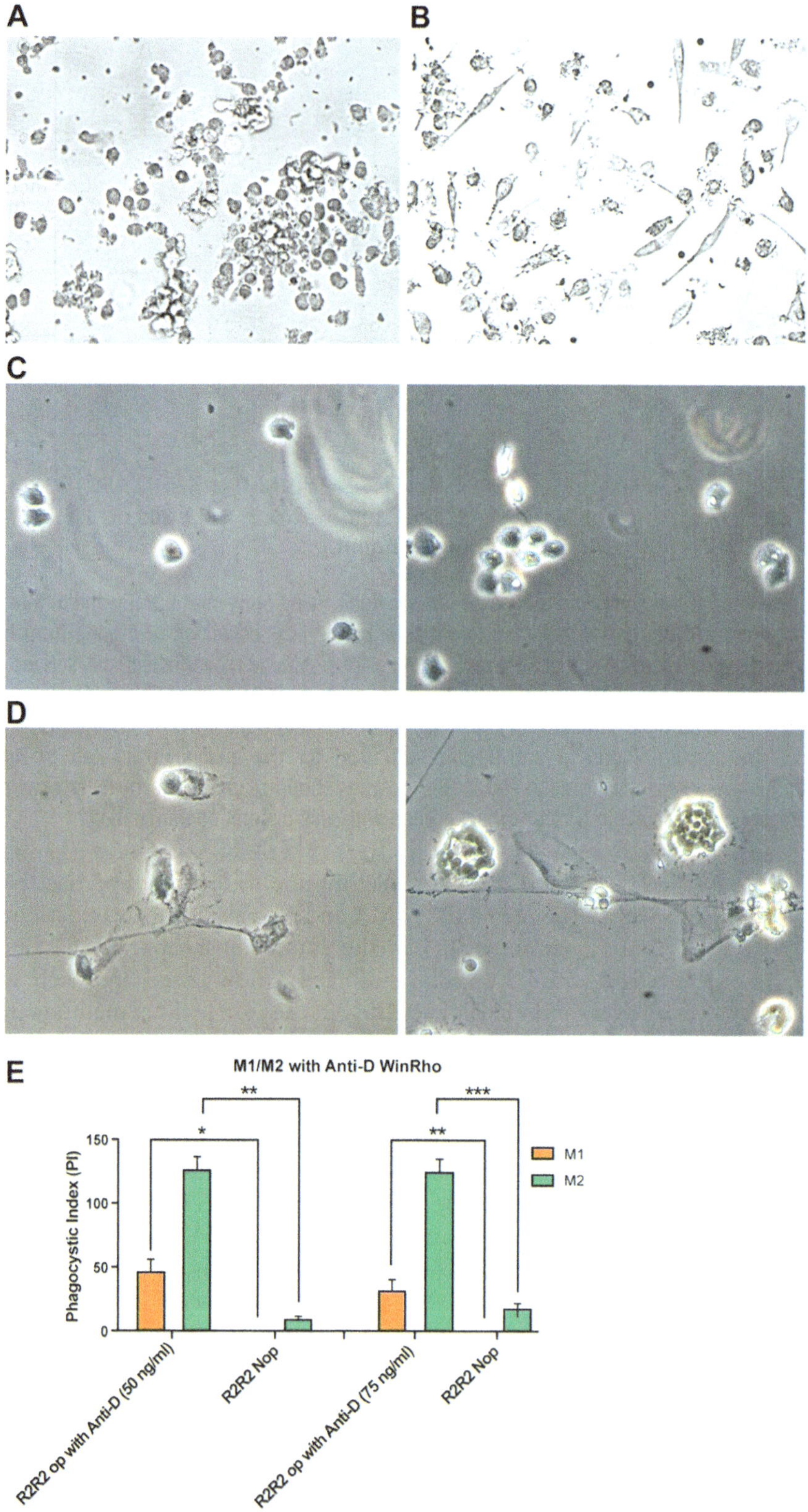

Fig. 2 Monocyte-macrophage assay (MOMA) using monocytes cultured to M1 or M2 macrophages. Images showing the differences in morphology of M1 vs. M2 macrophages. (**a**) Inflammatory M1 macrophages. (**b**)

2 Materials

2.1 Monocyte Monolayer Assay (MMA) Using Human Peripheral Blood Mononuclear Cells

1. Red blood cell storage/stabilization solution (e.g., ID-CellStab, Bio-Rad, 005650).
2. Fresh whole blood collected in acid-citrate-dextrose (ACD) tubes (BD 364606).
3. Fresh whole blood collected by venipuncture into a red-top for serum separation (no additive; BD 367820).
4. RPMI-1640 (e.g., Wisent, 350-000-CL), supplemented with 10% heat-inactivated FBS,1 mM GlutaPlus, 10 mM HEPES, and 1% penicillin/streptomycin. Store at 4 °C.
5. Ficoll Paque Plus, density 1.077 g/L (Cytiva,17-1440-03).
6. D-PBS, pH 7.4, without Ca2+/Mg2+ (Wisent Bioproducts, 311-425-CL).
7. cell strainer, 70 μm nylon (Falcon, 352350).
8. ACK lysis buffer (155 mM NH_4Cl, 0.1 mM EDTA, and 10 mM $KHCO_3$). Store at 4 °C.
9. Trypan Blue, 0.4% solution (Thermo Fisher Scientific, 15250061).
10. Manual cell counter (hemocytometer).
11. Chamber Slides (Lab-Tek II, 8-well, RS Glass Nunc 154534).
12. Coverslips (24 × 50 mm, #1 thickness; VWR, 48393-081).
13. Rh(D) positive R2R2 Red Blood Cells (RBCs) (Blood Collection Center, Canadian Blood Services; also, commercially available).
14. Anti-Rh(D): Commercial source of Rh immune globulin (e.g., WinRho. SDF CDN, Saol Therapeutics, 1003092).
15. Methanol.
16. Anti-Human Globulin (NOVACLONE, Immucor).
17. Elvanol mounting medium (made in-house; 15% (w/v) polyvinyl resin, 30% (v/v) glycerol in Dulbecco's PBS (D-PBS).
18. Light microscope capable of phase contrast microscopy.

Fig. 2 (continued) Anti-inflammatory M2 macrophages. Using 24-h buffy coat PBMCs. (**c**, **d**) Comparing results of phagocytosis of anti-D opsonized RBCs with M1 versus M2 macrophages. Using 48-hr buffy coat (*see* **Note 1**) (**c**) M1 macrophages with no opsonized RBCs (left side) and anti-D-opsonized RBCs (right side). (**d**) M2 macrophages with no opsonized RBCs (left side) and anti-D-opsonized RBCs (right side). (**e**) Graph showing comparison of M1 versus M2 phagocytosis of anti-D-opsonized RBCs. P values generated using Student's t-test: * < 0.05, ** < 0.01, ***,0.001. *Notes*: M1 and M2 macrophages have distinct morphology, with M1 being rounded while M2 have pseudopodia extensions, appearing more like fibroblasts. M2 macrophages have more robust phagocytic ability than do M1 macrophages

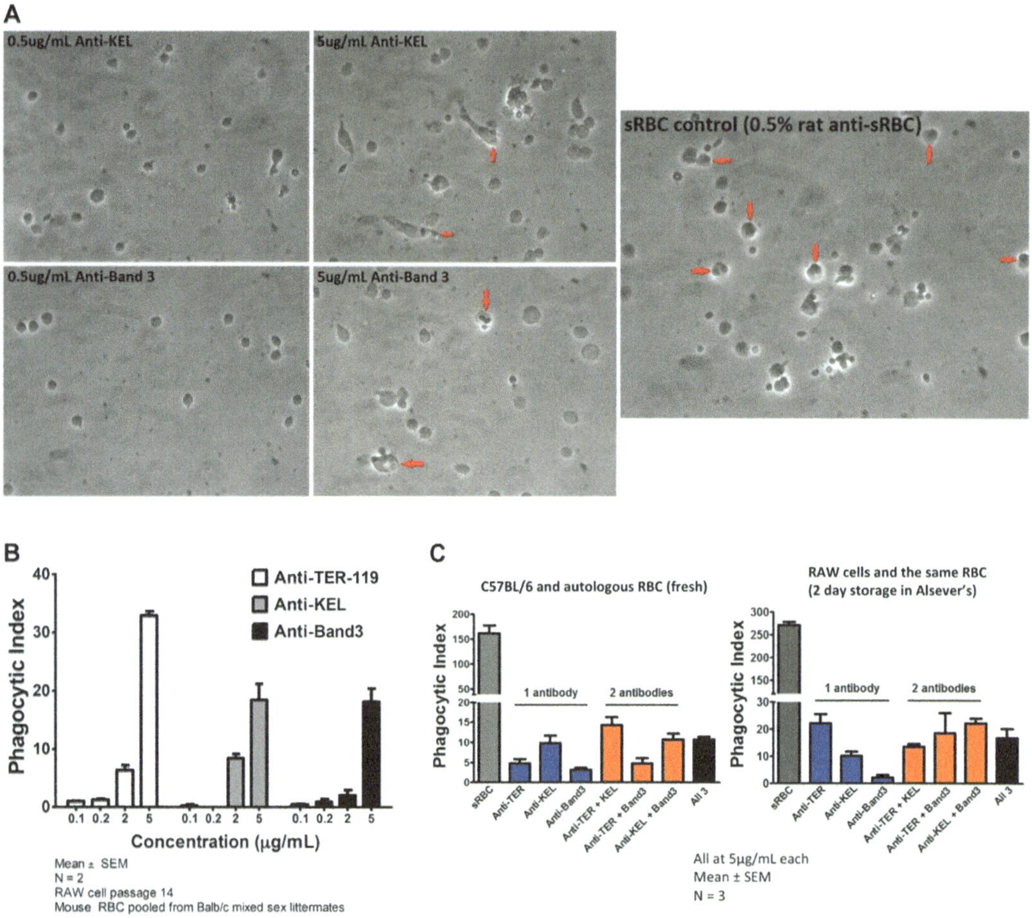

Fig. 3 Results of monocyte-macrophage assay using mouse PBMCs or RAW264.7 macrophage cell line. (**a**) BALB/c mouse PBMCs used to examine phagocytosis of autologous BALB/c RBCs with antibodies to mouse band-3 (34-3C) and mouse KEL (MIMA-8). Images are compared to phagocytosis when using sheep RBCs opsonized with anti-sheep RBCs (far right image). Red arrows indicate phagocytosed RBCs. (**b**) Bar graph summarizing phagocytosis when using RAW 264.7 and BALB/c RBCs opsonized with glycophorin-associated antigen (anti-TER-119), anti-band 3, or anti-KEL. (**c**) Bar graph showing phagocytosis using C57BL/6 mouse PBMCs and autologous RBCs opsonized with anti-TER-119, anti-band 3, or anti-KEL (left side), compared to RAW 264.7 phagocytosis (right side). *Notes*: RAW 264.7 macrophages give similar but slightly more robust and reproducible results. We routinely use 264.7 macrophages when testing mouse in vitro phagocytosis

2.2 MOnocyte-Macrophage Assay (MOMA) Using M1/M2 Macrophages

1. Poly-D-lysine, 0.1 mg/mL in water. Medstore, Cat # P6407.
2. Fresh whole blood collected in acid-citrate-dextrose (ACD) tubes (yellow-top tubes) or a buffy coat.
3. RPMI-1640 (Wisent, 350-000-CL), supplemented with 10% heat-inactivated FBS,1 mM GlutaMAX supplement, 1 mM HEPES, and 1% penicillin/streptomycin.

4. Monocyte isolation kit STEM-cells EasySep™ Human Monocyte Enrichment Kit without CD16 Depletion (STEMCELL Technologies, Cat # 19058).
5. Isolation medium: PBS Ca^{2+} and Mg^{2+} free + FBS 2% + 1 mM EDTA.
6. Human recombinant GM-CSF. STEMCELL Technologies. Cat # 78015.1.
7. Human recombinant M-CSF. STEMCELL Technologies. Cat # 78057.1.
8. Human recombinant IFN-gamma. STEMCELL Technologies. Cat # 78020.
9. LPS. Sigma Aldrich. Cat # L3024-5MG.
10. Human recombinant IL-4. STEMCELL technologies. Cat # 78045.1.
11. Accutase™. Cell detachment solution. STEMCELL Technologies. Cat #07920.
12. Cell scraper. Medstore. Cat # 83.3950.

2.3 MMA Using Monocytes Derived from Mouse PBMCs

1. Anticoagulant: ACD (acid-citrate-dextrose) (BD, cat. 364606).
2. Density gradient: Ficoll Paque Plus (GE Healthcare, cat. 17-1440-03).
3. Media: RPMI 1640 with 10% heat-inactivated FBS, 20 mM HEPES, and 0.01 mg/mL gentamicin.
4. 8-well chamber slides: LabTek, cat. no. 154534.
5. Phagocytes: Mouse PBMC from whole blood.
6. Red blood cells: 10% sheep RBC (sRBCs, MP Cat. 55876, available through Cedarlane).
7. Opsonizing antibody: rabbit IgG fraction to sRBC (MP Cat. 55806, available through Cedarlane).
8. Phagocytosis inhibition control (optional): 200 μg/mL mouse IgG (Sigma, Cat. 15381).
9. Run experiments with technical triplicates.

2.4 MOMA Using the Mouse RAW 264.7 Macrophage Cell Line

1. Media: RPMI 1640 with 10% heat-inactivated FBS, 20 mM HEPES, and 0.01 mg/mL gentamicin.
2. 8-well chamber slides: LabTek, cat. no. 154534.
3. Phagocytes: RAW 264.7 (American Type Culture Collection, ATCC) (80% confluency) (*see* **Note 1**).
4. Red blood cells: 10% sheep RBC (sRBCs, MP Cat. 55876, available through Cedarlane) (*see* **Note 2**).
5. Opsonizing antibody: rabbit IgG fraction to sRBC (MP Cat. 55806, available through Cedarlane) (*see* **Note 2**).

6. Phagocytosis inhibition control (optional): 200 μg/mL mouse IgG (from serum) (Sigma, Cat. 15381).
7. Run an experiment with technical triplicates.

3 Methods

3.1 Monocyte Monolayer Assay (MMA) Using Human Peripheral Blood Mononuclear Cells

3.1.1 Isolation of PBMCs

1. Obtain human whole blood from a donor or a patient in ACD tubes. Store the blood at room temperature (18–22 °C) for up to 36 h (*see* **Note 3**).
2. Transfer the whole blood ACD tubes to 50 mL Falcon tubes (approximately one 50 mL Falcon tube for every two ACD tubes). Add room temperature RPMI-1640 complete medium to the blood for a final volume of 35 mL.
3. Add 15 mL room temperature Ficoll Paque Plus to a new 50-mL Falcon tube.
4. Carefully layer the diluted whole blood on top of the Ficoll Paque Plus density gradient, minimizing mixing at the interface for optimal separation of blood (*see* **Note 4**).
5. Centrifuge the layered mixture at 700× *g* for 30 min with brakes OFF.
6. The density gradient centrifugation will separate the mixture into (from top to bottom: plasma, buffy coat [containing PBMCs], density gradient material (Ficoll Paque Plus), granulocytes, and red blood cells).
7. Aspirate and discard most of the top layer, which is plasma, and carefully retrieve the buffy coat (PBMCs) layer, avoiding bringing any additional material (*see* **Note 5**).
8. Transfer the retrieved PBMCs into a new 50-mL tube.
9. Wash the isolated buffy coat layer one time with pH 7.4 PBS solution for 10 min at 350× *g* with full brake ON inbetween washes.
10. Use a 70 uM cell strainer to eliminate any debris or unwanted material from the PBMCs into a 15-mL conical tube.
11. Wash twice with pH 7.4 PBS solution for 10 min at 350x g with full brake ON.
12. Lyse any RBCs carried over with ACK lysis buffer. Add 5–10 mL ACK lysis buffer, depending on pellet size, and incubate at room temperature for up to 3 min.
13. After incubation, top up with pH 7.4 PBS and centrifuge for 10 min at 350× *g* with full brake ON (*see* **Note 6**).
14. **Optional step.* Wash one more time. Perform this step if the number of RBCs is too high. Additional use of ACK lysis buffer should be avoided, if possible, as sometimes it may interfere with the reading of the assay (*see* **Notes 6** and 7).

15. Reconstitute PBMC pellet in 2–3 mL (use 0.5 mL per initial ACD tube) RPMI-1640 complete medium.
16. Count PBMCs using a hemocytometer in a 1:1 staining ratio with trypan blue by only counting the cells not stained with trypan blue. Reconstitute PBMCs to 2×10^6 cells/mL in RPMI-1640 complete medium (*see* **Note 8**).
17. Seed 400 μL (800,000 cells) using a micropipette into each well of the 8-well chamber slide and incubate at 37 °C, 5% CO_2 for at least 1.5 h in a humidified tissue culture incubator.

3.1.2 Pre-treatment of Adhered Monocytes (Only Needed If Trying to Test Inhibition or Enhancing Phagocytosis Properties of a Drug or Compound)

1. Reconstitute the test material in RPMI-1640 complete medium to the desired concentration.
2. Aspirate any non-adhered PBMCs from the wells using a micropipette and discard. Wash once with pH 7.4 PBS.
3. Add 400 μL of test material and incubate at 37 °C, 5% CO_2 for 1 h (*see* **Note 9**).

3.1.3 Opsonization of Testing Samples and Rh (D) + R2R2 Red Blood Cells

Rh(D) + R2R2 RBCs are used as a positive control for FcγR-mediated phagocytosis. R2R2 RBCs can be centrifuged at 870× *g* for 15 min with brakes ON and reconstituted in ID-CellStab (RBC storage/stabilization solution) and stored at 4 °C for up to a month (*see* **Note 10**).

1. Wash R2R2 RBCs in pH 7.4 PBS three times by centrifuging at 350× *g* for 5 min each time.
2. Opsonize the testing sample (e.g., patient or donor) RBCs using serum or plasma (*see* **Note 11**). A 5% RBC suspension for opsonization is recommended (e.g., 15 μL of packed RBCs in 300 μL antibody mixture). Also, opsonize the R2R2 RBCs with anti-Rh(D) 100 ng/mL.
3. Incubate at 37 °C, 5% CO_2 for 1 h. Intermittent reconstitution by mixing is recommended as RBCs settle at the bottom (e.g., vortex every 15 min).
4. Wash opsonized RBCs with pH 7.4 PBS three times by centrifugation at 350× *g* for 5 min each time (*see* **Note 12**).
5. To check if RBCs are opsonized successfully, perform an indirect antiglobulin test (IAT) by adding a secondary opsonizing anti-human antibody (anti-human globulin) to the primary opsonizing antibody (anti-Rh(D)) on the RBC surfaces. Hemagglutination or clumping of RBCs can be observed and interpreted as a successful opsonization.
6. Reconstitute washed opsonized R2R2 RBCs to 1.25% (v/v) using RPMI-1640 complete medium, for example, 1200 μL medium to 15 μL RBCs to achieve 1.25% (v/v) per well.

3.1.4 Fc Receptor-Mediated Phagocytosis

1. Aspirate pre-treatment test material (if added) or non-adhered cells (if not added) and discard, following the gentle aspiration and adding technique (*see* **Note 13**).
2. Gently wash wells one time with pH 7.4 PBS.
3. Add 400 μL of the appropriate 1.25% (v/v) opsonized RBCs mixture to each well of the triplicate.
4. Incubate at 37 °C, 5% CO_2 for 2 h. undisturbed.
5. After incubation, prepare two beakers with 100 mL pH 7.4 PBS in each one.
6. Remove the 8-well chambers using the manufacturer's adaptors. Dab off excess fluid on a paper towel while keeping slides moist.
7. Submerge the slide into the beaker containing 100 mL pH 7.4 PBS and gently wash it by moving it back and forth slowly (20–30 strokes) to remove any remaining non-phagocytosed RBCs.
8. Then submerge the slide in the second beaker and wash slowly for 20–30 strokes more.
9. Remove the slide from PBS and dab off the excess by touching the slide edge onto a paper towel. Air dry (*see* **Note 14**).
10. Fix by submerging in 100% methanol for 45 s, then air dry.
11. Mount the slide using an in-house made elvanol mounting medium and add coverslips (24 × 75 mm).
12. Allow it to dry overnight before quantification.

3.1.5 Quantification of Phagocytosis (Same for all the MMAs Described)

1. Using a phase contrast microscope and 40X objective lens, quantify phagocytosis using a manual cell counter (*see* **Note 15**).
2. Have two manual cell counters, one in each hand, to count phagocytosed RBCs in one and the total number of monocytes in the other (at least 300 monocytes should be counted per well).
3. Calculate the average phagocytic index (PI) per test (across technical triplicates) by dividing the number of phagocytosed RBCs by the number of total monocytes counted and multiplying by 100:

$$\frac{\text{Number of phagocytosed RBCs}}{\text{Number of total monocytes counted}} \times 100$$

4. Express the data as mean PI ± standard deviation (SD).

3.2 Monocyte-Macrophage Assay (MOMA) Using M1/M2 Macrophages

3.2.1 Day 0—Seeding of Monocytes

1. Prepare a 25 mL flask for each macrophage population. Add 5 mL poly-D-lysine to each and leave it in the hood for at least 1 h. (*see* **Note 16**).
2. Isolate PBMCs from buffy coat or patient samples, as usual (See Subheading 3.1.1).
3. After a pellet of PBMCs was generated, resuspend it in 10 mL of pre-warmed RPMI-1640 complete medium.
4. Determine the cell number and begin the monocyte isolation with the monocyte isolation kit. You will need at least 50×10^6 cells to run the kit (*see* **Note 17).**
5. Resuspend the cells at 50×10^6 cells/mL in isolation medium (*see* **Note 18**).
6. According to the cell number obtained, you should use the purple (0.25–2 mL) or gray (0.5–8.5 mL) magnet recommended in the STEM-cells kit.
7. Follow the kit instructions. Add the sample to the required propylene tube (5 mL or 14 mL).
8. Add enrichment cocktail to the sample (50 μL/mL of sample).
9. Mix and incubate at 2–8 °C for 10 min in an ice bucket.
10. Meanwhile, vortex magnetic particles for 30 s.
11. Add magnetic particles to the sample: 100 μL/mL of sample.
12. Mix and incubate at 2–8 °C for 5 min.
13. Top-up with isolation medium to 2.5 mL or 10 mL, accordingly.
14. Mix by pipetting up and down 2–3 times.
15. Place the tube (without lid) into the magnet and incubate at room temperature for 2.5 min.
16. Pick up the magnet and, in one continuous movement, invert the magnet and tube, pouring the cell suspension into a new tube, 5 mL or 14 mL.
17. Resuspend cells in RPMI-1640 medium and count them. Do this step as soon as possible.
18. Seed 1×10^6 monocytes into each flask previously coated with poly-D-lysine. Wash off residual poly-D-lysine with washing buffer or media. Bring to 5 mL final volume with RPMI-1640 if necessary (*see* **Note 18**).
19. Incubate at 37 °C, 5% CO_2, for at least 2 h.
20. Meanwhile, prepare M1 and M2 differentiation media. Prepare enough for day 0 (10 mL) and day 4 (2 mL) top-up.
    - M1 differentiation medium: RPMI-1640 + 2.5 ng/mL GM-CSF.
    - M2 differentiation medium: RPMI-1640 + 50 ng/mL M-CSF.

21. After the incubation time, wash each flask once with PBS and twice with complete RPMI-1640.
22. Add 10 mL of differentiation medium to each flask according to the cell type you want to differentiate.
23. Let cells differentiate for 6 days in the incubator at 37 °C, 5% CO_2. You will need to top up with differentiation medium on day 4, due to evaporation.

3.2.2 Day 4—Top-Up

1. Add 2 mL of each differentiation medium to the respective flask. Add medium directly to the flask (*see* **Note 19**).

3.2.3 Day 6—Macrophage Polarization

By day 6, monocytes are differentiated into macrophages, but they are not polarized yet to M1 or M2 cells; we will need to add additional cytokines for it.

1. Prepare M1 and M2 polarization media.
   - M1 polarization media: Prepare 5 mL of M1 polarization medium to add to the corresponding flask. The final concentrations should be as follows: 50 ng/mL IFN-gamma, 10 ng/mL LPS, and 2.5 ng/mL GM-CSF in RPMI-1640. *Note the flask at the end will have 15 mL of total volume (10 mL already in + 5 mL you are going to add), do the calculations accordingly.*
   - M2 polarization media: Prepare 5 mL of M2 polarization medium to add to the corresponding flask. The final concentrations should be as follows: 20 ng/mL IL-4 and 50 ng/mL M-CSF in RPMI-1640. *Note that the flask at the end will have 15 mL of total volume (10 mL already in + 5 mL you are going to add), do the calculations accordingly.*
2. Add 5 mL of M1 or M2 polarization medium to each flask.
3. Let the macrophages polarize for at least 2 days in the incubator at 37 °C, 5% CO_2 (*see* **Note 20**).

3.2.4 Day 8—Harvest and Flow Cytometry

1. Before you harvest the M1 or M2 macrophages, collect the supernatant into 1.5 mL tubes for further use (if needed).
2. Add 1 mL of Accutase to the flask and leave it in the incubator for 5 min.
3. To stop the reaction, add 3 mL of complete RPMI-1640.
4. Use a cell scraper to detach the cells from the bottom of the flask.
5. Watch the cells under the microscope and make sure there are no more cells attached to the bottom of the flask.
6. Collect the cells into a 15 mL tube.
7. Wash the cells in PBS 2 times.

8. Resuspend them in complete RPMI-1640 and count using the hemocytometer.
9. To analyze the quality and quantity of M1/M2 macrophages, you can run a flow cytometry assay (*see* **Notes 21** and **22**). Use 0.5×10^6 cells per tube and stain as follows:
   - M1: CD80+ CCR7+ CD206-.
   - M2: CD206+ CD209+ CD80-.

3.2.5 MOMA Using M1/M2 Macrophages

1. After obtaining the M1/M2 macrophages, count them using a hemocytometer in a 1:1 staining ratio with trypan blue.
2. Reconstitute M1/M2 to 1×10^6 cells/ mL in RPMI-1640 complete medium.
3. Seed 200 μL (200,000 cells) using a micropipette into each well of the 8-well chamber slide and incubate at 37 °C, 5% CO_2 for at least 1.5 h. in a fully humidified tissue culture incubator (*see* **Notes 23** and **24**).
4. Proceed with the next steps as a regular MMA (*see* Subheading 3.1.4) (*see* **Note 25**).

3.3 MMA Using Monocytes Derived from Mouse PBMCs

3.3.1 Blood Collection

1. Obtain ACD (acid-citrate-dextrose) from yellow cap collection tubes. Aliquot 200 μL into each 1.5 mL Eppendorf tube for blood collection (usually 1 Eppendorf per animal) and also 2x1mL Eppendorf containing ACD to pre-fill the syringes.
2. Perform cardiac puncture on animals using CO_2 as a method of euthanasia. Approximately 1 mL of blood is obtained per animal. Continue to mix the collected blood intermittently throughout the collection duration (*see* **Notes 25** and **26**).

3.3.2 PBMC Isolation

1. Transfer the blood from the Eppendorf tubes to a 50 mL Falcon tube using the P1000 pipette. Avoid transfer of blood clots if present (this would affect Ficoll isolation and lead to severe RBC contamination of the buffy coat).
2. Top volume up to 20 mL using RPMI media (e.g., dilution of the blood) and layer 10 mL of diluted blood over 3 mL Ficoll. Perform isolation in 2x15mL Falcon tube to use all the blood collected and maximize the PBMC yield.
3. Follow the general protocol for human PBMC isolation (*see* Subheading 3.1.1). In summary:
   (a) Spin at 700× *g* for 30 min (break OFF).
   (b) Discard plasma and collect the buffy coat layer (containing PBMC).
   (c) Wash 3 times using PBS.

4. Reconstitute cell concentration to 2,500,000 cells/mL, and seed 400 μL to obtain 1,000,000 cells/well (Can go as low as 800,000 cells/well if there are not enough cells).
5. Let PBMC adhere at 37 °C for 1-h and 30 min (*see* **Note 27**).

3.3.3 Opsonization

1. Depending on the size of the experiment, spin down 1-3 mL of the 10% RBCs (that's equivalent to 100–300 μL of an RBC pellet).
2. Wash 3x using PBS.
3. Opsonize using this ratio: 100 μL sRBC +300 μL PBS + 0.5% rabbit anti-sRBC (2 μL).
4. Incubate the sRBC at 37 °C for 1-h, invert to mix every 15 min.
5. After incubation, wash 3x using PBS.
6. Make 1.25% sRBC solution using RPMI media.
7. Add 400 μL of sRBC solution to each well and allow phagocytosis to occur at 37 °C for 2 h.

3.3.4 Fc Receptor-Mediated Phagocytosis

1. Follow the protocol in Subheading 3.1.4.

3.3.5 Quantification of Phagocytosis

1. See Subheading 3.1.5.

3.4 MOMA Using the Mouse RAW 264.7 Macrophage Cell Line

3.4.1 Macrophages

1. Warm media to 37 °C.
2. Check culture under microscope to ensure no contamination and check confluency (should be around 80%).
3. Remove media into 15 mL falcon tube, leave some media (~0.5 mL) in the plate.
4. Bend head of scraper to obtain a right angle (when still in sterile pouch). Scrap cells off plate. Discard scraper.
5. Collect cells into tube.
6. Centrifuge at 350× *g* for 10 min (setting 3).
7. Remove supernatant and resuspend pellet with 3-5 mL RPMI.
8. Count cells using hemocytometer: 50 μL trypan blue +40 μL PBS + 10 μL cells = 100 μL total (*cell counts* × *10* × *2500* = *cells/mL*).
9. Dilute cells to *125,000 cells/mL* (so that you have 50,000 cells/400 μL in each chamber).
10. Add 400 μL of macrophages into each chamber.
11. Incubate for at least 2 h for cell adherence.

3.4.2 Opsonization (Start at ~40 Minutes Post Macrophage Adherence)

1. Depending on the size of the experiment, spin down 1–3 mL of the 10% sheep RBC (that's equivalent to 100–300uL of sRBC pellet). 0.15% of opsonized sheep RBC needed for phagocytosis, so reverse-calculate how much sRBC you need.
2. Wash 3x using PBS.
3. Opsonize using this ratio: 100 μL sRBC +300 μL PBS + 0.5% rabbit anti-sRBC (2 μL).
4. Incubate the sRBC at 37 °C for 1-h, invert to mix every 15 min. *very important!!*.
5. After incubation, wash 3x using PBS.
6. Make 0.15% sRBC solution using RPMI media.
7. For example, for 3 full slides:
8. 3 slides × 8 wells × 400 μL/well × 1.1 (10% overestimation) = 10.56 mL total volume.
9. 10.56 mL × 0.15% = 0.0158 mL = 15.8 μL of sRBC pellet.
10. Add 400 μL of sRBC solution to each well and allow phagocytosis to occur at 37 °C for 30 min.

3.4.3 Methanol Fixing

1. After 30 min of phagocytosis, remove the chambers from the slide and dab away excess fluids.
2. Wash the slide by submerging it vertically into a 100 mL beaker containing PBS, and wash the slides by slowly moving the slide back and forth 30 times. Dab away excess PBS and allow to air dry.
3. Once the slide has completely dried (around 5 min), fix the slide by submerging into 100% methanol for 45 s.
4. Mount the slides using mountant and cover slips (*see* **Note 28**) Allow the mountant to dry overnight before counting slides.

3.4.4 Quantification

1. Phase contrast microscopy using a 40x objective lens. Manually quantify 300 phagocytes and the amount of phagocytosed sRBC. This can then be expressed as the phagocytic index (phagocytosed sRBC/phagocytes × 100), and with technical triplicates, data can be expressed as mean ± SEM.

3.5 Other Variations on the MMA

3.5.1 Use of Monocyte-Macrophage Cell Lines

The human monocyte cell line, THP-1, has been used extensively for phagocytosis assays [32–34]. This non-adherent cell line is usually differentiated to adherent macrophages by treatment with phorbol ester (PMA) prior to the phagocytosis assay [32]. Fcγ receptor IIIa is not usually expressed until the THP-1 cells are treated with PMA. Following PMA treatment, the full complement of Fcγ receptors is expressed on these cells [32]. However, to ensure expression of FcγRIIIa, THP-1 cells have been transfected to overexpress this receptor for use in phagocytosis assays [34]. The mouse macrophage cell line RAW264.7 has also been used by investigators to study erythrophagocytosis [31] (see Fig. 3 and Subheading 3.4).

3.6 Use of Flow Cytometry

Flow cytometry has been used to study antibody-opsonized RBC interaction with monocyte-macrophages [33, 35–37].

3.7 Use of Fluorescent-Labeled RBCs

Several studies have used fluorescently labeled RBCs in phagocytosis assays [33, 37], adapted for high throughput, such as plate reader-based assays or analysis of large numbers of monocyte/macrophages, such as flow cytometry [33]. The red fluorescent dye PKH26, which non-covalently but stably associates with the red cell membrane, is well-validated for such studies [33, 37]. One publication has reported success using PKH26 labeled RBCs and PMA-treated THP-1 cells to investigate the phagocytosis of RBCs opsonized with allo- or autoantibodies using flow cytometry [33]. A drawback of dye-labeling is that adherent vs phagocytosed red cells may not be distinguished readily; however, non-phagocytosed RBCs can be lysed to reveal only those fluorescent RBCs that have been partially or completely phagocytosed [34]. Use of the pH-sensitive pHrodo® dyes overcomes this limitation by only fluorescing under the acidic pH environment of the phagosome/lysosome compartment, so they can distinguish intracellular, phagocytosed RBC [38].

4 Notes

1. Passage RAW 264.7 cells every 4 days (1/15 split) in RPMI +10% FBS + 20 mM HEPES. 80% confluent 10 cm culture dish yields approximately 9×10^6 cells total.
2. Although antibodies specific to mouse RBC antigens, such as band 3, KEL or TER-119, or others can be used instead of the sheep RBC/anti-sheep RBC approach, more reproducible phagocytosis can be obtained using the sheep RBC system.
3. A minimum of 2 tubes, collected into acid-citrate-dextrose (ACD) anticoagulant, should be obtained to perform an autologous MMA, and these can be stored at room temperature overnight prior to the assay [13]. For an allogeneic MMA, buffy coat, collected into citrate-phosphate-dextrose (CPD), can be used if stored at RT no longer than 48 hrs after procurement. Buffy coats used after 48 h of RT storage give cleaner backgrounds with less platelet contamination. The expected amount of PBMCs that can be obtained from whole blood is approximately $1 \text{x} 10^6$ per mL of whole blood. It is important to take into consideration the number of controls and/or tests you intend to run to know how much whole

blood will be required. Alternatively, buffy coat PBMCs can be collected from multiple donors, pooled, and aliquots frozen for future allogeneic MMAs [17]. The optimal number of PBMCs to seed in every well is 800, 000 cells.

4. The 50-mL Falcon tube can be tilted at a 45° angle, and blood: RPMI mixture can be added dropwise by placing the pipette tip close to the density gradient and enabling the blood mixture to run down the side of the tube very slowly.
5. *Using plastic or glass Pasteur pipettes with a suction bulb to aspirate the interface containing the PBMCs. Use a circular motion along the edge of the tube to obtain the majority of the PBMCs without contamination with Ficoll, plasma, or low-density RBCs.*
6. Avoid using ACK lysis buffer since it makes the cells "sticky" and they tend to clog.
7. You may need to wash more than three times if hemolysis or red supernatant is observed.
8. *Cultured monocytes*: PBMCs from whole blood or buffy coat can be cultured for 7 or more days without added growth factors and will differentiate into macrophages. These culture-derived, or spontaneously differentiated macrophages, can be harvested using the protocol for M1/M2 macrophages (Subheading 3.2) and used for phagocytosis assays. Macrophages generated in this way will be heterogeneous [34, 35, 38, 39]; therefore, if done, one should first purify the monocytes using positive or negative selection.
9. Each treatment or test should be performed in technical triplicate, so it is recommended that three wells at a time be used when aspirating and adding solutions to avoid drying the wells.
10. Although R2R2 RBCs opsonized with a commercial anti-D such as WinRho provide a control with the highest expression of the D-antigen, any Rh-positive RBC could be substituted as long as the phagocytic index is moderately to strongly positive.
11. One can use plasma instead of serum, but we prefer to use freshly obtained serum, within one day, or that has been frozen and thawed on the day of testing. When using serum that is freshly taken and used within a couple of days, complement proteins would still be present to ascertain the optimal chance of seeing a positive result if the antibody can activate complement to enhance the phagocytosis.
12. Always wash an excess number of RBCs because they can be lost during the washes while aspirating the supernatant. The number of RBCs to be used is typically 1.25% per well. If, for example, the treatments are being done in triplicate with four treatments and one control, that would make a total of five

tests and fifteen wells (three wells per test). That would mean a total of 75 μL of RBCs is needed for opsonization. In that case, 150 μL of RBCs can be washed to account for any losses during the wash steps.

13. *When aspirating* or adding solutions to the chamber slides, be gentle so the tip of the pipette only touches a corner of the wells and does not disturb the weakly adhered cells.
14. Never touch the front of the slide with the paper towel or any other surface when dabbing the excess, it can result in monocytes being lost.
15. Although we use phase contrast microscopy to quantify the phagocytic indices, hematological stains can also be used with or without oil immersion.
16. Although you can use total PBMCs for this assay, we recommend using isolated monocytes for better results.
17. The minimum number of PBMCs you need to use the STEM-cells monocytes isolation kit is 50×10^6 cells. Take into consideration that you should obtain about 10% of monocytes from the original amount of PBMCs.
18. When finalizing the monocyte isolation step, resuspend the cells in RPMI-1640 as soon as possible, since EDTA contained in the isolation medium can be toxic to the cells over time.
19. The top-up step is necessary due to evaporation occurring in the incubator. Do not exchange the media because the cytokines secreted by the cells are important for their differentiation; just add the medium to the flask.
20. After the 2-day polarization, the M1/ M2 macrophages can be used for experimentation or kept in culture for up to 1 week.
21. You can distinguish M1 from M2 macrophages based on morphology (Fig. 2); however, it is important to confirm by flow cytometry for specific CD antigen expression.
22. The flow cytometry step is required just when you are setting up the procedure. Once you have confirmed you are getting M1 and M2 macrophages, you can omit this step. You should obtain around 90% of M1 (CD80+ CCR7+ CD206-) and above 85% of M2 (CD206+ CD209+ CD80-).
23. The seeding number of M1/M2 can be lowered by as many as 100, 000 cells per well if necessary.
24. We prefer doing the M1/M2 assays by culturing purified monocytes in T25 flasks. However, monocytes can be directly cultured and polarized in chamber slides by the following: Seed cells at 5×10^5 cells/mL and 400 μL/well in RPMI-1640 complete medium with a final cell number of 200,000 cells/well of 8-well chamber slides (Nunc Lab-Tek). After

plating and incubating at 37 °C, 5% CO_2, for at least 1 h, wash wells with PBS 1 time and followed by 2 times media wash. Follow the protocol outlined in Subheading 3.2.1 to prepare M1 and M2 differentiation media. Add 400 μL of either medium to each well, and let cells differentiate for 5 days. During the 5-day differentiation period, top-up the well with 100 μL of M1 or M2 differentiation media to account for evaporation on day 3 or day 4. Follow the protocol outlined in Subheading 3.2.3 to prepare M1 and M2 polarization media. For M1, add 200 μL of M1 polarization media to each well, with the final concentration 50 ng/mL IFN-gamma (STEMCELL Technologies), 10 ng/mL LPS (Sigma), and 2.5 ng/mL GM-CSF (STEMCELL Technologies) in RPMI-1640 complete. For M2, add 200 μL of M2 polarization media to each well, with the final concentration 20 ng/mL IL-4 (STEMCELL Technologies) and 50 ng/mL M-CSF (STEMCELL Technologies) in RPMI-1640 complete. After the 2-day polarization, the M1- or M2- macrophages can be used for experimentation or alternatively kept in culture (for up to 1 week).

25. Instead of primary blood-derived PBMCs, mouse peritoneal macrophages or bone marrow-derived macrophages could be used; however, PBMCs provide an easier approach for the MMA using primary mouse cells.

26. Depending on the age/size/strain of animals and how successful cardiac puncture is, the PBMC yield is around 3–5 × 10^6 per animal.

27. In the current protocol, PBMC-derived monocytes or differentiated macrophages are adhered directly to glass chamber slides prior to the MMA. Plastic and some types of glass may require coating, e.g., with cationic poly-lysine to promote attachment of monocytes/macrophages to enhance phagocytosis. Some investigators routinely use poly-L-lysine in their MMAs [17]. In fact, using our own chamber slide method, we noted that pre-coating the glass with poly-L-lysine substantially increased phagocytosis of IgG-opsonized RBC compared to untreated glass [1], and supplemental data]. It should be noted that there are two enantiomers of poly-lysine, poly-D-lysine, and poly-L-lysine. The "D" enantiomer is less degraded by cellular proteases and is what we use in our macrophage assay (see Subheading 3.2).

28. We use an in-house-made elvanol mountant, but any mountant would work.

Acknowledgments

I would like to acknowledge the many people who have worked on the MMA in the "Branch Lab" over the years. Thanks to Angie Mison, Cathy A. Branch, Darinka Sakac, Dr. Gregory Rampersad, Alison Foo, Yulia Katsman, Drew Kruspe, Madeleine Bareau, Cecile Chagneau, Laura Gromolard, Emma Duclaut, Emeralda Burke-Murphy, Megan Blacquiere, Mairead Holton, Shima Nahidi, and Tatiana Lipman. A special acknowledgment goes to Dr. Michael T. Gallagher who, with Dr. Donald R. Branch, developed the initial MMA in 1980 at the City of Hope National Medical Center, Duarte, California.

Conflict of Interest Statement The authors have no conflicts of interest to declare that are relevant to the content of this chapter.

References

1. Tong TN, Cen S, Branch DR (2019) The monocyte monolayer assay: past, present and future. Transfus Med Rev. 33(1):24–28. Epub 20180808. https://doi.org/10.1016/j.tmrv.2018.07.004
2. Branch DR, Gallagher MT, Mison AP, Sy Siok Hian AL, Petz LD (1984) In vitro determination of red cell alloantibody significance using an assay of monocyte-macrophage interaction with sensitized erythrocytes. Br J Haematol 56(1):19–29. https://doi.org/10.1111/j.1365-2141.1984.tb01268.x
3. Gallagher MT, Branch DR, Mison A, Petz LD (1983) Evaluation of reticuloendothelial function in autoimmune hemolytic anemia using an in vitro assay of monocyte-macrophage interaction with erythrocytes. Exp Hematol 11(1): 82–89
4. Branch DR, Gallagher MT (1985) Red blood cell mononuclear phagocyte assay. Vox Sang 48(5):323–324. https://doi.org/10.1111/j.1423-0410.1985.tb00191.x
5. Conley CL, Lippman SM, Ness PM, Petz LD, Branch DR, Gallagher MT (1982) Autoimmune hemolytic anemia with reticulocytopenia and erythroid marrow. N Engl J Med 306(5): 281–286. https://doi.org/10.1056/NEJM198202043060507
6. Alperin JB, Riglin H, Branch DR, Gallagher MT, Petz LD (1983) Anti-M causing delayed hemolytic transfusion reaction. Transfusion 23(4):322–324. https://doi.org/10.1046/j.1537-2995.1983.23483276867.x
7. Branch DR, Berkowitz LR, Becker RL, Robinson J, Martin M, Gallagher MT, Petz LD (1985) Extravascular hemolysis following the administration of cefamandole. Am J Hematol 18(2):213–219. https://doi.org/10.1002/ajh.2830180213
8. Branch DR, Gallahger MT (1986) Correlation of in vivo alloantibody significance or insignificance with an in vitro monocyte-macrophage phagocytosis assay. Br J Haematol 62(4): 783–785. https://doi.org/10.1111/j.1365-2141.1986.tb04106.x
9. Perez D, Cohen DW, Shulman IA, Branch DR (1986) Rhesus Du incompatibility in a newborn without hemolytic disease: a possible role for the mononuclear phagocyte system in the benign clinical course. Vox Sang 51(4): 341–343. https://doi.org/10.1111/j.1423-0410.1986.tb01983.x
10. Branch DR, Gallagher MT (1985) The importance of CO2 in short-term monocyte-macrophage assays. Transfusion 25(4):399–400. https://doi.org/10.1046/j.1537-2995.1985.25485273829.x
11. Nance SJ, Arndt P, Garratty G (1987) Predicting the clinical significance of red cell alloantibodies using a monocyte monolayer assay. Transfusion 27(6):449–452. https://doi.org/10.1046/j.1537-2995.1987.27688071692.x
12. Arndt PA, Garratty G (2004) A retrospective analysis of the value of monocyte monolayer assay results for predicting the clinical significance of blood group alloantibodies.

Transfusion 44(9):1273–1281. https://doi.org/10.1111/j.1537-2995.2004.03427.x

13. Tong TN, Burke-Murphy E, Sakac D, Pendergrast J, Cserti-Gazdewich C, Laroche V, Branch DR (2016) Optimal conditions for the performance of a monocyte monolayer assay. Transfusion 56(11): 2680–2690. Epub 20160821. https://doi.org/10.1111/trf.13766
14. Noumsi GT, Billingsley KL, Moulds JM (2015) Successful transfusion of antigen positive blood to alloimmunised patients using a monocyte monolayer assay. Transfus Med. 25(2):92–100. Epub 20150331. https://doi.org/10.1111/tme.12189
15. Karamatic Crew V, Poole J, Long S, Warke N, Colavecchia C, Burton N, Moulds M, Schlanser G, Wilson L, Noumsi G, Moulds JM, Moulds JJ, Daniels G (2008) Two MER2-negative individuals with the same novel CD151 mutation and evidence for clinical significance of anti-MER2. Transfusion 48(9):1912–1916. Epub 20080602. https://doi.org/10.1111/j.1537-2995.2008.01792.x
16. Tong TN, Branch DR (2017) Use of a monocyte monolayer assay to evaluate Fcgamma receptor-mediated phagocytosis. J Vis Exp. (119). https://doi.org/10.3791/55039. Epub 20170102. PubMed PMID: 28117787; PMCID: PMC5408648
17. Kipkeu BJ, Shyian ML, da Silveira CL, Duong TT, Yeung RSM, Binnington B, Branch DR, Acker JP, Holovati JL (2018) Evaluation of the functional properties of cryopreserved buffy coat-derived monocytes for monocyte monolayer assay. Transfusion 58(8):2027–2035. Epub 20180509. https://doi.org/10.1111/trf.14650
18. Michelis FV, Branch DR, Scovell I, Bloch E, Pendergrast J, Lipton JH, Cserti-Gazdewich CM (2014) Acute hemolysis after intravenous immunoglobulin amid host factors of ABO-mismatched bone marrow transplantation, inflammation, and activated mononuclear phagocytes. Transfusion. 54(3):681–690. Epub 20130705. https://doi.org/10.1111/trf.12329
19. Lemay AS, Tong TN, Branch DR, Huang M, Sumner C, Oldfield L, Hawes J, Cserti-Gazdewich CM, Lau W (2018) The first case of severe acute hemolytic transfusion reaction caused by anti-Sc2. Transfusion 58(11): 2506–2512. Epub 20181009. https://doi.org/10.1111/trf.14867
20. Tong TN, Blacquiere M, Sakac D, Burke-Murphy E, Yi Q, Callum J, Cserti-Gazdewich-C, Parmar N, Shehata N, Pavenski K, Lau W, Lin Y, Lieberman L, Branch DR, Pendergrast J (2020) The utility of a monocyte monolayer assay in the assessment of intravenous immunoglobulin-associated hemolysis. Transfusion. 60(12):3010–3018. Epub 20201022. https://doi.org/10.1111/trf.16131
21. Srivastava K, Albasri J, Alsuhaibani OM, Aljasem HA, Bueno MU, Antonacci T, Branch DR, Denomme GA, Flegel WA (2021) SCAR: The high-prevalence antigen 013.008 in the Scianna blood group system. Transfusion. 61(1):246–254. https://doi.org/10.1111/trf.16152. Epub 20201024. PubMed PMID: 33098316; PMCID: PMC9067365
22. Tong TN, Cserti-Gazdewich CM, Branch DR (2016) Value of MMA crossmatch? Transfus Med. 26(4):301–302. Epub 20160504. https://doi.org/10.1111/tme.12311
23. Branch DR, Sandhu G, Raos M (2021) Monocyte monolayer assay predictions of clinical outcome for serologically incompatible red blood cells is all about timing. Transfusion 61(8): 2516–2517. https://doi.org/10.1111/trf.16556
24. Branch DR, Holton MB, Ison T, Cote J, Dube C, Lau W (2021) Potentially clinically significant anti-Di(b) identified by monocyte monolayer assay before transfusion. Transfusion 61(1):331–332. https://doi.org/10.1111/trf.16114
25. Boligan KF, Sandhu G, Branch DR (2022) Methods to evaluate the potential clinical significance of antibodies to red blood cells. Curr Protoc 2(8):e504. https://doi.org/10.1002/cpz1.504
26. Cen SY, Holton MB, Binnington B, Denomme GA, Howie HL, Lebedev JN, Zimring JC, Branch DR (2020) IgG3 anti-Kell allotypic variation results in differential antigen binding and phagocytosis. Transfusion. 60(4): 688–693. Epub 20200113. https://doi.org/10.1111/trf.15663
27. Sandhu G, Lipman T, Bodnar M, Bienz MN, Branch DR (2023) Significant rosettes observed in monocyte monolayer assay due to complement-binding antibodies. Transfusion 63(7):1265–1266. Epub 20230428. https://doi.org/10.1111/trf.17384
28. Lipman T, Bienz MN, Pendergrast J, Cserti-Gazdewich C, Branch DR (2024) Unexpected difficulty in performance of a monocyte monolayer assay when using RBCs from a patient with sickle cell disease. Transfusion. 64(1): 4–5. Epub 20231116. https://doi.org/10.1111/trf.17605
29. Rampersad GC, Suck G, Sakac D, Fahim S, Foo A, Denomme GA, Langler RF, Branch DR (2005) Chemical compounds that target

thiol-disulfide groups on mononuclear phagocytes inhibit immune mediated phagocytosis of red blood cells. Transfusion 45(3):384–393. https://doi.org/10.1111/j.1537-2995.2005.04241.x

30. Li L, Noumsi GT, Kwok YY, Moulds JM, Scott MD (2015) Inhibition of phagocytic recognition of anti-D opsonized Rh D+ RBC by polymer-mediated immunocamouflage. Am J Hematol. 90(12):1165–1170. https://doi.org/10.1002/ajh.24211. Epub 20151117. PubMed PMID: 26440218; PMCID: PMC4738408

31. Loriamini M, Lewis-Bakker MM, Frias Boligan K, Wang S, Holton MB, Kotra LP, Branch DR (2023) Small molecule drugs that inhibit phagocytosis. Molecules. 28(2). https://doi.org/10.3390/molecules28020757. Epub 20230112. PubMed PMID: 36677815; PMCID: PMC9867408

32. Balola AHA, Mayer B, Bartolmas T, Salama A (2021) A fluorometric erythrophagocytosis assay using differentiated monocytic THP-1 cells to assess the clinical significance of antibodies to red blood cells. Vox Sang 116(10): 1106–1116. Epub 20210504. https://doi.org/10.1111/vox.13105

33. Gil Gonzalez L, Fernandez-Marrero Y, Norris PAA, Tawhidi Z, Shan Y, Cruz-Leal Y, Won KD, Frias-Boligan K, Branch DR, Lazarus AH (2022) THP-1 cells transduced with CD16A utilize Fcgamma receptor I and III in the phagocytosis of IgG-sensitized human erythrocytes and platelets. PLoS One 17(12): e0278365. https://doi.org/10.1371/journal.pone.0278365. Epub 20221214. PubMed PMID: 36516219; PMCID: PMC9749970

34. Healey G, Veale MF, Sparrow RL (2007) A fluorometric quantitative erythrophagocytosis assay using human THP-1 monocytic cells and PKH26-labelled red blood cells. J Immunol Methods. 322(1–2):50–56. Epub 20070228. https://doi.org/10.1016/j.jim.2007.01.024

35. Miksa M, Komura H, Wu R, Shah KG, Wang P (2009) A novel method to determine the engulfment of apoptotic cells by macrophages using pHrodo succinimidyl ester. J Immunol Methods 342(1–2):71–77. https://doi.org/10.1016/j.jim.2008.11.019. Epub 20090109. PubMed PMID: 19135446; PMCID: PMC2675277

36. Schwende H, Fitzke E, Ambs P, Dieter P (1996) Differences in the state of differentiation of THP-1 cells induced by phorbol ester and 1,25-dihydroxyvitamin D3. J Leukoc Biol 59(4):555–561

37. Montano F, Grinstein S, Levin R (2018) Quantitative phagocytosis assays in primary and cultured macrophages. Methods Mol Biol 1784:151–163. https://doi.org/10.1007/978-1-4939-7837-3_15

38. Safi W, Kuehnl A, Nussler A, Eckstein HH, Pelisek J (2016) Differentiation of human CD14+ monocytes: an experimental investigation of the optimal culture medium and evidence of a lack of differentiation along the endothelial line. Exp Mol Med 48(4):e227. https://doi.org/10.1038/emm.2016.11. Epub 20160415. PubMed PMID: 27080367; PMCID: PMC4855273

39. Tedesco S, Bolego C, Toniolo A, Nassi A, Fadini GP, Locati M, Cignarella A (2015) Phenotypic activation and pharmacological outcomes of spontaneously differentiated human monocyte-derived macrophages. Immunobiology. 220(5):545–554. Epub 20141223. https://doi.org/10.1016/j.imbio.2014.12.008

Chapter 43

Analysis of Galectin Binding to Blood Group Expressing Bacteria

Anu Paul, Hau-Ming Jan, Sasikala Muthusamy, Shang-Chuen Wu, Abraham B. Alton, William O. Scott, Carter J. Stowell, Ryan P. Jajosky, Dominique Paz, and Connie M. Arthur

Abstract

Microbial cell surfaces exhibit a remarkable diversity of complex carbohydrate structures, with most strains producing unique glycan coats distinct from those found on mammalian cells. However, some microbes employ carbohydrate-based molecular mimicry, potentially as a strategy to evade adaptive immune responses. This phenomenon is particularly intriguing in microbes capable of generating ABO blood group-like glycans. While molecular mimicry of host glycans may reduce adaptive immune recognition of specific host-like glycan epitopes expressed by bacteria, innate immune lectins known as galectins have been shown to recognize these glycan structures expressed by bacteria, suggesting that they may contribute to host defense against microbes that utilize molecular mimicry. Flow cytometry using fluorescently labeled galectins provides a powerful tool for examining galectin-bacteria interactions, including engagement of microbes that express blood group-like antigens. Herein, we describe the approaches used for investigating lectin–microbial interactions by flow cytometry.

Key words Human blood group B-glycan, Blood group glycan-expressing bacteria, Galectin-4, Thio-digalactoside inhibition, Bacteria flow cytometry

1 Introduction

Adaptive immunity has the unique ability to respond to a nearly infinite range of antigenic determinants [1]. However, tolerance mechanisms reduce immune reactivity to self. While this lowers the risk of autoimmunity, it creates a gap in immune repertoires against microbes that exploit molecular mimicry [2–4]. This is particularly evident with microbes that use glycans resembling blood group antigens [5, 6]. Blood group polymorphisms can create barriers to transfusion and transplantation due to the presence of anti-blood group antibodies [7–12]. While many of these antibodies arise from exposure during pregnancy or transfusion where they can cause

Sean R. Stowell and Connie M. Arthur (eds.), *Methods in Transfusion Medicine*, Methods in Molecular Biology, vol. 3053,
https://doi.org/10.1007/978-1-0716-5376-0_43,

significant complications in transfusion-dependent patients, as described in numerous studies [12–15], some develop spontaneously within the first few months of life. Regardless of how alloantibodies form, crossing alloimmune barriers during treatment of a variety of conditions can lead to a wide variety of patient complications, which has been documented in a number of studies [12–21]. This can be especially challenging for transfusion-dependent patients, including those with sickle cell disease, which are particularly prone to complications associated with alloantibody formation and associated complications [22–30].

While many blood group antigens reflect single amino acid polymorphisms, ABO(H) and other glycan antigens represent distinct carbohydrate structures that decorate the surface of red blood cells and other cell surfaces [7]. Bacterial cell surfaces are also decorated by diverse types of glycan structures [5, 6]. Recognition of the bacterial glycan structures by lectins and anti-glycan antibodies is at the center of host responses against invading pathogens. Occasionally, certain bacterial surface glycan structures strikingly resemble mammalian cell surface glycan structures. This phenomenon, termed as "molecular mimicry," is considered a major mechanism adapted by bacteria to evade host immunity. This is most pronounced for microbial glycans that resemble various blood group antigens, including ABO(H) blood group antigen-like structures. Initially, it was thought that the microbial genes responsible for synthesizing mammalian glycan-like structures arose via lateral gene transfer from eukaryotes. However, based on recent genetic evidence, convergent evolution rather than gene transfer is considered responsible for this phenomenon [2, 3].

Previous studies have demonstrated that immune lectins called galectins are capable of binding a variety of glycan determinants the resemble blood group antigens and killing bacteria that express glycans mimicking these mammalian host glycans [31–38]. Galectins are β-galactoside-binding lectins having a few evolutionarily conserved amino acids in the carbohydrate recognition domain (CRD) involved in ligand interaction [39, 40]. It was shown that human galectin-8 (Gal-8) can recognize, bind, and kill blood group glycan-expressing pathogen *E. coli* O86 [4]. The recognition of *E. coli* O86 by Gal-8 is entirely dependent on the carbohydrate–galectin interaction as evidenced by the loss of binding by Gal-8 pre-incubated with lactose, a disaccharide to which galectins specifically bind at their CRDs [31]. Subsequent studies have demonstrated that galectin engagement of microbes is not limited to Gal-8 or *E. coli* O86, with multiple galectins having now been shown to possess the ability to bind a variety of blood group-related antigens and kill microbes that use distinct forms of molecular mimicry [32, 33, 37–39, 41, 42].

This chapter will focus on the binding of human Gal-4 to bacteria that express glycan structures that resemble human blood group glycan structures. A few examples of bacteria that express blood group-like structures are *Escherichia coli* O86 (EC O86), *Streptococcus pneumoniae* 33F (SP33F), and *Providencia alcalifaciens* O5 (PAO5) (Fig. 1). We will also examine galectin binding using bacteria belonging to the same genus and species, but which differ at the strain level and lack blood group glycan expression.

2 Materials

2.1 Bacterial Culture for the Assay

2.1.1 Culturing E. coli and P. alcalifaciens Bacterial Strains

1. Bacterial glycerol stocks.
   (a) *E. coli* O86 and *E. coli* ΔwaaL mutant (provided by Peng George Wang from Georgia State University).
   (b) *Providencia alcalifaciens* O5 and *Providencia alcalifaciens* O19 (provided by Y. Knirel from the ND Zelinsky Institute of Organic Chemistry in Moscow, Russia).
2. LB broth-Lennox (Sigma-Aldrich, L3022).
3. Fisher brand™ Disposable Inoculating Loops and Needles, Catalog No.22-363-605.
4. Biosafety cabinet.
5. Bacteria culture tubes.
6. Shaking incubator.

2.1.2 Culturing S. pneumoniae Bacterial Strains

1. Bacterial glycerol stocks.
   (a) *Streptococcus pneumoniae* 33F and *Streptococcus pneumoniae* 2 (provided by Moon H. Nahm from the University of Alabama at Birmingham).
2. BD BBL™ Trypticase™ Soy Agar with 5% Sheep Blood (TSA II™) BD 221261.
3. Todd-Hewitt yeast broth (Bacto™ Todd-Hewitt Broth (BD Diagnostics, Supplier No: 249240) with 0.5% yeast extract).
4. Double Zip AnaeroPouch™-Bag (Mitsubishi Gas Chemical Company: Thermo Scientific™ R686010).
5. Fisher brand™ Disposable Inoculating Loops and Needles, Catalog No.22-363-605.
6. Biosafety cabinet.
7. Bacteria culture tubes.
8. Shaking incubator.

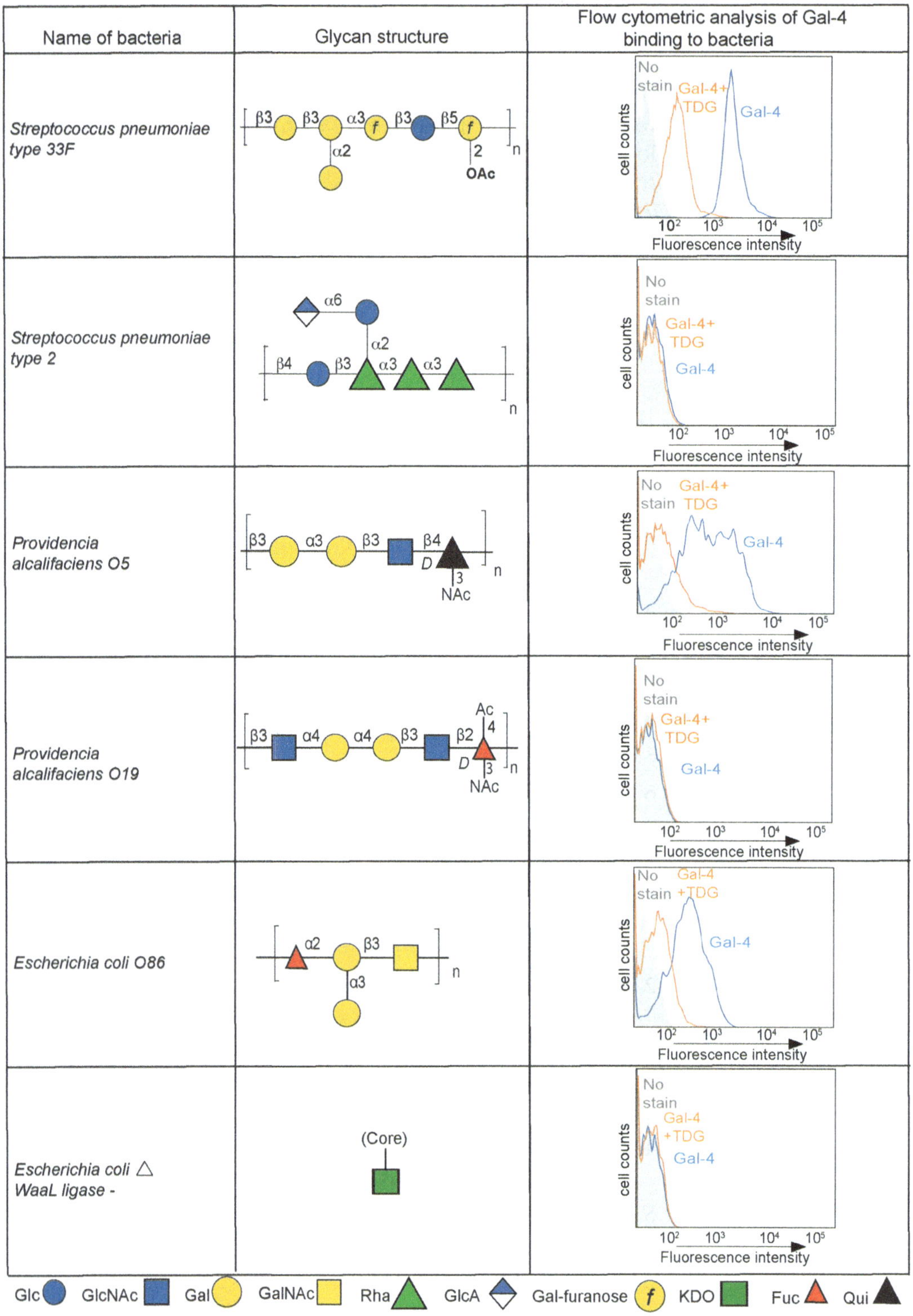

Fig. 1 Gal-4 recognizes bacteria expressing human blood group B antigen-like structure. In the first column, the names of bacteria used in the assay are given. In the second column, the glycan structure of the respective bacteria is given. In the third column, flow cytometric analysis of Gal-4 to SP 33F, SP 2, PAO5, PAO19, *Escherichia coli* O86, and *E. coli* O86-ΔWaaL with or without inhibition by TDG is shown. The outcome of incubation of Gal-4 alone is labeled blue. Gal-4 with TDG is labeled orange. Unstained control is labeled gray

2.2 Coupling of Human Gal-4 with Alexa Fluor 647-NHS Ester

1. Purified recombinant Gal-4.
2. UV-1800 Shimadzu Spectrophotometer.
3. Eppendorf Uvette disposable cuvettes (Fisher Scientific, 952010051).
4. Axygen 1.7 mL MaxyClear Snaplock Microcentrifuge tube Eppendorf tabletop centrifuge.
5. Disposable PD-10 desalting column (Cytiva, 17085101).
6. Alexa Fluor™ 647-NHS Succinimidyl Ester (Invitrogen: A37573).
7. Lactose (Monohydrate (ACS) GFS Chemicals: 46231).
8. End-over-end rotator.
9. Lactosyl-sepharose column.
10. 100 mM lactose in 1X PBS containing 14 mM 2-mercaptoethanol.
11. Amicon Ultra-4 centrifugal filters—Ultracel-10 K (Sigma-Aldrich).
12. Empty disposable PD-10 column (Cytiva, (17-0435-01).
13. 2-Mercaptoethanol (Sigma-Aldrich, M3148).

2.3 Pre-incubation of Gal-4 with Specific Sugars

1. (D-Galactopyranosyl)-β-D-thiogalactopyranoside (Biosynth, OG05033).

2.4 Galectin–Bacteria Interaction for Flow Cytometry Assay

1. PBS 1X.
2. Vortex mixer.
3. 4 °C cold room.

2.5 Flow Cytometry Assay

1. Cytek Iso-flow sheath fluid/BD FACS Flow sheath fluid.
2. Cytek Northern Lights or FACS Canto II flow cytometer (BD Biosciences).
3. Quality control beads for Cytek Northern Lights.
4. PBS.
5. 5 mL Polystyrene Round-Bottom Tubes (12 × 75 mm style) [Falcon].

2.6 Data Analysis

1. Data analyzing software: FlowJo version 10.

3 Methods

3.1 Bacteria Culture for the Assay

3.1.1 Culturing E. coli and P. Alcalifaciens Bacterial Strains

1. For culturing *E. coli* O86, *E. coli* ΔwaaL mutant, PAO5, and PAO19, inoculate bacteria from glycerol stock in 2 mL LB broth.
2. Incubate overnight at 37 °C.
3. From overnight culture, subculture to fresh 5 mL LB broth in bacteria culture tube.
4. Grow at 37 °C until mid-log phase (0.4–0.6 OD_{600}).

3.1.2 Culturing S. pneumoniae Bacterial Strains

1. Culture bacteria on trypticase soy agar II blood agar plates or in Todd-Hewitt yeast broth at 37 °C in 5% CO_2 using an Anaero-Pouch-MicroAero bag. This can also be completed in an incubator with 5% CO_2.
2. If culture was started on TSAII agar plates then once colonies are formed, transfer to Todd-Hewitt yeast broth and incubate at 37 °C with 5% CO_2 until reaching the exponential growth phase (i.e., 0.5–0.6 OD_{600}).

3.2 Coupling of Human Gal-4 with Alexa Fluor 647-NHS Ester

1. Recombinant galectins are purified according to the standard protocols described previously (*see* **Note 1**).
2. Remove lactose and 2-ME from galectin using a PD-10 desalting column.
3. Combine the OD_{280} positive fractions. The concentration of the protein should be at least 2 mg/mL for optimal coupling to occur.
4. Add lactose at a 100 mM concentration (36 mg/mL).
5. Add 50 μL volume of Alexa Fluor™ 647 (10 mg/mL) to 1 mL of galectin (2 mg/mL) solution.
6. Incubate at room temperature for 1 h while in rotator shaker.
7. For using the Alexa Fluor 647-coupled galectin for any functional assay, pass protein-label mixture over a PD-10 desalting column to remove lactose and unconjugated label.
8. Pool the protein fractions together.
9. To obtain an active fraction of Alexa 647-coupled galectin, pass the protein through 2 mL of packed lactosyl-sepharose column (*see* **Note 2**).
10. Wash the column using wash buffer, i.e., PBS with 14 mM 2-ME.
11. Elute the bound galectin using a buffer containing 100 mM lactose in PBS containing 14 mM 2ME.
12. Pass the eluted active galectin fraction containing lactose through PD-10 desalting column.

13. Collect the protein fractions and pool them together by concentration in an Amicon centrifuge.
14. Use spectrophotometer to determine the OD_{280}.
15. Calculate the actual concentration according to the manufacturer's protocol (*see* **Note 3**).

3.3 Pre-incubation of Gal-4 with Specific Sugar TDG

1. Calculate the concentration of Gal-4 and add 40 mM TDG to an equal volume of 2 μM Gal-4 (*see* **Note 4**).
2. Pre-incubate galectin with TDG or PBS on ice for 30 min with intermittent mixing.

3.4 Galectin–Bacteria Interaction for Flow Cytometry Assay

1. Bacteria grown to mid-log phase in LB broth is pelleted at 6000× *g* for 5 min.
2. Wash with cold PBS at 4 °C and spin at 6000× *g* for 5 min.
3. Resuspend the bacteria in PBS to 0.1 $OD_{600.}$
4. Incubate bacteria at 0.1 OD_{600} and 0.1 μM Alexa Fluor 647-labeled Gal-4, with or without thio-digalactoside, at a final volume of 200 μL at 4 °C for 10 min in the vortex shaker in cold room.
5. Spin down bacteria at 6000× *g* for 5 min.
6. Wash with PBS and spin at 6000× *g* for 5 min.
7. Resuspend in PBS and take the samples in FACS tubes for flow cytometric assay.

3.5 Flow Cytometry Assay and Analysis of Data

1. We use either FACS Canto II flow cytometer (BD Biosciences) or Cytek Northern Lights spectral flow cytometer for flow cytometric analysis. Herein, we describe the method for using the Cytek Northern Lights spectral flow cytometer. The Northern Lights instrument incorporates Cytek's powerful Full Spectrum Profiling™ (FSP™) technology in a one- to three-laser system.
2. Add sheath fluid to the tank.
3. Check the waste fluid level in the tank.
4. Turn on the Northern Lights and log in to Spectroflo.
5. Resuspend Spectroflo QC beads by inverting several times, then add 1 drop to 300 μL of sheath fluid.
6. Run daily QC before starting the experiment.
7. To run an experiment, go to acquisition, create a new experiment.
8. Follow all the prompts:
   (a) Name the experiment.
   (b) Select the fluorophores (add unlisted fluorophores in the library section).

(c) Select manual tube or 96-well U bottom plate.

(d) Add a reference group and the fluorophores.

(e) Add your samples and name them.

(f) Name the fluorophores.

(g) Choose your acquisition settings.

9. Before starting, make sure the tube button is showing if you want to run a tube. Put on a reference control, run the unstained sample, and then click Start.
10. Use log scales to set the Forward scatter (FSC) and Side scatter (SSC) gains to get the population centered on the chart. We have used the following settings: FSC gain 200, SSC gain 500, and FSC threshold 10,000.
11. Adjust the flow rate to medium.
12. Run samples one by one and click record.
13. Make sure that SIT Flush happens between samples or when you remove a manual tube.
14. Run the reference control for the fluorophore in use.
15. Go to "unmix" and determine appropriate auto-fluorescence extraction.
16. On the next screen, gate the negative and positive populations. Select the channel that has the highest fluorescent signal and then gate only on the strongest part of the positive signal.
17. Gate on the unstained population.
18. Unmix.
19. Select or create an unmixed worksheet for one of your samples.
20. Go back to Edit > Acquisition and select the worksheet that you want to show for your experimental samples. Of note, the reference groups must show the raw worksheet.
21. Select the stopping gate and the storage gate.
22. Run your samples.
23. After you collect the data, perform fluidics shutdown. Fluidics shutdown can be performed with the 40-tube rack in which the bottom left tube is 10% bleach, the tube to the right is distilled H_2O, the next tube is 30% Contrad, and the fourth tube is distilled H_2O. The software will inform you about when to turn off the machine.

3.6 Analyzing Data

The acquired data was processed using FlowJo version 10. (https://www.flowjo.com/solutions/flowjo).

4 Notes

1. Galectin purification protocols have been extensively covered previously. Readers are recommended to refer to these sources for detailed explanations on the purification of galectins [43].
2. Refer to methods for the preparation of lactosyl-sepharose.
3. For further information on correction factors for commonly used fluorophores, use the following link:https://tools.thermofisher.com/content/sfs/manuals/mp10168.pdf
4. It is ideal to also use an equal molar concentration of sucrose as a negative control for Gal-4 hapten-inhibition assay. This helps control for the potential stoichiometric effect of simply adding a hapten to the solution.

Conflicts of Interest

This work was funded by NIH P01HL171803, R01 HL165975, R01 HL135575, R01 HL154034, K99HL169746, and AABB Foundation Early-Career Scientific Research Grants. No other authors have conflicts of interest.

References

1. Chi H, Pepper M, Thomas PG (2024) Principles and therapeutic applications of adaptive immunity. Cell 187(9):2052–2078
2. Arthur CM et al (2015) Innate immunity against molecular mimicry: examining galectin-mediated antimicrobial activity. BioEssays 37(12):1327–1337
3. Elde NC, Malik HS (2009) The evolutionary conundrum of pathogen mimicry. Nat Rev Microbiol 7(11):787–797
4. Stebbins CE, Galan JE (2001) Structural mimicry in bacterial virulence. Nature 412(6848): 701–705
5. Arthur CM et al (2024) ABO blood groups and galectins: implications in transfusion medicine and innate immunity. Semin Immunol 74-75:101892
6. Reeves P (1995) Role of O-antigen variation in the immune response. Trends Microbiol 3(10): 381–386
7. Arthur CM, Stowell SR (2023) The development and consequences of red blood cell alloimmunization. Annu Rev Pathol 18:537–564
8. Jajosky R et al (2023) Prior immunization against an intracellular antigen enhances subsequent red blood cell alloimmunization in mice. Blood 141(21):2642–2653
9. Patel SR et al (2018) Marginal zone B cells induce alloantibody formation following RBC transfusion. Front Immunol 9:2516
10. Zerra PE et al (2021) Marginal zone B cells mediate a CD4 T-cell-dependent extrafollicular antibody response following RBC transfusion in mice. Blood 138(8):706–721
11. Jajosky RP et al (2023) Antibody-mediated antigen loss switches augmented immunity to antibody-mediated immunosuppression. Blood 142(12):1082–1098
12. Mener A et al (2018) Complement serves as a switch between CD4+ T cell-independent and -dependent RBC antibody responses. JCI Insight 3(22):e121631
13. Chonat S et al (2025) Complement is activated in patients with acute chest syndrome caused by sickle cell disease and represents a therapeutic target. Sci Transl Med 17(807):eadl4922
14. Pirenne F, Floch A, Diop S (2023) Alloimmunisation against red blood cells in sickle cell disease: transfusion challenges in high-income and low-income countries. Lancet Haematol 10(6):e468–e476

15. Jajosky RP et al (2025) CD47 regulates antigen modulation and red blood cell clearance following an incompatible transfusion. Front Immunol 16:1548548
16. Pirenne F, Yazdanbakhsh K (2018) How I safely transfuse patients with sickle-cell disease and manage delayed hemolytic transfusion reactions. Blood 131(25):2773–2781
17. Joseph A et al (2023) ABO Genotyping finds more A(2) to B kidney transplant opportunities than lectin-based subtyping. Am J Transplant 23(4):512–519
18. Halpin AM et al (2025) Multiplex bead immunoassay in ABO-A2-incompatible kidney transplantation. Am J Transplant 25(9):1884–1894
19. Tormey CA, Hendrickson JE (2019) Transfusion-related red blood cell alloantibodies: induction and consequences. Blood 133(17):1821–1830
20. Arthur CM et al (2022) Nonhuman glycans can regulate anti-factor VIII antibody formation in mice. Blood 139(9):1312–1317
21. Zerra PE et al (2017) Marginal zone B cells are critical to factor VIII inhibitor formation in mice with hemophilia a. Blood 130(23): 2559–2568
22. Yazdanbakhsh K, Provan D, Semple JW (2023) The role of T cells and myeloid-derived suppressor cells in refractory immune thrombocytopenia. Br J Haematol 203(1):54–61
23. Liu Y et al (2023) Hemolysis dictates monocyte differentiation via two distinct pathways in sickle cell disease vaso-occlusion. J Clin Invest 133(18)
24. Arthur CM et al (2021) Antigen density dictates RBC clearance, but not antigen modulation, following incompatible RBC transfusion in mice. Blood Adv 5(2):527–538
25. Chang DY et al (2023) The ongoing challenge of RBC alloimmunization in the management of patients with sickle cell disease. Presse Med 52(4):104211
26. Dean CL et al (2019) Challenges in the treatment and prevention of delayed hemolytic transfusion reactions with hyperhemolysis in sickle cell disease patients. Transfusion 59(5): 1698–1705
27. Patel SR et al (2018) Recipient priming to one RBC alloantigen directly enhances subsequent alloimmunization in mice. Blood Adv 2(2): 105–115
28. Chonat S et al (2020) Eculizumab for complement mediated thrombotic microangiopathy in sickle cell disease. Haematologica 105(12): 2887–2891
29. Chonat S et al (2018) Contribution of alternative complement pathway to delayed hemolytic transfusion reaction in sickle cell disease. Haematologica 103(10):e483–e485
30. Dumas G et al (2016) Eculizumab salvage therapy for delayed hemolysis transfusion reaction in sickle cell disease patients. Blood 127(8): 1062–1064
31. Stowell SR et al (2010) Innate immune lectins kill bacteria expressing blood group antigen. Nat Med 16(3):295–301
32. Jan HM et al (2024) Galectin-4 antimicrobial activity primarily occurs through its C-terminal domain. Mol Cell Proteomics 23(5):100747
33. Wu SC et al (2022) Innate immune Galectin-7 specifically targets microbes that decorate themselves in blood group-like antigens. iScience 25(7):104482
34. Leppanen A et al (2022) Examination of whole-cell galectin binding by solid phase and flow Cytometric analysis. In: Methods Mol Biol, vol 2442, pp 187–203
35. Stowell CP, Stowell SR (2019) Biologic roles of the ABH and Lewis histo-blood group antigens part I: infection and immunity. Vox Sang 114(5):426–442
36. Stowell SR, Stowell CP (2019) Biologic roles of the ABH and Lewis histo-blood group antigens part II: thrombosis, cardiovascular disease and metabolism. Vox Sang 114(6):535–552
37. Blenda AV et al (2022) Galectin-9 recognizes and exhibits antimicrobial activity toward microbes expressing blood group-like antigens. J Biol Chem 298(4):101704
38. Wu SC et al (2021) Full-length Galectin-3 is required for high affinity microbial interactions and antimicrobial activity. Front Microbiol 12: 731026
39. Wu SC et al (2023) Blood group a enhances SARS-CoV-2 infection. Blood 142(8): 742–747
40. Liu FT, Stowell SR (2023) The role of galectins in immunity and infection. Nat Rev Immunol 23(8):479–494
41. Ho AD et al (2022) An automated approach to assess relative galectin-glycan affinity following glycan microarray analysis. Front Mol Biosci 9: 893185
42. Wu SC et al (2023) Whole microbe arrays accurately predict interactions and overall antimicrobial activity of galectin-8 toward distinct strains of Streptococcus pneumoniae. Sci Rep 13(1):5324
43. Wu SC et al (2021) Generation and use of recombinant galectins. Curr Protoc 1(3):e63

Chapter 44

Western Blot Detection of Blood Group A and B Antigens

Katherine H. Tiemeyer, Akua A. Appah-Sampong, and Marie A. Hollenhorst

Abstract

Epidemiologic studies have demonstrated an association between ABO blood group status and risk of hemorrhage and thrombosis. However, the mechanisms that govern this association are not fully understood. ABO blood type is defined by the presence of carbohydrate antigens termed the A, B, and H antigens. These antigens can be found attached to glycoproteins and glycolipids of red blood cells, platelets, and endothelial cells; they can also modify plasma coagulation factors. Despite the prevalence and clinical significance of ABH antigens, the repertoire of proteins that carry these blood group antigens is not well established. This knowledge gap limits our ability to understand the reason for the association between ABO blood group status and risk of hemorrhage or thrombosis. In an effort to narrow that gap, we describe a Western blot method that can be used to determine whether a protein carries the blood group A and/or B antigens.

Key words Glycoproteins, Glycosylation, Blood Group Antigens, ABO Blood Group System, Western Blot

1 Introduction

The carbohydrate structures that dictate ABO blood group status are perhaps the most well-known human glycans. These oligosaccharide antigens, termed A, B, and H, covalently modify lipids and proteins on the surface of red blood cells, platelets, endothelial cells, and epithelial cells. When carried on glycoproteins, ABH antigens can be linked to the protein in one of two ways: via the nitrogen of asparagine residues (N-linked) or the oxygen of serine/threonine residues (O-linked). The H antigen serves as a biosynthetic precursor to both the A and B antigens, which differ only by a single monosaccharide [1, 2]. In blood type A individuals, α1,3-*N*-acetylgalactosaminyltransferase (A-glycosyltransferase) adds *N*-acetylgalactosamine (GalNAc) in an α1,3 linkage to the terminal galactose of the H antigen, whereas in blood type B individuals, α1,3-galactosyltransferase (B-glycosyltransferase) adds galactose

Sean R. Stowell and Connie M. Arthur (eds.), *Methods in Transfusion Medicine*, Methods in Molecular Biology, vol. 3053, https://doi.org/10.1007/978-1-0716-5376-0_44,

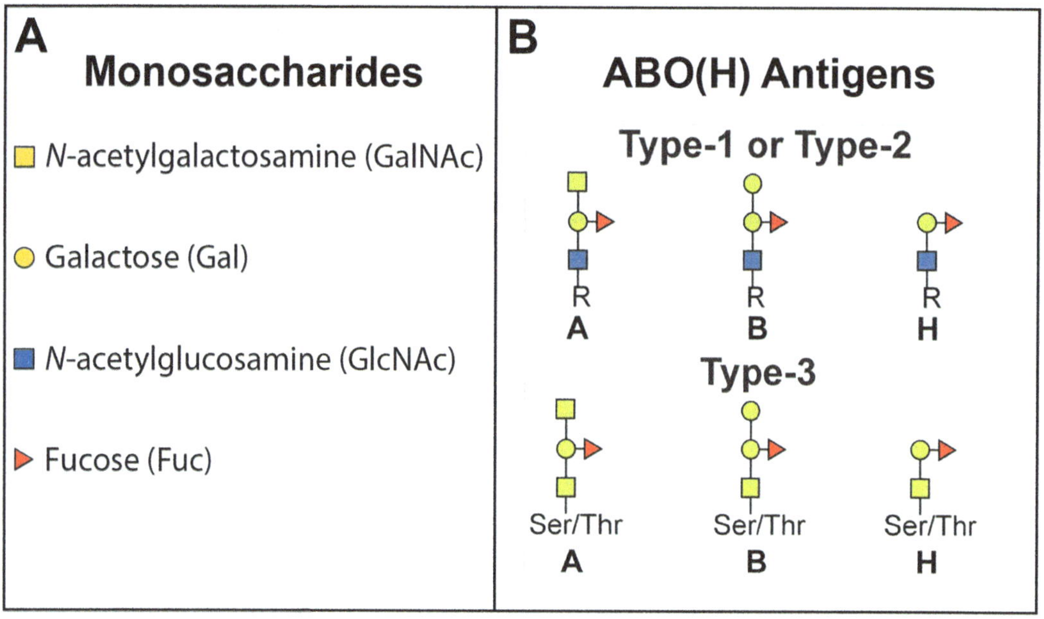

Fig. 1 Monosaccharide composition of ABO(H) blood group antigens. (**a**) ABO(H) blood group antigens are carbohydrate polymers composed of monosaccharides. Monosaccharides are depicted according to the Symbol Nomenclature for Glycan standards (SNFG) [19, 20]. (**b**) The A, B, and O blood groups are defined by the A, B, and H carbohydrate antigens, respectively. ABH antigens are classified into different types. Type-1 and type-2 ABH antigens are built upon a GlcNAc-Gal core, differing only with respect to the linkage between the two monosaccharides (β1,3 for type-1, β1,4 for type-2). Type-3 ABH antigens contain a GalNAc residue in place of the GlcNAc found in type-1 and type-2, and these antigens directly modify Ser/Thr residues. (Figure reproduced with permission from *Journal of Thrombosis and Haemostasis* [18])

(Gal) in an α1,3 linkage to the terminal galactose of the H antigen (Fig. 1) [1, 2].

While the immunogenicity of ABO(H) antigens has long been recognized as a property of significant clinical importance in transfusion and transplantation medicine, epidemiological studies detailing the association of ABO blood group with risks of bleeding and clotting have raised further questions regarding the physiological significance of these antigens. Multiple large cohort studies have shown that blood type O individuals are at higher risk of bleeding than those of non-O blood type [3, 4]. Similarly, non-O blood type predisposes to thrombosis [5, 6]. These observations can be partially attributed to differences in plasma levels of coagulation factors between O and non-O blood types. For example, von Willebrand factor (VWF), a glycoprotein that facilitates clot formation, exists at 25–30% higher plasma concentrations in individuals with non-O compared to those with O blood type [7]. A similar finding has been reported in plasma levels of Factor VIII (FVIII), another glycoprotein of critical importance for thrombus formation [8]. Still, recent data suggest that differences in plasma concentrations of VWF and FVIII alone are not sufficient to explain the hemostatic differences observed in O and non-O individuals. Further studies support the notion that the ABO(H) antigens on platelets or on other coagulation factors may modulate hemostasis and thrombosis [9–11].

Given the mounting evidence that ABO(H) antigens influence the molecular interactions that maintain hemostatic equilibrium, it is critical to establish the repertoire of human proteins that carry ABO(H) antigens to further untangle the association between ABO blood group and risk of hemorrhage and thrombosis. To date, only a handful of proteins have been reproducibly identified as carriers of ABO(H) antigens, primarily using immunoaffinity techniques for the identification and isolation of antigen-carrying proteins [12–16]. As a result, the interpretation of these data is limited by the sensitivity and specificity of the antibodies used. Furthermore, prior studies have often relied on non-standardized biological reagents (e.g., donor serum/plasma, antibodies that are no longer commercially available) and frequently lacked robust positive and negative controls. These limitations highlight the need for reliable and reproducible methods for detecting ABH antigens.

Here, we describe a method for immunoblot detection of ABH antigens using anti-A and anti-B antibodies that are routinely used for clinical ABO typing. Drawing inspiration from prior publications reporting the use of these antibodies as Western blot reagents, we have developed an optimized method that enables sensitive and specific detection of their respective antigens in human platelet lysates (Fig. 2) [15, 17]. We also describe positive and negative controls for anti-A and anti-B Western blots. Commercially available synthetic glycoproteins carrying A, B, or H antigens are robustly detected at nanogram amounts which serve as immunoblot positive control samples. In addition, we define a method for enzymatic conversion of A and B antigens to O(H) antigens through the cleavage of the immunogenic determinant monosaccharide. These enzymes (informally referred to as "Azyme" and "Bzyme") effectively abolish the reactivity with anti-A and anti-B antibodies and serve as a powerful tool for the validation of ABH status.

We have previously employed this method to identify human platelet glycoprotein Ibα as a carrier of ABO(H) glycans, but myriad applications exist [18]. We expect that this protocol could be applied to other human tissue lysates to identify ABH antigen-carrying proteins. Coupled with immunoprecipitation or protein purification, one could easily assess ABH status of any protein of interest. This method could also be used to qualitatively determine the relative abundance of ABH antigens on proteins across different biological samples: for example, to assess the variability in expression across different blood donors. Taken together, these methods describe a standardized and reproducible protocol for detecting ABH antigens by immunoblot.

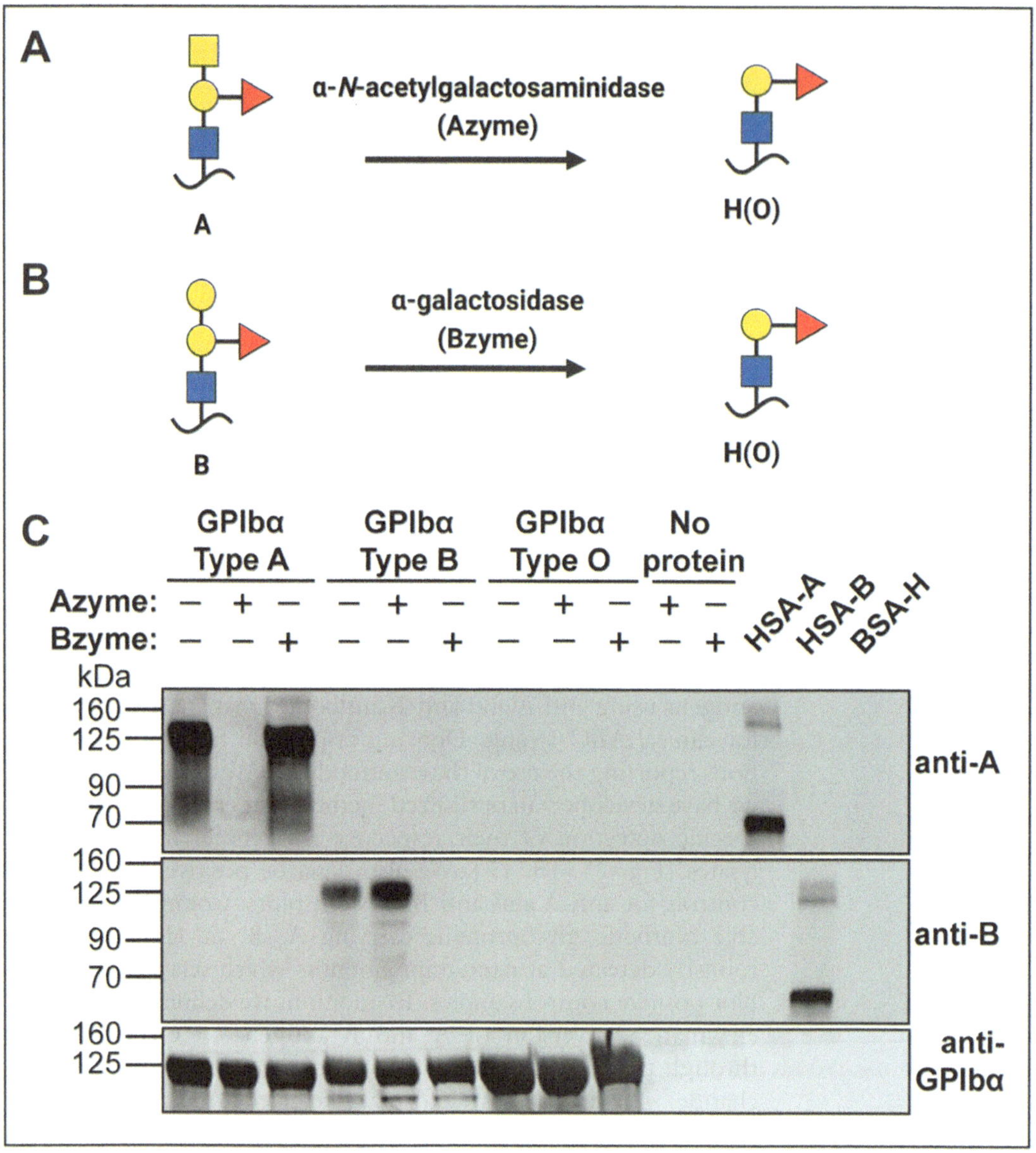

Fig. 2 Enzymatic conversion of A and B antigens to O(H) antigen. (**a**) Schematic representation of α-*N*-acetylgalactosaminidase ("Azyme") hydrolysis of the terminal GalNAc of the A antigen to yield the H antigen. (**b**) α-galactosidase ("Bzyme") hydrolysis of the terminal Gal of the B antigen to yield the H antigen. (**c**) Glycoprotein Ibα ectodomain purified from human platelets of blood type A, B, or O was untreated or treated with Azyme or Bzyme. The resulting proteins were analyzed by Western blot with anti-A and anti-B antibodies. The following synthetic glycoproteins were used as controls: human serum albumin covalently modified with A antigen (HSA-A), human serum albumin covalently modified with B antigen (HSA-B), and bovine serum albumin covalently modified with the H antigen (BSA-H). Blue square, *N*-acetylglucosamine (GlcNAc); yellow square, *N*-acetylgalactosamine (GalNAc); yellow circle, galactose (Gal); red triangle, fucose (Fuc). (Figure reproduced with permission from *Journal of Thrombosis and Haemostasis* [18])

2 Materials

2.1 Glycosidase Treatment of Glycoproteins Carrying Human Blood Group A or B Antigens

2.1.1 α-N-acetyl-galactosaminidase ("Azyme") Used for Hydrolysis of the Terminal N-acetylgalactosamine (GalNAc) of the A Antigen to Yield the H Antigen

- Azyme: GalNAcEXO, G1-NA1-020, Genovis (*see* **Note 1**).
- 20 mM Tris–HCl, pH 7.4.
- Biological sample containing glycoprotein (s) known or hypothesized to carry the human blood group A antigen (*see* **Note 2**).

2.1.2 α-Galactosidase ("Bzyme") Used for Hydrolysis of the Terminal Galactose (Gal) of the B Antigen to Yield the H Antigen

- Bzyme: α-galactosidase from green coffee bean, G8507, Sigma-Aldrich (*see* **Note 1**).
- 50 mM sodium phosphate buffer, pH 6.5.
- Biological sample containing glycoprotein(s) known or hypothesized to carry the human blood group B antigen (*see* **Note 2**).

2.2 Western Blot Detection of Human Blood Group A or B Antigens (see Fig. 3)

- Criterion Gel Electrophoresis Cell, #1656001, Bio-Rad.
- 4–12% Criterion XT Precast Bis-Tris gel, #3450123, 3450124, 3450125, Bio-Rad.
- Trans-Blot Turbo, #1704150, Bio-Rad.
- XT MOPS Buffer, #1610788, Bio-Rad.
- 4× Laemmli Sample Buffer, #1610747, Bio-Rad.
- 2-Mercaptoethanol, #1610710, Bio-Rad.
- Chameleon Duo Pre-Stained Protein Ladder, P/N 92860000, Li-COR.
- Intercept (PBS) Blocking Buffer, P/N 927-90001, Li-COR.
- Revert 700 Total Protein Stain, P/N 926-11011, Li-COR.
- Ortho Clinical Diagnostics ABO Blood Group Reagents, Bio-Clone: Anti-A, Cat# 23-287-450, Ref# 210520, Thermo Fisher Scientific (RRID: AB_2909591).
- Ortho Clinical Diagnostics ABO Blood Group Reagents, Bio-Clone: anti-B, Cat# 23-287-451, Ref#210521, Thermo Fisher Scientific (RRID: AB_2909591).
- Bio-Rad ChemiDoc MP Imaging System, #12003154.

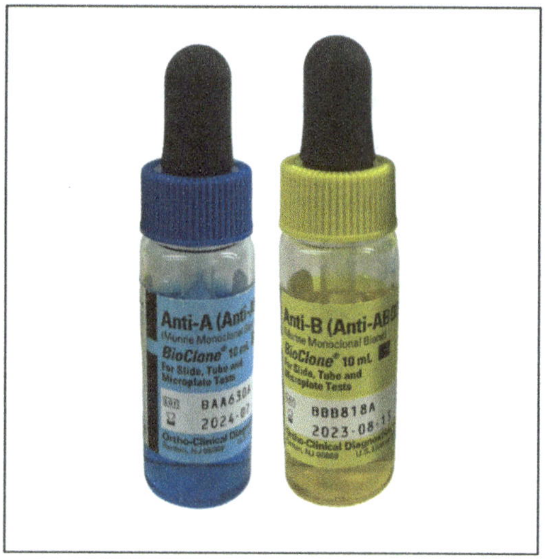

Fig. 3 Representative images of anti-A and anti-B reagents. Pictured are the Anti-A and Anti-B BioClone reagents produced by Ortho Clinical Diagnostics (now QuidelOrtho). These reagents are commercially available through Fisher Scientific

3 Methods

3.1 Glycosidase Treatment of Glycoproteins Carrying Human Blood Group A or B Antigens

3.1.1 α-N-acetyl-galactosaminidase ("Azyme") for Hydrolysis of the Terminal GalNAc of the A Antigen to Yield the H Antigen

1. Treat glycoprotein with 1 unit of GalNAcEXO per μg of glycoprotein (*see* **Note 3**).
2. Bring sample to the desired final volume using 20 mM Tris–HCl, pH 7.4 (*see* **Note 4**).
3. Incubate at 37 °C for 2 h.

3.1.2 α-Galactosidase ("Bzyme") for Hydrolysis of the Terminal Gal of the B Antigen to Yield the H Antigen

1. Treat glycoprotein with 32 mU of α-galactosidase per μg of glycoprotein (*see* **Note 5**).
2. Bring sample to the desired final volume using 50 mM sodium phosphate buffer, pH 6.5 (*see* **Note 4**).
3. Incubate at 37 °C overnight.

3.2 Western Blot Detection of Human Blood Group A or B Antigens

1. Prepare samples for sodium dodecyl sulfate-polyacrylamide gel electrophoresis (SDS-PAGE) by adding 4× Laemmli sample buffer, containing 10% 2-mercaptoethanol, diluted 1:4 (*see* **Note 6**).

2. Boil samples at 95 °C for 5–10 min to denature proteins.
3. Briefly spin down samples in a tabletop centrifuge.
4. Load gel according to previously determined loading scheme (*see* **Note 7**).
5. Separate glycoprotein(s) by SDS-PAGE using a 4–12% Criterion XT Precast Bis-Tris gel in 1× XT MOPS buffer at 200 V until the dye front has reached the bottom of the gel (*see* **Note 8**).
6. Transfer protein to a 0.2 μm nitrocellulose membrane for immunoblotting using a Trans-Blot Turbo (Bio-Rad) transfer system according to the manufacturer's protocol.
7. Perform total protein staining with Revert 700 Total Protein Stain according to the manufacturer's protocol (*see* **Note 9**).
8. Block in Intercept (PBS) blocking buffer (Li-COR) overnight at 4 °C with gentle shaking (*see* **Note 10**).
9. Incubate in anti-A murine monoclonal blend *OR* anti-B murine monoclonal blend (Ortho Clinical Diagnostics) diluted 1:10 in Intercept (PBS) Blocking Buffer containing 0.2% Tween-20 for 1 h at room temperature with gentle shaking (*see* **Note 11**).
10. Wash 4 times for 5 min in phosphate-buffered saline (PBS) containing 0.1% Tween-20.
11. Incubate in goat anti-mouse IgM IRDye 800CW diluted to 1: 15,000 in Intercept (PBS) Blocking Buffer containing 0.4% Tween-20 for 1 h at room temperature with gentle shaking.
12. Wash 4 times for 5 min in phosphate-buffered saline (PBS) containing 0.2% Tween-20.
13. Rinse blot briefly in phosphate-buffered saline (PBS) after the last wash.
14. Image blot at 800 nm on imaging system of choice (e.g., Bio-Rad ChemiDoc MP, Li-COR Odyssey DLx).

4 Notes

1. The terms "Azyme" and "Bzyme" are informal terms used to describe enzymes that hydrolyze the terminal monosaccharides defining the A and B antigens, respectively.
2. The protocol described was validated on purified glycoprotein samples [18], but researchers may consider adapting it for other types of samples, such as cell lysates.
3. GalNAcEXO is *Akkermansia muciniphila* exo-α-*N*-acetylgalactosaminidase, expressed in *E. coli*.

4. Final volumes can range, e.g., 10–63 μL [18].
5. The α-galactosidase from green coffee beans (Sigma-Aldrich) is supplied as an ammonium sulfate suspension. The following protocol should be followed prior to use: Centrifuge the suspension at 10,000 × g for 10 min at 4 °C. Discard the supernatant, and then resuspend the pelleted enzyme in an equal volume of 50 mM sodium phosphate buffer, pH 6.5, to reach a final concentration of 45.6 units/mL.
6. The 4× Laemmli sample buffer may settle at the bottom of sample tubes. Gently pipette the samples up and down for more even distribution.
7. The following synthetic glycoproteins can be used as controls: human serum albumin covalently modified with A antigen and human serum albumin covalently modified with B antigen (Dextra Laboratories).
   (a) Blood Group A-human serum albumin (6-atom spacer), NGP9305, Dextra
   (b) Blood Group B-human serum albumin (6-atom spacer), NGP9323, Dextra
8. The specific gel system and running buffers should be optimized to achieve the best separation of the sample(s) of interest.
9. While we report using Revert total protein staining immediately following protein transfer to a nitrocellulose membrane, researchers should test the optimal timing of Revert staining relative to other blotting steps. Depending on the emission wavelengths of the secondary detection reagent(s) used, it will be important to ensure there is no bleed-through from overlapping channels between detection reagents.
10. A 1-h blocking step at room temperature may also be employed.
11. While we report using Ortho Clinical Diagnostics ABO Blood Group BioClone Reagents for A and B antigen detection, the Grifols Diagnostics Solutions Anti-A (ABO1) ref#210520 and Anti-B (ABO2) ref#210521 reagents may also be used. In our experience, several commercially available anti-A and anti-B antibodies were not as sensitive or specific as the aforementioned clinical reagents. For detection of the H antigen, *Ulex europaeus* agglutinin I (UEA-I) lectin can be used via lectin blotting. However, it should be noted that UEA-I may also recognize non-H antigen structures.

Acknowledgments

MH was supported by NIH K99HL156029 and a National Bleeding Disorder Foundation Career Development Award. KT was supported by Yale MSTP NIH T32GM136651.

Conflict of Interest This work was funded by the Brigham and Women's Department of Medicine Goldberg Scholarship to Nurture Scientific Careers in Academic Medicine (to MH) and an International Society of Thrombosis and Haemostasis Fundamental Research Career Development Award (to MH). The authors have no conflicts of interest to declare that are relevant to the content of this chapter.

References

1. Jajosky RP, Wu SC, Zheng L et al (2022) ABO blood group antigens and differential glycan expression: perspective on the evolution of common human enzyme deficiencies. iScience 26(1):105798. https://doi.org/10.1016/j.isci.2022.105798
2. Varki A, Cummings RD, Esko JD et al (2022) Essentials of glycobiology, 4th edn. Cold Spring Harbor Laboratory Press. Accessed 22 Feb 2023. http://www.ncbi.nlm.nih.gov/books/NBK579918/
3. Mehic D, Hofer S, Jungbauer C et al (2020) Association of ABO blood group with bleeding severity in patients with bleeding of unknown cause. Blood Adv 4(20):5157–5164. https://doi.org/10.1182/bloodadvances.2020002452
4. Moeller A, Weippert-Kretschmer M, Prinz H, Kretschmer V (2001) Influence of ABO blood groups on primary hemostasis. Transfusion 41(1):56–60. https://doi.org/10.1046/j.1537-2995.2001.41010056.x
5. Wu O, Bayoumi N, Vickers MA, Clark P (2008) ABO(H) blood groups and vascular disease: a systematic review and meta-analysis. J Thromb Haemost 6(1):62–69. https://doi.org/10.1111/j.1538-7836.2007.02818.x
6. He M, Wolpin B, Rexrode K et al (2012) ABO blood group and risk of coronary heart disease in two prospective cohort studies. Arterioscler Thromb Vasc Biol 32(9):2314–2320. https://doi.org/10.1161/ATVBAHA.112.248757
7. Jenkins PV, O'Donnell JS (2006) ABO blood group determines plasma von Willebrand factor levels: a biologic function after all? Transfusion 46(10):1836–1844. https://doi.org/10.1111/j.1537-2995.2006.00975.x
8. O'Donnell J, Laffan MA (2001) The relationship between ABO histo-blood group, factor VIII and von Willebrand factor. Transfus Med 11(4):343–351. https://doi.org/10.1046/j.1365-3148.2001.00315.x
9. Pujol-Moix N, Martinez-Perez A, Sabater-Lleal M et al (2019) Influence of ABO locus on PFA-100 collagen-ADP closure time is not totally dependent on the von willebrand factor. Results of a GWAS on GAIT-2 project phenotypes. IJMS. 20(13):3221. https://doi.org/10.3390/ijms20133221
10. Fei DJ (2019) ABO on platelets goes beyond transfusion. Blood 133(12):1274–1275. https://doi.org/10.1182/blood-2019-02-898791
11. Dunne E, Qi QM, Shaqfeh ES et al (2019) Blood group alters platelet binding kinetics to von Willebrand factor and consequently platelet function. Blood 133(12):1371–1377. https://doi.org/10.1182/blood-2018-06-855528
12. Curtis BR, Edwards JT, Hessner MJ, Klein JP, Aster RH (2000) Blood group A and B antigens are strongly expressed on platelets of some individuals. Blood 96(4):1574–1581. https://doi.org/10.1182/blood.V96.4.1574
13. Stockelberg D, Hou M, Rydberg L, Kutti J, Wadenvik H (1996) Evidence for an expression of blood group A antigen on platelet glycoproteins IV and V. Transfus Med 6(3):243–248. https://doi.org/10.1111/j.1365-3148.1996.tb00075.x
14. Hou M, Stockelberg D, Rydberg L, Kutti J, Wadenvik H (1996) Blood group A antigen expression in platelets is prominently associated with glycoprotein Ib and IIb. Evidence for an

A_1/A_2 difference. Transfus Med 6(1):51–59. https://doi.org/10.1046/j.1365-3148.1996.d01-52.x

15. Tasaki M, Yoshida Y, Miyamoto M et al (2009) Identification and characterization of major proteins carrying ABO blood group antigens in the human kidney. Transplantation 87(8): 1125–1133. https://doi.org/10.1097/TP.0b013e31819e0054
16. Wang X, Zhang F, Jiang Y et al (2021) Highly individual- and tissue-specific expression of glycoprotein group A and B blood antigens in the human kidney and liver. BMC Immunol 22(1): 66. https://doi.org/10.1186/s12865-021-00456-2
17. Matsui T, Fujimura Y, Nishida S, Titani K (1993) Human plasma alpha 2-macroglobulin and von Willebrand factor possess covalently linked ABO(H) blood group antigens in subjects with corresponding ABO phenotype. Blood 82(2):663–668. https://doi.org/10.1182/blood.V82.2.663.663
18. Hollenhorst MA, Tiemeyer KH, Mahoney KE et al (2023) Comprehensive analysis of platelet glycoprotein Ibα ectodomain glycosylation. J Thromb Haemost. https://doi.org/10.1016/j.jtha.2023.01.009
19. Varki A, Cummings RD, Aebi M et al (2015) Symbol nomenclature for graphical representations of glycans. Glycobiology 25(12): 1323–1324. https://doi.org/10.1093/glycob/cwv091
20. Neelamegham S, Aoki-Kinoshita K, Bolton E et al (2019) Updates to the symbol nomenclature for glycans guidelines. Glycobiology 29(9):620–624. https://doi.org/10.1093/glycob/cwz045

Chapter 45

Flow Cytometric Examination of Galectin Binding to Red Blood Cells

Hau-Ming Jan, Hsien-Ya Lin, Dominique Paz, Vivien C. Lee, Rebecca C. Hale, Katelyn Sturgis, Carter J. Stowell, Wenhui Li, and Shang-Chuen Wu

Abstract

Lectins have the capacity to interact with cell surface carbohydrates, where they can influence various cellular processes. While early studies utilized lectin-induced cell agglutination to assess general binding characteristics, flow cytometry offers a more precise and quantitative method for measuring lectin interactions with specific cell populations. This technique is particularly valuable in studying galectins, a family of lectins that exhibit distinct binding preferences to red blood cells (RBCs) based on their blood type. This approach enables the determination of each lectin's binding specificity toward cell surface blood group antigens and other carbohydrate modifications without the potential confounding effects that differences in quaternary structure might have on their agglutination capabilities. We describe herein the production of fluorescently labeled galectins to analyze their specificity toward RBCs obtained from individuals with different blood types using flow cytometry.

Key words Flow cytometry, Red blood cells, Fluorescence staining, Galectin

1 Introduction

Lectins, a diverse group of carbohydrate binding proteins found in various organisms, are characterized by their ability to agglutinate specific target cells, a phenomenon that proved useful for studying both the lectins themselves and the distinct features of glycans recognized by distinct lectins on a cell's surface [1, 2]. By observing the unique agglutination patterns produced by lectins from different sources, early studies were able to characterize these proteins based on their distinct binding properties [2, 3]. These agglutination studies not only provided insight into the various glycoforms present on different cell types but also laid the groundwork for hapten-based lectin inhibition studies, which offered further

Sean R. Stowell and Connie M. Arthur (eds.), *Methods in Transfusion Medicine*, Methods in Molecular Biology, vol. 3053, https://doi.org/10.1007/978-1-0716-5376-0_45,

understanding of the relative affinity of different lectins for particular glycan structures [3–6].

The agglutination of cells through cell surface carbohydrate engagement is not unique to lectins, as IgM antibodies targeting carbohydrates can also induce agglutination. This phenomenon played a crucial role in the discovery of ABO blood group antigens, where anti-A or anti-B antibodies were observed to spontaneously agglutinate RBCs from blood group A or blood group B individuals, respectively [7]. This test remains in use today for determining blood group status, with patient antibodies being tested against a panel of RBCs with known blood types. Additional screening for antibodies against non-ABO blood group antigens is also conducted, as individuals can develop antibodies against a wide variety of RBC alloantigens, which has been studied through numerous preclinical and in vitro model systems that have provided insight into the pathways that govern alloantibody formation following exposure through transfusion or pregnancy [8–11]. Although a number of studies have suggested that anti-ABO antibodies and alloantibodies against other antigens likely develop through different mechanisms and may influence transfusion outcomes in distinct ways [11–15], together they can lead to serious transfusion complications, partially due to the harmful effects of hemolysis on patient outcomes that have been illustrated in numerous studies [16–28]. Indeed, the accumulation of antibodies against various blood group antigens can complicate future transfusions, potentially leading to increased morbidity and mortality, as demonstrated in a variety of studies particularly in transfusion-dependent patient populations [29–35].

Plant lectins can serve as valuable tools in blood typing and transfusion compatibility assessments. Their ability to specifically bind to distinct features of carbohydrate-based blood group antigens makes them particularly useful in resolving blood typing discrepancies, especially when dealing with specific blood group subtypes that may not be easily identified through conventional methods [7]. However, recent research has shed light on potential limitations of plant lectin-based approaches, particularly in the context of transplantation where accurate subtyping is critical [36]. Despite this, lectins continue to be used to test blood group status of individuals when commonly employed antibody-based approaches are inadequate.

The ability of lectins to differentiate between RBCs based on blood type is not exclusive to plants. Among metazoan lectins, galectins exhibit distinct binding patterns toward RBCs based on blood group status [37]; however, galectin interactions with RBCs are more nuanced compared to plant lectins [38, 39]. While some plant lectins exclusively recognize RBCs of a specific blood type, most galectins can recognize all RBCs but preferentially agglutinate those from certain blood types [40–44]. This subtlety in binding patterns makes it challenging to discern key differences between galectin family members using agglutination assays alone. Moreover, varying quaternary structures of galectins, which can influence their agglutination abilities, further complicate the assessment of galectin interactions with cell surfaces when relying on agglutination assays alone. As a result, while agglutination-based assays are simple and provide an excellent initial approach to assessing lectin-RBC interactions, this strategy does not fully capture the intricate features of galectin-RBC interactions.

To address the limitations of agglutination-based approaches, a wide variety of studies have employed various biochemical strategies in studying galectin-glycan interactions, including the use of glycan microarrays, which have provided valuable insights into the biochemical features of galectins responsible for their specificity for carbohydrate ligands [38–41, 45–51]. However, these techniques often fail to accurately represent features of the cell surface that may influence lectin interactions. While several strategies can be used to overcome this limitation, such as analyzing cell interactions in solid-phase assays [41, 52], flow cytometry offers a straightforward method for examining lectin interactions with the cell surface [40]. We will describe the production, labeling, and use of galectins to investigate their interactions with RBCs through flow cytometric analysis.

2 Materials

2.1 Preparation of Galectin Using E. coli

1. pET-28b(+) vector that contains galectin gene (Gal-4, Gal-4N, Gal-4C).
2. BL-21(DE3) *Escherichia coli.*
3. LB-Kanamycin Solution: LB-Kanamycin Solution was prepared by supplementing standard Luria-Bertani (LB) broth with the 50 μg/mL of the antibiotic kanamycin.
4. Glycerol stock of transformed bacteria.
5. Isopropyl β- d-1-thiogalactopyranoside (IPTG).
6. Centrifuge (6000 × g).
7. Bacterial lysis buffer (*see* **Note 1**):
   - 60 μL of lysozyme stock solution (100 mg/mL; dissolved Lysozyme from chicken egg white, lyophilized powder, [Sigma Aldrich] in sterile H_2O).
   - 60 μL ribonuclease A stock solution (10 mg/mL) (Sigma-Aldrich).
   - 60 μL DNase 1 (10 mg/mL) (Sigma-Aldrich).

- 60 mL PBS with 14 mM beta-mercaptoethanol, pH 7.4, and mix well.
- 2 Pierce™ protease inhibitor tablets (EDTA free; Thermo Fisher Scientific).

8. Sonicator.
9. Centrifuge (20,000 × g).
10. Lactosyl-Sepharose column.
11. Phosphate buffered saline (PBS).
12. Lactose.
13. Amicon ultra-15 centrifugal filter units.

2.2 Preparation of Fluorescent Alexa Fluor 647-Labeled Galectin

1. PD-10 desalting column.
2. Phosphate buffered saline (PBS).
3. Galectin protein solution.
4. Lactose.
5. Alexa Fluor 647 NHS Ester (Lumiprobe, 46820).
6. Aliquot containers.
7. Centrifuge (3400 × g).
8. Amicon ultra-15 centrifugal filter units.
9. Lactosyl-Sepharose column.

2.3 Preparation of RBC Samples

1. Phosphate buffered saline (PBS).
2. Red blood cells (RBCs) with Blood group A, B, and H antigens.
3. Alexa Fluor 647-labeled protein.
4. Thio-Digalactoside (TDG).

2.4 Flow Cytometry Analysis

1. FACS Canto II flow cytometer (BD Biosciences).
2. Sheath fluid.
3. Waste containers.
4. BD FACSDiva software.
5. Flow cytometer sample holder.
6. FlowJo software (version 10).
7. Single-stained controls.
8. Red blood cells (RBCs) with Blood group A, B, and H antigens.
9. Statistical software: GraphPad Prism 10.

3 Methods

3.1 Preparation of Galectin Using E. Coli

1. Cloning and transformation:
   (a) Clone the galectin gene into a pET-28b(+) vector and transform it into BL21(DE3) *Escherichia coli*. Here, we use the DNA sequences of Galectin 4 (Gal-4), N-terminal domain of Galectin 4 (Gal-4N), and C-terminal domain of Galectin 4 (Gal-4C) to express the corresponding proteins.
   (b) Positive clones can be stored at −80 °C as glycerol stocks.
2. Bacterial culture and induction:
   (a) Inoculate 100 mL of LB-Kanamycin solution with a loopful of glycerol stock of the transformed bacteria. Incubate overnight at 37 °C with shaking.
   (b) Inoculate six flasks containing 1 L LB-Kanamycin broth each with 10 mL of the overnight culture.
   (c) Incubate at 37 °C with shaking until OD600 reaches 0.6–0.8.
   (d) Add IPTG to a final concentration of 1 mM and incubate at 16 °C for 20 h with shaking.
3. Harvesting bacterial pellets:
   (a) Centrifuge the culture at 6000 × g for 30 min at 4 °C.
   (b) Collect bacterial pellets and store at −20 °C if not processing immediately.
4. Bacterial lysis:
   (a) Resuspend bacterial pellets in cold bacterial lysis buffer with 14 mM β-mercaptoethanol.
   (b) Sonicate the suspension on ice with a 5 s ON, 5 s OFF cycle for 30 min at 60% intensity.
   (c) Centrifuge the lysate at 20,000 × g for 30 min at 4 °C.
5. Galectin purification:
   (a) Load the supernatant onto a lactosyl-sepharose column equilibrated with PBS.
   (b) Wash the column with 10 column volumes of PBS containing 14 mM β-mercaptoethanol.
   (c) Elute the galectin with 100 mM lactose in PBS containing 14 mM β-mercaptoethanol.
   (d) Concentrate the eluted protein using Amicon Ultra-15 centrifugal filter units.

3.2 Preparation of Fluorescent Alexa Fluor 647-Labeled Galectin (see Note 2)

1. Removing lactose and beta-mercaptoethanol from galectin:
   (a) Equilibrate a PD-10 desalting column with five column volumes of PBS.
   (b) Load the galectin solution onto the prepared PD-10 desalting column.
   (c) Elute galectin with PBS to remove lactose and β-mercaptoethanol.
   (d) Collect the eluate containing purified galectin.
2. Preparing galectin solution:
   (a) Dilute the galectin protein to 2 mg/mL in 1 mL of PBS.
   (b) Add 36 mg of lactose to the 1 mL of PBS to achieve a final concentration of 100 mM lactose.
   (c) Mix thoroughly until the lactose is completely dissolved.
3. Preparing Alexa-647 NHS ester solution:
   (a) Dissolve 25 mg of Alexa Fluor 647 NHS ester in 2.5 mL of PBS to make a 10 mg/mL solution.
   (b) Aliquot the solution into 50 μL portions and store at −80 °C until use.
4. Labeling galectin with Alexa-647:
   (a) Add 50 μL of the 10 mg/mL Alexa Fluor 647 NHS ester solution to 1 mL of 2 mg/mL galectin solution that contains 100 mM lactose.
   (b) Mix gently and incubate at room temperature, in the dark for 1 h.
5. Removing unreacted dye:
   (a) Pass the reaction mixture through a PD-10 desalting column to remove any unreacted Alexa-647 NHS ester.
   (b) Collect the labeled galectin eluate.
6. Purifying active galectin:
   (a) Load the labeled galectin solution onto a lactosyl-sepharose column.
   (b) Wash the column with 5 column volumes of PBS.
   (c) Elute the active protein fraction using 100 mM lactose.
7. Concentrating labeled galectin:
   (a) Use an Amicon Ultra-15 centrifugal filter unit to concentrate the labeled galectin to a final volume of 800 μL.
   (b) Centrifuge at 3400 × g at 4 °C for 20 min, or until the volume reaches 800 μL.

8. Final purification:
   (a) Pass the labeled galectin through a pre-equilibrated PD-10 column to remove residual lactose.
   (b) Determine the concentration of purified, labeled galectin by measuring absorbance at 280 nm (A280) using a spectrophotometer, with correction for Alexa Fluor 647 absorbance at 650 nm (A650).

3.3 Preparation of RBC Samples

1. Resuspension and washing:
   (a) Resuspend RBCs in PBS and wash twice with PBS at 4 °C.
2. Staining with fluorescent proteins:
   (a) Incubate 1 μL packed RBCs with 0.1 μM Alexa Fluor 647-labeled galectin with or without 25 mM thiodigalactoside (TDG) at 4 °C for 20 min.
3. Post-incubation washing:
   (a) Wash the stained cells twice with 200 μL PBS and resuspend them in PBS for flow cytometry analysis.

3.4 Flow Cytometry Analysis (see Note 3)

3.4.1 Instrument Setup

1. Preparation:
   (a) Turn on the FACS Canto II flow cytometer and allow it to warm up for at least 30 min before running samples.
   (b) Ensure that the sheath fluid and waste containers are correctly positioned and filled or emptied as needed.
2. Empirically optimize settings:
   (a) Set up the flow cytometer software (BD FACSDiva) to recognize the specific fluorophores used in the experiment.
   (b) Adjust the photomultiplier tube (PMT) voltage settings for each fluorescence channel to optimize signal detection and minimize background noise.
   (c) Set the appropriate forward scatter (FSC) and side scatter (SSC) thresholds to exclude debris and ensure only RBCs are analyzed.

3.4.2 Data Acquisition

1. Sample loading:
   (a) Vortex the RBC samples gently to ensure even suspension of cells.
   (b) Load the samples into the flow cytometer sample holder.
2. Start the flow cytometer and run the samples at a low flow rate to ensure optimal data collection and avoid coincident events. Monitor the event rate and adjust the sample concentration if necessary to achieve an event rate within the recommended range (*see* **Note 4**).

3. Acquire data for at least 10,000 events per sample.
4. Save the data files in the appropriate format (e.g., FCS format) for subsequent analysis.

3.4.3 Data Processing

1. Use FlowJo software (version 10) for data analysis.
2. Create a forward scatter (FSC) versus side scatter (SSC) plot to distinguish RBCs from debris and other cell types. Apply gates to select the RBC population based on size and granularity. Create additional gates to analyze specific subsets of RBCs based on fluorescence intensity.
3. Median fluorescence intensity (MFI) was measured to quantify galectin binding to the RBC surface. The percentage of positive cells was determined by applying a threshold defined by the negative control.
4. Analyze the binding of fluorescently labeled galectin to RBCs. Compare the binding affinity of galectin to different blood group antigens (A, B, O) with and without the inclusion of TDG (a specific inhibitor of galectin binding).
5. Generate histograms and scatter plots to visualize the binding patterns and quantify the differences between samples.

3.4.4 Data Interpretation

1. Graphical representation: Use FlowJo to generate overlay histograms to visualize the data. Compare the fluorescence intensity distributions between different samples and experimental conditions.
2. Statistical analysis: Perform statistical tests to determine the significance of differences in fluorescence intensity or percentage of positive cells between groups (*see* **Note 5**).
3. Summarize the findings in a comprehensive report, including graphical representations and statistical analysis. Discuss the implications of the results in the context of RBC properties and interactions, particularly focusing on the binding specificity of galectins to glycan structures on RBCs (Fig. 1 and Table 1).

4 Notes

1. Preparation of bacterial lysis buffer: Prepare bacterial lysis buffer fresh and always keep it on ice to maintain its effectiveness and prevent degradation of components.
2. Galectin labeling with Alexa-647 NHS ester: During the reaction of galectin with Alexa-647 NHS ester, the presence of lactose is crucial. Lactose prevents the labeling of amine active residues in galectin, thereby preserving the carbohydrate binding ability of galectin during the NHS labeling process.

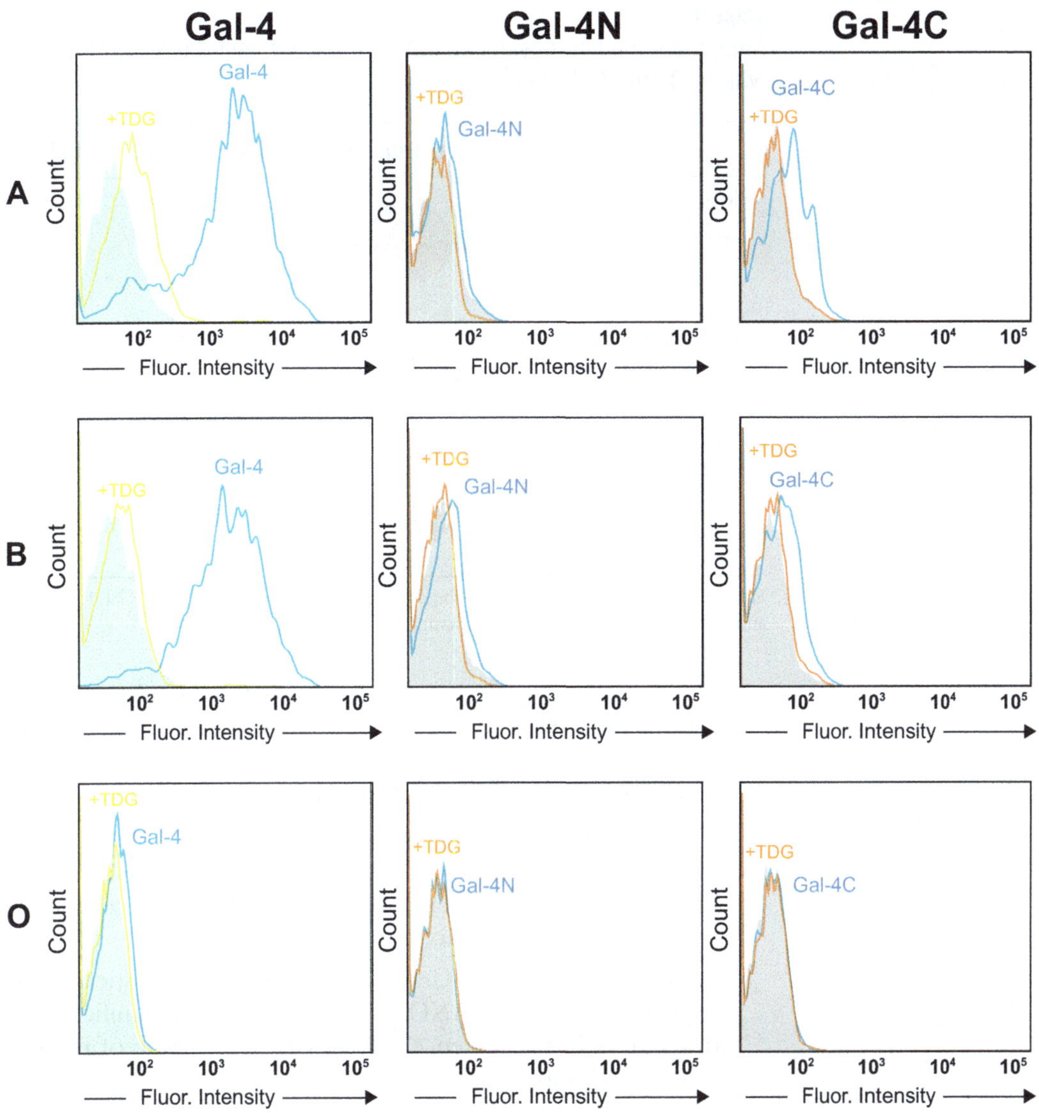

Fig. 1 Differential Binding of Gal-4, Gal-4N, and Gal-4C to RBCs from Blood Groups A, B, and O. Flow cytometric analysis of Gal-4, Gal-4N, and Gal-4C binding to RBCs of blood groups A, B, or O, with and without the inclusion of TDG, as indicated. The histograms show the fluorescence intensity corresponding to galectin binding. The outcome of incubation with each galectin alone is shown in blue, indicating galectin binding to RBCs. TDG inhibition is shown in orange, demonstrating its competitive inhibitory effect on galectin binding. Unstained control samples, which establish the baseline fluorescence of the RBCs without any galectin, are labeled in gray. This analysis highlights the differential binding specificity of Gal-4, Gal-4N, and Gal-4C to various blood group antigens on the RBCs. (This research was originally published in Molecular & Cellular Proteomics. Jan and Wu et al. [47]. © 2024 The Authors)

Table 1
Differential Binding Specificity of Gal-4, Gal-4N, and Gal-4C to RBCs with A, B, and O Antigens

	Blood group antigens	Gal-4	Gal-4N	Gal-4C
Blood group A	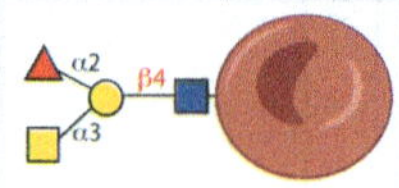	++++	+	++
Blood group B	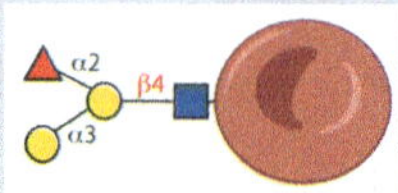	++++	+	++
Blood group O	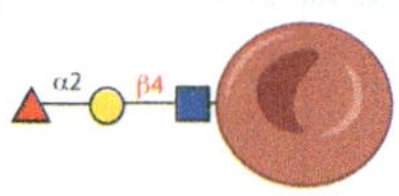	+	++	++

Simplified visual representation of the differential binding specificity of Gal-4, Gal-4N, and Gal-4C to red blood cells containing A, B, and O antigens

3. Flow cytometry analysis is a critical part of examining red blood cells (RBCs) for various parameters such as size, granularity, intracellular content, and surface glycan epitopes. This section provides instructions on setup, data acquisition, and analysis using flow cytometry.
4. Flow cytometry data acquisition: For optimal data acquisition in flow cytometry, an event rate of 500–2000 events per second is suggested to ensure accurate and reliable results.
5. Statistical analysis: Use GraphPad Prism 10 for statistical analysis, such as *t*-tests and ANOVA, to determine the significance of differences in fluorescence intensity or percentage of positive cells between groups.

Conflict of Interest

This work was funded by NIH K99HL169746 and AABB Foundation Early-Career Scientific Research Grants. No other authors have conflicts of interest.

References

1. Tsaneva M, Van Damme EJM (2020) 130 years of plant lectin research. Glycoconj J 37(5):533–551
2. Van Damme EJ (2014) History of plant lectin research. Methods Mol Biol 1200:3–13
3. Rudiger H, Gabius HJ (2001) Plant lectins: occurrence, biochemistry, functions and applications. Glycoconj J 18(8):589–613
4. Sharon N, Lis H (2004) History of lectins: from hemagglutinins to biological recognition molecules. Glycobiology 14(11):53R–62R

5. Sharon N (2008) Lectins: past, present and future. Biochem Soc Trans 36(Pt 6): 1457–1460
6. Stanley P, Sundaram S (2014) Rapid assays for lectin toxicity and binding changes that reflect altered glycosylation in mammalian cells. Curr Protoc Chem Biol 6(2):117–133
7. Jajosky RP et al (2023) ABO blood group antigens and differential glycan expression: perspective on the evolution of common human enzyme deficiencies. iScience 26(1):105798
8. Arthur CM, Stowell SR (2023) The development and consequences of red blood cell alloimmunization. Annu Rev Pathol 18:537–564
9. Jajosky R et al (2023) Prior immunization against an intracellular antigen enhances subsequent red blood cell alloimmunization in mice. Blood 141(21):2642–2653
10. Jajosky RP et al (2023) Antibody-mediated antigen loss switches augmented immunity to antibody-mediated immunosuppression. Blood 142(12):1082–1098
11. Mener A et al (2018) Complement serves as a switch between CD4+ T cell-independent and -dependent RBC antibody responses. JCI Insight 3(22)
12. Adam I et al (2025) ABO-A antibody induction in mice is T cell-dependent, estrogen-independent, and modulated by CD22. Am J Transplant 25(6):1180–1192
13. Bansal N et al (2024) ABO-incompatible heart transplantation-evolution of a revolution. J Heart Lung Transplant 43(9):1514–1520
14. Mener A et al (2018) Complement component 3 negatively regulates antibody response by modulation of red blood cell antigen. Front Immunol 9:676
15. Arthur CM et al (2017) Antigen density dictates immune responsiveness following red blood cell transfusion. J Immunol 198(7): 2671–2680
16. Arthur CM et al (2021) Antigen density dictates RBC clearance, but not antigen modulation, following incompatible RBC transfusion in mice. Blood Adv 5(2):527–538
17. Jajosky RP et al (2024) Dynamics of antibody engagement of red blood cells in vivo and in vitro. Front Immunol 15:1475470
18. Hod EA et al (2010) Use of mouse models to study the mechanisms and consequences of RBC clearance. Vox Sang 99(2):99–111
19. Zimring JC et al (2007) Nonhemolytic antigen loss from red blood cells requires cooperative binding of multiple antibodies recognizing different epitopes. Blood 110(6):2201–2208
20. Hod EA, Zimring JC, Spitalnik SL (2008) Lessons learned from mouse models of hemolytic transfusion reactions. Curr Opin Hematol 15(6):601–605
21. Zimring JC, Spitalnik SL (2015) Pathobiology of transfusion reactions. Annu Rev Pathol 10: 83–110
22. Merle NS et al (2019) P-selectin drives complement attack on endothelium during intravascular hemolysis in TLR-4/heme-dependent manner. Proc Natl Acad Sci USA 116(13): 6280–6285
23. Ghosh S et al (2013) Extracellular hemin crisis triggers acute chest syndrome in sickle mice. J Clin Invest 123(11):4809–4820
24. Meuleman MS, Roumenina LT, Grunenwald A (2023) Complement involvement in sickle cell disease. Presse Med 52(4):104205
25. Roumenina LT, Bartolucci P, Pirenne F (2019) The role of complement in post-transfusion hemolysis and hyperhemolysis reaction. Transfus Med Rev 33(4):225–230
26. Merle NS et al (2019) Complement activation during intravascular hemolysis: implication for sickle cell disease and hemolytic transfusion reactions. Transfus Clin Biol 26(2):116–124
27. Chonat S et al (2020) Role of complement in alloimmunization and hyperhemolysis. Curr Opin Hematol 27(6):406–414
28. Liepkalns JS et al (2013) Resistance of a subset of red blood cells to clearance by antibodies in a mouse model of incompatible transfusion. Transfusion 53(6):1319–1327
29. Viayna E et al (2022) Red cell alloimmunization is associated with increased health care costs, longer hospitalizations, and higher mortality. Blood Adv 6(20):5655–5658
30. Vidler JB et al (2015) Delayed haemolytic transfusion reaction in adults with sickle cell disease: a 5-year experience. Br J Haematol 169(5):746–753
31. Dean CL et al (2019) Challenges in the treatment and prevention of delayed hemolytic transfusion reactions with hyperhemolysis in sickle cell disease patients. Transfusion 59(5): 1698–1705
32. Chonat S et al (2018) Contribution of alternative complement pathway to delayed hemolytic transfusion reaction in sickle cell disease. Haematologica 103(10):e483–e485
33. Dean CL et al (2019) Multiple hemolytic transfusion reactions misinterpreted as severe

vaso-occlusive crisis in a patient with sickle cell disease. Transfusion 59(2):448–453

34. Nickel RS et al (2016) Impact of red blood cell alloimmunization on sickle cell disease mortality: a case series. Transfusion 56(1):107–114
35. Thein SL et al (2020) Hemolytic transfusion reactions in sickle cell disease: underappreciated and potentially fatal. Haematologica 105(3):539–544
36. Joseph A et al (2023) ABO genotyping finds more A(2) to B kidney transplant opportunities than lectin-based subtyping. Am J Transplant 23(4):512–519
37. Liu FT, Stowell SR (2023) The role of galectins in immunity and infection. Nat Rev Immunol 23(8):479–494
38. Wu SC et al (2023) Blood group A enhances SARS-CoV-2 infection. Blood 142(8): 742–747
39. Arthur CM et al (2024) ABO blood groups and galectins: implications in transfusion medicine and innate immunity. Semin Immunol 74-75:101892
40. Stowell SR et al (2008) Galectin-1, −2, and −3 exhibit differential recognition of sialylated glycans and blood group antigens. J Biol Chem 283(15):10109–10123
41. Stowell SR et al (2008) Differential roles of galectin-1 and galectin-3 in regulating leukocyte viability and cytokine secretion. J Immunol 180(5):3091–3102
42. Hirabayashi J et al (2002) Oligosaccharide specificity of galectins: a search by frontal affinity chromatography. Biochim Biophys Acta 1572(2–3):232–254
43. Abbott WM, Hounsell EF, Feizi T (1988) Further studies of oligosaccharide recognition by the soluble 13 kDa lectin of bovine heart muscle. Ability to accommodate the blood-group-H and -B-related sequences. Biochem J 252(1):283–287
44. Feizi T et al (1994) The adhesive specificity of the soluble human lectin, IgE-binding protein, toward lipid-linked oligosaccharides. Presence of the blood group A, B, B-like, and H monosaccharides confers a binding activity to tetrasaccharide (lacto-N-tetraose and lacto-N-neotetraose) backbones. Biochemistry 33(20): 6342–6349
45. Wu SC et al (2021) Full-length Galectin-3 is required for high affinity microbial interactions and antimicrobial activity. Front Microbiol 12: 731026
46. Wu SC et al (2022) Innate immune Galectin-7 specifically targets microbes that decorate themselves in blood group-like antigens. iScience 25(7):104482
47. Jan HM et al (2024) Galectin-4 antimicrobial activity primarily occurs through its C-terminal domain. Mol Cell Proteomics 23(5):100747
48. Blenda AV et al (2022) Galectin-9 recognizes and exhibits antimicrobial activity toward microbes expressing blood group-like antigens. J Biol Chem 298(4):101704
49. Wu SC et al (2023) Whole microbe arrays accurately predict interactions and overall antimicrobial activity of galectin-8 toward distinct strains of Streptococcus pneumoniae. Sci Rep 13(1):5324
50. Stowell SR et al (2014) Microbial glycan microarrays define key features of host-microbial interactions. Nat Chem Biol 10(6): 470–476
51. Stowell SR et al (2010) Innate immune lectins kill bacteria expressing blood group antigen. Nat Med 16(3):295–301
52. Leppanen A et al (2022) Examination of whole-cell galectin binding by solid phase and flow cytometric analysis. Methods Mol Biol 2442:187–203

Chapter 46

Analysis of Erythrocyte Membrane Alloantigens

Kashyap R. Patel, Ryan P. Jajosky, Caitlin L. Cepeda, Vivien C. Lee, and Connie M. Arthur

Abstract

Red blood cell (RBC) transfusion is a critical medical intervention for managing various diseases marked by anemia. However, this treatment carries the risk of alloimmunization, which can result in hemolysis following an incompatible RBC transfusion. Exposure to RBC alloantigens on fetal RBCs can likewise induce a maternal alloimmune response in the setting of pregnancy. Antibody-mediated immunosuppression (AMIS) is currently the only known method to actively prevent alloimmunization following allogeneic RBC exposure. While the mechanism of AMIS remained enigmatic for many years, recent studies suggest that passively administered antibodies may, in part, prevent de novo alloimmunization by inducing the removal of the target antigen from the RBC surface. Although antibody-mediated antigen removal can be detected indirectly by flow cytometry, western blot analysis of the target antigen provides a more definitive assessment of antigen removal following antibody engagement. We will describe the methods used to isolate RBC membrane proteins and analyze the levels of antigen using western blot techniques by employing the Hen egg lysozyme, Ovalbumin, and Duffy (HOD) model system as an example.

Key words Erythrocyte membrane protein, Ghost RBC, Western blot, Antigen modulation

1 Introduction

Red Blood Cell (RBC) transfusion is a critical medical intervention, not only in the emergent setting for patients experiencing acute blood loss but also in the management of patients with chronic conditions, such as sickle cell disease and thalassemia [1, 2]. However, the development of alloantibodies following allogenic RBC exposure can increase the risk of hemolytic transfusion reactions (HTRs) [3–5]. While antibodies directed against ABO blood group antigens are the most frequent immunological barrier to transfusion and transplantation, and likely have important implications in the evolution of innate immune factors that protect blood group positive individuals from microbes that decorate themselves in blood group antigens [6–9], alloantibody formation against high frequency antigens or the generation of complex alloantibody

Sean R. Stowell and Connie M. Arthur (eds.), *Methods in Transfusion Medicine*, Methods in Molecular Biology, vol. 3053,
https://doi.org/10.1007/978-1-0716-5376-0_46,

profiles against a variety of antigens can also increase the length of time required to procure compatible blood, prolonging anemia, and associated complications [10–16]. Alloantibodies that form against RBC alloantigens, either due to transfusion or pregnancy, can also cross the placenta and induce anemia in the developing fetus, resulting in hemolytic disease of the fetus and newborn (HDFN) [17–23]. Transfusion-dependent patients, in particular, such as patients with sickle cell disease, can also experience delayed hemolytic transfusion reactions (DHTRs) and other complications arising from challenges procuring compatible blood in a timely manner [2, 11, 16, 24, 25], which can cause significant complications as DHTRs in particular can be masked by similarities in presentation to the underlying disease [26].

Modern blood banking techniques have reduced the number of HTRs caused by incompatible transfusions [27, 28]. ABO testing and screening for other alloantibodies ensure the appropriate matching to blood products for ABO and RBC-induced alloantibodies. Currently, the International Society of Blood Transfusion (ISBT) recognizes 45 blood group systems containing >300 antigens [29]. Phenotyping of donor RBC units to facilitate alloantigen matching can be performed by serological or molecular methods [30]. Serological methods are based on incubating antibodies with RBCs and then detecting hemagglutination. Newer molecular techniques based on genotyping donors can support high-throughput predictions of RBC antigen expression [31, 32].

Despite the discovery of RBC alloantigens and the ability of fetal RBCs to generate a maternal alloimmune response, mechanisms of alloimmunization against RBC alloantigens, both as a result of pregnancy and following transfusion, have remained relatively unknown [33]. This limited understanding has been partly due to the lack of adequate animal models capable of faithfully recapitulating key elements of this process [3, 33, 34]. However, many studies have now demonstrated through the use of distinct models, key features of the immune response to RBC antigens [21, 35–40]. Recent studies have defined a number of key features of RBC alloimmunization, including the roles of innate immune cells, B cells, T cells, and cytokines that appear to differentially govern the development of alloantibodies following transfusion [41–47]. Similar pathways may be involved in alloimmunization against other intravascularly delivered therapeutics, such as platelets and clotting factor replacements [48–51]. However, a variety of studies have demonstrated that each alloantigen appears to engage unique pathways [39, 52–54], highlighting the importance of identifying common nodes when seeking to actively target the development of alloantibodies in at-risk patients [55].

While alloantigen matching protocols have been implemented to reduce the likelihood of alloimmunization [31, 56–58], few options exist for targeted prevention of alloantibody formation following alloantigen exposure during pregnancy. This is especially important when considering that the paternal blood type is rarely known prior to pregnancy, making efforts focused on the prevention of alloantigen exposure impractical. Given the risk of developing alloantibodies during pregnancy and the potential complications of maternal alloimmunization on a developing fetus, strategies capable of actively inhibiting alloimmunization are needed. Through a combination of epidemiological and basic science studies, the possibility of inhibiting de novo alloantibody formation through passive administration of antibodies directed against the most common offending antigen, RhD, was realized [59]. This process, termed antibody-mediated immunosuppression (AMIS), has significantly reduced the incidence of anti-D antibody formation in RhD negative mothers carrying a RhD positive fetus [23].

While AMIS has proven effective in preventing RhD alloimmunization, its application remains limited to this specific antigen, leaving alloimmunization to other antigens during pregnancy largely unaffected. The inability to extend the success of anti-D to other alloantigens stems partly from an incomplete understanding of the underlying mechanism of AMIS. Various theories have been proposed to explain how passively administered antibodies prevent new antibody formation, including steric hindrance, inhibitory Fc receptor engagement, rapid RBC removal, and, more recently, antibody-induced antigen loss [18, 19, 22, 60, 61]. Except for active immune suppression through inhibitory Fc receptors, these mechanisms are generally thought to function by reducing the availability of antigen to corresponding antigen-specific B cells and recent studies have provided key insight into factors that may regulate antibody-induced antigen removal [17, 60, 62, 63]. Recent utilization of preclinical models has allowed a number of studies to provide significant insight into the various consequences of antibody engagement that may contribute to the inhibition or augmentation of an alloimmune response following allogeneic RBC exposure [18, 20, 22, 36, 53, 64–68].

Despite the putative role of antibody-induced antigen loss in AMIS, antigen loss can be challenging to detect. Among approaches for examining antigen levels, western blot analysis is a practical and widely used method for directly examining antigen levels beyond flow cytometry, offering an effective strategy to analyze complex protein mixtures, including RBC membrane proteins. This technique, which involves detergent-free hypotonic lysis of RBCs to generate a membrane fraction, has been successfully employed in various studies [45, 69, 70] to characterize RBC membrane protein variations in Alzheimer's disease, elucidate the role of complement in alloimmunization, and identify mouse RBC autoantigens in autoimmune hemolytic anemia. Here, we describe

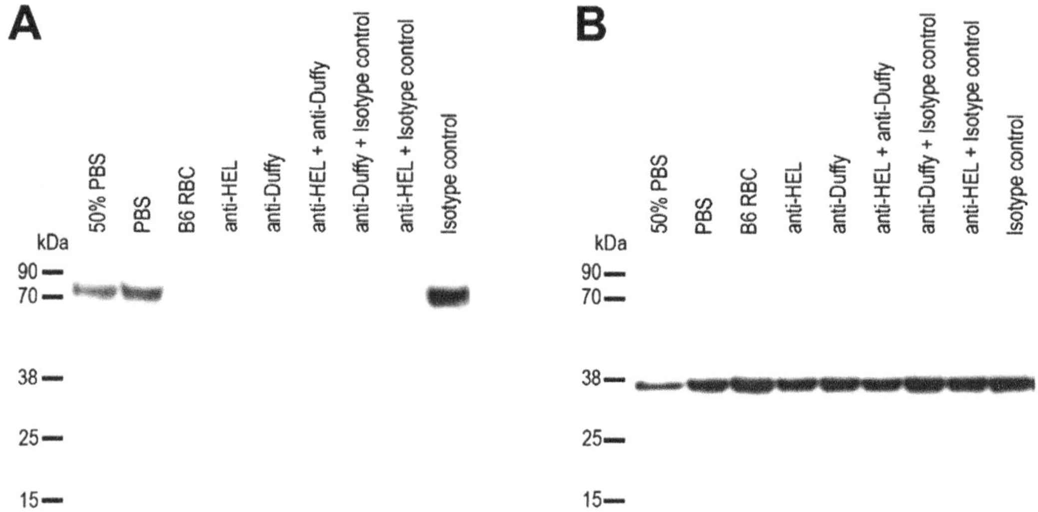

Fig. 1 Western blot analysis of red blood cell (RBC) membrane proteins. (**a**) Blot showing a band corresponding to HOD (Hen egg lysozyme, Ovalbumin, and Duffy) antigen when probed for Hen egg lysozyme (HEL). Each lane contains RBC membrane proteins isolated by hypotonic lysis after 48 h post HOD RBC transfusion in B6 mice passively immunized with various antibodies indicated on top of the blot. Reduced signal observed when mice are passively immunized with anti-HEL or anti-Duffy mouse IgG1 and IgG2a antibodies, respectively. (**b**) The same blot is stripped and re-probed with anti-GAPDH antibody to confirm equal sample loading in each well. (Image was adapted from a first version published in *Blood*. Jajosky et al. [68])

the use of western blot analysis to examine the modulation of the HOD (Hen egg lysozyme, Ovalbumin and Duffy) antigen when studying AMIS [68] (Fig. 1).

2 Materials

2.1 Preparation of Ghost RBCs

1. B6 mice transfused with FVB HOD RBCs and passively immunized with anti-HOD antibodies.
2. Sterile 1.5 mL and 2 mL polypropylene tubes.
3. Murine whole blood collection tools based on approved IACUC (Institutional Animal Care and Use Committee) protocol.
4. Anticoagulant Citrate Dextrose (ACD-A) Solution.
5. Centrifuge with adjustable brakes and capable of holding 2 mL, 15 mL, and 50 mL tubes.
6. Phosphate buffered saline (PBS) pH 7.4, without calcium and magnesium.
7. RBC lysis buffer: 5 mM disodium hydrogen monophosphate, pH 7.4.

8. RBC lysis buffer with protease and phosphatase inhibitor—weigh and add protease and phosphatase inhibitor to make 1% w/v solution (Thermo Fisher Scientific) (*see* **Note 1**).

2.2 Western Blot

1. Bicinchoninic acid (BCA) assay kit.
2. 4× Laemmli Sample Buffer (non-reducing).
3. Heat block.
4. SDS-polyacrylamide Bis-Tris gel (4–20% polyacrylamide gradient).
5. Tris-MOPS SDS-PAGE running buffer: 50 mM Tris Base, 50 mM MOPS, 0.1% SDS, 1 mM EDTA, pH 7.0.
6. Polyvinylidene difluoride membrane.
7. Western blotting sponge pads and filter paper.
8. Western blot transfer buffer: 25 mM Tris Base, 192 mM glycine, 0.1% SDS, 20% methanol, pH 8.3.
9. Methanol.
10. Western blot transfer apparatus.
11. PBST: PBS with 0.05% Tween 20.
12. Western blot blocking buffer: 5% skimmed milk in PBST (*see* **Note 2**).
13. Orbital shaker.
14. Peroxidase conjugated anti-HEL antibody (Rockland, 200-4375S) diluted 1:1000 in western blot blocking buffer.
15. Mouse anti-GAPDH antibody (Abcam, ab125247) diluted 1: 5000 in western blot blocking buffer.
16. Peroxidase conjugated anti-mouse IgG (R&D Biosystem, HAF007).
17. Enhanced chemiluminescence (ECL) western blot substrate (Thermo Fisher Scientific).
18. Blot stripping buffer: 25 mM Glycine, 1% SDS, pH 2.0.
19. Western blot imaging system.

3 Methods

3.1 Preparation of Murine RBC Membrane Fraction

1. Collect whole blood in a sterile 1.5 mL tube by an appropriate IACUC-approved method from a B6 mouse transfused with FVB HOD RBCs and passively immunized with anti-HOD antibodies. Approximately 500 μL of whole blood can be collected from the face-bleed method of an adult mouse (*see* **Note 3**).

2. Immediately add sterile ACD-A solution to the whole blood at a whole blood to ACD-A ratio of approximately 10:1 (V/V) to prevent coagulation.
3. Centrifuge whole blood at 800× *g* for 10 min at 25 °C with brakes turned off to separate cells from plasma and anticoagulant.
4. Aspirate and discard the top layer of plasma without disturbing the packed RBC pellet.
5. Transfer 200 μL of packed RBCs to a 50 mL conical bottom tube and add 20 mL cold PBS. Gently invert the tube a few times to resuspend the RBC pellet.
6. Centrifuge the tube at 800× *g* for 10 min at 4 °C with brakes set on low. Carefully aspirate and discard the supernatant without disturbing the pellet.
7. Resuspend the pellet in 20 mL cold PBS and repeat the wash twice, for a total of three times, to remove contaminating plasma proteins.
8. After removing supernatant from the last wash, collect the 50 μL of the cell pellet from the 50 mL tube and transfer the cells to a fresh 2 mL tube and store on ice for the following procedure.
9. Add 1800 μL cold RBC lysis buffer to the tube and gently lyse the cells by inverting the tube a few times. Centrifuge the tube at 16,000× *g* for 30 min at 4 °C with brakes set on low.
10. Aspirate and discard the 1800 μL supernatant without disturbing the pellet (*see* **Note 4**).
11. Add 1800 μL cold RBC lysis buffer and resuspend the pellet by pipetting. Centrifuge the tube at 16,000× *g* for 10 min at 4 °C with brakes set on low. Aspirate and discard the 1800 μL supernatant without disturbing the pellet. Wash the pellet by repeating this step three more times for four washes (*see* **Note 5**).
12. Wash the RBC membrane pellet with 1800 μL cold RBC lysis buffer containing protease and phosphatase inhibitor. Centrifuge the sample at 16,000× *g* for 10 min at 4 °C with brakes set on low. Aspirate and discard the supernatant.
13. Resuspend pellet in 100 μL cold PBS and store at −80 °C.

3.2 Western Blot

1. Thaw the RBC membrane samples by leaving them on ice and dilute the sample twofold in PBS. Determine total protein concentration with bicinchoninic acid (BCA) assay by following the suggested manufacturer's protocol (*see* **Note 6**). Use 40 μg RBC membrane protein for western blot analysis.
2. Heat 40 μg membrane protein on a heat block for 5 min at 80 °C after adding Laemmli sample buffer (non-reducing).

3. Resolve the sample on an SDS-polyacrylamide Bis-Tris gel (4–20% polyacrylamide gradient) in the presence of Tris-MOPS running buffer for 1 h at 150 V of constant voltage (*see* **Note 7**).
4. Soak the gel, filter paper, PVDF membrane, and sponge pads in western blot transfer buffer for at least 10 min prior to starting the transfer. Pre-wet the PVDF membrane in 100% methanol before transferring it into the blotting buffer.
5. Assemble the western blotting apparatus and transfer the resolved proteins from the gel onto the PVDF membrane according to the manufacturer's protocol.
6. Wash the membrane with 10 mL PBST for 5 min to remove excess transfer buffer. Add the membrane to 10 mL blocking buffer and incubate for 1 h on an orbital shaker.
7. Remove the blocking buffer and add 10 mL peroxidase conjugated anti-HEL antibody diluted 1:1000 in blocking buffer. Incubate at 4 °C for 18 h on an orbital shaker.
8. Remove the antibody solution and wash the membrane with 10 mL PBST by incubating for 5 min on an orbital shaker. Change the wash buffer three more times, each time adding fresh 10 mL PBST followed by 5 min incubation.
9. Remove the membrane from the wash buffer and add 6 mL ECL western blot substrate to cover the whole membrane. Incubate for 5 min and capture an image using an imaging system capable of detecting chemiluminescence (*see* **Note 8**).
10. Wash off the ECL western blot substrate by washing the membrane with 10 mL PBST and 5 min incubation on an orbital shaker. Repeat the wash two more times.
11. Transfer the membrane into a western blot stripping buffer and incubate on an orbital shaker for 10 min.
12. Remove the western blot stripping buffer and wash the membrane with 10 mL PBST and 5 min incubation on an orbital shaker. Repeat the wash two more times.
13. Re-block the membrane with blocking buffer as previously described and stain the membrane with 1:5000 diluted anti-GAPDH antibody in blocking buffer for 18 h at 4 °C on an orbital shaker.
14. Remove the antibody solution and wash the membrane with 10 mL PBST by incubating for 5 min on an orbital shaker. Change the wash buffer three more times, each time adding fresh 10 mL PBST followed by 5 min incubation.
15. Add 10 mL peroxidase conjugated anti-mouse IgG diluted 1:1000 in blocking buffer. Incubate at 25 °C for 1 h on an orbital shaker.

16. Wash the unbound antibodies with 10 mL PBST by incubating for 5 min on an orbital shaker. Change the wash buffer three more times, each time adding fresh 10 mL PBST followed by 5 min incubation.
17. Re-image the membrane by following the procedure described in **step 9**.
18. Quantify the intensity of the observed bands (*see* **Note 9**).

4 Notes

1. Prepare fresh RBC lysis buffer with protease and phosphatase inhibitor immediately before use.
2. Prepare fresh western blot blocking buffer immediately before use.
3. Minimum volume requirement for western blot analysis of RBC membrane fraction is 50 μL packed murine RBC, corresponding to approximately 120 μL whole blood.
4. The cell membrane pellet can be difficult to distinguish from the cytoplasm of RBC. Tilt the tube at a 45° angle and aspirate from the top of the supernatant.
5. After four washes with RBC lysis buffer, the pellet should have minimal hemoglobin. If the pellet appears red, then proceed with additional washes following the same centrifugation speed and time until the pellet turns visibly white.
6. A twofold dilution at a minimum is required to bring the membrane protein concentration within the linear range of the assay. The expected range of protein concentration is 1 to 2 mg/mL.
7. Precast gels compatible with the available SDS-PAGE gel running system can be used to ensure migration homogeneity and reproducibility.
8. Exposure time must be adjusted to detect possible faint bands.
9. Band intensity can be quantified with image analysis software such as ImageJ.

Acknowledgments

This work was funded by NIH P01HL171803, R01 HL165975, R01 HL135575, R01 HL154034, K08HL171877, and AABB Foundation Early-Career Scientific Research Grants. No other conflicts of interest to report.

References

1. Pirenne F, Floch A, Diop S (2023) Alloimmunisation against red blood cells in sickle cell disease: transfusion challenges in high-income and low-income countries. Lancet Haematol 10(6):e468–e476
2. Pirenne F, Yazdanbakhsh K (2018) How I safely transfuse patients with sickle-cell disease and manage delayed hemolytic transfusion reactions. Blood 131(25):2773–2781
3. Zimring JC, Spitalnik SL (2015) Pathobiology of transfusion reactions. Annu Rev Pathol 10: 83–110
4. Narbey D et al (2017) Incidence and predictive score for delayed hemolytic transfusion reaction in adult patients with sickle cell disease. Am J Hematol 92(12):1340–1348
5. Dean CL et al (2019) Challenges in the treatment and prevention of delayed hemolytic transfusion reactions with hyperhemolysis in sickle cell disease patients. Transfusion 59(5): 1698–1705
6. Storry JR, Olsson ML (2009) The ABO blood group system revisited: a review and update. Immunohematology 25(2):48–59
7. Wu SC et al (2023) Blood group a enhances SARS-CoV-2 infection. Blood 142(8): 742–747
8. Blenda AV et al (2022) Galectin-9 recognizes and exhibits antimicrobial activity toward microbes expressing blood group-like antigens. J Biol Chem 298(4):101704
9. Jan HM et al (2024) Galectin-4 antimicrobial activity primarily occurs through its C-terminal domain. Mol Cell Proteomics 23(5):100747
10. Roumenina LT, Bartolucci P, Pirenne F (2019) The role of complement in post-transfusion hemolysis and hyperhemolysis reaction. Transfus Med Rev 33(4):225–230
11. Merle NS et al (2019) Complement activation during intravascular hemolysis: implication for sickle cell disease and hemolytic transfusion reactions. Transfus Clin Biol 26(2):116–124
12. Chonat S et al (2019) Challenges in preventing and treating hemolytic complications associated with red blood cell transfusion. Transfus Clin Biol 26(2):130–134
13. Merle NS et al (2019) P-selectin drives complement attack on endothelium during intravascular hemolysis in TLR-4/heme-dependent manner. Proc Natl Acad Sci USA 116(13): 6280–6285
14. Chang DY et al (2023) The ongoing challenge of RBC alloimmunization in the management of patients with sickle cell disease. Presse Med 52(4):104211
15. Falguiere C et al (2023) Delayed hemolytic transfusion reaction in children with sickle cell disease: first 5-year retrospective study in mainland France. Haematologica 108(3):889–894
16. Thein SL et al (2020) Hemolytic transfusion reactions in sickle cell disease: underappreciated and potentially fatal. Haematologica 105(3):539–544
17. Brinc D, Lazarus AH (2009) Mechanisms of anti-D action in the prevention of hemolytic disease of the fetus and newborn. Hematology Am Soc Hematol Educ Program 2009:185–191
18. Yu H et al (2014) Antibody-mediated immune suppression of erythrocyte alloimmunization can occur independently from red cell clearance or epitope masking in a murine model. J Immunol 193(6):2902–2910
19. Sullivan HC et al (2018) Anti-RhD reduces levels of detectable RhD antigen following anti-RhD infusion. Transfusion 58(2): 542–544
20. Bernardo L et al (2015) IgG-mediated immune suppression to erythrocytes by polyclonal antibodies can occur in the absence of activating or inhibitory Fcgamma receptors in a full mouse model. J Immunol 195(5): 2224–2230
21. Stowell SR et al (2013) Alloantibodies to a paternally derived RBC KEL antigen lead to hemolytic disease of the fetus/newborn in a murine model. Blood 122(8):1494–1504
22. Stowell SR et al (2015) Anti-KEL sera prevents alloimmunization to transfused KEL RBCs in a murine model. Haematologica 100(10):e394–e397
23. Stowell SR (2016) Working together to block alloimmunization. Blood 128(8):1029–1030
24. Vidler JB et al (2015) Delayed haemolytic transfusion reaction in adults with sickle cell disease: a 5-year experience. Br J Haematol 169(5):746–753
25. Pirenne F, Pondarre C (2023) Alloimmunization and hyperhemolysis in sickle cell disease. Hematology Am Soc Hematol Educ Program 2023(1):653–659
26. Chonat S et al (2025) Complement is activated in patients with acute chest syndrome caused by sickle cell disease and represents a therapeutic target. Sci Transl Med 17(807):eadl4922
27. Storch EK et al (2019) Review of current transfusion therapy and blood banking practices. Blood Rev 38:100593

28. Hendrickson JE, Tormey CA, Shaz BH (2014) Red blood cell alloimmunization mitigation strategies. Transfus Med Rev 28(3):137–144
29. Gassner C et al (2022) International Society of Blood Transfusion Working Party on Red Cell Immunogenetics and Blood Group Terminology Report of Basel and three virtual business meetings: update on blood group systems. Vox Sang 117(11):1332–1344
30. Quirino MG et al (2019) Methods for blood group antigens detection: cost-effectiveness analysis of phenotyping and genotyping. Hematol Transfus Cell Ther 41(1):44–49
31. Cone Sullivan JK, Gleadall N, Lane WJ (2022) Blood group genotyping. Clin Lab Med 42(4): 645–668
32. Raos M et al (2022) The role of serological and molecular testing in the diagnostics and transfusion treatment of autoimmune haemolytic anaemia. Blood Transfus 20(4):319–328
33. Hod EA, Zimring JC, Spitalnik SL (2008) Lessons learned from mouse models of hemolytic transfusion reactions. Curr Opin Hematol 15(6):601–605
34. Hod EA et al (2010) Use of mouse models to study the mechanisms and consequences of RBC clearance. Vox Sang 99(2):99–111
35. Thomas TA et al (2023) Reticulocytes in donor blood units enhance red blood cell alloimmunization. Haematologica 108(10):2639–2651
36. Jash A et al (2024) Complement C3 and marginal zone B cells promote IgG-mediated enhancement of RBC alloimmunization in mice. J Clin Invest 134(8):e167665
37. Maier CL et al (2023) Storage differentially impacts alloimmunization to distinct red cell antigens following transfusion in mice. Transfusion 63(3):457–462
38. Arthur CM et al (2021) Antigen density dictates RBC clearance, but not antigen modulation, following incompatible RBC transfusion in mice. Blood Adv 5(2):527–538
39. Arthur CM et al (2022) Clodronate inhibits alloimmunization against distinct red blood cell alloantigens in mice. Transfusion 62(5): 948–953
40. Patel SR et al (2018) Recipient priming to one RBC alloantigen directly enhances subsequent alloimmunization in mice. Blood Adv 2(2): 105–115
41. Tamagne M et al (2021) Whole-blood CCR7 expression and chemoattraction in red blood cell alloimmunization. Br J Haematol 194(2): 477–481
42. Pal M et al (2021) Hemolysis inhibits humoral B-cell responses and modulates alloimmunization risk in patients with sickle cell disease. Blood 137(2):269–280
43. Godefroy E et al (2015) TIGIT-positive circulating follicular helper T cells display robust B-cell help functions: potential role in sickle cell alloimmunization. Haematologica 100(11):1415–1425
44. Yazdanbakhsh K, Shaz BH, Hillyer CD (2017) Immune Regulation of sickle Cell Alloimmunization. ISBT Sci Ser 12(1):248–253
45. Mener A et al (2018) Complement component 3 negatively regulates antibody response by modulation of red blood cell antigen. Front Immunol 9:676
46. Godefroy E et al (2016) Altered heme-mediated modulation of dendritic cell function in sickle cell alloimmunization. Haematologica 101(9):1028–1038
47. Mener A et al (2018) Complement serves as a switch between CD4+ T cell-independent and -dependent RBC antibody responses. JCI Insight 3(22):e121631
48. Zerra PE et al (2017) Marginal zone B cells are critical to factor VIII inhibitor formation in mice with hemophilia A. Blood 130(23): 2559–2568
49. Arthur CM et al (2022) Nonhuman glycans can regulate anti-factor VIII antibody formation in mice. Blood 139(9):1312–1317
50. Zerra PE et al (2020) Fc gamma receptors and complement component 3 facilitate anti-fVIII antibody formation. Front Immunol 11:905
51. Arthur CM et al (2016) CD8+ T cells mediate antibody-independent platelet clearance in mice. Blood 127(14):1823–1827
52. Arneja A et al (2016) Interleukin-6 receptor-alpha signaling drives anti-RBC alloantibody production and T-follicular helper cell differentiation in a murine model of red blood cell alloimmunization. Haematologica 101(11): e440–e444
53. Jash A et al (2021) Antibodies to low-copy number RBC alloantigen convert a tolerogenic stimulus to an immunogenic stimulus in mice. Front Immunol 12:629608
54. Jajosky R et al (2023) Prior immunization against an intracellular antigen enhances subsequent red blood cell alloimmunization in mice. Blood 141(21):2642–2653
55. Zerra PE et al (2021) Marginal zone B cells mediate a CD4 T-cell-dependent extrafollicular antibody response following RBC transfusion in mice. Blood 138(8):706–721
56. Vichinsky EP et al (1990) Alloimmunization in sickle cell anemia and transfusion of racially unmatched blood. N Engl J Med 322(23): 1617–1621
57. Chou ST et al (2013) High prevalence of red blood cell alloimmunization in sickle cell

disease despite transfusion from Rh-matched minority donors. Blood 122(6):1062–1071

58. Wolf J et al (2024) Red cell specifications for blood group matching in patients with haemoglobinopathies: an updated systematic review and clinical practice guideline from the international collaboration for transfusion medicine guidelines. Br J Haematol 206(1):94–108
59. Reali G (2007) Forty years of anti-D immunoprophylaxis. Blood Transfus 5(1):3–6
60. Cruz-Leal Y et al (2024) Trogocytosis drives red blood cell antigen loss in association with antibody-mediated immune suppression. Blood 143(9):807–821
61. Jajosky RP et al (2024) Dynamics of antibody engagement of red blood cells in vivo and in vitro. Front Immunol 15:1475470
62. Cruz-Leal Y, Lazarus AH (2021) Could antigen loss be a potential mechanism to explain antibody-mediated immune suppression? Transfusion 61(4):1004–1006
63. Cruz-Leal Y, Marjoram D, Lazarus AH (2017) Prevention of hemolytic disease of the fetus and newborn: what have we learned from animal models? Curr Opin Hematol 24(6):536–543
64. Liu J et al (2016) Antigen modulation as a potential mechanism of anti-KEL immunoprophylaxis in mice. Blood 128(26):3159–3168
65. Maier CL et al (2018) Antibody-mediated immune suppression by antigen modulation is antigen-specific. Blood Adv 2(21):2986–3000
66. Shinde P et al (2020) IgG subclass determines suppression versus enhancement of humoral alloimmunity to Kell RBC antigens in mice. Front Immunol 11:1516
67. Mener A et al (2019) Antibody-mediated immunosuppression can result from RBC antigen loss independent of Fcgamma receptors in mice. Transfusion 59(1):371–384
68. Jajosky RP, Patel KR, JWL A, Zerra PE, Chonat S, Ayona D, Maier CL, Morais D, Wu SC, Luckey CJ, Eisenbarth SC, Roback JD, Fasano RM, Josephson CD, Manis JP, Chai L, Hendrickson JE, Hudson KE, Arthur CM, Stowell SR (2023) Antibody-mediated antigen loss switches augmented immunity to antibody-mediated immunosuppression. Blood 142(12):1082–1098
69. Mohanty JG et al (2010) Alterations in the red blood cell membrane proteome in alzheimer's subjects reflect disease-related changes and provide insight into altered cell morphology. Proteome Sci 8:11
70. Barker R N et al (1993) Identification of murine erythrocyte autoantigens and cross-reactive rat antigens. Immunology 78 (4):568–573

Chapter 47

Extraction and Quantification of Skin Immune Cells and Skin Lipids

Ruth Choa, Lillian Sun, and Taku Kambayashi

Abstract

We have recently shown that the immune system, specifically T cells stimulated by the skin-derived cytokine thymic stromal lymphopoietin, can promote total body adipose loss. This effect is caused by the regulation of lipid metabolism in the skin, whereby T cells induce the release of a lipid-rich substance called sebum. The adoptive transfer of thymic stromal lymphopoietin-stimulated T cells can also induce adipose loss and sebum secretion, making this approach applicable to cellular therapies for metabolic and dermatologic diseases. The skin is the body's largest organ system and provides a critical barrier surface that senses and protects the host from the outside environment. Sebocytes within the skin secrete sebum, a lipid-rich substance that coats the skin and protects it against water, pathogens, and sun damage while also regulating the skin immune landscape and microbiome. Methods to quantify and characterize sebum production are needed to better investigate the role of sebum in skin immunobiology. Here, we describe a protocol that we developed to extract lipids from mouse fur followed by thin layer chromatography analysis of the various lipid classes. We also describe a protocol to maximally extract immune cells from the skin for flow cytometric analysis, which has previously been limited by low cell numbers. These methods will be useful to study skin immunobiology including, but not limited to, its impact on sebum secretion.

Key words Sebum, T cells, Skin immune cells, Skin lipids, Thin layer chromatography

1 Introduction

The skin is the largest barrier surface in the body, interfacing between the outside world and the rest of the body. In addition to its thermoregulatory roles, the skin both senses our environment and mediates protection from it [1]. Sebum contributes to all components of the skin barrier including the mechanical, chemical, immunologic, and microbiome barriers. The acidic nature of sebum prevents bacterial and viral skin penetration, inhibits expression of bacterial colonization factors, and functions as a delivery vehicle for secreted antimicrobial peptides such as defensins, cathelicidins, and RNAses [2–4]. Fatty acid components of sebum such as sapienic acid and oleic acid are directly cytotoxic to bacteria and

Sean R. Stowell and Connie M. Arthur (eds.), *Methods in Transfusion Medicine*, Methods in Molecular Biology, vol. 3053, https://doi.org/10.1007/978-1-0716-5376-0_47,

fungi [5]. Skin resident memory T cells rely on sebum as a nutritional source [6] while skin innate lymphoid cells (ILCs) and invariant natural killer T cells (iNKTs) are activated to secrete inflammatory cytokines in response to changes in sebum composition [7, 8]. Sebum composition also critically dictates commensal microbiota composition, which is critical for preventing skin colonization by pathogenic bacteria [9, 10] and educating the cutaneous immune system [11, 12].

It has recently been shown that the immune system can regulate skin lipid production [13]. Thymic Stromal Lymphopoietin (TSLP) is a barrier site cytokine that is produced by the skin and can stimulate whole body loss of adipose tissue by promoting the loss of lipids at the skin as sebum, a lipid-rich substance produced by skin sebocytes [13]. TSLP activates T cells to secrete interleukin-4 and 13 (IL-4/13) which act directly on skin sebocytes to increase cell lipogenesis, turnover, and holocrine secretion of sebum [13, 14]. The loss of lipids as sebum causes the body to undergo white adipose tissue lipolysis as it replenishes the lipids being lost at the skin. Transfer of TSLP-activated T cells into TSLP naïve mice also results in adipose loss and increased sebum production [13], suggesting that adoptive cell therapy methods can be used to target the TSLP-sebum axis. In this chapter, we describe methods to study skin immune cells and their impact on sebum secretion and composition.

First, we developed a method to optimize extraction of immune cells from the skin. There are many different methods reported for extracting lymphocytes from the skin. It is intuitive that different protocols of lymphocyte extraction would lead to differential extraction of cells. This differential extraction can affect the absolute number of cell populations and the frequencies of specific cell populations. For example, reported frequencies of regulatory T cells as a fraction of CD4 T cells vary as much as 15–60% in naïve ear skin [15–17]. Absolute numbers vary even more from method to method. Given this variability in the efficiency of T cell isolation from skin tissue, we sought to optimize a protocol that would maximize extraction of viable T cells from ear skin. We compared techniques for mechanical dissociation of ear skin as well as different concentrations of DNase. Many published methods instruct the fine mincing of ear tissue prior to digestion. However, we surprisingly found that reversing the order, i.e., mincing after digestion, doubled the number of live cells, and increased the number of $TCRb^+$ cells from ear tissue by tenfold (Fig. 1). In addition, we found that using a DNase I concentration of 500 mg/mL, compared to 100 mg/mL, in the digestion solution yielded double the number of $CD4^+$ T cells (Fig. 1).

Next, we developed a method to study skin sebum production using thin layer chromatography (TLC). Various methods exist to study skin sebaceous gland biology. Hematoxylin and eosin staining

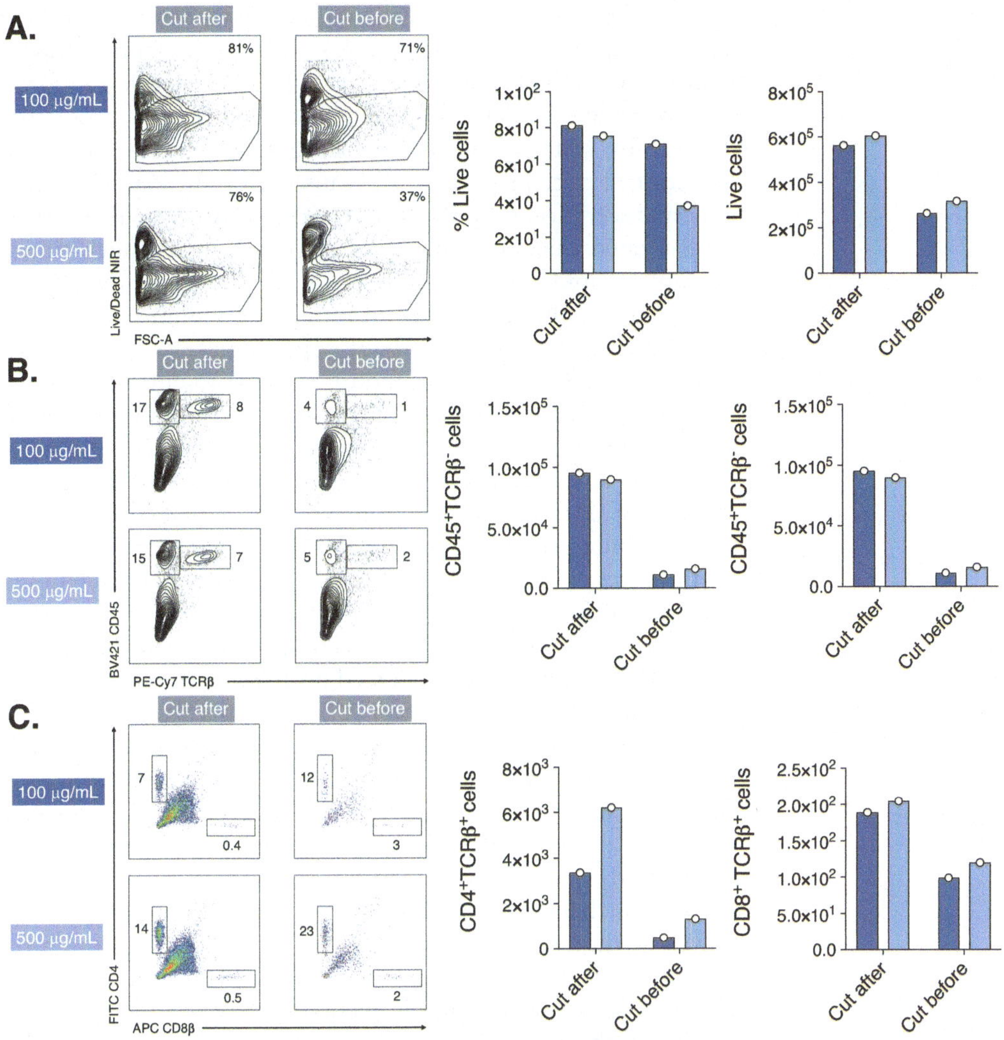

Fig. 1 Sample flow cytometric data following isolation of lymphocytes from the skin. Flow cytometric plots and quantification of cells of skin cut after (left plots) or before (right plots) digestion with DNase at 100 mg/mL (top plots) or 500 mg/mL (bottom plots) are shown for (**a**) total live cells, (**b**) TCRb$^-$ or TCRb$^+$ CD45$^+$ cells, and (**c**) CD4$^+$ or CD8$^+$ CD45$^+$TCRb$^+$ cells

of sebaceous glands allows for quantification of sebocyte cell number and size. Additional stains with Oil Red O, which stains neutral lipids, and Nile Red, which stains both neutral and polar lipids, can be used to quantify lipid content within sebocytes [18]. However, the issue with these histologic methods is that they do not capture the actual secretion of sebum from sebocytes. Sebum is released from sebocytes via a process called holocrine secretion, whereby mature sebocytes die and release their intracellular lipid contents up the hair follicle [19]. Thus, simply looking at sebocyte size or lipid content does not provide information about holocrine secretion rate. Larger sebocyte size with higher lipid content may be an inaccurate proxy for actual increased secretion and release of sebum. For example, mice treated with TSLP develop a "greasy fur" appearance, visibly displaying increased sebum production, however by histological analysis, have smaller sebaceous glands than control mice [13]. This is because TSLP increases the rate of holocrine secretion such that the sebocyte turnover rate is faster in TSLP-treated mice and sebocytes do not have as much time to accumulate lipid intracellularly as the lipids are being expulsed extracellularly. Other methods of measuring sebum have included visual grading or using absorbent paper, tapes, or glass slides to photometrically quantify the amount of lipid present on the surface of a skin area [20]. However, these methods only work well for hairless skin areas on humans and do not work well for mouse models. In addition, these methods can quantify total skin lipids but do not differentiate between different sources of skin lipids which include sebocytes, which produce ~80% of skin lipids, or keratinocytes, which produce ~20% of skin lipids [21]. Lipidomics with high performance liquid chromatography and mass spectrometry (MS) is a newer method that can identify specific lipid species and provide comprehensive detailed profiling of the skin lipid composition at very high resolution [22]. It is particularly useful for probing a change in a specific lipid species in response to a certain treatment. However, MS tends to be expensive and time-consuming and so may not be the best method for high through-put sample processing. Also, depending on the lipid species being investigated, it may be time and effort-intensive to develop a MS method for that certain lipid. Therefore, a skin lipid isolation and analysis method that is low-cost, easy to use, and high through-put, yet can still distinguish between lipid classes derived from sebum vs. keratinocyte lipids is needed.

The method for lipid isolation described here allows for analysis of lipid classes by thin layer chromatography (TLC). It relies on chemical extraction of lipids from mice fur followed by separation of lipid classes on a gel by polarity. The gel is then developed and imaging analysis programs such as ImageJ can be used to quantify various lipid classes. Classes of lipids that can be evaluated include squalene, cholesterol esters, wax esters, triglycerides, free fatty acids, and free cholesterol. The quantification of wax esters can help determine the amount of sebum, since they are present in sebum but not in keratinocyte lipids. This method is relatively high-throughput, inexpensive, and easy to use.

2 Materials

2.1 Immune Cell Isolation from Skin

1. Donor mice.
2. Ice bucket, ice.
3. Scissors.
4. Blunt tweezers.
5. Pointed tweezers.
6. 24-well plate.
7. RPMI-1640 (Gibco, henceforth RPMI-0).
8. RPMI-1640 supplemented with 10% FBS (RPMI-10).
9. Liberase TL (Roche).
10. DNAse I, grade II (Roche).
11. 1.7 mL microcentrifuge tubes.
12. Bulb transfer pipette.
13. 70 mm cell strainer.
14. 50 mL conicals.
15. Centrifuge.
16. Incubator.
17. Pipette.
18. Pipette tips.

2.2 Lipid Extraction from Fur

1. Mice.
2. Clippers.
3. 20 mL glass vials.
4. 4 mL glass vials.
5. Scale.
6. Centrifuge.
7. Glass beaker.
8. Chloroform.
9. Methanol.
10. Acetone.
11. Ultrasonic water bath.
12. Syringes.
13. Syringe filters.
14. N_2 gas evaporator.
15. Pipette.
16. Pipette tips.

2.3 Thin Layer Chromatography

1. Pencil.
2. Ruler.
3. TLC plates (Sigma-Aldrich).
4. TLC nonpolar lipid mixture standard (Matreya).
5. Oleyl Oleate wax ester standard.
6. Glass TLC tanks.
7. Glass beakers.
8. Hexane.
9. Isopropyl diether.
10. Acetic acid.
11. Benzene.
12. Cupric sulfate.
13. Phosphoric acid.
14. Baking oven.
15. Pipette.
16. Pipette tips.

2.4 TLC Analysis

1. Adobe photoshop.
2. ImageJ.
3. Prism or R.

3 Methods

3.1 Immune Cell Isolation from Skin

1. Fill ice bucket with ice.
2. Prepare 1 mL digest solution per mouse in a conical tube.
   (a) Serum-free RPMI.
   (b) 250 mg/mL Liberase TL (from −20 °C frozen stock at 5 mg/mL in PBS).
   (c) 500 mg/mL DNase I (from −20 °C frozen stock of 10 mg/mL in PBS).
3. Label a 24-well plate, 2 wells/mouse.
4. Add 460 mL digest solution to these wells.
5. Place a 24-well plate on ice.
6. Euthanize mice.
7. Cut both ears from each mouse along the line where fur begins, using blunt tweezers and scissors.
8. Place 1 ear in each of the two wells allocated per mouse, keeping the plate on ice.

9. Repeat in batches as needed until ears have been collected from all mice, taking care to place the tissues on ice as soon as possible after euthanasia. This will help maintain the cell viability.
10. Split (separate) each ear into dorsal and ventral sides, pulling apart using a pair of pointed tweezers.
11. Place both halves of the ear dermis side down back into the well, ensuring the tissue lays flat and that the dermis side maintains good contact with the digest solution. This is critical for complete digestion.
12. When all ears have been split, place the plate in an incubator set to 37 °C for 1 h and 45 min.
13. After the digest is complete, place the 24-well plate back on ice.
14. Add 460 mL of RPMI containing 10% FBS to each well to quench the reaction.
15. For each sample:
    (a) Transfer both ears of each mouse from the two separate wells into labeled 1.7 mL tubes.
    (b) Use a transfer pipette to transfer the liquid from one of the wells into the 1.7 mL tube.
    (c) Use sharp scissors to quickly mince tissue for ~30 s and transfer liquid to a labeled 15 mL conical tube.
    (d) Transfer the liquid from the second well to wash the 1.7 mL tube and transfer into the same 15 mL conical tube.
    (e) Add 2 mL of serum-free RPMI to the 15 mL conical tube.
    (f) Use a transfer pipette to pipette up and down vigorously ~30 times.
    (g) Pass through a 70 mm cell strainer into a labeled 50 mL tube.
    (h) Wash filter with 6 mL of serum-free RPMI into the same tube.
    (i) Place the 50 mL conical tube on ice.
16. Centrifuge samples at 1200 rpm for 5 min at 4 °C.
17. Aspirate supernatant.
18. Resuspend pellet in 450 mL of RPMI containing 10% FBS.
19. Cells are now ready for in vitro assays, antibody staining, and flow cytometry.

3.2 Lipid Extraction from Fur

1. Euthanize mice.
2. Shave an equal area of back fur from all mice (either 2.5 cm × 5 cm or 3 cm × 3 cm works well; do not spray fur with ethanol). The direction of shaving should be from the tail toward the head.

3. Place the fur into labeled 20 mL glass vials with 1 vial per mouse sample. Fur can either be used directly in the next proceeding step of lipid extraction or stored at −20 °C for up to 1 month for lipid extraction later.
4. Label the 4 mL glass vials with sample names. Weigh the empty 4 mL vials.
5. Spin down the fur in the 20 mL glass vials at 2000 rpm for 7 min at room temp in the centrifuge so that all the fur is at the bottom of the 20 mL glass vials.
6. Make a 2:1 volume ratio of chloroform:methanol in a glass beaker. Add 2 mL of chloroform:methanol mixture to each fur sample in the 20 mL glass vials, making sure to submerge the fur.
7. Cap the 20 mL glass vials tightly and place them into a water bath sonicator for 6 min. After 6 min, remove the samples from the water bath and dry the outside of each 20 mL glass vial with a paper towel.
8. Cap the syringes with syringe filters. Transfer 1.6 mL of chloroform:methanol from each 20 mL glass vial to a syringe and syringe filter into the corresponding 4 mL glass vial for each sample. Make sure to transfer the same amount of liquid from each sample.
9. Next, add 2 mL of acetone to the fur in the 20 mL glass vials.
10. Cap the 20 mL glass vials tightly and place them into a water bath sonicator for 6 min. After 6 min, remove the samples from the water bath and dry the outside of each 20 mL glass vial with a paper towel.
11. Transfer 1.6 mL of acetone from each 20 mL glass vial to the syringes and syringe filter into the corresponding 4 mL glass vial for each sample. Make sure to transfer the same amount of liquid from each sample to the syringe. There should be approximately 3.2 mL of total liquid containing chloroform, methanol and acetone in each 4 mL glass vial.
12. Place the 4 mL vials onto a nitrogen evaporator to dry (*see* **Note 1**).
13. Weigh the dried 4 mL tubes, subtract the empty vial weight to get the lipid weight.
14. Resuspend the dried lipids in 0.25 mL of chloroform/methanol (4:1, %volume/volume v/v) for loading onto TLC plates. Sample vials can be wrapped in parafilm and stored at −80 °C for up to 2 weeks or can be used directly for TLC.

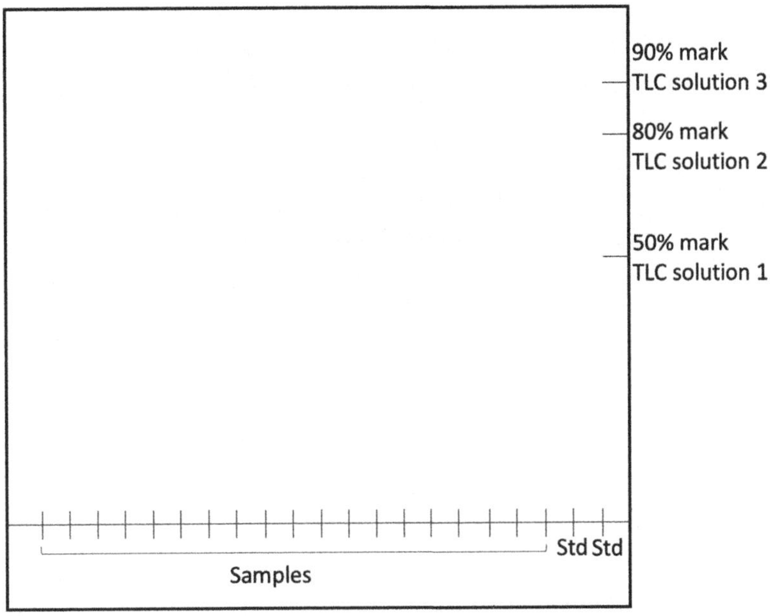

Fig. 2 Example TLC plate layout. The bottom horizontal line is drawn 1.5 cm up from the bottom of the plate. Dash marks for standards (std) and samples are drawn. Dash marks indicating the height to which the three TLC solutions are run are drawn on the side of the plate at 50%, 80% and 90% up the plate height

3.3 Thin Layer Chromatography (TLC)

1. Spotting the TLC plate (*see* Fig. 2 for example plate layout) (*see* **Notes 2** and **3**).
   (a) With a pencil, draw a horizontal line across the bottom of the plate, 1.5 cm up from the bottom edge of the plate.
   (b) Mark dashes along the right edge of the plate at 50%, 80%, and 90% of the plate height up from the bottom horizontal line.
   (c) Mark out evenly spaced dashes along the bottom horizontal line for all the samples (one dash per sample), making sure to also include dashes for the lipid standards (TLC nonpolar lipid mixture and Oleyl oleate wax ester).
   (d) Carefully pipette 5 mL of each sample drop by drop on the designated dashes at the bottom line. Touch the pipette tip to the plate and let the fluid release naturally onto the spot without pushing down on the plunger to keep the spot small. Allow each droplet to dry before adding more sample to the same spot.
   (e) Pipette 1 mL of standards to the designated dashes.
2. Preparing the TLC solutions:
   (a) Make 100 mL of each TLC solution (three total) in separate beakers and pour separately into each TLC tank:
      (i) Solution 1: 80:20:1 hexane:isopropyl diether: acetic acid.

(ii) Solution 2: 1:1 hexane: benzene.

(iii) Solution 3: 100% hexane.

3. Running the TLC plate (*see* **Note 4**):

   (a) Gently place the TLC plate in TLC solution 1 (80:20:1 hexane:isopropyl diether:acetic acid). Make sure that the solution height does not surpass that of the bottom horizontal line where the samples are spotted.

      (i) Allow the solution to run up to the 50% mark on the plate. Make sure to place the lid on the TLC tank or else the solution will evaporate quickly.

   (b) Carefully take out the plate from the tank and let it air dry for 15 min.

   (c) Next, place the TLC plate in TLC solution 2 (1:1 hexane: benzene).

      (i) Allow the solution to run up to the 80% mark. Make sure to place the lid on the TLC tank.

   (d) Carefully take out the plate from the tank and let it air dry for 15 min.

   (e) Finally, place the TLC plate in TLC solution 3 (100% hexane).

      (i) Allow the solution to run to the 90% mark (top of plate). Make sure to place the lid on the TLC tank.

   (f) Carefully take out the plate from the tank and let it air dry for 15 min.

4. Spray the plate uniformly with a solution of 10% cupric sulfate and 8% phosphoric acid diluted in water (should be a bright blue solution) and let it air dry for ~10 min (preheat the oven to 120 °C during this time).

   (a) To make ~200 mL of 10% cupric sulfate with 8% phosphoric acid solution combine the following:

      (i) 31.6 g cupric sulfate.

      (ii) 172.8 mL DI water.

      (iii) 8 mL phosphoric acid.

5. Bake the TLC plate at 120 °C for 20 min to visualize the lipid species. *See* Fig. 3 for an example of lipid classes seen by TLC.

6. Allow the TLC plate to cool for 5 min.

7. Take a photograph or scan the TLC plate to create a jpeg file that can be analyzed.

3.4 TLC Analysis

1. Open the jpeg file in Adobe Photoshop and threshold the image by setting the background level of brightness.

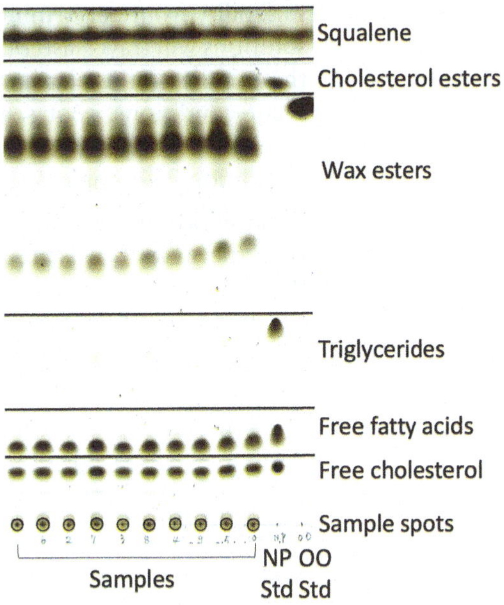

Fig. 3 Example TLC plate after development and oxidation of lipid species for visualization. Shown is an example of a developed TLC plate following cupric sulfate/phosphoric acid treatment and baking. Lipid classes that can be visualized include free cholesterol, free fatty acids, triglycerides, wax esters, cholesterol esters, and squalene. The standards nonpolar lipid mixture (NP Std, visualizes free cholesterol, free fatty acids, and triglycerides) and oleyl oleate (OO Std, visualizes wax esters) can be used to determine where the various lipid classes appear

2. Open the thresholded image in ImageJ and use the "integrated intensity" feature to quantify the intensity of each lipid band for each sample (*see* **Notes 5** and **6**).
3. Compare intensities of lipid bands for each lipid class between samples by using Prism or R.

4 Notes

1. When placing samples on the nitrogen evaporator, place a pipette tip on the tip of the nitrogen evaporator sample needle. Lower the sample needle slowly into the 4 mL glass vial containing the sample, making sure not to touch the liquid sample itself and making sure that the nitrogen gas is not too strong to cause significant spraying of the liquid sample, as this can cause loss of sample. It may take several hours or overnight for the samples to evaporate.
2. When spotting samples on the TLC plate, make sure to alternate samples from different conditions to decrease sample

variability from performing TLC (when running the TLC, the solutions will travel faster up the edges of the plate compared to the middle of the plate). For example, if there are two treatment conditions, spot samples from right to left: Condition 1—sample 1; Condition 2—sample 1; Condition 1—sample 2; Condition 2—sample 2, etc.

3. When spotting the samples on the TLC plate, it is important to keep the spot of the sample as small as possible and make sure that the samples do not touch each other. This prevents contamination between the samples.
4. It is possible to run a total of up to four TLC plates at a time in each TLC tank solution by placing the TLC plates against each other back-to-back (glass sides facing each other) and then leaning two TLC plates each against each side of the TLC tank wall. Ensure that the gel side of the TLC plates does not contact the other plates.
5. Triglycerides are usually only seen in fur from mice eating a high-fat diet. Mice eating normal chow have very few triglycerides in their fur.
6. There are often two bands seen for wax esters seen by TLC, one band that is more polar (lower band on the plate) and one that is less polar (higher band on the plate). Oleyl oleate is less polar and migrates to the higher wax ester band. To quantify total wax esters in a sample, analyze the intensity for each wax ester band separately and add them together.

Conflicts of Interest

The authors have no conflicts of interest to declare that are relevant to the content of this chapter.

References

1. Eyerich S, Eyerich K, Traidl-Hoffmann C, Biedermann T (2018) Cutaneous barriers and skin immunity: differentiating a connected network. Trends Immunol 39:315–327
2. Rippke F, Schreiner V, Schwanitz HJ (2002) The acidic milieu of the horny layer: new findings on the physiology and pathophysiology of skin pH. Am J Clin Dermatol 3:261–272
3. Lee DY et al (2008) Sebocytes express functional cathelicidin antimicrobial peptides and can act to kill propionibacterium acnes. J Invest Dermatol 128:1863–1866
4. Borkowski AW, Gallo RL (2011) The coordinated response of the physical and antimicrobial peptide barriers of the skin. J Invest Dermatol 131:285–287
5. Lovászi M, Szegedi A, Zouboulis CC, Törőcsik D (2017) Sebaceous-immunobiology is orchestrated by sebum lipids. Dermatoendocrinol 9: e1375636
6. Pan Y et al (2017) Survival of tissue-resident memory T cells requires exogenous lipid uptake and metabolism. Nature 543:252–256
7. de Jong A (2015) Activation of human T cells by CD1 and self-lipids. Immunol Rev 267:16–29
8. Kim BS (2015) Innate lymphoid cells in the skin. J Invest Dermatol 135:673–678

9. Byrd AL, Belkaid Y, Segre JA (2018) The human skin microbiome. Nat Rev Microbiol 16:143–155
10. Iwase T et al (2010) Staphylococcus epidermidis Esp inhibits Staphylococcus aureus biofilm formation and nasal colonization. Nature 465: 346–349
11. Nakatsuji T, Cheng JY, Gallo RL (2021) Mechanisms for control of skin immune function by the microbiome. Curr Opin Immunol 72:324–330
12. Lunjani N, Ahearn-Ford S, Dube FS, Hlela C, O'Mahony L (2021) Mechanisms of microbe-immune system dialogue within the skin. Genes Immun 22:276–288
13. Choa R et al (2021) Thymic stromal lymphopoietin induces adipose loss through sebum hypersecretion. Science 373:eabd2893
14. Choa R et al (2024) Thymic stromal lymphopoietin induces IL-4/IL-13 from T cells to promote sebum secretion and adipose loss. J Allergy Clin Immunol 154(2):480–491
15. Harrison OJ et al (2019) Commensal-specific T cell plasticity promotes rapid tissue adaptation to injury. Science 363:eaat6280
16. Tanaka Y, Yokoyama Y, Kambayashi T (2023) Skin-derived TSLP stimulates skin migratory dendritic cells to promote the expansion of regulatory T cells. Eur J Immunol 53: e2350390
17. Zarin P et al (2023) Treg cells require Izumo1R to regulate γδT cell-driven inflammation in the skin. Proc Natl Acad Sci USA 120: e2221255120
18. Hinde E et al (2013) A practical guide for the study of human and murine sebaceous glands in situ. Exp Dermatol 22:631–637
19. Niemann C, Horsley V (2012) Development and homeostasis of the sebaceous gland. Semin Cell Dev Biol 23:928–936
20. Firooz A, Rajabi-Estarabadi A, Zartab H (2017) Agache's Measuring the Skin: Non-invasive Investigations, Physiology, Normal Constants. Springer International Publishing Switzerland, pp 133–142 https://doi.org/10.1007/978-3-319-32383-1
21. Pappas A (2009) Epidermal surface lipids. Dermatoendocrinology 1:72–76
22. Camera E, Ludovici M, Galante M, Sinagra JL, Picardo M (2010) Comprehensive analysis of the major lipid classes in sebum by rapid resolution high-performance liquid chromatography and electrospray mass spectrometry. J Lipid Res 51:3377–3388

Chapter 48

Defining the Role of Marginal Zone B Cells in RBC Alloimmunization

James W. McCoy, Sungwoong Kim, Zahra Naseh, Megan Fuller, Sumaiya Dickens, Montana Jackson, Toni Chanroo, and Patricia E. Zerra

Abstract

Red blood cell (RBC) transfusions are critical for treating a range of hematologic and surgical conditions but carry the risk of alloimmunization, particularly in chronically transfused individuals such as those with sickle cell disease. The development of alloantibodies complicates subsequent transfusions, increases the likelihood of hemolytic reactions, and can undermine curative interventions like bone marrow transplantation. Although current preventive strategies, including extended antigen matching, have reduced alloimmunization rates, they are not universally effective. Recent findings using the HOD mouse model, which expresses hen egg lysozyme, ovalbumin, and the human Duffy antigen, highlight a pivotal role for marginal zone (MZ) B cells in initiating alloantibody responses. Depletion of MZ B cells markedly impairs both IgM and IgG production, suggesting an alternative immune activation pathway independent of conventional germinal center responses driven by T follicular helper and follicular B cells. Additionally, transfused RBC immunogenicity appears to be modulated by antigen-intrinsic factors such as storage duration, emphasizing the influence of antigen-specific properties on immune outcomes. These insights reveal a complex interplay between cellular and antigenic determinants in shaping alloimmune responses. Advanced tools like flow cytometry and immunohistochemistry have proven indispensable in dissecting these mechanisms and hold promise for guiding the development of more effective strategies to prevent RBC alloimmunization.

Key words Red blood cell transfusion, Alloimmunization, Marginal zone B cells, Marginal Zone B Cell Depletion, HOD mouse model, Immunohistochemistry, Flow cytometry

1 Introduction

Red blood cell (RBC) transfusions are among the most frequently performed medical interventions, yet they carry the significant risk of alloimmunization, an immune response in which the recipient develops antibodies against non-self RBC alloantigens [1–3]. This process can complicate future transfusions and increase the

James W. McCoy and Sungwoong Kim have contributed equally to this work.

Sean R. Stowell and Connie M. Arthur (eds.), *Methods in Transfusion Medicine*, Methods in Molecular Biology, vol. 3053, https://doi.org/10.1007/978-1-0716-5376-0_48,

likelihood of severe hemolytic reactions, particularly in patients who require chronic transfusion support, such as those with sickle cell disease (SCD). The presence of alloantibodies not only makes it more difficult to find compatible blood units but can also exacerbate underlying anemia, elevate morbidity and mortality [2, 4–8], and compromise the efficacy of curative treatments like hematopoietic stem cell transplantation and gene therapy, which often rely on extensive transfusion support. While strategies such as matching for common alloantigens have helped reduce alloimmunization rates [9], they remain insufficient in fully preventing these responses [10, 11]. Therefore, identifying shared immune mechanisms that drive alloantibody formation across diverse antigens is essential for developing more effective and broadly applicable prevention strategies.

Traditionally, alloantibody formation has been attributed to downstream immune processes involving $CD4^+$ T follicular helper (TFH) cells [12] and follicular (FO) B cells [13–17] within germinal centers (GCs), which drive high-affinity, long-lived antibody responses [18, 19]. Although therapeutic efforts targeting FO B-cell and TFH responses are promising, defining immune pathways that are triggered before their activation may allow for earlier intervention and prevention of downstream immune amplification. Recent studies have highlighted marginal zone (MZ) B cells as key early initiators of alloimmunization, independent of conventional germinal center pathways (Fig. 1). For example, in the KEL RBC model expressing the clinically relevant human KEL antigen, MZ B cells are both necessary and sufficient to drive IgG alloantibody formation in a $CD4^+$ T-cell-independent manner [20]. These findings prompted an investigation into whether similar pathways are engaged by other alloantigens. Using the HOD model, which expresses hen egg lysozyme (HEL), ovalbumin (OVA), and the human Duffy antigen, we found that MZ B cells are also essential for initiating alloimmunization [21]. HOD RBCs localize to the splenic marginal sinus, colocalizing with MZ B cells, and depletion of these cells significantly impairs both IgM and IgG responses. However, unlike KEL, HOD-induced alloantibody formation requires $CD4^+$ T-cell help, indicating engagement of a distinct immune pathway. Together, these results suggest that while MZ B cells serve as a common early checkpoint across multiple alloantigen models, the downstream immune trajectory may diverge depending on the specific antigen involved. This underscores the potential of targeting MZ B cell-mediated pathways as a complementary strategy to modulate RBC alloimmunization at its earliest stages.

To interrogate these complex interactions, advanced immunological tools such as flow cytometry and fluorescent microscopy have proven indispensable. Flow cytometry enables detailed phenotypic and quantitative analyses of immune cell populations,

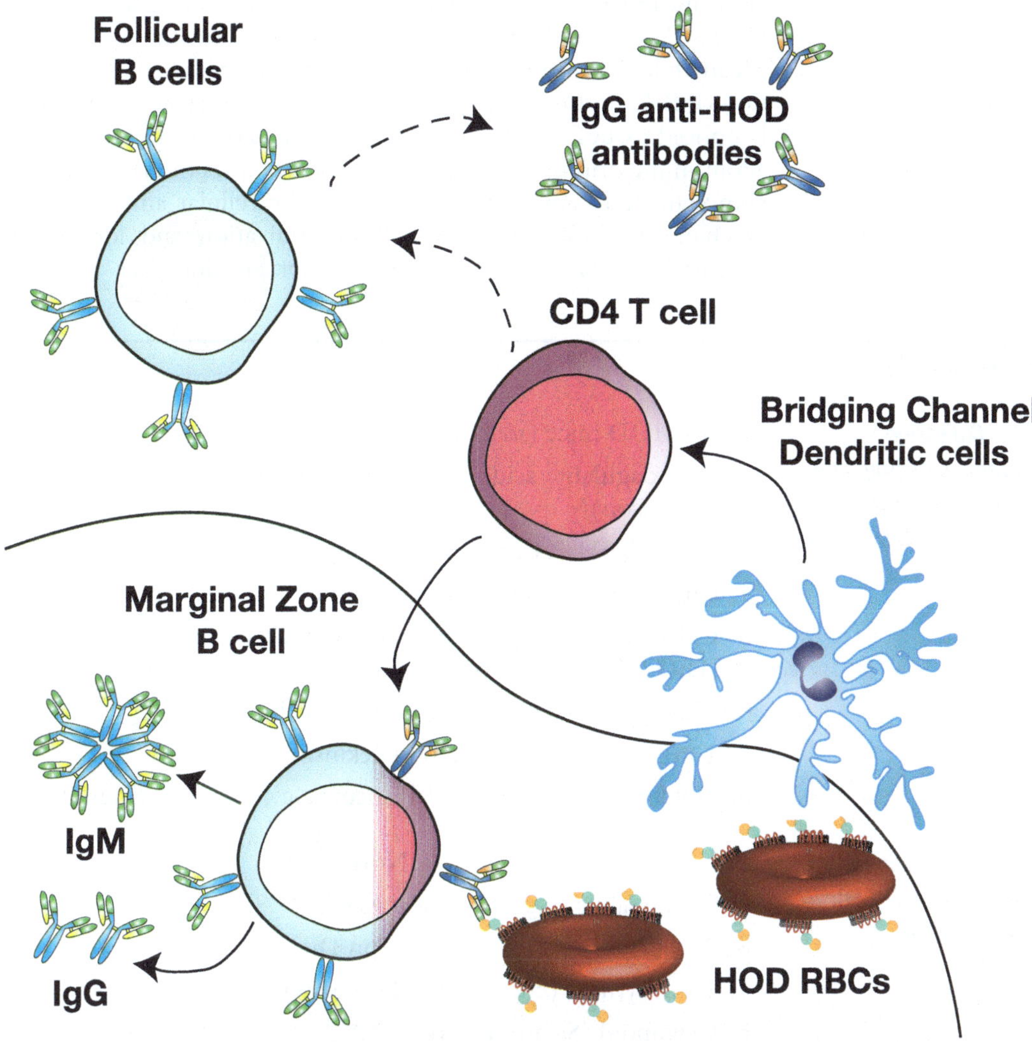

Fig. 1 Schematic Illustration of Cellular Interactions Driving Antibody Responses to HOD RBCs. This figure depicts the proposed cellular interactions involved in the alloantibody response to HOD RBCs. Transfused HOD RBCs localize within the splenic marginal zone, where they are captured by MZ B cells and dendritic cells. MZ B cells contribute to early antibody responses by directly secreting IgM and IgG antibodies. Bridging channel dendritic cells extend into the follicle and interact with CD4 T cells, facilitating their activation. Within the follicle, CD4 T cells provide help to follicular (FO) B cells, which undergo germinal center reactions and contribute to the production of high-affinity IgG anti-HOD antibodies. This schematic highlights the coordinated roles of innate-like and adaptive immune cells in shaping the alloimmune response to transfused RBCs. (This research was originally published in *Blood* [21] with permission from *Blood*, the Journal of the American Society of Hematology)

allowing researchers to monitor dynamic changes in MZ B cells, CD4$^+$ T cells, and other relevant subsets following transfusion. Meanwhile, immunohistochemistry (IHC) provides spatial resolution of RBC-immune cell interactions within the spleen and other lymphoid tissues, revealing key patterns of colocalization that drive alloimmune priming. Together, these techniques offer a powerful, complementary approach to dissecting the cellular and molecular mechanisms underlying RBC alloimmunization and identifying potential targets for early therapeutic intervention.

2 Materials

2.1 Collection, Storage, Labeling, and Transfusion of DiO-Labeled B6-HOD RBCs

1. B6-HOD mice (*see* **Note 1**).
2. Anticoagulant acid citrate dextrose (ACD) (e.g., Becton Dickinson).
3. 1X PBS, pH 7.4 (e.g., Cytiva, Sterile).
4. Citrate phosphate dextrose adenine (CPDA-1) (e.g., Fenwal).
5. CellTracker, 3, 39-dihexadecyloxacarbocyanine perchlorate (DiO; Molecular Probes).
6. 27½-gauge needle (e.g., Becton Dickinson).
7. 1 mL syringe (e.g., Becton Dickinson).
8. Goldenrod 5.5 mm animal lancet (e.g., Braintree Scientific).

2.2 Cryosectioning of Spleen for HOD RBC Colocalization Analysis

1. C57BL/6, H-2^b mice (*see* **Note 1**).
2. Sterile saline (e.g., Fresenius Kabi).
3. 27½-gauge needle (e.g., Becton Dickinson).
4. 1 mL syringe (e.g., Becton Dickinson).
5. Cryomold (Sakura Finetek USA).
6. 2-methylbutane (Isopentane, e.g., Sigma-Aldrich).
7. Dry ice.
8. Tissue-Tek O.C.T. Compound (OCT) (Sakura Finetek USA).
9. Leica CM 1850 Cryostat (or suitable equipment).
10. Slides, glass (e.g., Fisher Scientific).
11. Acetone (e.g., Sigma-Aldrich).

2.3 Immunohistochemistry (IHC) Staining of Spleen Sections

1. PAP pen (Electron Microscopy Sciences).
2. 1X Phosphate-buffered saline (PBS), pH 7.4 (e.g., Cytiva, Sterile).
3. Glass pipette (e.g., Fisher Scientific).
4. Vacuum pump.

5. 5% Blocking buffer (5% Fetal bovine serum (FBS) or bovine serum albumin (BSA) in PBS, e.g., Thermo Fisher Scientific).
6. Humidification chamber (Electron Microscopy Sciences).
7. Fisherbrand Multi-Platform Shaker (or suitable equipment).
8. Alexa Fluor 647 Rat anti-Mouse IgD (Biolegend).
9. PE Rat anti-Mouse CD1d antibody (BD Biosciences).
10. Prolong Gold antifade mounting media (Thermo Fisher Scientific).
11. Cover slip (e.g., Sigma-Aldrich).

2.4 MZ B Cell Depleting Antibody IP Injections (Day −4 and −2)

1. C57BL/6, H-2^b mice (*see* **Note 1**).
2. 1X PBS, pH 7.4 (e.g., Cytiva, Sterile).
3. 5 mL Macro centrifuge tubes (e.g., Celltreat).
4. CD11a antibody (anti-Mouse LFA-1α) (clone M17/4, Bio X Cell).
5. CD49d antibody (anti-Mouse/Human VLA-4) (clone PS/2, Bio X Cell).
6. CD11a Isotype control Rat IgG2a antibody (clone 2A3, Bio X Cell).
7. CD49a Isotype control Rat IgG2b antibody (clone LTF2, Bio X Cell).
8. 27½-gauge needle (e.g., Becton Dickinson).
9. 1 mL syringe (e.g., Becton Dickinson).

2.5 Transfusing B6-HOD RBCs (Day 0)

1. DiO-labeled HOD RBCs (*see* Subheadings 2.1 and 3.1).
2. 27½-gauge needle (Becton Dickinson).
3. 1 mL syringe (Becton Dickinson).

2.6 Collection of Splenocytes for MZ B Cell Depletion Assessment (Day +1, +5, +7, and +14)

1. MZ B cell-depleted C57BL/6, H-2^b mice (*see* Subheadings 2.4 and 3.4).
2. Isoflurane (Piramal Critical Care).
3. Styrofoam dissection station.
4. Surgical scissors and forceps (e.g., Sigma-Aldrich).
5. Ethanol, 70% (e.g., Sigma-Aldrich).
6. 50 mL conical tube (e.g., MIDSCI).
7. R10 Medium (10% FBS in RPMI 1640, e.g., Sigma-Aldrich).
8. Cell strainer, 70 μm (e.g., Sigma-Aldrich).
9. 1 mL syringe (e.g., Becton Dickinson).
10. Sigma red cell lysis buffer (e.g., Sigma-Aldrich).
11. 1X PBS, pH 7.4 (e.g., Cytiva, Sterile).

2.7 Cell Counting and Flow Cytometry Staining

1. Trypan blue (e.g., Sigma-Aldrich).
2. Cell counting slide (Nexcelom).
3. Nexcelom Cellometer Auto T4 (or suitable equipment).
4. 1X PBS, pH 7.4 (e.g., Cytiva, Sterile).
5. 96-well plate (e.g., Corning).
6. Zombie NIR Fixable Viability Kit (Biolegend).
7. FACS buffer (1% BSA in PBS).
8. Mouse Fc block (e.g., BD Bioscience).
9. Alexa 700 Rat anti-Mouse B220 (clone RA3-6b2, Biolegend).
10. Pacific Blue Rat anti-Mouse CD21 (clone 7G6(RUO), Biolegend).
11. APC Rat anti-Mouse CD23 antibody (clone B3B4, Biolegend).

2.8 Flow Crossmatch (Day +3, +5, +7, +14, and +21)

1. Experimental C57BL/6, H-2^b mice (*see* Subheadings 2.4–2.5 and 3.4–3.5).
2. Anticoagulant acid citrate dextrose (ACD) (e.g., Becton Dickinson).
3. 1 mL Eppendorf tube (VWR Micro Centrifuge Tube).
4. 1X PBS, pH 7.4 (e.g., Cytiva, Sterile).
5. DPBS (Dulbecco's Phosphate Buffered Saline) (Sigma).
6. 96-well U-bottom plate (Cat# 268152, Thermo Scientific).
7. APC Goat anti-Mouse IgG (Jackson ImmunoResearch Laboratories).
8. FITC Goat anti-Mouse IgM (Jackson ImmunoResearch Laboratories).
9. PE Goat anti-Mouse IgG1 (Jackson ImmunoResearch Laboratories).
10. Alexa Fluor 488 Goat anti-Mouse IgG2b (Jackson ImmunoResearch Laboratories).
11. PE Host Goat anti-Mouse IgG2c (Jackson ImmunoResearch Laboratories).
12. PerCP Goat anti-Mouse IgG3 (Jackson ImmunoResearch Laboratories).
13. FACS buffer (1% BSA in PBS).

3 Methods

3.1 Collection, Storage, DiO-Labeling, and Transfusion of DiO-Labeled B6-HOD RBCs

1. Collect 2100 μL of whole blood from B6-HOD mice via cheek bleed into a 50 mL conical tube containing 300 μL of ACD (1: 8 ratio of ACD to blood; *see* **Notes 2**, **3**, and **4**).
2. Wash the blood twice with 1× phosphate-buffered saline (PBS) by centrifugation at 300× *g* for 10 min at 4 °C; *see* **Note 5**.

3. If the use of stored RBCs is desired, adjust the packed RBCs to 75% hematocrit using 14% CPDA-1 and store at 4 °C in the dark for 7 to 10 days. Following storage, remove the supernatant and proceed with the experiment.
4. Transfer 1 mL of packed RBCs to a light-protected microcentrifuge tube and add 50 μL of DiO dye.
5. Incubate the RBC/DiO mixture in a 37 °C water bath for 30 min, gently swirling every 5 min.
6. Wash the labeled RBCs three times by adding 10 mL of PBS, mixing gently by inversion or rocking, and centrifuging at 300× *g* for 10 min at 4 °C.
7. To confirm labeling efficiency, dilute 1 μL of washed packed RBCs in 800 μL of FACS buffer and analyze by flow cytometry.
8. Prepare the transfusion mixture by diluting 50 μL of DiO-labeled packed RBCs per mouse in PBS to a final volume of 300 μL (*see* **Note 6**).
9. Inject each mouse via the lateral tail vein with 300 μL of the labeled RBC suspension using a 27gauge ½-inch needle attached to a 1 mL syringe.

3.2 Cryosectioning of Spleen for HOD RBC Colocalization Analysis

1. Transfuse recipient mice (MZ B cell-depleted or isotype control-treated) with either PBS or DiO-labeled HOD RBCs (*see* **Note 3**).
2. Twenty-four hours post-transfusion, euthanize mice with isoflurane followed by cervical dislocation (*see* **Note 7**).
3. Sterilize the dissection area with 70% ethanol and secure the mouse on a Styrofoam platform.
4. Using sterile scissors and forceps, perform a midline incision, separate the skin, and remove the lower fur.
5. Excise the spleen with a clean set of instruments and immediately embed it in O.C.T. compound within a cryomold (*see* **Note 8**).
6. Freeze the mold in chilled isopentane placed within a dry ice bath (*see* **Note 9**).
7. Store embedded tissues at −80 °C until cryosectioning.
8. Mount frozen spleens onto a cryostat chuck using O.C.T. and allow the sample to solidify on dry ice (*see* **Note 10**).
9. Section spleens at 5–7 μm thickness at −20 °C and collect the sections on microscope slides.
10. Fix the slides in −20 °C acetone for 20 min, then either proceed with staining or store them at −80 °C. Thaw stored slides at room temperature for ~20 min before use.

3.3 Immuno-histochemical (IHC) Staining of Spleen Sections

1. Use a hydrophobic barrier (PAP) pen to encircle the tissue section and let it dry completely.
2. Wash slides three times (1–2 min each) by adding PBS inside the hydrophobic barrier using a pipette; aspirate with a glass pipette or vacuum.
3. Add 100 μL of 0.5% blocking buffer to each slide and incubate in a humid chamber for 2 h at room temperature.
4. Remove excess buffer and add 100 μL of primary antibody cocktail: Alexa Fluor 647 Rat anti-Mouse IgD and PE Rat anti-Mouse CD1d (1:100 in blocking buffer). Incubate for 2 h at room temperature.
5. Wash slides three times in PBS on a shaker (10 min each).
6. Mount with ProLong Gold antifade reagent in the dark (*see* **Note 11**).
7. After curing, examine slides using fluorescence or confocal microscopy. (Refer to Fig. 2 for representative colocalization images.)

3.4 MZ B Cell Depleting Antibody IP Injections (Day −4, and −2)

1. Label three 5 mL Eppendorf tubes: "PBS," "Depleting AB," and "Isotype Control AB" (*see* **Note 3**).
2. For depletion, prepare 250 μL containing 100 μg each of anti-CD11a and anti-CD49d in PBS.
3. For the isotype control, prepare 250 μL with 100 μg each of Rat IgG2b and Rat IgG2a in PBS.
4. For the PBS group, add 250 μL of PBS alone.
5. Inject 250 μL of the respective solution intraperitoneally using a 27½-gauge needle and a 1 mL syringe.

3.5 Collection, Storage, and Transfusion of B6-HOD RBCs (Day 0)

1. Prepare the donor RBC injection mixture as outlined in Subheading 3.1, **steps 1–3**.
2. Prepare the transfusion mixture by diluting 50 μL of packed RBCs per mouse in PBS to a final volume of 300 μL.
3. Inject each mouse via the lateral tail vein with 300 μL of the RBC suspension using a 27-gauge ½-inch needle attached to a 1 mL syringe.

3.6 Collection of Splenocytes for MZ B Cell Depletion Assessment (Day +1, +5, +7, and +14)

1. Euthanize the mouse using isoflurane followed by cervical dislocation.
2. Disinfect the surgical area with 70% ethanol and perform a midline dissection.
3. Excise the spleen using sterile tools and place it into a 50-mL conical tube containing ice-cold R10 buffer.

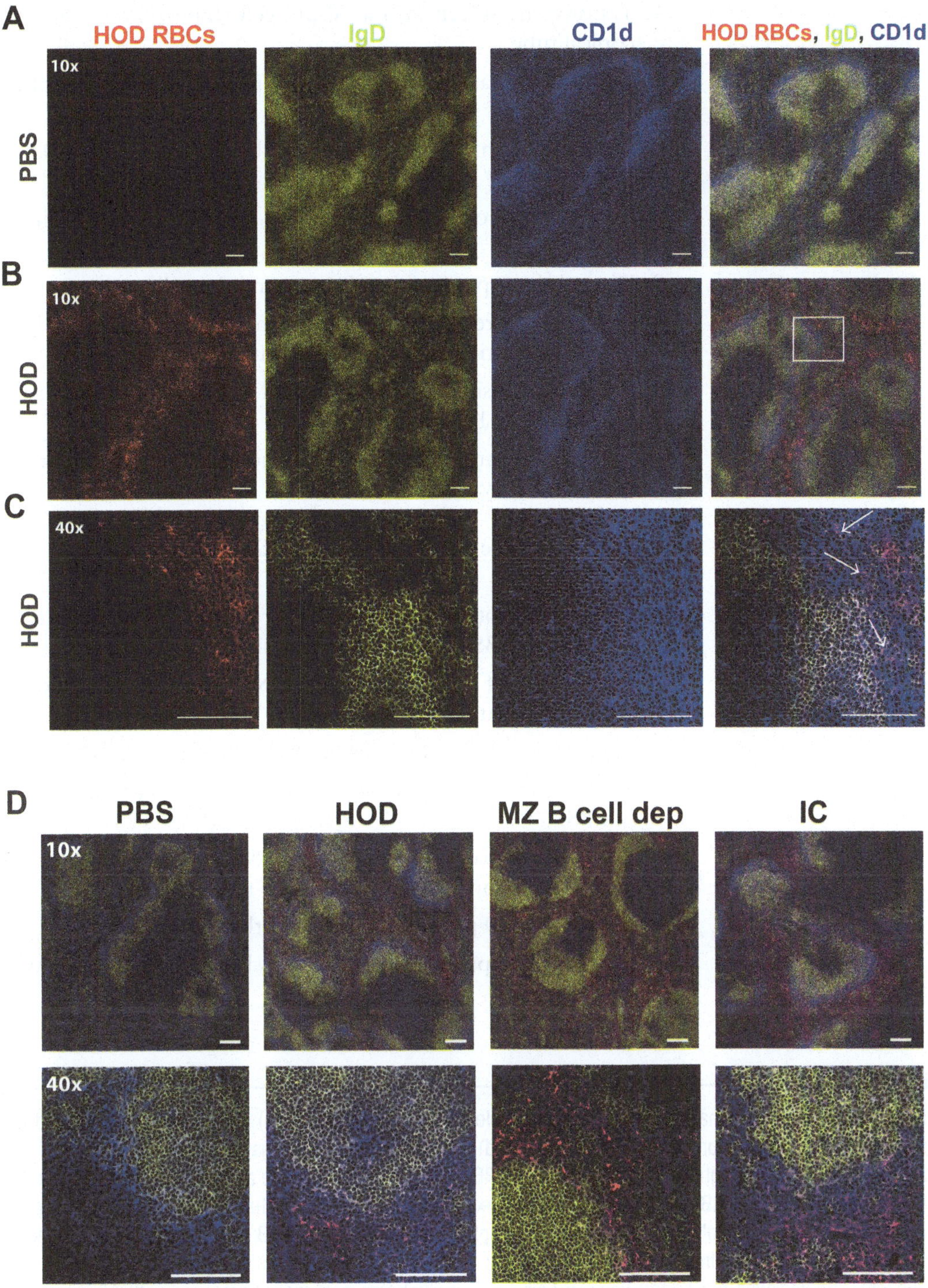

Fig. 2 HOD RBCs colocalize with marginal zone B cells in the splenic marginal sinus following transfusion. DiO-labeled HOD red blood cells (RBCs) were transfused into HOD-negative B6 recipients and tracked by immunofluorescence microscopy 24 h post-transfusion. Spleens were harvested and stained to visualize follicular (FO) B cells (IgD; yellow) and marginal zone (MZ) B cells (CD1d; blue) (**a**–**b**). Representative

4. Transfer the spleen into a 70-μm cell strainer over a 50-mL conical tube.
5. Gently dissociate cells using the blunt end of a 1-mL syringe plunger.
6. Rinse with 5 mL increments of R10 buffer, collecting ~20 mL total volume.
7. Keep samples on ice and centrifuge at 300× *g* for 15 min at 4 °C.
8. Discard the supernatant and resuspend the pellet.
9. Lyse residual red cells by adding 2 mL of Sigma red cell lysis buffer, incubating at room temperature for 5 min.
10. Quench the lysis by adding 18 mL of PBS and centrifuge again at 300× *g* for 10 min at 4 °C.
11. Carefully discard the supernatant and proceed to staining for flow cytometry.

3.7 Cell Counting and Flow Cytometry Staining

1. Resuspend splenocytes in 600 μL of PBS per sample and mix gently.
2. Take an aliquot for viability using trypan blue (10 μL of cells +180 μL of PBS + 10 μL of trypan blue).
3. Load 20 μL of stained cells onto a Nexcelom slide and determine viability using a Cellometer.
4. Transfer 4 × 10^6 viable cells per well into a 96-well plate.
5. Centrifuge at 300× *g* for 5 min at 4 °C and wash in 200 μL of PBS.
6. Add 50 μL Zombie NIR viability dye (1:100 in PBS) and incubate at room temperature for 20 min in the dark.
7. Wash with 150 μL FACS buffer and then centrifuge.
8. Block Fc receptors with 50 μL Fc block (1:100) in FACS buffer.

Fig. 2 (continued) low-magnification images of spleens from PBS-treated (**a**) and HOD RBC-transfused (**b**) mice show the localization of transfused RBCs (red) within the marginal sinus (**c**). A magnified view of the boxed region in (**b**) highlights colocalization of HOD RBCs with MZ B cells (white arrows). To assess MZ and FO B cell contributions to RBC localization, DiO-labeled HOD RBCs were transfused into control, MZ B cell-depleted, or FO B cell-depleted mice (D). Despite depletion of either MZ or FO B cells, HOD RBCs continued to localize within the marginal sinus, suggesting that initial RBC localization is independent of these B cell subsets. Imaging was performed using a Leica SP8 multiphoton confocal microscope with 10× or 40× objectives as indicated. Scale bars, 100 μm. Representative images are shown from experiments independently reproduced two to three times, with three mice per group per experiment. (This research was originally published in *Blood* [21] with permission from *Blood*, the Journal of the American Society of Hematology)

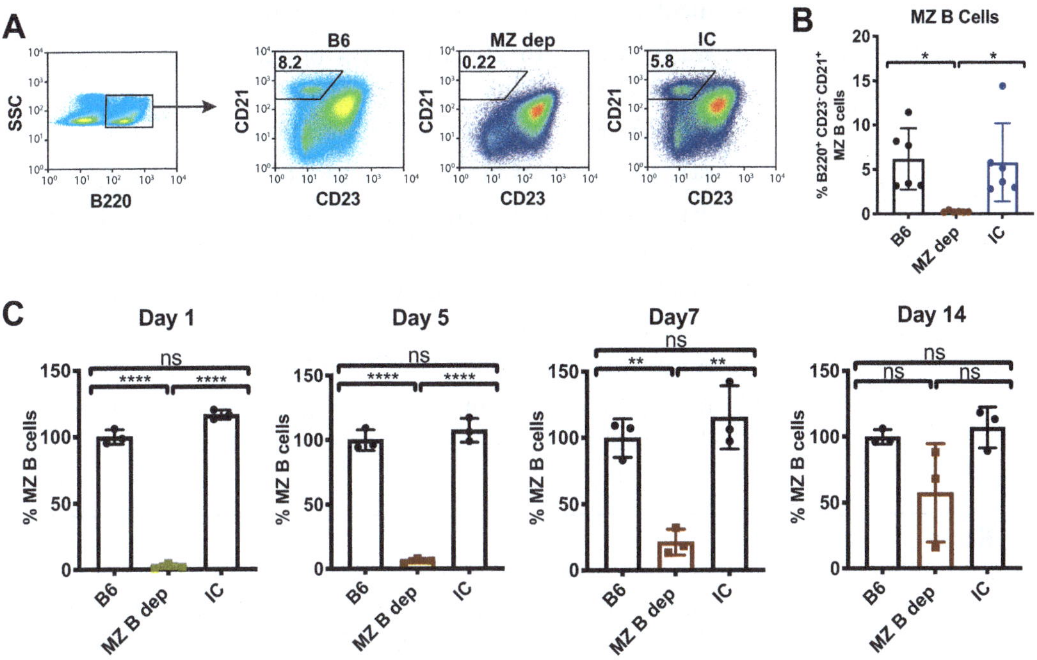

Fig. 3 Kinetics and efficiency of marginal zone (MZ) B cell depletion following antibody treatment. (**a**) Gating strategy used to identify B220$^+$ CD23$^-$ CD21^{hi} MZ B cells in splenocytes. (**b**) Quantification of MZ B cells in B6 mice treated with PBS (B6), MZ B cell-depleting antibodies (MZ dep), or isotype control antibodies (IC), showing effective depletion in MZ dep-treated mice. (**c**) Time-course analysis of MZ B cell frequencies following antibody treatment. Quantification of B220$^+$ CD23$^-$ CD21^{hi} MZ B cells was performed on days 1, 5, 7, and 14 post-treatment in mice treated with PBS (B6), MZ B cell-depleting antibodies (MZ B dep), or IC. The data demonstrate sustained depletion of MZ B cells over time in MZ dep-treated mice, with repopulation of MZ B cells on Day 14. (This research was originally published in *Blood* [21] with permission from *Blood*, the Journal of the American Society of Hematology)

9. Add 50 μL of antibody cocktail (anti-B220, anti-CD21, anti-CD23; all 1:100 dilution).
10. Incubate on ice for 30 min in the dark.
11. Wash cells three times in FACS buffer and centrifuge.
12. Resuspend in 200 μL of PBS and analyze by flow cytometry (*see* Fig. 3).

3.8 Flow Crossmatch (Day +3, +5, +7, and +14)

1. Collect blood from B6-HOD or C57BL/6 mice using a lancet into 1 mL Eppendorf tubes containing ACD (1:8 ratio to blood).
2. Dilute the mixture in 12 mL cold 1× PBS in a 15-mL conical tube.
3. Wash samples twice in 1× DPBS (centrifuge at 1200 rpm, 10 min, brake setting 6).
4. In a 96-well U-bottom plate, add 10 μL of test plasma and 2 μL of packed RBCs per well.

5. Incubate at room temperature for 15 min.
6. Wash twice with 200 μL FACS buffer, flicking the plate to remove supernatant.
7. Add 25 μL of antibody cocktail (1:100 in FACS buffer):
   (a) Panel 1: anti-mouse APC IgG, FITC IgM, PE IgG1.
   (b) Panel 2: anti-mouse Alexa Fluor 488 IgG2b, PE IgG2c, and PerCP IgG3.
8. Incubate for 30 min at 4 °C or 15 min at room temperature, protected from light.
9. Wash twice with 200 μL FACS buffer.
13. Resuspend cells in 100 μL FACS buffer and store at 4 °C in the dark until analysis by flow cytometry (*see* Fig. 4).

4 Notes

1. Mice used as recipients are female C57BL/6, H-2^b mice purchased from Charles River Laboratories. Transgenic HOD mice served as RBC donors [22, 23]. Mice 8 to 12 weeks of age at the start of the experiment are housed in sterilized cages on an auto-watering rack under controlled conditions.
2. This representative suggested volume is for blood sufficient to transfuse 10 recipient mice.
3. All procedures must be conducted within a biosafety cabinet to ensure the sterility of all reagents and injection materials.
4. 50 μL of packed RBCs (pRBCs) are needed per mouse, and you should assume half will be lost in the DiO-staining procedure. Therefore, plan to collect twice the number of pRBCs needed in your experiment.
5. When centrifuging RBCs, use the brake to decelerate slowly to avoid disturbing the pellet.
6. Take the total packed RBCs and multiply by 5, then add this amount of PBS to the pRBCs.
7. The timing of splenic harvest may vary depending on the aim of the experiment.
8. When placing the spleen in the cryomold, ensure it is centered and properly aligned, with its longer side parallel to the longer side of the cryomold. Adjust the orientation based on your intended sectioning direction and purpose.
9. Slowly submerge the cryomold containing the spleen horizontally into isopentane, keeping the open part of the mold facing upward to prevent the O.C.T. compound from spilling out.
10. Ensure that the frozen spleen embedded in the O.C.T. compound is firmly secured on the cryostat mount.

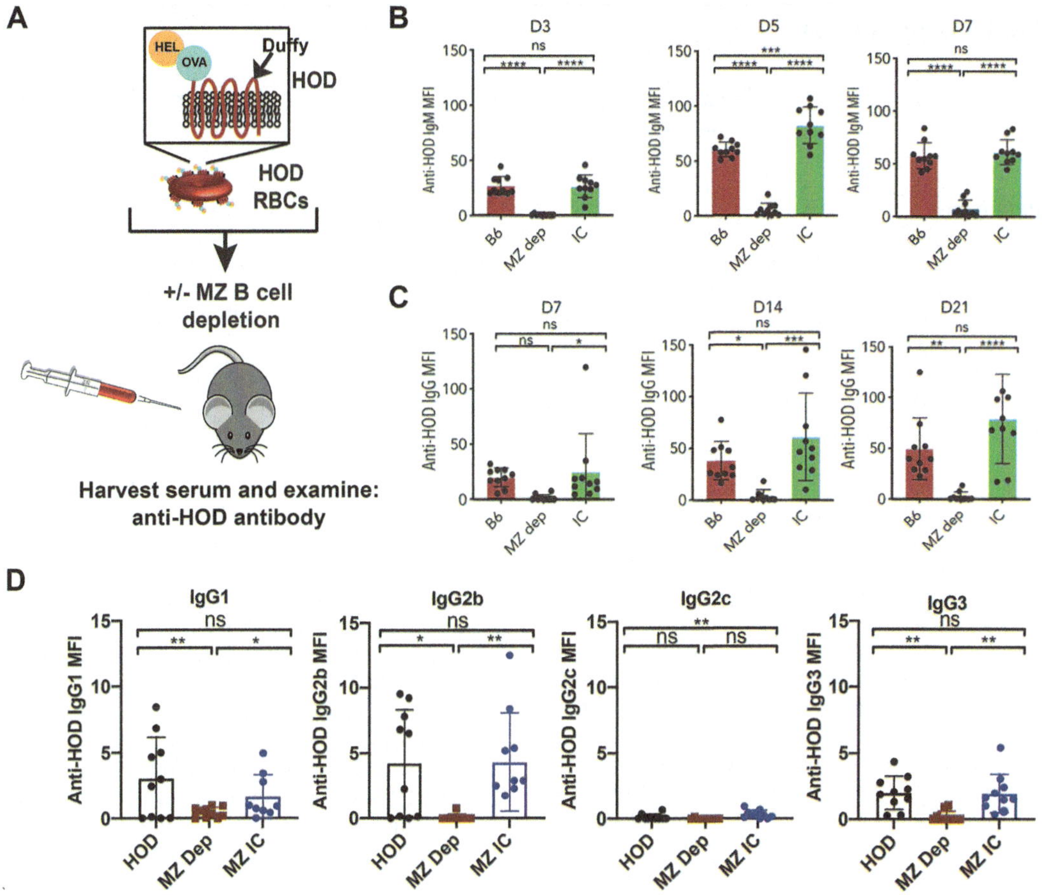

Fig. 4 MZ B cell depletion inhibits anti-HOD alloantibody formation. (**a**) Schematic of the experimental design: B6 mice received PBS, MZ B cell-depleting antibodies, or isotype control antibodies, followed by transfusion with HOD RBCs. (**b–c**) Quantification of anti-HOD IgM (**b**) and IgG (**c**) alloantibody formation 7, 14, and 21 days post-transfusion in mice treated with PBS (red), MZ B cell-depleting antibodies (blue), or isotype control antibodies (green). (**d**) Anti-HOD IgG subclass distributions were evaluated 14 days post-transfusion using flow crossmatch to compare responses among PBS, MZ B cell-depleted, and isotype control-treated recipients. Data are representative of two independent experiments, with 5 mice per group. $P < 0.0001$ (), $P < 0.0005$ (*), $P < 0.006$ (), $P < 0.04$ (*); unpaired Student's t-test or one-way ANOVA with Tukey's post hoc test. D3, day 3; D5, day 5; D7, day 7; D14, day 14; D21, day 21; MFI, mean fluorescence intensity; ns, not significant. (This research was originally published in *Blood* [21] with permission from *Blood*, the Journal of the American Society of Hematology)

This prevents movement during sectioning, which could lead to uneven sectioning or sample loss.

11. Transfer a small amount of mounting medium into a microcentrifuge tube and centrifuge at 2000 rpm for 5 min to remove any bubbles. Carefully apply a sufficient amount of mounting medium onto the sample, ensuring the tissue is fully covered and no bubbles form during the transfer. Bubbles can create blind spots during imaging.

Conflicts of Interest

The authors have no conflicts of interest to declare that are relevant to the content of this chapter.

References

1. Ambruso D et al (1987) Experience with donors matched for minor blood group antigens in patients with sickle cell anemia who are receiving chronic transfusion therapy. Transfusion 27(1):94–98
2. Vichinsky EP et al (1990) Alloimmunization in sickle cell anemia and transfusion of racially unmatched blood. N Engl J Med 322(23): 1617–1621
3. Yazdanbakhsh K, Ware RE, Noizat-Pirenne F (2012) Red blood cell alloimmunization in sickle cell disease: pathophysiology, risk factors, and transfusion management. Blood 120(3): 528–537
4. Rosse WF et al (1990) The cooperative study of sickle cell disease transfusion and alloimmunization in sickle cell disease. Blood 76(7): 1431–1437
5. Narbey D et al (2017) Incidence and predictive score for delayed hemolytic transfusion reaction in adult patients with sickle cell disease. Am J Hematol 92(12):1340–1348
6. Vidler JB et al (2015) Delayed haemolytic transfusion reaction in adults with sickle cell disease: a 5-year experience. Br J Haematol 169(5):746–753
7. Habibi A et al (2016) Delayed hemolytic transfusion reaction in adult sickle-cell disease: presentations, outcomes, and treatments of 99 referral center episodes. Am J Hematol 91(10):989–994
8. Chonat S et al (2020) Eculizumab for complement mediated thrombotic microangiopathy in sickle cell disease. Haematologica 105(12): 2887
9. Hillyer CD et al (2008) Integrating molecular technologies for red blood cell typing and compatibility testing into blood centers and transfusion services. Transfus Med Rev 22(2): 117–132
10. Chou ST et al (2013) High prevalence of red blood cell alloimmunization in sickle cell disease despite transfusion from Rh-matched minority donors. Blood 122(6):1062–1071
11. Yee ME et al (2017) Red blood cell minor antigen mismatches during chronic transfusion therapy for sickle cell anemia. Transfusion 57(11):2738–2746
12. Attanavanich K, Kearney JF (2004) Marginal zone, but not follicular B cells, are potent activators of naive CD4 T cells. J Immunol 172(2): 803–811
13. Tangye SG et al (2013) The good, the bad and the ugly—TFH cells in human health and disease. Nat Rev Immunol 13(6):412–426
14. You Y et al (2011) Marginal zone B cells regulate antigen capture by marginal zone macrophages. J Immunol 186(4):2172–2181
15. Martin F, Kearney JF (2002) Marginal-zone B cells. Nat Rev Immunol 2(5):323–335
16. Cinamon G et al (2008) Follicular shuttling of marginal zone B cells facilitates antigen transport. Nat Immunol 9(1):54–62
17. Malkiel S et al (2009) The loss and gain of marginal zone and peritoneal B cells is different in response to relapsing fever and Lyme disease Borrelia. J Immunol 182(1):498–506
18. Webb LM, Linterman MA (2017) Signals that drive T follicular helper cell formation. Immunology 152(2):185–194
19. Vinuesa CG et al (2016) Follicular helper T cells. Annu Rev Immunol 34(1):335–368
20. Patel SR et al (2018) Marginal zone B cells induce alloantibody formation following RBC transfusion. Front Immunol 9:2516
21. Zerra PE et al (2021) Marginal zone B cells mediate a CD4 T-cell–dependent extrafollicular antibody response following RBC transfusion in mice. Blood 138(8):706–721
22. Mener A et al (2018) Complement serves as a switch between CD4+ T cell–independent and–dependent RBC antibody responses. JCI Insight 3(22):e121631
23. Stowell SR et al (2013) Antigen modulation confers protection to red blood cells from antibody through Fcγ receptor ligation. J Immunol 191(10):5013–5025

Chapter 49

A Flow Cytometric Method of Determining CD71+ Erythroid Cells in Neonatal Whole Blood

Wenhui Li, William O. Scott, Dominique Paz, Rebecca C. Hale, and Connie M. Arthur

Abstract

The neonatal immune system exhibits a unique composition and function, rendering neonates particularly susceptible to infections and inflammatory conditions such as necrotizing enterocolitis (NEC). A distinct feature of neonatal immunity is the abundance of $CD71^+$ erythroid cells (CECs), which are significantly more prevalent in neonates than in adults and possess immunosuppressive properties that can modulate neonatal immune responses. However, their quantification and functional analysis have been challenging given the small volume of blood typically available for assessment.. In this study, we present a comprehensive 24-color flow cytometry panel optimized to detect and quantify $CD71^+CD235a^+$ cells in minimal volumes of neonatal whole blood. This panel enables precise enumeration of CECs and detailed characterization of other key immune cell subsets, including T cells, monocytes, and natural killer cells. Additionally, our method allows for the functional assessment of CECs, such as evaluating Arginase 2 levels, to better understand their immunomodulatory roles. This approach provides a robust tool for dissecting the neonatal immune landscape and offers valuable insights into how CECs may impact other immune populations. Ultimately, this approach lays the groundwork for further research into the mechanisms behind neonatal vulnerability to infections and inflammation, potentially guiding the development of targeted therapeutic strategies.

Key words Neonatal immune system, CD71+ erythroid cells, Immunosuppressive properties, Arginase II activity, Necrotizing enterocolitis

1 Introduction

The neonatal immune system exhibits unique characteristics that distinguish it from that of adults, reflecting an immature yet rapidly developing immune landscape. This immature immune status renders neonates particularly vulnerable to infections and inflammatory conditions, such as necrotizing enterocolitis (NEC) [1–4]. Among neonates admitted to neonatal intensive care units (NICUs), 18–35% are diagnosed with anemia, and this rate increases to 70% in extremely preterm neonates weighing less

Sean R. Stowell and Connie M. Arthur (eds.), *Methods in Transfusion Medicine*, Methods in Molecular Biology, vol. 3053, https://doi.org/10.1007/978-1-0716-5376-0_49,

than 1000 grams at birth [5–7]. Building on the foundation of a number of preclinical models designed to characterize how recipient immune factors and a variety of distinct pathways impact the development of alloantibodies and affects various transfusion-related complications [8–13], recent studies have revealed that both anemia and transfusion can influence intestinal immune responses and systemic inflammation [2, 4]. These findings indicate that anemia may act as a priming factor, predisposing the developing intestine to transfusion-induced inflammation during a critical period of development [2, 4, 14]. These clinical challenges underscore the need for a deeper understanding of neonatal immune regulation and its key cellular players.

$CD71^+$ erythroid cells (CECs), a subset of immature red blood cells, have recently emerged as an important component of the neonatal immune system [15–17]. These cells, which account for approximately 1% of circulating cells in healthy adults [18], are significantly more abundant in neonates where they can comprise up to 10% of circulating cells in human neonates [19]. CECs are known to exhibit immunosuppressive properties [20, 21], through mechanisms such as Arginase 2 production [22], which may help prevent excessive inflammation during this critical period of immune development. However, the high abundance of CECs in neonates may also contribute to increased susceptibility to infections or influence the progression of conditions such as anemia and NEC.

Despite their biological significance, quantifying and functionally characterizing circulating erythroid cells in neonatal blood remains technically challenging due to their fragility and low abundance relative to mature red blood cells [23]. To address this, we developed a robust 24-color multi-parameter flow cytometry panel optimized for small volumes of neonatal whole blood. This panel enables the reliable detection and quantification of $CD71^+CD235a^+$ cells, which can be further subdivided into $CD45^+CD71^+CD235a^+$ and $CD45^-CD71^+CD235a^+$ subsets, populations that may possess distinct immunomodulatory potentials [24]. Importantly, functional markers such as Arginase2, expressed in nucleated cells, are incorporated to assess immunosuppressive capacity.

In addition to identifying CECs, the panel provides comprehensive immunophenotyping of key immune cell subsets and functional profiles, including T cells, monocytes, macrophages, and natural killer cells, offering a broader view of the neonatal immune landscape. Moreover, the panel is modular and can be adapted to suit specific research objectives, making it a versatile tool for exploring neonatal immunity and CEC functionality.

While this study focuses on the quantification of CECs and other immune cell subsets, the methodology we have developed can be extended in future investigations to examine potential interactions between CECs and immune cells. Such studies may yield critical insights into the immunological crosstalk underlying neonatal immunity and its relevance to conditions such as NEC, infections, and responses to transfusion therapies.

In summary, this study presents a comprehensive and adaptable flow cytometric framework for characterizing CECs and immune cell subsets in neonatal whole blood, laying a strong foundation for future research into their roles and interactions in neonatal health and disease.

2 Materials

2.1 Preparation of Flow Cytometry Panel

1. BD Horizon™ Brilliant Stain Buffer (Cat No. 563794, BD, USA).
2. Antibodies:
   (a) CD71-BV421.
   (b) CD235a-PE-Cy7.
   (c) CD45-APC-fire 810.
   (d) Anti-Arg2.
   (e) CD14-Spark Blue.
   (f) CD86-PE-fire 640.
   (g) CD206-PE-Dazzle 594.
   (h) CD183-BV711.
   (i) CX3CR1-PE.
   (j) CD3- Per-CP.
   (k) CD4- AF-700.
   (l) CD8-BV570.
   (m) CD25 PE-Dazzle 594.
   (n) CD19-BV750.
   (o) CD20-PE-fire 810.
   (p) CD16-Spark NIR 685.
   (q) CD56-BV605.
   (r) Live/Dead-Zombie Yellow.
   (s) Anti-Arg2 antibody [EPR9473] (ab225989).
3. Alexa Fluor® 488 Conjugation Kit (Fast)—Lightning-Link® (ab236553).
4. Human Tru-stain FcX™ (Cat No. 422305, BioLegend, USA).
5. True-stain monocyte blocker (Cat No. 426102, BioLegend, USA).
6. Ultra-Comp Beads.

7. PBS (store at 4 °C): 137 mM sodium chloride (NaCl), 0.43 mM sodium dihydrogen phosphate (NaH_2PO_4), 2.7 mM potassium chloride (KCl), 12 mM sodium bicarbonate ($NaHCO_3$), 5 mM 4-(2-hydroxyethyl)-1-piperazineethanesulfonic acid (HEPES), 1 mM magnesium dichloride hexahydrate ($MgCl_2 \times 6H_2O$).

2.2 Human Neonatal Blood Preparation

1. Neonatal blood coated with CPDA.
2. PBS (store at 4 °C): 137 mM sodium chloride (NaCl), 0.43 mM sodium dihydrogen phosphate (NaH_2PO_4), 2.7 mM potassium chloride (KCl), 12 mM sodium bicarbonate ($NaHCO_3$), 5 mM 4-(2-hydroxyethyl)-1-piperazineethanesulfonic acid (HEPES), 1 mM magnesium dichloride hexahydrate ($MgCl_2 \times 6H_2O$).
3. RBC lysis buffer (Cat No. 420302, BioLegend, USA).
4. 1.5 mL Eppendorf tube.

2.3 Cell Staining for Flow Cytometry Analysis

5. Brilliant staining buffer (Cat No. 566349, BD, USA).
6. Icemaker.
7. Vortex, Mini 120 V.
8. Bench centrifuge.
9. Multichannel pipette 20–200 μL.
10. 96-well plate.
11. Full-spectrum flow cytometer (CyTEK NL-3000, Serial No. 0419).

2.4 Flow Cytometry Analysis

12. Compensation beads (Cat No. 01-2222-42).
13. QC beads (SpectroFlo® QC Beads, Cat No. SKU B7-10001).
14. Full-spectrum flow cytometer (CyTEK NL-3000, Serial No 0419).
15. FlowJo software.

3 Methods

3.1 Preparation of Flow Cytometry Panel

3.1.1 Preparation of Single-Stained Beads

To enable accurate compensation and spectral unmixing, prepare single-stained compensation controls using compensation beads or cells for each fluorophore listed below. For each fluorescent antibody, proceed with the following steps:

1. Label a 1.5 mL microcentrifuge tube with the name of the fluorophore (e.g., "BV421" s, *see* **Note 1**).

2. Add one drop (or 50 μL) of compensation beads (e.g., Ultra-Comp eBeads or equivalent) into the tube with 100 μL.
3. Dilute the conjugated antibody corresponding to the listed fluorophore according to the manufacturer's recommended dilution (typically 1:50 to 1:400 dilution). Add 1 μL of the antibody to the beads.
4. Vortex gently to mix and incubate at room temperature for 15–20 min, protected from light.
5. After incubation, add 1 mL of PBS containing 1% BSA to wash the beads.
6. Centrifuge at 500× *g* for 5 min, aspirate the supernatant, and resuspend the pellet in 300–500 μL of PBS with 1% BSA for acquisition.

3.1.2 Preparation of Control Live/Dead Cell Stain

1. Aliquot approximately 100 μL of lysed neonatal whole blood (prepared as described in Subheading 3.2) into two 1.5 mL microcentrifuge tubes labeled "Live" and "Dead."
2. Place the "Dead" tube in a 56 °C water bath for 20 min to induce cell death, then remove and allow to cool to room temperature for 5–10 min.
3. In parallel, place the "Live" tube at room temperature without treatment.
4. Combine equal volumes from both tubes ("Live" and "Dead") to create a mixed control containing both live and dead cells.
5. Centrifuge and remove the PBS supernatant from the cells.
6. Stain "Live," "Dead," and Combined ("Live" and "Dead") cells with the appropriate dilution of Zombie Yellow Live/Dead stain for 15 min in PBS at room temperature in the dark (*see* **Notes 2** and **3**).
7. Following staining, wash once with PBS and resuspend for flow cytometry analysis.

3.1.3 Antibody Master Mix Preparation

1. Label a 1.5 mL Eppendorf tube as "antibody mix."
2. Prepare a cocktail of all antibodies listed below by adding the recommended volume of each antibody according to optimized titration (*see* **Note 4**).
3. Dilute the antibodies in Brilliant buffer to bring the total volume of the mix to accommodate staining for one sample (typically 50 μL per test).
4. Gently vortex the tube to mix thoroughly.
5. Store on ice and protect from light until use.
6. Antibodies to include in the box CD71-BV421, CD235a-PE-Cy7, CD45-APC-fire 810, CD14-Spark Blue

550, CD3-PerCP, CD86-PE-fire 640, CX3CR1-PE, CD56-BV605, CD183-BV711, CD45RA-BV510, CD66b-APC-Cy7, CD4-AF700, CD16-Spark NIR 685, CD19-BV750, CD8-BV570, MHC Class II-BV650, CD163-BV480, CD25-BV785, CD206-PE-Dazzle 594, CD62L-PerCP-Cy5.5, CD20-PE-fire 810, and CD69-AF647.

3.2 Cell Preparation

3.2.1 Washing Neonatal Whole Blood

1. Aliquot 60 μL of fresh neonatal whole blood into a 1.5 mL microcentrifuge tube.
2. Add 200 μL of PBS to the blood sample to dilute it.
3. Centrifuge the tube at 500× *g* for 2 min using a soft spin setting to preserve fragile cells.
4. Carefully aspirate and discard the supernatant without disturbing the pellet.

3.2.2 RBC Lysis

1. Prepare 1× RBC lysis buffer by diluting 10× lysis buffer 1:10 in distilled water (e.g., 1 mL of 10× buffer +9 mL ddH_2O). Allow the solution to equilibrate to room temperature before use.
2. Add 1 mL of RBC lysis buffer to the pellet.
3. Gently pipette up and down to mix and ensure even contact with all cells.
4. Incubate at room temperature for 5 min to lyse red blood cells.
5. Centrifuge at 500× *g* for 5 min to pellet the remaining cells.
6. Aspirate the supernatant, being careful not to disturb the cell pellet.
7. Resuspend the pellet in 60 μL of PBS in preparation for antibody staining and transfer to a 96-well plate.

3.3 Cell Staining

3.3.1 Surface Staining

1. Add the optimized volume/dilution of Zombie Yellow Dye to 60 μL of live/dead control (*see* **Notes 3** and **5**) for each sample.
2. Incubate all samples for 15 min at room temperature in the dark.
3. Wash once with 200 μL of PBS. Centrifuge at 40× *g* for 2 min for plates.
4. Carefully remove the supernatant.
5. Add 25 μL of Fc block (1:100). Incubate for 10 min in the dark at room temperature.
6. Add 25 μL of stain "mix" to each sample.
7. Incubate the samples in the dark at room temperature for 20 min.
8. Centrifuge samples at 400× *g* for 2 min for plates.
9. Remove the supernatant by carefully pipetting.

3.3.2 Intracellular Staining

1. Thoroughly resuspend cells and add 100 μL of fixation/permeabilization solution per well for microwell plates (*see* **Note 6**) for 20 min at 4 °C.
2. Wash cells two times in 1× BD Perm/Wash™ buffer (*see* **Note 7**) and pellet.
3. Thoroughly resuspend fixed/permeabilized cells in 50 μL of BD Perm/Wash™ buffer containing anti-Arginase 2 antibody.
4. Incubate at 4 °C for 30 min in the dark.
5. Wash the cells twice with 250 μL of 1× BD Perm/Wash™ buffer per wash when using microwell plates.
6. After the final wash, resuspend the cells in staining buffer in preparation for flow cytometric analysis.

3.4 Flow Cytometry Analysis

3.5 Data Collection

1. Perform quality control (QC) to ensure the flow cytometer is functioning properly.
2. Load and run the reference control to establish spectral signatures for unmixing.
3. Load and run experimental samples for collection.

3.6 Gating Strategy

Flow cytometry data were analyzed using FlowJo software to identify CECs, monocytes, T cells, neutrophils, B cells, and NK cells, along with their respective marker expression profiles (*see* **Note 8**). CECs were defined as $CD71^{+}CD235a^{+}$ cells and further categorized into $CD45^{+}$ and $CD45^{-}$ subsets. Arginase-2 expression was also evaluated within these populations (Fig. 1).

4 Notes

1. Repeat this procedure for each of the following fluorophores: CD71-BV421, CD235a-PE-Cy7, CD45-APC-fire 810, CD14-Spark Blue 550, CD3-PerCP, CD86-PE-fire 640, CX3CR1-PE, CD56-BV605, CD183-BV711, CD45RA-BV510, CD66b-APC-Cy7, CD4-AF700, CD16-Spark NIR 685, CD19-BV750, CD8-BV570, MHC Class II-BV650, CD163-BV480, CD25-BV785, CD206-PE-Dazzle 594, CD62L-PerCP-Cy5.5, CD20-PE-fire 810, and CD69-AF647.
2. To accurately gate live versus dead cells using a fixable viability dye, prepare a control sample containing both live and heat-killed cells. This control enables proper compensation and verification of viability dye performance. To establish proper

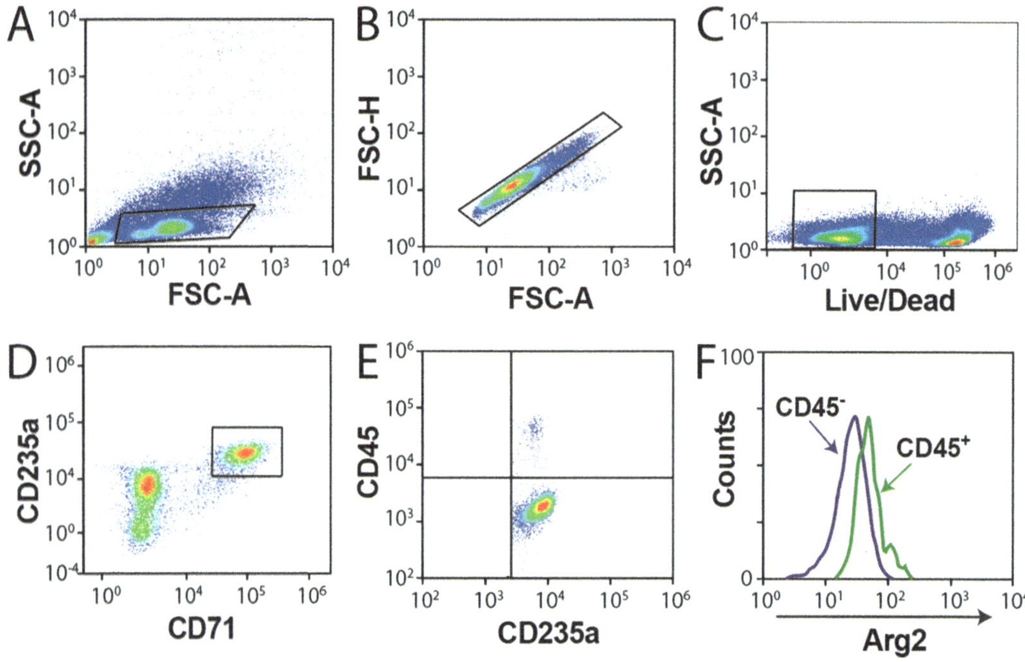

Fig. 1 A sequential flow cytometry gating strategy for CD71+ CD235a+ cells and their expression of Arginase 2. (**a**) Total events are first gated based on forward scatter (FSC-A) and side scatter (SSC-A). (**b**) Single cells are identified using FSC-H vs FSC-A to exclude doublets. (**c**) Live cells are selected by gating out Zombie Yellow-positive (dead) cells. (**d**) Among live single cells, CD71 and CD235a expression are used to identify erythroid cells ($CD71^{+}CD235a^{+}$). (**e**) Within the $CD71^{+}CD235a^{+}$ population, CD45 expression is used to distinguish $CD45^{-}$ late erythroid progenitors and CD45+ hematopoietic progenitors. (**f**) Arginase-2 expression was assessed in the $CD71^{+}CD235a^{+}$ population to evaluate functional characteristics related to immune regulation. Arg:Arginase 2

gating for live and dead cell populations during flow cytometry analysis, a Live/Dead control sample was prepared using the heat-kill method.

3. Recommended dilutions fall between 1:100 and 1:1000. A titration between these concentrations prior to staining in your assay is recommended for optimal staining. The buffer used for Zombie Yellow stain should be free of Tris buffer and protein supplements such as BSA and FBS.

4. Titration is required for each antibody. To titrate an antibody for flow cytometry, prepare serial dilutions of the fluorochrome-conjugated antibody (e.g., 1:50, 1:100, 1: 200,1:400, 1:800) in PBS. Aliquot ~1–5 × 10^5 cells per well in a 96-well V-bottom plate, optionally adding Fc block to reduce nonspecific binding. Add 50 μL of each antibody dilution to the corresponding wells and incubate for 20–30 min at 4 °C in the dark. Wash the cells twice with PBS, resuspend in 200 μL of buffer, and analyze on a flow cytometer. Determine

the optimal dilution by identifying the lowest concentration that provides the maximum signal with minimal background staining.

5. Staining for viability is completed separately from other cell staining, as the buffers for viability staining and antibody staining are not compatible.
6. The wells should always have at least 50 μL (or the starting amount) of the sample; as we started with 50 μL (or the starting amount), prepare accordingly.
7. To prevent cell aggregation, vortex the sample gently before adding the Fixation/Permeabilization solution.
8. Monocytes were gated as $CD3^{-}CD19^{-}$ live singlets and identified based on CD14 and HLA-DR expression. They were further classified into classical ($CD14^{++}CD16^{-}$), intermediate ($CD14^{+}CD16^{+}$), and non-classical (CD14^low$CD16^{+}$) subsets. Their functional profile was assessed using markers such as CD86 (activation), CD206 (M2-like polarization), and CX3CRl (inflammation/migration). T cells were defined as $CD3^{+}CD19^{-}$, and their subsets were analyzed using CD4 and CD8 expression. Further profiling included CD45RA to distinguish naïve ($CD45RA^{+}$) from memory ($CD45RA^{-}$) T cells. Regulatory T cells (Tregs) were identified within the $CD4^{+}$ population as $CD25^{+}$ cells. B cells were identified as $CD3^{-}CD45^{+}CD19^{+}CD20^{+}$. Neutrophils were gated as $CD3^{-}CD19^{-}$ cells and identified based on low CD14 and high CD16 expression, with further characterization using CD62L and CD66b. NK cells were defined as $CD3^{-}CD14^{-}CD19^{-}$ and characterized by CD56 and CD16 expression to distinguish CD56bright$CD16^{-}$ and CD56dim$CD16^{+}$.

Acknowledgments

This work was funded by NIH grants P01HL171803, R01 HL165975, R01 HL135575, and R01 HL154034. No other authors have conflicts of interest.

References

1. Bazacliu C, Neu J (2019) Necrotizing Enterocolitis: long term complications. Curr Pediatr Rev 15(2):115–124
2. Arthur CM et al (2019) Anemia induces gut inflammation and injury in an animal model of preterm infants. Transfusion 59(4): 1233–1245
3. Paul DA et al (2011) Increased odds of necrotizing enterocolitis after transfusion of red blood cells in premature infants. Pediatrics 127(4):635–641
4. MohanKumar K et al (2019) A murine neonatal model of necrotizing enterocolitis caused by anemia and red blood cell transfusions. Nat Commun 10(1):3494
5. Christensen RD et al (2006) Thrombocytopenia among extremely low birth weight

neonates: data from a multihospital healthcare system. J Perinatol 26(6):348–353
6. Castle V et al (1986) Frequency and mechanism of neonatal thrombocytopenia. J Pediatr 108(5 Pt 1):749–755
7. Andrew M et al (1987) Clinical impact of neonatal thrombocytopenia. J Pediatr 110(3): 457–464
8. Jajosky R et al (2023) Prior immunization against an intracellular antigen enhances subsequent red blood cell alloimmunization in mice. Blood 141(21):2642–2653
9. Zerra PE et al (2021) Marginal zone B cells mediate a CD4 T-cell-dependent extrafollicular antibody response following RBC transfusion in mice. Blood 138(8):706–721
10. Jajosky RP et al (2025) CD47 regulates antigen modulation and red blood cell clearance following an incompatible transfusion. Front Immunol 16:1548548
11. Patel SR et al (2018) Marginal zone B cells induce alloantibody formation following RBC transfusion. Front Immunol 9:2516
12. Jajosky RP et al (2024) Dynamics of antibody engagement of red blood cells in vivo and in vitro. Front Immunol 15:1475470
13. Jajosky RP et al (2023) Antibody-mediated antigen loss switches augmented immunity to antibody-mediated immunosuppression. Blood 142(12):1082–1098
14. DeSimone RA et al (2023) Associations of donor, component, and recipient factors on hemoglobin increments following red blood cell transfusion in very low birth weight infants. Transfusion 63(8):1424–1429
15. Elahi S et al (2013) Immunosuppressive CD71+ erythroid cells compromise neonatal host defence against infection. Nature 504(7478):158–162
16. Dunsmore G et al (2019) Lower abundance and impaired function of CD71+ erythroid cells in inflammatory bowel disease patients during pregnancy. J Crohns Colitis 13(2): 230–244
17. Zhao L et al (2018) Late-stage tumors induce anemia and immunosuppressive extramedullary erythroid progenitor cells. Nat Med 24(10):1536–1544
18. Li W, William N, Acker JP (2023) Donor sex, pre-donation hemoglobin, and manufacturing affect CD71+ cells in red cell concentrates. Transfusion 63(3):601–609
19. Elahi S et al (2020) CD71(+) erythroid cells in human neonates exhibit immunosuppressive properties and compromise immune response against systemic infection in neonatal mice. Front Immunol 11:597433
20. Zhao GJ et al (2022) CD71(+) erythroid cell expansion in adult sepsis: potential causes and role in prognosis and nosocomial infection prediction. Front Immunol 13:830025
21. Miller D et al (2018) CD71+ erythroid cells from neonates born to women with preterm labor regulate cytokine and cellular responses. J Leukoc Biol 103(4):761–775
22. Delyea C et al (2018) CD71(+) erythroid suppressor cells promote fetomaternal tolerance through arginase-2 and PDL-1. J Immunol 200(12):4044–4058
23. Li W, Acker JP (2022) Development and validation of a sensitive flow cytometric method for determining CECs in RBC products. Clin Chim Acta 530:119–125
24. Li W, Acker JP (2026) CD71+ red blood cells mediate increased erythrophagocytosis and reduce monocyte number in a monocyte suspension assay. Scand J Immunol 103(2): e70087. https://doi.org/10.1111/sji.70087

Chapter 50

Defining the Role of Marginal Zone B Cells in FVIII Inhibitor Development

Sungwoong Kim, James W. McCoy, Zahra Naseh, Megan Fuller, Sumaiya Dickens, Montana Jackson, Toni Chanroo, and Patricia E. Zerra

Abstract

The formation of factor VIII (FVIII) inhibitors in hemophilia A patients involves complex immune responses, including the activation of CD4 T cells and B cells. Marginal zone (MZ) B cells, an innate-like B cell population in the spleen, play a key role in the early stages of inhibitor development by rapidly responding to blood-borne antigens. These cells are uniquely positioned to capture and present FVIII to CD4 T cells, initiating a robust immune response that can lead to the formation of neutralizing antibodies. This chapter explores the critical role of MZ B cells in FVIII inhibitor development, focusing on their function in antigen presentation and their potential as therapeutic targets to prevent inhibitor formation. Using immunohistochemistry (IHC) and flow cytometry, we investigate the interactions between MZ B cells, CD4 T cells, and other immune components in the spleen, providing a deeper understanding of the molecular mechanisms underlying FVIII inhibitor development. By elucidating these immune interactions, we aim to inform the development of novel strategies to mitigate FVIII inhibitor formation in hemophilia A patients.

Key words Hemophilia A, Recombinant Human FVIII, FVIII Inhibitors, Marginal Zone B Cells, Marginal Zone B Cell Depletion, Immunohistochemistry, Flow Cytometry

1 Introduction

Hemophilia A is a genetic bleeding disorder resulting from a deficiency in factor VIII (FVIII), a crucial protein in the blood coagulation cascade. This X-linked recessive disorder affects approximately 1 in 5000 male births worldwide, leading to spontaneous bleeding episodes and prolonged bleeding following injuries or surgeries [1]. The standard treatment for hemophilia A involves the administration of exogenous FVIII concentrates to replace the deficient protein and restore hemostasis. However, a significant complication of FVIII replacement therapy is the development of neutralizing antibodies, known as inhibitors, against the administered FVIII [2–5]. These inhibitors render the treatment

Sean R. Stowell and Connie M. Arthur (eds.), *Methods in Transfusion Medicine*, Methods in Molecular Biology, vol. 3053, https://doi.org/10.1007/978-1-0716-5376-0_50,

ineffective by binding to and neutralizing the activity of FVIII, creating a challenging clinical scenario [5, 6]. Inhibitor development occurs in approximately 20–40% of patients with severe hemophilia A and is a major cause of morbidity [7, 8].

The formation of FVIII inhibitors involves complex immune responses, including both conventional T and B cell-mediated mechanisms [9, 10] (Fig. 1). FVIII is recognized as a foreign antigen by the immune system, leading to the activation of T cells, which provide help to B cells. B cells then differentiate into plasma cells that produce anti-FVIII antibodies, targeting various epitopes on the FVIII molecule and neutralizing its coagulant function. CD4 T cells, particularly T follicular helper cells, interact with follicular B cells to initiate germinal center reactions, leading to the production of high-affinity antibodies and the generation of B cell memory.

For germinal center reactions to occur, antigenic material must be transported to the B-cell follicle. Recent research suggests that this transport process is highly regulated, enabling the immune system to distinguish between foreign and self-antigens [11–14]. In the bloodstream, cells located within the marginal sinus of the spleen, which lies at the interface of the red and white pulp, are particularly well-positioned to perform this surveillance [15, 16]. Among these cells, marginal zone (MZ) B cells play a crucial role in the immune response (Fig. 1). These innate-like B cells, located in the marginal zone of the spleen, act as first responders to blood-borne antigens, efficiently capturing and presenting them to T cells [11–14] (Fig. 2). MZ B cells are particularly adept at rapidly differentiating into antibody-secreting cells upon antigen encounter, contributing significantly to the immune response against FVIII.

MZ B cells uniquely recognize and respond to FVIII, and their ability to facilitate antigen transport to dendritic cells (DCs) enhances CD4 T-cell activation [12, 14, 17, 18]. Recent data suggest that MZ B cells, in collaboration with other components of the marginal sinus, may play a pivotal role in the formation of FVIII inhibitors [19]. In particular, the spleen's MZ macrophages (MZMs) work alongside MZ B cells to respond to blood-borne antigens and help trigger immune responses [20–24]. Thus, MZ B cells may serve as early regulators of inhibitor formation following FVIII exposure, making them a potential target for novel therapeutic strategies aimed at preventing inhibitor development [19].

To investigate the role of MZ B cells in FVIII inhibitor formation, various immunological techniques are employed. Immunohistochemistry (IHC) is used to visualize and localize specific antigens within tissue sections, allowing for the identification of MZ B cells and their interactions with other immune cells in the spleen. Flow cytometry enables detailed analysis of cell surface markers and intracellular proteins, facilitating the characterization

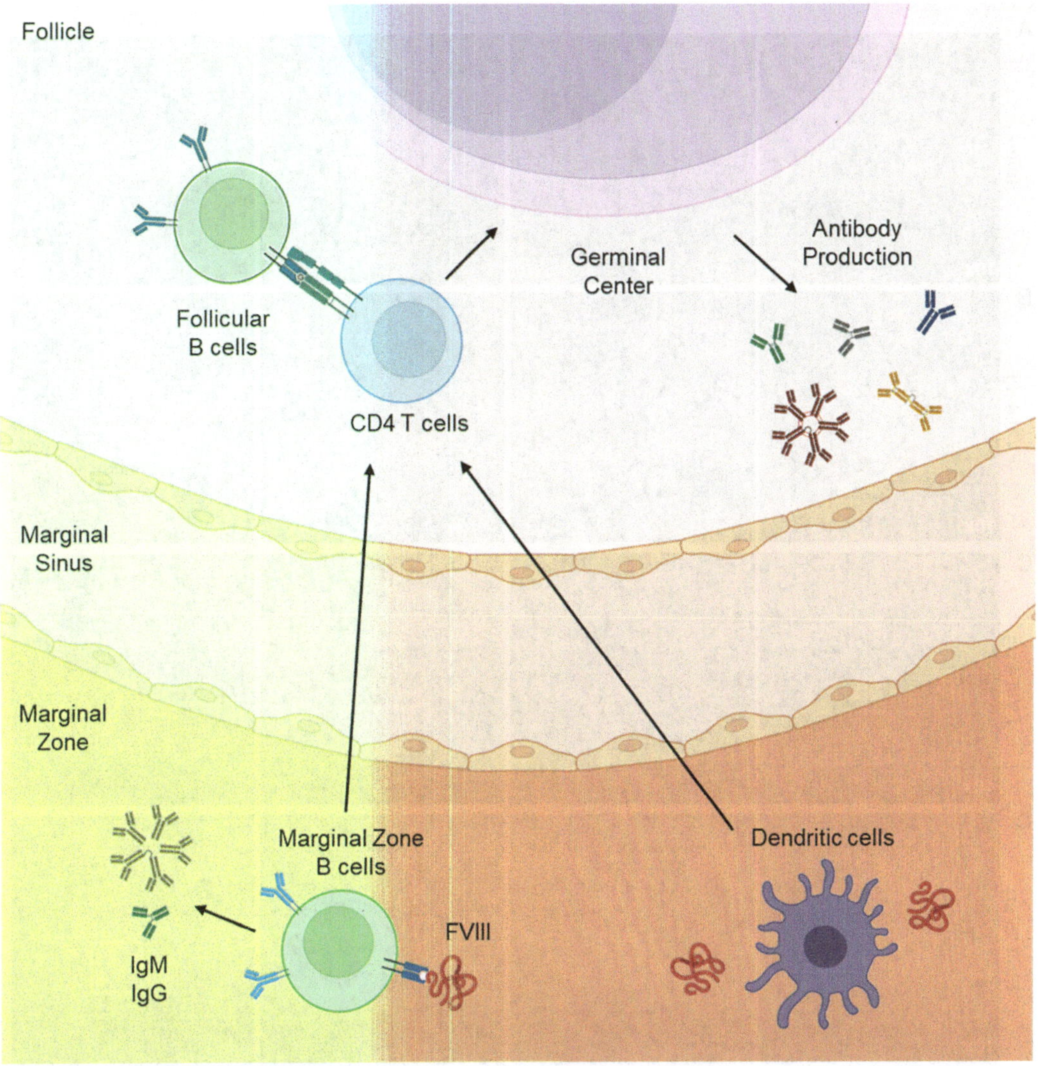

Fig. 1 A Sequential Model for Antibody Production Against Factor VIII Through Marginal Zone B Cell and CD4 T Cell Development. This figure illustrates the process of antibody production against Factor VIII, highlighting the roles of MZ B cells and CD4 T cells. Initially, MZ B cells and dendritic cells in the spleen's marginal zone capture and process the Factor VIII antigen. These antigen-presenting cells then transfer antigen fragments into the B-cell follicle. Within the follicle, MZ B cells present the antigen to CD4 T cells, leading to their activation and proliferation. Activated CD4 T cells, in turn, provide necessary signals to germinal center B cells to initiate the germinal center reaction. This process includes hypermutation and selection, resulting in the production of high-affinity antibodies specifically targeting FVIII

of MZ B cells and their functional properties, including antigen presentation and their role in T-cell activation.

In this chapter, we will delve into the intricate processes underlying FVIII inhibitor formation, with a particular focus on the contributions of MZ B cells. We will describe experimental approaches to assess MZ B cell involvement, including the use of

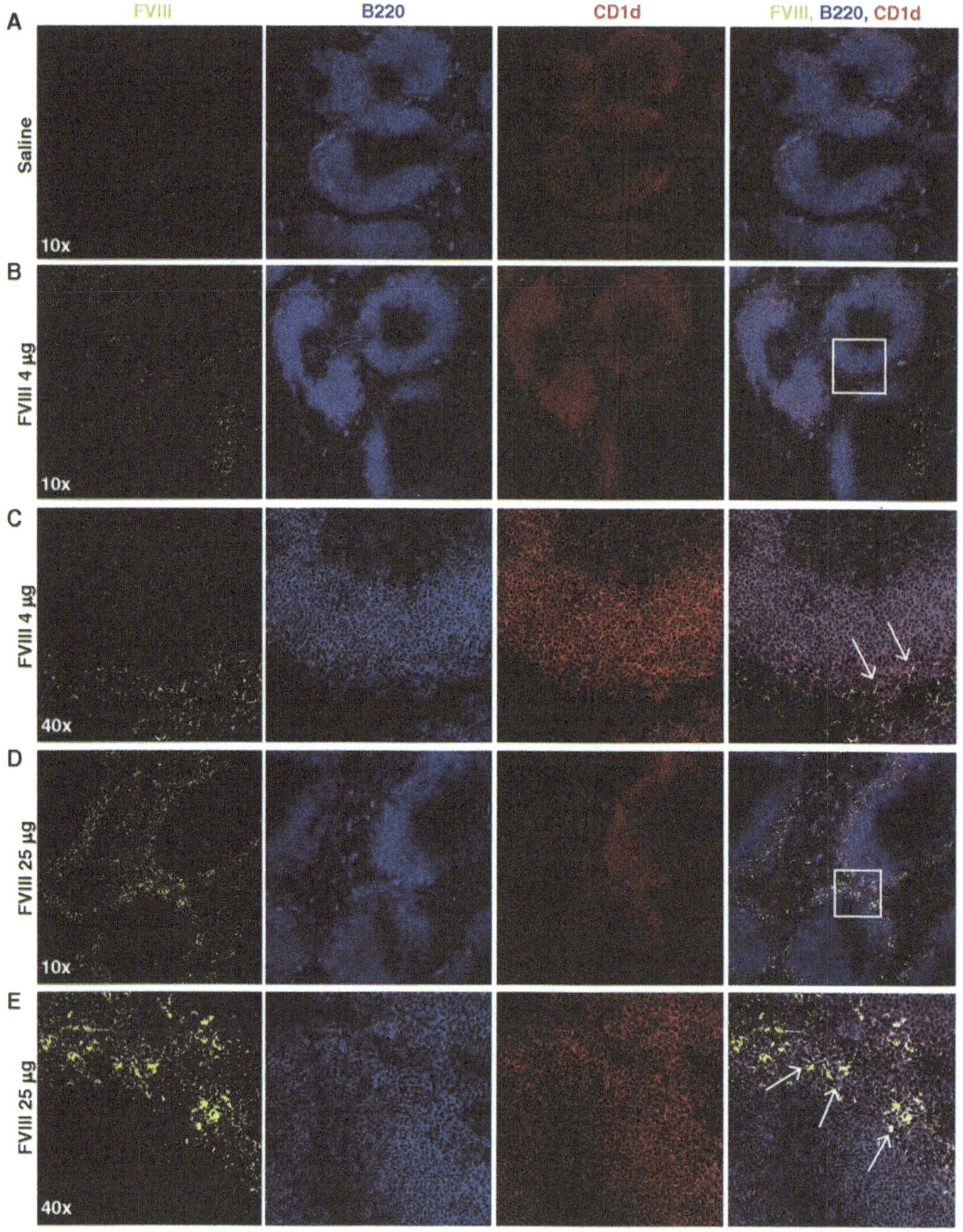

Fig. 2 Localization of FVIII in the Marginal Sinus of the Spleen with MZ B Cells. FVIII-deficient TKO mice were injected with saline (**a**), 4 mg of FVIII (**b**, **c**), or 25 mg of FVIII (**d**, **e**), and spleens were harvested 15 min post-injection. Frozen spleen sections were stained with polyclonal sheep anti-FVIII-FITC (yellow), B220-PE-CF594 (blue), and CD1d-PE (red). Images were obtained using a Leica SP8 multiphoton confocal microscope at 10× and 40× magnification. The white box indicates the area magnified at 40×. Arrows denote the colocalization of FVIII and CD1d, identifying MZ B cells. (This research was originally published in *Blood* [19] with permission from *Blood*, the Journal of the American Society of Hematology)

immunohistochemistry (IHC) to visualize MZ B cell localization, their interactions with other immune cells (Fig. 2), and MZ B cell depletion studies using CD11a and CD49d antibody-mediated depletion (Fig. 3). Through these methods, we aim to better understand how MZ B cells contribute to FVIII antigen processing and inhibitor formation, offering insights for new therapeutic strategies to mitigate inhibitor development in hemophilia A patients.

2 Materials

2.1 Cryosectioning of Spleen for MZ B Cell Depletion Assessment

1. TKO mice (*see* **Note 1**).
2. Recombinant Human FVIII (rhFVIII) (*see* **Note 2**).
3. Sterile saline (e.g., Fresenius Kabi).
4. 27 ½ inch needle (e.g., Becton Dickinson).
5. 1 mL Syringe (e.g., Becton Dickinson).
6. Cryomold (Sakura Finetek USA).
7. 2-methylbutane (Isopentane, e.g., Sigma-Aldrich).
8. Dry ice.
9. Tissue-Tek O.C.T. Compound (O.C.T.) (Sakura Finetek USA).
10. Leica CM 1850 Cryostat (or suitable equipment).
11. Glass slides (e.g., Fisher Scientific).
12. Acetone (e.g., Sigma-Aldrich).

2.2 IHC Staining of Spleen Tissue

1. PAP pen (Electron Microscopy Sciences).
2. 1X Phosphate-buffered saline (PBS), pH 7.4 (e.g., Cytiva, Sterile).
3. Glass pipette (e.g., Fisher Scientific).
4. Vacuum pump.
5. 5% Blocking buffer (5% Fetal bovine serum (FBS) or bovine serum albumin (BSA) in PBS, e.g., Thermo Fisher Scientific).
6. Humidification chamber (Electron Microscopy Sciences).
7. Fisherbrand Multi-Platform Shaker (or suitable equipment).
8. Sheep anti-Human FVIII polyclonal antibody (HTI, Essex Junction, VT).
9. FITC Rabbit anti-Sheep IgG secondary antibody (Sigma-Aldrich).
10. PE-CF594 Rat anti-Mouse B220 antibody (BD Biosciences).
11. PE Rat anti-Mouse CD1d antibody (BD Biosciences).
12. Deionized water.

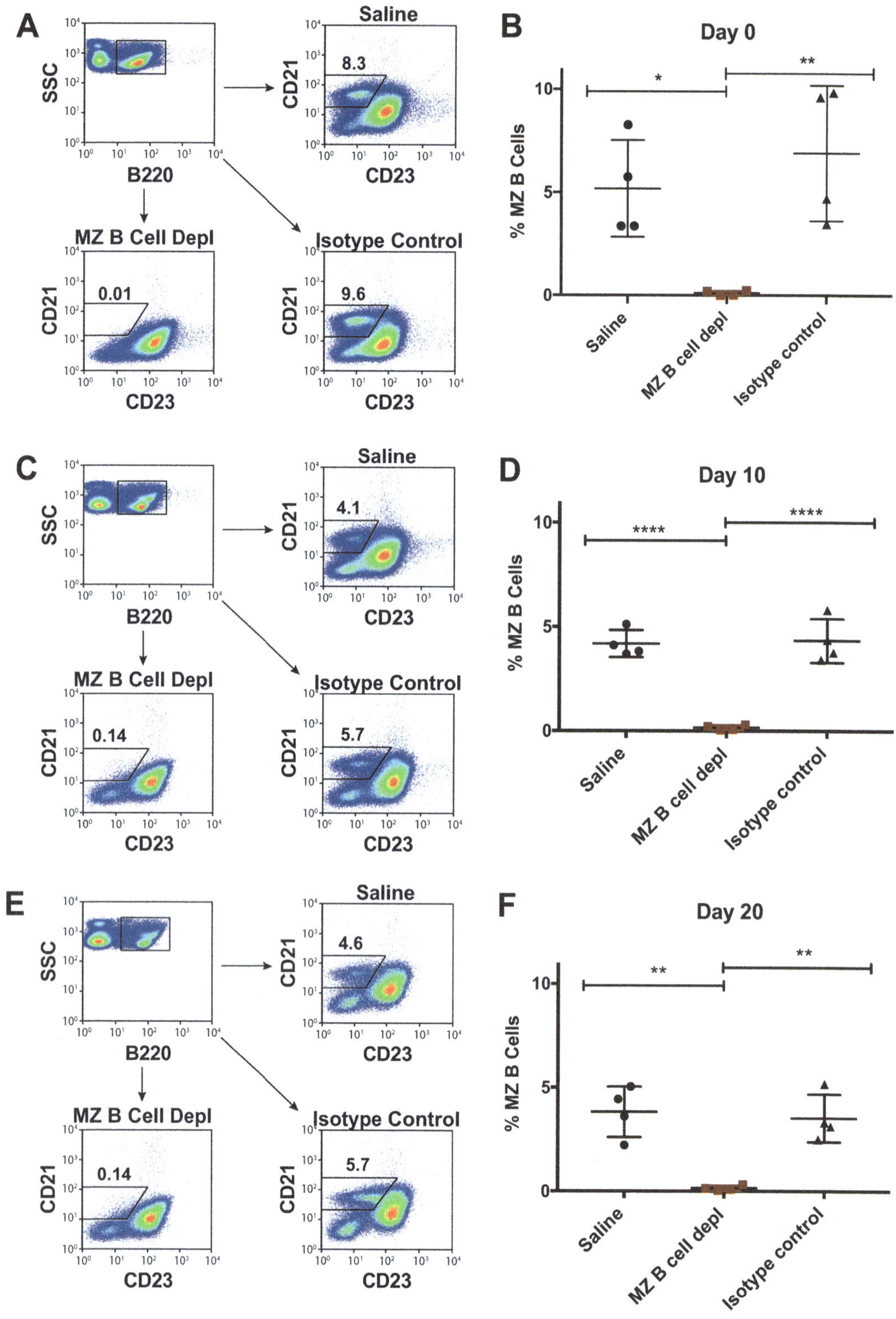

Fig. 3 Depletion of MZ B Cells in Mice with Hemophilia A. Mice with hemophilia A were administered MZ B-cell-depleting antibodies on days −4, −2, +10, and +20. Flow cytometry was performed on splenocytes from representative mice to confirm successful depletion. Shown are representative flow cytometry plots of

13. Prolong Gold antifade mounting media (Thermo Fisher Scientific).
14. Cover slip (e.g., Sigma-Aldrich).

2.3 Depleting Antibody IP Injections (Day −4, −2, +10, and +20)

1. TKO mice.
2. 1X PBS, pH 7.4 (e.g., Cytiva, Sterile).
3. 5 mL macro centrifuge tubes (e.g., Celltreat).
4. CD11a antibody (anti-Mouse LFA-1α) (clone M17/4, Bio X Cell).
5. CD49d antibody (anti-Mouse/Human VLA-4) (clone PS/2, Bio X Cell).
6. CD11a isotype control rat IgG2a antibody (clone 2A3, Bio X Cell).
7. CD49a iotype control rat IgG2b antibody (clone LTF2, Bio X Cell).
8. 27 ½ inch needle (e.g., Becton Dickinson).
9. 1 mL syringe (e.g., Becton Dickinson).

2.4 Recombinant Human FVIII Injection (Day 0, +7, +14, and +21)

1. TKO mice.
2. Recombinant Human FVIII (rhFVIII).
3. Sterile saline (e.g., Fresenius Kabi).
4. 27 ½-inch needle (e.g., Becton Dickinson).
5. 1 mL syringe (e.g., Becton Dickinson).

2.5 Collection of Splenocytes for MZ B Cell Depletion Assessment (Day +1, +11, and +21)

1. TKO mice.
2. Isoflurane (Piramal Critical Care).
3. Styrofoam dissection station.
4. Surgical scissors and forceps (e.g., Sigma-Aldrich).
5. Ethanol, 70% (e.g., Sigma-Aldrich).
6. 50 mL conical tube (e.g., MIDSCI).
7. R10 Medium (10% FBS in RPMI 1640, e.g., Sigma-Aldrich).

Fig. 3 (continued) $B220^+CD21^{hi}CD23^{lo/-}$ cells following the injection of saline, MZ B-cell-depleting antibody (MZ B cell depl), or isotype control antibody on days 0 (**a**), +10 (**c**), and +20 (**e**). Quantitative analysis of $B220^+CD21^{hi}CD23^{lo/-}$ cells (% MZ B cells) following the administration of saline, MZ B-cell-depleting antibody, or isotype control antibody on days 0 (**b**), +10 (**d**), and +20 (**f**). Error bars indicate standard deviation (SD). Horizontal lines represent the mean of each group. Statistical significance is indicated as $^*P < 0.03$, $^{**}P < 0.003$, $^{****}P < 0.0001$, determined by 1-way ANOVA with post hoc Tukey test. SSC, side scatter. (This research was originally published in *Blood* [19] with permission from *Blood*, the Journal of the American Society of Hematology)

8. Cell strainer, 70 μm (e.g., Sigma-Aldrich).
9. 1 mL syringe (e.g., Becton Dickinson).
10. Sigma red cell lysis buffer (e.g., Sigma-Aldrich).
11. 1X PBS, pH 7.4 (e.g., Cytiva, Sterile).

2.6 Cell Counting and Flow Cytometry Staining

1. Trypan blue (e.g., Sigma-Aldrich).
2. Cell counting slide (Nexcelom).
3. Nexcelom Cellometer Auto T4 (or suitable equipment).
4. 1X PBS, pH 7.4 (e.g., Cytiva, Sterile).
5. 96-well plate (e.g., Corning).
6. Zombie NIR Fixable Viability Kit (Biolegend).
7. FACS buffer (1% BSA in PBS).
8. Alexa 700 Rat anti-Mouse B220 (clone RA3-6b2, Biolegend).
9. Pacific Blue Rat anti-Mouse CD21 (clone 7G6(RUO), Biolegend).
10. APC Rat anti-Mouse CD23 antibody (clone B3B4, Biolegend).
11. Mouse Fc block (e.g., BD Bioscience).

3 Methods

3.1 Cryosectioning of Spleen for Assessment of FVIII Localization

1. Administer 1, 2, 4, or 25 μg of FL-rhFVIII or saline to TKO mice via retro-orbital injection (*see* **Note 3**).
2. Fifteen minutes after FVIII administration, euthanize the mouse using isoflurane followed by cervical dislocation.
3. Secure the mouse onto a Styrofoam dissection station and sterilize the surgical area with 70% ethanol.
4. Using designated scissors and forceps for skin and fur removal, make a midline incision, separate the skin, and remove the lower fur.
5. With a separate set of scissors and forceps, carefully excise the spleen.
6. Immediately place the spleen into a cryo-mold and fill it with O.C.T. (*see* **Note 4**).
7. Freeze the spleen by submerging the mold in cold isopentane placed in a glass beaker within a dry ice bucket (*see* **Note 5**).
8. Store the frozen spleen at −80 °C until ready for cryosectioning and IHC.
9. Mount the frozen spleen onto a cryostat chuck using O.C.T. and place the chuck on dry ice to solidify (*see* **Note 6**).

10. Section the spleen using a cryostat (set to −20 °C and 5–7 μm thickness) and transfer sections onto slides.
11. Fix slides in acetone at −20 °C for 20 min by immersing them in a pre-chilled acetone container.
12. Use the slides immediately or store them at −80 °C. If stored, thaw at room temperature for ~20 min before proceeding.

3.2 IHC Staining of Spleen Tissue

1. Use a PAP pen to draw a hydrophobic barrier around the tissue and allow it to dry completely.
2. Wash slides three times in PBS by placing them on a paper towel, adding PBS inside the barrier using a pipette, incubating for 1–2 min, and removing PBS with a glass pipette or vacuum.
3. Add 100 μL of 5% blocking buffer to each sample and incubate for 2 h at room temperature in a humidification chamber.
4. Remove excess liquid and add 100 μL of primary antibody cocktail (anti-Human FVIII, 1:100 dilution in blocking buffer) to each sample, incubating for 1 h at room temperature in a humidification chamber.
5. Wash slides three times in PBS for 10 min using a shaker.
6. Add 100 μL of secondary antibody (FITC Rabbit anti-Sheep IgG, 1:100 dilution in blocking buffer) and incubate for 1 h at room temperature in a humidification chamber.
7. Wash slides three times in PBS for 10 min on a shaker.
8. Add 100 μL of tertiary antibody (PE-CF594 Rat anti-Mouse B220 and PE Rat anti-Mouse CD1d, 1:100 dilution in blocking buffer) and incubate for 2 h at room temperature in a humidification chamber.
9. Wash slides three times in PBS for 10 min on a shaker.
10. Remove excess liquid and mount slides using Prolong Gold antifade mounting media in the dark (*see* **Note 7**).
11. After the mounting media has completely cured, examine the samples using fluorescence or confocal microscopy. Figure 2 displays the colocalization of recombinant human FVIII with MZ B cells in the spleen as observed by confocal microscopy.

3.3 MZ B Cell Depleting Antibody IP Injections (Day −4, −2, +10, and +20)

1. Label three 5 mL Eppendorf tubes as "PBS," "Depleting AB," and "Isotype Control AB" (*see* **Note 3**).
2. Prepare the depleting antibody solution by adding 100 μg each of anti-CD11a and anti-CD49d to the "Depleting AB" tube, then add PBS to bring the total volume to 250 μL.
3. Prepare the isotype control solution by adding 100 μg each of Rat IgG2b and Rat IgG2a to the "Isotype Control AB" tube, and then add PBS to bring the total volume to 250 μL.

4. Add 250 μL of PBS to the "PBS" tube.
5. Using a 27 ½ gauge needle attached to a 1 mL syringe, inject each mouse intraperitoneally (IP) with 250 μL of either the MZ-depleting antibody cocktail, the isotype control, or PBS alone (*see* **Note 8**).

3.4 Recombinant Human FVIII Injection (Day 0, +7, +14, and +21)

1. Administer FL-hrFVIII (2 or 4 μg) in a total volume of 100 μL sterile saline via retro-orbital injection on Day 0, +7, +14, and +21 (*see* **Notes 3** and **8**).

3.5 Collection of Splenocytes for MZ B Cell Depletion Assessment (Day +1, +11, and +21)

1. Euthanize the mouse using isoflurane followed by cervical dislocation.
2. Secure the mouse onto a Styrofoam dissection station and sterilize the area with 70% ethanol.
3. Make a midline incision using designated scissors and forceps, separate the skin, and remove the lower fur.
4. Carefully excise the spleen using a separate set of sterile instruments.
5. Immediately place the spleen into the cap of a 50 mL conical tube containing ice-cold supplemented R10 medium.
6. Transfer the spleen and buffer into a 70 μm cell strainer placed atop a 50 mL conical tube.
7. Gently crush the spleen through the strainer using the blunt end of a 1 mL syringe (*see* **Note 9**).
8. Rinse the filter by adding ice-cold R10 medium in 5 mL increments, allowing the suspension to collect in the tube until reaching a total volume of ~20 mL.
9. Cap the tube, place it on ice, and repeat for all samples.
10. Centrifuge at 300 × g for 15 min at 4 °C to pellet the splenocytes.
11. Discard the supernatant and gently resuspend the pellet in the residual buffer.
12. Add 2 mL of red cell lysis buffer and incubate at room temperature for 5 min (*see* **Note 10**).
13. Add 18 mL of PBS, then centrifuge at 300 × g for 10 min at 4 °C.
14. Carefully discard the supernatant.

3.6 Cell Counting and Flow Cytometry Staining

1. Resuspend the cells in 600 μL of PBS per harvested mouse.
2. Mix gently and take a small sample for cell counting, keeping the remaining cells on ice.

3. Prepare a 1:20 trypan blue staining mixture by adding 10 μL of cells to 180 μL of PBS, and then add 10 μL of trypan blue.
4. Load 20 μL of the stained cell mixture onto a Nexcelom counting slide and determine viability using the Cellometer.
5. Transfer 4×10^6 live cells into designated wells of a 96-well plate.
6. Centrifuge at 300 × g for 5 min at 4 °C to pellet the cells.
7. Wash the pellet by resuspending it in 200 μL PBS, then pellet again by centrifugation.
8. Add 50 μL of Zombie NIR dye (1:100 dilution) and incubate at room temperature for 20 min in the dark.
9. Wash with 150 μL of FACS buffer and centrifuge.
10. Vortex briefly and then add 50 μL of mouse Fc block (1:100 dilution) in FACS buffer.
12. Add 50 μL of antibody cocktail (Alexa 700 Rat anti-mouse B220, Pacific Blue Rat anti-Mouse CD21, APC Rat anti-Mouse CD23, each at 1:100 dilution).
11. Incubate on ice for 30 min, protected from light.
12. Wash three times with FACS buffer, centrifuging between washes.
13. Resuspend cells in 200 μL of FACS buffer.
14. Analyze samples using flow cytometry. Figure 3 presents the results for the assessment of MZ B cell depletion via flow cytometry.

4 Notes

1. Factor VIII knockout (TKO) mice on a C57BL/6 background were used for all experiments [25]. These mice have a complete deletion of the F8 coding sequence, resulting in the absence of detectable F8 messenger RNA in the C57BL/6 strain. Male and female mice, aged 8 to 12 weeks at the time of the first injection, were housed in sterilized cages on an automatic watering rack under controlled conditions.
2. Full-length recombinant human FVIII (FL-rhFVIII) was generously donated by Hemophilia of Georgia.
3. All procedures must be conducted within a biosafety cabinet to ensure the sterility of all reagents and injection materials.
4. When placing the spleen in the cryomold, ensure it is centered and properly aligned, with its longer side parallel to the longer side of the cryomold. Adjust the orientation based on your intended sectioning direction and purpose.

5. Slowly submerge the cryomold, containing the spleen, horizontally into isopentane, keeping the open part of the mold facing upward to prevent the O.C.T. compound from spilling out.
6. Ensure the frozen spleen embedded in the O.C.T. compound is firmly secured on the cryostat mount. This prevents movement during sectioning, which could lead to uneven sectioning or sample loss.
7. Transfer a small amount of mounting medium into a microcentrifuge tube and centrifuge at 2000 rpm for 5 min to remove any bubbles. Carefully apply a sufficient amount of mounting medium onto the sample, ensuring it is fully covered and no bubbles form during the transfer. Bubbles can create blind spots during imaging.
8. Ensure all injection solutions are thoroughly mixed and free of bubbles in the syringe before injecting into mice to prevent complications.
9. Ensure the tissue is strained smoothly and evenly to minimize damage to single cells and maximize cell yield.
10. RBC lysis buffer capacity varies by brand. Test your specific RBC lysis buffer beforehand to ensure that it does not cause excessive damage to splenocytes before conducting experiments.

Conflict of Interest

The authors have no conflicts of interest to declare that are relevant to the content of this chapter.

References

1. Dunn AL, Abshire TC (2006) Current issues in prophylactic therapy for persons with hemophilia. Acta Haematol 115(3–4):162–171
2. Kempton CL, White GC (2009) How we treat a hemophilia A patient with a factor VIII inhibitor. Blood 113(1):11–17
3. Ehrenforth S et al (1992) Factor VIII inhibitors in haemophiliacs. Lancet 340(8813):253
4. Lollar P (2004) Pathogenic antibodies to coagulation factors. Part one: factor VIII and factor IX. J Thromb Haemost 2(7):1082–1095
5. Ehrenforth S et al (1992) Incidence of development of factor VIII and factor IX inhibitors in haemophiliacs. Lancet 339(8793):594–598
6. Meeks SL et al (2007) Antihuman factor VIII C2 domain antibodies in hemophilia A mice recognize a functionally complex continuous spectrum of epitopes dominated by inhibitors of factor VIII activation. Blood 110(13): 4234–4242
7. Aledort L (2004) Comparative thrombotic event incidence after infusion of recombinant factor VIIa versus factor VIII inhibitor bypass activity. J Thromb Haemost 2(10):1700–1708
8. Kempton CL, Meeks SL (2014) Toward optimal therapy for inhibitors in hemophilia. Blood 124(23):3365–3372
9. Ramiscal RR, Vinuesa CG (2013) T-cell subsets in the germinal center. Immunol Rev 252(1):146–155
10. De Silva NS, Klein U (2015) Dynamics of B cells in germinal centres. Nat Rev Immunol 15(3):137–148

11. Attanavanich K, Kearney JF (2004) Marginal zone, but not follicular B cells, are potent activators of naive CD4 T cells. J Immunol 172(2): 803–811
12. Snapper C et al (1993) Comparative in vitro analysis of proliferation, Ig secretion, and Ig class switching by murine marginal zone and follicular B cells. J Immunol (Baltimore, Md.: 1950) 150(7):2737–2745
13. Group, T.t.R.A.t.P.S. (1997) Leukocyte reduction and ultraviolet B irradiation of platelets to prevent alloimmunization and refractoriness to platelet transfusions. N Engl J Med 337(26): 1861–1870
14. Cerutti A, Cols M, Puga I (2013) Marginal zone B cells: virtues of innate-like antibody-producing lymphocytes. Nat Rev Immunol 13(2):118–132
15. Mebius RE, Kraal G (2005) Structure and function of the spleen. Nat Rev Immunol 5(8):606–616
16. Weill J-C, Weller S, Reynaud C-A (2009) Human marginal zone B cells. Annu Rev Immunol 27(1):267–285
17. Zandvoort A, Timens W (2002) The dual function of the splenic marginal zone: essential for initiation of anti-TI-2 responses but also vital in the general first-line defense against blood-borne antigens. Clin Exp Immunol 130(1): 4–11
18. Ferguson AR, Youd ME, Corley RB (2004) Marginal zone B cells transport and deposit IgM-containing immune complexes onto follicular dendritic cells. Int Immunol 16(10): 1411–1422
19. Zerra PE et al (2017) Marginal zone B cells are critical to factor VIII inhibitor formation in mice with hemophilia A. Blood 130(23): 2559–2568
20. Navarrete A et al (2009) Splenic marginal zone antigen-presenting cells are critical for the primary allo-immune response to therapeutic factor VIII in hemophilia A. J Thromb Haemost 7(11):1816–1823
21. You Y et al (2011) Marginal zone B cells regulate antigen capture by marginal zone macrophages. J Immunol 186(4):2172–2181
22. Bergtold A et al (2005) Cell surface recycling of internalized antigen permits dendritic cell priming of B cells. Immunity 23(5):503–514
23. Karlsson MC et al (2003) Macrophages control the retention and trafficking of B lymphocytes in the splenic marginal zone. J Exp Med 198(2):333–340
24. Li H et al (2015) Interferon-induced mechanosensing defects impede apoptotic cell clearance in lupus. J Clin Invest 125(7):2877–2890
25. Chao BN et al (2016) Characterization of a genetically engineered mouse model of hemophilia A with complete deletion of the F8 gene. J Thromb Haemost 14(2):346–355

Index

A

B

C

Sean R. Stowell and Connie M. Arthur (eds.), *Methods in Transfusion Medicine*, Methods in Molecular Biology, vol. 3053, https://doi.org/10.1007/978-1-0716-5376-0,

D

E

F

G

H

O

P

R

S

T

U

W